PATIENT CARE STANDARDS
Nursing process, diagnosis, and outcome

PATIENT CARE STANDARDS
Nursing Process, Diagnosis, and Outcome

SUSAN MARTIN TUCKER, R.N., B.S.N., P.H.N.
Director of Nursing, Kaiser Permanente Medical Center,
East San Fernando Valley,
Panorama City, California

MARY M. CANOBBIO, R.N., M.N.
Assistant Clinical Professor, School of Nursing,
Cardiovascular Clinical Specialist, Division of Cardiology,
University of California, Los Angeles,
Los Angeles, California

ELEANOR VARGO PAQUETTE, R.N., B.S.
Coordinator of Staff Development, Department of Education and Training,
Kaiser Permanente Medical Center,
Los Angeles, California

MARJORIE FYFE WELLS, R.N., B.S.
Director of Illness Prevention Clinic,
Senior Citizen's Guild,
Ann Arbor, Michigan

FOURTH EDITION
with 245 illustrations

The C. V. Mosby Company
ST. LOUIS · WASHINGTON, D.C. · TORONTO · 1988

A TRADITION OF PUBLISHING EXCELLENCE

Editor: Don E. Ladig
Assistant editor: Audrey Rhoades
Project manager: Kathleen L. Teal
Manuscript editor: Judith Bange
Designer: Rey Umali
Production: Teresa Breckwoldt, Ginny Douglas

FOURTH EDITION

Copyright © 1988 by The C.V. Mosby Company

All rights reserved. No part of this publication may be reproduced, stored in a retrieval system, or transmitted, in any form or by any means, electronic, mechanical, photocopying, recording, or otherwise, without prior written permission from the publisher.

Previous editions copyrighted 1975, 1980, 1984

Printed in the United States of America

The C.V. Mosby Company
11830 Westline Industrial Drive, St. Louis, Missouri 63146

Library of Congress Cataloging in Publication Data

Patient care standards.

  Bibliography: p.
  Includes index.
  1. Nursing—Standards. I. Tucker, Susan Martin.
[DNLM: 1. Nursing Care—standards.
2. Patient Care Planning—standards. WY 100 P297]
RT85.5.P38   1988   610.73′0218   87-24843
ISBN 0-8016-5133-6

TS/VH/VH   9 8 7 6 5 4 3 2   01/D/050

CONTRIBUTORS

Diane Cooper, R.N., M.N.
Lecturer, School of Nursing,
University of California,
Los Angeles, California

Diana R. Danmeyer, R.N., F.N.P., M.N.
Parent-Child Clinical Nurse Specialist,
Clinical Educator, Kaiser Permanente Medical Center,
Panorama City, California;
Assistant Clinical Professor,
School of Nursing,
University of California,
Los Angeles, California

S. Lorraine Daskal, R.N., B.S.N.
Clinical Educator,
Department of Education and Training,
Kaiser Permanente Medical Center,
Los Angeles, California

Ezelia R. Goode, R.N., B.S.N.
Clinical Educator,
Department of Education and Training,
Kaiser Permanente Medical Center,
Los Angeles, California

Christine F. Rodemich, R.N., B.S.N., M.S.N.
Assistant Professor of Allied Health,
Glendale Community College,
Glendale, California

Renata A. Szlakiewicz-Jones, R.N., M.N.
Clinical Educator,
Department of Education and Training,
Kaiser Permanente Medical Center,
Los Angeles, California

Sarah Mottram Vaughan, B.S.N., M.S.N.
Pediatric Clinical Specialist,
Southern Connecticut State University,
New Haven, Connecticut

Mickie D. Welsh, R.N., M.S.N.
Lecturer, School of Nursing,
University of California,
Los Angeles, California

Ellen R. Whalen, R.N., M.S.N.
Department Administrator,
Coronary Care and Postcoronary Care Unit,
Kaiser Permanente Medical Center,
Bellflower, California

Mary E. Willmann, R.N.
Pediatric Clinician,
Utilization Review Coordinator,
Kaiser Permanente Medical Center,
Los Angeles, California

CONSULTANTS

Barbara Boylan-Lewis, R.N., B.S.N. M.A.
Enterostomal Therapist,
Catherine McAuley Health Center,
Ann Arbor, Michigan

Francis Chung, Pharm.D.
Pharmacist Specialist—Oncology,
Kaiser Permanente Medical Center,
Los Angeles, California

Paula Gillette, R.N.
Clinical Specialist,
Department of Gynecologic Oncology,
University of California, Irvine Medical Center,
Irvine, California

Betty Gudmundson, R.N., B.S.N.
Education Coordinator—Orthopedics,
St. Joseph Mercy Hospital,
Ann Arbor, Michigan

Patricia O'Brien, R.N., M.S.N., P.N.P.
Pediatric Clinical Nurse Specialist,
Yale–New Haven Hospital,
Program Instructor,
Yale University School of Nursing,
New Haven, Connecticut

Janet M. Tornow, R.D.
Fostoria, Ohio

Barbara Verner, R.N., B.S.N.
Supervisor of Obstetrics and Gynecology,
Kaiser Permanente Medical Center,
Los Angeles, California

ACKNOWLEDGMENT

Steven E. Beebe
Medical Illustration and Graphic Art
Glendale, California

PREFACE

By applying the nursing process, nurses assess, diagnose, treat, and evaluate patient care through clinical reasoning. This reflects the current and dynamic state of the art and science of nursing practice, which contrasts with the past when nursing practice was totally dependent on physicians' orders to perform patient care activities. Although nurses continue to carry out physicians' orders (dependent functions), there is a broader scope of practice encompassing independent activities related to the nursing process, theory testing, and research, as well as collaborative interdependent medical and nursing practice. As changes occur in the health care industry with the focus on decreasing inpatient length of stays, same-day surgery, prospective payment, and capitation plans, it is essential to maintain safe and consistent standards of practice that ensure positive patient outcomes within any health care delivery system. The Joint Commission on Accreditation of Hospitals is in the process of developing outcome standards on which member hospitals will measure their performance. This change from evaluating processes to outcomes can only be in the best interest of our client, the patient. *Patient Care Standards* has undergone a major revision in this fourth edition to reflect these dynamic changes in clinical nursing practice. The format for each of the standards has changed as well, to meet in part these needs as well as those of the health care industry and the consumer in the assurance of quality patient care.

The first chapter has been revised to include specific nursing diagnoses and care for the physiologic and psychobehavioral patterns, as well as some general care standards that relate to multi–body system conditions. The subsequent chapters are divided into body systems, and the related standards are preceded by an extensive assessment tool.

To assist the nurse in the nursing process, each standard has been divided into sections. The following describes the components of most of the standards.

Title. The medical condition, surgical intervention, procedure, or pharmacologic agent that is the basis for the standard is identified.

Definition. A brief description of the condition, surgical procedure, disease, or condition is given.

Assessment

Observations/findings. Defining characteristics, as well as objective and subjective signs and symptoms, are presented. Generally for medical conditions the observations/findings listed are what one would most expect to see. In contrast those listed for surgical procedures are provided as a patient-monitoring guide to prevent complications and promote a positive outcome.

Laboratory/diagnostic studies. Condition-appropriate studies are identified, as well as some laboratory values and trends.

Potential complications. Potential condition/procedure–related complications are identified. Nursing interventions are directed toward preventing these complications.

Medical management. Major therapeutic interventions are listed, as well as those functions requiring a physician's order.

Nursing diagnoses/goals/interventions

Nursing diagnoses. Nursing diagnoses are listed in a priority sequence and are those most commonly associated with the condition. They are related to the etiologies or other factors from the assessment data to assist the nurse in understanding the reason or rationale for performing the intervention. North American Nursing Diagnosis Association (NANDA)–approved nursing diagnoses are used except on rare occasions, and these exceptions are clearly identified in a footnote.

Goals. Patient-centered goals direct the plan of care and form the outcome criteria and standards on which evaluation of care is based. Goals for convalescing and ongoing or chronic conditions often become discharge criteria.

Interventions. Nursing care activities are prioritized under the specific nursing diagnosis. They describe actions to perform in order to achieve the specific identified goal and to prevent complications. Some *rationales* are linked with the intervention when it is of utmost importance.

Evaluation. Summary statements reflect goal attainment and provide an indicator of the quality and appropriateness of care resulting in a positive patient outcome. Outcome statements relating to cognitive, affective, and psychomotor skills based on patient education are identified under the nursing diagnosis "knowledge deficit."

As with past editions, *Patient Care Standards* can be used by the bedside nurse for reference when caring for the hospitalized patient; the primary nurse, case manager, team leader, or clinical specialist can use them as a guide to patient care planning and patient/family education; the nursing administrator and nurse manager should find them valuable in assuring the quality and appropriateness of care. They should prove to be a valuable study aid for the student nurse as a concise overview of standards of care related to a specific patient condition. They should also be useful to nurses who come in contact with clients outside the acute care hospital, including skilled nursing and extended care facilities, as well as public health nurses, home health nurses, and those engaged in discharge planning, utilization review, quality assurance, patient teaching, and ambulatory outpatient care facilities. Staff development educators should find the standards helpful in the identification of nursing performance problems that are resolved by planned educational experiences.

Patient Care Standards is presented to promote continuity, consistency, and quality care and to promote the delivery of safe, effective, and appropriate care by guiding nurses in the implementation of the nursing process using nursing diagnoses and by providing a tool to evaluate the outcome of patient care.

Susan Martin Tucker
Mary M. Canobbio
Eleanor Vargo Paquette
Marjorie Fyfe Wells

CONTENTS

1 General Care and Nursing Diagnoses, 1

Standards of Care Related to Nursing Diagnoses, 1
Impairment of skin integrity, actual or potential, 1
Alteration in oral mucous membrane, actual or potential, 1
Activity intolerance, actual or potential, 2
Impaired physical mobility, 2
Potential for injury, 3
Alteration in nutrition, 3
Sleep pattern disturbance, 5
Alteration in bowel elimination; alteration in urinary elimination patterns, 5
Potential for spiritual distress, 6
Potential alteration in body temperature, 7
Alteration in comfort: pain, chronic or acute, 8
Knowledge deficit, 9

Standards of Care Related to Behavioral Dysfunctions/Nursing Diagnoses, 10
Disturbance in self-concept: body image, self-esteem, role performance, personal identity, 10
Anxiety, 14
Hopelessness, 16
Dysfunctional grieving, 18
Ineffective individual coping, 19
Potential for violence: self-directed or directed at others, 20
Alteration in thought processes, 23
Impaired social interaction, 24

Other Aspects of General Care, 29
General preoperative care/teaching, 29
Care of patient in recovery room, 30
Assessment of the aging patient, 31
Emotional care of the dying patient, 32
Enteral nutrition, 34
Total parenteral nutrition (TPN), 51
Care of patient with central venous catheter, 55
Alteration in nutrition: less than body requirements, 59
Intravenous continuous drip narcotics, 64
Transcutaneous electrical nerve stimulation (TENS), 65

2 Cardiovascular System, 67

Cardiovascular assessment, 67
Peripheral vascular assessment, 73
Venous thrombosis, 74
Vein ligation and stripping, 76
Chronic arterial insufficiency, 77
Carotid endarterectomy, 80
Aortofemoral bypass graft, 81
Hypertensive crisis, 83
Angina pectoris, 85
Myocardial infarction (MI), 87
Vasodilator drugs, 89
Infective endocarditis, 93
Valvular heart disease, 94

Pericarditis, 98
Pericardiocentesis, 99
Cardiac tamponade, 100
Heart failure, 101
Shock syndrome, 104
Cardiac surgery (open-heart procedure), 108
Post–cardiac injury syndrome, 114
Cardiac rehabilitation, 115
ECG rhythms, 119
Pacemaker insertion, 134
Cardiac catheterization, 138
Percutaneous transluminal angioplasty (PTCA), 138
Hemodynamic monitoring, 141
Intraaortic balloon counterpulsation: balloon pump, 145
Shock trousers: pneumatic trousers (MAST), 148
Cardioversion (synchronized shock), 150
Defibrillation (direct current countershock), 150
Anticoagulant therapy, 151
Digitalis therapy, 154

3 *Hematologic System,* 157

Hematologic assessment, 157
Pernicious anemia (hyperchromic macrocytic anemia), 161
Iron deficiency anemia (hypochromic, microcytic anemia), 163
Hemolytic anemia, 165
Aplastic anemia, 168
Polycythemia, 173
Thrombocytopenia, 175
Acute leukemia, 177
Bone marrow transplantation (BMT), 181
Disseminated intravascular coagulation (DIC), 196
Multiple myeloma, 198
Hodgkin's disease, 202
Malignant lymphoma, 205
Splenectomy, 206
Lymphangiography, 208
Bone marrow study, 209
Pheresis, 209
Blood transfusions, 218

4 *Respiratory System,* 219

Respiratory assessment, 219
Therapeutic bronchoscopy, 224
Thoracentesis, 225
Aspiration of secretions, 226
Oxygen therapy, 227
Humidity and aerosol therapy, 229
Chronic obstructive pulmonary disease (COPD), chronic obstructive lung disease (COLD), 230
Asthma, 233
Bronchitis, 236
Bronchiectasis, 238
Emphysema, 239
Pulmonary rehabilitation, 242
Pneumonia, 243
Pulmonary edema, 245

Pulmonary embolism, 247
Pulmonary tuberculosis, 248
Sarcoidosis, 250
Pneumothorax, 252
Tension pneumothorax, 254
Hemothorax, 255
Thoracic empyema, 256
Atelectasis, 257
Pleural effusion, 258
Flail chest, 260
Respiratory failure, 261
Adult respiratory distress syndrome (ARDS), 263
Laryngectomy: radical neck dissection, 266
Thoracotomy, lobectomy, pneumonectomy, 269
Chest tubes, 271
Artificial airways, 272
Tracheostomy, 275
Continuous mechanical ventilation, 277
Intermittent positive pressure breathing (IPPB), 280
Incentive spirometer, 281

5 *Neurologic System*, 283

Neurologic assessment, 283
Diagnostic procedures, 288
Care of patient with altered consciousness, 288
Seizures, 291
Cerebrovascular disruptions, 293
Cerebrovascular accident (CVA), 296
Brain tumors, 300
Craniocerebral trauma, 302
Spinal cord injuries, 304
Surgical intervention of central nervous system, 307
Alzheimer's disease, 309
Parkinson's disease, 310
Multiple sclerosis (disseminated sclerosis), 313
Myasthenia gravis, 315
Myasthenia gravis crisis, cholinergic crisis, 317
Amyotrophic lateral sclerosis (ALS), 319
Guillain-Barré syndrome (acute infectious polyneuritis; polyradiculitis), 321
Neurologic infections, 323
Substance abuse (drug abuse and intoxication), 325
Lumbar puncture (spinal tap), 329
Hypothermia: care of patient, 329
Intracranial pressure (ICP) monitoring, 330
Increased intracranial pressure (ICP), 331
Bowel training, 332
Skull tongs (halo traction), 333
Care of patient on a circle bed, 333
Stryker frame, 334
General rehabilitative care of neurologic patient, 334
Paraplegia, 335
Quadriplegia, 336

6 *Digestive System*, 339

Gastrointestinal assessment, 339

Esophagus, 342

Esophageal trauma, 342
Esophageal stricture, esophagitis, achalasia, diverticulosis, 343
Bleeding esophageal varices, 344
Hiatal hernia with esophageal reflux, 346
Esophageal carcinoma, 347
Esophageal surgery, 349
Care of patient with Celestin tube, 350
Endoscopy: esophageal, gastric, duodenal, 352
Care of patient with Sengstaken-Blakemore tube or Linton tube, 352

Stomach, 354

Peptic ulcer disease (gastric and duodenal), 354
Gastric bleeding, 355
Gastric surgery, 357
Dumping syndrome, 358
Surgical intervention for obesity, 359
Gastric carcinoma, 364
Care of patient with nasogastric tube, 365
Care of patient with upper GI ostomy, tube, or prosthetic valve, 367

Intestines, 370

Irritable bowel syndrome: regional enteritis (Crohn's disease) and ulcerative colitis, 370
Peritonitis, 372
Short bowel syndrome, 373
Intestinal obstruction, 374
Intestinal carcinoma, 376
Paralytic ileus, 377
Diverticular disease of colon, 378
Intestinal surgery, 380
Continent ileostomy (Kock's pouch), 382
Ileoanal reservoir, 386
Care of patient with naso-oral intestinal tube (Cantor or Miller-Abbott tube), 388
Abdominal herniorrhaphy, 390
Ostomy management and care, 391
Colostomy irrigation, 393
Rectal surgery, 393

Gallbladder, 394

Biliary obstruction (stones, infection), 394
Biliary surgery, 396
Care of patient with T tube, 397
Transhepatic biliary decompression catheter, 398

Liver, 399

Cirrhosis: portal, postnecrotic, biliary, 399
Viral hepatitis, 401
Continuous peritoneal-jugular shunt for ascites (LeVeen shunt), 403
Care of patient undergoing paracentesis for ascites, 405
Hepatic surgery, 406
Portacaval-splenorenal shunts for portal hypertension, 407
Hepatic carcinoma, 410
Liver biopsy, 412

Pancreas, 413

Acute and chronic pancreatitis, 413
Pancreatic surgery, 414
Pancreatic carcinoma, 417

7 Endocrine System, 419

Endocrine assessment, 419
Hypothyroidism: myxedema, 424
Hyperthyroidism: thyroid crisis (storm, thyrotoxic crisis), 427
Thyroidectomy, 430
Hypoparathyroidism, 432
Hyperparathyroidism, 434
Parathyroidectomy, 436
Diabetic ketoacidosis, 437
Hyperosmolar hyperglycemic nonketotic coma, 440
Teaching the diabetic patient, 442
Hypoglycemia, 450
Hypopituitarism, 453
Hypophysectomy, 454
Central diabetes insipidus, 456
Adrenocortical insufficiency, 457
Cushing's syndrome, 460
Primary aldosteronism, 462
Pheochromocytoma, 464
Adrenalectomy, 465
Corticosteroid therapy, 467

8 Musculoskeletal System, 470

Musculoskeletal assessment, 470
Rheumatoid arthritis, 472
Orthopedic sepsis: acute pyogenic arthritis, acute osteomyelitis, 474
Osteosarcoma, 475
Systemic lupus erythematosus (SLE), 476
Progressive systemic sclerosis (scleroderma), 479
Gouty arthritis, 480
Osteoporosis, 481
Low back pain, 482
Fractures, 483
Maxillomandibular fixation, 485
Spinal surgery, 487
Fracture or dislocation of cervical spine, 489
Ankylosing spondylitis, 491
Chemonucleolysis, 492
Hip surgery, 493
Total joint arthroplasty: hip, knee, ankle, shoulder, elbow, wrist, finger, 495
Amputation of leg: above or below knee, 499
Arthroscopic surgery of knee, 501
External fixation for complicated fractures, 502
Digital replantation, 504
Compartmental syndrome, 506
Tissue pressure monitoring, 507
Open menisectomy, 509
Bunionectomy, 510
Traction, 511
Care of patient in traction, 513
Care of patient in cast, 514
Crutch-walking procedure, 516
Exercise terminology, 517
Continuous passive motion device, 517

9 *Genitourinary System,* 518

Genitourinary assessment, 518
Urinary tract infection (UTI), 522
Gonorrhea, 524
Urinary incontinence, 526
Surgery for female urinary incontinence, 528
Artificial urinary sphincter, 531
Acute urinary retention, 534
Neurogenic bladder, 537
Care of patient with indwelling urethral catheter, 540
Urinary diversion, 542
Polycystic kidney disease, 548
Glomerulonephritis, 551
Renal calculi/urolithiasis, 553
Renal failure, 557
Peritoneal dialysis, 562
Hemodialysis, 567
Nephrectomy, 571
Renal transplant: care of recipient, 575
Prostatic hypertrophy, 579
Prostatectomy, 580
Penile implant, 584
Torsion of spermatic cord, 588
Orchiopexy, 589
Orchiectomy for testicular tumor, 591

10 *Female Reproductive System,* 594

Female reproductive system assessment, 594
Pelvic inflammatory disease (PID), 596
Toxic shock syndrome (TSS), 597
Genital herpes, 598
Premenstrual syndrome (PMS), 599
Menopause and climacteric, 599
Hydatidiform mole, 600
Choriocarcinoma, 601
Dilation and curettage (D & C), 601
Cold-knife conization of cervix, 602
Abortion: saline or prostaglandin infusion, 603
Tubal ligation (abdominal), 604
Tubal pregnancy and salpingectomy, 605
Total abdominal hysterectomy and bilateral salpingo-oophorectomy (TAH-BSO), 606
Radical hysterectomy, 608
Vulvectomy, 609
Pelvic exenteration, 612
Care of patient receiving radium (cesium) therapy sealed in a mould, afterloader, colpostat, or Ernst applicator, 614
Modified radical mastectomy, 616

11 *Integumentary System,* 618

Integumentary system assessment, 618
Decubitus (pressure) ulcer, 619
Cellulitis, 621
Herpes type I viral infection, 622
Herpes zoster (shingles), 623
Care of patient with burns, 625

12 *Optic and Auditory Systems,* 631

Optic System, 631
Eye assessment, 631
Glaucoma: adult onset, 632
Eye surgery, 633
Visually impaired patient, 635
Contact lens removal, 637
Instillation of eye drops/ointments, 637

Auditory System, 638
Ear assessment, 638
Meniere's syndrome (endolymphatic hydrops), 639
Stapedectomy, 640
Myringotomy with tube insertion, 641
Tympanoplasty: types I through V, 642
Auditory-impaired patient, 643

13 *Oncology,* 646

Oncology assessment, 646
Cancer detection and prevention, 651
  General, 651
  Skin cancer, 652
  Cancer of head and neck, 652
  Lung cancer, 653
  Cancer of esophagus and stomach, 654
  Colorectal cancer, 655
  Renal, pelvis, and bladder cancer and cancer of ureter and urethra, 656
  Testicular cancer, 657
  Prostate cancer, 658
  Breast cancer, 658
  Vaginal cancer, 660
  Ovarian cancer, 660
  Cervical cancer, 661
  Uterine cancer (endometrial), 662
  Leukemia, 662
  Hodgkin's disease, 663
Antineoplastic chemotherapy, 666
Complications in chemotherapy, 684
  Myelosuppression, 684
  Nausea and vomiting, 690
  Stomatitis/mucositis, 692
  Diarrhea, 694
  Constipation, 695
  Gonadal dysfunction, 696
  Cardiotoxicity, 696
  Pulmonary toxicity, 697
  Urologic toxicity, 698
  Hyperuricemia, 699
  Neurotoxicity, 700
  Hepatotoxicity, 701
  Alopecia, 702
  Dermatologic toxicity, 703
  Extravasation, 704
Radiotherapy, 705
Unsealed radioactive chemotherapy, 709

14 Perinatal/Neonatal Standards, 711

Mother, 711

Antepartum assessment, 711
Pregnancy-induced hypertension (PIH; preeclampsia), 713
Eclampsia, 716
Hyperemesis gravidarum, 717
Amniocentesis, 718
Care of diabetic mother during last trimester of pregnancy, 719
Care of diabetic mother during labor and delivery, 720
Premature ruture of membranes (PROM), 721
Placenta previa, 722
Abruptio placentae, 723
Prolapsed umbilical cord, 724
Preterm (premature) labor, 725
Care of mother in first stage of labor, 728
Care of mother during delivery: second stage of labor, 732
Oxytocin infusion: augmentation or induction of labor, 733
Fetal distress, 734
Care of mother on fetal monitor, 735
Nonstress test (NST), 737
Contraction stress test (CST), 738
Postpartum care, 739
Cesarean delivery, 743
Breast-feeding, 747
Postpartum hemorrhage, 749

Newborn, 751

Care of newborn, 751
Care of premature infant, 755
Small for gestational age (small for date, low birth weight, intrauterine growth retardation, dysmaturity), 757
Large for gestational age (dysmaturity, high birth weight), 758
Postterm infant (postmaturity), 759
Infant of diabetic mother (IDM), 759
Hyperbilirubinemia, 761
Phototherapy, 762
Exchange transfusion, 763
Umbilical catheterization, 765
Neonatal sepsis, 765
Infants of addicted mothers, 767
Necrotizing enterocolitis (NEC), 769
Congenital syphilis, 770
TORCH infections, 771
Respiratory distress syndrome (hyaline membrane disease), 773
Meconium aspiration syndrome, 774
Care of newborn with endotracheal tube, 775
Care of newborn on a ventilator, 776
Bronchopulmonary dysplasia, 777
Intermittent gavage feeding, 778
Family-centered care of high-risk infant, 779

15 Pediatrics, 781

Basic Standards of Care, 781

Infant age-group care, 781
Toddler age-group care, 784
Preschool-age child care, 784

School-age child care, 785
Adolescent age-group care, 788

Respiratory System, 788
Croup: laryngotracheobronchitis, 788
Epiglottitis, 793
Pertussis: whooping cough, 795
Pneumonia, 796
Asthma, 798
Bronchiolitis, 800
Cystic fibrosis, 802

Gastrointestinal System, 805
Cleft lip repair, 805
Cleft palate repair, 806
Tracheoesophageal fistula, 808
Tracheoesophageal fistula repair, 810
Pyloric stenosis, 812
Ruptured (perforated) appendix, 813
Hirschsprung's disease: aganglionic megacolon, 815
Abdominoperineal pull-through procedure, 817
Gastroenteritis, 819
Diet for control of diarrhea, 820
Oral rehydration therapy, 821
Incarcerated inguinal hernia, 821
Intussusception, 822

Central Nervous System, 822
Hydrocephalus, 822
Ventricular shunt insertion, 823
Myelomeningocele, 825
Meningitis, 828

Genitourinary System, 830
Acute glomerulonephritis, 830
Nephrosis (nephrotic syndrome), 832

Hematology, 834
Acute leukemia, 834
Sickle cell crisis, 837

Endocrine System, 839
Diabetes mellitus (insulin dependent/type 1), 839
Failure to thrive (FTT), 841

Cardiovascular System, 844
Congenital heart defects, 844
Congenital heart surgery, 850
Congestive heart failure (CHF), 857
Pediatric digitalis therapy, 859
Temporary artificial pacemaker, 860

Other Aspects of Pediatrics, 860
Child abuse, 860
Anorexia nervosa, 862
Vital signs, 865
Nutrition, 866
Drugs, 868

Bibliography, 869
Appendixes
   A Medical-Surgical Care, 876
   B Guidelines for Patient Care Planning, 883

CHAPTER 1

General Care and Nursing Diagnoses

Standards of Care Related to Nursing Diagnoses

The standards of care in this section are the basic nursing functions required for all patients regardless of medical diagnosis. They are included to assist the nurse in selecting appropriate interventions for the following nursing diagnoses, on which the nurse may act independently. The nursing diagnoses included here were accepted in 1986 by the North American Nursing Diagnosis Association (NANDA). This is a partial listing of NANDA-approved nursing diagnoses.

IMPAIRMENT OF SKIN INTEGRITY, ACTUAL OR POTENTIAL

A state in which an individual's skin is altered or at risk of becoming altered

Assessment

Observations/findings

Debilitating diseases
Neuromuscular dysfunction
Cardiopulmonary impairment
Normal skin
Pruritis, abrasions, discoloration
Dryness, turgor
Redness over bony prominences
Color, cleanliness
Odor, integrity
Immobolizing devices

GOAL: *Patient's skin integrity will be maintained clean, dry, and intact*

Interventions

Bathe daily: complete or partial bed bath, tub, or shower using warm water and mild soap
   Provide privacy and avoid chilling
   Massage skin with mild lanolin-based lotions to increase circulation and maintain integrity
   Dry skin thoroughly
Assess perineal and perianal areas as needed; observe for excoriation, vaginal discharge, and pain; apply lotions or cornstarch to area as needed
Assess feet and hands; observe nail beds and observe for signs of rash, dryness, or skin breaks
   Soak in warm soap and water, dry well, and apply lotion prn
   Cleanse and trim nails prn
Assess condition of hair; observe for matting, tangles, signs of alopecia, lice, and cradle cap scales and dryness
   Comb hair daily and shampoo as needed
   Apply baby oil and massage into scalp; leave on 1 hr for scales, then gently shampoo and comb
   Apply alcohol to release tangles
   Style for comfort and easy care
Assess male patient for shaving needs
   Apply warm towels to face prior to shaving
   Rinse skin well and apply lotion after shaving
Maintain physical comfort
Change bed linen daily and prn; keep linen neat, dry, wrinkle-free, and clean
Provide adequate warmth
Change position frequently: small changes of body parts prevent pressure and fatigue

ALTERATION IN ORAL MUCOUS MEMBRANE, ACTUAL OR POTENTIAL

A state in which the oral cavity is disrupted or at risk of being disrupted

Assessment

Observations/findings

Mucous membranes, tongue, gums
   Moisture, integrity
   Swelling, bleeding
   Lesions, odor
   Tongue size
Teeth
   Cleanliness, odor
   Integrity, caries
   Sensitive to heat or cold
   Presence of dentures
NPO
Nasogastric tube
Wired jaws

GOAL: *Patient's oral cavity will be maintained clean, moist, and odor-free*

Interventions

Assess mucous membrane, tongue, and gums
Observe for moisture, cleanliness, integrity, edema, color, bleeding, and odor
Assess teeth for cleanliness, integrity, sensitivity to heat or cold, presence of dentures, and sordes
Brush teeth bid and prn with toothpaste, powder, baking soda, or mouthwash
Rinse with water or mouthwash
Apply petroleum jelly, lip balm, or glycerin-lemon mixture for dryness
Remove dentures and cleanse bid with toothpaste or powder and running water; protect from breakage and place in marked denture cup when not in use
Cleanse mouth with equal parts of hydrogen peroxide and water prn for sordes

ACTIVITY INTOLERANCE, ACTUAL OR POTENTIAL

A physiologic and/or psychologic state in which an individual expresses or demonstrates an inability to endure normal or increased activity

Assessment

Observations/findings

Response to activity
  Respiratory: dyspnea, shortness of breath, tachypnea
  Cardiovascular: decreased or increased pulse rate, altered rhythm, altered blood pressure
  Weakness, pallor, cyanosis
  Vertigo, confusion
Complains of fatigue, altered sleep patterns
General malaise
Ability and incentive to perform activity
Medical disease or condition
Medications, age, nutritional state
Environmental conditions: sensory overload, deprivation

GOAL: *Patient will be assisted with identifying factors that cause intolerance and progress toward optimum levels of activity for age, physical and psychologic limits, and medical disease process*

Interventions

Physical

Assess body systems for possible cause of inactivity
  Disturbance in oxygen maintenance
  Fluid or electrolyte imbalance
  Deficiencies in nutrition
  Neuromuscular disorders
Observe patient for pain and insufficient rest/sleep
Monitor side effects of all medications and diagnostic studies
Assess patient's tolerance to activity
  Explain procedure, activity, or treatment
  Monitor resting vital signs
  Have patient perform activity at own rate
  Monitor vital signs immediately and again in 3 min
  Discontinue activity if any of the following occur: chest pain, dyspnea, cyanosis, vertigo, confusion, hypotension, failure of systolic pressure increase, increased diastolic pressure, decreased respiratory rate, continuing tachycardia
  Reduce energy expenditure where possible
Increase activity slowly to increase tolerance; assist as needed
Coordinate care to allow for rest periods
Provide a safe environment
Maintain and increase strength with active or passive range-of-motion (ROM) exercises
Encourage self-care activities as soon as able
Provide adaptive devices to assist in activities of daily living (ADLs) as needed: padded eating utensils, long-handled tongs, etc.

Psychologic

Assess patient for presence of depression or lack of incentive, and assess for maladaptive behaviors
Explain importance of activity to tolerance
Involve patient in care plan and short-term goal setting
Acknowledge and praise attempted or completed tasks
Discuss, and assist patient with identifying, possible incentives to increase activity
Assist patient with identifying past coping behaviors that were successful

IMPAIRED PHYSICAL MOBILITY

A state in which an individual experiences or is at risk of experiencing a reduction or limitation in physical activity

Assessment

Observations/findings

Neuromuscular dysfunction: paralysis, muscular dystrophy or sclerosis, spinal cord injury
Musculoskeletal impairment: fracture, dislocation, surgery, atrophy, lupus erythematosus, amputations
Respiratory, cardiovascular conditions

Debilitating disease: cancer, renal, endocrine dysfunction
Pain, edema
Immobilizing devices
Assistance required
Mobilization devices required, weight-bearing limits
Coordination and muscle strength
Range of motion ability
Age, medications, emotional state

GOAL: *Patient's mobility will be maintained at optimum level for age, diagnosis, and physical limitations*

Interventions

Assess body systems for cause of immobility
Assess patient's mobility tolerance and motivation
Monitor vital signs prior to sitting up or ambulating
Following activity monitor vital signs at 3 min and at 15 min
   Observe for hypotension, hypertension, tachycardia, bradycardia, tachypnea, or bradypnea
   Observe for cyanosis, dyspnea, shortness of breath, and peripheral or neurovascular changes
Perform active or assist with and teach passive ROM exercises q4h; note tolerance and motivation
Maintain body alignment while in bed
Provide bed cradle as needed
Prevent footdrop or contractures with foot board
Support dependent limbs as needed with pillows or immobilizing devices; avoid pillow under knee
Avoid long periods in any one position: frequent small changes prevent pressure, discomfort, and fatigue
Maintain casts, braces, traction, or prosthetic devices in correct position to avoid discomfort or pressure
Progress in mobility slowly as tolerated and ordered
Assist patient as needed with sitting up, dangling, standing, and ambulation
Initiate and teach use of mobilizing devices as needed: crutches, walker, wheelchair, sling, Ace bandage

POTENTIAL FOR INJURY

A state in which a person is at risk of physical harm because of perceptual or environmental problems, lack of mental acuity, or age

Assessment

Observations/findings

Neuromuscular dysfunction
Sensory/cerebral impairment
Mobility impairment
Debilitating disease
Environmental hazards
Mobilizing devices
Age, occupation
Medical history
Accident history

GOAL: *Patient will demonstrate knowledge and understanding of potential hazards where possible and practice prevention measures or will be protected from injury as needed*

Interventions

Assess patient's mental, visual, and auditory acuity
Monitor neuromuscular status, age, and medication history
Assess ability to perform ADLs, exercises, and to ambulate
Maintain safe environment
Orient patient to surroundings
Provide needed equipment and maintain within easy reach; avoid clutter
Maintain side rail, bed position, and use of restraints policy as written
No smoking in room
Maintain clean and comfortable room
Assist patient with ADLs and teach use of safety rules of mobilizing devices as needed
Explain all treatments, procedures, and care
Provide adequate lighting
Instruct patient on safety precautions at home
Maintain electrical and hospital equipment in good repair
Maintain safe medication administration
Administer medications according to policy
Understand and monitor side effects
Instruct patient to take medications as prescribed on discharge and explain side effects to report to physician
Advise patient to avoid over-the-counter (OTC) medication unless prescribed by physician
Provide safety teaching according to maturational age
Home hazards
Fire, flammable items
Floors, stairs, ramps
Tubs, showers, pools
Lighting
Chemicals, medications

ALTERATION IN NUTRITION

A state in which a person experiences or is at risk of experiencing alteration of normal weight according to age and body build

TABLE 1-1. Height and Weight Tables for Adults with Desirable Weights for Persons Age 25 and Over

Men					Women				
Height		Small frame (lb)	Medium frame (lb)	Large frame (lb)	Height		Small frame (lb)	Medium frame (lb)	Large frame (lb)
Feet	Inches				Feet	Inches			
5	2	128-134	131-141	138-150	4	10	102-111	109-121	118-131
5	3	130-136	133-143	140-153	4	11	103-113	111-123	120-134
5	4	132-138	135-145	142-156	5	0	104-115	113-126	122-137
5	5	134-140	137-148	144-160	5	1	106-118	115-129	125-140
5	6	136-142	139-151	146-164	5	2	108-121	118-132	128-143
5	7	138-145	142-154	149-168	5	3	111-124	121-135	131-147
5	8	140-148	145-157	152-172	5	4	114-127	124-138	134-151
5	9	142-151	148-160	155-176	5	5	117-130	127-141	137-155
5	10	144-154	151-163	158-180	5	6	120-133	130-144	140-159
5	11	146-157	154-166	161-184	5	7	123-136	133-147	143-163
6	0	149-160	157-170	164-188	5	8	126-139	136-150	146-167
6	1	152-164	160-174	168-192	5	9	129-142	139-153	149-170
6	2	155-168	164-178	172-197	5	10	132-145	142-156	152-173
6	3	158-172	167-182	176-202	5	11	135-148	145-159	155-176
6	4	162-176	171-187	181-207	6	0	138-151	148-162	158-179

Weights at ages 25-59 based on lowest mortality.
Weight in pounds according to frame (in indoor clothing weighing 5 pounds, shoes with 1-inch heels).

Weights at ages 25-59 based on lowest mortality.
Weight in pounds according to frame (in indoor clothing weighing 3 pounds, shoes with 1-inch heels).

Metropolitan Life Insurance Co., New York, 1983.

EFFECT OF SOME DRUGS ON NUTRITIONAL STATUS

Aspirin	Malabsorption of folate
	Excretion of vitamin C
Barbiturates	Malabsorption of thiamin, vitamin B_{12}
	Excretion of vitamin C
Corticosteroids	Malabsorption of calcium, zinc, phosphorus
Hydralazine	Excretion of pyridoxine
Methotrexate	Malabsorption of vitamin B_{12}, folate, fat
Mineral oil	Malabsorption of fat-soluble vitamins, calcium, phosphorus
Neomycin	Malabsorption of major nutrients
Oral contraceptives	Possible decreased absorption of vitamin C, B complex vitamins, magnesium, zinc
Penicillin	Loss of potassium
Tetracycline	Malabsorption of calcium, iron, magnesium, pyridoxine
	Excretion of vitamin C, riboflavin, niacin, folic acid
Thiazides	Excretion of potassium, magnesium, zinc, riboflavin

From Long, B.C., and Phipps, W.J.: Essentials of medical-surgical nursing: a nursing process approach, St. Louis, 1985, The C.V. Mosby Co.

MEDICATIONS TO BE TAKEN WITH FOOD

Aminophylline	Nitrofurantoin (Macrodantin)
Chlorothiazide (Diuril)	Phenylbutazone (Butazolidin)
Ferrous sulfate	Phenytoin (Dilantin)
Indomethacin (Indocin)	Prednisolone
Metronidazole (Flagyl)	Reserpine (Serpasil)
	Triamterene (Dyrenium)

From Long, B.C., and Phipps, W.J.: Essentials of medical-surgical nursing: a nursing process approach, St. Louis, 1985, The C.V. Mosby Co.

Assessment

Observations/findings

Normal weight for age and size
Weight loss or gain
Prescribed diet, fluid intake (oral, parenteral)
Medical/surgical condition
NPO, nasogastric aspiration
Tube feedings, total parenteral nutrition (TPN)
Anorexia, dysphagia, dentures, ability to chew and feed self
Nausea, pain, discomfort
Nutritional status or history (anorexia nervosa, bulimia)

Medication history
Diagnostic tests, chemotherapy
Activity level
Emotional status
Cultural/ethnic preferences

GOAL: *Patient's nutritional status will be maintained to meet body requirements*

Interventions

Assess cause(s) for alterations in weight
Provide prescribed diet and fluids
Measure and record intake as needed
Encourage patient to eat and drink as prescribed
Assist patient in selection of beneficial foods according to order and need
Serve meals attractively and maintain pleasant surroundings
Place patient in comfortable position for eating
Promote small, frequent meals as needed
Assist with feeding or feed as necessary
Report alterations in eating or drinking patterns to physician
Administer oral hygiene before and after meals
Wash face and hands before and after meals
Assess medications for side effects causing decreased salivation (diuretics)
Discuss and explain types of food needed to produce weight loss or gain
Encourage activity to tolerance
Weigh patient as needed at same time with same clothing and scale
Maintain tube/parenteral feedings as ordered
Assess cultural/ethnic food preferences and provide where possible
Deal with causes of stress or depression that may contribute to overeating or lack of desire to eat
Withhold or restrict fluid intake as ordered

SLEEP PATTERN DISTURBANCE

A state in which a person experiences or is at risk of experiencing alterations in quantity or quality of rest/sleep because of environmental or biologic factors

Assessment

Observations/findings

Impaired cardiopulmonary function
Elimination dysfunction
Impaired metabolism, pregnancy
Immobilizing devices
Pain, discomfort, restlessness
Environmental changes
Medications
Depression, anxiety, fear
Debilitating diseases
Dreams, interrupted sleep
Inappropriate fatigue
Sensory deprivation

GOAL: *Patient's normal pattern of rest and sleep will be improved or will be maintained to optimum level, and a healthy balance of rest and activity will be provided*

Interventions

Assess and identify cause(s) of sleep disturbance
Assess patient's normal rest/sleep pattern
Control environmental disturbances, noise
Maintain quiet environment: close doors, pull drapes and dividers; decrease incoming stimuli
Provide night lights, soft music
Coordinate nursing functions to allow for rest periods and less interruptions during night
Limit visitors during rest periods and limit fluid intake where possible after 6 PM
Maintain balance of daytime activity and rest
Increase activity to tolerance
Limit sleep during daytime and stimulate wakefulness as required
Involve in unit and diversional activities
Provide comfort measures
Maintain warm, clean, comfortable bed
Provide needed equipment within easy reach
Encourage usual sleeping aids
Administer hs care as close to bedtime as possible
Administer hs sedative prn; obtain repeat order from physician as needed

ALTERATION IN BOWEL ELIMINATION; ALTERATION IN URINARY ELIMINATION PATTERNS

A state in which a person experiences or is at risk of experiencing alterations in elimination, bowel or urinary due to physiologic, psychologic, or metabolic factors

Assessment

Observations/findings

Gastrointestinal (GI)/renal dysfunction
Medication history
Age
Neuromuscular dysfunction
Anomalies

Pain, anxiety, fear
Fluid volume imbalance
Pregnancy, lack of privacy
Mental, visual acuity
Bowel elimination
    Nutritional status, diet, roughage intake
    Presence or absence of bowel sounds
    Normal elimination patterns: frequency, amount, color, consistency
    Tube feedings, TPN
    Type of present stool: formed, loose, hard
    Laxative use
    Activity level
    Distention, flatus, impaction
    Perianal irritation
    Hemorrhoids, fissures
    Paralytic ilius, malabsorption/dumping syndrome, surgical intervention
    Ostomy, ileoanal reservoir
Urine elimination
    Normal urinary pattern, frequency, amount, color
        Presence of urethral catheter
        Dehydration, fluid intake
        Nocturia, dribbling, incontinence, hesitancy
        Perineal irritation
        Estrogen deficiency, prostatic enlargement
Cystitis: dysuria, frequency, urgency, hematuria
Fecal impaction
Presence of ostomy

GOAL: *Patient's elimination will be maintained to optimum level within parameters of age and disease process*

Interventions

Assess cause(s) of altered elimination patterns
Assess normal elimination pattern
Bowel elimination
    Assess daily defecation routine and maintain pattern as much as possible
    Provide natural stimulants (coffee, prune juice) as allowed
    Maintain privacy
    Monitor and record daily bowel movements; monitor for melena as needed
    Initiate diet changes, if allowed, to maintain normal consistency
    Increase activity and fluid intake as allowed
    Provide natural laxatives initially, if allowed, before administering laxative or enema
    Instruct patient to avoid use of laxatives routinely
    Explain that medications can often cause diarrhea or constipation
    Initiate relaxing techniques to assist in defecation as needed
    Reduce rectal pain/discomfort from hemorrhoids through use of lubricants, increased exercise, cool compresses, stool softeners, suppositories
    Administer perianal care after each defecation
Urine elimination
    Assess cause(s) of impaired elimination
    Measure fluid intake and urine output as ordered or if deemed necessary
    Observe color, frequency, amount, and consistency
    Monitor for sugar, acetone, blood, and pH as ordered
    Monitor for residual urine as ordered
    Observe for frequency, urgency, dysuria, and distention
    Administer perineal care following urination
    Provide privacy
    Increase fluid intake, if allowed, to maintain hydration
    Institute voiding measures as needed: running water, leaning forward
    Maintain bedpan within easy reach
    Monitor indwelling urethral catheters for patency, correct position of collection unit, and infection; teach self-catheterization as needed
    Provide daily meatal care according to hospital policy
    Administer antibiotics as ordered

POTENTIAL FOR SPIRITUAL DISTRESS

A state in which a person experiences or is at risk of experiencing a disturbance in religious, intellectual, cultural, ethical, or moral beliefs

Assessment

Observations/findings

Anxiety, fear, grief, depression, guilt, hopelessness
Isolation, loss of faith, anger
Loss of body part or function
Terminal, debilitating disease
Barriers to religious practice
Conflicts of condition vs. religious beliefs
Self-destructive behavior
Requests prayers of others and religious symbols

GOAL: *Patient's spiritual beliefs and practices will be promoted and maintained*

Interventions

Assess cause(s) of spiritual distress, utilizing the following principles

Patient's belief in divine power, its existence, and credibility
Meaning of religion; description or relationship of divine power
Means of communicating with divine power
Effect of beliefs on personal life
Sense of identity, worth, and purpose
Relationship with others: value, need, changes caused by illness
Meaning of illness or suffering in relation to belief
Important features of religious faith
   Assistance with fear, pain
   Source of strength, hope, love
Religious practices, symbols, medals, garments

Provide a quiet, private atmosphere for expressions of faith, self, and meaning of life
Listen with attention, understanding, and compassion
Be available and sensitive to patient's need to express feelings
Talk with, not at, patient
Be cognizant of your nonverbal behavior, biases, preconceptions, and judgments
Do not impose your beliefs on patient
Accurately interpret and clarify meanings expressed and behavior observed
Assist patient with facing reality; explore experience of illness and meaning of suffering
Encourage self-awareness and mobilization of internal strengths and resources
Assist patient through uncompleted developmental stages to attain trust, hope, love, forgiveness, and purpose in life
Assist patient with exploring life situations and discovering practical solutions to problems
Allow and encourage free choice and decision making
Praise successes: physical, emotional, and spiritual
Convey to patient that he is important and what he does with his life matters
Use touch therapeutically when providing daily care: stroking, holding hands, and grooming
Provide pleasant view and special pictures
Control odors and smoking as necessary
Provide articles necessary for religious practice: special clothing, rosary, books, etc.
Arrange religious symbols for easy viewing
Arrange for favorite music: recordings and tapes
Read favorite, comforting passages from Bible, Koran, Torah, Book of Mormon, poetry, other meaningful works
Share in prayers or special practices when appropriate
Provide uninterrupted time for meditation, silence, and prayer
Arrange for communion, anointment, and other practices
Arrange easy access for communication with loved ones, chaplain, priest, rabbi, or minister
Provide special foods, meals, and periods of fasting as needed
Consider needs in special situations
   Birth: baptism or circumcision
   Medical procedures: amputation, burial, transfusions
   Note schedule for holy days
   Religious observances
   Anointment
   Laying-on of hands
   Healing services
   Confession
   Communion
   Holy days
   Restrictions or needs in diet or appearance
   Not cutting or shaving of hair
   Use of special clothing
Death
   Rite for anointing the sick
   Bathing and placement of body
   Positioning of extremities
   Other special practices

POTENTIAL ALTERATION IN BODY TEMPERATURE

A state in which a person is at risk for failure to maintain body temperature within the normal range

Assessment

Observations/findings

Medications causing vasoconstriction or dilation
Altered metabolic rate
Inappropriate clothing
Illness or trauma affecting thermal regulation
Tachycardia: full, bounding vs. weak, thready
Tachypnea
Hyperemia
Diaphoresis
Chills, headache, malaise
Restlessness, thirst, dehydration
Delerium, convulsions, tremors, hyponatremia
Convulsions

GOAL: *Patient's body temperature will remain normal or return to normal without residual problems*

Interventions

Monitor vital signs to identify hyperthermia
Administer antipyretics and/or sedatives as ordered

Explain coding procedure to patient
Administer alcohol sponge bath or cooling tub bath as ordered
Apply cold, wet sheets or ice packs as ordered; limit to 20 to 30 min at one time
Administer medication as ordered to prevent shivering
Monitor temperature q10 min during procedure
Discontinue cooling measures when temperature is 1° F above normal
Dry skin thoroughly (avoid friction) and provide clean, dry linen
Reduce physical activity and urge fluids (oral or parenteral) as ordered and tolerated
Administer antibiotics and antipyretics as ordered
Reinstitute cooling measures as needed
Maintain cool room temperature

ALTERATION IN COMFORT: PAIN, CHRONIC OR ACUTE

A state in which a person experiences discomfort in response to painful stimuli

Assessment

Observations/findings

Trauma: surgery, accidents
Carcinoma, any body system dysfunction
Inflammation, immobility, pressure points
Diagnostic tests
Pregnancy
Previous history of pain, surgery, or illness
Family history, age, religion, role, reward structure, experience with pain
Medication history
Subjective data
  Location, type, severity, intensity of pain; use rating scale 0 to 10: 0 for no pain and 10 for worst possible pain
  Medication used or other comfort measures
  Effect pain has on appetite, sleep, activity, and emotions
  Coping patterns used to relieve pain
Objective data
  Acute pain
    Pain up to 6 month's duration
    Disease or injury accounting for pain
    Healing will take place; pain will subside
  Chronic pain
    Over 6 month's duration
    Recurrent or ongoing pathology
    Benign, with adequate coping
    Intractable, with ineffective coping
  Activation phase
    Increased BP, P, and R
    Pallor, dilated pupils
    Increased muscle tension
    Cold perspiration
    Raised hairs on body
  Rebound phase: occurs if origin of pain is brief and intense
    P slower than prepain state
    BP lower than prepain state
  Adaptation phase: occurs if pain occurs frequently or is of long duration
    May take several hours to occur
    Mild increase in BP and P
  Stress reaction: occurs when pain persists for many days
    Increased production of 17-ketosteroids
    Increased production of eosinophils
    Increased susceptibility to infection
    Anger, irritability
    Tone of voice, speed of speech
    Vocalization: groan, whimper, cry, sob
    Facial expressions: clenched teeth, fist, lips
    Withdrawal
    Person is unable to verbalize (child, older aphasic, etc.)
    Pulling at painful part, abdominal rigidity
    Fetal position
    Unrelieved crying, moaning
    Restlessness
    Anorexia, insomnia
    Tachycardia, tachypnea

GOAL: *Patient will express or demonstrate minimal discomfort or absence of acute pain and identify positive coping behaviors for chronic pain*

Interventions

Develop trusting relationship
  Encourage patient to talk about himself
  Be a good listener
  Avoid judgmental statements
  Be truthful and consistent
  Accept pain as patient sees it
  Follow through on commitments to patient
  Initiate contacts with patient
  Assist patient with understanding his pain
  Explain relationship to pathology
  Estimate duration of pain when possible
  Explain painful procedures
Involve patient in care; allow some control over daily activities where possible
Encourage pain reduction techniques as appropriate:

rocking movements, external warmth, visual focal point with breathing patterns, effleurage

KNOWLEDGE DEFICIT

A state in which a person experiences a lack of cognitive knowledge or psychomotor skills that alters or may alter health maintenance

Assessment
Observations/findings
PATIENT

Verbalization or exhibition of lack of knowledge or skill
Failure to comply with prescribed health care
Past medical history
Marital status, role
Occupation, age, sex
Socioeconomic, cultural background
Ethnic values
Willingness, ability, and readiness to learn
Level of comprehension
Stressors, coping behaviors

NURSE

Ability to teach
Security in knowledge of material to be taught
Insight into individual needs of patient
Perception of expressed and unexpressed needs of patient
Ability to assess patient's readiness to learn
Awareness of own strengths and weaknesses
Security in approach to patients
Ability to be flexible in approach to patients
Ability to listen and *hear*
Ability to present information in a calm, unhurried, logical, and interesting manner

PRINCIPLES OF LEARNING

Desire to learn must be present before learning can take place
Each individual learns at own pace
Environment must be free from stress, discomfort, pain, or distracting factors
Information is best learned if it is meaningful, organized, and relevant
Individual will learn only if he sees value of information

PRINCIPLES OF TEACHING

Present information in small segments
Use language that is easily understood
Teach from a well-organized plan
Allow time for questions
Obtain feedback after each segment is presented
Continue with plan only when understanding is ensured
Maintain eye contact during presentation
Present information step by step and obtain a return demonstration when teaching a procedure
Use as many audiovisual aids as possible
   Films
   Slides
   Booklets
   Diagrams
   Procedure pictures
   Procedure equipment
Offer praise when learning takes place
Understand teaching plan that is most effective when initiated as soon after admission as possible, predicated on patient's condition and readiness

ASSESSMENT OF PATIENT'S LEARNING NEEDS

Utilize "knowledge deficit" nursing diagnosis of appropriate standards
Incorporate individual learning needs, either as expressed by patient or as observed by nurse
Assess needs daily or as condition changes and learning takes place
Communicate plan to all members of nursing team via conferences and nursing care plan

ESTABLISHMENT OF GOALS FOR LEARNING

Utilize information obtained in assessment
Set goals according to priority, patient's needs, and readiness to learn
Set small, specific, and realistic goals to provide patient with a sense of accomplishment
Write goals in nursing care plan

IMPLEMENTATION OF THE PLAN

Decide on a plan of action
   Who will do the teaching?
   How will the information be presented?
   When is the best time?
   What tools will be needed to augment the presentation?
   How will feedback be obtained?

GOAL: *Patient and/or significant other will demonstrate understanding of skill and/or information needed*

Interventions
Presentation

Present information about
   Orientation to hospital setting

Disease process
Procedures or surgery to be performed
Medications
Treatments
What to expect from staff and what is expected of patient
Prepare for information, question-and-answer sessions
On the spot, unplanned, according to patient's needs
Concerned with feelings, behavior, fears, or anxieties
Present teaching and learning skills and procedures patient must know how to perform
Obtain feedback
Be certain learning has taken place
Return demonstration
Questions
Correction of misconceptions
Reinforcement of teaching as needed

Evaluation

Establish whether learning has taken place
Observable change in patient's behavior
Patient's ability to perform a procedure or skill
Patient's ability to answer questions correctly
Communicate information to nursing care plan and/or patient's chart as to whether learning has taken place

Standards of Care Related to Behavioral Dysfunctions/Nursing Diagnoses

The standards of care in this section are also related to specific nursing diagnoses that were accepted in 1986 by NANDA. This section has been included to assist the nurse in the clinical setting by providing suggestions for interventions in those cases where patients present problematic behavior. As with the first section of this chapter, inclusion of all approved nursing diagnoses/behavioral dysfunctions is beyond the scope of this section; however, reference is made to many diagnoses that are related to one another either etiologically or by defining characteristics. Those diagnoses that have broad application and that are often seen in association with physical illness have been presented.

The primary aim of the nursing diagnosis is clear direction for nursing intervention. Individualization of nursing care plans is desirable to optimize health; hence the psychosocial aspects of patient care need inclusion if this is to be accomplished.

Diagnosis of behavioral dysfunctions may be used in the psychiatric–mental health setting, though its primary purpose is to facilitate the generalist in acute care, long-term care, and home health care areas in providing quality services. The term *behavioral dysfunction* does not imply mental illness, and for this reason there has been no attempt to define this concept here.

The psychiatric/mental health nurse frequently refers to the *American Psychiatric Association's Diagnostic and Statistical Manual, Third Edition (DSM III)*. The manual consists of a holistic, multiaxial coding system that is atheoretic and offers specific behavioral criteria that must be met before a psychiatric diagnostic label is assigned to a patient. Many mental health nurses prefer to use this reliable tool and feel that nursing needs to further develop its use. A separate nursing taxonomy of behavioral dysfunctions, however, can be coordinated with the use of the *DSM III*. Nursing diagnosis more clearly guides the practice of nursing and fosters development as an independent autonomous profession.

Behavioral dysfunction standards, as they relate to nursing diagnosis, will be a useful tool for the nurse in formulating care plans. An extensive list of suggested interventions is provided. It is hoped that the nurse will select those interventions that seem appropriate to the individual patient's care. The "defining characteristics" portion will enable the nurse to select the most relevant diagnosis. The "description" includes a brief definition of the diagnosis and possible etiology, which is not meant to be theoretically based.

The following is a partial listing of 1986 NANDA-approved nursing diagnoses related to behavior.

DISTURBANCE IN SELF-CONCEPT: BODY IMAGE, SELF-ESTEEM, ROLE PERFORMANCE, PERSONAL IDENTITY

Description

Self-concept is the dynamic organization of the personality structure of an individual that develops out of experience, especially through early interactions with significant others, and serves as the fundamental frame of reference for the individual's perceptions and beliefs. As such, the self-concept remains fairly stable over time and yet is influenced by biopsychosocial phenomena. Any threat to the self-concept, as in illness of any sort, will generate anxiety. The self-system is made up of various components. Specifically, NANDA has included body image, self-esteem, role performance, and personal identity to be considered in nursing assessment.

Body Image
Description

An individual's body image is a component of the self system that is a dynamic cognitive, perceptual organization of the physical self, which is influenced by cultural, social, and psychologic variables. It involves the conscious and unconscious perceptions of the physical self as they relate to sexuality, appearance, health, age, body functioning, body boundary, and integrity of the physical self. A person's body image develops and changes throughout life, though a relatively consistent body image is present by school age. Disturbance in body image may occur developmentally, as in adolescence and old age. Other disturbances may occur situationally, as in an accident, surgery, chronic debilitating illness, terminal illness, stroke, or psychiatric disorder. Any alteration in body image involves grief work. Resolution of the grief work relates to acceptance of the change. An individual's perception of the altered body image and perception of the importance of the body part involved seem to be the most significant variables influencing acceptance, rather than the concrete change, actual disability, or actual loss.

Defining characteristics of altered body image

Denial of physical change or illness
Refusal to look at body part
Inability to touch body part
Hiding or overexposing of body part
Refusal to perform ADLs
Social withdrawal and alienation
Excessive fear of rejection by others: individual feels stigmatized
Regression
Excessive anger or open hostility
Identity concerns (sexual and role performance)
Depersonalization: unreality and instability of personal identity
Diffuse body boundary: merging with physical or social environment
Self-destructive behavior
Loss of self-esteem
Shame and guilt
Nursing diagnoses often associated with disturbance in body image: social isolation, potential for self-directed violence, ineffective individual and family coping, sensory-perceptual alteration, altered thought process, alteration in comfort, altered sexual patterns, sexual dysfunction, dysfunctional grief, and powerlessness

GOALS: *Patient will*
Verbalize physical change, loss, or disability
Discuss altered body image with staff and significant others
Begin grief work
Identify and express feelings: positive and negative
Initiate self-care activities
Seek knowledge or information about disability or change
Use resources for support

Interventions

Determine patient's perception of change in body image and subsequent threat to self
Encourage verbalization of emotions such as anger, fear, frustration, and anxiety about altered functioning or lost body part
Encourage patient to look at and touch changed or lost body part
Assist family in adapting to change through providing resources, encouraging verbalization, and including in care of family member
Encourage discussion of physical changes in simple, direct, and factual manner
Assess own attitudes and values related to wholeness and physical appearance
Give realistic feedback about loss or change
Discuss sexual concerns openly and honestly
Encourage patient to participate in all therapeutic modalities offered in treatment
Give positive feedback for attempts to enhance and integrate new body image
Allow patient to progress at own rate; do not force independent functioning or allow for too much dependency
Help patient discriminate between internal stimuli and those that come from environment
Use active listening for nonverbal clues as well as verbal statements
Assess previous adaptive and maladaptive responses to stressors and illness
Assess for self-destructive behavior
Display empathy rather than sympathy
Provide patient and family with hospital and community resources
Discuss options available, such as cosmetic procedures, mechanical devices, and rehabilitative services
Teach patient and family the stages of grief and importance of grief work

Evaluation

Patient
    Completes grief work
    Verbalizes an acceptance of altered body functioning or loss
    Realistically plans for future role functioning
    Incorporates prosthesis, stoma, or device into changed body image
    Verbalizes an interest and willingness to rejoin and resume social interactions and activities
    Utilizes hospital and community support systems

Self-Esteem

Description

Self-esteem is the set of evaluative attitudes toward the self that are associated with personal satisfaction and effective functioning. It gradually develops through exposure to the environment and the social milieu. Self-esteem is a judgment about one's worth and reflects the degree of self-respect and confidence one has at a given point in time. Self-esteem is not fixed, and is greatly influenced by the interactions one has with significant others.

Defining characteristics of low self-esteem

Negative labeling such as "I am bad," "I'm weak"
Self-destructive behavior
Unassertive behavior: passive and dependent or hostile and controlling
Inflated self-importance
Reliance on medications and/or alcohol
Lack of insight and self-awareness
Marked resistance to change and/or overinvestment with the familiar
Lack of interest in personal hygiene and grooming
Tendency to view the world in a negative light, which reflects lack of trust
Overachieves in an attempt to be perfect and please and/or does not participate, so fails
Difficulty with giving and receiving compliments or realistic constructive criticism
Lack of interest in environment: does not initiate
Has experienced multiple losses
Overreliance on external reinforcement
Reluctance to share feelings
Relates repeated negative interpersonal experiences
Nursing diagnoses often associated with disturbance in self-esteem: social isolation, impaired social interaction, hopelessness, powerlessness, self-care deficit, self-directed potential for violence, anticipatory and dysfunctional grieving, rape trauma syndrome, ineffective individual and family coping, anxiety, altered sexuality patterns, alteration in nutrition, posttrauma response, and potential for noncompliance

GOALS: *Patient will*
Verbalize several positive aspects of self
Demonstrate interest in appearance and attend to personal hygiene and grooming
Display only mild anxiety when faced with changes in routine
State needs without expressing excessive fear of rejection
Act assertively out of personal choice with use of "I" statements
Complete tasks
Discuss alternatives in action

Interventions

Provide for success experiences by introducing tasks at patient's level of functioning
Assess for possible alcohol or drug dependency
Communicate acceptance of patient and show genuine concern by spending unstructured, undemanding time
Explore patient's feelings and give validation for their expression
Provide for positive feedback on accomplishments
Explore alternative approach or coping strategies
By giving observations, comment on positive attributes
Explore with patient his current strengths
Encourage group interaction and explore possible support groups for aftercare
Assist with grooming and hygiene when necessary
Help patient list past success experiences
Teach assertive techniques: use of "I" statements, ability to say "no," body posture, eye contact, tone of voice, personal space, tactics for negotiation
Teach difference between assertion and nonassertion; aggressive and passive behaviors
Practice role playing
Discuss activities that might increase self-esteem

Evaluation

Patient
  Verbalizes realistic appreciation of self, including attributes and limitations
  Presents a positive personal appearance that reflects good grooming and hygiene
  Initiates approach strategies to potentially threatening events or changes in environment
  Demonstrates appropriate assertive behavior in social interactions
  Reports a minimal level of interpersonal anxiety
  Displays no overt self-destructive behaviors
  Effectively communicates needs

Role Performance

Description

Roles stem from societal expectations of performance. Roles have identifiable patterns of behavior as specified by society and are influenced by developmental issues, situational transitions, family dynamics, culture, norms, and social position. The significant roles one chooses become incorporated into the individual's self-concept and how effectively the individual performs given roles will influence self-esteem.

Defining characteristics of disturbance in role performance

Change in self-perception of role
Change in other's perception of role
Role conflict
Lack of appropriate role models
Change in usual number of responsibilities
Change in physical capacity to perform role
Lack of knowledge of role
Change in social system
Change in personal values and expressive behaviors
Nursing diagnoses often associated with disturbance in role performance: alteration in cardiac output, alteration in comfort, ineffective individual and family coping, alteration in family process, dysfunctional grieving, altered growth and development, altered health maintenance and impaired home maintenance management, knowledge deficit, alteration in parenting, powerlessness, sexual dysfunction, social isolation, alteration in thought process, and impaired mobility

GOALS: *Patient will*
State specific behaviors necessary for mastery of role
Demonstrate ability to perform specific role functions
Verbalize knowledge of expected role behaviors
Identify areas of ambivalence and conflict in reciprocal and related role obligations
Verbalize behaviors necessary to integrate multiple role responsibilities
Clarify and validate role expectations with significant others
Begin grief work over lost or altered role functioning

Interventions

Assess nature and degree of disturbance in role performance
Assess patient's and significant other's perceptions of role disturbance
Assess cultural and economic factors
Determine number and types of roles within family structure
Assist patient and family with clarifying expected roles and those that must be relinquished or altered
Assist patient with verbalizing realistic expectations of role and concrete behaviors necessary to implement performance
Support grief work if lost role has occurred
Determine if patient is in role that is compatible with sexual orientation, sexual functioning, and self-concept
Provide role model for patient or resources to reference groups that supply new models
Assist in role rehearsal through role playing

Evaluation

Patient
　Verbalizes realistic perception and acceptance of new, lost, or altered role
　Demonstrates role mastery
　Develops with family or significant other specific behavioral strategies for assimilating role-specific changes in existing system

Personal Identity

Description

Personal identity is the coherent sense of self as a unique and separate identity that develops through successful resolution of developmental issues. Identity rests on the ability to distinguish self from others and the environment.

Defining characteristics of disturbance in personal identity

Disturbance in body image
Sex role disturbance
Gender identity confusion
Pathologic symbiotic relationships
Undifferentiated or fused family
Dissociative states
Developmental crisis such as adolescence
Delirium or dementia
Functional psychotic states: schizophrenia, bipolar disorder
Severe anxiety and/or panic
Hypnagogic states
Nursing diagnoses often associated with alteration in personal identity: disabling ineffective family coping, impaired gas exchange, posttrauma response, sensory-perceptual alteration, sexual dysfunction, sleep pattern disturbance, social isolation, altered thought process, altered tissue perfusion, hyperthermia, hopelessness

GOALS: *Patient will*
State satisfaction with gender, sexual behavior, and sexual preference choice
Participate in the real or actual environment
Maintain adequate balance of nutrition, hydration, elimination, and rest

Communicate effectively with others
Remain oriented to person, time, place, and situation
Verbalize developmental issues that affect personal identity
Identify actual threats to the self system
Report anxiety is at mild level

Interventions

Assist patient with identifying actual threats to self from misinterpretation of perceived threat
Provide accurate information about threat
Provide calm, structured environment
Direct activities that support reality issues: simple and concrete
Use simple, direct, and concise statements
Assess for altered homeostatis due to physiologic disequilibrium
Assess developmental issues: age, crisis, regression
Encourage verbalization of anxiety concerning sexual identity and sexual preference; be nonjudgmental
Assess for loss of contact with reality: hallucinations and/or delusions
Do not argue with delusions; do not reinforce; look for needs they might satisfy and find more appropriate manner of meeting them
Objectively point out your reality when hallucinations are present; help patient focus on here and now; decrease stimuli and help reduce level of anxiety
Use anxiety-reducing interventions
Teach principles of normal growth and development
Refer to psychiatric unit or psychotherapy as necessary

Evaluation

Patient
  States ability to define and identify self
  Maintains contact with reality
  Verbalizes realistic plan to meet actual threats to self
  Acknowledges and accepts developmental changes into new personal identity

ANXIETY

Description

Anxiety is a feeling of apprehension due to a real or perceived threat to some significant value that is held essential to the individual's self-concept and sense of personal security. Anxiety differs from fear in that fear usually involves a reaction to a definable and specific danger, though anxiety often accompanies fear. It is essential for the nurse to assess the level of anxiety so as to intervene appropriately.

Mild Anxiety

Description

Mild anxiety is normal anxiety that motivates an individual on a daily basis wherein the ability to perform and problem solve is enhanced.

Defining characteristics of mild anxiety

Slight discomfort
Restlessness
Mild insomnia
Mild change in appetite
Irritability
Repetitive questions
Attention-seeking behaviors
Increased alertness
Increased perception and problem solving
Easily angered
Focus on future problems
Fidgety movements
All of the NANDA nursing diagnoses may be associated with anxiety in one of its levels

GOALS: *Patient will*
Verbalize increased insight
Learn new task or material

Interventions

Watch for signs of increasing anxiety
Help client channel energy constructively
Use prn medication sparingly
Encourage problem solving
Provide accurate and factual information
Be aware of defense mechanisms used
Assist in identifying successful coping skills
Maintain a calm, unhurried manner
Teach client that mild anxiety is a normal part of living
Teach relaxation exercises and techniques

Evaluation

Patient
  Utilizes capabilities of effective coping to solve potential or actual threat
  Increases knowledge of self and or situation
  Reports an enhancement of self-esteem

Moderate Anxiety

Description

Moderate anxiety is anxiety that now interferes with new learning by narrowing the perceptual field so that the individual grasps less but is able to attend with direction by others.

Defining characteristics of moderate anxiety

Progression of mild anxiety
Selectively attentive to environment
Concentrates on individual tasks only
Moderate subjective discomfort
Increase in amount of time spent on problem situation
Voice tremors
Change in voice pitch
Tachypnea
Tachycardia
Tremulousness
Increased muscle tension
Nail biting, finger drumming, toe tapping, or foot swinging

GOALS: *Patient will*
Attend to threat with assistance by care giver
Utilize ways of reducing anxiety

Interventions

Maintain calm, unhurried manner when dealing with patient
Speak in calm, firm, reassuring manner
Use short, simple sentences
Avoid becoming anxious, angry, or defensive
Listen to patient with respect and interest
Offer some physical contact with patient; touch patient's hand or arm
Administer tranquilizers and sedatives as ordered
Assist patient with labeling and recognizing anxiety
Assist patient with identifying and describing feelings and the source of distress
   Do not probe
   Allow patient to cry
   Allow for verbal expression of anger
Assist patient with correcting events that precipitated anxiety
Encourage participation in diversional activities
   Reading
   Watching television
   Listening to the radio
   Writing letters
   Physical activity: walking
   Visiting with relatives or friends
Assist patient with identifying coping mechanisms that will reduce anxiety and with using those that have been successful in the past
Teach patient to use relaxation techniques with assistance
Encourage patient to engage in activities using large muscle groups
Establish and maintain familiar routines
Teach patient the importance of establishing daily exercise to control stress level
Continue with mild anxiety care

Evaluation

Patient perceives threat realistically and has diminished anxiety level

Severe Anxiety

Description

During an episode of severe anxiety the perceptual field is narrowed to the point that the individual is unable to problem solve or learn. The focus is on small or scattered details, and communication patterns are disrupted. The patient may exhibit many aborted attempts to reduce anxiety and usually verbalizes great subjective distress.

Defining characteristics of severe anxiety

Sense of impending doom
Excessive muscle tension (headache, muscle spasms)
Diaphoretic
Respiratory changes
   Sighing
   Hyperalimentation
   Hyperventilation
   Dyspnea
   Dizziness
GI changes
   Nausea, vomiting
   Heartburn
   Belching
   Anorexia
   Diarrhea or constipation
Cardiovascular changes
   Tachycardia
   Palpitations
   Precordial discomfort
Greatly reduced range of perception
Inability to learn
Inability to concentrate
Sense of isolation
Difficult or inappropriate verbalization
Purposeless activity
Hostility

GOALS: *Patient will*
Verbalize a decrease in behavioral, affective, and physiologic symptoms of anxiety
Display ability to concentrate and attend with assistance to the immediate environment

Utilize coping strategies to reduce anxiety level with assistance
Identify thoughts or perceptions that preceded the severe anxiety

Interventions

Isolate patient in quiet and safe environment
Provide frequent to constant contact and care
Administer medications as ordered
Assist and/or make decisions for patient; do not ask patient to do this entirely for self
Observe for signs of increasing agitation
Do not touch patient without permission
Assure patient that he will be safe
Assess for safety in the immediate environment

Evaluation

Patient demonstrates that anxiety level has been reduced to moderate level

Panic

Description

Anxiety has escalated to the level that the individual is now a danger to self and/or others and may become immobilized or strike out in a random fashion.

Defining characteristics of panic

Severe hyperactivity or immobility
Extreme sense of isolation
Loss of identity; personality disintegration
Severe shakiness and muscular tension
Inability to communicate in complete sentences
Distortion of perception and unrealistic appraisal of environment and/or threat
Disorganized behavior in attempting to escape
Assaultive

GOAL: *Patient will not harm self or others*

Interventions

Remain with patient; call for assistance
Remove as many physical and psychologic stressors from environment as possible
Speak in a calm, reassuring manner using low voice tones
Tell patient that you (staff) will not allow him to harm self or others
Isolate patient in quiet, safe area
Continue with severe anxiety care

Evaluation

Anxiety level decreases to moderate level

HOPELESSNESS

Description

Hopelessness is a subjective state in which an individual sees limited or no alternatives or personal choices available and is unable to mobilize energy on his own behalf. It is a state of extreme powerlessness (either trait or situational) in which the individual remains apathetic and socially withdrawn.

Defining characteristics of hopelessness

Terminal illness
Moderate to severe depression
Passivity and helplessness
Regression and dependency
Apathy or excessive crying
Resignation and powerlessness
Hypersomnia or insomnia
Severe weight loss (greater than 10 lb)
Loss of self-esteem
Loss of energy and interest in usual activities
Loss of will to live
Loss of belief in transcendent being
Inability to externalize anger
Loss of ability to care for self and meet basic needs
Nursing diagnoses often associated with hopelessness: altered cardiac output, ineffective breathing pattern, alteration in comfort (chronic pain), impaired verbal communication, dysfunctional grieving, impaired physical mobility, alteration in nutrition, powerlessness, disturbance in self-concept, sleep pattern disturbance, social isolation, altered thought process, altered tissue perfusion, potential for self-directed violence, self-care deficit, ineffective individual coping, spiritual distress

GOALS: *Patient will*
Verbalize personal influence in current situation
Initiate self-care
Verbalize belief system or sustaining values
Externalize anger appropriately
Initiate social interaction
Establish adequate nutrition and rest
Verbalize positive feelings about self
Display no morbid or self-destructive thoughts or actions

Interventions

Maintain a kind but firm attitude in all patient care activities
Maintain adequate hydration and nutrition
Measure intake and output as ordered or if indicated

Allow patient to wear own clothes when possible

Involve patient in decision-making process when formulating care plan

Help patient set small, realistic goals

Give positive reinforcement for independent functioning

Assist patient with identifying areas over which he has control

If appetite is poor and patient is eating insufficiently, offer soft, nutritious foods that are easily chewed; include high-protein between-meal snacks and a variety of liquids such as milk shakes, custards, and eggnog

Maintain liquids and foods within easy reach

Offer frequent small amounts

Discourage intake of nonnutritive items such as coffee and foods high in refined sugar

Encourage intake of water

Serve food attractively and at proper temperature

Provide foods that patient prefers; assist with menu selection

Do not give patient choice of not eating by asking, "Do you feel like eating?" Offer foods, saying, "I have something for you to eat"

Administer stool softeners or laxatives as ordered

Encourage intake of foods rich in fiber

Reinforce and assist grooming efforts and personal hygiene; encourage male patient to shave and female patient to apply makeup and style hair

Encourage patient to do things for self in order to feel better rather than waiting to feel better first before doing things for self

Assist with positioning in bed, sitting, and ambulation

Offer positive recognition for increased activity level

Provide noncompetitive activities (handicrafts, sewing, simple puzzles) prior to progressing to competitive activities such as board games

Promote planned rest periods during the day based on physical condition

Discourage sleeping all day or remaining in bed

Decrease environmental and other stimuli at night to promote sleep

    Promote bedtime rituals

    Avoid stressful conversation

    Avoid caffeine-containing substances

    Avoid exercise prior to bedtime

    Offer back rub and warm milk

    Do not encourage dependence on hypnotics, especially those that suppress REM (rapid eye movement) sleep

Continually assess for suicide potential

If patient expresses plan for suicide, ask for details of plan

Support all verbalization of feelings, especially anger

Report suicidal ideation to attending physician

Observe closely for any self-destructive behavior as mood-elevating medications take effect or if patient demonstrates a sudden change in affect or behavior

Plan time to sit with patient; do not act rushed and remain comfortable during silent periods; do not require patient to always talk

Do not discourage patient from crying; remain with and support patient unless patient requests privacy

Do not belittle patient's statements or offer inappropriately cheerful remarks or platitudes such as "Everything's going to be all right"

Be sure reassurances are realistic and are meant for patient, not nurse

Assess your own feelings of powerlessness and helplessness

Avoid agreement with self-deprecating statements and cast doubt on their validity, but do not argue with patient

Reinforce positive statements about self and others; do not be overcomplimentary

If patient expresses feelings of guilt, assist him with exploring their origin and with exploring associated feelings of anger and resentment

Respect denial of illness if patient is unable to accept it; do not force reality on patient

Assist and support gradually increasing amounts of independent self-care

Provide for physical exericse at patient's level of tolerance

Maintain a clean orderly environment

Ask if visit by religious or spiritual support person is desired

Administer antidepressants as ordered

    Be aware of lag time of up to 2 weeks before they take effect

    Familiarize yourself with side effects; most common are anticholinergic

    Beware of possible "cheeking" medication or hoarding at bedside: antidepressants are lethal

Evaluation

Patient

    Demonstrates relief of symptoms of moderate and severe depression

    Reaches acceptance stage of death and dying if terminal illness is present

    Utilizes problem solving to increase individual capabilities

    Verbalizes source of hope

Participates fully in own treatment
Verbalizes no self-destructive thoughts
Establishes social network for support

DYSFUNCTIONAL GRIEVING

Description

Grief is an individual's response to the loss of a person, object, or concept that is highly valued; uncomplicated grief is a healthy, adaptive response. Its absence may well signal dysfunctional behavior. Engel defines the sequence of events in normal grief as follows: shock and disbelief, developing awareness, restitution, and resolution. Nursing care primarily revolves around facilitating this natural response to loss by (1) providing for privacy, (2) seeing that the bereaved does not experience abandonment, (3) supporting the verbalization of feelings and concerns, (4) facilitating saying "good-bye" through permitting viewing and touching of the body and supporting cultural/religious rituals, and (5) promoting socialization and interaction with significant others. Grief work may last up to 2 years. The stages of grief do not always go in order and may be repeated.

Anticipatory grief is the initiation of the process of grieving before the significant loss actually takes place.

Dysfunctional grieving represents a distortion of normal grief in which the process is either delayed, prolonged, or exaggerated.

Defining characteristics of dysfunctional grief

Excessive, protracted grief
Delayed response or denial of loss
Lasting patterns of ineffective functioning
Emergence of unresolved past losses as if they just occurred
Absence of anticipatory grief due to denial or sudden loss
Unabated searching
Excessive self-blame and guilt
Introjection of illness through physical symptoms similar to those of the deceased
Anniversary symptoms
Severe depression
Intense separation anxiety
Social withdrawal
Prolonged and stressful anticipatory grief with excessive ambivalence
Self-destructive behaviors
Nursing diagnoses often associated with dysfunctional grief: disturbance in self-concept, alteration in family process, impaired home maintenance management, hopelessness, alteration in parenting, powerlessness, self-care deficit, sexual dysfunction, social isolation, potential for self-directed violence, spiritual distress

GOALS: *Patient will*
Realistically accept loss
Actively work through grief stages by verbally expressing feelings and by nonverbal expression of emotions
Involve self in social network
Resume self-care, former interests, and responsibilities when possible
Seek new relationships and interests
Work through past losses as they apply to current situation

Interventions

Identify significance of loss or multiple losses
Discuss ambivalence
Be aware of stage of grief and support patient's expression of grief
Use active listening and permit verbalization of anger
Observe for suicidal ideation
Facilitate discussion of positive and negative aspects of loss
Facilitate exploration of support groups
Provide opportunities for social interaction
Teach patient and significant other about grief process
If individual attempts to consistently deny grief, plan to spend time each shift talking about loss, but avoid confrontation during discussion if patient changes subject and shifts reference; take cues from patient; be available to reopen subject when patient initiates conversation; use times of silence to convey support by offering your presence nonverbally
Assure individual that all feelings are normal, including anger, hatred, and feelings of desertion, guilt, or betrayal
Expect individual to meet responsibilities and give positive reinforcement for resuming role responsibilities
Withdraw attention (negative reinforcement) if individual does not fulfill responsibilities for own care, which he is capable of doing
Assist individual with identifying ways of adapting life-style to accommodate the loss
Be aware that it is acceptable to share your feelings with individual as long as these activities serve to support patient through his grief and are not expressions of unresolved loss on your part
If you become uncomfortable with your own unre-

solved feelings of loss, have another nurse who is comfortable talk with individual

Evaluation

Patient
- Relates realistically to both the pleasures and the disappointments of the lost relationship
- Establishes new and meaningful relationships and interests
- Displays no exaggerated or distorted emotional reactions to the deceased or loss
- Engages in constructive, meaningful life-style (pre-crisis level of functioning)
- For anticipatory grief: maintains a constructive and meaningful relationship with the dying significant other without displaying characteristics of dysfunctional grief

INEFFECTIVE INDIVIDUAL COPING

Description

Ineffective coping is the impairment of adaptive behaviors and problem-solving abilities of a person in meeting life's demands and roles. Adaptive behaviors can be viewed as those that enable an individual to identify stressors and resolve the stress response. All crises are considered stressors and result when an event such as loss, transition, or challenge is perceived as a threat to self that may overwhelm the individual, leaving him vulnerable and unable to function effectively. Crises are time limited (resolved within 6 to 8 weeks), and are coped with either adaptively or maladaptively. During crisis, anxiety rises and personal safety and security is perceived as endangered. The individual struggles to reach a state of psychic equilibrium through learned coping strategies. If these coping mechanisms are ineffective in resolving the present situation, lasting impairment in functional ability may result. This further reduces coping strategies. Successful resolution of a crisis can potentiate growth and enhance self-esteem and coping ability or, as mentioned above, leave an individual feeling powerless. There are three types of crises: maturational, situational, and social. Examples of these follow:

Maturational (anticipated, normative): birth, life stages (e.g., adolescence, marriage, children leaving home, menopause)

Situational (unanticipated): hospitalization and illness, death of significant person, job loss, divorce, birth of premature infant or infant with defects

Social (unanticipated): violent crimes; war; fire, flood, or earthquake; civil riots

Defining characteristics of ineffective individual coping

Situational, maturational, or social crisis
Multiple losses and/or life changes
Inability to meet role expectations
Alteration in social interaction
Excessive or inappropriate use of defense mechanisms
Depression and low self-esteem
Excessive somatic complaints and/or psychophysiologic disorders
Excessive use of prescribed tranquilizers
Overeating
Excessive smoking or alcohol intake
Inability to problem solve
Loss of control
Escalating anxiety levels
Ineffective individual coping can be associated with most approved nursing diagnoses, since any illness or disorder may represent a threat large enough to precipitate a crisis

GOALS: *Patient will*
- *Obtain realistic perception of event or stressor*
- *Develop an awareness of emotional responses to stressor*
- *Develop adaptive, long-term coping responses that reduce stress*
- *Develop plans and actions that foster problem solving and use of personal and community resources*
- *Utilize constructive outlets for anger and aggression*

Interventions

Understand that patient may not know what the problem is
Assist patient with clearly identifying precipitating event
Explore major changes that have occurred in previous 2 weeks
Ask patient how he feels and help patient to put a label on the emotion
Assist patient with identifying
- How problem affects his life and future
- How problem is affecting family or significant other
- If other factors could be influencing the way he sees problem

Assist patient with identifying strengths and coping skills
- Ask if anything like this has happened to him before
- Ask how past crises were handled
- Inquire as to how patient usually decreases tension and anxiety

Ascertain if patient has tried to use any of the same anxiety-reducing methods this time
    If not, attempt to explore possible reasons or blocks to using prior coping skills
    If they were tried and were unsuccessful, ask what kept them from working
    Assist patient with exploring and identifying what else he thinks might work
Assist patient with identifying nature and strength of situational supports; collect data about current and potential sources of support
    Persons with whom patient lives
    Persons with whom patient is close
    Friends or best friend
    Persons available to help
    Persons whom patient trusts and feels are understanding
    Community services
Assist patient with planning alternative solutions utilizing patient's own coping skills and situational and environmental supports
Offer suggestions of other adaptive coping strategies
Confront self-defeating and destructive behavior in a factual and nonjudgmental manner; make observations about amount of alcohol intake, use of tranquilizers, or overindulgence in food or cigarette smoking
Acknowledge patient's feelings about crisis
Assist patient with sorting out feelings and validating them as acceptable and normal
Assist patient with exploring alternative coping skills
Assist patient with testing role playing or rehearsing new approaches to problem
Present self as role model for open and direct communication, innovative thinking, flexibility, and self-awareness
Give positive reinforcement for all adaptive coping skills utilized in situation
Teach relaxation techniques
Teach psychologic and physiologic effects of chronic stress

Evaluation

Patient
    Returns to precrisis level of functioning
    Develops an adequate response repertoire
    Displays no symptoms of excessive anxiety or lasting physiologic responses to stress
    Increases self-esteem
    Acknowledges increased confidence to solve future problems effectively

POTENTIAL FOR VIOLENCE: SELF-DIRECTED OR DIRECTED AT OTHERS

Description

A potential for violence is characterized by aggressive behavior with the potential for harming self or others.

Potential for Violence: Self-Directed—Suicide

Description

Self-directed violence is characterized by any activity that has negative consequences for the individual's physical or mental well-being.

Defining characteristics of suicidal behavior

Low self-esteem
Major loss
Terminal illness or major disability
Lack of future orientation
Lack of impulse control; history of substance abuse
Severe depression
Agitation and increased restlessness
Excessive guilt
Hopelessness; person feels like a failure
Moderate or greater levels of anxiety
Powerlessness
Verbal statements concerning thoughts of death
    "I just can't cope with life anymore"
    "My family would be better off without me"
Decreased verbal communication with family and/or significant others
Gives needed things away
Makes a will
Checks on life insurance
Refuses to spend money for new possessions
Diminished ability to care for self
Writes letters saying "goodbye" or asking for forgiveness
Nursing diagnoses often associated with a selfdirected potential for violence: ineffective coping by family and individual, disturbance in self-concept, anxiety, fear, hopelessness, powerlessness, spiritual distress

GOALS: *Patient will*
    Acknowledge that significant others and/or staff has heard a cry for help
    Verbalize feelings rather than acting them out
    Make a "no suicide" contract with health care giver
    Define a source of hope in environment

Interventions

Maintain a safe environment to protect patient from injury
- Attempt to place in room with shatterproof windows
- Do not leave patient alone until full assessment of intent is made
- Remove patient's personal belongings that might prove to be harmful—drugs, razors, glass objects, cords, belts, panty hose, neckties—and explain to patient that you are doing this to remove potential danger from area
- Assure adequate staffing on unit, especially during intershift report and meal breaks; understand that most hospital suicides occur at this time
- Check site of incision, drains, and drainage tube insertion sites and document
- Consider reducing amounts of drugs (e.g., morphine, heparin) piggybacked into main IV lines
- Face IV pump or controller-regulating mechism away from patient and out of reach
- Note IV rate of flow and level in bottle each time you enter room
- Give medication in liquid form rather than tablets, which may be saved or concealed

Remember that no one can prevent a person intent on suicide from harming self

Understand that relationship building is more essential than removing hazards from immediate environment

Observe for sudden changes in patient's mood

Have same nurse each shift if possible

Ask patient for details of suicide plan

Do not withhold patient's thoughts of suicide from staff

Notify physician of patient's intent to commit suicide

Be aware that as depression lessens, patient may acquire energy needed to carry out a suicide plan

Be aware that previous attempts at suicide increase the risk for a repeated attempt

Remember that the more violent the plan, the more likely it is that the patient will commit suicide

Encourage patient to talk about feelings

Encourage communication with significant others who are viewed as supportive or as a potential means of support by patient

Avoid overly cheerful remarks

Do not change subject if patient begins to discuss his self-destructive thoughts

Assist patient with identifying alternatives to problem (see care plans for coping and anxiety)

Be aware of your own anxiety when caring for patient; understand that everyone has some fantasy of suicide at some point in time

Be aware that patient's dependency as well as your responsibility for preventing self-destructive behaviors in patient can be frustrating and burdensome; use support of peers to talk out own feelings

Encourage diversional activities that will promote outlet for angry feelings

Assist family with identifying and sharing their feelings with staff

Write down and give patient, family, and significant others phone numbers to contact (physician, suicide prevention center, hot lines, etc.)

Be certain that family and significant others can identify patient's cries for help and know to stay with patient at these times while calling for assistance

Evaluation

Patient will
- Demonstrate ability to manage stressors without resorting to violence against self
- Develop discharge plans with staff
- Express satisfaction with current life situation
- Demonstrate increased self-esteem

Potential for Violence: Directed at Others—Excessive Hostility or Assaultive Behavior

Description

A potential for violence directed at others is characterized by the acting out of anger, hostility, or resentment in such a manner that it brings threat or harm to others in a socially unacceptable context. Hostility may be considered different from anger in that it is viewed as destructive, whereas anger can be seen as constructive. Anger is often justified and can be a healthy response to threatening, fearful, or frustrating situations. Expressing anger may enhance self-esteem and give an individual a sense of power in a situation. Expressing anger appropriately involves the creative use of energy. Unexpressed anger tends to pile up and create a negative and resentful individual who often vents anger inappropriately or not at the original source. Aggressive behavior is hostility acted out and may involve significant danger to others. There are important ethical and legal issues involved in managing aggressive behavior. It is the responsibility of the nurse to become familiar with those issues within the institution. Aggression indicates that behavior is out of control, and it is the responsibility of the staff to protect the patient and others from harm, not to punish.

Defining characteristics of actual or potential acting out of violence or assaultive behavior

Verbal abuse
Rising agitation, pacing
Low self-esteem
Lack of impulse control, history of substance abuse
Panic
Resistance to hospitalization or treatment
Psychosis: loss of contact with reality (delusions and/or hallucinations)
Intoxication by drugs or alcohol
Increased voice volume: shouting, swearing
Destruction of property
Nursing diagnoses associated with potential for violence directed at others: disturbance in self-concept, alteration in thought processes, sensory-perceptual disturbance, anxiety, powerlessness, ineffective individual coping

GOALS: *Patient will*
Demonstrate appropriate expression of anger rather than destructive, hostile acting out of aggression
Verbalize feelings of anger, frustration, and anxiety immediately and directly
Display decreased agitation
Demonstrate awareness of escalating anxiety and causative factors
Demonstrate coping skills to lesson frustration
Experience a sense of reality

Interventions

Call patient by name; speak in calm, firm, and reassuring manner
Do not approach an openly hostile, aggressive patient by yourself; obtain assistance from another staff member
Act interested in what patient has to say
Do not invade personal space
Do not touch patient
Direct patient to calm and control self
Remove others from immediate area
Do not threaten, argue, or respond with hostility
Move around room while speaking with patient
Watch patient's eyes: body part that will be attacked will be observed by patient
State that you cannot allow patient to harm self or anyone in environment
Do not leave patient alone
Be aware of your own feelings and behavior
   Maintain and communicate control to patient
     Do not become personally insulted or demonstrate anger at patient's behavior
     Do not give in to patient's inappropriate demands
     Have another nurse remain with patient if you become upset or defensive
Decrease environmental stimulation
Give patient as much control over his own area as is safely possible
Focus on patient's feelings
Avoid pat reassurances and overgeneralizations
Use the same terms patient uses: "upset," "frustrated," "ticked off"
Avoid use of physical restraint unless patient is also using physical violence
Make every attempt to talk patient out of intended assaultive behavior
Apply mechanical restraints only if absolutely necessary and according to policy of institution
Offer medication
Administer chemical restraint (medications) according to institutional policy
When incident has passed
   Assist patient with identifying and discussing feelings
   Assist patient with identifying what triggered loss of control
   Assist patient with identifying alternative ways of expressing emotion and relieving tension
Be aware of importance of staff continuing with routine patient care activities
Manage emotional reactions of other patients to the incident
Involve patient in activities to promote release of energy and feelings: large muscle movement
Understand that rejection of patient by staff can increase patient's anxiety and perpetuate anger
Teach difference between assertive and agressive behavior

Evaluation

Patient
   Verbalizes alternative ways of dealing with aggressive feelings in conflict situations
   Utilizes energy of anger constructively
   Remains in reality
   Demonstrates nondestructive ways of interacting with others and environment
   Displays effective coping strategies in reducing anxiety and in assessing potentially threatening situations
   Develops increased self-awareness and increased self-esteem

ALTERATION IN THOUGHT PROCESSES

Description

An alteration in thought processes is a disruption in cognition that may alter an individual's perception of reality, problem-solving ability, orientation, memory, comprehension, recognition, and ability to attend to the environment. This alteration results in ineffective coping, inappropriate use of language, and resulting emotional consequences. This condition may be chronic and progressive or acute and reversible.

Defining characteristics of altered thought processes

Memory deficits
Hypervigilance or hypovigilance
Confusion
Disorientation
Distractibility
Compromised decision making
Delusions
Disordered sequencing of thought
Loss of abstract reasoning
Inability to problem solve
Loss of intellectual functioning
Inability to define reality
Bizarre thinking as noted by use of language
Exaggerated emotional responses: lability, apathy or blunted affect, inappropriate affect
Nursing diagnoses often associated with alteration in thought process: anxiety, ineffective breathing pattern, alteration in cardiac output, impaired verbal communication, ineffective individual coping, alteration in family process, fear, hopelessness, hyperthermia, impaired physical mobility, posttrauma response, sensory-perceptual alteration, sleep pattern disturbance, social isolation, ineffective thermoregulation, alteration in tissue perfusion, potential for violence

GOALS: *Patient will*
  Verbalize a sense of reality
  Maintain awareness of safety issues in environment
  Verbalize coherently to others
  Assume responsibility for self-care
  Alert staff to changes in physiologic functioning
  State anxiety level is at mild level
  Seek validation of perceptions
  Participate in decision making or care plan

Disorientation

Description

Disorientation is the inability to correctly identify self in relation to time, place, or person.

Defining characteristics of disorientation

Chronic, dementia
Acute, delirium
Psychomotor agitation
Insomnia
Excessive fear
Visual hallucinations
Aggressive behavior
Purposeless activity
Reversible causes such as the following: alcohol intoxication, altered cerebral blood flow, dehydration, electrolyte imbalance, high fever, infection, metabolic disturbance, sleep pattern disturbance, toxic reactions, head trauma, malnutrition, sensory deprivation or overload, overmedication, etc.
Irreversible causes such as the following: senile dementia, chronic progressive neurologic conditions, neoplasms that present with the following behaviors: psychomotor agitation or retardation, disinterest in personal care, confabulation, "sundowner's" syndrome, short-term memory loss, inability to concentrate, loss of intellectual abilities, delusions, lability of affect and concrete thinking

GOALS: *Patient will*
  Verbalize present location
  Verbalize correct time, day, and date
  Demonstrate personal identity by correctly identifying self, age, personal characteristics, and recognizing family and significant others
  Know correct year and month
In situations in which chronic, progressive dementia exists, it may be appropriate to lower expectations and goals to the following: patient will
  Correctly identify self
  Initiate self-care activities
  Recognize safety hazards in environment
  Decrease agitation
  Sleep through night

Interventions

Assess causative factors and possible etiology of disorientation (acute and reversible delirium versus chronic and irreversible dementia)
Treat acute delirium as a medical emergency
Protect patient from self-injury with attention to equipment at bedside
Provide soft restraints or restraint jacket to prevent unescorted wandering
Cover adequately to avoid unintentional physical exposure
Wear clearly visible name tag
Introduce self to patient prior to giving care
Relate date, time of day, and recent activities

Speak in kind tone using short, simple sentences
Give one direction at a time
Adjust lighting to prevent shadows and distortions
Leave a night light on
Assist patient in self-care activities
Maintain a therapeutic environment; orient patient to room, display familiar items, place personal items in accessible place, display clock and calendar, keep equipment and possessions in same place
Post list of daily activities in clear view
Label bathroom and other areas with large-lettered signs or use a color code to help patient identify personal items and room
Encourage ambulation when possible
Encourge socialization
Provide radio, TV, newspapers
Address patient by name
Tell patient when you do not understand his statements
Do not point out deficits of behavior
Do not laugh at misinformation or misperceptions
Provide repetitive schedules
Encourage independence
Encourage visits from family and significant others
    Assess patient's response to visitors
    Assist family with their emotional reactions
    Help family in goal setting that is realistic
Provide tasks that do not require new learning
Give positive reinforcement in participation in activities
Provide same staff when possible

Evaluation

Patient
    Maintains orientation to time, place, and person
    Demonstrates increased cognitive functioning
    Remains in reality
    Maintains safety consciousness

Compromised Decision Making

Description

Compromised decision making is lack of ability to make independent decisions or to choose among alternatives.

Defining characteristics of compromised decision making

Impaired or poor judgment
Poor impulse control
Diminished self-confidence
Inability to see more than one solution to a problem
Division of world into black and white issues
Inability to choose among alternative actions
Impaired relationship with others due to excessive dependency

GOALS: *Patient will*
    Make contribution to treatment plan
    Seek increasing responsibility for own activity and behavior
    Verbalize alternative solutions to problems

Interventions

Assess any physical condition that may affect decision making or cognition
Assist patient with clearly identifying a problem
Decrease anxiety (see anxiety care plan)
Assist patient with identifying potential alternatives
Encourage patient to write down pros and cons of each alternative
Assist patient with identifying previous successfully made decisions
Encourage verbalization and recognition of factors that hinder decision making
Reassure patient that it is acceptable to make mistakes
Remind patient that any decision will have negative aspects
Encourage patient to make simple choices first
    Choice of activity
    Selection on menu
    Time of procedures
Explain importance of not making decisions based on preferences of others
Reinforce patient's verbalization of independent opinions, thoughts, and decisions
Assist and reinforce progression to more complex decision making
Point out resources that are available for decision to be made
Teach assertive communication techniques
Assist with appropriate action once decision has been made

Evaluation

Patient
    Makes realistic judgments
    Assumes responsibility in major areas of life once relinquished

IMPAIRED SOCIAL INTERACTION

Description

Impaired social interaction is the state in which an individual participates in an insufficient quantity, excessive quantity, or ineffective quality of social exchanges. Satisfying social interaction implies functional communication. An individual communicates effectively by speaking directly from the first-person pronoun, using descriptive terminology in which the verbal and nonverbal contents of the message are congruent. A few examples of utilizing dysfunctional communication are when blaming, excusing, placating, or changing the subject occur. When communications are unsuccessful, they compromise a sense of belonging, caring, self-esteem, and mutuality, and thus social interaction is impaired.

Communication is viewed as a dynamic process and therefore has no beginning or ending point per se. Both verbal and nonverbal messages are conveyed and received. Some of the significant variables that may influence communication are past experience, attitudes, values, anxiety, culture, status, position, and role. Communication involves a sequence of sender, message, receiver, and feedback. Disruptions may occur in one or more parts of the sequence.

Defining characteristics of impaired social interaction

Message inappropriate to content
Inconsistent nonverbal messages
Absent or inappropriate feedback loop
Lack of assertive skills
Controlling and manipulative behavior
Withdrawal or avoidance of social interaction
Excessive interpersonal dependency
Low self-esteem
Verbal communication does not match nonverbal message
Inability to form meaningful, intimate relationships
Developmental issues
Poorly defined status or position
Cultural discrepancy or language barrier
Exaggerated emotional responses
Socioeconomic disparity
Cognitive and/or perceptual disturbance
Physical disability or stigma
Excessive interpersonal anxiety
Nursing diagnoses often associated with impaired social interaction: anxiety, impaired verbal communication, altered growth and development, hopelessness, powerlessness, disturbance in self-concept, altered sexuality patterns, altered thought process, alteration in family process, ineffective individual and family coping, social isolation

GOALS: *Patient will*
Verbalize satisfaction in social interaction
Report decreased interpersonal anxiety
Recognize when manipulative, demanding, dependent, or withdrawn behavior interferes with social interaction

Manipulative Behavior
Description

Manipulative behavior involves controlling the behavior of others to achieve one's goals: passive behavior gets needs met indirectly through others; aggressive behavior is directed against or toward others in an attempt to get one's own needs met. These two ways of interacting are utilized when an individual feels powerless to meet his own needs through assertive interaction.

Defining characteristics of manipulative behavior

Lack of insight toward problems and/or denial of problems
Inability to express anger openly
Changes subject of conversation or activity of group
Cries or acts helpless when confronted
Attention-seeking behavior such as monopolizing conversations in both social and therapeutic interactions
Constantly seeks approval and recognition
Overly solicitous and ingratiating
Attempts to gain special attention or privileges
Demonstrates anger, and feels hurt, deserted, and unworthy when above attempts are denied
Reports confidential information to others
Attempts to use others' weaknesses against them; plays one person against the other
Consistently breaks rules and routines and disrupts procedures
Intellectualizes and rationalizes problems away
Projects blame onto others
Views self as uniquely special and deserving
Attempts to get others to rescue him by being helpless and boosting others' self-esteem by relying on them to fix the problem

GOALS: *Patient will*
Recognize manipulatory patterns
Control impulses to achieve immediate gratification of needs
Identify needs met through manipulation of others

Interventions

Assess needs that patient is trying to meet through manipulation
Decrease manipulation of staff
  Avoid discussing yourself and other staff members with patient

Assign consistent staff when possible
Develop plan of care with other staff and communicate to all involved with patient's care
Communicate frequently with other staff to ensure continuity and consistency of approach
Point out manipulative behavior to patient if patient states
"You're the only one who understands . . ."
"You're the only one who cares about me"
"You're the only one I can talk to"
Caution staff to not attempt to be liked or to be patient's favorite nurse
Do not accept favors or gifts, which foster a personal relationship
Be matter of fact in interactions with patient
Avoid angry, negative, and punitive responses to patient when patient is being manipulative
Offer limited choices (e.g., "Would you like to ambulate now or at 9 o'clock?")
Be direct in interactions; do not bargain or rationalize
Assist patient in recognizing his own patterns of manipulative behavior by providing nonthreatening similar examples
Point out relationship between need to control and inability to achieve self-control
Encourage identification of alternate and appropriate behaviors for meeting needs; use role playing
Give verbal and nonverbal positive reinforcement when patient functions without being manipulative
Encourage and support verbalization about feelings, medical conditions, and/or surgery and current treatment; listen nonjudgmentally
Build trust through consistency and keeping promises
Assure patient that if limits are set, that it is because you care and that caring and limit setting are neither mutually exclusive nor opposites
Involve patient in his own plan of care without allowing patient to dictate aspects of care

Evaluation

Patient
Verbalizes satisfaction with improved social interaction
Demonstrates ability to define and meet needs without manipulative behavior
Actively participates in planning own care

Demanding Behavior

Description

Demanding behavior occurs in syndromes involving anxiety, fear, helplessness, inadequacy, inferiority, hostility, manipulation, and dependent behavior. The individual believes he is incapable of fulfilling his own needs or having his needs met by making requests in a direct, matter-of-fact manner. Attempts are then made to coerce others to meet these needs by making requests with forceful and manipulative behavior with implied threat.

Defining characteristics of demanding behavior

Makes frequent requests
Constant attention seeking
Attempts to coerce others to meet needs
Asks others to do what he is capable of doing
Displays helplessness when making requests
Displays anger when requests are not met immediately
Detains staff with subsequent requests after initial request has been met
May be domineering, sarcastic, or ridiculing
May use threats if requests are not met
Does not use proper channels of communication: goes over nurses' authority by talking to supervisors, etc.

GOALS: *Patient will*
Verbalize a sense of control over environment
Communicate assertively
Utilize proper channels of communication
Recognize negative impact on others when demanding behavior is utilized

Interventions

Be aware that dynamics between staff and patient create and maintain the problem situation
Be aware that staff's responses to patient will influence whether or not patient continues to be demanding; avoid displaying annoyance or anger with patient's request; understand that such a display perpetuates patient's demands
Be aware that depersonalization due to hospitalization promotes anxiety and contributes to patient's perception of lack of control and self-esteem
Assess unfilled needs of patient
Involve patient in deciding how needs will be met
Assist patient with identifying demanding behaviors
Relate to patient your own responses to his demanding behavior in nonemotional tone of voice
Assist patient with developing alternative behavior by
Asking directly for what is wanted
Taking responsibility for behavior by using the personal pronoun "I" before a request
Becoming more aware of responses and associated feelings when requests are not met immediately

Reinforcing independently made direct questions
Do not refuse or ignore request
Give reasons why requests cannot be met
Anticipate realistic requests and meet them rapidly
Allow patient as much control as possible in own care
Spend time with patient when he is not demanding; set up a regular schedule of checking in with patient that is independent of his using the call light
Give full attention to patient during verbal interactions and recognize positive qualities in order to promote self-esteem
Demonstrate interest and be attentive to patient as a person
Allow opportunity for appropriate ventilation of feelings regarding annoyances and restrictions; feeling of powerlessness
If you tell patient that you will be back in 20 minutes, be sure that you are
Avoid withdrawing from patient by insensitive mechanistic actions

Evaluation

Patient
  Displays a positive regard for assertive social interactions
  Makes realistic requests of staff in situations that patient is unable to meet by self or without help

Withdrawn Behavior
Description

Withdrawn behavior is an attempt to avoid interaction with others and thus avoid relatedness; it is a defense against anxiety that is related to a stressor or threat. The range of behavior can be from disinterest in others to severe withdrawal with an accompanying increase in primary process thinking. This may ultimately lead to autistic behavior of delusions and hallucinations as the individual withdraws more from the environment and attends to internal thoughts and stimuli.

Defining characteristics of withdrawn behavior

Dull, flat, or inappropriate affect/mood
Apathetic
Depressed
Absence of spontaneity
Inappropriate response to environmental stimuli
Excessive fear and increasing levels of anxiety
Decreased or absent verbalization
Decreased motor activity or agitation
Lack of awareness of surroundings
Inattention to grooming and personal habits
Inappropriate social behavior, including open masturbation, obscene language, handling of excreta
Regression: may assume fetal position
Disturbance in thought content, such as delusions
Disturbance in perception, such as hallucinations

GOALS: *Patient will*
  Report only mild anxiety in social interactions
  Respond appropriately to environmental stimuli
  Initiate social interactions
  Assist with basic self-care and grooming
  Have adequate nutrition and fluid intake

Interventions

Communicate with patient in a positive, accepting manner
Plan time to sit with patient
Consider touching patient's hand if a negative response is not anticipated
Avoid attempts to ororoverbalize with patient
Remain comfortable during silent periods
Avoid asking questions that require "yes" or "no" answers
Expect patient to respond to conversation
Provide reality-orientated conversation focusing on the here and now; avoid generalizations and abstract concepts
Allow sufficient time for patient to respond
Avoid placing patient in private room
Administer phenothiazines and antidepressants as ordered
Measure intake and output if indicated
Assist with meeting basic needs: eating, drinking, elimination, bathing, and ambulation
Assist and teach ROM exercises and turn q2h if bedridden
Maintain skin integrity
Use television and/or radio in room
Provide newspapers and magazines
Involve patient in plan of care
Assist patient with indentifying alternate and appropriate behaviors
Orient patient to time, place, and person; use clock and calendar in room
Give positive reinforcement for self-care activities
Be aware that logical arguments only increase delusional thought content
Encourage and support verbalization of feelings about concrete issues: medical condition, menu, etc.
Decrease anxiety level (see anxiety care plan)
Provide a regular schedule of activities (routines)

Ask patient to look at you when you are speaking to him

Share with patient that you do not see or hear hallucinatory material

Use empathy: "That must be frightening"

Gradually introduce patient to more people in environment

Evaluation

Patient
  Reports a satisfying social interaction with nurse
  Identifies increased self-esteem
  Responds with positive and appropriate affect to social interaction
  Remains in reality
  Initiates and completes self-care activities

Dependent Behavior

Description

Dependent behavior includes impaired decision making; a tendency to lean on others for guidance, direction, support, protection, and advice; and a compelling need to relate with a stronger person in order to cope with stressors.

Defining characteristics of dependent behavior

Constantly seeks attention
Whines
Seems helpless when making a request
Refuses to make decisions
Asks others to do what he could do himself
Feels no responsibility for
  Decisions
  Behaviors
  Feelings
  Thoughts
Lacks initiative
Low self-esteem
Procrastinates
Passive
Low frustration tolerance
Lacks social skills
Few adaptive coping skills
Lacks problem-solving skills
Moderate interpersonal anxiety
Moderate to severe depression
Covert expressions of anger
Repeated hospitalizations; many physical complaints
Substance abuse and/or dependency
Inability to define or express needs appropriately

GOALS: *Patient will*
  Verbalize needs and feelings openly and directly
  Initiate activities and social interactions
  Identify reliance on medications and/or alcohol
  Relinquish reliance on physical symptoms in order to stay in "sick role"

Interventions

Assess for suicidal thoughts or behaviors
Assess patient's dependence on drugs and/or alcohol
Maintain consistent approach
  Set limits for unrealistic and inappropriate requests
  Use calm, firm tone of voice when speaking
  Do not display anger or frustration toward patient
Do not reward attention-seeking behavior
Meet dependency needs at first while gradually assisting patient in becoming more independent in stages: (1) do for patient; (2) do with patient; (3) allow patient to take lead while you provide support; (4) provide positive reinforcement for independent behaviors
Avoid making simple decisions for patient
Offer alternative choices
Investigate physical symptoms reported by patient but do not encourage "sick role" behavior
Assist patient with verbalizing and identifying strengths
Do not be the only one the patient can talk with; involve other staff with patient
Avoid feelings of sympathy; do not give phone number to patient or allow him to call you at work or home
Assist patient with identifying consequences of behavior, including indecisiveness
Assist patient with expressing anger in open and direct manner when his demands or requests are not met
Positively reinforce expression of genuine feelings
Refer to self-help groups when appropriate
Teach about physical and/or phychologic dependency that occurs with continued use of tranquilizers and/or alcohol

Evaluation

Patient
  Assumes responsibility for major areas of life
  Resumes appropriate role functioning
  Reports satisfying social interactions
  Makes decisions independently
  Copes with stressors without using tranquilizers and/or alcohol

Other Aspects of General Care

GENERAL PREOPERATIVE CARE/TEACHING

Assessment
Observations/findings

EMOTIONAL STATUS

Understanding of operative, preoperative, and postoperative procedures
Ability to verbalize fears and anxieties
Relationship, response, and behavior of patient and family
Family's knowledge of operative procedure

PHYSICAL STATUS

Nutritional and hygienic state
Elimination habits
Medications being taken
Medical background
    Diseases
    Surgery
Socioeconomic background
Allergies
Physical handicaps, limitations
Signs of infection
Mental, visual, auditory acuity

LEGAL STATUS

Informed consent signed for operation
Physician's preoperative orders complete
Identification bands on and correct
Patient's willingness to receive blood noted
Environmental understanding
    Use of equipment in room
    Use of call bell
    Purpose and use of side rails

Interventions

Maintain NPO after midnight or as ordered
Take and record BP, T, P, R, and weight; report abnormalities to physician
Check and record allergies
Verify ordered laboratory work on chart; report abnormalities to physician
Check that surgical preparations are correct and noted
Check that patient showers with antibacterial soap hs and as ordered
Give enemas as ordered
Complete bowel preparation if ordered
See that electrocardiogram (ECG) and chest x-ray examinations are done and read if ordered
Complete history and physical
Complete blood type and cross match; note number of units available
Give preoperative medications; make sure side rails are up after injection
Insert nasogastric tube and/or indwelling bladder catheter if ordered
Initiate parenteral fluids if ordered
Have patient void prior to leaving for operating room
Remove dentures, contact lenses, nail polish, makeup, prosthesis, and/or valuables prior to leaving for operating room; religious medals may be pinned to gown
Have chart complete and ready; have patient addressograph plate and/or Kardex ready with chart

Preoperative teaching
Emotional

Reinforce physician's explanation of surgical procedure
Answer questions as honestly as possible
Allow time for and encourage verbalization of fears and anxieties
Avoid standard clichés such as "Don't worry," "Everything is just fine," "I know how you feel"
Listen to and *hear* patient
Avoid rushing through explanations
Accept patient's behavior unless it is unsafe; avoid judging it or trying to change it
Involve family or significant other in care and instructions when possible

Physical

Explain all procedures, the reason for them, and their importance
    Preoperative
        Enema
        Skin preparation
        NPO
        Laboratory work
    Postoperative
        Parenteral fluids
        Vital signs
        Dressings
        Pain and availability of medications
        Nasogastric and other tubes
        Indwelling bladder catheter
        Intermittent positive pressure breathing (IPPB), incentive spirometer
        Avoid touching incision

Teach patient, using return demonstration, how to
   Turn, cough, and deep breathe, depending on surgical procedure
   Support incision during coughing
   Deep breathe hourly postoperatively
   Exercise actively and how passive ROM exercises will be done
   Sit up, get up, and ambulate; chair sitting should be avoided
Explain importance of progressive care
   Early ambulation
   Self-care encouraged as soon as patient is able
Discuss with patient and family purpose of recovery room
   Visiting policies
   Type of care
   Length of stay if applicable
   Possibility of placement in intensive care unit (ICU) if needed or indicated
Explain other hospital policies as indicated
   Visiting hours
   Number of visitors
   Location of waiting rooms
   How physician will contact them after operation

CARE OF PATIENT IN RECOVERY ROOM

Assessment
Observations/findings
GENERAL ANESTHESIA

Level of consciousness
   Unconscious
      No cough or gag reflex
      Endotracheal tube
      Airway
   Semiconscious
      Endotracheal tube out
      Oral or nasal airway
      Partial return of reflexes
   Awake; return of reflexes
Respiration
   Rate
   Rhythm
   Depth
   Quality
Laryngospasm
Endotracheal tube or airway present
   Position
   Adequate ventilation
Pulse
   Rate
   Rhythm
   Quality
Blood pressure
   Hypotension
   Hypertension
   Normal
Parenteral infusion
   Flow rate
   Type of solution
   Site
   Patent vein
   Medications
Pain
   Amount
   Tolerance
Skin
   Color
      Normal
      Flushed
      Cyanotic
      Pallid
   Condition
      Dry
      Moist
      Hot
      Cold
Nail beds: color
   Normal
   Cyanotic
Return of reflexes
Type of surgery performed
Site of incision
   Dry
   Bleeding
   Drainage
   Drains
Dressing
   Dry
   Intact
Drainage tubes: patency and connections
   Nasogastric tube
   Nephrostomy
   Indwelling urethral catheter
   Chest tubes
Past medical history
   Diabetes
   Cardiac problems
   Asthma
   Emphysema

SPINAL ANESTHESIA
Monitor each item under general anesthesia section; also check legs for the following

Mobility
Color
Temperature
Return of sensation

Interventions

Maintain patent airway
  Endotracheal tubes, nasal and oral airways
    Suction prn
    Support
      Pulmonator
      IPPB
  Inadequate airway
    Hyperextend neck
    Bring chin forward
    Turn head to one side
    Insert oral or nasal airway
    Notify anesthesiologist of respiratory impairment
Take initial BP, P, and R and report to anesthesiologist
Moniter q15 min and prn until stable
  BP, R, and apical pulse
  Level of consciousness
  Return of reflexes
  IV site
  Site of incision
  Drainage tubes and equipment
  Movement of extremities
Maintain NPO
Maintain parenteral fluids as ordered
Measure intake and output
Administer oxygen and IPPB as ordered
Restrain arms when necessary
Reinforce dressing prn; notify physician if drainage is excessive
Administer blood and blood components as ordered
Administer all medications as ordered
Perform passive ROM exercises to extremities if allowed
Position to maintain optimal ventilation and comfort
Maintain pain management; administer narcotics in one-fourth, one-third, or one-half doses until patient has reacted fully
Keep warm and dry; cover with warm blankets if necessary
Remain with patient if restless
  Turn patient's head to one side at first sign of vomiting
  Suction as needed
Administer oral hygiene q1h to 2h; keep mouth and tongue moist
Monitor rectal or axillary temperature q1h to 4h
Assist and teach patient to turn, cough, and deep breathe q1h to 2h when reactive
Auscultate chest for breath sounds q30 min
Maintain quiet environment; avoid discussions over patient's bed
Discharge to room when
  Patient is fully reactive
  Patient is moving extremities well
  Vital signs have been stable for 1 hr
  Patient is medicated for pain and vital signs are stable
  Dressings have been checked and no bleeding or excessive drainage is noted
  All drainage tubes are functioning
  Patient has been seen by anesthesiologist and approval has been given

ASSESSMENT OF THE AGING PATIENT

aging *Part of the continuum of life; effects vary widely from one individual to the next; does not progress at a uniform rate and at any given time patient may exhibit only a few of the characteristics (Disease should not necessarily be equated with aging, although when one health problem is identified, others must be suspected, since multiple disease conditions are a primary characteristic of advancing years.)*

Normal Variations during the Aging Process

Assessment
Observations/findings

General
  Height less than ½ inch less than during youth
  Steady weight loss in men over 65 years old (weight gain in women)
  Ears and nose appear large in relation to size of face
  Wrinkling and sagging of skin
  Loss of hair pigmentation and thinning of hair
Eyes
  Dry and lusterless
  Discoloration of sclera
  Arcus senilis (opaque ring near edge of cornea)
  Diminished pupil size
  Pale brown discoloration in iris
  Diminished peripheral vision
Ears: hearing loss
  Initial loss of high-frequency tones
  Suspiciousness and irritability may or may not be present
Mouth
  Loss of taste perception
  Recession of gums if not edentulous

Breasts: pendulous, elongated, and/or flaccid
Respiratory system
  Decreased tidal volume
  Decreased peripheral perfusion
  Tracheal deviation if upper dorsal scoliosis present
Cardiovascular system
  Decreased resting heart rate (and cardiac output)
  Easily palpable arterial pulse
Gastrointestinal system
  Diminished salivation and gastric acid secretion
  Constipation
Genitourinary system
  Nocturnal micturition frequent
  Incontinence
  Difficult in initiating and ending the stream in male (due to prostatic hypertrophy)
Female reproductive system
  Narrowing and shortening of vagina
  Diminished vaginal lubrication
  Dyspareunia
  Long-term estrogen therapy effects
    Uterine bleeding
    Mastalgia
    Weight gain
    Fluid retention
    Hypertension
  Uterine contractions with orgasm may be uncomfortable
Male reproductive system
  Decrease in size and firmness of testes
  Enlarged prostate gland
  Decrease in amount and viscosity of seminal fluid
  Increased diameter of penis
  Longer duration of excitement and plateau or orgasmic phases; resolution phase may last 12 to 24 hr
  Libido and sense of satisfaction usually do not change
Musculoskeletal system
  Decrease in quick voluntary movements
  Decrease in muscle mass; not necessarily associated with loss of strength
  Osteoarthritic changes in joints
    Heberden's nodes at distal finger joints
    Bouchard's nodes at proximal finger joints
  Dupuytren's contracture of lateral fingers, preventing full extension
  Osteoporosis: kyphosis may be an early indication
  Broad-based stance
Skin
  Thinning of skin over back of hands
  Decreased activity of sebaceous and sweat glands; may result in "dry skin"
  Thinning and/or loss of scalp, pubic, and axillary hair
  Small, scattered scarlet growths (senile telangiectasis)
  Paler skin with increased pigment deposition (freckles)
  Local or general skin areas lacking pigmentation (vitiligo); increases with age
  Hyperkeratosis, or warts with raised pale, brown, or black epidermal overgrowth usually located over long axis of skin creases
    Cutaneous skin tags (acrochordons) around lower neck, axillary area; usually soft and flesh colored and on pedicles
Neurologic system
  Decrease in conduction velocity of some nerves
  Diminished sense of smell
  Diminished sense of position
  Decreased tactile sense
  Deep tendon reflexes may be decreased
  Diminished sensitivity to hot and cold extremes in temperature

Interventions

Face patient in such a way that nurse's lips and eyes are clearly seen
Avoid shouting
Use high-wattage lamp to reflect off printed forms; avoid reflecting light in patient's eyes
Repeat questions, instructions, and explanation if memory, hearing, or learning disability is present
  Learning that involves unlearning is most difficult
  Level of intelligence remains unchanged
Encourage use of items of marked textural difference if tactile sense is impaired
Use color contrasts if vision perception is diminished
Address patient by his preferred name
Use lower tone and/or pitch of voice
Be aware of own nonverbal communication through face and body stance
Administer medications judiciously
  Absorption, detoxification, and excretion of drugs is diminished; lower dosage levels and decreased frequency of administration may be indicated
  Assess need for analgesia carefully, since sensitivity to pain is usually decreased

EMOTIONAL CARE OF THE DYING PATIENT

Nurse self-assessment/interventions

To care for the dying patient, the nurse must
  Learn about self and own feelings concerning dying

Look at own cultural background
Examine own exposure to death
   Family and friends
   Reactions to these experiences
Be honest about feelings: anxiety, depression, avoidance, coping mechanisms
Examine how nurse sees own death
Share feelings about death with others; initiate open discussion to better understand behavior
Learn to listen; realize that all patient's questions do not require answers—often patient will answer own questions if nurse does not provide "pat" answers
Explore feelings about life: respect, discontent, etc.
Recognize own power in controlling patient and his responses to care
   Avoid using this power as threat to patient
   Use it to give respectful, humane care
Consider effect patient has on nurse; examine how nurse sees him as an individual human being
Consider the following in caring for the dying patient
   Be aware of what physician has told patient; avoid conflicting statements
   Realize that decision to tell patient of outcome of disease lies with physician and family
   Be honest in dealing with patient who has not been told of impending death (ask patient what he thinks or feels about the question "Am I going to die?")
Communicate situations and conversations with patient to others on the staff; provide continuity and avoid discrepancies in emotional care

Family assessment/interventions

Realize that family or significant other will need support during patient's illness
   Do not judge actions or behavior of family
      Realize that family may have gone through a lot with a long illness and are no longer able to cope
      Understand that a change in family structure is occurring
         Emotional: loss of a loved member
         Financial: long illnesses become a burden
   Be aware that preillness relationships and/or problems will continue
   Assist family in grieving process
      Understand that they, too, will go through the stages of dying
      Be aware that timing of stages is very often not the same as patient's
      Understand that family very often may not reach stage of acceptance
      Work with family past denial stage so that they can let patient know the truth, thus permitting open and frank communication with patient
   Assist family in making plans, both intermediate and long-term
   Help family see patient's need to live as normally as possible as long as possible
   Assist family in making arrangements for home care when possible and desirable for patient
      Teach methods of care that will be required
      Arrange help through social service department and community resources

Patient assessment/interventions

Realize patient needs compassionate, consistent, and realistic care during terminal illness
Be aware that he is sensitive to feelings of others
   Understand that patient will avoid discussion of his death and feelings if he senses others are unable to talk of dying
   Be aware that he will very often discuss feelings with nursing staff rather than with the physician
Provide needed hope, human contact, and caring
   Understand that hope must be realistic; patient needs treatment for alleviation of pain rather than getting well
   Do not avoid patient during any of the stages of dying
   Realize that patient needs continuous caring by all members of staff
Be aware that patient has many fears
   Explain all procedures and nursing functions
   Discuss fears with patient
      The unknown
      Loss of control of body and behavior
      Pain: patient needs explanation of availability of different drugs and therapies such as radiation or surgery
      Helplessness: patient needs general nutrition, some activity, and deep breathing every day, which usually help initially
Understand that patient needs to have each day be as comfortable, good, and productive as possible

Care during the Stages of Dying
DENIAL AND SHOCK
Assessment
Observations/findings

Ignoring or distorting reasons given for illness
Refusal to participate in care
Refusal to follow directions of physician or staff

Interventions

Recognize that this mechanism will be utilized after patient is told of impending death
Do not interfere with this mechanism unless it becomes destructive (patient refuses further treatment and care)
Spend time with patient to show that he will not be left alone
Do not support denial; conversations should include reality
Continue to teach and encourage self-care and special procedures

ANGER
Assessment
Observations/findings

Abusive language
Refusal of care
Refusal of nutrition and self-care
Negative criticism of staff
Striking out
  Not permitting others close to him
  Throwing objects
  Removing IV leads, etc.
  Calling for nurse and then asking why nurse is there

Interventions

Recognize that patient is not angry with nurse personally
Do not allow physically harmful behavior to continue
  Spend time with patient and discuss his anger
  Encourage verbalization of anger
Plan care with patient
Question how patient evaluates care being given
Continue to question and discuss patient's anger

BARGAINING
Assessment
Observations/findings

Statements such as "I hope I live until. . . ," "If only I could . . ."

Interventions

Realize patient needs time to accept death and needs this mechanism
Spend time with patient
Discuss importance of events and people

DEPRESSION
Assessment
Observations/findings

Apathy
Decreased ability to concentrate
Insomnia
Inability to wake up
Crying
Constant fatigue
Poor appetite
Lack of interest in people or environment

Interventions

Recognize that patient is beginning to separate himself from life
Do not attempt to cheer patient
Be available to sit quietly and if appropriate hold patient's hand
Accept crying and do not interrupt
Realize that patient may only want most beloved person to be with him

ACCEPTANCE
Assessment
Observations/findings

Devoid of feelings
Absence of emotional affect
Peacefulness
Less pain and discomfort, usually

Interventions

Plan care to allow person with whom patient is comfortable to care for him
Realize that patient may not want to be alone

ENTERAL NUTRITION

Provision of nutritional support to meet nutritional requirements via a nasogastric tube, orogastric tube, esophagostomy, gastrostomy, duodenostomy, or jejunostomy; preferred for the patient who has a functional GI tract, but is unable to consume an adequate nutritional intake, or when oral intake is contraindicated; may be indicated in the following clinical conditions: physical impairments (e.g., obstructive lesions of the esophagus or pharynx, following radical head and neck surgery, fractured facial bones); neurologic conditions associated with impaired swallowing and oropharyngeal trauma; increased metabolic needs due to trauma, burns or sepsis, or the presence of an endotracheal tube (Jejunostomy is indicated for patients with obstruction of the stomach, duodenum, and proximal jejunum.)

Assessment
Observations/findings

Dietary history
  Intolerance to lactase

Food allergies, dietary restrictions
Medical history
   Chronic renal disease
   Liver disorders
   Diabetes mellitus
   Heart disease
Cerebrovascular accident (CVA)
   Coma
Respiratory
   Respiratory distress
   Aspiration
   Coughing
   Choking
   Cyanosis
   Increased respiratory rate
   Decreased breath sounds
   Rales at lung bases
Skin and mucous membranes
   Skin irritation and/or breakdown, nares, ostomy tube
   Poor skin turgor
   Dry mucous membranes
   Diaphoresis
Level of consciousness
   Coma
   Change in mental status
Gastrointestinal
   Nausea
   Vomiting
   Diarrhea
   Abdominal distention
   Decreased or absent bowel sounds
   Abdominal cramping
   Constipation
   Esophageal reflux
   Gastric residual
   Tube placement: stomach, duodenum, jejunum, esophagus

Laboratory/diagnostic studies

Serum electrolytes
Serum osmolality
Serum glucose
Urine glucose
Urine specific gravity
BUN
Serum creatinine
Serum albumin
Serum transferrin

Potential complications

Hypernatremia
Hyperchloremia
Azotemia
Dehydration
Hyperglycemia
Nausea
Vomiting
Aspiration
Diarrhea
Constipation
Gastric retention
Fluid overload
Gastric rupture
Dumping syndrome
   Weakness
   Diaphoresis
   Lightheadedness
   Tachycardia
   Cramping
Tube displacement
Intraperitoneal leakage and leakage of fluid around catheter (associated with gastrostomy and jejunostomy tubes)

Medical management

Treatment of underlying disease process
Desired route
Tube selection
Type of formula (concentration and rate)
Intermittent or continuous feed
Antidiarrheal agents
Laxatives
Insulin
Intake and output
Daily weights
Daily laboratory studies

Nursing diagnoses/goals/interventions

ndx: Alteration in bowel elimination: diarrhea related to rapid rate of infusion, high osmolality of formula, lactose intolerance, and/or bacterial contamination of feeding solution

GOAL: *Patient will resume usual bowel elimination pattern*

Record color, odor, amount, and frequency of stool
Measure intake and output q8h
Test stool for occult blood
Weigh patient daily at same time with same clothing and scale
Assess for signs and symptoms of dehydration
   Poor skin turgor
   Decreased urine output
   Increased urine specific gravity
   Dry mucous membranes

Text continued on p. 48.

TABLE 1-2. Observation of Fluid and Electrolyte Imbalances

Imbalances	Causes	Neuromuscular system	GI system
ELECTROLYTE IMBALANCES			
Hyperkalemia (potassium excess)	Excessive administration of potassium chloride Decreased renal excretion, as in renal failure, hypovolemia, potassium-sparing diuretics Trauma to tissues such as burns and crush injuries (will release intercellular potassium and result in hyperkalemia) Aldosterone insufficiency Respiratory or metabolic acidosis Banked blood	Weakness, flaccid paralysis, twitching, hyperreflexia, paresthesia or numbness and tingling sensations, (usually affect the face, tongue, hands, and feet), apathy, confusion	Diarrhea, intestinal colic, nausea
Hypokalemia (potassium deficit)—cont'd	Increased renal loss (diuretics; diuresis phase following burns; diabetic acidosis, Cushing's syndrome; nephritis) Hypomagnesium Inadequate intake of potassium Acid base imbalance: alkalosis; loss from vomiting, diarrhea, excess use of laxatives, GI suction or fistulas, steroid administration	Muscular cramps, paresthesias, muscular weakness to flaccid paralysis, fatigue, mental confusion, hyporeflexia, drowsiness, apathy, irritability, tetany, coma	Anorexia, nausea and vomiting, abdominal distention, paralytic ileus

Respiratory system	Cardiovascular system	Renal system	Skin and mucous membranes	Blood gas values	Interventions
Respiratory paralysis and involvement of muscle of phonation	Bradycardia, lethal dysarrhythmias and cardiac arrest ECG changes: tall peaked T waves, shortened QT interval, disappearance of P waves, widening of QRS complex, flat to absent P wave and asystole				Observe patient for changes in heart rate, rhythm, and ECG pattern Be aware that cardiac arrest can occur Restrict potassium-containing foods, fluids, and salt substitutes Monitor serum potassium levels Do not give calcium if patient is on digitalis, since it potentiates the effect of digitalis Avoid potassium-containing medications such as potassium penicillin Administer IV glucose, insulin, and sodium bicarbonate as ordered (helps shift potassium into the cells) Administer cation-exchange resins as ordered (helps to remove potassium by way of the GI tract) Peritoneal or hemodialysis may be ordered if other therapy fails
Respiratory muscle weakness, paralysis of the diaphragm, shallow respirations, apnea, and death may result	Irregular rhythm, ECG: flat or inverted T wave, appearance of U wave, short and depressed ST segment, peaking of P waves, QT interval prolonged, circulatory failure, hypotension and systolic arrest Effectiveness of digitalis enhanced (to the point of toxicity)				Monitor serum potassium and report significant changes Observe for signs and symptoms of metabolic alkalosis Watch for signs of digitalis toxicity in patients receiving digitalis (blurred vision, nausea and vomiting) Monitor rate of IV administration of potassium Monitor intake and output (report changes)

Continued.

TABLE 1-2. Observation of Fluid and Electrolyte Imbalances—cont'd

Imbalances	Causes	Neuromuscular system	GI system
Hypokalemia (potassium deficit)—cont'd			
Hypocalcemia (calcium deficit)	Inadequate intake of calcium Decreased absorption from intestine Hypoparathyroidism Vitamin D deficiency Rapid dilution of the plasma by intravenous calcium-free solutions Chronic renal failure Chronic malabsorption syndrome Neoplastic diseases Hypomagnesemia Cushing's syndrome Acute pancreatitis Hyperphosphatemia Extreme stress situations Excessive citrated blood, alkalosis	Muscle tremors, paresthesias, especially numbness or tingling, skeletal muscle cramps, abdominal spasms and cramps Hyperactive reflexes Convulsions Positive Trousseau's sign Positive Chvostek's sign Emotional depression or confusion	Paralytic ileus GI bleeding
Hypercalcemia (calcium excess)—cont'd	Hyperparathyroidism Prolonged immobilization (causes calcium displacement from bone to blood) Hypophosphatemia Metastatic carcinoma Alkalosis Thyrotoxicosis Vitamin D overdose	Generalized muscle weakness Depressed or absent deep tendon reflexes (DTRs) Drowsiness Lethargy Headaches Loss of muscle tone Ataxia Mental confusion	Anorexia Nausea Vomiting Constipation Epigastric pain Polydipsia

Respiratory system	Cardiovascular system	Renal system	Skin and mucous membranes	Blood gas values	Interventions
					Encourage intake of food and fluids rich in potassium (e.g., orange juice, bananas, bouillon, meat broths, colas, tea, leafy vegetables)
					Observe for changes in heart rate, rhythm, and ECG pattern
					Determine source of potassium losses
	Dysrhythmias Hypotension Prolonged QT interval with normal T wave on ECG				Monitor rate, rhythm, and ECG pattern Administer calcium gluconate or calcium chloride 10% as ordered Monitor serum calcium levels every 12 to 24 hr Report calcium deficit to physician Monitor PT and platelet levels Observe for signs and symptoms of tetany Provide dietary calcium (i.e., cheese, cream, milk, yogurt) Administer vitamin D as ordered Monitor prothrombin and platelet levels Check for bleeding from any source (calcium aids in blood clotting) Monitor use of laxatives and antacids (those containing phosphate affect calcium metabolism)
	Bradycardia Hypertension ECG: QT interval shortened, T waves inverted Ventricular arrhythmias Enhanced effectiveness of digitalis	Development of renal calculi, kidney stones Polyuria			Assess for possible causes Administer loop diuretics to increase excretion of calcium Administer corticosteroids and mithramycin as ordered (lowers serum calcium concentration) Administer antacids cautiously: some contain calcium

Continued.

TABLE 1-2. Observation of Fluid and Electrolyte Imbalances—cont'd

Imbalances	Causes	Neuromuscular system	GI system
Hypercalcemia (calcium excess)—cont'd	Addison's disease Multiple myeloma Skeletal muscle paralysis Cardiac failure Prolonged thiazide diuretic therapy Excessive calcium intake Parathyroid tumor Sarcoidosis	Impairment of memory Slurred speech Personality or behavior changes Stupor or coma Pathologic fractures may occur Flank or deep bone pain	
Hypernatremia (sodium excess)	Primary aldosteronism: excessive steroids (Cushing's disease) Excessive IV Administration of large amounts of sodium chloride solution without water replacement Renal failure (with sodium retention) Neurohypophyseal dysfunction (as in diabetes insipidus) High-protein diets with minimal fluid intake Diabetes mellitus Excessive ingestion of sodium chloride Decreased water intake, severe vomiting or diarrhea Inadequate circulation of blood to the kidneys (congestive heart failure; CHF) Cirrhosis of the liver	Sodium ↑, water ↓ CNS depression (lethargy to coma), muscle weakness, muscle rigidity, muscle tremors	
Hyponatremia (sodium deficit)—cont'd	Inappropriate ADH syndrome Excessive intake of hypotonic fluids Severe malnutrition Vomiting Diarrhea GI drainage from suction or fistulas	Headache Vertigo Anxiety Muscle weakness and cramps Lassitude, apathy, confusion Hyperreflexia	Anorexia, nausea, vomiting, diarrhea, cramping

Respiratory system	Cardiovascular system	Renal system	Skin and mucous membranes	Blood gas values	Interventions
					Position and move patient carefully to prevent pathologic fractures
					Administer isotonic fluids as ordered
					Encourage fluid intake of 2000 to 3000 ml a day
					Monitor intake and output
					Avoid dietary intake of calcium (dairy products and green leafy vegetables)
					Monitor serum calcium levels
					Observe for changes in heart rate, rhythm, and ECG pattern
					Observe for symptoms of digitalis toxicity
Sodium ↑; water ↑ (increase in extracellular fluid volume); may cause pulmonary edema: shortness of breath, coughing, cyanosis, increased respiratory rate	Sodium ↑, water ↓: postural hypotension Sodium ↑, water ↑: elevated blood pressure; pitting edema		Increased sodium with decrease in fluid intake: observe for signs and symptoms of dehydration (dry mucous membranes, flushed skin, elevated temperature)		Sodium ↑, water ↓: Increase po fluid intake Administer IV fluids as ordered Instill water with or between tube feedings Sodium ↑, water ↓: Administer diuretics as ordered Restrict Na intake Restrict fluid intake Monitor intake and output q8h Weigh daily Monitor vital signs q8h Check urine for specific gravity
Hyperpnea	Hypotension Orthostatic hypotension Tachycardia Thready peripheral pulse or loss of peripheral pulse, collapsed neck veins	Decreased urine output Oliguria to anuria	Flushed, dry, hot skin Fever Loss of skin turgor		Administer IV normal saline solution as ordered (monitor rate carefully) Monitor serum sodium and potassium levels Administer sodium orally as ordered Maintain intake and output q8h

Continued.

TABLE 1-2. Observation of Fluid and Electrolyte Imbalances—cont'd

Imbalances	Causes	Neuromuscular system	GI system
Hyponatremia (sodium deficit)—cont'd	Severe diaphoresis Trauma such as surgery or burns Small bowel obstruction and peritonitis Renal disease Administration of sodium-removing diuretics Water intoxication (IV therapy, tap water enemas)		
Hypermagnesemia (magnesium excess)	Renal failure Adrenal insufficiency Excessive ingestion of magnesium-containing medications Diabetic ketoacidosis (with severe water loss) Hyperparathyroidism	Drowsiness, lethargy, loss of deep tendon reflexes Respiratory depression, coma, and cardiac arrest	Nausea
Hypomagnesemia (magnesium deficit)—cont'd	Acute pancreatitis Malabsorption syndrome (nontropical sprue or steatorrhea) Diarrhea, vomiting Excessive calcium intake Primary hyperparathyroidism and other hypercalcemic states Alcoholism Bowel resection, small bowel bypass, or inherited intestinal defects Gastrointestinal fistulas Excessive renal secretion Nasogastric suctioning Diabetic ketoacidosis Toxemia of pregnancy	Neuromuscular irritability Tremors, tetany, increased reflexes, clonus Convulsions Disorientation Agitation, depression Hallucinations Athetoid or choreiform movements, convulsions, clonus, positive Babinski's sign, positive Chovstek's sign, and positive Trousseau's sign Paresthesias of feet and legs	Anorexia Nausea

Respiratory system	Cardiovascular system	Renal system	Skin and mucous membranes	Blood gas values	Interventions
					Weigh daily
					Encourage foods and fluids high in sodium (milk, meat, eggs, fruit juices, bouillon)
					Use normal saline for all irrigations
Depressed respirations	Hypotension Bradycardia, weak pulse, prolonged QT interval on ECG Heart block				Avoid use of all magnesium-containing medications (e.g., Maalox, Mylanta and milk of magnesia) Monitor vital signs and level of consciousness q1h Encourage fluid intake Administer IV calcium gluconate as ordered Monitor serum magnesium levels q6h Observe for flushing of skin and diaphoresis
	Tachycardia Hypotension Atrial or ventricular premature contractions Nonspecific T wave changes				Administer magnesium sulfate as ordered When administering IV magnesium sulfate, observe patient carefully Monitor for signs and symptoms of high serum magnesium Check for loss of patellar reflex q5 min Monitor respiratory rate q5 min Observe for increased thirst, flushing of skin, diaphoresis, anxiety, or drowsiness Notify physician immediately if patient develops loss of patellar reflex, hypotension, or flushing of face Take precautions against seizures Monitor blood pressure, pulse, and neuro signs q4h

Continued.

TABLE 1-2. Observation of Fluid and Electrolyte Imbalances—cont'd

Imbalances	Causes	Neuromuscular system	GI system
Hypomagnesemia (magnesium deficit) —cont'd			
ACID-BASE IMBALANCES			
Respiratory alkalosis; deficit of H_2CO_3 Decreased P_{CO_2}	Fever, bacteremia, shock Hyperthyroidism Severe pain Hyperventilation caused by hysteria, intentional overbreathing, brain trauma, or ventilators Overdose of epinephrine or salicylates CNS disturbances (meningitis, encephalitis, brainstem injury) Pulmonary embolism Interstitial lung diseases, CHF Hypoxia due to high altitude or severe anemia	Syncope, vertigo, headache, muscle spasm and weakness Tingling in fingers and face Tetany, convulsions, or coma may develop	
Respiratory acidosis (excess H_2CO_3, elevated P_{CO_2})—cont'd	Hypoventilation Emphysema Chronic obstructive pulmonary disease (COPD) Pneumonia Asthma Pickwickian syndrome Barbiturate poisoning Brain trauma with pressure on medulla Neuromuscular disorder (Guillian-Barré myasthenia gravis) Spinal cord trauma Airway occlusion Pneumothorax Atelectasis Postanesthesia Inadequate mechanical ventilation	Anxiety, weakness, headache Depression of CNS Disorientation and coma	Nausea and vomiting may occur

Respiratory system	Cardiovascular system	Renal system	Skin and mucous membranes	Blood gas values	Interventions
					Watch for signs and symptoms of digitalis toxicity (a deficit in magnesium may precipitate or aggravate digitalis toxicity)
					Monitor serum magnesium levels q6h
					Observe for diarrhea
Rapid respirations	Arrhythmias may occur			pH: increased Pco$_2$: decreased HCO$_3$: normal	Implement measures to treat underlying problem
					If alkalosis is caused by anxiety, attempt to calm and reassure patient
					Encourage breathing into a paper bag and/or other breathing techniques
					Administer sedatives as ordered
Distressed respirations Cyanosis	Rapid pulse Ventricular fibrillation may occur			pH: decreased Pco$_2$: increased HCO$_3$: increased	Maintain patent airway
					Place patient in semi-Fowler's position
					Suction nasal and/or pharyngeal airways and trachea as necessary
					Avoid sedation
					Monitor heart rate and rhythm
					Administer oxygen at flow rate ordered
					Monitor fluid and electrolyte levels
					Monitor arterial blood gasses
					Assess for signs and symptoms of respiratory distress
					Administer sodium bicarbonate as ordered
					Maintain mechanical ventilation as ordered
					Perform chest physiotherapy and postural drainage as ordered

Continued.

TABLE 1-2. Observation of Fluid and Electrolyte Imbalances—cont'd

Imbalances	Causes	Neuromuscular system	GI system
Metabolic alkalosis (base bicarbonate excess)	Ingestion of large amounts of sodium bicarbonate (e.g., baking soda or antacids) Vomiting Prolonged gastric suction Diarrhea Potassium-free IV solutions Transfusion Alkalosis Adrenocortical hormone use Excess infusion of parenteral bicarbonate	Hypertonicity, tetany, tremors, convulsions, sensorium changes, irritability, disorientation	
Metabolic acidosis (base bicarbonate deficit)	Diabetic ketoacidosis Prolonged starvation Alcohol abuse Renal failure Vomiting of GI contents Systemic infections Salicylate intoxication Severe diarrhea Abnormal intake of exogenous acids (e.g., ammonium chloride and ferrous sulfate)	Muscle weakness Headache CNS depression, disorientation, stupor, coma	Nausea, vomiting, diarrhea
FLUID IMBALANCES			
Hypervolemia (extracellular fluid volume excess)	Excess sodium intake Malnutrition Excessive ADH secretion Oliguria phase of renal disease Excessive administration of IV fluids CHF Chronic liver disease with portal hypertension	Behavior change, loss of attention, confusion and aphasia; convulsions, coma, and death may follow	Anorexia Nausea and vomiting Constipation Thirst
Hypovolemia (extracellular fluid volume deficit)	Decreased fluid intake Anorexia Excessive output: vomiting, diarrhea, wounds, burns, excessive diaphoresis Uncontrolled diabetes leading to osmotic diuresis	Behavior change, apathy, restlessness, disorientation, lethargy, muscle weakness, tingling of extremities	Anorexia, nausea and vomiting Diarrhea Constipation Abdominal cramps and distention Thirst

General Care and Nursing Diagnoses

Respiratory system	Cardiovascular system	Renal system	Skin and mucous membranes	Blood gas values	Interventions
Shallow, slow respirations	Sinus tachycardia Arrhythmias			pH: increased Pco$_2$: normal or slightly increased HCO$_3$: increased	Monitor accurate intake and output Monitor vital signs q8h Perform neuro check q8h Take seizure precautions Irrigate gastric suction with isotonic solutions Avoid excessive amounts of NaHCO$_3$ Avoid sedatives or hypnotics Administer medications, treatments, and fluids as ordered by physician
Kussmaul's respirations (rapid, deep breathing) Shortness of breath on exertion	Cardiac arrhythmias Bounding pulse Increased blood pressure			pH: decreased Pco$_2$: normal HCO$_3$: decreased	Monitor accurate intake and output Monitor serum electrolyte levels Monitor blood gas levels Observe for signs of hyperkalemia Monitor vital signs q4h Perform neuro checks q4h Seizure precautions Administer medications, treatments, and fluids as ordered by physician
Dyspnea, orthopnea, rales, productive cough	Observe for symptoms of pulmonary edema: Dyspnea, orthopnea, coughing, cyanosis Increased respiratory rate Edema Distended neck vein Increased CVP readings Auscultation of S$_3$	Oliguria	Skin warm, moist, and flushed		Monitor accurate intake and output Weigh daily Monitor vital signs q4h Monitor IV fluid rate carefully Explain reason for restricted fluid intake Observe for signs and symptoms of CHF Restrict sodium intake Administer diuretics as ordered
	Hypotension (postural systolic hypotension) Rapid heart rate Collapsed neck veins Decreased CVP readings	Oliguria Concentrated urine	Poor skin turgor, flushed skin, dry mucous membranes, furrows on tongue		Monitor intake and output Monitor vital signs q8h Administer IV fluids as ordered Encourage po intake, if allowed

Continued.

TABLE 1-2. Observation of Fluid and Electrolyte Imbalances—cont'd

Imbalances	Causes	Neuromuscular system	GI system
Hypovolemia (extracellular fluid volume deficit)—cont'd	Antidiuretic hormone (ADH) insufficiency Diuretic phase of renal disease Excessive use of diuretics		

Review laboratory results; report abnormalities to physician
Review current medications (e.g., antibiotics) for possible side effects
Assess for intolerance to feeding solution q4h
Report untoward reactions to physician immediately
   Abdominal distention
   Nausea
   Vomiting
   Cramping
Auscultate bowel sounds q4h
Report hyperactive or hypoactive bowel sounds to physician
Check for gastric residual q4h
Notify physician if residual is greater than 100 ml (replace residual)
Avoid rapid rate of infusion
   Initiate tube feeding slowly at half-strength concentration
   Increase rate according to patient tolerance
   Regulate flow rate using enteral pump (some IV infusion pumps can be adapted to deliver enteral feedings)
   Place time tape on formula bag or bottle; monitor rate q1h
   Suggest change in method of feeding and/or formula
   Give formula at room temperature
   Administer antidiarrheal agents as ordered
Avoid excessive osmolality of formula
   Contact physician regarding change in formula
   Administer enteral feedings at approximate serum osmolality
   Administer dilute strength and/or decrease volume per physician order
Intervene for lactose intolerance
   Contact physician regarding change to lactose-free formula
   Delete all milk products from diet
Avoid bacterial contamination

Wash hands thoroughly prior to preparation of formula
Allow formula to hang for no longer than 4 to 6 hr
Refrigerate unused formula
Rinse feeding container and gavage set between feedings
Flush tube with water when feeding is disconnected
Change feeding container and gavage set daily

ndx: Ineffective airway clearance related to aspiration of feeding solution

GOAL: *Patient will have a decreased risk of aspiration and maintain clear airways*

Ensure correct placement of tube in stomach q4h (with small-bore tube, x-ray examination may be necessary to confirm placement)
Confirm by radiograph placement of all intestinal tubes
Keep head of bed elevated 30 degrees at all times
Clamp tube feeding when patient must be placed flat
Check for residual q4h for continuous feed feeding and before each intermittent or bolus feed
Report to physician if residual is 100 ml or more and hold feeding
Replace aspirate: prevents loss of gastric juices and electrolytes
Assess patient for cramping, bloating, and nausea
Auscultate bowel sounds q4h
Monitor vital signs T, P, R, and BP q4h
Inflate cuff if cuffed tracheostomy tube, and keep inflated for 1 hr following feeding
Assess for signs and symptoms of aspiration; report findings to physician
   Shortness of breath
   Fever
   Cough
   Discolored tracheal aspirate
   Increased respiratory rate
   Cyanosis

Respiratory system	Cardiovascular system	Renal system	Skin and mucous membranes	Blood gas values	Interventions
					Set up 24-hr schedule for fluid intake Administer plasma or albumin as ordered Assist patient when moving from lying to sitting or standing position

Diminished breath sounds
Rales
Prior to removal of orogastric or nasogastric tube, irrigate and clamp or pinch tube to minimize risk of aspiration as tube is being withdrawn

***ndx*:** Fluid volume deficit related to insufficient fluid intake and abnormal fluid loss associated with high osmolality of enteral feeding

GOAL: *Patient will maintain normal hydration as evidenced by good skin turgor, moist mucous membranes, urine specific gravity within normal limits, and balanced intake and output*

Assess q8h for signs and symptoms of fluid volume deficit
Report the following to physician
   Poor skin turgor
   Descreased urine output
   Dry mucous membranes
   Weight loss greater than 0.5 kg/day
   Decreased blood pressure
   Increased urine specific gravity
Measure intake and output q8h
Weigh patient daily at same time with same clothing and scale
Increase free water via feeding tube as prescribed
Thereafter, flush feeding tube with 30 to 50 ml of water q4h to 6h
Check urine specific gravity q8h
Administer hypertonic formulas using half-strength concentration
Change hypertonic formula to isotonic formula
Document baseline mental status
Assess mental status q4h; report changes to physician
Monitor continuous feedings q1h
Use enteral pump to regulate rate of feedings
Monitor urine or serum glucose q6h as ordered

***ndx*:** Alteration in bowel elimination: constipation related to formula composition and inadequate water intake

GOAL: *Patient will resume usual bowel elimination pattern*

Ensure administration of high-residue formula
Increase free water via feeding tube as prescribed
Flush feeding tube with 30 to 50 ml of water q4h to 6h
Administer stool softener as prescribed
Give 4 to 6 oz of prune juice daily through tube, if allowed
Review medications (e.g., narcotics) for possible side effects
Encourage physical activity within limits
Assist with ambulation
Assist patient to chair twice a day
Change position q2h
Check for fecal impaction
Allow for adequate time in bathroom or with commode/bedpan
Provide privacy for patient
Monitor bowel elimination pattern

***ndx*:** Impairment of skin integrity: irritation or breakdown related to pressure from feeding tube and/or drainage from ostomy tube insertion site

GOAL: *Patient will not exhibit signs of skin irritation or breakdown*

Use small-bore feeding tube when possible
Position tube to prevent undue pressure on nares
Reposition tube and change tape daily
Cleanse and lubricate nares q4h and prn
Provide oral care q4h and prn
Provide skin care at insertion site of ostomy tube
Assess tube insertion site q8h for tenderness, redness, and drainage

Report abnormalities to physician
Change ostomy site dressing q2d and prn
Cleanse site with soap and water
Apply stoma adhesive around tube at insertion site
Cover site with Op-Site or similar dressing
Secure ostomy tube
Report continuous leakage around tube to physician

ndx: Disturbance in self-concept related to change in body appearance resulting from nasal or ostomy tube

GOAL: *Patient will verbalize need for tube feedings and will begin to participate in self-care*

Assess level of anxiety and understanding of need for tube feedings; if feasible, select and/or change to a feeding tube that is tolerated physically and psychologically by patient
Encourage patient to express feelings about the way he feels and looks
Reassure patient that feelings are appropriate
Continue to be sensitive to patient's needs and feelings
Assess for readiness to begin self-care
Instruct patient and/or significant other regarding feeding procedure
Provide emotional support and positive feedback for participation in self-feeding
Provide opportunity for questions and reinforce instructions as necessary
Continue to support coping efforts
Provide referrals as necessary (social service, dietitian, support groups, clergy)
Encourage ambulation if not contraindicated
Provide small amounts of favorite foods orally, if allowed

ndx: Knowledge deficit related to purpose and administration of tube feedings, complications, nasal tube and enterostomy care, and/or activity

GOAL: *Patient and/or significant other will demonstrate understanding of home care and follow-up instructions through interactive discussion and actual return demonstration*

Purpose and administration of tube feedings

Explain that all necessary nutrients—protein, fats, carbohydrates, vitamins, and minerals—will be supplied by tube feeding
Discuss formula selection and reason for same
Instruct patient and/or significant other in formula preparation, storage, and feeding schedule
Instruct patient and/or significant other in administration of formula and medications via feeding tube

Complications

Discuss signs and symptoms of feeding intolerance: nausea, vomiting, diarrhea, cramping, bloating; discuss importance of reporting signs and symptoms to physician
Explain reasons for administration of feeding with patient upright
Demonstrate procedure for checking placement of feeding tube
Discuss signs and symptoms of possible aspiration: coughing, choking, difficulty in breathing, elevated temperature; discuss importance of reporting signs and symptoms to physician
Discuss importance of flushing tube with water following each feeding
Demonstrate urine and/or serum glucose checking procedure; discuss importance of reporting abnormalities to physician
Discuss measures to prevent constipation
Contact home health nurse if tube is blocked, broken, or dislodged

Nasal tube and enterostomy care

Demonstrate taping of tube to prevent slipping
Demonstrate cleansing and lubrication of nares; explain that this should be done q4h and prn
Teach importance of maintaining good oral hygiene
Demonstrate ostomy care
Discuss importance of reporting redness, drainage, foul odor, or tenderness around stoma to physician
Teach patient how to remove and insert ostomy feeding tube per physician order (esophagotomy and gastrostomy tubes may be removed after several weeks and inserted only for feedings)

Activity

Instruct patient to increase activity/exercise as desired and tolerated
Discuss benefits of exercise
  Promotes feeling of well-being
  Increases gastric motility

Evaluation

Patient
  Tolerates tube-feeding volume, concentration, and formula as prescribed
  Evacuates soft-formed stool every other day
  Has good skin color, turgor, and moist mucous membranes

Maintains weight
Demonstrates administration of tube feedings
Demonstrates serum and/or glucose testing
Has no fever or cough; tracheal aspirate is clear
Shows no evidence of skin breakdown
Demonstrates dressing change and application of skin barrier to ostomy site
States is coping with imposed restrictions

TOTAL PARENTERAL NUTRITION (TPN)

Infusion of necessary nutrients—amino acids, fat, trace elements, carbohydrates, vitamins, and electrolytes—through a peripheral or central vein; peripheral or central venous nutrition may be chosen when the enteral route is not available because of mechanical or functional abnormalities of the GI tract; clinical conditions that may indicate the need for parenteral nutrition are short bowel syndrome, ileus, malabsorption, pancreatitis, hypermetabolic states (trauma, sepsis), and altered metabolic states (acute renal failure, hepatic insufficiency)

Assessment

Observations/findings

Insertion site
  Pain
  Warmth
  Redness
  Edema
  Drainage at insertion site
  Leakage at insertion site
Fever
Leukocytosis
Glucose intolerance

Laboratory/diagnostic studies

Potassium
Phosphorus
Magnesium
Blood glucose
Calcium
Sodium
Chloride
Blood urea nitrogen (BUN)
Prothrombin time (PT)
White blood cell count (WBC)
Liver enzymes
Bilirubin
Serum albumin
Transferrin

Potential complications

Mechanical
  Pneumothorax (with subclavian vein catheterization)
  Air embolism
  Catheter and venous thrombosis
Septic: catheter sepsis (bacterial or fungal)
Metabolic
  Hyperglycemia
  Hyperosmolar nonketotic coma
  Hypoglycemia
  Fatty acid deficiency
  Electrolyte abnormalities
  Liver dysfunction
  Mineral and trace elements deficiency

Medical management

Route of administration
X-ray examination to determine placement of central line
Keep vein open with isotonic solution until catheter placement is confirmed
Rate of flow
Increase or decrease in rate of solution
Fat emulsion
Daily weights
Urine glucose
Blood glucose monitoring
Administration of insulin
Intake and output
Daily laboratory studies

Nursing diagnoses/goals/interventions

ndx: Potential for infection related to invasive procedure and delivery of high concentrations of glucose parenterally

> GOAL: *Patient will not exhibit signs or symptoms of infection as evidenced by temperature within normal limits and absence of redness, warmth, pain, and swelling at insertion site*

Peripheral venous nutrition

Wash hands thoroughly prior to insertion of IV needle or catheter
Select distal veins in upper extremities
Clip or shave hair at site according to hospital policy
Prepare site with povidone-iodine swab and allow to air dry
Apply povidone-iodine ointment to catheter site
Cover site with sterile dressing
Observe for signs and symptoms of phlebitis and/or infiltration

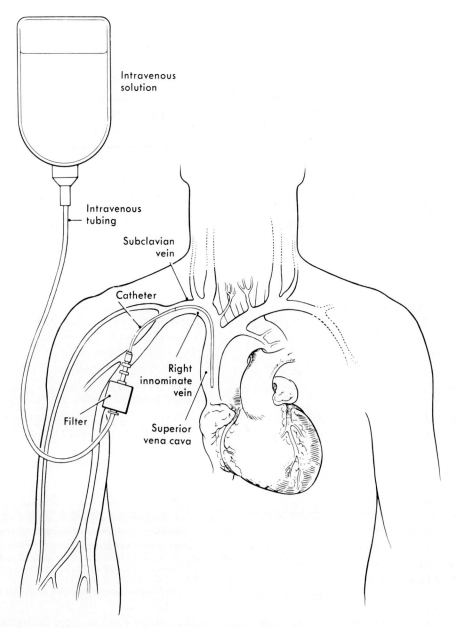

FIGURE 1-1. Total parenteral nutrition administered through a central line.

Remove catheter or needle if phlebitis or infiltration is present
Rotate catheter site q48h to 72h or according to hospital policy
Tape IV tubing securely
Monitor catheter site every hour
Change IV tubing q24h or according to hospital policy
Use 0.22 μm filter on amino acid dextrose line
Use strict aseptic technique when assembling and changing administration set
Monitor vital signs T, P, and R q4h; report elevation of temperature to physician
Monitor blood glucose as ordered
Check urine for glucose as ordered, usually q6h (glucosuria may indicate impending sepsis)
Ensure that final amino acid concentration does not exceed 10% dextrose
Ensure continuous infusion of fat emulsion when 10% dextrose is infused peripherally
Keep TPN solution refrigerated until ready to be used
Allow solution to hang no longer than 24 hr
Never piggyback medications other than fat emulsion via TPN line
Securely tape needle used for piggybacking fat emulsion

Central venous nutrition

Assist physician with insertion of central line catheter
Ensure catheter insertion under sterile conditions
Ensure proper site preparation
Change central line dressing using sterile technique
Prepare site with povidone-iodine and allow to air dry
Apply povidone-iodine ointment to catheter site
Cover site with sterile dressing
Observe site for signs of sepsis: erythema, swelling, tenderness, drainage at insertion site
Monitor vital signs T, P, and R q4h; report temperature elevation to physician
Monitor blood glucose as ordered
Check urine for glucose as ordered, usually q6h (glucosuria may indicate impending sepsis)
Monitor catheter site q1h
Tape tubing securely
Do not use stopcocks on TPN line
Change IV tubing q24h or according to hospital policy
Use 0.22 μm filter on amino acid dextrose line
Use strict aseptic technique when assembling and changing administration set
Allow solution to hang no longer than 24 hr
Never use line for piggybacking medications, central venous pressure (CVP) readings, or aspiration of blood for laboratory studies

ndx: Potential for complications: metabolic abnormalities, pneumothorax, air embolism, or adverse reactions to amino acid and/or fat emulsion therapy*

GOAL: *Patient will not experience complications from parenteral nutritional therapy*

Metabolic abnormalities

Monitor for signs and symptoms of hyperglycemia
   Polyuria
   Glycosuria: elevated blood sugar
   Polydipsia, polyphagia
   Dimmed, blurred vision
Hypoglycemia
   Tachycardia
   Cold sweat
   Posterior occipital headache
   Irritability, jitteriness
   Lethargy
   Blood glucose level <60 mg/dl
Perform urine and/or serum testing q6h
Measure vital signs q4h
Assess neurologic status q8h
Monitor intake and output q8h
Weigh patient daily at same time with same clothing and scale
Initiate TPN solution slowly
Increase rate per patient tolerance and physician order
Do not increase rate to catch up
Monitor flow rate of solution using infusion control device
Do not interrupt infusion for more than 1 hr q8h
Ensure patency of line
For hyperglycemia, administer insulin as ordered
For hypoglycemia, administer IV 50% dextrose as ordered
Taper solution before discontinuing
Review medications that may affect glucose metabolism
Assess for possible sepsis
Monitor for signs and symptoms of fluid overload
   Pedal or sacral edema
   Rapid weight gain: 1 lb (0.45 kg) or more a day
   Pitting edema
   Increased blood pressure
   Bounding pulse
Monitor for signs and symptoms of fluid deficit

---

*Not a NANDA-approved nursing diagnosis.

Poor skin turgor
Dry mucous membranes
Tachycardia
Hypotension
Weight loss

Review all routine laboratory tests for abnormalities

Assess for signs and symptoms of fatty acid deficiency, alopecia, brittle nails, desquamating dermatitis, decreased immunity, thrombocytopenia, and delayed wound healing

Report abnormalities to physician

Pneumothorax

Ausculate chest for breath sounds q1h

Assess respiratory status q1h and report signs and symptoms to physician
Sudden onset of sharp chest pain
Coughing secondary to pleural irritation
Dyspnea, cyanosis, hypotension

Obtain baseline BP, apical pulse, T, and R

Keep vein open with isotonic solution until chest x-ray examination confirms correct placement of central line

Air embolism

Assess for signs and symptoms of air embolism, dyspnea, tachycardia, cyanosis, and hypotension

Place patient in head-down position during subclavian or jugular vein insertion

Use Luer-Lok connections on all central line tubing

Securely tape all tubing connections

Use air-eliminating filters when possible

Clamp catheter or assist and teach patient to perform Valsalva maneuver during tubing changes

Reaction to TPN

Assess patient for dyspnea, chest abdominal or back pain, fever, flushing, chills, headache, decreased blood pressure, cyanosis, diaphoresis, and/or urticaria

Stop infusion and report untoward reactions to physician

Monitor and report elevated triglyceride levels and/or elevated liver function tests

ndx: Knowledge deficit related to purpose of TPN, complications associated with therapy, and/or expected outcome

GOAL: *Patient and/or significant other will demonstrate understanding of TPN therapy and its management through interactive discussion and return demonstration*

Provide patient and/or significant other with instructions regarding
Reasons for TPN
Importance of therapy
Expected outcome
Need for protection of IV site
Need for prevention of tension on central venous catheter
Importance of intake and output measurement
Signs and symptoms to report to nurse and/or physician
Excessive urination
Chills
Elevated temperature
Feeling of warmth
Shortness of breath
Excessive thirst
Leakage of fluid at catheter site
Pain or tenderness at catheter site
Swelling at catheter site

Home total parenteral nutrition: provide patient and/or significant other with the following instructions regarding
Type of solution
Schedule for infusion
Obtaining the solution
Storage of solution
Inspection of solution
Procedure for changing central line dressing
Frequency of dressing change
Supplies needed
Where to obtain supplies
Cleansing of site
Observation of site
Procedure for flushing catheter
Purpose of flushing
Frequency of flushing
Solution used for flushing
Changing injection site cap
Frequency of change
Clamping of catheter prior to cap change
Signs and symptoms to report to physician
Elevated temperature
Rapid weight loss
Rapid weight gain
Increased fatigue
Shortness of breath
Tightness in chest
Redness, swelling, or drainage at insertion site
Glucose present in urine

Instruct patient regarding
Amount of physical activity allowed
Need to keep follow-up appointments

Resources for assistance as needed
Importance of avoiding crowds and persons with infections
How to recognize and handle possible complications: air embolism, blood backup, catheter injury

Ensure that patient and/or significant other demonstrates
    Handwashing technique
    Preparation and infusion of TPN solution
    Use of infusion pump
    Clamping catheter
    Flushing catheter
    Changing injection site cap
    Central line dressing change
    Care of catheter insertion site
    Measuring and recording intake and output
    Testing urine for sugar and acetone
    Taking and recording temperature

Evaluation

Vital signs are within normal limits
There are no signs of infection, redness, swelling, or drainage at insertion site
Central line catheter remains patent
Skin turgor is good
Patient has gained previous weight loss and weight has stabilized
Laboratory tests are within normal limits
Patient demonstrates
    Handwashing technique
    Changing tubing
    Use of infusion pump
    Clamping, flushing, and cap change
    Dressing change and care of insertion site
Patient verbalizes comfort with above procedures
Patient states action to take if complications occur

TABLE 1-3. Regulation of IV Drip Rates

Amount/hr (ml)	Amount/8 hr (ml)	Amount/24 hr (ml)	Drops/min
PEDIATRIC MICRODRIP (60 DROPS/ML)			
4	30	90	4
5	40	120	5
6	50	150	6
8	60	180	8
9	70	210	9
10	80	240	10
12	100	300	12
14	110	330	14
18	150	450	18
22	180	540	22
25	200	600	25
30	250	750	30
37	300	900	37
ADULT IV SET (10 DROPS/ML)			
125	1000	3000	21
100	800	2400	16
90	720	2160	15
80	640	1920	13
70	560	1680	11
60	480	1440	10
50	400	1200	8
40	320	960	6
30	240	720	5
ADULT IV SET (15 DROPS/ML)			
125	1000	3000	30
100	800	2400	25
90	720	2160	22
80	640	1920	20
70	560	1680	17
60	480	1440	15
50	400	1200	12
40	320	960	10
30	240	720	7

CARE OF PATIENT WITH CENTRAL VENOUS CATHETER

central venous catheter *A venous catheter inserted into the superior vena cava through the subclavian, internal, or external jugular vein; can be used for monitoring of venous pressure, infusion of medications, TPN, and rapid infusion of fluid and blood products, and blood withdrawal*

Insertion of catheter

Auscultate chest for breath sounds
Obtain baseline BP, apical pulse, T, and R
Provide emotional support
    Explain procedure to patient
    Reinforce physician's explanation of procedure
Prepare to assist physician with insertion of central venous catheter
    Maintain sterile technique
    Shave hair from insertion site
    Prepare skin around insertion site with povidone-iodine solution
    Establish and maintain a sterile field throughout insertion
Place patient in supine or Trendelenburg position if subclavian or jugular vein is used as insertion site
Administer isotonic IV solution at a keep-open rate until position of catheter is verified by chest x-ray examination
Apply sterile occlusive dressing to catheter insertion site; label with date and time of insertion
Obtain chest x-ray film

Postinsertion assessment

Observations/findings

Chest, shoulder, or neck pain
Edema in catheterized arm
Neck vein distention
Redness, swelling, or drainage at insertion site
Temperature elevation
Elevated WBC
Occlusion of central line
Rejection of catheter
Air embolization
Accumulation of serous fluid around site

Potential complications

Infection at site
Venous thrombosis
Catheter migration
Catheter embolus
Occlusion of catheter
Extravasation
Septicemia
Pneumothorax
Hemothorax
Hematoma
Cardiac tamponade
Cardiac arrhythmias

Postinsertion care

Immediate care

Observe patient for signs of pneumothorax until chest x-ray film is read
    Auscultate chest for breath sounds q30 min for two times and then qh; report diminished or absent breath sounds to physician
    Report respiratory distress and presence of chest pain to physician
Prepare for insertion of chest tubes if pneumothorax is present

Ongoing care

Check BP, T, P, and R q4h
Auscultate chest for breath sounds q8h
Administer parenteral fluids as ordered
    Maintain a closed system
    Keep system free of air
    Have a rubber-tipped hemostat available to clamp catheter if necessary
    Maintain a continuous drip of parenteral solutions at all times unless obtaining a CVP reading or aspirating a blood specimen
Change dressing daily
    Inspect catheter insertion site for signs of infection, redness, tenderness, drainage, and edema
    Cleanse skin around insertion site with povidone-iodine solution
    Apply bacteriostatic ointment to catheter insertion site; avoid antibiotic ointment
    Apply sterile occlusive dressing
    Secure tubing to skin in order to prevent tension on catheter
Measure intake and output q8h
Send tip of catheter to laboratory for culture when catheter is removed

Patient teaching/discharge outcome

See standard of care for primary condition
Ensure that patient and/or significant other knows and understands
    Purpose of central catheter
    Importance of not touching catheter and tubing
    Importance of reporting any difficulty in breathing, sudden chest pain at insertion site, or fever to nurse
    When to flush catheter
    When to change dressing
    Type and amount of parenteral solutions to be infused daily
    Need to keep solution refrigerated (bring to room temperature prior to administration)
    Where to purchase solution and supplies needed
    Name of medication, dosage, time of administration, and side effects
    Need to avoid crowds and persons with infections
Ensure that patient and/or significant other demonstrates
    Handwashing technique
    Dressing change
        Inspect catheter insertion site for redness, tenderness, drainage, or swelling
        Clean skin around insertion site with povidone-iodine solution
        Apply bacteriostatic ointment to insertion site
        Apply sterile occlusive dressing
    Flushing catheter
    Administration of parenteral solutions and/or medications as ordered by physician
    Use of infusion pump if necessary

Multilumen Subclavian Catheters

Three separate subclavian catheters contained in one sheath; allows infusion of incompatible drugs simultaneously—the solutions do not mix but exit via a separate lumen; the catheters vary in length, gauge, and volume

Postinsertion assessment
Observations/findings

See Care of Patient with Central Venous Catheter (p. 56)

Potential complications

See Care of Patient with Central Venous Catheter (p. 56)

Postinsertion care

Use larger-gauge lumen for administration of blood products or blood withdrawal (i.e., 16-gauge CVP readings can be taken from distal lumen only)
Reserve one lumen for TPN use only
Keep occlusive clamp available at bedside

Site care

Observe site q1h
Inspect site for redness, drainage, swelling, leakage of fluid, or loose sutures
Notify physician if any of the above occur
Change dressing qd for gauze dressing, q5d for transparent dressng or when nonocclusive
Cleanse site with povidone-iodine solution
Apply povidone-iodine ointment to catheter insertion site
Apply occlusive gauze or transparent dressing

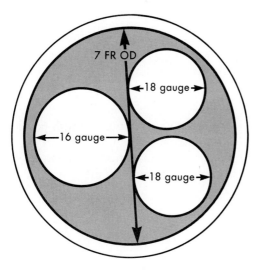

FIGURE 1-2. Multilumen catheter. French polyurethane catheter featuring three internal lumens: 18-gauge proximal, 18-gauge middle, and 16-gauge distal. (Redrawn from Recker, D.H., and Metzler, D.J.: Crit. Care Nurse 4(3):92, 1984.)

Maintaining patency of lumens

Flush each catheter lumen with heparin q12 if catheter lumen not in use
Flush after each intermittent medication infusion or blood sampling
Change Luer-Lok intermittent injection site cap q3d or according to hospital policy
Cap change should coincide with heparin flush

Blood withdrawal

Collect blood specimen for laboratory studies as ordered
Stop infusion through other lumens
Perform procedure using sterile technique
Aspirate and discard the first 3 ml
Withdraw amount of blood needed for laboratory studies
Flush with normal saline, then heparin solution 3 ml
Resume infusion through other lumens

Patient teaching/discharge outcome

See Care of Patient with Central Venous Catheter (p. 56)

Long-Term Venous Access Devices
SILASTIC ATRIAL CATHETER

A central line catheter (single or double lumen) tunneled subcutaneously and inserted by cutdown into the central venous system by way of the cephalic or internal jugular vein; procedure is performed under fluroscopy, using sterile technique; a Dacron cuff anchors catheter subcutaneously

Postinsertion assessment
Observations/findings

See Care of Patient with Central Venous Catheter (p. 56)

Potential complications

See Care of Patient with Central Venous Catheter (p. 56)

Postinsertion care

Clamp catheters with occlusive clamp only
Administer TPN as ordered by physician
Administer antibiotics as ordered by physician
Administer blood and blood products as ordered by physician

Blood withdrawal

Collect blood specimen for laboratory studies as ordered

Stop infusion through both lumens
Perform procedure using sterile technique
Aspirate and discard first sample
  Adult: 5 ml
  Child: 3 ml
Aspirate amount of blood needed for laboratory studies
Flush with normal saline, then heparin solution 5 ml
Resume infusion through other lumen

Site care

Change transparent dressing q5d or when nonocclusive
Inspect catheter insertion site for redness, drainage, or edema
Cleanse insertion site with povidone-iodine solution
Apply povidone-iodine ointment to catheter insertion site
Apply sterile transparent dressing
Secure IV tubing to prevent tension on catheter
Obtain order to remove site sutures within 7 days

Maintaining patency of catheter lumens

Flush each catheter lumen with heparin q12h if lumen is not in use
Flush after each intermittent medication infusion or blood sampling
Change injection site caps q3d or according to hospital policy
Use small-gauge (25-gauge or 22-gauge 1-inch) needle when entering injection site caps for flushing, etc.

Patient teaching/discharge outcome

See Care of Patient with Central Venous Catheter (p. 56)
Ensure that patient and/or significant other demonstrates
  Handwashing technique
  Method of changing dressing
  Technique for heparinizing the catheter
  Method of changing injection site caps
  Administration of parenteral solution as ordered
  Administration of medications as ordered
  Use of infusion pump
Ensure that patient and/or significant other knows and understands
  Need to notify physician if any of the following occur
    Inability to flush catheter
    Broken catheter
    Swelling, redness, drainage at insertion site
    Dislodged catheter
    Burning sensation during flushing
    Fever of 100° F (37.8° C) or above
  Instructions regarding Activity
    Resume activity as tolerated
    Shower daily
    Change transparent dressing after shower if wet
    May swim, if allowed

IMPLANTED PORT

Implantation of an infusion port under the skin to provide vascular access for patients requiring repeated infusion of drugs, TPN, blood products, and other fluids; the system consists of an implantable silicone catheter and an implantable stainless steel portal with a self-sealing septum; the IV system is inserted into the superior vena cava or right atrium via the subclavian or internal jugular vein with the portal placed over the third or fourth rib

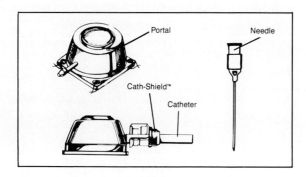

FIGURE 1-3. Parts of Port-A-Cath® implantable drug delivery system. (Courtesy Pharmacia Deltec, Inc., St Paul, Minn.)

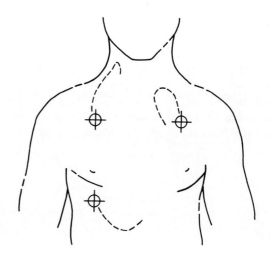

FIGURE 1-4. Some commonly used locations for placement of Port-A-Cath® portal and catheter. (Redrawn from Patient information Port-A-Cath® [booklet], Pharmacia Deltec, Inc., St. Paul, Minn.)

Postinsertion assessment

Observations/findings

Accumulation of serous fluid around implant site

Aching discomfort to acute pain in shoulder, neck, or arm on ipsilateral or contralateral side

Supraclavicular or neck swelling

Venous dilation

Redness, swelling, tenderness, and drainage at site

Device rotation palpate skin over device and check for possible rotation or migration of portal

Device extrusion

Potential complications

See Care of Patient with Central Venous Catheter (p. 56)

Postinsertion care

Site care

Always access the device, portal septum area, using sterile technique

Cleanse skin over portal septum area with providone-iodine solution

Accessing the system

Use special noncore needles to access the device (regular needle cannot be used)

Do not leave needle open to air while it is in the portal, as it may cause air embolus

Attach extension tubing or stopcock to needle; allows patient movement without dislodging needle and facilitates changing of syringe or connections

Prime needle and extension tube with normal saline prior to use

Maintaining patency of the device

Flush system with 5 ml of normal saline prior to administration of any drugs, than flush the heparin

Always leave system filled with heparinized saline after each use

For intermittent use, flush catheter q4 weeks

Avoid reflux when withdrawing needle from septum; press down on portal while maintaining positive injection pressure

Dressing/tubing/needle change

Change dressing and tubing q48h or according to hospital policy

Provide site care

Apply povidone-iodine ointment to needle site

Place sterile rolled gauze between skin and needle for support

Apply sterile transparent dressing over needle, gauze, and extension tube

Tape needle securely to skin

Administer TPN as ordered by physician

Administer antibiotics as ordered by physician

Administer blood and blood products as ordered by physician

Follow hospital protocol for administration of chemotherapeutic agents

Blood sampling

Flush system with 5 ml of normal saline to ensure patency of line

Withdraw 3 ml of blood and discard

Aspirate amount of blood needed for laboratory studies

Flush with normal saline 20 ml, then heparinized saline 5 ml or according to hospital policy

Patient teaching/discharge outcome

Ensure that patient and/or significant other demonstrates
  Handwashing technique
  Technique for accessing the system, always cleansing skin around site with povidone-iodine solution
  Technique for expelling all air from syringe, tubing, and needle (bandage or dressing to site is not required)
  Technique for flushing the system
  Administration of parenteral solution as ordered
  Administration of medications as ordered; use of infusion pump

Ensure that patient and/or significant other knows and understands
  Instructions regarding activity
    Resume activity as tolerated
    Shower daily
    May swim, if allowed
    Carry special identification card
  Need to notify physician if any of the following occur:
    Inability to flush system
    Movement of portal; appearance of bruising, swelling, redness, or tenderness at portal site
    Fever of 100° F (37.8° C) or above

ALTERATION IN NUTRITION: LESS THAN BODY REQUIREMENTS

malnutrition *Nutritional intake is insufficient to meet requirements; lack of evaluation and early treatment of nutritional needs are contributing factors of malnutrition occurring in hospitalized patients; can cause delayed healing of wounds, an in-*

ELECTRONIC INFUSION DEVICES			
Nonvolumetric devices:	Deliver solution in drops/min	Drop rate–calibrated infusion pumps:	Are designed to count drops and are set in terms of gtts/min; move solution through the line by application of positive pressure
Volumetric devices:	Deliver a specific volume in a given time as shown in ml/hr		
Drop rate–calibrated infusion controllers:	Regulate infusion rate by gravity by electronically counting or measuring drops (controllers that set the rate in drops/min are now considered obsolete)	Volumetric infusion pumps:	Rate setting adjustment is calibrated in ml/hr rather than drops/min; pump output pressure limits are established by manufacturer and can range as high as 25 psi
Volumetric infusion controllers:	Count the volume in each drop; permit flow rate to be set in ml/hr rather than gtt/min (Controllers *do not* add pressure to the line to overcome resistance to flow)	Variable pressure limit volumetric infusion pumps:	Are designed to provide only the pressure needed for specific clinical situations; allow nurse to set pressure limit based on clinical considerations
Infusion pumps:	Apply positive pressure to the line to overcome flow; most deliver solution to a vein at an average pressure of psi (pounds per square inch) *(Pressure can increase if a line is occluded partially or totally)*		

creased risk of sepsis, pulmonary complications, and an increased hospital stay; in addition, treatments such as radiation therapy and chemotherapy may be poorly tolerated by the patient with malnutrition; the following three forms of malnutrition are generally recognized

marasmus *A diet low in calories and protein but providing a balanced deficit; patient experiences weight loss and fat and muscle depletion; visceral protein status may appear normal*

kwashiorkor *A diet adequate in calorie intake but limited in protein; patient experiences depletion of the visceral protein stores and depression of the cellular immune response*

marasmic kwashiorkor *Protein calorie malnutrition (a diet low in protein and calories); the type of malnutrition commonly seen in the seriously ill hospitalized patient; patient experiences weight loss, depletion of visceral protein stores, decreased fat and muscle stores, and decreased cellular immune response*

Assessment

Observations/findings

DIETARY HISTORY

Recent weight loss or gain
Anorexia
Sitophobia
Inadequate food or nutrient intake
Excessive food or fluid intake
Body weight 20% above or below ideal for height and body build
Fad or chronic weight loss diets
Loss of taste or smell
Food allergies
Food sensitivities
Vomiting, diarrhea, constipation
Inadequate intake of fiber
Increased intake of fat, sodium, sugar, and/or alcohol
Involuntary weight loss with adequate food intake
Difficulty in swallowing
Difficulty in chewing

MEDICAL HISTORY

GI surgery
   Obstruction and prolonged ileus
   GI cancer
Inflammatory bowel disease
   Short bowel syndrome
   Fistulas
   Pancreatitis
   Abscesses
   Radiation enteritis
   Gastric ulcers
Chronic illnesses
   Heart disease
   Diabetes mellitus
   Renal disease
   Cerebrovascular accident (CVA)
   Hepatitis
   Coma
Increased metabolic requirements
   Burns
   Infection
   Pregnancy
   Lactation
   Fever
   Trauma
   Hyperthyroidism
Long-term drug therapy
   Anticonvulsants
   Antacids
   Saline cathartics
   Antibiotics
   Anticoagulants
   Antiinflammatory agents
   Diuretics
   Chemotherapeutic agents
   Immunosuppressants
   Chelating agents
   Corticosteroids
   Alcohol
   Hypoglycemic agents
   Laxatives
   Antihistamines
   Psychotropic drugs
   Oral contraceptive agents

SOCIAL/ECONOMIC HISTORY

Lives alone and/or eats alone
Elderly
Immobility
Limited income
Lack of cooking facilities at home

Level of education
Ethnic, religious, cultural beliefs
Substance abuse

PHYSICAL ASSESSMENT

General appearance
   Pale
   Thin
   Wasted
   Emaciated
   Low body weight <80% for height, build, and sex
Hair
   Sparce
   Dull
   Dry
   Depigmented
   Fine, straight
   Easily plucked
Eyes
   Dull
   Dry
   Bitot's spots
   Red or pale conjunctiva
   Xerosis
   Retinal hemorrhage
Mouth
   Redness and swelling of mouth and lips
   Cheilosis
   Angular fissures and scars
Tongue
   Swollen
   Magenta colored
   Smooth
   Hypertrophic
   Atropic papillae
Gums
   Swollen
   Bleed easily
   Recession of gums
   Pale
Teeth
   Cavities
   Mottled appearance
Face
   Depigmentation
   Skin dark over cheeks and under eyes
   Swollen face
Glands
   Thyroid enlargement
   Parotid enlargement

Skin
   Dryness of skin (xerosis)
   Pale
   Flaky dermatitis
   Lacks fat under skin
   Petechiae
   Follicular hyperkeratosis
   Soreness
Nails
   Spoon shaped
   Brittle
   Ridged
Musculoskeletal system
   Muscle atrophy
   Hemorrhages into muscles
   Calf tenderness
   Weakness
Cardiovascular system
   Tachycardia
   Cardiomegaly
   Arrhythmias
   Systolic blood pressure, decreased
GI system
   Hepatomegaly
   Splenomegaly
Neurologic system
   Mental irritability
   Confusion
   Loss of position and vibratory sense
   Decrease and loss of ankle and knee reflexes
Respiratory system: shortness of breath

Laboratory/diagnostic studies

Hemoglobin decreased
Hematocrit decreased
Serum albumin decreased
Serum transferrin decreased
Urinary creatinine excretion decreased
Total lymphocyte count decreased
Impaired cellular immune functions (manifested by delayed hypersensitivity reactions to skin tests [e.g., PPD] mumps, Candida)
   BUN elevated
   Cholesterol decreased
   Total iron binding capacity, serum electrolytes
   Serum iron
   Serum folate
Height and weight index; anthropometric measurements
   Triceps skinfold thickness (TST)
      Estimates degree of subcutaneous fat, midarm circumference (MAC), and midarm muscle circumference (MAMC)
      Reflects degree of muscle depletion due to catabolism in malnourished patient

Potential complications

Infection
Poor tissue healing
Interference with blood clotting
Impaired immune response
Anemia
Dehydration
Obesity

Medical management

Treatment of underlying disease process
Medication orders
Change in medications as necessary
Parenteral nutrition
Enteral nutrition
Urine glucose
Daily weights
Intake and output
Blood glucose monitoring

Nursing diagnoses/goals/interventions

ndx: Alteration in nutrition: less than body requirements related to anorexia

GOAL: *Patient will consume nutrients to meet energy requirements and will maintain or regain weight for height and body build*

Administer antiemetics as ordered
Eliminate unpleasant odors and sights from environment
Encourage small amounts of food q2h; alternate with liquids
Determine patient's food preferences
Discuss importance of consuming adequate nutrients
Arrange with significant others to bring favorite foods from home
Provide protein/calorie–rich foods and supplements
Avoid drinking fluids with meals
Provide oral care before and after each meal and q4h
Offer small amounts of cold liquids q2h: flavored gelatin liquid, ginger ale, cola
Ensure period of rest prior to eating
Serve all foods in pleasant, attractive environment
If possible, arrange for family member to have meals with patient
Administer analgesics 1 hr prior to eating per physician's order

Avoid unpleasant or painful procedures prior to meals
Instruct patient to use spices and sauces to help improve taste and smell of foods
Instruct patient to avoid rich, fried, or greasy foods
Record intake and output q8h
Weigh patient daily at same time with same clothing and scale

ndx: Alteration in nutrition: less than body requirements related to dysphagia and difficulty in chewing

GOAL: *Patient will increase oral intake of nutrients to maintain weight for height and body build*

Assess cough/gag reflex and ability to swallow
Assist patient to sitting position prior to eating
Encourage rest period before meals to prevent fatigue
Provide patient with foods that are easy to chew or swallow (e.g., custards, applesauce, pureed foods)
Allow adequate time for meals
Instruct patient to chew and swallow slowly (for CVA patient, place food at back of tongue and on side of face he can control)
Provide high-protein drinks as a supplement
Offer small feedings q2h
Weigh patient daily at same time with same clothing and scale
Measure intake and output q8h
Monitor calorie count for 72 hr
Determine protein and calorie needs of patient
Instruct patient to flex head slightly, which will aid in swallowing
Ensure that food does not remain in cheek pouches
Provide oral care before and after each meal and q4h
Instruct patient to avoid spicy, acid, too hot, or too cold foods
Avoid harsh or coarse foods
Minimize distractions during eating
Serve food attractively in pleasant environment
Reheat food as necessary
Crush pills and give with gelatin or puddings

ndx: Alteration in nutrition: less than body requirements related to malabsorption of nutrients and increased nutrient losses (diarrhea)

GOAL: *Patient will consume nutrients to effect stabilization of weight or weight gain as indicated*

Discuss dietary restrictions
    Avoid foods and fluids that are poorly digested or act as irritants to GI tract
        Foods high in milk fat: patient may have milk intolerance (deficiency of lactase)
        Foods with high fiber content
        Spicy foods
        Flatus-forming foods (e.g., onions, cabbage, baked beans, chili, broccoli)
        Foods and fluids containing caffeine (coffee, tea, soft drinks, chocolate)
Encourage patient to chew food thoroughly
Administer medications as ordered
Assess for response and reactions to medications
    Anticholinergics
    Antispasmodics
    Bulk-forming agents
    Antidiarrheal agents
    Cholestyramine (to bind bile salts)
    Steroid therapy (to reduce inflammation)
    Pain medications
    Sedatives
    Antibiotics
    Vitamins
Monitor serum electrolytes, clotting studies, serum albumin, Hgb, and Hct
Observe for occult blood in stool
Monitor intake and output
Observe for fluid volume deficit or excess (p. 46)
Check BP, T, P, and R q4h
Document amount of vomitus
Maintain NPO as ordered
Administer total parenteral nutrition (TPN) as ordered (p. 51)
Administer blood transfusion as ordered
Identify factors that may contribute to diarrhea
Monitor character, amount, color, and frequency of stools
Assess for presence of abdominal cramping, flatus, or abdominal distention
Ausculate abdomen for bowel sounds q2h to 4h; report increase or decrease to physician
Implement measures to promote rest
Instruct patient to avoid smoking (nicotine has stimulant effect on GI tract)
Avoid alcoholic beverages
Avoid taking temperature rectally (excessive diarrhea may cause excoriation of rectum)
Assess skin integrity q shift
Weigh patient daily at same time with same clothing and scale
Provide high-protein, high-calorie supplement
Provide oral care q4h
Assist patient with identifying and managing stress
Obtain dietary consultation as necessary

ndx: Alteration in nutrition: less than body requirements related to inability to procure, plan, and prepare a nutritious diet

GOAL: *Patient will obtain necessary nutrients to maintain or regain weight for height and body build*

Assess current daily food intake
Assess food and fluid likes and dislikes
Discuss problems with prescribed diet
Review financial resources
Determine availability of cooking facilities at home
Instruct patient and/or significant other about kinds and amounts of foods that meet nutritional requirements
Instruct patient regarding specific dietary restrictions
Have patient select a balanced diet from a selective menu
Give positive reinforcement
Discuss methods of food procurement
- Have friend or volunteer service purchase and/or prepare food; utilize Meals on Wheels
- Have supermarket deliver food
- Consult senior citizens' center for assistance
- Consult dietary service, social service, or community health nurse as indicated

ndx: Knowledge deficit related to factors that contribute to inadequate nutrition, complications of insufficient nutritional intake, and/or lack of understanding of dietary needs

GOAL: *Patient and/or significant other will demonstrate understanding of reasons for dietary modifications and ways to maintain an optimal nutritional status through interactive discussion*

Factors that contribute to inadequate nutrition

Discuss basic underlying disease process that may be a contributing factor
Discuss how to increase dietary intake to meet increased metabolic needs
List medications that may interfere with absorption and utilization of nutrients
Discuss importance of alcohol avoidance

Complications of insufficient nutritional intake

Discuss the potential for
- Vitamin deficiencies
- Loss of weight
- Anemia
- Increased susceptibility to infection
- Slow healing of wounds
- Poor tolerance to therapy (i.e., radiation therapy, chemotherapy)

List physical signs and symptoms
- Weakness
- Fatigue
- Dizziness
- Soreness of mouth
- Hair falls out easily
- Muscle tenderness

Lack of understanding of dietary needs

Discuss the basic food groups
State reasons for dietary modifications
Explain how to plan meals using prescribed dietary plan
Discuss purpose of prescribed vitamin supplementation
 List foods that are high in protein and calories
 Discuss management of TPN (p.51) or enteral nutrition (p. 34)

Evaluation

Patient verbalizes increase in intake of food
Nutritional intake meets calorie and protein requirements
Patient maintains ideal body weight or gains weight as indicated
Patient has no nausea, vomiting, or diarrhea
Skin tugor is good
Laboratory values (BUN, serum albumin, Hgb, Hct, lymphocytes, electrolytes, cholesterol) are within normal levels
Oral mucous membrane is intact
Patient verbalizes knowledge of nutritional needs
Patient demonstrates ability to obtain, plan, and prepare a nutritious diet
Patient can explain reasons for dietary restrictions

INTRAVENOUS CONTINUOUS DRIP NARCOTICS

Indications

Inability to provide pain relief by other routes
Bleeding, pain, or tissue damage from intramuscular or subcutaneous routes
Rectal and oral routes contraindicated (e.g., in terminally ill patients)

Assessment

Observations/findings

Dosage necessary for maximum pain relief and minimum side effects
Side effects
- Drowsiness
- Mood changes

Mental cloudiness
Respiratory depression
Increased P_{ACO_2}
Decreased GI motility
Nausea
Vomiting
Alterations of endocrine and autonomic nervous systems

Desired effects
Analgesia
Alertness
Increased coherence
Decreased anxiety
Improved coping ability
Improved relationships with others
Improved cardiac function
  Decreased tachycardia
  Modulation of BP
Regular respiratory rhythm

Interventions

Choose narcotic based on minimum toxicity
Dilute solution dependent on dosage required for analgesia and amount of fluid per hour that is therapeutic for patient
Titrate hourly drip rate to level of analgesia desired without untoward effects
Regulate drip carefully with controller or pump as indicated
Involve patient in plans; encourage communication about how patient feels
Monitor BP, P, R, and level of consciousness qh while dosage is being adjusted
Monitor BP, P, R, and level of consciousness q2h when optimum dosage is achieved
Check arterial blood gases as ordered
Initiate flow sheet with vital signs and dosage per hour as indicated

TRANSCUTANEOUS ELECTRICAL NERVE STIMULATION (TENS)

Transmission of an electrical impulse to the body from a battery-powered device through electrodes attached to the skin; pain is relieved by production of a pleasant tingling, tapping, or massaging sensation

Indications

Postoperatively
During labor and delivery
Acute injuries
Chronic conditions

Contraindications

Cardiac pacemaker
Significant arrhythmias
Myocardial infarction (MI)
Cardiac monitoring (creates artifact)
First trimester of pregnancy
Use over carotid sinus nerves, eyes, or laryngeal and pharyngeal muscles

Assessment

Observations/findings

Muscle spasm
Increased pain
Nausea
Headache
Skin irritation
Sensations produced
  Tingling
  Pleasure
  Itching
  Burning
  Pricking
Unit function
  No stimulation
  Cuts in and out
Unit settings
  Rate: 2 to 200 pulses/min (hertz [Hz])
  Pulse width: 0 to 500 μsec
  Amplitude

Interventions

Assist patient in placing electrodes according to recommendations of manufacturer
Maintain electrodes in total contact with skin
Change electrode positions prn to prevent skin irritation
Observe patient for appropriate pain relief
Adjust rate and pulse width settings to prevent unpleasant sensations
Maintain electrodes in place
Activate unit in response to pain
For skin irritation
  Remove electrodes
  Expose to air
  Apply skin cream
  Reposition electrodes away from irritation
  Change type of electrode if necessary
For nausea
  Reposition electrodes
  Vary rate, pulse width, and amplitude
For headache
  Turn down pulse width dial
  Turn down amplitude

Use shorter stimulation period
　　Place electrodes farther apart
　　Vary rate
If problems are not resolved
　　Try different TENS device
　　Discontinue using TENS
Refer patient for assistance by TENS specialist if available
Refer patient to pain clinic for assistance

Patient teaching/discharge planning

Ensure that patient and/or significant other knows and understands
　　Mechanisms of rate, pulse width, and amplitude adjustments
　　Appropriate sensations to be achieved
　　How to adjust settings to
　　　　Achieve maximum pain relief
　　　　Avoid unpleasant sensations
　　　　Avoid muscle spasm and pain exacerbation
　　Need to change electrode placement prn
　　Skin care to maintain skin integrity
　　Need to wear TENS all day: on 2 hr, off 1 hr—total stimulation of 6 to 8 hr
　　Need to wear TENS all night if sleep is interrupted (turn unit on if awakened by pain)
　　Need to maintain a record of settings that work

CHAPTER 2

Cardiovascular System

CARDIOVASCULAR ASSESSMENT

Subjective Data

Pain
  Onset
  Duration
  Location
  Radiation
  Description
Indigestion
Weakness
Fatigue
Fainting
Syncope
Shortness of breath with or without activity or on waking at night
Dyspnea on exertion (DOE)
Palpitations
Paroxysmal nocturnal dyspnea (PND)
Fever
Cough, wheezing, hemoptysis
Edema of extremities
Cyanosis
Nausea
Numb, cold extremities
Changes in vision
Headaches

Objective Data

General appearance
  Color
  Assumed position
  Respirations
Vital signs
  Arterial pulses
    Rate
    Rhythm
    Equality
    Presence
    Absence
  Respirations
    Rate
    Character
    Type
    Temperature
  Neck veins
    Distention
    Pressure
    Pulsation
  BP
    Position and extremity
    Pulse pressure
  Pulsus paradoxus
  Pulsus alternans
  Urinary output
    Amount
    Character
    Color
  Precordium (Figure 2-3)
    Point of maximal impulse (PMI)
    Lifts
    Bulges
    Pulsations
    Thrills
    Symmetry
    Cardiac border
  Heart sounds (Figure 2-4)
    Intensity
    Pitch
    Duration
    Timbre
    Origin
    Frequency of S_1, S_2
    Presence of S_3, S_4
    Murmurs
  Breath sounds
    Location
    Description
      Decreased
      Vesicular
      Bronchial
      Wheezes
      Rhonchi
      Rales
      Rubs

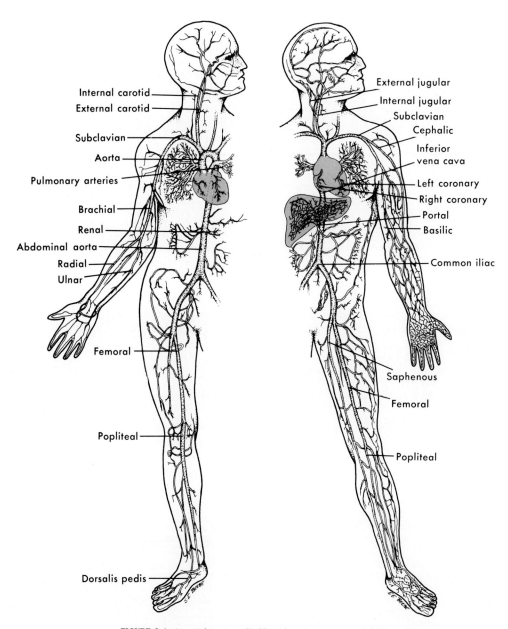

FIGURE 2-1. Arterial system *(left)* and venous system *(right).*

Cardiovascular System

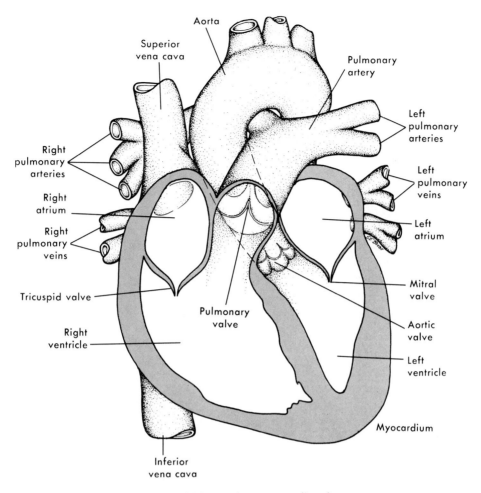

FIGURE 2-2. Circulatory system (heart).

Skin
   Color
   Temperature
   Turgor
   Diaphoresis
   Dryness
Extremities
   Appearance
   Color
   Temperature
   Capillary filling time
   "Clubbing"
   Nail shape
   Description of lesions
Central nervous system (CNS)
   Level of consciousness
   Neuro signs
   Reflexes
   Response to pain

Pertinent Background Information
CONCURRENT DISEASES OR CONDITIONS

Hypertension
Obesity
Diabetes
Pulmonary conditions
   Pneumonia
   Emphysema
   Cor pulmonale
Renal conditions

PSYCHOLOGIC RESPONSES

Response to stress
Methods of coping
Response to pain
Relationships with others
Recent stressful life events

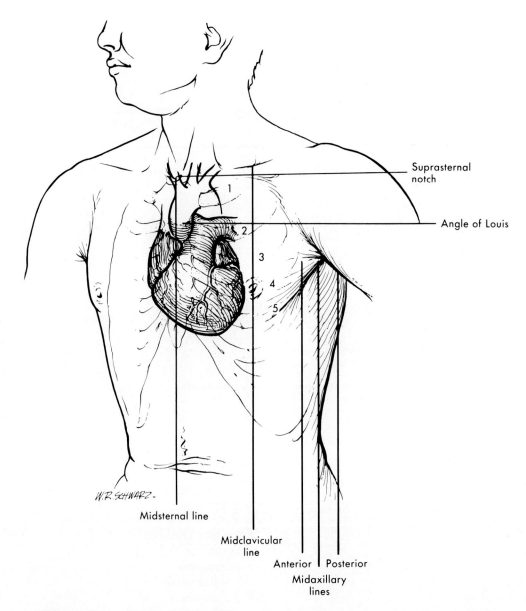

FIGURE 2-3. Chest wall landmarks. (From Malasanos, L., et al.: Health assessment, ed. 3, St. Louis, 1986, The C.V. Mosby Co.)

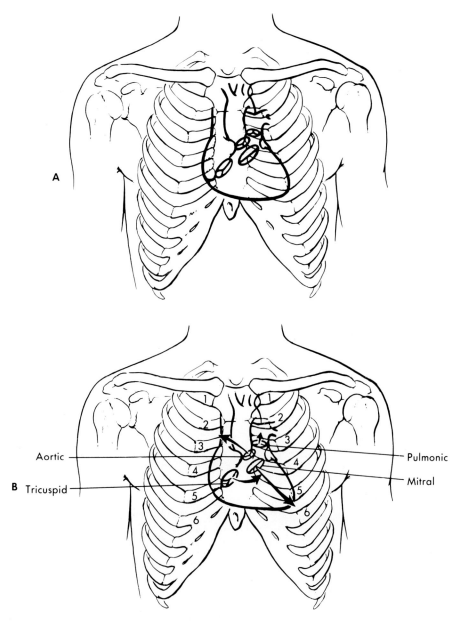

FIGURE 2-4. **A,** Anatomic location of heart valves. **B,** Transmission of closure sounds from heart valves. (From Malasanos, L., et al.: Health assessment, ed. 3, St. Louis, 1986, The C.V. Mosby Co.)

PREVIOUS MEDICAL HISTORY

Systemic infections
   Rheumatic fever
   Endocarditis
   Kawasaki disease
Coronary artery disease
   Myocardial infarction (MI)
   Angina
   Heart failure
Heart murmur
Congenital heart disease
Cardiovascular surgery
Thromboembolism
Occlusive vascular disease
Pulmonary conditions
Renal conditions

FAMILY HISTORY

Heart disease
Hypertension
Diabetes
Obesity
Arterial and venous diseases
Cerebrovascular accident (CVA)
Kidney disease

SOCIAL/CULTURAL HISTORY

Cultural orientation
Educational level
Smoking
Alcohol use
Exercise and activity levels
Occupation (sedentary or active)
Sleep patterns
Leisure activities
Environmental factors
Economic resources
Social support resources
   Marital status
   Number of siblings, children

MEDICATION HISTORY

Prescription medication
   Digitalis preparations
   Antihypertensives
   Anticoagulants
   Diuretics
   Birth control pills
Over-the-counter medication
   Aspirin
   Cold and flu remedies
   Sleeping pills

Diagnostic Aids

LABORATORY STUDIES

Enzyme profile
   Serum glutamic oxaloacetic transaminase (SGOT)
   Creatine phosphokinase (CPK-MB)
   Lactic acid dehydrogenase (LDH)
Lipid profile
Electrolyte profile
Cholesterol value
Triglyceride value
Complete blood cell count (CBC)
Erythrocyte sedimentation rate (ESR)
Hemoglobin (Hgb)
Hematocrit (Hct)
Clotting profile
Prothrombin time (PT)
Partial thromboplastin time (PTT)
Heparin time
Glucose level
Urinalysis

ELECTROCARDIOGRAM

P wave
PR interval
Q wave
ST segment
T wave
U wave
Axis calculation

OTHER PROCEDURES

Noninvasive

Radiologic studies
   Chest x-ray examination
   Fluoroscopy
Echocardiography
   M-mode
   Two-dimensional
   Doppler
Treadmill (stress test)
Holter monitor
Nuclear studies
   Thallium uptake
   Computerized tomography (CT) scan
   Multigated cardiac blood pool imaging (MUGA)
   Magnetic resonance imaging (MRI)

Invasive

Arterial pressure
Digital subtraction angiography (DSA)
Digital vascular imaging (DVI)
Cardiac catheterization
Coronary angiography

Ventriculography
Electrophysiologic studies: His bundle recordings

PERIPHERAL VASCULAR ASSESSMENT

Subjective Data

Pain
   Initiating factors: onset
     Continuous exercise
     Rest
     Amount of exercise tolerated
   Provoking factor: change in environmental temperature
   Alleviating factors
     Rest
     Exercise
     Effect of prescribed medication
   Location
     Calf
     Foot
Edema of extremity(ies)
Redness, pallor, cyanosis
Numb, cold extremities
Transient ischemic attack (TIA)
Abdominal or back pain

Objective Data

General appearance
   Color
   Assumed position
Age
Vital signs: BP, T, P, and R
Pulses
   Rate
   Equality
   Rhythm
   Amplitude
     4+: strong, bounding (normal)
     3+: easily palpable
     2+: difficult to palpate
     1+: weak, thready
     0: absent
   Bruits
     Carotid
     Subclavian
     Femoral
Skin
   Temperature
   Tissue loss
     Ulceration
     Gangrene
   Lesions

Color
   Pale; increased pallor with walking, with elevation
   Mottled
   Cyanosis
   Redness (rubor); increased in dependent position
Hair loss
Opacification of nails
Lower extremities
   Cold feet
   Intermittent claudication
     Pain: calves: thighs, buttocks
     Onset with continuous exercise
     Relieved by rest
   Pain with rest
   Tissue loss
Upper extremities
   Digital ischemia
   Fingertip ulcerations
   Gangrene
   Allen test (positive)
Abdomen
   Pulsatile abdominal mass
   Bruits
Capillary filling time
   Normal: <3 sec
   Abnormal: >3 sec

Pertinent Background Information
CONCURRENT DISEASES OR CONDITIONS

Hypertension
Diabetes
Obesity
Heart failure
Renal conditions

PREVIOUS MEDICAL HISTORY

Thrombophlebitis
Cerebrovascular disease
Cornonary artery disease
Aneurysm

FAMILY HISTORY

Premature deaths
Cerebrovascular diseases
Atherosclerosis

MEDICATION HISTORY

Over-the-counter: aspirin
Prescribed medications
   Digoxin
   Antihypertensives

Anticoagulants
Antiinflammatory
Steroids
Birth control pills
Fibrinolytics
Vasodilators

SOCIAL HISTORY

Smoking, tobacco use
Alcohol use
Occupation (sedentary or active)
Environmental factors
Exercise and activity levels
Leisure activities

Diagnostic Aids

NONINVASIVE

Segmental limb systolic pressure (SLPs)
  Normal
    Lower extremities
      Midthigh: 16 mm Hg
      Upper third of leg: 3 to 12 mm Hg
      Above ankle: 1 to 18 mm Hg
      Foot: 0.2 to 1 mm Hg
    Upper extremities
      Upper arm: 4 to 16 mm Hg
      Elbow: 3 to 12 mm Hg
      Wrist: 1 to 10 mm Hg
      Hand: 0.2 to 2 mm Hg
Phlebography (venography)
Intermittent claudication determination
Doppler flow velocity tracings
Plethysmography
Radioactive fibrinogen uptake
Infrared thermography (IRT)
Carotid phonoangiogram (CPG)
Stress testing
Allen test
  Radial
  Ulnar

INVASIVE

Radionuclide studies
Digital subtraction angiography (DSA)
Angiography

VENOUS THROMBOSIS

An abnormal vascular condition associated with thrombus formation within a blood vessel, which develops as a result of stasis, hypercoagulability, or damage to the internal lining of the vein; can occur in superficial or deep veins; the following are terms used to describe venous disorders that reflect thrombus (clot) formation

phlebitis *Inflammation of a vein*
phlebothrombosis (venous thrombosis) *Intraluminal thrombus with minimal or no inflammatory component; these have a greater tendency to embolize*
thromboembolism *Phenomenon of thrombus dislodgment and migration*
thrombophlebitis *An acute condition characterized by thrombus and inflammation in deep or superficial veins*

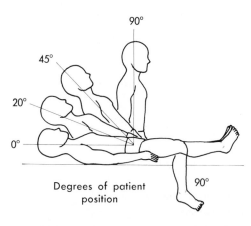

FIGURE 2-5. Degrees of patient position.

Assessment

Observations/findings

Extremity
  Pain
    Heaving feeling
    Tenderness
    Cramping
    Calf pains with dorsiflexion of foot (Homan's sign)
  Redness
  Taut, shiny skin
  Swelling and edema
  Increased size compared with nonaffected extremity
  Increased skin temperature
  Peripheral pulses: present, absent
Elevated temperature

Laboratory/diagnostic studies

Phlebography (venography)
Doppler Ultrasound
Phlethysmography
Fibrinogen uptake test

Potential complications

Pulmonary embolism
MI
CVA

Medical management

Medications
    Anticoagulant therapy: heparin, warfarin (p. 151)
    Fibrinolytic agents: streptokinase
    Antiplatelet agents
    Analgesics
Surgical management
    Thrombectomy
    Procedures to prevent distal embolization
        Extravascular vena cava interruption
        Intracaval filter (Mobin-Udden umbrella, Kimray-Greenfield filter)

Nursing diagnoses/goals/interventions

ndx: Alteration in comfort: pain related to inflammatory process

GOAL: *Patient will verbalize pain relief*

Maintain bed rest, limit self-care activities
Elevate affected limb above level of right atrium
Apply warm, moist compresses as ordered; avoid burning edematous skin
Use bed cradle over affected extremity
Provide support or antiembolic stockings
Administer analgesics as ordered

ndx: Alteration in tissue perfusion: peripheral related to interruption of venous flow

GOAL: *Patient will demonstrate improved venous blood flow to extremities*

Maintain complete bed rest during acute phase (4 to 7 days)
Position patient comfortably; avoid position that restricts venous return
Elevate affected limb above level of right atrium
    Avoid use of pillows
    Never gatch knees without raising foot of bed
Check circulation of affected extremity q4h
Check pulses in all extremities q4h; use Doppler sensor if pulse seems absent
Measure and record size of affected limb qd
Do not wash or massage affected extremity
Provide support or antiembolic stockings
Administer anticoagulation and fibrolytic therapy as ordered
Check laboratory values as indicated

PTT q4h to 12h to maintain 1½ to 2½ times control
PT qd to maintain level 1½ to 2½ times control
Instruct patient to avoid smoking
Implement progressive exercise program as ordered
    Ambulate as ordered
    Alternate with bed rest
    Never dangle
    Ambulate 10 min qh while awake or as ordered
    Apply stockings prior to ambulating
    Avoid standing for long periods; alternate position by standing on toes, then on heels
    Exercise toes and change weight distribution q10 to 15 min
Elevate legs 10 min qh when sitting
    Do not constrict circulation in groin area
    Flex calf muscles and perform quadriceps contractions 10 min qh
    Avoid crossing legs at knees
Build exercise tolerance by increasing walking distance each day; continue after discharge, increasing distance to 1 to 2 miles

ndx: Potential for impaired gas exchange related to embolization of thrombus

GOAL: *Patient will maintain adequate ventilation*

Observe for signs of pulmonary embolism: chest pain, dyspnea, tachypnea, hemoptysis, pallor
Auscultate chest for breath sounds q4h
Maintain bed rest during acute phase
Avoid exercising and massaging affected extremity during acute phase
Administer anticoagulant therapy as ordered
Encourage patient to turn, cough, and deep breathe q2h to 4h
Obtain and monitor Po_2 and Pco_2 as ordered

ndx: Potential alteration in skin integrity related to venous stasis and fragility of small blood vessels

GOAL: *Patient will maintain skin integrity*

Administer daily hygiene measures
    Observe skin for redness, breakdown, or ulcerations
    Use small amount of mild soap
    Rinse well
    Dry gently but thoroughly; avoid vigorous rubbing
    Do not allow skin to remain wet
Use bed cradle for affected extremity
Do not wash or massage affected extremity
Assist and teach patient as appropriate to make small changes in position

Perform active or passive range-of-motion (ROM) exercises with unaffected extremities

ndx Knowledge deficit regarding disease process

GOAL: *Patient and/or significant other will demonstrate increased understanding of disease process and self-care management through interactive discussion and actual return demonstration*

Plan exercise program that includes aerobic activities, such as swimming
Explain importance of not smoking
Discuss skin care
   Avoid use of harsh soaps
   Do not rub or massage extremity
   Keep extremity warm and avoid exposure to extremes in temperature
Explain need to avoid use of constrictive clothing such as garters, girdles, underwear with elastic groin bands, and knee-high or ankle stockings with elastic tops
Discuss symptoms of recurrence to report to physician (see Observations/Findings, p. 74)
Discuss medications: name, dosage, time of administration, purpose, and side effects
Explain need to avoid taking over-the-counter medications without checking with physician
Discuss anticoagulant precautions if appropriate (p. 151)
Discuss symptoms of complications to report to physician
   Pulmonary emboli
   MI
   CVA
   Renal problems
Explain importance of ongoing outpatient care
Demonstrate application of support or antiembolic stockings
Demonstrate deep-breathing exercises

Evaluation

Patient
   Verbalizes relief from pain, swelling, or redness
   Demonstrates adequate tissue perfusion
      Pulses are palpable
      Extremities are warm with normal color
   Demonstrates effortless breathing; performs self-care activities without signs of shortness of breath (SOB)
   Verbalizes increased knowledge level and home care management

VEIN LIGATION AND STRIPPING

Ligation of the saphenous vein and stripping (removal) from the groin to the ankle

Assessment
Observations/findings

Color, warmth, and sensation of affected extremity
Edema or heaviness of affected extremity
Dilation of leg veins
Leg cramps when standing

Potential complications

Thrombophlebitis (p. 74)
Phlebitis
Leg ulcers
Hemorrhage

Medical management

Diet
Medications: analgesics

Nursing diagnoses/goals/interventions

ndx Alteration in tissue perfusion: peripheral related to inadequate venous return and/or immobility

GOAL: *Patient will demonstrate improved peripheral circulation*

Maintain bed rest
   Elevate legs as ordered
   Do not gatch knee
   Avoid dangling
Check color, warmth, and sensation of affected extremity qh for 6 hr; report any change to physician
Apply elastic bandages from toes to groin; leave in place for 24 hr
Remove elastic bandages or stockings as ordered
   Reapply q8h and prn
   Avoid constriction
   Keep snug and wrinkle free
   Check frequently for slippage, especially after ambulation
Assist with ambulation within 24 hr as ordered
Increase activity as ordered
   Ambulate with assistance
   Do not allow chair sitting (patient must be either walking or in bed)
   Perform active and/or passive ROM exercises to unaffected extremities q4h and dorsiflexion of foot of affected extremity

ndx: Alteration in comfort: pain related to surgical incision

GOAL: *Patient will verbalize absence of discomfort*

Evaluate source of pain
   Postoperative
   Constructive dressings
   Bleeding
   Local site infection
Check bandages for bleeding qh; report excessive bleeding to physician
Check dressings for signs of wound infection; report to physician
   Low-grade temperature
   Swelling, redness, pain, purulent drainage
Reinforce and/or change dressings as ordered
Check BP, T, P, and R q4h as indicated
Administer analgesics as indicated

ndx: Knowledge deficit regarding home management

GOAL: *Patient and/or significant other will demonstrate knowledge and skills in self-care management through interactive discussion*

Discuss possibility of varicosities recurring
Explain importance of avoiding constriction of venous blood return in extremities
   Do not wear tight garters or girdles
   Avoid crossing legs
   Walk rather than sitting or standing
   Wear full-length support hose, elastic stockings, or bandages as ordered
   Elevate legs while sitting
   Sleep with legs elevated
Explain importance of skin care
   Keep legs and feet warm and dry
   Avoid chilling
   Apply lotion prn to legs, but do not massage
Explain need to maintain normal weight for age and height and reduce if overweight
Explain need to check with physician before taking oral contraceptives
Discuss signs and symptoms of wound infection and bleeding to report to physician
   Redness
   Pain
   Drainage
   Edema
Explain importance of ongoing outpatient care

Evaluation
Patient
   Demonstrates improved tissue perfusion
     Peripheral pulses are palpable
     Extremities are warm with normal color
   Verbalizes absence of discomfort
   Verbalizes knowledge regarding self-care to minimize recurrence of varicosities

CHRONIC ARTERIAL INSUFFICIENCY

Inadequate blood flow in arteries caused by occlusive atherosclerotic plaques or emboli, damaged or diseased vessels, aneurysms, hypercoagulability states, or heavy use of tobacco

Assessment
Observations/findings

Pain
   Foot, calf, thigh, or buttocks
   Sharp and viselike
   Cramping
   Tired feeling in legs
   Usually occurs during exercise; decreases when exercise stops (intermittent claudication)
   May occur at rest, especially at night, accompanied by very hot or cold feeling
   Increases with elevation of legs
Diminished to absent pedal and popliteal pulses
Extremities
   Numbness
   Hair loss
   Skin glossy, thin, smooth, cold, discolored, atrophied
   Nails thickened: accumulation of cornified material
   Pigmentation, rashes
   Pallor
     Increased with elevation of extremity
     Decreased with extremity below heart level
   Rubor
   Swelling
   Delayed venous filling in dependent position

Laboratory/diagnostic studies

Doppler ultrasonography
Plethysmography
Angiography

Potential complications

Peripheral ischemia, necrosis
Cellulitis
Gangrene

Medical management

Medications
    Thrombolytic enzymes: urokinase, streptokinase
    Antiplatelets: aspirin, dipridamole
    Pentoxifylline (Trental)
Low-saturated fat, low-cholesterol diet
Percutaneous transluminal angioplasty
Laser thermal angioplasty
Surgical management
    Arterial reconstruction
        Arterial revascularization
        Endarterectomy
        Bypass graft surgery
        Femoropopliteal reconstruction: femoropopliteal bypass (Figure 2-6), profundoplasty
    Lumbar sympathectomy
    Amputation of limb

Nursing diagnoses/goals/interventions

ndx: Alteration in tissue perfusion related to interruption of arterial flow

GOAL: *Patient will have increased arterial blood flow to extremities*

Check arterial pulses; determine pulse volume qid
Auscultate for bruits
Elevate head of bed; use 4- to 6-inch block as ordered
Position patient comfortably; avoid use of knee gatch
Protect affected extremity
    Place bed cradle over affected area
    Use heel guards (sheepskin) or white cotton socks
    Avoid use of heating devices on lower extremities
Keep patient warm
    Have patient wear socks when in bed or walking
    Use cotton blankets next to patient
    Use flannel or cotton bedclothes
    Use extra blankets if required
    Avoid chilling
Assist patient with getting out of bed as ordered; avoid one position, sitting or standing, for long periods of time
Encourage scheduled walking exercise program; with increased pain, stand until pain eases, then continue walking
Sit with feet dependent
Perform active or passive ROM exercises to all extremities q4h to 6h
Turn patient q2h while on bed rest
Change patient's position slightly q20 to 30 min
Avoid raising lower extremity above heart level
Instruct patient to avoid use of nicotine
Administer medications as ordered

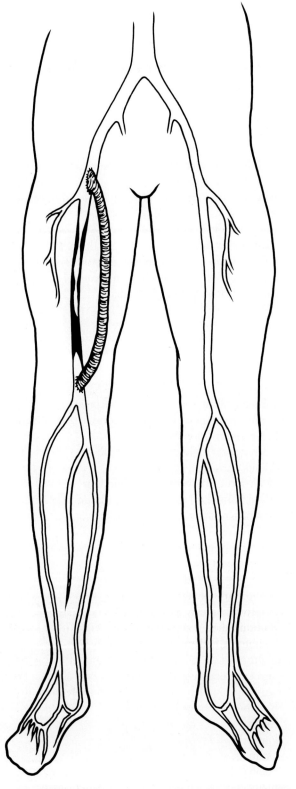

FIGURE 2-6. Femoropopliteal bypass graft to revascularize right lower limb. (From Guzzetta, C., and Dossey, B.: Cardiovascular nursing: bodymind tapestry, St. Louis, 1985, The C.V. Mosby Co.)

ndx: Alteration in comfort level: pain related to peripheral ischemia

GOAL: *Patient is able to identify strategies to control pain*

Assist patient with identifying activities that precipitate or aggravate pain; with understanding nature of pain
Instruct patient to stand or dangle at side of bed to obtain relief from ischemic pain
Encourage regular exercise program but instruct patient to stop and rest before claudication occurs
Administer analgesics as indicated
Initiate alternative pain relief measures
  Relaxation techniques: meditation, deep breathing
  Guided imagery
  Biofeedback
Involve patient in decision making regarding measures to reduce pain
Assess effectiveness of pain relief measure(s)

ndx: Impairment of skin integrity, actual or potential, related to impaired circulation

GOAL: *Patient will regain and maintain skin integrity*

Administer daily hygiene measures
  Observe skin for signs of scaling, breaks, or cuts
  Use small amount of mild soap
  Rinse well
  Dry gently but thoroughly; avoid vigorous rubbing
  Apply lanolin-based lotions; do not allow skin to remain wet
Check skin color and temperature in both legs qid
Maintain care of ulcer areas as ordered
  Administer soaks, medications, and dressings as ordered
  Avoid use of adhesive tapes directly on skin
  Avoid use of tight, constrictive socks or hose; use cotton socks
Maintain diet of preference, including foods high in vitamins B complex and C

ndx: Knowledge deficit regarding disease process

GOAL: *Patient and/or significant other will demonstrate increased understanding of disease process and self-care management through interactive discussion*

Discuss nature of disease process and precipitating risk factors (see risk factor profile, p. 87)
Explain importance of care of legs and feet
  Inspect legs, feet, and toes daily for blisters, skin breaks, and discolored areas
  Wash daily with mild soap, dry well, and apply lanolin-based lotion, but do not leave skin wet
  Clean small cuts or abrasions with soap and water; protect from further injury
  Report cuts or skin breaks that do not begin healing in 2 to 3 days to physician
  Trim toenails straight across
  Do not cut, file, or use over-the-counter medications on corns or calluses
  Avoid exposing legs to extremes in temperature; wear warm coverings in cold weather and avoid exposure to sunshine
  Do not apply direct heat to legs, such as hot water bottles or electric pads; wear cotton or woolen socks to warm feet
Explain need to avoid injury to legs and feet
  Always wear well-fitting shoes or slippers; never go barefoot
  Wear well-fitting, correct-size stockings
  Avoid tight-fitting or constrictive clothing such as garters, girdles, underwear with elastic legs, and knee-high or ankle stockings with elastic tops
  Avoid crossing legs
  Avoid scratching legs or feet
  Turn on lights when getting up at night to avoid bumps
  Sleep with bed level or head elevated
  Avoid tight-fitting covers over legs and feet
Explain importance of exercise program
  Walk to tolerance; increase time each week until able to walk without pain for 30 to 60 min; may initially experience decreased ability
  Walk until pain increases, stop and stand still to decrease pain, then continue to walk
  Do not sit or raise legs above heart level to decrease pain
  Remember that same distance walked in one direction must also be walked on return
Explain need to avoid smoking or other tobacco use
Discuss symptoms of recurrence to report to physician (see Observations/Findings, p. 77)
Explain importance of maintaining diet as ordered: low-calorie, low-cholesterol, low-fat
Explain importance of eating foods that are high in protein and vitamins B complex and C
Discuss medications: name, dosage, time of administration, purpose, and side effects
Explain need to avoid taking over-the-counter medications without checking with physician
Explain importance of ongoing outpatient care

Evaluation

Patient
  Demonstrates improved tissue perfusion
    Peripheral pulses are palpable
    Extremities are warm with normal color
  Demonstrates that skin integrity is maintained
  Verbalizes that comfort level is achieved; utilizes a variety of strategies effective in reducing pain level
  Verbalizes increase knowledge level regarding disease process, risk factors, and home care management

CAROTID ENDARTERECTOMY

Surgical removal of atherosclerotic plaques or thrombus from the carotid artery to increase blood flow

Assessment

Observations/findings

Respiratory distress
  Bradypnea
  Tachypnea
  Cyanosis
  Tracheal deviation to opposite side
  Laryngeal edema
  Stridor
Neurologic deficit
  Cerebral ischemia
    Decreasing BP, increasing P and R
    Dizziness
    Altered level of consciousness
    Confusion
    Disorientation
    Memory loss
  Unequal reaction of pupils to light
  Unequal handgrips
  Inability to protrude tongue
  Muscle weakness of mouth on operative side
  Dysphagia
Altered speech
  Slurred
  Indistinct
Arrhythmias

Potential complications

Seizure activity
Hemorrhage
Shock
Embolism
Infection
CVA (p. 296)

Medical management

Parenteral fluids
Medications
  Antihypertensive
  Vasopressor

Nursing diagnoses/goals/interventions

ndx: Potential alteration in tissue perfusion: cerebral related to interruption of arterial flow

GOAL: *Patient will maintain adequate cerebral blood flow*

See Care of Patient in Recovery Room (p. 30)
Maintain bed rest in quiet environment; position with head elevated 30 to 45 degrees
Check and compare temporal pulses q15 min for four times, then q2h to 4h
Mark pulse site on skin
Note rate and volume
Check neuro signs qh
Check BP, R, and apical pulse q1h to 2h for 24 hr; report increase or decrease to physician immediately
Check rectal temperature q2h to 4h for 24 hr
Administer medications as ordered
Check incision qh for bleeding and edema
Report excessive bleeding or edema to physician
Reinforce dressing prn
Control pain as ordered; apply ice collar to neck as ordered
Provide emotional support
  Gentle reassurance
  Means of communicating; phrase questions for "yes" or "no" answers
Continue with immediate postoperative care and decrease frequency of nursing functions as patient's condition improves
Ambulate as ordered; check and report any altered gait
Change dressing prn
Continue checking neuro signs q8h

ndx: Potential for injury: respiratory distress

GOAL: *Patient will demonstrate normal ventilation*

Maintain patent airway
  Perform oropharyngeal suctioning only if ordered
  Assist and teach patient to turn and deep breathe q1h to 2h
Avoid coughing
Auscultate chest for breath sounds q1h to 2h
Report complaints of severe hoarseness, sore throat, or dysphagia to physician

Monitor oxygen saturation via arterial blood gases or ear oximetry as indicated

ndx: Potential for injury: cranial nerve injury (CN VII, X, XI, XII) related to surgical trauma

GOAL: *Patient will not experience sensory motor dysfunction*

Check facial nerve function
  Ability to smile and speak
  Facial asymmetry
Check for vagal nerve function
  Ability to swallow
  Loss of gag reflex, hoarseness
  Bradycardia
Check for accessory nerve function: ability to move and raise arms and shoulders
Check for hypoglossal function: ability to protrude tongue and swallow

ndx: Knowledge deficit regarding self-care management

GOAL: *Patient will demonstrate knowledge and skills in self-care management through interactive discussion and actual return demonstration*

Explain importance of activity
  Exercise to tolerance
  Avoid bending from waist
  Plan rest periods
  Avoid lifting or straining
Explain importance of observing neurologic status
  Monitor
    Vision
    Gait
    Speech
    Muscle weakness
  Report changes to physician immediately
Demonstrate care of incision
Discuss signs of wound infection
  Redness
  Pain
  Drainage
  Edema
Discuss diet
Explain importance of ongoing outpatient care

Evaluation

Patient
  Demonstrates adequate cerebral blood flow as evidenced by
    Mental alertness and orientation
    Absence of dizziness
    Equal and reactive pupils
    Normal motor-sensory function
  Demonstrates effortless breathing
  Verbalizes knowledge and skills in self-care management

AORTOFEMORAL BYPASS GRAFT

Surgical resection of an aortic aneurysm and insertion of a graft conduit to deliver blood to the femoral vessels, bypassing diseased segments

Assessment

Observations/findings

Marked increase or decrease in BP, P, and R
Decreased arterial pressure or central venous pressure (CVP)
Signs of arterial graft occlusion of lower extremities (lower limb ischemia)
  Mottled or pale skin
  Skin cool to touch
  Absence of pulses
Site of incision
  Redness
  Pain
  Swelling

Potential complications

Embolism to extremities, cerebrum, or heart
Cardiac
  MI
  Congestive heart failure (CHF)
  Arrhythmias
Hemorrhage
Shock
Renal failure
  Decreased urine output
  Specific gravity <1.030
Bowel ischemia
  Diarrhea with or without blood
  Abdominal tenderness
  Leukocytosis
  Metabolic acidosis
Spinal cord ischemia
  Paraplegia
  Paraparesis
Prosthetic graft infection
  Purulent wound drainage
  Low-grade fever without chills
  Sepsis
  Graft occlusion

Local hemorrhage
Septic embolization: cellutitis
Sinus tract infection

Laboratory/diagnostic studies

Doppler: systolic ankle pressure
White blood cell count (WBC), chemistries, electrolyes

Medical management

Hemodynamic monitoring: pulmonary artery pressure (PAP), arterial pressure
Cardiac monitor
Medications
Anticoagulation therapy
Antibiotic therapy
Vasodilators
Ankle-to-brachial systolic pressure index (0.95 mm Hg or more)

Nursing diagnoses/goals/interventions

ndx Potential alteration in tissue perfusion related to interruption of arterial flow

GOAL: *Patient will have increased arterial blood flow to lower extremities*

Maintain bed rest; elevate head 30 to 45 degrees
   Do not gatch knees
   Avoid sharp hip flexion
Check and compare pedal pulses q15 min for four times, then q4h; mark pulse site on skin
Check lower extremities for color, warmth, and sensation q15 min for 4 hr, then q4h
Check and compare ankle-to-brachial systolic pressure index (ratio) as ordered; report if less than 1 mm Hg
Provide antiembolic stockings or elastic bandages as ordered; remove, reapply, or rewrap q8h
Do not massage or apply heat to lower extremities
Ambulate as ordered; no chair sitting
Administer daily skin care
   Observe for signs of breaks or drainage
   Avoid use of adhesive tapes to sensitive skin of distal lower extremity
Protect affected extremity
   Place bed cradle over affected area
   Use sheepskins

ndx Potential for infection related to arterial prosthetic graft procedure

GOAL: *Patient will demonstrate absence of infectious process*

Check for signs of infection of incision (see Observations/Findings, p. 81)
Check T q4h
Check dressing q1h to 2h
   Observe for healing process
   Reinforce prn
   Report excessive drainage to physician
Administer prophylactic antibiotic as ordered
Avoid prolonged use of urinary catheters, nasogastric tubes, or pressure catheter that may cause transient bacteremia
Use strict aseptic technique in dressing change, venipressure, or suctioning procedures
If graft infection occurs
   Administer antibiotic therapy as ordered
   Perform irrigation of graft and wound as ordered
   Prepare for surgical intervention as ordered
      Graft removal
      Revascularization
      Amputation

ndx Potential for complications*

GOAL: *Patient will not demonstrate signs of complications*

Cardiac complications

Monitor ECG, arterial pressures, PAP, CVP qh; report changes to physician
Check BP, R, and apical pulse q4h for 48 hr
Record description of chest pain; report increase or significant change to physician
Administer antihypertensive, antiarrhythmic drugs as indicated
Obtain ECG rhythm strip during episodes of chest pain
Obtain isoenzymes (CPK-MB) as indicated
Monitor potassium levels

Bowel ischemia

Maintain NPO, usually for first 12 hr or until bowel sounds are present
Progress diet as tolerated and ordered after nasogastric tube removal
Connect nasogastric tube to intermittent suction as ordered
Auscultate abdomen q2h to 4h
Measure abdominal girth for distention q8h
Report increased distention to physician

---

*Not a NANDA-approved nursing diagnosis.

Renal failure

Administer parenteral fluids with electrolytes as ordered
Measure intake and output
    Use indwelling urethral catheter as ordered
    Measure output qh
    Report output of less than 30 to 50 ml/hr to physician

Hemorrhage

Check for signs of bleeding q4h to 8h
    Hematoma in groin area
    Bleeding of skin incision
    Retroperitoneal bleeding: signs of hypovolemia—low CVP and pulmonary capillary wedge pressure (PCWP), decreased urine output, severe back pain
Monitor laboratory studies q4h to 8h

ndx Knowledge deficit regarding home care management

GOAL: *Patient and/or significant other will demonstrate knowledge and skills in self-care management through interactive discussion and actual return demonstration*

Explain importance of exercise and activity
    Avoid sitting or standing without moving for long periods
    Do not cross legs
    Exercise slightly beyond tolerance
Explain importance of maintaining planned rest periods
Demonstrate correct application of antiembolic stockings or elastic bandages
Discuss care of legs and feet
    Do not wear constrictive clothing: girdles, garters, etc.
    Avoid extreme heat and cold
    Keep feet warm
    Exercise feet and legs as ordered
Demonstrate care of incision
Discuss signs of wound infection
    Redness
    Pain
    Swelling
    Drainage
Explain importance of not smoking
Discuss symptoms of recurrence to report to physician
Explain importance of ongoing outpatient care

Evaluation

Patient
    Demonstrates improved tissue perfusion
        Graft is patent
        Peripheral pulses are palpable
        Extremities are warm with normal color
        Ankle-to-brachial pressure index is normal or improved
    Demonstrates absence of graft infection
        Temperature is normal
        Graft is patent
        Skin integrity is maintained
    Demonstrates absence of complications
    Verbalizes increase knowledge level regarding home care management

HYPERTENSIVE CRISIS

Sudden severe elevation of BP (systolic greater than 200 mm Hg, diastolic greater than 120 mm Hg) with mean arterial pressure greater than 150 mm Hg

Assessment

Observations/findings

Severe occipital headache radiating frontally
    Neck stiffness, soreness
    Palpitations
    Pallor
    Diaphoresis
Tachycardia or bradycardia
Diplopia
Vertigo
Anxiety
Nausea, vomiting
Tinnitus
Muscle twitching
Seizure activity
Epistaxis
Distended neck veins
Narrowed pulse pressure
Hypertensive encephalopathy
    See Neurologic Assessment (p. 283)
    Confusion
    Irritability
    Stupor
    Somnolence
    Coma

Laboratory/diagnostic studies

Serum
    Electrolytes, chemistries
    Aldosterone
    Cholesterol, triglycerides
    Thyroid

Urine
　Steroids; catecholamines; renin
　Urinalysis: BUN, uric acid
　24 hr VMA
　Aldosterone
Electrocardiogram (ECG)
　Cardiomegaly
　Ischemia
Chest x-ray examination
　Increased cardiothoracic ratio
CT scan
　Cerebral tumor
　Cerebral ischemia
　Encephalopathy

Potential complications

Cardiac arrhythmias
MI (p. 87)
Renal failure (p. 557)
Heart failure (p. 101)
CVA (p. 296)

Medical management

Admission to intensive care unit (ICU)
Cardiac monitor
Hemodynamic monitoring: arterial pressure
Medications
　Antihypertensives
　Diuretics
　Beta blockers
　Anticonvulsants
　Sedatives
　Antiemetics

Nursing diagnoses/goals/interventions

ndx: Potential for injury related to severe, acclerated, or malignant hypertension

GOAL: *Patient will demonstrate return of BP to within safe limits*

Maintain bed rest; elevated head of bed, shock blocks, or circle bed may be ordered
Check BP on admission in both arms: lying, sitting, and with arterial pressure monitor if available
Check BP, R, apical pulse, and neuro signs q5 to 10 min
　Use same arm for BP each time
　Use Doppler sensor if indicated
Monitor arterial pressure as ordered
Maintain parenteral fluids with medications as ordered
Administer medications as ordered
　Antihypertensives: IV, IM
　　Observe for side effects or toxic effects of each medication
　　Monitor IV medications continuously
　　Titrate according to prescribed BP parameters as ordered
　Anticonvulsants
　Sedatives
　Diuretics
　Antiemetics
Observe for sudden hypotension; report to physician immediately
Place on cardiac monitor; record ECG rhythm strip q4h to 6h and prn
Measure intake and output
　Check output qh, noting amount and color of urine
　Report output of less than 30 ml/hr
Monitor electrolytes, BUN, creatinine as ordered
Check specific gravity and perform urinalysis as ordered
Weigh patient daily at same time with same clothing, and scale
Maintain seizure precautions
Maintain quiet environment
Keep NPO if nausea and/or vomiting is present
Maintain low-calorie, low-sodium diet as ordered
Restrict fluids as ordered
Do not allow smoking or use of nicotine products
Continue with immediate care and decrease frequency of nursing functions as patient's condition improves
Maintain progressive ambulation
　Patient in circle bed (p. 333)
　Patient in regular bed
　　Elevate head of bed slowly in beginning, then take BP
　　Progress to dangling for 10 min as ordered if BP is stable
　　Take BP while sitting up
　　Have patient stand at bedside and take BP, then have patient take small steps when ordered
Observe at all time for orthostatic hypotension
　Pallor
　Diaphoresis
　Faintness
　Loss of consciousness
Ambulate to tolerance; avoid fatigue

ndx: Potential for injury related to encephalopathy

GOAL: *Patient will be free of injury*

Maintain safety precautions as indicated
　Side rails up
　Bed in low position
　Soft restraints
　Posey jackets
Monitor level of consciousness (LOC): orientation to person, place, and time

Neuro check q5 to 10 min on admission, progressing to q2h to 4h as indicated
Notify physicians of any sudden changes in LOC, pupillary responses, or movement of extremities
Maintain seizure precautions: oral airway at bedside
Orient patient to environment as needed

ndx: Alteration in comfort related to (biologic) increased vascular pressure and emotional (anxiety)

GOAL: *Patient will demonstrate that comfort level has been achieved*

Maintain quiet, low-lighted environment
Evaluate source of discomfort
Limit activities
Provide and maintain periods of rest
Avoid smoking or use of nicotine products
Induce analgesia and sedation as ordered
Administer comfort measures as indicated
  Ice packs
  Reassurance and frequent simple explanation
  Position of comfort; assist with turning gently, using pull sheet as indicated
Instruct to avoid Valsalva maneuver
Avoid constipation

ndx: Knowledge deficit regarding disease process and self-care

GOAL: *Patient and/or significant other demonstrate increased understanding of disease process and self-care management through interactive discussion and actual return demonstration*

Explain nature of disease and purpose of treatment and procedures
Explain importance of quiet, nonstressful environment
Discuss medications: name, dosage, time of administration, purpose, and side effects or toxic effects
Explain need to avoid taking over-the-counter medication without checking with physician
Discuss symptoms of recurrence or progression of disease to report to physician
  Headache
  Dizziness
  Faintness
  Nausea, vomiting
Explain importance of decreasing weight or maintaining stable weight
Explain importance of not smoking
Explain need to avoid fatigue and heavy lifting
Explain importance of planned daily exercise program and rest periods

Explain need for low-calorie, low-sodium diet as ordered
Explain importance of maintaining proper fluid intake; amount allowed and limitations such as caffeinated coffee and tea, and alcohol
Explain to avoid constipation and straining
Demonstrate taking and recording of BP and P if indicated

Evaluation

Patient
  Demonstrates return of BP to acceptable limits
  Demonstrates absence of injury potential
    Patient is alert and oriented
    There are no neurologic deficits
  Verbalizes absence of discomfort
  Appears calm
  Verbalizes knowledge and skills in self-care management

ANGINA PECTORIS

Chest pain or discomfort due to myocardial ischemia, which is the result of an imbalance between myocardial oxygen supply and demand (While angina pectoris most commonly occurs in the setting of coronary atherosclerosis, it may occur in patients with normal coronary arteries.)

Assessment
Observations/findings

Chest pain or pressure: mild to severe aching; sharp, tingling, or burning sensation or pressure; described as heavy, squeezing, heartburn, or tight chest lasting 5 to 30 min
Precipitating factors
  Physical or emotional stress
  Exposure to temperature extremes such as cold
  Following a heavy meal
Alleviating factors
  Termination of precipitating factors
  Taking nitroglycerin (NTG) tablets
Associated signs and symptoms
  Sweating
  Lightheadedness
  Palpitations
  Shortness of breath
Anxiety
Indigestion
Skin: pallor, diaphoresis
Respiration: shortness of breath
Cardiac: tachycardia; pulsus alternans; atrial and/or ventricular gallops (S_3 S_4)

Laboratory/diagnostic studies

Cardiac enzymes: CPK-MB, SGOT, SGPT

Electrocardiographic (ECG) changes recorded during episodes of pain: ST segment depression; T wave changes (Figure 2-7)

Exercise stress test (EST): during chest pain—horizontal ST segment or down-sloping of 1 mm or less; failure of systolic blood pressure to rise or drop; ST elevations

Thallium 201 scintigraphy: ischemic areas appear as "cold" areas, reflecting reduced thallium uptake; when ischemia is relieved, "cold" areas show normal thallium uptake

Radionuclide blood pool imaging with technetium 99m

Potential complications

Myocardial infarction
Heart failure

Medical management

BP, T, R, and apical pulse q4h to 6h and prn
Medications
    Nitrates
    Beta-adrenergic blocking agents
    Calcium antagonist
    Analgesics, sedatives
Diet: low saturated fat, low cholesterol, low sodium

Nursing diagnoses/goals/interventions

ndx Alteration in comfort: pain related to myocardial ischemia

GOAL: *Patient will verbalize absence of chest discomfort*

Maintain rest during episodes of pain
Record description of pain and activity prior to onset
Administer nitrates as ordered
Administer oxygen as indicated
Maintain diet as ordered; if chest pain occurs during eating, advise small feedings rather than two or three large meals
Avoid constipation; administer mild laxatives or stool softeners

ndx Knowledge deficit regarding disease process

GOAL: *Patient and/or significant other will demonstrate increased understanding of disease process and management of chest discomfort through interactive discussion*

Discuss nature of angina pectoris: etiology, risk factors involved, and importance of modification (see boxed material on p. 87)
Discuss management and nature of chest pain; assist in identifying precipitating factors
Discuss allowances and limitations
    Avoid isometric-type activity: heavy lifting and pushing
    Exercise regularly; encourage regular home exercise program (p. 118)
    Avoid sexual activities when fatigued; if chest pain occurs during sexual activity, stop and take nitrates if ordered; if pain persists or extreme fatigue occurs, report symptoms to physician

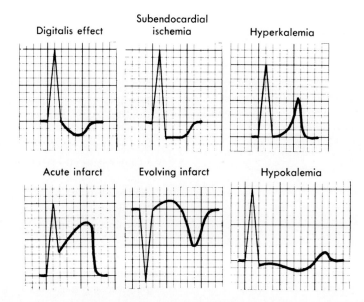

FIGURE 2-7. ST-T segment changes. (From Goldberger, A.L., and Goldberger, E.: Clinical electrocardiography: a simplified approach, ed. 3, St. Louis, 1986, The C.V. Mosby Co.)

CARDIOVASCULAR RISK FACTOR PROFILE	
Family history of heart disease	Elevated serum level of lipids and fats
Sex: Males (35-55) Females (>50 or after menopause)	Diabetes mellitus Physical inactivity; sedentary life-style
Hypertension	Stress
Smoking	For women <50 years:
Overweight/obesity	use of estrogen (i.e., birth control pills) and smoking

Self-management during episodes of pain
    Stop activity and rest
    Take nitrates as ordered
    Report to physician if pain persists longer than 20 min or diaphoresis and SOB appears
Diet as ordered; avoid caffeine intake
Explain importance of controlling any coexisting diseases that may aggravate atherosclerotic process: hypertension, diabetes, hyperlipidemia
Explain importance of weight control; avoid obesity
Explain role that stress plays in aggravating heart disease; need to identify stress-producing factors; methods of stress management using relaxation techniques
Discuss name of medications, dosage, times of administration, purpose, and side effects

Evaluation

Chest discomfort is achieved
    Patient verbalizes absence of pain
    Patient appears relaxed and verbalizes a sense of calm
Patient verbalizes understanding of precipitating factors contributing to chest discomfort
Patient verbalizes appropriate actions to take for pain control

MYOCARDIAL INFARCTION (MI)

Occlusion of the coronary artery and its branches, resulting in myocardial ischemia and necrosis

Assessment

Observations/findings

Severe, crushing chest pain
    Precordial
    Substernal
    Unrelated to exertion or respiration
Diaphoresis
Skin
    Cold
    Clammy
    Pale
Shortness of breath
Faintness
Indigestion
Decreased BP
Tachycardia
Elevated temperature
Anxiety
Restlessness
Behavioral responses
    Denial
    Depression
Heart sounds
    S_3 gallop
    Pericardial friction rub
    Murmurs

Laboratory/diagnostic studies

Elevated enzymes
    Creatine phosphokinase (CPK-MB, CPK)
    LDH
    SGOT
    Elevated ESR
    Elevated WBC
ECG changes (Figure 2-7)
    ST segment elevation
    Q waves
Echocardiography: ventricular wall motion abnormalities
Radionuclide blood pool studies
    Localization of infarct area
    Ventricular function
Angiography

Potential complications

Heart failure
Cardiogenic shock
Extension of MI
Pulmonary/systemic emboli
Pericarditis
Rupture
    Ventricular
    Papillary muscle
Ventricular septal defect
Valvular dysfunction
Ventricular aneurysm
Postmyocardial infarction syndrome (Dressler's)

Medical management

Coronary care unit (CCU) admission
Oxygen therapy: 2 to 4 L/min

Parenteral fluids
Diet: low saturated fat, low sodium, low cholesterol
Cardiac monitor
Medications
    Pain management
    Sedatives
    Antiarrhythmics
    Beta-adrenergic blocking agents
    Vasodilators
    Anticoagulants
    Calcium antagonist
Intraaortic balloon pump (IABP)
Hemodynamic monitoring
Myocardial reperfusion
    Percutaneous transluminal coronary angiography
    Streptokinase infusion
Surgical reperfusion: coronary artery bypass graft

Nursing diagnoses/goals/interventions

ndx: Alteration in comfort: pain related to myocardial ischemia or necrosis

GOAL: *Patient will verbalize absence of chest pain*

Maintain bed rest; position patient comfortably
Record description of pain and factors that aggravate pain; determine if influenced by respiration
Administer oxygen as ordered
Administer drug therapy as ordered; assess and record response
Check BP
Initiate nonpharmacologic measures to relieve pain: relaxation techniques; guided imagery; quiet, restful environment

ndx: Potential alteration in cardiac output related to loss of myocardial contractility

GOAL: *Patient will demonstrate stable or improved cardiac output*

Maintain bedrest
Assess for and report signs of decreased cardiac output
    Decreased BP, increased heart rate
    Decreased urine output
    Fatigue and weakness
    Cool, pale, clammy skin
Check BP, T, R, and apical pulse q2h to 4h and prn
Place patient on cardiac monitor; check rhythm strips q4h to 6h and prn
Administer oxygen therapy as ordered
Auscultate breath sounds q4h to 6h
Auscultate heart sounds q4h to 6h
Monitor serial serum enzymes as ordered
Monitor PAP, PCWP, or CVP as ordered
Take serial 12-lead ECG as ordered
Monitor intake and output q2h to 4h
Maintain parenteral fluids as ordered
Administer medications as ordered
Maintain diet as ordered; avoid iced drinks and chilled foods
Avoid Valsalva maneuver, such as straining; use stool softeners or laxatives

ndx: Anxiety related to perceived or actual threat of biologic integrity

GOAL: *Patient will demonstrate reduced anxiety level*

Initiate comfort measures such as a quiet, restful environment and relaxation techniques
Minimize contact with stressful stimuli such as other anxious patients
Use calm, reassuring voice
Discuss and orient patient to CCU environment and equipment
Administer sedation as indicated
Give simple explanations regarding care and procedures
Encourage expression of feelings; permit crying

ndx: Knowledge deficit regarding disease process

GOAL: *Patient and/or significant other will demonstrate increased understanding of disease process and health management through interactive discussion*

Review physician's explanation of heart condition
    Extent of infarction
    Associated complications
        Arrhythmias
        Angina
        Postmyocardial infarction syndrome
        Heart failure
    Nature of disease process
        Risk factors involved and methods of modification
        Precipitating factors of angina
Explain importance of planned rest periods
Explain importance of activity limitations as related to healing process; that healing takes approximately 6 to 8 weeks
Explain importance of controlling any coexisting disease that may aggravate recovery
    Hyperlipidemia
    Hypertension
    Diabetes

Explain importance of weight control

Explain stress management: need to control stress-producing events and activities

Explain limitations and allowances of activity
- Check with physician for walking and exercise limitations
- Avoid or modify activity following heavy meals, alcohol consumption, periods of emotional stress, or in extremes of temperature

Explain importance of encouraging independence in self-care activities

Explain importance of communication with significant other

Explain need to deal with feelings about possible role change and sexual activity

Discuss signs and symptoms of an extending MI vs. angina
- Extending MI: chest pain, shortness of breath, perspiration, weakness not relieved by medication or rest, pain not always associated with physical exertion
- Angina: chest pain or pressure is usually relieved by rest and/or vasodilators; pain is usually associated with physical or emotional strain

Explain importance of calling physician if chest pain lasts longer than 20 min (if pain is associated with other symptoms, call physician immediately)

Explain importance of maintaining low-sodium, low-cholesterol, low-lipid, and low-calorie diet as ordered

Explain need to avoid use of caffeine products such as coffee, certain teas, and cola drinks

Explain need to avoid use of tobacco products such as cigarettes, cigars, and chewing tobacco

Explain importance of dietary limitations (if no specific diet is ordered, limit intake of eggs, cream, butter, and foods high in animal fat; modify or restrict salt intake)

Explain need to rest after meals (avoid exercising up to 2 hr after heavy meals)

Explain name of medications, dosage, time of administration, purpose, and side effects

Explain need to avoid taking over-the-counter medications without checking with physician

Explain need to avoid constipation and straining

Explain need to avoid sitting in same position for long periods

Explain need to exercise at regular intervals; encourage home exercise program (p. 118)

Explain importance of checking with physician with regard to resuming sexual activity, traveling, and driving automobile

Explain need to avoid isometric-type activity: heavy lifting and pushing

Explain need to monitor daily activities (space activities with periods of rest; stop when fatigued; avoid rushing)

Evaluation

Comfort level is achieved; patient verbalizes absence of pain

Anxiety level is redirected; patient appears relaxed and verbalizes sense of calm

Cardiac output remains stable or improved
- Vital signs and urine output are within normal values
- Patient demonstrates hemodynamic stability
- Patient is able to perform activities of daily living

Knowledge level is increased
- Patient verbalizes increased understanding of disease process and health care management
- Patient verbalizes appropriate actions regarding pain management and medications

VASODILATOR DRUGS

Pharmacologic agents that improve cardiac performance through relaxation of blood vessels; effect occurs through direct action on vascular smooth muscles or indirectly through interference with the neurogenic process (Table 2-1)

Assessment
Observations/findings

Arterial pressure
Heart rates
Hemodynamic measurements
- Cardiac output (CO)
- Pulmonary capillary wedge pressure (PCWP)
- Pulmonary artery diastolic pressure (PADP)
- Systemic vascular resistance (SVR)
- Left ventricular end diastolic pressure (LVEDP)

Arrhythmias
Liver function
Laboratory studies
- Drug levels
- Electrolytes

Clinical indications
- CHF
- Cardiogenic shock
- Angina
- Hypertension

TABLE 2-1. Potential Complications of Vasodilator Drugs Commonly Used for the Treatment of Heart Failure

Nitroprusside	Phentolamine	Nitroglycerin, nitrates	Hydralazine	Prazosin	Nifedipine	Captopril
Hypotension	Hypotension	Hypotension	Hypotension	Hypotension	Hypotension	Hypotension
Nausea, vomiting	Nausea, vomiting	Headache	Nausea, vomiting	Nausea, vomiting	Nausea	Proteinuria
Mental confusion	Tachycardia	Methemoglobinemia	Drug fever	Fluid retention	Headache	Loss of taste
Cyanide poisoning		Tolerance	Skin rash	Weight gain	Fluid retention	Neutropenia
Thiocyanate toxicity			Lupus syndrome	Tachyphylaxis	Chest pain	
Lactic acidosis			Fluid retention			
Hypothyroidism			Weight gain			
Vitamin B_{12} deficiency			Peripheral neuropathy			
Methemoglobinemia						

Modified from Bassie, B.M., and Chatterjee, K.: Med. Clin. North Am. 63(1):34, 1979.

Sodium Nitroprusside

A drug that causes relaxation of arterial and venous smooth muscle; decreases venous return and LVEDP; used in treatment of hypertensive crisis to lower BP and in CHF and cardiogenic shock to reduce preload; reduces SVR to decrease afterload

Hemodynamic effects

CO: increases
BP: decreases
SVR: decreases
LVEDP: decreases
Heart rate (HR): increases

Method of administration

IV
  Onset of action: immediate
  Duration: effect stops within 10 min of stopping infusion

Usual dosage

IV: 0.5 to 10 μg/kg/min
NOTE: Given in intensive care area where continuous hemodynamic monitoring can be done; may be given alone or with dopamine

Acute care

Obtain baseline readings prior to administration
  CO
  SVR
  PADP
  PCWP
  BP
  HR
Determine parameters to be achieved
Wrap IV solution in foil because of light sensitivity
Change solution q4h; dilute medication with 5% dextrose in water—do not use saline or bacteriostatic water for reconstitution
Check arterial pressure and/or cuff BP q5 min when beginning infusion, then q15 min as ordered
Infuse solution using automatic infusion pump
Check for side effects that may indicate overdosage
  Headache, dizziness, ataxia
  Loss of consciousness
  Restlessness
  Diaphoresis
  Weak pulse
  Palpitations
  Dyspnea
  Nausea, vomiting
Secure IV site; check for tissue sloughing and necrosis

Nitrates

Drugs that cause arterial and venous dilation, reduce venous return, and cause a decrease in LVFP and PAP; used in treatment of CHF and angina pectoris

Hemodynamic effects

CO: no change; decreases
BP: decreases
SVR: no change
LVEDP: decreases
HR: increases

Methods of administration

Oral
Sublingual
Topical (ointment)

Usual dosage

Nitroglycerin tablets

Sublingual: gr $1/400$, $1/200$, $1/150$, $1/100$
   Onset of action: 1 to 2 min
   Duration: 30 min

Nitroglycerin ointment 2%

Topical: 1 to 2 inches
   Onset of action: 15 to 30 min
   Duration: 4 to 6 hr

Isosorbide dinitrate

Oral: 5 to 30 mg
   Onset of action: 15 min
   Duration: 90 min
Chewable: 5 to 10 mg
   Onset of action: 2 to 5 min
   Duration: 3 to 4 hr
Sublingual: 2.5 to 10 mg
   Onset of action: 30 min
   Duration: 4 hr

Side effects

Headaches: varying intensity
Dizziness
Tachycardia
Orthostatic hypotension
Flushing
Palpitations
Nausea, vomiting
Hypersensitivity reaction

Patient teaching/discharge planning

Ensure that patient and/or significant other knows and understands

Name of medication, purpose, dosage, and side effects
Need to avoid sudden changes in body position (e.g., standing up)
Need to lie down if dizziness occurs
That patient may take aspirin or acetaminophen if headaches occur; need to report to physician if not relieved
Need to take medication on time; importance of not interrupting dose (prn nitrates may be taken prophylactically prior to anticipated stress-producing activity, e.g., long walks, climbing stairs or hills)
Need to avoid alocoholic beverages
That cotton be removed from medication container
Need to store medications in cool dark place in airtight container (drugs lose potency when exposed to light, moisture, and heat)
Need to check expiration date and replace supply q3 months

Procedure for sublingual administration

Read label carefully; do not confuse with oral or chewable tablets
A burning sensation indicates fresh tablets
Wet tablet with saliva and place under tongue; stop activity and rest until tablet is absorbed or pain relieved
If tablet is taken for angina, may repeat q5 min for maximum of 3 doses; keep record of doses taken
If no relief occurs within 15 min, notify physician or go to nearest emergency room

Procedure for topical administration

Clean area of skin to be used; remove any traces of previous application
Select hairless or shaved area of skin for best absorption of medication: upper arms, chest, thigh, abdomen, forehead, back
Use applicator paper that comes with ointment for accurate dose measurement (doses may come in ½ inch, 1 inch, 1½ inch applications)
Apply applicator paper with measured ointment over skin area; do not rub or spread ointment into skin; leave paper attached to ointment
Cover applicator paper with plastic wrap and secure with tape to protect clothing and promote absorption

Procedure for chewable tablets

Read label carefully; do not confuse chewable tablets with oral or sublingual ones
Chew tablets thoroughly before swallowing

Procedure for oral administration
    Read label carefully; do not confuse with chewable or sublingual tablets
    Take on empty stomach 30 min before meals or 1 to 2 hr after meals

Hydralazine

A drug that causes vascular smooth muscle relaxation; action is principally arterial; used in treatment of hypertension and in CHF by reducing afterload

Hemodynamic effects

CO: increases
BP: decreases
SVR: decreases
LVEDP: no change
HR: increases

Methods of administration

Oral
    Onset of action: 20 to 45 min
    Duration: 3 to 6 hr
IV
    Onset of action: 5 to 15 min
    Duration: 2 to 6 hr
IM
    Onset of action: 10 to 30 min
    Duration: 2 to 6 hr

Usual dosage

CHF
    Orally: 50 to 100 mg tid/qid
Hypertension
    Orally: 10 to 50 mg qid
    IM: 20 to 40 mg q4h to 6h
    IV: 20 to 40 mg q4h to 6h

Side effects

Headache
Dizziness
Tachycardia
Arrhythmias
Angina
Palpitations
Sodium retention
Nausea, vomiting, diarrhea
Lupus erythematosus
    Fever
    Rash
    Muscle and/or joint aches

Prazosin

A drug that causes arterial and venous relaxation by blocking alpha-adrenoreceptors; reduces systemic arterial pressure and venous return; used in treatment of hypertension and in CHF to decrease afterload

Hemodynamic effects

CO: increases
BP: decreases
SVR: decreases
LVEDP: decreases
HR: no increase

Methods of administration

Oral
    Onset of action: 2 hr
    Duration: up to 24 hr
    Usual dosage
        Initial dose: 1 mg tid
        Maintenance dose: 3 to 20 mg/day
        Maximum dose: 20 mg/day

Side effects

Dizziness
Headache
Drowsiness, weakness
Orthostatic hypotension
Depression
Palpitations
Blurred vision
Dry mouth
Nausea, vomiting
Abdominal cramps
Constipation
Priapism
Syncope

Nifedipine

A potent arterial vasodilator with mild negative inotrophic effect used in treatment of coronary artery spasm (Prinzmetal's variant angina), stable and unstable angina, and hypertension; acts as an afterload reducing agent in CHF

Hemodynamic effects

CO: increases
BP: decreases
SVR: decreases
LVEDP: decreases
HR: increases

Method of administration

Oral
Usual dosage
  CHF: 10-20 mg tid
  Stable angina; Prinzmetal's: 10 mg bid to qid
    (maximum 80 mg/24 hr)
  Unstable angina: 10 mg q24 h
    (maximum 60 mg/24 hr)
  Hypertension: 10 mg bid

Side effects

Dizziness
Lightheadedness
Swelling of ankles and feet
Flushing
Headache
Nausea

Captopril

An inhibitor of angiotension-converting enzyme that results in arteriolar dilation and diminished sympathetic activity

Hemodynamic effects

CO: increases
BP: decreases
SVR: decreases
LVEDP: decreases
Heart rate: no change

Method of administration

Oral
  Onset of action: 60 to 90 min
  Duration of action: 6 to 12 hr
Usual dosage
  CHF: 12.5 bid/tid
  Hypertension: 25 mg tid; may increase up to 450 mg/day

Side effects

Skin rash with or without itching
Fever
Dizziness
Lightheadedness
Swelling of face, mouth, and hands
Irregular pulse

Patient teaching/discharge outcome

Ensure that patient and/or significant other knows and understands
  Name of medication, purpose, dosage, and side effects
  That patient may develop dizziness with first dose; if loss of consciousness occurs, need to notify physician to reduce dosage
  Need to lie down if dizziness occurs
  Need to avoid sudden changes in body position (e.g., standing up)
  Importance of not discontinuing medication because of side effects; need to notify physician

INFECTIVE ENDOCARDITIS

An infectious process involving the endothelium of the heart, including the cardiac valves

Assessment

Observations/findings

Recurrent temperature elevation
  Acute: 102° to 104° F (39° to 40° C)
  Subacute: 102° F (39° C)
Alternating chills and diaphoresis
Malaise
Arthralgia
Petechia
  Conjunctiva
  Oral mucous membrane
  Legs
Osler's nodes
"Cafe au lait" complexion
Anorexia
Weight loss
Headache
Embolism: spleen, kidneys, extremities, lungs
Splenomegaly
Systolic heart murmurs

Laboratory/diagnostic studies

Positive blood cultures
Normocytic, normochromic anemia
Elevated ESR
Leukocytosis
Echocardiogram: presence of vegetation or abscesses
Electrocardiogram: atrial fibrillation or flutter

Potential complications

Cardiac
  Abscesses
  Valvular heart disease
  Heart failure
  Myocarditis

Embolization
   Cerebral
   Renal
   Splenic
   Coronary
Mycotic aneurysms

Medical management

Parenteral therapy
Medications
   IV antibiotics
   Antipyretics: salicylates
   Analgesics
   Anticoagulation

Nursing diagnoses/goals/interventions

ndx: Alteration in nutrition: less than body requirements

GOAL: *Patient will receive nutrients to maintain body function*

Weigh daily
Maintain diet as ordered
Offer high-calorie supplemental feedings

ndx: Diversional activity deficit related to prolonged hospitalization (4 to 6 weeks)

GOAL: *Patient will engage in identified inpatient diversional activities*

Encourage patient to explore diversional activities such as reading, puzzles, and out-of-hospital passes
Initiate occupational therapy if indicated
Encourage daily structured exercise program

ndx: Potential alteration in fluid volume: excess related to cardiac factor

GOAL: *Patient will avoid complications of fluid excess*

Weigh daily
Auscultate chest for breath and heart sounds q4h to 6h
Check BP, T, R, and apical pulse q4h
Measure intake and output
Restrict sodium and fluids as ordered
Administer medications as ordered (e.g., diuretics)
Maintain activity as tolerated
Avoid fatigue; maintain planned rest periods
Assist and teach patient to turn, cough, and deep breathe q4h to 6h when on bed rest

ndx: Potential alteration in thought processes related to cerebral embolization

GOAL: *Patient will demonstrate absence of complications of embolic episodes*

Observe for signs of embolization each shift and prn; report positive signs to physician immediately
Administer anticoagulant therapy as ordered
Instruct patient about need to continue with anticoagulants, if ordered, to prevent future embolic episode

ndx: Knowledge deficit regarding to disease process

GOAL: *Patient and/or significant other will demonstrate increased understanding of disease process and self-care management through interactive discussion*

Discuss symptoms of recurrence to report to physician
   Fatigue
   Elevated temperature
   Chills
   Weight loss
   Just not feeling well
Explain need to avoid persons with infections, especially upper respiratory infection (URI), and to report symptoms (e.g., cold, flu, cough) to physician
Explain importance of avoiding fatigue; need to plan rest periods before and after activity
Explain importance of reporting to physician any event that may predispose to bacteremia
   Dental or gum therapy
   Surgical procedures
   Medical procedures
   Childbirth
   Trauma
   Furuncles
Explain need to maintain good oral hygiene: daily care and regular visits to dentist
Explain importance of ongoing outpatient care
Discuss name of medication, dosage, times of administration, purpose, and side effects
Explain significance of prophylactic antibiotic therapy prior to procedures that predispose to bacteremia (see Table 2-2)

Evaluation

Nutritional status is improved and maintained
There are no complications
Patient demonstrates understanding of home care activities

VALVULAR HEART DISEASE

An acquired or congenital disease involving the heart valves being maintained in a closed or open position; most common types are aortic or mitral stenosis and aortic or mitral regurgitation (Table 2-3)

TABLE 2-2. Recommended Antibiotic Coverage for Endocarditis Prophylaxis

Drug	Dosage
Penicillin For most patients: orally	Adults: 2 g of penicillin V 1 hr prior to procedure; then 1 g 6 hr after initial dose Children less than 60 lb: 1 g of penicillin V 1 hr prior to procedure; then 500 mg 6 hr after initial dose
Erythromycin For those patients allergic to penicillin; may also be selected for those receiving oral penicillin as continuous rheumatic fever prophylaxis	Adults: erythromycin 1 g orally 1 hr prior to procedure; then 500 mg 6 hr after initial dose Children: 20 mg/kg orally 1 hr prior to procedure; then 10 mg/kg 6 hr after initial dose
Ampicillin plus gentamicin For those patients at higher risk of infective endocarditis (especially those with prosthetic heart valves) who are not allergic to penicillin	Adults: ampicillin 1-2 g plus gentamicin 1.5 mg/kg IM or IV both given 30 min before procedure; then penicillin V 1 g orally 6 hr after initial dose Children: ampicillin 50 mg/kg plus gentamicin 2 mg/kg IM or IV, both given 30 min before procedure; then penicillin V 500 mg for children under 60 lb (1 g for children over 60 lb) orally 6 hr after initial dose
Vancomycin IV and erythromycin orally For higher-risk patients (especially those with prosthetic heart valves) who are allergic to penicillin	Adults: vancomycin 1 g IV over 60 min, begun 60 min before procedure; no repeat dose is necessary Children: vancomycin 20 mg/kg IV over 60 min before procedure; no repeat dose is necessary

Modified from the American Heart Association, Circulation 56:139A, 1978.

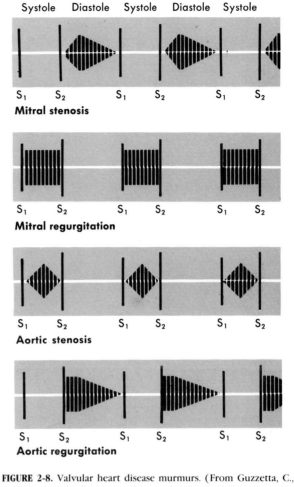

FIGURE 2-8. Valvular heart disease murmurs. (From Guzzetta, C., and Dossey, B.: Cardiovascular nursing: bodymind tapestry, St. Louis, 1985, The C.V. Mosby Co.)

Assessment
Observations/findings

NOTE: Observations and care listed are for moderate to severe forms of valvular heart disease
Fatigue
Malaise
Shortness of breath
DOE
Anorexia
PND
Palpitations

Laboratory/diagnostic studies
ECG
    Atrial, ventricular hypertrophy
    Arrhythmias: atrial fibrillation, flutter
    Conduction defects: bundle branch blocks
Echocardiogram: decreased excursion of leaflets
Chest x-ray examination
    Cardiomegaly
    Pulmonary vascular congestion
    Valve calcification
Cardiac catheterization

TABLE 2-3. Common Valvular Disorders: Adult Onset

Aortic stenosis	Mitral stenosis	Aortic regurgitation	Mitral regurgitation
OBSERVATIONS			

DOE
Syncope
Fatigue
Angina pectoris
Decreased pulse pressure
Carotid pulse
  Slow with long upstroke
  Small quality to pulse
	DOE
	Fatigue
	Decreased tolerance to exercise
	Orthopnea
	PND
	Cough
	Hemoptysis
		Dyspnea
		Awareness of strong pulsations of heart
		Excessive sweating
		Skin warm, flushed, and damp
		Dizziness
		Neck pain
		Head bobbing (DeMusset's sign)
		Pulses
		  Visible arterial pulsations in neck
		  Bisferiens pulse
		  Water-hammer (Corrigan's) pulse
		Widened pulse pressure to greater than 80 mm Hg
			Dyspnea
			Fatigue
			Exercise intolerance
			Orthopnea
			Palpitations

Apical impulse: strong, sustained during systole
Systolic thrill
Heart sounds
  Moderate: crescendo-decrescendo, rough, harsh systolic murmur heard over aortic area
Decreased aortic second sound
	Apical impulse: tapping quality
	
	Heart sounds
	  Loud first heart sound; low-pitched rumbling diastolic murmur with an opening snap heard at apex
		Apical impulse: forceful, sustained, displaced downward and outward
		Heart sounds
		  Decrescendo: high-pitched blowing heard at left sternal border
		  Systolic ejection sound
		  Diastolic murmur
			Apical impulse; large, laterally displaced
			
			Heart sounds
			  Holosystolic systolic murmur heard at apex
			  First heart sounds diminished
			  Splitting of second heart sound
			  Third heart sound

POTENTIAL COMPLICATIONS			
	Endocarditis Systemic emboli: brain, extremities, abdomen	Endocarditis	Endocarditis Rupture of chordae tendineae; systemic emboli
DIAGNOSTIC FINDINGS			

ECG
  Left ventricular hypertrophy (LVH)
  Conduction defects
    Left anterior hemiblock
    Left bundle branch block (LBBB)
    Complete heart block
  Arrhythmias: atrial fibrillation
	ECG
	  P waves notched or peaked in I, II, III, and AVF
	  Atrial fibrillation
	  Right ventricular hypertrophy (RVH)
		ECG
		  Normal
		  Septal Q waves V_5V_6
		  LVH
			ECG
			  Nonspecific ST segment and T wave abnormalities
			  LVH
			  P waves abnormalities
			  Atrial arrhythmias: premature atrial contractions (PAC's), atrial fibrillation

Chest x-ray examination: enlargment of LV; calcification of aortic valve	Chest x-ray examination: enlargement of LA, RV, right atria (RA), and pulmonary trunk; calcification of mitral valve	Chest x-ray examination: enlargement of LV; dilation of aorta	Chest x-ray examination: enlargement of LA, LV
Hemodynamic changes: elevated left atrial (LA) and LV pressures	Hemodynamic changes: elevated pressures—LA, pulmonary artery (PA), and RV	Hemodynamic changes: elevated left ventricular end-diastolic pressure (LVEDP)	Hemodynamic changes: elevated LA and PA pressures and PCWP

Potential complications

Embolism
    Brain
    Lungs
Left ventricular (LV) failure
Right ventricular (RV) failure
Infective endocarditis
Rupture of papillary muscles or chordae tendineae
Pulmonary edema

Medical management

Medications
    Antibiotics
    Inotropics
    Vasodilators
    Diuretics
    Analgesics
    Anticoagulants
Cardiac monitoring
Hemodynamic monitoring
Surgical management
    Commissurotomy
    Valvotomy
    Valvuloplasty
    Valve replacement

Nursing diagnoses/goals/interventions

ndx: Alteration in cardiac output related to valvular insufficiency (preload)

GOAL: *Patient will demonstrate adequate cardiac output*

Maintain bed rest as ordered; elevate head of bed 30 to 40 degrees
Check BP, T, and R with apical pulse q4h
Auscultate breath sounds q4h to 6h
Auscultate heart sounds q6h to 8h
Monitor cardiac rhythm for changes from baseline
Administer parenteral therapy with electrolytes as ordered
Administer inotropic medication as ordered
Measure intake and output
Maintain diet as ordered; serve small, frequent feedings
Maintain activity as tolerated
    Avoid fatigue; maintain planned rest periods
    Perform active or passive ROM exercises to extremities qid
Provide emotional support; encourage communication with significant other

ndx: Alteration in fluid volume excess related to cardiac decompensation

GOAL: *Patient will demonstrate stable fluid balance*

Auscultate breath sounds q4h to 6h
Assess for increase or decrease in jugular venous pressure
Administer diuretics and vasodilator therapy as ordered
Measure intake and output
Restrict sodium and fluids as ordered
Monitor electrolytes, chemistries, Hgb, and Hct

ndx: Knowledge deficit regarding disease process

GOAL: *Patient and/or significant other will demonstrate increased understanding of disease process and health management through interactive discussion*

Explain nature and cause of disease process
Explain importance of reporting signs and symptoms of
    Heart failure
        Increased fatigue
        Tachypnea
        Orthopnea
        Cough
    Infective endocarditis
        Elevated temperature
        Malaise and anorexia
        Chills alternating with diaphoresis
Explain importance of reporting to physician any event that may predispose to bacteremia
    Dental or gum manipulation
    Genitourinary procedures
    Drainage of abscesses
    Presence of skin boils
    Gynecologic procedures
        Childbirth
        Dilation and curettage (D & C)
        Therapeutic abortion
        Tubal ligation
Explain importance of notifying dentist, urologist, and gynecologist of valvular disease
Explain importance of medical counseling for women in need of contraceptives
Explain importance of medical counseling for women desiring pregnancy prior to conception
Explain need to maintain good oral hygiene
    Daily care
    Regular visits to dentist
Explain need to avoid fatigue; to plan rest periods before and after activity

Explain importance of prophylactic antibiotic therapy when ordered (Table 2-2)
Discuss name of medication, dosage, times of administration, purpose, and side effects
Explain need to avoid taking over-the-counter drugs without checking with physician
Explain importance of ongoing outpatient care

Evaluation

Cardiac output is maintained
Fluid balance is regained
Knowledge base is achieved

PERICARDITIS

An inflammatory process involving the parietal and visceral layers of the pericardium and outer myocardium

Assessment
Observations/findings

Substernal chest pain
   Precordial
   May radiate to shoulder or neck
   Severe, sharp
   Increases with inspiration
   Relieved by sitting up and leaning forward
Increased systemic venous pressure
Pericardial friction rub: scratchy sound in time with heartbeat
Difficult respirations
Elevated temperature
Chills alternating with diaphoresis
Restlessness
Nausea
Muscle aches
Anxiety
Fatigue
Orthopnea
Paricardial effusion

Laboratory/diagnostic studies

ECG
   Concave, elevated ST segment (early stage)
   T wave inversion (late stage)
   Arrhythmias
Leukocytosis (increased WBC)
Increased ESR
Chest x-ray examination: symmetrically enlarged cardiac silhouette
Echocardiogram: presence of pericardial effusion

Potential complications

Cardiac tamponade
Heart failure

Medical management

Medications
   Nonsteroidal antiinflammatory agents: indomethacin
   Analgesics-antipyretics: aspirin
   Corticosteroids
Pericardiocentesis
Surgical procedures
   Pericardial window
   Pericardiectomy

Nursing diagnoses/goals/interventions

ndx: Alteration in comfort: pain related to pericardial friction rub

GOAL: *Patient will verbalize absence of chest discomfort*

Assess and record quality of chest pain
Maintain bed rest
   Elevate head 45 degrees
   Provide padded overbed table
Administer pain medications as ordered

ndx: Anxiety related to perceived or actual threat to biologic integrity

GOAL: *Patient will demonstrate reduced anxiety level*

Provide emotional support
   Remain with patient if anxious
   Encourage communication with significant other
Explain procedures and treatments thoroughly
Ensure quiet environment; reduce external stimuli
Use calm, reassuring voice

ndx: Potential alteration in cardiac output: decreased related to alteration in preload

GOAL: *Patient will demonstrate stable cardiac output*

Monitor for signs of cardiac tamponade
   Narrowing pulse pressure
   Pulsus paradoxus
Check BP, T, R, and apical pulse q4h
   Maintain cooling measures for elevated temperature
   Keep patient warm and dry
Assist and teach patient to turn, cough, and deep breathe q4h
Auscultate chest for breath sounds q4h

Auscultate heart sounds q6h to 8h
Administer parenteral therapy as ordered
Administer nonsteroidal inflammatory medication
Measure intake and output
Prepare for pericardiocentesis when ordered

ndx Knowledge deficit regarding disease process

GOAL: *Patient and/or significant other will demonstrate increased understanding of disease process and management of chest discomfort through interactive discussion*

Discuss symptoms of recurrence to report to physician
　Increasing fatigue
　Elevated temperature
　Difficult respirations
　Chest pain
Explain need to avoid persons with infections, especially URI, and to report symptoms (e.g., cold, flu, cough) to physician
Explain need to avoid fatigue; alternate periods of activity with rest
Explain importance of ongoing outpatient care
Discuss medications: name, dosage, time of administration, purpose, and side effects
Explain need to avoid taking over-the-counter medications without checking with physician

Evaluation

Chest pain is relieved
Anxiety level is reduced
Patient verbalizes home care management
Patient demonstrates hemodynamic stability

PERICARDIOCENTESIS

Withdrawal of blood or fluid from the pericardial sac via percutaneous needle puncture (Figure 2-9)

Preparation

Reinforce physician's explanation of procedure
Obtain signed consent
Maintain NPO 6 to 8 hr prior to procedure when possible
Elevate head of bed 20 to 30 degrees as ordered
Obtain 12-lead ECG and rhythm strip; connect ECG unipolar lead to needle using aligator clip
Administer oxygen by mask or cannula as ordered
Obtain and record baseline arterial pressures, as well as paradoxic pulse and pulse pressure
Maintain parenteral fluids as ordered
Obtain necessary equipment as ordered
　ECG machine
　Needles: No. 16 spinal
　Syringes
　Three-way stopcock
Administer medications as ordered
　Atropine
　Lidocaine
　Sedatives
Maintain defibrillator and emergency drugs at bedside
Provide emotional support

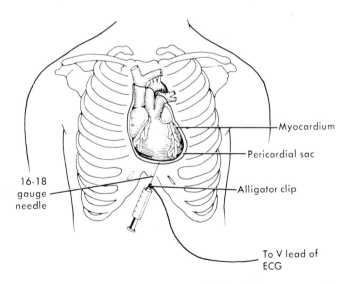

FIGURE 2-9. Periocardiocentesis. (From Budassi, S.A., and Barber, J.: Emergency nursing: principles and practice, St. Louis, 1980, The C.V. Mosby Co.)

Assessment during and following procedure

Observations/findings

Level of consciousness
ECG
  ST elevations
  Increased PR interval
Arterial pressure
CVP
Right atrial pressure (RAP)
Pericardial aspirate
  Amount
  Color
  Turbidity
  Blood
Respirations

Potential complications

Puncture of coronary artery, ventricle, or lung
Arrhythmias
Ventricular fibrillation
Laceration of lung
Cardiac tamponade

Postprocedure care

Maintain bed rest
Check BP, R, and apical pressure q15 min for 1 hr, then q4h as ordered
Monitor arterial pressures; check for decreased pulse pressure or pulsus paradoxus q15 min for 1 hr, then q4h as ordered
Administer oxygen as ordered
Maintain NPO as ordered
Auscultate heart sounds q2h to 4h
Observe for recurrence of tamponade; be prepared to repeat pericardiocentesis or surgical intervention
Continue ongoing care for specific disease process

CARDIAC TAMPONADE

Rapid accumulation of fluid or blood within the pericardial cavity, which results in restriction of diastolic filling

Assessment

Observations/findings

Distended neck veins with inspiratory rise in venous pressure (Kussmaul's sign)
Decreased BP; narrowing pulse pressure; pulsus paradoxus > 10 mm Hg
Decreased heart sounds
Pericardial friction rub
Anxiety and restlessness
Tachypnea
Skin
  Cyanotic
  Dusky
  Pale
Posture: patient sits upright or leans forward
Abdominal pain
Peripheral pulses: weak, absent
Hemodynamic findings
  Decreased CO
  Elevated CVP
  Lowered left atrial pressure (LAP)

Laboratory/diagnostic studies

Echocardiogram: pericardial effusion
ECG
  Tachycardia
  Low voltage
  Widespread ST elevations
  T wave changes
Chest x-ray examination: enlarged cardiac silhouette (globular shape)
Blood pooling scanning

Potential complications

Heart failure
Cardiogenic shock
Cardiac arrest

Medical management

NPO
Parenteral fluids
Pericardiocentesis
BP and apical pulse and respiration rate q15 to 30 min
Medications
  Cardiotonics
  Corticosteroids
  Antiarrhythmics
Twelve-lead electrocardiogram
Maintain defibrillator and emergency drugs at bedside

Nursing diagnoses/goals/interventions

ndx: Alteration in cardiac output related to restricted ventricular filling

GOAL: *Patient will demonstrate hemodynamic stability*

Maintain bedrest; elevate head of bed 45 degrees
Place patient on cardiac monitor; check rhythm strip qh
Auscultate for pulsus paradoxus q1h to 2h
Monitor hemodynamics; check pressures q15 to 30 min

RAP
PCWP, CVP
Cardiac output

ndx: Alteration in comfort related to chest discomfort

GOAL: *Patient will verbalize absence of chest discomfort*

Assess quality and characteristics of chest pain
Maintain bed rest in position of comfort
Administer pain medication as ordered
Provide emotional support
Remain with patient

Evaluation

Patient demonstrates normal cardiac output
Patient demonstrates return to baseline clinical status
Comfort level is achieved

HEART FAILURE

Inability of the heart to increase cardiac output sufficiently to meet the body's metabolic demand

Assessment

Observations/findings
GENERAL

Fatigue
Effort intolerance
Anorexia
Cachexia
Nausea and/or vomiting
Tachypnea
Dyspnea
Nocturia
Tachycardia
Pulsus alternans
Gallop rhythms (S_3, S_4)
Peripheral cyanosis
Anxiety
Restlessness
Rales, rhonchi
Cheyne-Stokes respiration
Respiratory assessment
Drug toxicity
   Digitalis toxicity
   Hypokalemia
Arrhythmias

LEFT VENTRICULAR FAILURE

Shortness of breath
Restlessness
Dyspnea, exertional and/or at rest
PND
Orthopnea
Tachypnea
Cough: dry, unproductive
Hemoptysis
Elevated BP
Tachycardia
Ventricular gallop: S_3
Hypoxemia
Rales, rhonchi
Cyanosis

RIGHT VENTRICULAR FAILURE

Increased venous pressure
Distended neck veins
Edema; firm, pitting
   Peripheral extremities
   Sacrum
   Genitalia
Ascites
Right upper quadrant abdominal pain
Hepatosplenomegaly
Weight gain
Decreased urine output
Anorexia

Laboratory/diagnostic studies
GENERAL

Serum
   Hct, Hgb
   BUN, creatinine
   Electrolytes
      Hyponatremia
      Hyperkalemia
      Hypokalemia
   Bilirubin: hyperbilirubinemia
   Enzymes: SGOT, SGPT, LDH
   PT
   Albumin
   Glucose
   Arterial blood gases
Urine
   Specific gravity
   Protein
   Creatinine
   Sodium
ECG
Chest x-ray examination
Echocardiogram
MUGA
Hemodynamic monitoring
Pulmonary function tests

LEFT VENTRICULAR FAILURE

ECG: left ventricular hypertrophy (LVH), left atrial hypertrophy (LAH), arrhythmias
Increased PCWP
Decreased CO
Chest x-ray examination
 Redistribution of pulmonary flow to upper lobes
 Kerly B lines
 Pleural effusion
 Increased cardiac shadow
Pulmonary function tests
 Decreased vital capacity (VC), residual volume, and total lung capacity

RIGHT VENTRICULAR FAILURE

ECG: right ventricular hypertrophy (RVH), right atrial hypertrophy (RAH)
Elevated RV pressure, PAP, and PWP
Elevated CVP
Chest x-ray examination
 Generalized enlargement of cardiac shadow

Potential complications

Pulmonary edema
Pulmonary infarction
Cardiogenic shock

Medical management

Bed rest
Low-sodium diet
Medications
 Diuretics
 Digitalis
 Vasodilators
 Inotropic drugs
Oxygen therapy
Cardiac monitor
Hemodynamic monitoring
IABP

Nursing diagnoses/goals/interventions

ndx: Alteration in cardiac output related to mechanical factors (preload, afterload, or contractility)

GOAL: *Patient will demonstrate improved cardiac output*

Maintain bed rest
Elevate head of bed 30 to 60 degrees; lean patient forward on padded overbed table
Check BP, R and apical pulse as ordered or q1h to 2h
Check RAP, PAP, and PCWP q2h to 4h as ordered
Monitor cardiac output q2h to 4h as ordered
Administer positive inotropic drugs as ordered
 Digitalis
 Dobutamine
 Amrinone
 Milrinone
Monitor for signs of drug toxicity
Maintain quiet environment
Restrict activities as ordered
Provide bedside commode
Plan care to avoid fatigue
 Maintain rest periods between procedures
 Have patient rest before and after meals
 Maintain planned rest periods
Provide emotional support; offer simple explanations

ndx: Alteration in fluid volume: excess related to increased systemic venous congestion and/or RV failure

GOAL: *Patient will demonstrate stable fluid balance*

Auscultate chest for breath and heart sounds as ordered or q2h to 4h
Maintain parenteral fluids by microdrip when ordered; avoid rapid and excessive hydration
Administer diuretics and vasodilator therapy as ordered
Measure intake and output
 Record urine output qh; if less than 30 ml/hr, report to physician
 Estimate diaphoretic fluid loss
Weigh patient daily at same time with same clothing and scale; report increase of 500 g/day or greater
Monitor BUN and electrolytes
Observe for effect and toxicity of diuretic
Maintain sodium-restricted diet as ordered
Maintain fluid restrictions; assist patient with planning distribution of fluids over waking hours

ndx: Ineffective breathing pattern related to tracheobronchial secretions

GOAL: *Patient will demonstrate bilateral excursion and breath sounds*

Maintain body position best suited to promote optimum ventilation
Auscultate chest for breath sounds as ordered or q1h to 2h; report adventitious, decreased, or absent breath sounds
Maintain patent airway
 Assist and teach patient to turn, cough, and deep breathe q1h to 2h if congested, 2h to 4h if not congested

Perform postural drainage, percussion, and vibration as indicated
Check respirations q1h to 2h; note quality and rate
Administer humidified oxygen per nasal cannula as ordered
Allow no smoking
Administer sedation and bronchodilators as ordered

***ndx*:** Potential alteration in skin integrity related to edema

GOAL: *Patient will maintain skin integrity*

Check skin and bony prominences for signs of redness, scaling, breaks, or ulcerations qid
Turn and reposition q2h
Administer skin care q2h
Keep skin dry when diaphoretic
Provide antiembolic support stockings
Give back rubs with massage to bony prominences q2h to 4h, using lanolin-based lotion
Prevent and eliminate pressure and friction; position pillows or other supports between pressure areas to avoid two skin areas touching
Assist patient out of bed frequently or as ordered
Initiate decubitus care at first signs of tissue breakdown or ulceration (p. 619)
Use suggested preventive devices
  Alternating pressure mattress
  Air pressure beds (Clinitron)

***ndx*:** Alteration in nutritional status: less than body requirements related to impaired absorption of nutrients secondary to low cardiac output

GOAL: *Patient will obtain sufficient nutrients to maintain body function*

Observe daily for signs of malnutrition
  Dry body weight 20% or more under the ideal for age, height, and frame
  Decreased triceps skinfold measurements
  Stomatitis
  Anorexia
  Increasing fatigue and weakness
  Decreased serum albumin, transferrin, iron-binding capacity, BUN
  Lack of interest in food
Weigh patient daily at same time with same clothing and scale
Administer oral hygiene q2h to 4h
Administer medications to relieve nausea and/or vomiting
Maintain diet as ordered
Do not force patient to eat
Tempt appetite with food preferences compatible with diet restrictions and cultural values
Serve small, frequent meals
Supplement with high-calorie foods as ordered
Initiate caloric count if nutritional status fails to improve
Obtain dietary consultation to evaluate nutritional status and to assist in selection of foods
Initiate tube feedings or parenteral nutrition as indicated

***ndx*:** Knowledge deficit regarding disease process and home care management

GOAL: *Patient and/or significant other demonstrate understanding of disease process and self-care management through interactive discussion*

Explain nature and cause of disease process
Explain importance of maintaining daily activity plan
  Alternate exercise and other activities with rest periods
  Avoid fatigue
Explain importance of maintaining prescribed diet and fluid amounts; need to avoid food high in sodium
Explain need to avoid persons with infections, especially, URI
Explain importance of daily weights—at same time and with same amount of clothing
Explain symptoms of early heart failure to report to physician
  Decreased exercise tolerance
  Shortness of breath
  DOE
  PND
  Persistent cough
  Swelling of extremities
  Sudden weight gain of more than 3 lb (6.6 kg) in a 24 hr period
  Increased nocturia
Explain importance of not smoking
Discuss medications: name, dosage, time of administration, purpose, and side effects (see Vasodilator Drugs, p. 89; Digitalis Therapy, p. 154)
Explain importance of avoiding extreme temperature changes
Explain importance of ongoing care

Evaluation

Patient
  Will have improved cardiac output as evidenced by
    Vital signs within acceptable limits for age

CO, LVEDP, and PCWP within acceptable limits
Increased activity tolerance
Demonstrates improved ventilation as evidenced by
Effortless breathing
Lung clear on auscultation
Po_2 and Pco_2 levels within normal limits
Exhibits no signs of fluid overload as evidenced by
Absence of edema
Weight loss, return to baseline
Verbalizes an increased knowledge level regarding disease process, diet, medications, and activity allowances and limitations
Demonstrates maintenance of skin integrity as evidenced by
Intact skin
Warm and dry skin with normal color
Demonstrates adequate nutritional status as evidenced by
Dry body weight that is normal for age and body build
Improved appetite
Good skin turgor, increased muscle mass
Improved energy to perform ADLs

SHOCK SYNDROME

A clinical syndrome in which blood flow to the tissues is insufficient to sustain normal cell metabolism, resulting in a generalized decrease in perfusion to vital body function (see boxed material and Table 2-4)

hypovolemic shock *Deficient return of venous blood to the heart due to external losses of blood plasma or extracellular fluid or internal sequestration of plasma*

vasogenic (warm shock) *Shock syndrome that results in massive vasodilation from an increase in total vascular capacity; most common form is sepsis, but may occur as a result of other factors, including anaphylactic reactions*

cardiogenic shock *Shock due to inadequate tissue perfusion that results from impaired LV function*

Assessment
Observations/findings
HYPOVOLEMIC SHOCK

Syncope
Vertigo
Restlessness
Anxiety
Decreased or falling BP: determined by patient's baseline pressure
Narrowed pulse pressure
Hemodynamic studies
  Interaarterial pressure
    Early: normal
    Late: decreased
  Decreased PAP, PCWP
  Decreased CO
  Decreased CVP (<3 cm H_2O pressure)
Flat neck veins
Collapsed peripheral veins
Tachycardia: weak, thready pulse
Tachypnea: shallow respirations
Extreme weakness
Altered levels in mental status
  Lethargy
  Semiconsciousness
  Coma

TABLE 2-4. Early and Late Signs of Shock Syndrome

	Early	Late
Blood pressure	↓ Pulse pressure ↑ Diastolic pressure	↓ Systolic pressure
Urine output	↓ Urine sodium concentration ↑ Urine osmolality	↓ Urine volume
Acid-base changes	↑ Respiratory alkalosis Metabolic alkalosis	Metabolic acidosis
Tissue perfusion	Slight restlessness Occasionally warm, dry skin	Cold, clammy skin Cloudy sensorium

From Shock, 1976, The Upjohn Company. Reproduced with permission of The Upjohn Company.

SHOCK SYNDROME: CAUSES/ETIOLOGIES

HYPOVOLEMIC SHOCK

Loss of blood volume (hemorrhage, GI bleeding; wounds)
Loss of plasma volume (dehydration, burns, peritonitis)

CARDIOGENIC SHOCK

Acute myocardial infarction
Other causes (pulmonary emboli, cardiac surgery, tamponade)

VASOGENIC SHOCK

Sepsis
Immune-mediated (anaphylaxis)
Deep anesthesia effects

Circumoral pallor
Conjunctival pallor
Lip cyanosis
Skin
  Pale
  Cool
  Clammy
  Cyanotic
  Mottling of extremities
Subnormal temperature
Excessive thirst
Nausea, vomiting
Renal status
  Urinary output below 30 ml/hr
  Elevated serum creatinine
  Elevated serum urea nitrogen
  Low urine sodium (<20 mEq/L)
Internal or external circulating blood volume loss
  Hemorrhage
    Postsurgical
    Gastrointestinal (GI)
    Following trauma
  Plasma volume losses
    Burns
    Excessive diarrhea, vomiting

VASOGENIC SHOCK

Fainting
Vertigo
Restlessness
Anxiety
Early stage
  Normal or slightly decreased BP
  Decreased or normal peripheral vascular resistance
  Hemodynamics
    Decreased or normal PCWP
    Normal CO
  Warm skin
  Tachycardia: bounding pulse
Late stage
  Decreased BP
  Increased peripheral vascular resistance
  Decreased CO
  Decreased PCWP
  Metabolic acidosis
  Tachycardia
Excessive thirst
Nausea, vomiting
Tachypnea: see Respiratory Assessment (p. 219)
Temperature
  Subnormal
  Elevated

Altered level of consciousness
  Lethargy
  Semiconsciousness
  Coma
Skin
  Pale
  Cool
  Clammy
  Cyanotic
Renal status
  Urinary output below 30 ml/hr
  Elevated serum creatinine
  Elevated serum urea nitrogen
Wounds
  Swelling, redness
  Abnormal secretions
  Generalized uticaria, pruritus

CARDIOGENIC SHOCK

Restlessness
Anxiety
Decreased or falling BP; determined by patient's baseline pressure
Intraarterial hypotension: systolic pressures <90 mm Hg
Left ventricular pressures
  Increased LVEDP
  Increased LAP
  Increased PCWP
Cardiac output
  2.2 L/min
  Decreased ejection fraction
  Decreased cardiac index
Decreased SVR
Elevated RV filling pressures
  Presence of jugular vein distention
  Increased CVP: above 15 cm H_2O pressure
  Positive hepatojugular reflex
Tachycardia
  Thready radial pulse
  Irregular or absent peripheral pulses
Presence of S_3, S_4 gallops or murmurs
Respiratory distress
  Tachypnea
  Orthopnea
  Hypoxia
Alteration in level of consciousness
  Apathy
  Lethargy
  Semiconsciousness
  Coma
Skin

Pale
Cool
Clammy
Cyanosis
Temperature
  Subnormal
  Elevated
Excessive thirst
Nausea, vomiting
Renal status
  Urinary output below 20 ml/hr
  Elevated serum creatinine
  Elevated serum urea nitrogen
ECG changes
  Ischemic changes
  Arrhythmias
  Ventricular fibrillation
Pain
  Chest
  Abdominal

Laboratory/diagnostic studies
HYPOVOLEMIC SHOCK

Electrolytes
Chemistries
Arterial blood gases

VASOGENIC SHOCK

Cultures
  Blood
  Sputum
  Urine
WBC
ESR
Chest x-ray examination
Clotting profile

CARDIOGENIC SHOCK

Serum
  Arterial blood gases
  Chemistries
  Electrolytes
  Drug levels
  Cardiac enzymes
Chest x-ray examination
MUGA
Echocardiogram
Radionuclide ventriculography

Potential complications
HYPOVOLEMIC SHOCK

Heart failure

VASOGENIC SHOCK
Adult respiratory distress syndrome (p. 263)
Disseminated intravascular coagulation (p. 196)

CARDIOGENIC SHOCK

Metabolic acidosis
  Increased serum lactate levels
  Decreased pH
Electrolyte imbalances
Myocardial ischemia: elevated enzymes
Heart failure
Pulmonary edema
Adult respiratory distress syndrome (p. 263)
  Diminished breath sounds
  Pulmonary congestion
Acidosis
Electrolyte imbalance

Medical management

Admission to cardiac intensive care unit
Cardiac monitor
Hemodynamic monitoring
Assisted mechanical ventilation
Oxygen therapy
Medications
  Vasodilators, sodium nitroprusside
  Sympathomimetics: dopamine, dobutamine
  Osmotic diuretics
  For vasogenic shock: epinephrine, anthihistamine, hydrocortisone
Parenteral therapy
  Blood replacement
  Plasma volume expanders
  Fluid challenges
Vascular support
  IABP

Nursing diagnoses/goals/interventions

ndx: Alteration in tissue perfusion related to hypovolemia

GOAL: *Patient will maintain tissue perfusion and cellular oxygenation*

Maintain complete bed rest; flat supine position; position extremities to faciliate circulation
Maintain parenteral therapy as ordered: whole blood, plasmanate, volume expanders
Measure intake and output qh
Connect indwelling urethral catheter to closed gravity drainage system; notify physician if urinary output is less than 30 ml/hr
Measure all body fluid loss; estimate loss in dressings or perineal pads

Administer medications as ordered
Assess for effects of drug therapy and signs of toxicity
Maintain NPO or clear liquid as ordered
Check R, apical pulse, and femoral pulse q15 min and prn
Monitor PAP and PCWP qlh to 2h as ordered
Monitor intraarterial pressure qlh to 2h; check peripheral arm BP q15 min if arterial line is not in place
Monitor cardiac output as ordered
Check CVP reading qh and prn
Check rectal temperature qh
Administer oxygen as ordered prn; assisted ventilation may be required
Apply pressure to control bleeding if necessary
   Pressure dressing
   Direct pressure
   Gastric tube with balloon
   Traction to urethral catheter
Apply shock trousers as ordered; patient may arrive in trousers (p. 148)
Prepare medications to control bleeding if ordered
   Vitamin K
   Protamine sulfate
Prepare for surgery
   Resuturing of the bleeding site
   Removal of ruptured organ or resection of bleeding site
   See General Preoperative Care/Teaching (p. 29)
Avoid routine nursing functions during acute phase
Keep patient warm and dry
Provide emotional support
Remain with patient
Maintain esthetic environment
Maintain quiet, nonstressful environment

ndx: Alteration in cardiac output: decrease related to factors affecting preload, afterload, and myocardial contractility

GOAL: *Patient will demonstrate improved cardiac output*

Maintain position best suited to promote optimum ventilation; elevate head of bed 30 to 60 degrees; assisted ventilation may be indicated
Avoid routine nursing functions
Maintain complete bed rest
Maintain NPO
Initiate IV; maintain an open vein
Monitor ECG continuously
Measure intake and output qh
   Maintain parenteral fluids as ordered
Connect indwelling urethral catheter to closed gravity drainage system; notify physician if urinary output is less than 30 ml/hr
Check BP, R, apical pulse, and femoral pulse q15 min and prn
Monitor LAP, PAP, and PCWP qlh to 2h as ordered
Monitor intraarterial pressure qlh to 2h as ordered
Monitor cardiac output as ordered
Calculate systemic vascular resistance as ordered

$$\frac{\text{Mean aortic pressure} - \text{Mean right atrial pressure (mm Hg)}}{\text{Cardiac output (L/min)}}$$

Check CVP reading qh and prn
Check axillary temperature qh
Administer oxygen as ordered prn
Administer medications as ordered
   To decrease afterload and O_2 consumption
      Vasodilators
      Corticosteroids
      Adjust flow rate according to BP response
   To increase myocardial contractility and reduce peripheral vascular resistance (PVR)
      Sympathomimetics
      Vasodilators
      Adjust flow rate according to BP response
Administer digitalis preparations as ordered
Administer plasma volume expanders as ordered; adjust flow rate according to PAP and PCWP readings
Administer IV medications as ordered
Administer pain management as ordered
Administer oral hygiene qh; keep mouth moist
Keep patient warm and dry
Auscultate heart sounds q2h to 4h
Prepare for intraaortic balloon counterpulsation as ordered
Provide emotional support
Resume normal hygiene measures as tolerated; maintain planned rest periods
Avoid constipation, straining, or rectal stimulation; give stool softeners or laxatives as ordered

ndx: Gas exchange: impaired related to hypoventilation and/or decreased cardiac output

GOAL: *Patient will maintain adequate ventilation*

Auscultate chest for decreased or adventitious breath sounds qlh to 2h
Monitor arterial blood gases via intraarterial line as ordered
Administer oxygen as ordered
Suction as ordered to ensure patient airway
Assist and teach patient to cough and deep breathe qlh to 2h

ndx: Anxiety/fear related to actual or potential biologic threat

GOAL: *Patient will exhibit decrease in anxiety level*

Explain all procedures and treatments
Remain with patient to offer reassurance
Maintain quiet, nonstressful environment
Allow family or significant other to remain with patient as condition permits
Encourage verbalization of needs and fears of dying
Maintain calm and reassuring manner

Evaluation

Patient
- Demonstrates improved cardiac output as evidenced by
  - Vital signs within normal limits
  - CO and PCWP within normal limits
  - Improved mentation
- Demonstrates improved ventilation as evidenced by
  - Effortless breathing
  - Clear lungs
  - Po_2 and Pco_2 levels within normal limits
- Verbalizes decrease in anxiety level

CARDIAC SURGERY (OPEN-HEART PROCEDURE)*

cardiac surgery Care depends on whether the operation is an open-heart procedure, requiring use of the cardiopulmonary bypass machine, or a closed-heart procedure, requiring use of the cardiopulmonary bypass machine, or a closed-heart procedure, which does not always require use of the bypass machine

Classification of Cardiac Surgery
CLOSED-HEART SURGERY

Patent ductus arteriosus (PDA)
Coarctation of aorta
Palliative pulmonary shunts
  Blalock/Taussig
  Potts
  Glenn
Closed mitral commissurotomy

---

*The standard for postoperative care of the patient with open-heart surgery can be utilized in either the open-heart or closed-heart procedure. The patient with closed-heart surgery will usually require less specialized equipment with decreased frequency of nursing functions; however, he may have complications that would also be seen in the patient with open-heart surgery (e.g., atelectasis and hypertension).

OPEN-HEART SURGERY

Atrial septal defect (ASD)
Ventricular septal defect (VSD)
Transposition of great vessels
Tetralogy of Fallot
Truncus arteriosus
Tricuspid atresia
Aortic stenosis
Coronary artery bypass graft (CABG)
Ventricular aneurysm
Mitral commissurotomy
Mitral valve replacement
Aortic valve replacement
Aortic aneurysm
Fontan procedures for complex congenital heart defects

Preoperative Care
Assessment
Observations/findings

Level of consciousness
See Respiratory Assessment (p. 219)
Emotions
  Anxiety: adaptive vs. maladaptive
  Euphoria
  Depression
  Denial
  Fear
BP, T, P, and R
Skin
  Color
  Turgor
  Temperature
Peripheral circulation
Heart sounds
  Murmurs
  Rubs
  Gallops
Breath sounds: abnormal
  Decreased breath sounds
  Rales
  Rhonchi
  Wheezes
Smoking history
Weight and height
Activity tolerance
Medications being taken
  Cardiac medications
  Anticoagulants/antiplatelets
  Antiarrhythmics
  Birth control pills

Laboratory/diagnostic studies

ECG: acute changes, increase in arrhythmias
  12-lead
  Rhythm strip
Chest x-ray examination
  Cardiomegaly
  Pulmonary vascular congestion
CBC: Hgb, Hct
Blood type and cross match
Coagulation studies: PT, PTT, and platelets
Electrolytes
BUN
Creatine
Urinalysis
Pulmonary function
  VC
  Tidal volume
  Minute ventilation

Preoperative teaching

Involve family or significant other in care and instructions
Reinforce physician's explanation regarding
  Operative procedure
  Location, type, and length of incision(s)
  Length of time anticipated for recovery
Explain preoperative procedures
  Skin preparation: shaving, antiseptic bath or shower
  Visits from anesthesiologist and respiratory therapist
Check if dental clearance was given (dental checks should be done 10 to 14 days prior to operation)
Explain and review postoperative procedures and routines of CCU or ICU
  How special unit will differ from regular unit
  Types of noises to be experienced
  Visiting privileges
  Usual length of stay in unit
  Pain to be experienced and availability of medications as needed
  Method of communication while intubated
  Disorientation that may occur resulting from medications and/or lack of sleep
Evaluate patient's awareness, emotional status, and fears regarding
  Surgical procedure
  Heart-lung machine
  Short- and long-term outcomes
  Possible disabilities
  Previous surgical experiences
Report any *acute* changes in emotional status
  Anxiety
  Depression
  Fear of dying
Instruct patient on simple relaxation techniques such as guided imagery
Introduce patient to unit staff who will be caring for him postoperatively
When possible, introduce patient and family to CCU or ICU, explaining equipment to be used
  Cardiac monitor
  Hemodynamic monitor
  Drainage tubes
  Pacing wires, pacemaker
  Respirator
  Nebulizer
  Oxygen administration
  IV therapy
    Blood transfusions
    Replacement fluids
Review postoperative medications, particularly those that will be long term, such as anticoagulants
Review procedures for and stress importance and purpose of
  Turning
  Coughing
  Deep breathing
  Incentive spirometry
  Foot and leg exercises
Practice these procedures 1 to 2 days before operation
Withhold medications as ordered (e.g., anticoagulants)
Refer to spiritual advisor or social service worker as indicated

Postoperative Care
Assessment
Observations/findings
GENERAL

Neurologic: level of consciousness
Pulmonary
  Respirations
    Quality
    Rate
    Character
  Breath sounds: equal or decreased
    Dullness
    Rales
    Rhonchi
  Chest drainage
    Amount
    Quality
    Color

Cardiovascular
  Hemodynamic parameters
    Arterial BP
    HR, rhythm
    LAP, LVEDP, PCWP
    CVP
  Heart sounds
    Rubs
    Murmurs
  Arterial pulses
    Quality
    Rate
    Rhythm
    Equality
  Skin
    Color
    Turgor
    Temperature
  ECG: check for presence of acute changes or arrhythmias
  Pacemaker: settings
Renal
  Intake and output
  Urine output
    Amount
    Color
    Specific gravity
    Osmolality
  Electrolytes
  BUN, creatinine
Gastrointestinal
  Nasogastric tube drainage
    Amount
    Color
  Absence or presence of bowel sounds
  Abdominal tone
    Flat
    Distended
    Tenderness
  Incision(s), location
    Midsternotomy
    Submammary
    Leg

VALVE REPLACEMENT

Type of valve replaced
  Heterograft
  Mechanical
  Homograft
Valve sounds: normal
  Mechanical: opening, closing clicks
  Heterograft, homograft: produces no clicks
Valve dysfunction: occurrence of new regurgitant-type murmur
  Obstruction
  Perivalvular leak
  Rupture
Anticoagulation therapy (p. 151)
Endocarditis

CORONARY ARTERY GRAFT

Graft site
  Saphenous vein
  Mammary artery

CONGENITAL HEART DISEASE REPAIR

Type of repair: palliative, correction
Use of conduits, grafts, baffles

Laboratory/diagnostic studies

CBC, chemistries, platlet function
Arterial blood gases
Chest x-ray examination

Potential complications
GENERAL

Cardiovascular
  Arrhythmias
    Premature ventricular contractions (PVCs)
    Ventricular tachycardia
    Atrial fibrillation
    Atrial flutter
    Asystole
    Complete heart block
    Elevated PAP, LAP, and PCWP
    Low CO syndrome
      Restlessness
      Lethargy
      Skin: cool, pale, peripheral cyanosis
    Tachycardia
    Decreased arterial pressure
    Decreased urine output
    Increased PCWP and LAP
    Increased SVR
  Hypertension
  Hemorrhage
    Increased drainage through chest tubes
    Presence of bright red drainage
    Adults: blood loss >150 ml/hr
    Children: blood loss >5 ml/kg/hr
    Decreased Hct
    Hypotension
  Pericarditis

Cardiac tamponade
Shock
  Cardiogenic
  Hypovolemic
Heart failure
Endocarditis
Postpericardiotomy syndrome
Venous thrombosis
Pulmonary
  Atelectasis
  Pneumonitis
  Respiratory acidosis
  Pleural effusions
  Tension pneumothorax
  Respiratory failure
Neurologic
  Altered level of consciousness
  Postpump psychosis
    Restlessness
    Agitation
    Confusion
    Combativeness
    Visual and auditory disturbances
    Transient perceptual disorientation
  Cerebral embolism (CVA, p. 296)
Renal
  Electrolyte imbalance
    Hyponatremia
    Hypokalemia
  Metabolic
    Acidosis
    Alkalosis
  Hypovolemia
    Decreased BP
    Tachycardia
    Low PAP
    Oliguria
Gastrointestinal
  Stress ulcers
  Paralytic ileus
Systemic infection: elevated temperature

VALVE REPLACEMENT

Disintegration of prosthesis
Vegetations from resected valve

MITRAL VALVE REPLACEMENT

Brain embolism
Supraventricular tachyarrhythmias
  Atrial tachycardia
  Rapid atrial fibrillation
Low CO syndrome

TRICUSPID VALVE REPLACEMENT/AORTIC VALVE REPLACEMENT

Conduction defects
Subendocardial necrosis

CORONARY ARTERY BYPASS GRAFT

Acute myocardial infarction
Ventricular arrhythmias
  PVC
  Ventricular tachycardia
Low CO syndrome
Graft failure
  Angina

CONGENITAL HEART DISEASE REPAIR

Conduction defects
Atrial arrhythmias
Conduit obstruction
Patch leaks

Medical management

Admission to cardiac intensive care unit
Oxygen therapy with mechanical assisted ventilation
Cardiac monitor
Hemodynamic monitoring
Medications
  Narcotics, analgesics
  Antihypertensives
  Antiarrhythmics
  Introtropic agents
    Dopamine
    Dobutamine
    Digoxin
  Vasodilators
  Anticoagulants
  Electrolytes
Parenteral therapy
  Blood replacement
  Plasma expanders
  Colloids
Pacemaker insertion
Intraaortic balloon pump (IABP)

Nursing diagnoses/goals/interventions (adults)

ndx Impaired gas exchange related to hypoventilation, atelectasis, and/or ventilation/perfusion abnormalities

GOAL: *Patient will maintain adequate oxygenation and ventilation*

Maintain patent airway
Administer oxygen and assisted ventilation as ordered

Elevate head of bed to 45 degrees; supine position
Check quality and rate of R
Check FIO_2 tidal volume to yield arterial Po_2 of about 100 mm Hg
Measure arterial blood gases as ordered; observe for and report signs of respiratory alkalosis or acidosis
Auscultate chest for diminished or adventitious breath sounds q1h to 2h
Suction q1h to 2h
Oxygenate 1 to 2 min prior to and following procedures
Watch for and record any arrhythmias during procedure
Assist and teach patient to turn; percuss chest and reposition q2h
Assist and teach patient to turn, cough, and deep breathe q1h to 2h in absence of endotracheal tube
Use high-humidity face mask after extubation
Perform chest x-ray examination q4h to 6h as ordered

ndx: Alteration in cardiac output: decreased related to mechanical factors (altered preload, afterload, contractility, heart rate)

GOAL: *Patient will demonstrate improved cardiac output*

Maintain bed rest with head of bed elevated 45 degrees
Check BP, apical pulse, and peripheral pulses q15 to 30 min for 2h, then qh as ordered, reporting
  Systolic BP: drop of 20 mm Hg
  Systolic <80 or >180
  Diastolic BP >100
  Decreased amplitude in pulses
  Pulse rate <60 or >100 beats/min
Connect pressure lines: arterial PA, LA, and venous; record pressures q1h to 2h
Calculate CO and SVR as ordered
Check temperature on admission, q1h × 6, then q4h
Initiate rewarming procedures
  Blankets
  Heat lamp
Auscultate chest for heart sounds q2h to 4h
Monitor urine output q1h; report outputs <30 ml/h
Administer fluids, blood products, and medications as ordered
Perform laboratory studies q4h to 6h as ordered
  Cardiac enzymes, CPK-MB, SGOT, LDH
  Electrolytes and potassium levels (checked more frequently)
  Hgb, Hct

Initiate IABP as ordered
Avoid valsalva maneuvers, such as constipation
  Bedside commode
  Stool softeners
  Mild laxative
For arrhythmias
  Take and record ECG rhythm strips qh; measure rate plus PR, QRS, and QT intervals
  Watch for and record any arrhythmias during procedure and report to physician
  Monitor for fluid and electrolyte disturbances
  Perform blood studies q4h to 6h or as indicated: electrolytes, potassium
  Connect pacemaker when ordered; check rate and milliamperes (MA)
  Administer antiarrhythmic agents as ordered
  Administer medications to correct electrolyte imbalances and/or hypoxia

ndx: Injury potential: hemorrhage related to surgically induced fibrinolysis and/or inadequate reversal of heparin

GOAL: *Patient will demonstrate adequate hemostasis*

Monitor for clinical signs of excessive bleeding
Perform blood studies q4h to 6h as ordered
  Hgb, Hct
  Coagulation: PT, PTT, platlet count
Measure chest drainage qh; report drainage in excess of 150 to 200 ml/hr
Administer transfusions, platlets, and plasma expanders as ordered
Administer drugs to correct coagulopathy
  Protamine sulfate
  6-aminocaproic acid (Amicar)
  Epsilon aminocaproic acid (EACA)
  Vitamin K
Check dressings q1h to 2h
  Note drainage, amount, color, and consistency
  Change as indicated

ndx: Ineffective breathing pattern related to pleural effusion

GOAL: *Patient will demonstrate fully expanded lung: bilateral equal excursion, breath sounds*

Connect chest tubes to drainage and suction as ordered; check patency and record amount and color q1h to 2h and prn
Auscultate chest for diminished breath sounds q1h to 2h

Assist patient to cough and deep breathe q1h to 2h

Assist and encourage patient to use incentive spirometry

Administer oxygen therapy as ordered

ndx Potential for infection

GOAL: *Patient will demonstrate absence of infection*

Observe suture sites for local redness, drainage, and swelling

Check rectal, oral, or axillary temperature q2h as indicated

Change incisional dressings daily

Administer antibiotics as ordered

Change IV and pressure lines and dressings as ordered
- IV: q48h
- Arterial: q4d
- Central: q3d to 4d

Remove urethral catheter when patient awakens or as soon as possible

Obtain laboratory studies as indicated
- CBC with differential
- Blood and urine cultures

ndx Alteration in fluid volume: excess related to physiologic effects of cardiopulmonary bypass and extravascular fluid shifts

GOAL: *Patient will demonstrate a stable fluid balance*

During rewarming check RAP, LAP, and PAP q5 min, then q30 to 60 min

Maintain parenteral fluids as ordered
- Limit fluid intake as ordered
- Titrate according to LAP, PCWP, and CVP

Know approximate fluid allowances
- CABG: 2000 ml/24 hr
- Valve replacement: 1000 to 1500 ml/24 hr
- Congenital heart defect surgery after bypass
  - 60 ml/kg for first 10 kg body weight
  - 30 ml/kg for next 10 kg body weight
  - 15 ml/kg for remainder of weight

Maintain NPO

Connect indwelling catheter to closed urinary drainage system

Measure intake and output qh; record color and specific gravity of urinary drainage

Weigh patient q8h as ordered (weight change of 1 kg indicates loss or gain of 2.2 lb)

Maintain diet progression from clear liquid to regular diet; restrict sodium as ordered—2 g sodium

ndx Alteration in thought process related to biophysiologic changes (cerebral hypoxia, age, metabolic alterations, CNS depressants, sleep deprivation)

GOAL: *Patient will regain baseline level of consciousness*

Check LOC and neuro signs q15 to 30 min for 2 hr, then qh or as indicated

Deal with any personality or psychologic changes
- Use reality orientation
- Offer explanations to all procedures
- Administer sedatives as ordered
- Reorient patient to time of day and surroundings
- Use simple, clear sentence structure
- Anticipate needs
- Maintain quiet environment; minimize external stimuli as much as possible
- Remain with patient

Allow family to visit and participate in care when possible

Provide assurance of daily progress

Maintain patient safety; use soft restraints

ndx Knowledge deficit regarding health care and follow-up management care

GOAL: *Patient and/or significant other will demonstrate adequate knowledge and skills to support needed self-care activities through interactive discussion and actual return demonstration*

Explain nature and type of operative procedure

Explain precautions and complications associated with surgery

Discuss body image changes and changes in sexuality

Explain importance of limitations and allowances as related to preoperative status

Discuss need to become independent; avoid being overprotective

Explain need to ambulate to tolerance; to avoid excessive physical exertion

Explain need to maintain a progressive activity program (p. 116)

Explain need to avoid fatigue

Explain need to avoid sitting for long periods of time

Explain that sexual activity may be contraindicated for 2 to 4 weeks; need to check with physician when feasible to resume

Discuss medications: name, dosage, time of administration, purpose, and side effects

Explain need to avoid taking over-the-counter medication without checking with physician

Discuss diet as ordered and explain need to avoid overeating
  Refer to dietition for specific diets
  Restrict salt intake
Explain need to weigh daily if ordered
Discuss symptoms to report to physician
  Shortness of breath
  Swelling of hands and legs
Explain importance of wearing medical alert band if patient has (is taking)
  Prosthetic valve
  Pacemaker (p. 134)
  Anticoagulants (p. 151)
Explain need to avoid persons with infections, especially URI
Discuss symptoms of wound infection to report to physician
  Elevated temperature
  Rapid, irregular pulse
  Chills
  Anorexia
  Redness
  Pain
  Swelling
  Drainage
Care of incision
Importance of ongoing care
Importance of contacting spiritual advisor or social worker as necessary

Valve replacement

Explain importance of anticoagulation therapy
  Mechanical valves: life-long therapy
  Heterografts: 3 to 6 months as ordered
Explain importance of reporting to physician signs and symptoms of endocarditis
  Elevated temperature
  Chills, diaphoresis
  Anorexia
Explain importance of reporting to physician any event that may predispose to bacteremia
  Dental and gum manipulation
  Genitourinary procedures
  Gynecologic procedures (D & C)
  Childbirth
  Skin boils, infective acne
Explain importance of notifying all physicians, dentists, urologists, and obstetricians of valve replacement
Explain need to maintain good oral hygiene
  Daily care
  Regular visits to dentist
  (NOTE: Patient should wait 6 weeks after surgery before seeing a dentist)
Explain significance of prophylactic antibiotic therapy prior to procedures that predispose to bacteremia

Evaluation

Patient
  Demonstrates adequate ventilation as evidenced by
    Effortless breathing
    Absence of respiratory complications
    Clear, equal, and bilateral breath sounds
    Po_2 and Pco_2 within normal limits
  Demonstrates improved cardiac output as evidenced by
    Vital signs within normal limits
    CO, LVEDP, and PCWP within acceptable limits
    Increased activity tolerance
  Demonstrates stable hemostasis as evidenced by
    Progressive decline in chest tube drainage
    Stable or improved Hct, Hgb
  Shows no sign of infection
  Demonstrates baseline level of consciousness
  Exhibits no signs of fluid overload
    Absence of edema, no jugular venous distention (JVD)
    Weight loss, return to baseline
  Verbalizes understanding of clinical status and demonstrates skills and understanding in home health management

POST–CARDIAC INJURY SYNDROME

A group of signs and symptoms that occur following injury to the myocardium or pericardial cavity, which are thought to be due to the immune response or hypersensitivity reaction to pericardial injury

postcardiotomy *Following cardiac surgery (usually 7 to 10 days after surgery)*
postmyocardial infarction syndrome *(Dressler's syndrome) A late-appearing autoimmune response to myocardial necrosis; symptoms usually appear 3 to 6 weeks following MI*

Assessment
Observations/findings

Elevated temperature
Diaphoresis
Chest discomfort or pain
Pericardial friction rub
Dyspnea

Malaise
Arthralgias
Anxiety
    Worry
    Fear of consequences

Laboratory/diagnostic studies

Leukocytosis
Increased ESR
Chest x-ray examination: pleural effusions
Echocardiogram: pericardial effusion

Potential complications

Pericarditis
Cardiac tamponade

Medical management

Medications
    Aspirin
    Indomethacin
    Corticosteroids

Nursing diagnoses/goals/interventions

ndx: Alteration in comfort related to chest discomfort and fever

GOAL: *Patient demonstrates that comfort level has been achieved*

Maintain bed rest as ordered
    Elevate head of bed 45 degrees
    Provide padded overbed table
Check BP, T, R, and apical pulse q4h
Auscultate heart sounds q6h to 8h
Administer medications as ordered
    Analgesics
    Antiinflammatory agents
    Antipyretics
Maintain diet as ordered
Provide emotional support; explain procedures, treatment

ndx: Anxiety related to knowledge deficit

GOAL: *Patient will demonstrate reduced anxiety level*

Explain that syndrome commonly occurs following trauma or injury to heart and pericardial cavity and may clear up without specific treatment
Explain symptoms to report to physician
    Elevated temperature
    Chest pain
    Chills, diaphoresis
    Difficult respirations

Explain need to avoid fatigue to alternate periods of activity with rest
Discuss name of medication, dosage, times of administration, purpose, and side effects

Evaluation

Patient
    Demonstrates that comfort level has been achieved; activity returns to normal
    Demonstrates reduced level of anxiety
        Verbalizes insight into causes of symptoms and appropriate actions to take for signs and symptoms
        Appears calm

CARDIAC REHABILITATION

*Physical and psychologic restoration of the patient with heart disease to an enjoyable and productive life as efficiently as possible; suggested for patients with angina, cardiomyopathy, pacemakers, and congenital heart disease and for patients recovering from myocardial infarction, valve surgery, and coronary artery bypass surgery**

Inpatient Program

Assessment

Observations/findings

CRITERIA FOR TERMINATING

Symptoms during activity and/or 30 min following activity or exercise session
    Severe dyspnea
    Chest pain
    Vertigo
    Diaphoresis
    Fatigue
    Leg claudication
    Disorientation or confusion
    Palpitations
Heart rate
    Increase greater than 20 to 25 beats/min during activity or exercise
    Appearance of irregular rhythm
On telemetry: during exercise and rest periods
    ST elevation of 3 mm or more
    ST segment depression of 2 mm
    Multiple premature ventricular beats (PVCs)

---

*Definition from Guidelines for Cardiac Rehabilitation Centers, 1985, copyright the American Heart Association Greater Los Angeles Affiliate.

Atrioventricular (AV) block
Paroxysmal atrial tachycardia
BP
   Drop of 15 to 20 mm Hg when patient stands
   Decrease in pulse pressure
   Increase in systolic-diastole pressures: greater than 20 mm Hg

Medical management

Prescription for inclusion to program
Prescription for activity order

Interventions

MI
   Maintain bed rest for first 3 to 4 days except for use of bedside commode
   Progress to chair rest
   Avoid prolonged bed rest
CABG
   Maintain bed rest for first 1 to 2 days postoperatively or as ordered by physician
   Start activity levels within 24 hr or as ordered by physician

Activity progression program

Follow physician's orders for progressive activity program
Initiate program using a predeveloped in-hospital exercise program (e.g., Table 2-5)
Evaluate patient's progress on a daily basis and plan activity levels for the day (done by rehabilitation team and/or charge nurse and physician)
Increase activity levels gradually until discharge date
Avoid exercises
   After meals; allow 1 hr
   In the presence of arrhythmias
   In the presence of CHF
Begin exercise program while patient is on telemetry
Record and report any signs or symptoms of shortness of breath, fatigue, or nausea if they occur during or up to 24 hr following exercise
Obtain the following baseline information prior to activity
   On telemetry
      ECG rhythm strip, noting rate and rhythm
      Resting BP, P, and R, noting rate, rhythm, and quality

TABLE 2-5. Cardiac Rehabilitation Program: Inpatient Activity (Myocardial Infarction)*

Level	Self-care activities	Position	Exercises	Repetitions	Education
Level I (1 to 1.5 MET†)	1. Absolute bedrest, complete bed bath 2. Begin feeding self while sitting with head of bed elevated to 45 degrees and arms supported 3. Turn self	1. Supine Advance to: Supine 2. Supine	a. Passive ROM: all extremities (excluding shoulders in acute MI) b. Active exercises: all extremities except shoulders as tolerated Deep breathing exercises: all levels	5 times 3 times	
Level II (1.5 to 2.5 MET [except bedside commode])	4. Bedrest 5. Feed self, wash face and hands, brush teeth, and shave in bed 6. Bedside commode (3 MET) 7. Up in chair 20-30 minutes bid 8. Light recreational activity such as reading, writing	3. Supine	Active plantar and dorsiflexion ankle exercises qid		
Level III (1.5 to 3 MET)	9. In bed, patient assists with self bath (not legs or back) 10. Stand patient and take vital signs	4. Supine	a. Advance active exercises to include neck rotation and shoulder flexion to 90 degrees as tolerated	5 times	Begin education a. Energy conservation b. Body mechanics

Adapted from Guidelines for cardiac rehabilitation centers, June 1985, copyright the American Heart Association Greater Los Angeles Affiliate.
*Recommended levels and times are for average patients and must be individualized.
†MET = metabolic equivalent; the amount of oxygen consumed per kilogram of body weight per minute at rest. Approximately 3.5 cc/kg/min.

TABLE 2-5. Cardiac Rehabilitation Program: Inpatient Activity (Myocardial Infarction)—cont'd

Level	Self-care activities	Position	Exercises	Repetitions	Education
Level III—cont'd	11. May walk to bathroom with help 12. Walk to chair and sit 15 to 30 minutes tid		b. Active exercises: all limbs including shoulder flexion to 180 degrees	5 times	c. Concepts of heart anatomy and physiology
		Sitting	c. Knee extension and hip flexion	3 times	
		Advance to:			
		5. Supine	a. Active exercises: all extremities	7 times	
		Sitting	b. Knee extension and hip flexion	7 times	
		Sitting	c. Shoulder flexion to 90 degrees	7 times	
Level IV (3 MET)	13. Same bath 9 14. Begin dressing self (gown and pajamas) 15. If vital signs stable, see 10, walk to bathroom for toilet use only 16. Sit in chair 2 to 3 times a day 30 to 60 min with assistance	6. Supine Sitting 7. Supine	a. Exercise 5a b. Exercise 5b Instruct patient to perform independent exercise 3 times a day (patient to take own pulse)	7 times 7 times 5 times	d. Begin instruction in self heart rate measurement e. Discuss inpatient activity: importance of pacing, rest, relaxation f. Dietary assessment and referral if appropriate g. Begin discussion of: Signs and symptoms Risk factor Medication Warning signs Sexual counseling Activity progress
Level V	17. Sponge bathe self, sitting in bathroom (nurse bathes back) 18. Up in room and chair ad lib 19. Ambulate in hall 5 to 10 min with telemetry bid		Active exercises 5a, b, c walk slow pace one half length of corridor (50 feet) with telemetry		
Level VI (3 to 4 MET)	20. Sit down shower 21. Wash hair while seated 22. Shave, apply makeup in sitting position 23. Sit for meals 24. Full bathroom privileges 25. Up and about in room 26. Ambulate in hall 5 to 10 min bid with telemetry	8. Supine 9. Sitting 10. Walk 11. Ascend 12.	Active exercise 5a Active exercise 5b Increase distance walked as tolerated using moderate pace Three to six stair steps as tolerated May transport to cardiac rehabilitation center for low level activity or test	5 to 7 times 7 times	Complete home instruction a. Diet b. Medications c. Activity allowances and limitations
Level VII (4 to 5 MET)	27. Same as level VI with addition of walking in hall 150 feet, advancing as tolerated 28. Evaluate any special requirements for home activities	13.	Continue stairs and ambulation as tolerated		
Level VIII	29. Same as level VI and VII, advancing in frequency, distance, and time	14.	Establish progressive home activity program		

Off telemetry
  Resting BP, P, and R, noting rate, rhythm, and quality
Assist patient with performing activity
Obtain peak exercise heart rate
Obtain the following information during and 2 min following exercise
  On telemetry
    ECG rhythm strip toward end of activity, noting rate, rhythm, and ST segment changes or arrhythmias
    Postexercise heart rate
  Off telemetry
    BP and heart rate at 1 and 2 min intervals at end of exercise and at any signs of fatigue, pain, or shortness of breath
Observe and report patient's tolerance

Patient teaching/discharge outcome

Ensure that patient and/or significant other knows and understands
  Normal function of the heart
  Nature and causes of coronary heart disease
  Importance of identifying risk factors and need to modify or eliminate personal risk factors profile
    Family history of heart disease
    Patient history of heart disease
    Diabetes
    High blood pressure
    Overweight
    High cholesterol and/or triglyceride level
    Smoking
    Sedentary job and/or life-style
    Stressful life-style
  Dietary restrictions and limitations
  Importance of maintaining weight control
  Importance of verbalizing any questions and feelings regarding presence of heart disease
  Importance of verbalizing any feelings of anxiety and fear regarding sexual impotency, return to work, and death
  Warning signs and symptoms of overexercising to report to physician
    Excessive fatigue
    Chest discomfort
    Muscle pain
    Dizziness
    Shortness of breath
    Palpitations
  Physician's explanation of prescribed exercise program, allowances, and limitations
  Need to avoid isometric (static) activities and/or exercises (e.g., pushing heavy objects, doing push-ups, or carrying heavy objects)
  Importance of taking and recording heart rate before and following exercise, noting rate and rhythm
  Importance of reporting heart rate increase of greater than 20 to 25 beats/min
  Recommended limitations and allowances for first 2 weeks following discharge
    Avoid heavy lifting and pushing
    Refrain from extensive housework and gardening
    Avoid sitting in same position for longer than 2 hr
    Plan regular rest periods for at least twice a day
    Avoid vigorous arm and shoulder exercises, especially those that require arms to be held above shoulders (e.g., washing windows or painting house)
    Space activities, alternating activity with rest period
    Avoid exercising at the following times
      After meals; wait 1 hr
      When feeling very tired
      When suffering from a cold or other illness
    Stop activity at onset of warning signs and rest
  Importance of avoiding sexual activity for at least 2 weeks (check with physician when feasible to resume; once resumed, avoid after eating heavy meals, drinking alcoholic beverages in excess, or becoming emotionally stressed)
  Need to avoid travel by car, bus, airplane, or train without first checking with physician
  That all walking or exercise activities must be preceded by warm-up exercises (i.e., stretching and knee bends)

Prescribed Exercise Program

INITIAL POSTDISCHARGE ACTIVITIES FOR CARDIOVASCULAR RECONDITIONING

Continue predischarge activities; actively exercise all extremities, including shoulder flexion and knee extension
Distance walking

Week after discharge	Total distance (mile)	Time (min)
1	0.25	8 to 10
2	0.25	5
3	0.5	15
4	1.0	30

Adjust speed and time to maintain heart rate at less than 100 beats/min

Exercise Record: Target heart rate: _____ beats/min

Date	Resting heart rate	Distance	Time	Peak heart rate	Comment
1-3-88	80	¼ mile	5 min	100	No complaints

Record all exercise sessions, noting distance, time, and resting and peak heart rates (see chart above)
Follow all exercise sessions with a cooling down period

CARDIOVASCULAR RECONDITIONING PROGRAM

Ordered approximately 6 to 8 weeks following discharge (done by physician)
Follow prescription for exercise determined by treadmill stress test prior to start of program

ECG RHYTHMS

Rhythms of Sinus Origin

Rhythms originating in the sinus (sinoatrial; SA) node (Located in the right atrium near the opening of the superior vena cava, the sinus node functions as the normal pacemaker of the heart.)

NORMAL SINUS RHYTHM (Figure 2-12)
Assessment
Observations/findings

Rhythm: regular
Rate: 60 to 100 beats/min

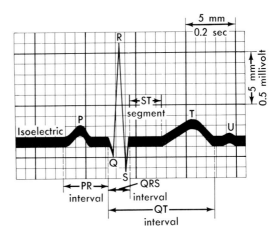

FIGURE 2-10. Normal ECG complex.

P wave: normal configuration, one before each QRS
PR interval: 0.12 to 0.20 sec
QRS complex: 0.06 to 0.10 sec

Medical management

None indicated

SINUS BRADYCARDIA (Figure 2-13)

A sinus rhythm of less than 60 beats/min; etiology— may be normal or occur in response to drugs or increased vagal tone

Assessment
Observations/findings

Faintness
Dizziness
Syncope
Rhythm: regular

TABLE 2-6. Meaning and Significance of ECG Intervals*

Description	Duration	Significance of disturbance
PR interval: from beginning of P wave to beginning of QRS complex; represents time taken for impulse to spread through the atria, AV node and His bundle, the bundle branches and Purkinje fibers, to a point immediately preceding ventricular activation	0.12 to 0.20 sec	Disturbance in conduction, usually in AV node, His bundle, or bundle branches but can be in atria as well
QRS interval: from beginning to end of QRS complex; represents time taken for a depolarization of both ventricles	0.06 to 0.10 sec	Disturbance in conduction in bundle branches and/or in ventricles
QT interval: from beginning of QRS to end of T wave; represents time taken for entire electrical depolarization and repolarization of the ventricles	0.36 to 0.44 sec	Disturbances usually affecting repolarization more than depolarization such as drug effects, electrolyte disturbances, and rate changes

From Andreoli, K., et al.: Comprehensive cardiac care: a text for nurses, physicians, and other health practitioners, ed. 4, St. Louis, 1979, The C.V. Mosby Co.
*Heart rate influences the duration of these intervals, especially that of the PR and QT intervals.

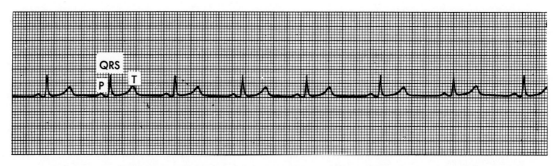

FIGURE 2-11. Cardiac cycle. Basic cardiac cycle (P = QRS = T). (From Goldberger, A.L., and Goldberger, E.: Clinical electrocardiology: a simplified approach, ed. 3, St. Louis, 1986, The C.V. Mosby Co.)

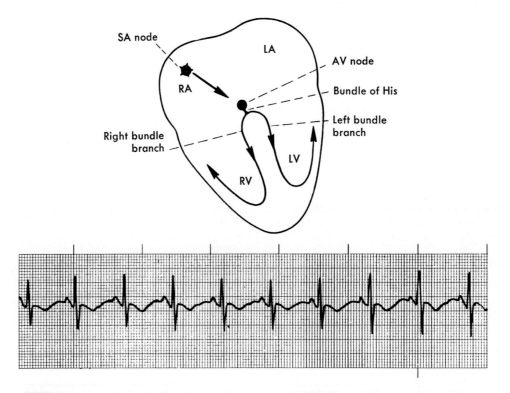

FIGURE 2-12. Normal sinus rhythm. (From Andreoli, K.: Comprehensive cardiac care: a text for nurses, physicians, and other health practitioners, ed. 5, St. Louis, 1983, The C.V. Mosby Co.)

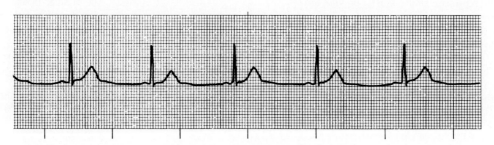

FIGURE 2-13. Sinus bradycardia. (From Andreoli, K., et al.: Comprehensive cardiac care: a text for nurses, physicians, and other health practitioners, ed. 5, St. Louis, 1983, The C.V. Mosby Co.)

Rate: below 60 beats/min
P wave: normal configuration, one before each
　QRS
　PR interval: 0.12 to 0.20 sec
　QRS complex: 0.06 to 0.10 sec

Medical management

Medications
　Atropine
　Isoproterenol
　Pacing: atrial, ventricular

Interventions

Check BP and apical pulse q4h and prn
Monitor cardiac activity; check rhythm strips q6h to 8h and prn
Administer oxygen therapy as ordered

Patient teaching

Ensure that patient and/or significant other knows and understands
　How to take radial pulse
　Pacemaker insertion (p. 134), if appropriate

SINUS TACHYCARDIA (Figure 2-14)

A sinus rhythm of greater than 100 beats/min; causes—drugs, exercise, emotions, fever, increased sympathetic stimulation

Assessment

Observations/findings

Fatigue
Shortness of breath
Rhythm: regular
Rate: 100 to 160 beats/min
P wave: normal configuration, one before each QRS
PR interval: 0.12 to 0.20 sec
QRS complex: 0.06 to 0.10 sec

Medical management

Treatment of underlying disease
Carotid sinus massage

Interventions

Administer medications as ordered
Maintain bed rest as indicated
Check BP, R, and apical puse q4h to 6h and prn
Administer oxygen therapy as ordered

SINUS ARRHYTHMIA (Figure 2-15)

An irregular sinus rhythm that is normally found in children and young adults; causes—respiratory variation

Assessment

Observations/findings

Rhythm: irregular
Rate: 60 to 90 beats/min; may increase with inspiration and decrease with expiration
P wave: normal configuration, one before each QRS complex
PR interval: 0.12 to 0.20 sec
QRS complex: 0.06 to 0.10 sec

Medical management

None indicated

SINUS ARREST (Figure 2-16)

A rhythm in which a sinus impulse is not generated; causes—may be drug induced, coronary artery disease, increased vagal tone

Assessment

Observations/findings

Dizziness
Syncope
Rhythm: irregular during periods of arrest

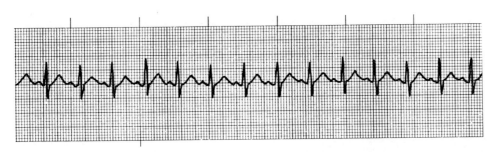

FIGURE 2-14. Sinus tachycardia. (From Andreoli, K., et al.: Comprehensive cardiac care: a text for nurses, physicians, and other health practitioners, ed. 5, St. Louis, 1983, The C.V. Mosby Co.)

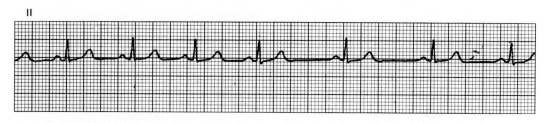

FIGURE 2-15. Sinus arrhythmia. (From Conover, M.B.: Exercises in diagnosing ECG tracings, ed. 3, St. Louis, 1984, The C.V. Mosby Co.)

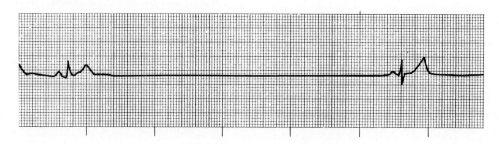

FIGURE 2-16. Sinus arrest. (From Andreoli, K., et al.: Comprehensive cardiac care: a text for nurses, physicians, and other health practitioners, ed. 5, St. Louis, 1983, The C.V. Mosby Co.)

Rate: 60 to 90 beats/min
P wave: absent during periods of arrest
PR interval: absent during periods of arrest
QRS complex: absent during periods of arrest

Potential complications

Ventricular standstill

Medical management

Medications: atropine
Cardiac pacing
Parenteral fluids
Cardiopulmonary resuscitation (CPR)

Interventions

Monitor cardiac activity; check rhythm strips q4h to 6h and prn
Maintain bed rest as indicated
Check BP, R, and apical pulse q4h to 6h and prn
Administer oxygen therapy as indicated

Rhythms of Atrial Origin

Supraventricular or atrial rhythms that originate outside the SA node and above the bundle of His

PREMATURE ATRIAL CONTRACTIONS (PACs) (Figures 2-17 and 2-18)

premature atrial beats *Ectopic beats generated outside the SA node; causes—anxiety, ingestion of tobacco, caffeine, electrolyte imbalance, hypoxia, drug toxicity*

Assessment

Observations/findings

Palpitations: skipped beats
Anxiety
Dizziness
Atrial flutter
Rhythm: irregular in presence of PACs
Rate: may be normal or irregular in presence of ectopic beats
P wave: premature P wave is distorted; may be inverted or fused on preceding T wave
PR interval: may be prolonged
QRS complex: abnormal conduction in ectopic beat; no QRS will follow in blocked P wave

Laboratory/diagnostic studies

Holter examination

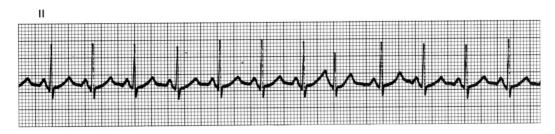

FIGURE 2-17. Premature atrial contraction. (From Conover, M.B.: Exercises in diagnosing ECG tracings, ed. 3, St. Louis, 1984, The C.V. Mosby Co.)

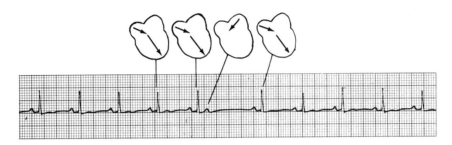

FIGURE 2-18. Nonconducted premature atrial contraction (PAC). (From Conover, M.B.: Understanding electrocardiography: arrhythmias and the 12-lead ECG, ed. 4, St. Louis, 1984, The C.V. Mosby Co.)

Medical management

Treatment of underlying disease none indicated for occasional PACs
Medications: antiarrhythmics

Interventions

Monitor cardiac activity; check rhythm strips q4h to 6h and prn
Check BP, R, and apical pulse q6h to 8h
Restrict caffeine and nicotine as ordered

ATRIAL FLUTTER (Figure 2-19)

A rapid, regular ectopic atrial rhythm with characteristic "flutter" waves; causes—most forms of cardiac disease

Assessment

Observations/findings

Tachycardia
Tachypnea
Palpitations
Shortness of breath
Rhythm
   Atrial: regular
   Ventricular: may be regular or irregular

Rate
   Atrial: 250 to 350 beats/min
   Ventricular: 100 to 150 beats/min
   PR interval: unmeasurable
   P wave: absent; rhythm shows F waves in sawtooth shape
   QRS complex: usually normal

Potential complications

CHF
Shock

Medical management

Treatment of underlying disease
Cardioversion
Carotid massage
Medications
   Antiarrhythmics
   Digitalis preparations
Atrial pacing
12-lead ECG

Interventions

Monitor cardiac activity; check rhythm strips q4h to 6h and prn

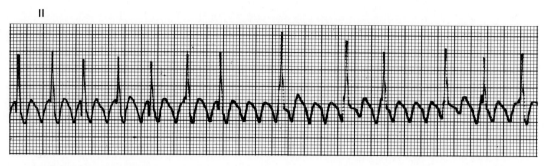

FIGURE 2-19. Atrial flutter. (From Conover, M.B.: Exercises in diagnosing ECG tracings, ed. 3, St. Louis, 1984, The C.V. Mosby Co.)

Check BP, R, and apical pulse q2h to 4h
Maintain bed rest as indicated
Administer oxygen therapy as ordered

ATRIAL FIBRILLATION (Figure 2-20)

A rapid, irregular, ectopic atrial rhythm with characteristic "fibrillatory" activity; causes—coronary artery disease (CAD), valvular heart disease, hypertension, increased left atrial size in the elderly

Assessment
Observations/findings

Palpitations
Faintness
Tachycardia
Irregular pulse
Pulse deficit (apical and radial pulses)
Chest discomfort
Rhythm: irregular
Rate
  Atrial: 350 beats/min
  Ventricular: 90 to 100 beats/min
PR interval: unmeasurable
P wave: absent; rhythm shows f waves that are seen as undulations
QRS complex: usually normal

Potential complications

Mural thrombi
CHF
Shock

Medical management

Medications: antiarrhythmics
Cardioversion
12-lead ECG

Interventions

Monitor cardiac activity; check rhythm strips q4h to 8h and prn
Check BP, R, and apical pulse q4h to 6h and prn
Administer oxygen therapy as ordered

PAROXYSMAL ATRIAL TACHYCARDIA (PAT) (Figure 2-21)

An ectopic atrial rhythm that is regular and may start and stop abruptly; causes—precipitated by sympathetic stimulation (e.g., emotion, caffeine, tobacco, fatigue, excessive alcohol intake)

Assessment
Observations/findings

Palpitations
Shortness of breath
Lightheadedness
Hypokalemia
Chest pain or discomfort
Abdominal discomfort
Tachycardia of short or prolonged duration
Rate: 150 to 200 beats/min
P wave: normal or buried in QRS or T wave; may not be visible
PR interval: usually normal
QRS complex: usually normal

Laboratory/diagnostic studies

Holter examination

Potential complications

CHF
Shock
Rhythm: usually regular

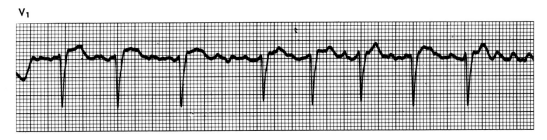

FIGURE 2-20. Atrial fibrillation. (From Conover, M.B.: Exercises in diagnosing ECG tracings, ed. 3, St. Louis, 1984, The C.V. Mosby Co.)

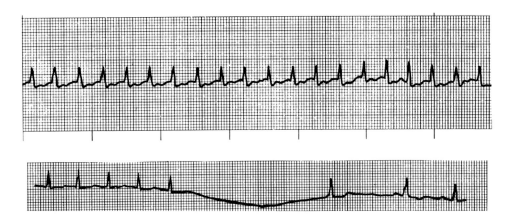

FIGURE 2-21. Paroxysmal atrial tachycardia (PAT). (From Andreoli, K., et al.: Comprehensive cardiac care: a text for nurses, physicians, and other health practitioners, ed. 5, St. Louis, 1983, The C.V. Mosby Co.)

Medical management

Carotid massage
Medications
    Antiarrhythmics
    Vagotonic preparations
Cardioversion
Atrial or ventricular pacing
12-lead ECG

Interventions

Monitor cardiac activity; check rhythm strips q4h to 6h and prn
Administer oxygen therapy as ordered
Check BP, R, and apical pulse q2h to 4h
Maintain bed rest as indicated
Check serum potassium level if patient is taking digitalis preparations
Maintain quiet environment

Rhythms of Ventricular Origin

Rhythms that occur as either escape or reentry (overdrive) rhythms arising within the ventricles

PREMATURE VENTRICULAR CONTRACTIONS (PVCs)
(Figures 2-22 and 2-23)

Premature beats arising in the ventricles below the bundle of His; may be a forerunner of ventricular tachycardia and ventricular fibrillation; causes—increased sympathetic stimulation (e.g., caffeine, tobacco, emotion), most forms of heart disease, electrolyte imbalance

Assessment
Observations/findings

Palpitations
Precordial pain
Dizziness
Faintness

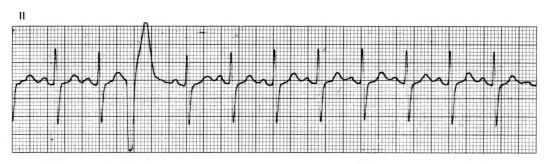

FIGURE 2-22. Premature ventricular contraction (PVC). (From Conover, M.B.: Exercises in diagnosing ECG tracings, ed. 3, St. Louis, 1984, The C.V. Mosby Co.)

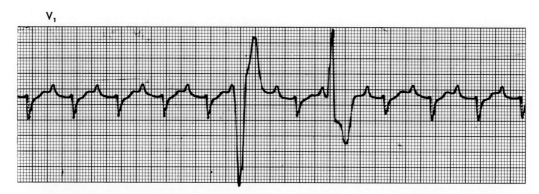

FIGURE 2-23. Multifocal premature ventricular contractions (PVCs). (From Conover, M.B.: Exercises in diagnosing ECG tracings, ed. 3, St. Louis, 1984, The C.V. Mosby Co.)

Momentary loss of consciousness
Rhythm: irregular
Rate
  Atrial: normal
  Ventricular: rapid
P wave: does not precede premature beat; premature beat is usually followed by complete compensatory pause
PR interval: unmeasurable
QRS complex: premature beat is wide and bizarre in appearance, lasting longer than 0.12 sec

Laboratory/diagnostic studies

Holter examination

Potential complications

Ventricular tachycardia
Ventricular fibrillation

Medical management

Treatment of underlying disease
Medications: antiarrhythmics

12-lead ECGs for
  Multifocal PVCs
  R on T phenomenon
  Coupling or paired PVCs
  Six or more PVCs/min

Interventions

Monitor cardiac activity; check rhythm strips q4h to 6h and prn; report if more than 6 PVCs/min or if they occur close to preceding T waves
Check BP, R, and apical pulse q4h to 6h and prn
Administer oxygen therapy
Restrict caffeine, nicotine, and hot and cold fluids

VENTRICULAR TACHYCARDIA (Figure 2-24)

Three or more consecutive PVCs; causes—ischemic heart disease, significant chronic heart disease, drug toxicity

Assessment

Observations/findings

Anxiety
Palpitations

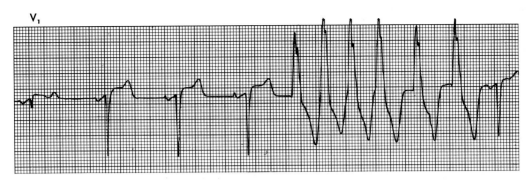

FIGURE 2-24. Ventricular tachycardia. (From Conover, M.B.: Exercises in diagnosing ECG tracings, ed. 3, St. Louis, 1984, The C.V. Mosby Co.)

Dizziness
Precordial discomfort
Cyanosis
Confusion
Syncope
Altered level of consciousness
Rhythm: usually regular
Rate: ventricular; 150 to 200 beats/min
P wave: absent; may be retrograde to atria
PR interval: unmeasurable
QRS complex: wide and bizarre in configuration, lasting more than 0.12 sec

Potential complications

Heart failure
Ventricular fibrillation

Interventions
Immediate care

Apply direct current (DC) countershock (p. 150)
Administer medications as ordered: lidocaine bolus and/or drip
Initiate CPR as indicated
Initiate parenteral fluids as ordered
Take 12-lead ECG as ordered
Check BP, R, and apical pulse q15 to 30 min as indicated
Administer oxygen as indicated

Ongoing care

Monitor cardiac activity; check rhythm strips q4h to 6h and prn
Check BP, R, and apical pulse q4h to 6h and prn
Administer medications as ordered
 Antiarrhythmics
 Sedatives
Maintain bed rest as indicated

VENTRICULAR FIBRILLATION (Figure 2-25)

Disorganized electrical activity of ventricles, which leads to abrupt cessation of effective blood flow; causes—severe heart disease, drug toxicity

Assessment
Observations/findings

Anxiety
Palpitations
Dizziness
Cyanosis
Precordial pain
Nausea, vomiting
Shortness of breath
Altered level of consciousness
Absence of pulse
Rhythm: irregular
Rate: 210 beats/min or greater
P wave: not seen; absent atrial activity
QRS complex: wide undulations; wandering, irregular baseline

Interventions
Immediate care

Cough CPR if patient is awake and able to cough
Apply DC countershock (p. 150)
Administer CPR; usually indicated
Give medications as ordered
Give parenteral fluids as ordered
Take 12-lead ECG as ordered
Administer oxygen with assisted ventilation as ordered
Check BP, R, and apical pulse q15 to 30 min

Ongoing care

Monitor cardiac activity; check rhythm strips q2h to 4h and prn
Check BP, R, and apical pulse q1h to 2h and prn

Maintain bed rest as indicated
Keep defibrillator and emergency cart at bedside until condition stabilizes

TORSADES DE POINTES (POLYMORPHOUS VENTRICULAR TACHYCARDIA) (Figure 2-26)

Atypical ventricular tachycardia occurring in the setting of delayed repolarization (prolonged QT interval); causes—drug toxicity such as quinidine, electrolyte imbalance

Assessment
Observations/findings

Palpitations
Faintness
Syncope
Rhythm: regular or irregular
Rate: ventricular, 150 to 300 beats/min
PR interval: not measurable
QRS complex: wide and bizarre in configuration, lasting >0.12 sec; amplitude and direction of QRS complex will vary
QT interval during baseline rhythm: >0.46 sec or >33% of baseline
T wave during baseline: very broad and flat

Potential complications

Ventricular fibrillation
Sudden death

Medical management

Correction of underlying cause if identifiable (e.g., drug toxicity: quinidine, procainamide, amiodarone)
Correction of electrolyte imbalance: hypokalemia, hypomagnesemia
Medications (avoid drugs that prolong QT intervals, e.g., isoproterenol)
Overdrive pacing: rate set at 80 to 120 beats/min
Cardioversion
Left stellate ganglionectomy

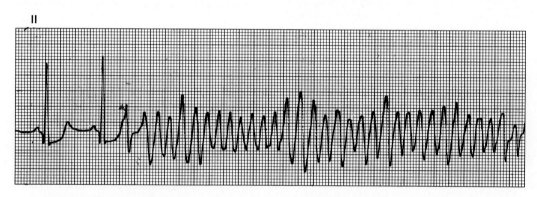

FIGURE 2-25. Ventricular fibrillation. (From Conover, M.B.: Exercises in diagnosing ECG tracings, ed. 3, St. Louis, 1984, The C.V. Mosby Co.)

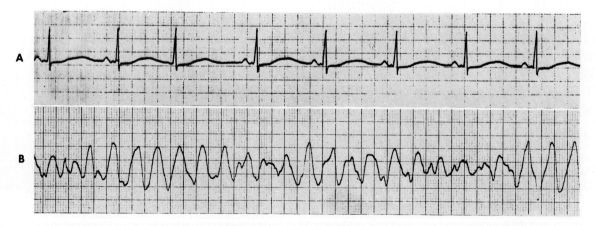

FIGURE 2-26. Torsade de pointes. Sinus rhythm. T waves are flat, and QT interval is prolonged. (Courtesty Dr. Daniel H. Schwartz. From Goldberger, E.: Textbook of clinical cardiology, St. Louis, 1982, The C.V. Mosby Co.)

Interventions

Monitor cardiac activity; check rhythm strips q4h to 6h and prn
Check BP, P, and apical pulse q4h to 6h and prn

Atrioventricular (AV) Block

A conduction disturbance involving the AV junction, which normally functions as a bridge between the atria and ventricles

FIRST-DEGREE AV BLOCK (Figure 2-27)

A consistent delay; causes—digoxin toxicity, ischemic heart disease, hyperkalemia

Assessment

Observations/findings

Rhythm: regular
Rate: 60 to 90 beats/min
P wave: normal configuration; one before each QRS
PR interval: prolonged, greater than 0.20 sec
QRS complex: 0.06 to 0.10 sec

Medical management

Medications
    Atropine
    Isoproterenol

Interventions

Monitor cardiac activity; check rhythm strips q4h to 6h and prn
Check BP, R, and apical pulse q4h to 6h and prn
Discontinue use of digitalis preparation or quinidine as ordered
Check serum levels of digitalis preparation and potassium as indicated
Observe for changes in PR interval and measure

SECOND-DEGREE AV BLOCK

An AV conduction disturbance characterized by nonconducted P waves and classified as type I or type II; causes—digoxin toxicity, ischemic heart disease

Assessment

Observations/findings

Rhythm: regular
Rate
    Atrial: rapid or slow
    Ventricular: may be slow
P wave: may show one or more nonconducted P waves
PR interval: may be prolonged, greater than 0.28 sec
QRS complex: 0.06 to 0.10 sec

Laboratory/diagnostic studies

Serum drug levels
His bundle recording

Potential complications

Angina
Heart failure
Complete AV block

Medical management

Medications
    Atropine
    Isoproterenol
Temporary cardiac pacing

Interventions

Monitor cardiac activity; check rhythm strips q2h to 4h
BP, R, and apical pulse q4h to 6h and prn

MOBITZ TYPE I (WENCKEBACH'S PHENOMENON) (Figure 2-28)

Causes—digoxin toxicity, inferior wall myocardial infarction (MI), rheumatic fever

Assessment

Observations/findings

Rhythm
    Atrial: regular
    Ventricular: will vary according to degree of block
Rate

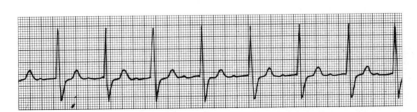

FIGURE 2-27. First-degree AV block. (From Conover, M.B.: Understanding electrocardiography: arrhythmias and the 12-lead ECG, ed. 4, St. Louis, 1984, The C.V. Mosby Co.)

Atrial: regular
Ventricular: will vary according to degree of block
P wave: may have multiple P waves before each QRS
PR interval: becomes progressively prolonged (greater than 0.28 sec) until one P wave is blocked; cycle will then be repeated
QRS complex: 0.06 to 0.10 sec; PR interval will shorten until P wave is blocked and no QRS will follow

Medical management

Medications
   Atropine
   Isoproterenol

Interventions

Withdraw use of digitalis preparation as ordered
Check serum levels of digitalis preparation and potassium as indicated

MOBITZ TYPE II (Figure 2-29)

Causes—digitalis toxicity, anterior MI

Assessment

Observations/findings

Dizziness
Weakness
Rhythm
   Atrial: regular
   Ventricular: will vary according to degree of block

Rate
   Atrial: 60 to 90 beats/min
   Ventricular: will vary according to degree of block
P wave: may have multiple P waves before each QRS
PR interval: remains constant and may be greater than 0.20 sec
QRS interval: usually normal, but may be widened or distorted as in bundle-branch block

Potential complications

Complete AV block

Medical management

Cardiac monitor
Medications
   Atropine
   Isoproterenol
Temporary or permanent cardiac pacing

THIRD-DEGREE HEART BLOCK (COMPLETE)
(Figure 2-30)

Causes—chronic conduction defect disease, digoxin toxicity, ischemic heart disease, congenital heart disease

Assessment

Observations/findings

Bradycardia
Syncope
Increased systolic pressure

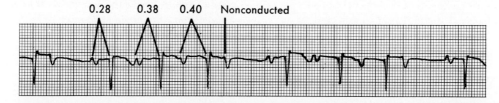

FIGURE 2-28. Second-degree AV block: Mobitz type 1 (Wenckebach's phenomenon) with narrow QRS complex. (From Conover, M.B.: Understanding electrocardiography: arrhythmias and the 12-lead ECG, ed. 4, St. Louis, 1984, The C.V. Mosby Co.)

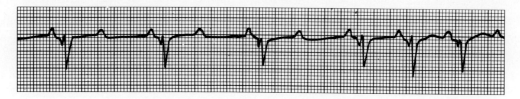

FIGURE 2-29. Second-degree AV block: Mobitz type II. (From Conover, M.B.: Exercises in diagnosing ECG tracings, ed. 3, St. Louis, 1984, The C.V. Mosby Co.)

Altered level of consciousness
Angina
Seizure activity
Rhythm: regular; atrial and ventricular rhythms act independently of each other
Rate
 Atrial: 60 to 90 beats/min
 Ventricular: 25 to 45 beats/min
P wave: multiple P waves that occur independently of QRS
PR interval: unmeasurable
QRS complex
 Normal if impulse originates above bifurcation of bundle of His
 Greater than 0.12 sec if impulse originates below bifurcation

Potential complications

Heart failure
Shock
Ventricular fibrillation

Medical management

Transvenous cardiac pacing
Medications
 Atropine
 Isoproterenol
12-lead ECG

Interventions

Monitor cardiac activity; check rhythm strips q2h to 4hr and prn
Check BP, R, and apical pulse q2h to 4h and prn
Administer oxygen therapy as ordered
Maintain bed rest as indicated

Bundle-Branch Block (Figure 2-31)

An intraventricular conduction disturbance involving one or more of the three fascicles of conduction: right bundle branch, left anterior, left posterior bundle branch; causes—many forms of chronic heart disease, congenital heart disease, Chagas' disease, infection

Assessment

Observations/findings

Rhythm: usually regular
Rate: usually regular; may be fast or slow
P wave: normal
PR interval: 0.12 to 0.20 sec
QRS complex: greater than 0.12 sec; complex is distorted

Laboratory/diagnostic studies

His bundle recordings

Medical management

No treatment specified
12-lead ECG

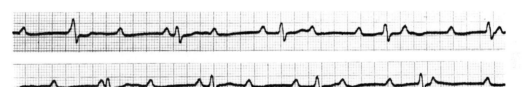

FIGURE 2-30. Third-degree (complete) AV block. (From Andreoli K., et al.: Comprehensive cardiac care: a text for nurses, physicians, and other health practitioners, ed. 5, St. Louis, 1983, The C.V. Mosby Co.)

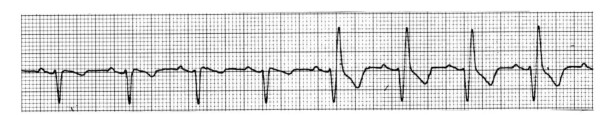

FIGURE 2-31. Bundle-branch block (BBB). (From Conover, M.B.: Exercises in diagnosing ECG tracings, ed. 3, St. Louis, 1984, The C.V. Mosby Co.)

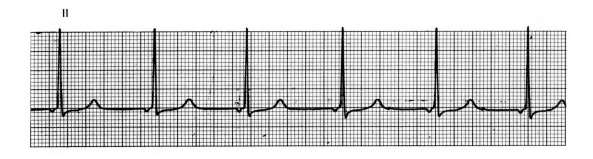

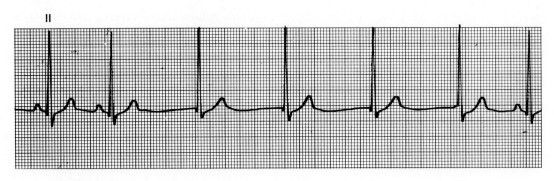

FIGURE 2-32. Junctional escape rhythms. (From Conover, M.B.: Exercises in diagnosing ECG tracings, ed. 3, St. Louis, 1984, The C.V. Mosby Co.)

Interventions

Check if patient is taking digitalis preparations or any antiarrhythmics and notify physician

Monitor cardiac activity as indicated; check rhythm strips q4h to 8h

Atrioventricular Junctional Rhythms

Arrhythmias that originate at the AV junction; may include premature, escape, and accelerated junctional tachycardia; causes—digitalis toxicity, MI, hypoxia, hyperkalemia, tricuspid valve surgery, rheumatic fever

AV JUNCTIONAL ESCAPE (Figure 2-32)

Assessment

Observations/findings

Dizziness
Faintness
Heart block
Rhythm: regular
Rate: 40 to 60 beats/min
P wave: may precede or follow QRS; may be inverted
PR interval: not measurable
QRS complex: 0.06 to 0.10 sec; may be slightly abnormal

Medical management

Treatment of underlying disease
Medications
  Atropine
  Isoproterenol
Ventricular pacing
12-lead ECG as ordered

Interventions

Monitor cardiac activity; check rhythm strips q4h to 6h
Check serum levels of digitalis preparation and potassium as indicated

Wolff-Parkinson-White Syndrome (Ventricular Preexcitation) (Figure 2-33)

Preexcitation of the ventricles over an accessory AV pathway; cause—congenital heart disease

Assessment

Observations/findings

Rhythm: regular
Rate: regular
P wave: normal configuration; one before each QRS

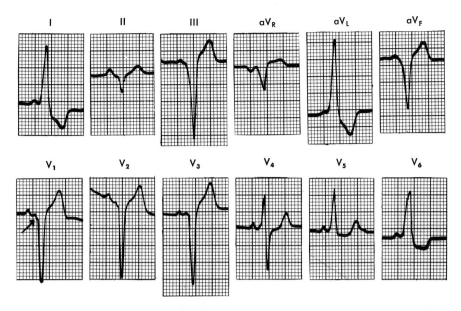

FIGURE 2-33. Characteristic triad of Wolff-Parkinson-White (WPW) pattern: wide QRS complex, short PR interval, and delta wave (arrow in lead V_1). (From Goldberger, A.L., and Goldberger, E.: Clinical electrocardiography: a simplified approach, ed. 3, St. Louis, 1986, The C.V. Mosby Co.)

PR interval: less than 0.12 sec
QRS complex: when following shortened PR interval, complex is widened and distorted, exhibiting delta waves

Laboratory/diagnostic studies

Holter examination
Electrophysiologic studies

Potential complications

Atrial tachycardia
Atrial fibrillation

Medical management

Valsalva maneuver; eyeball pressure
Medications as ordered
   Calcium channel–blocking agents
   Beta-adrenergic–blocking agents
Cardioversion

Interventions

Monitor cardiac activity as indicated; check rhythm strips q4h to 6h; report any changes in rhythm to physician

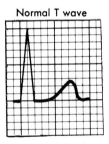

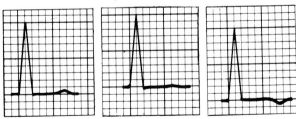

FIGURE 2-34. Miscellaneous ECG changes. (Flattening of T wave or slight T wave inversion are abnormal but relatively nonspecific changes. (From Goldberger, A.L., and Goldberger, E.: Clinical electrocardiography: a simplified approach, ed. 3, St. Louis, 1986, The C.V. Mosby Co.)

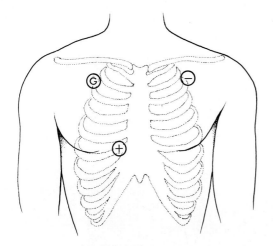

FIGURE 2-35. MCL. Modified V_1 monitoring lead.

ECG Rhythms: Nursing Diagnoses/Goals/Interventions (General)

ndx: Anxiety related to altered heart action

GOAL: *Patient will exhibit decreased anxiety level*

Provide continuous explanation for various monitoring devices in use and procedures
Promote physical rest to decrease cardiac workload
Administer sedation as ordered

ndx: Knowledge deficit regarding disease process

GOAL: *Patient and/or significant other will demonstrate increased understanding of disease process and self-care management through interactive discussion and actual return demonstration*

Explain purpose of treatment and equipment
Reinforce physician's explanation of rhythm disturbance and associated symptoms to report
Explain need to exercise to tolerance and/or as ordered
Explain purpose and demonstrate method of taking pulse
Explain dietary restrictions as ordered; need to avoid caffeine and nicotine
Discuss medications: name, dosage, time of administration, purpose, and side effects
Need to avoid taking over-the-counter medications without checking with physician
Importance of ongoing outpatient care
Pacemaker care when indicated

PACEMAKER INSERTION

pacemaker An electronic device used to electronically stimulate the myocardium to control or maintain the heart rate

Preprocedure teaching

Reinforce physician's explanation of procedure
    How pacemaker functions
        To optimize cardiac function
        To restore and/or maintain AV synchronization
    Indications
        To control bradyarrhythmias
        To control tachyarrhythmias
        To control ventricular fibrillation
    Type or mode to be used
        Temporary
        Permanent
    Method of insertion
        Transvenous
        Transthoracic
        Epicardial
Ensure that patient and/or significant other knows and understands
    Procedure, duration of procedure, where it will be performed (operating room vs. procedure room), equipment that will be used (e.g., fluoroscopy), and type of anesthesia
Importance of restricting activities for 4 to 6 hr in order to avoid lead dislodgment
Importance of performing passive ROM exercises to extremities postoperatively
Importance of being closely monitored postoperatively
Signs and symptoms of pacemaker malfunction
    Faintness
    Dizziness
    Dyspnea
    Twitching
        Pectoral muscles
        Abdominal muscle
    Hiccups
    Chest pain

Postprocedure assessment

Observations/findings
TEMPORARY PACEMAKER (Figure 2-36)

Heart rate based on preset pacemaker setting
Pacemaker unit (Figure 2-37)
    Firing at preset rate
    Output threshold (milliamperes)
    Sensing needle
    Terminal connections
Electrical grounding
ECG pattern (Figure 2-38)
    Pacemaker artifact
    Capturing
    Patient's underlying rhythm
Battery failure
    Loss of capture

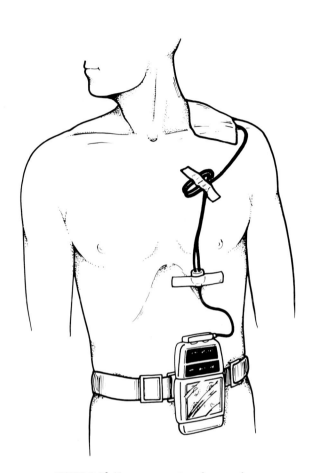

FIGURE 2-36. Temporary external pacemaker.

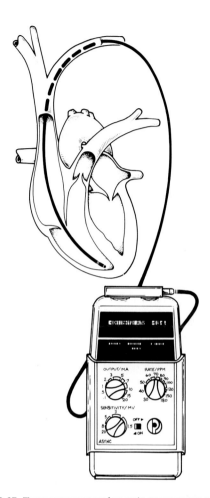

FIGURE 2-37. Temporary pacemaker unit: transvenous approach.

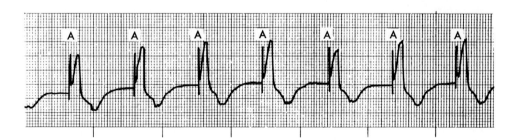

FIGURE 2-38. Ventricular pacemaker. *A,* Pacemaker spikes. (From Andreoli, K., et al.: Comprehensive cardiac care: a text for nurses, physicians, and other health practitioners, ed. 5, St. Louis, 1983, The C.V. Mosby Co.)

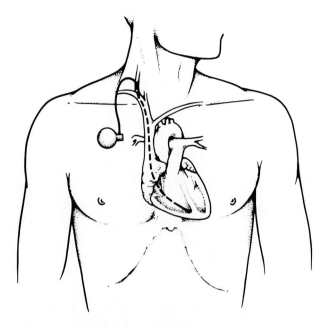

FIGURE 2-39. Permanent pacemaker.

Failure to sense
Sensing needle: not moving

PERMANENT PACEMAKER

Pacemaker unit (Figure 2-39)
   Heart rate: based on preset pacer rate
   Location of pulse generator
   Mode
     Dual chamber: sensed or paced
       Ventricular inhibited (demand): VVI
       AV sequential: DVI
       Atrial triggered: VDD
       Universal: DDD
   Programmable
     Pacer rate
     Output (milliamperes)
     Sensitivity (to PQRS complex)
     Mode
       Atrial
       Ventricular

Potential complications

Pacemaker dysfunction
   Decreased BP
   Pallor or cyanosis
   Decreased urinary output
   Bradycardia
   Fatigue
   Shortness of breath
   ECG pattern changes
   Absent pacemaker artifact
   No ventricular response, absence of QRS complex after pacemaker artifact
   Competition; presence of pacemaker response complex and patient's own complex
   Runaway pacemaker; pacemaker artifact appears at several hundred per minute
Catheter dislodgment
   Change in QRS configuration
   Loss of artifact on ECG
   Failure to sense
   Hiccups
   Muscle twitching: chest, abdomen
Stokes-Adams syndrome
   Hypotension
   Vertigo
   Fainting
   Convulsions
   Coma
Cardiac arrhythmias
   PVCs
   Ventricular tachycardia
Site of insertion
   Discoloration
   Pain
   Swelling
   Bleeding
Perforation
Infection
   Elevated temperature
   Tachycardia
Cardiac tamponade

Medical management

Cardiac monitor
Parenteral fluids
Pacemaker
   Heart rate setting
   Threshold (milliamperes)

Nursing diagnoses/goals/interventions

ndx: Potential for injury related to pacemaker dysfunction, displacement or breakage of pacing catheter, infection, or bleeding

GOAL: *Patient will demonstrate clinical stability and absence of complications*

Maintain bed rest as ordered; assist patient with assuming position of comfort during immediate postoperative period
Place patient on cardiac monitor

Check BP, T, and R q4h; check apical pulse q1h to 2h for 7 hr, then q4h
For temporary pacemaker
  Check settings: output, sensing, and rates
  Immobolize and secure extremity
Check rhythm strips on return to unit, q4h, and prn, noting pacemaker function and rate
Check site of insertion q2h to 4h; report any excessive bleeding to physician
Maintain parenteral fluids as ordered
Administer medication as ordered
  Antiarrhythmics
  Pain management
Avoid electrical hazards
Continue with immediate postoperative care and decrease frequency of nursing functions as patient's condition improves
Increase activity as tolerated and ordered
Change dressing daily as ordered, using aseptic technique

Temporary pacemaker

Ground all equipment
Secure all terminal connections
Avoid use of electrical equipment such as shavers
Insulate exposed pacemaker wires by enclosing pacemaker and connections with rubber glove
Avoid wetting pacemaker
Apply soft restraints prn

Permanent pacemaker

Avoid exposure to electrical equipment that causes electromagnetic interference (EMI) such as diathermy and ungrounded equipment
Ground all equipment
Apply soft restraints prn

ndx: Potential for noncompliance related to knowledge deficit

  GOAL: *Patient and/or significant other will demonstrate understanding of self-care management through interactive discussion and actual return demonstration*

Permanent pacemaker

Ensure that patient and/or significant other knows pacemaker model, date of insertion, location of pacer generator, and pacer rate
Demonstrate method of caring for pacemaker
Demonstrate changing of dressing
Demonstrate taking of pulse for 1 min; give patient range of normal rates and instruct him to report to physician if pulse is less than set range (i.e., < than 5 beats/min below set rate)
Explain need for emotional support
Deal with behavioral changes such as denial
Discuss living with pacemaker; help patient adjust to any limitations and explain that pacemaker will eliminate feelings of faintness and fatigue
Discuss signs of pacemaker failure
  Pulse < 60 beats/min or < 5 beats/min below set rate
  Dizziness
  Faintness
  Palpitations
  Hiccups
  Chest pain
Discuss method of reporting pacemaker failure
  Telephone monitoring
  Notifying physician
Discuss signs of infection around pacemaker generator
  Fever
  Heat
  Pain
  Swelling
Discuss medications: name, dosage, times of administration, purpose, and side effects
Explain need to avoid taking over-the-counter medication without checking with physician
Discuss diet as ordered
Explain importance of ongoing outpatient care: pacemaker clinic, use of transtelephonic system
Explain need to maintain activities as ordered
  Avoid traveling for at least 3 months after insertion
  Discuss type of employment and make adjustments in work accordingly
  Resume sexual activity as tolerated
  Avoid engaging in body contact sports such as baseball, football, and basketball
Explain need to wear nonrestrictive clothing over site of pacemaker
Discuss electrical safety
  Avoid working with radar or electrical equipment such as diathermy motors that may cause electromagnetic interference
  Ground home appliances so that they have little or no effect on permanent pacemakers
  Wear medical alert band
  Carry pacemaker card with information regarding type of pacemaker, set rate, date of implantation, and name of physician
  Inform dentist of pacemaker prior to any extensive dental work

Evaluation

Anxiety level is reduced
Patient demonstrates an understanding of home health care
   Demonstrates pulse taking
   Verbalizes electrical sources that may interfere with pacemaker function
   Verbalizes signs of pacemaker failure and actions to take
There are no complications

CARDIAC CATHETERIZATION

An invasive cardiac procedure; assists in detection and localization of intracardiac problems, determines intracardiac measurements, and shows visualization of the cardiac chambers; performed with patient under local anesthesia

Preprocedure teaching

Involve family or significant other in care and instruction
Reinforce physician's explanation of purpose of procedure
Review routine preparation for procedure
   Leg shave and preparation
   Medication for sedation may be ordered
   No food or water 6 to 12 hr before procedure as ordered
Explain sensations to be experienced during procedure
   Palpitations
   Warm, flushed feeling during injection of dye
   Desire to cough
   Feeling of falling when rotated from side to side
Explain sensations to be expected following procedure
   Soreness at insertion site
   Possible backache from lying on table for 1 to 3 hr
   Fatigue
Stress importance of bed rest and immobility of extremity after procedure

Postprocedure assessment

Observations/findings

Hematoma at site of insertion
   Neck
   Antecubital fossa
   Inguinal
Vasospasm of affected extremity
   Numbness
   Tingling
   Cyanosis
   Loss of pulse
Chest pain

Potential complications

Ventricular arrhythmias
Syncope
Allergic reaction to dye
Nausea, vomiting
Difficulty in breathing
Shortness of breath
Tachycardia
Edema of face and hands
Decrease or fall in BP
Thrombus
Thrombophlebitis
Cardiac perforation
Increased myocardial ischemia
Infection
Cardiac tamponade

Postprocedure care

Maintain bed rest for 6 to 8 hr following procedure or as ordered
   Elevate head of bed 20 to 30 degrees
   Keep extremity immobile for 2 to 4 hr after procedure as ordered
   Maintain sandbag over puncture site as ordered
Check BP, T, R, apical pulse, and peripheral pulses, noting quality q15 min for four times, then qh for 4 hr, then as ordered
Take 12-lead ECG as ordered
Monitor cardiac activity as ordered; check rhythm strips q4h and prn
Inspect dressing at site of insertion q2h to 4h, noting amount and color of drainage; change qd and prn
Reinforce dressing as necessary
Inspect surrounding skin
   Redness or discoloration
   Swelling
   Irritation
Control pain as ordered
Ambulate as tolerated
Instruct patient to report any signs of pain, swelling, or discoloration of puncture site
Continue ongoing care for underlying disease process

PERCUTANEOUS TRANSLUMINAL ANGIOPLASTY (PTCA)

A nonsurgical procedure utilizing a balloon-tipped catheter to dilate coronary arteries stenosed by atherosclerotic plaques

Preprocedure teaching

Involve family or significant other in care and instruction
Reinforce physician's explanation of purpose for procedure, desired outcome, and associated risks
Explain need to follow directions regarding administration and withholding of medications
Encourage verbalization and questions
Evaluate patient's awareness and emotional status: fears of procedure and possible necessity of cardiac surgery
Explain that procedure is similar to cardiac catheterization
Review routine preparation for procedure
    Skin prepared for coronary bypass surgery
    Medication for sedation may be ordered
    No food or water 24 hr before procedure
Explain sensations to be expected
    During procedure
        Palpitations
        Warm, flushed feeling during injection of dye
    Following procedure
        Soreness at insertion site
        Possible backache from lying on table for 3 to 5 hr
        Fatigue
Stress importance of bed rest and immobility of extremity after procedure
Explain and review postprocedure procedures
    Need to be admitted to CCU for 24 hr for observation
    Routines of CCU
    Visiting privileges
    Equipment to be used
        Temporary pacing electrode
        Cardiac monitor
        Swan-Ganz catheter
        Oxygen administration
        IV therapy
NOTE: Cardiac surgical team must be on standby during procedure; see Cardiac Surgery for brief explanation of differences in patient care following cardiac surgery
Administer medications as ordered
    Salicylates and dipyridamole may be ordered 2 days prior to procedure
    Nitrates
    Beta-blocking agents may be decreased
    Calcium antagonists

Preparation

Obtain informed consent
Maintain NPO 24 hr prior to procedure
Withhold anticoagulation therapy 1 to 2 days prior to procedure

Postprocedure assessment

Observations/findings

Chest pain or pressure
ECG changes
    ST elevations, depressions
    Ventricular arrhythmias
Shortness of breath
Skin
    Pale
    Diaphoretic
Decreased BP
Hematoma at site of insertion
Vasospasm of affected extremity
    Numbness
    Tingling
    Cyanosis
    Loss of pulse
Arrhythmias
Behavorial response
    Anxiety
    Fear

Laboratory/diagnostic studies

CBC
Coagulation studies
Type and cross match
Serum electrolytes
Cardiac enzymes
12-lead ECG
Exercise stress test
Cardiac catheterizations
Thallium cardiac imaging

Potential complications

Coronary artery spasm during catheterization: balloon inflation
Venous thrombosis
MI
Rupture or dissection of coronary artery
    Cardiac tamponade
    MI
    Shock
    Cardiac arrest
Hemorrhage at cannulation site

Medical management

Admission to CCU for 24 to 48 hr
Bed rest in flat position for 6 to 8 hr
Cardiac monitor
Parenteral fluids
Medications
    Nitrates
    Analgesics
    Antiarrhythmics
    Anticoagulants

Nursing diagnoses/goals/interventions

ndx: Potential alteration in tissue perfusion: peripheral related to hematoma, thrombus formation, and/or infection secondary to arterial cannulation

GOAL: *Patient will maintain tissue perfusion and cellular oxygenation*

Maintain bed rest for 6 to 8 hr following procedure as ordered
Observe cannulation site for swelling, tenderness, discoloration, warmth, and drainage
Keep extremity immobile for 2 to 4 hr after procedure
Check, T, R, and peripheral pulses, noting quality, q15 min for four times, then qh for 6 hr, then as ordered
Observe for diminished pulses in extremity distal to cannulation site; report decreased or absent pulses immediately to physician
Inspect dressing at site of insertion q2h to 4h, noting amount and color of drainage
Maintain 5 to 10 lb sandbag over cannulation site
Reinforce dressing as necessary
Inspect surrounding skin
    Redness or discoloration
    Swelling
    Irritation
Administer medications as ordered
    Antiplatelets
    Anticoagulants
Maintain parenteral therapy as ordered
Obtain laboratory studies as ordered
    Cardiac enzymes
    Coagulation studies
    CBC
    Blood cultures

ndx: Potential alteration in cardiac output related to possible complications of PTCA

GOAL: *Patient will demonstrate no signs of low cardiac output syndrome*

Maintain bed rest with head of bed elevated 15 degrees
Check BP, R, and apical pulse q15 min for four times, then q30 min for four times, then qh for 6 hr, then as ordered
Monitor cardiac activity; check rhythm strips q4h and prn
Obtain 12-lead ECG as ordered
Obtain 12-lead ECG during episodes of chest pain; observe for and report any signs of ischemic change
Auscultate chest for heart and lung sounds q4h for 24 hr
Measure intake and output; report output of less than 30 ml/hr

ndx: Anxiety related to knowledge deficit and perceived threat to biologic integrity

GOAL: *Patient will demonstrate reduced anxiety level*

Reinforce physician's explanation of postprocedure results
Discuss allowances and limitations of activity
    Avoid heavy lifting and pushing
    Ambulate at regular intervals
Explain importance of calling physician if chest pain occurs, lasting longer than 20 min
Discuss medications: name, dosage, time of administration, purpose, and side effects
Explain importance of taking antiplatelet medications as ordered
Explain importance of ongoing outpatient care
Refer to standard for angina pectoris for patient teaching regarding
    Chest pain
    Risk factors
    Exercise, activities

Evaluation

Patient
    Maintains adequate peripheral tissue perfusion
        Pulse is full and bounding
            Cannulation site: color is good; there are no signs of tenderness or swelling
    Maintains good cardiac output
        Vital signs are stable
        Urine output is good
        Mentation is clear
    Demonstrates reduced level of anxiety
        Verbalizes insights into need for procedures
        Knows signs and symptoms to report
        Appears calm

HEMODYNAMIC MONITORING

Method of evaluating filling pressure of left ventricle, cardiac output, and intraarterial pressure (Figure 2-40)

pulmonary artery pressure (PAP) and pulmonary capillary wedge pressure (PCWP) *An indirect method of measuring left ventricular filling pressure; measures cardiac output and obtains mixed venous sampling using a Swan-Ganz catheter (Figures 2-41 to 2-43)*

Preprocedure teaching

Reinforce physician's explanation of procedure, duration, and equipment that will be used

Explain importance of immobilizing extremity

Attach cardiac monitor to patient; record baseline rhythm strip

Equipment preparation

Check integrity of balloon for double- and triple-lumen catheters before insertion; record amount of air needed for inflation

Position transducer to level of right atrium

Calibrate all equipment prior to insertion
   Transducer
   Recording display unit
   Monitor

Have 100 mg IV bolus of lidocaine and defibrillator at bedside during insertion

Be aware that insertion must be done under sterile conditions

Assessment

Observations/findings

Normal pressures
RA: 5 mm Hg
PA: 25 to 30/10 to 15 mm Hg
PCWP: 10 to 12 mm Hg

DURING INSERTION

Ventricular irritability
Pneumothorax (with subclavian insertion)
Laceration of lung apex

POSTINSERTION

Catheter insertion site
   Infection
      Inflammation
      Redness
      Thrombosis

TABLE 2-7. Problems Associated with Pressure Wave Forms

Observations	Etiologic factors	Interventions
Loss of wave form on oscilloscope	Displacement of catheter	Reposition patient; notify physician
Loss of PAP; PCWP is displayed on monitor	Self-wedging	Instruct patient to cough
		Obtain x-ray examination
Loss of PCWP	Displaced into PAP; balloon rupture	Use diastolic of PAP
Decreased amplitude of wave form	Damping due to	
	Clot in catheter	Flush lines: *Do not force if resistance is met*
	Air bubbles	Check all connections for air leaks; flush air bubbles
	Kinking of catheter	Notify physician
	Occluded catheter	Reposition patient; have patient cough
	Tip against artery wall	
Loss of PCWP; no resistance with inflation	Rupture of balloon	Seal off balloon lumen: *Do not allow any injection of air*
Air bubbles in pressure lines	Air leak in system	Check all connections and secure
Damping of wave form		
Inaccurate reading		
Artifacts and inadequate pressure readings	Respiratory interference	Record pressure at end exhalation
	Handling of pressure equipment during readings	Check for possible interference with tubing during readings
	Inaccurate calibration of equipment	Check for possible interference with tubing during readings
	Faulty equipment	Check electrical system for grounding
		Check calibration of and level to RA of transducer
		Check all equipment for proper functioning

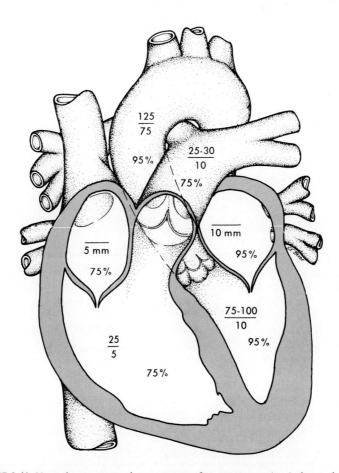

FIGURE 2-40. Normal pressures and percentages of oxygen saturation in heart chambers and great vessels.

Tenderness
Swelling
Edema
Endocarditis
Septicemia

Potential complications

Decreased circulation
　Numbness, absence of pulses to distal extremity
　Coolness, pallor, cyanosis of extremity
Blood loss
　Decreased BP
　Blood in tube and at insertion site
Pulmonary infarction (for pulmonary catheters)
　Chest pain
　Dyspnea
　Hemoptysis
　Tachypnea
　Arrhythmias
　　PVCs
　　Ventricular tachycardia
Embolus (air or thromboembolus)

Tachypnea
Dyspnea
Chest pain
Catheter displacement
　Loss of waveform
　Dampening of waveform
Rupture of balloon
　Absence of resistance to inflation
　Failure of PA line to wedge
　Blood backup in balloon line

FLUSH SYSTEM

For continuous flush via pressure transfer pack
Pressure maintained at 300 mm Hg or as ordered by manufacturer
Heparinized solution (500 U/500 ml 0.9 normal saline solution or 1 unit of heparin/ml of solution)

PRESSURE LINES

Patency
Complications
　Air bubbles

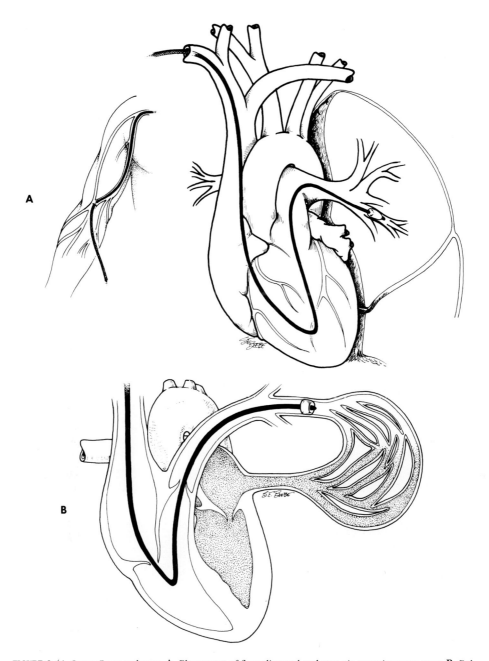

FIGURE 2-41. Swan-Ganz catheter. A, Placement of flow-directed catheter via superior vena cava. B, Balloon inflated and wedged in pulmonary artery.

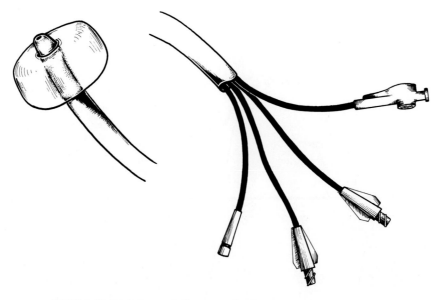

FIGURE 2-42. Triple-lumen, balloon-tipped pulmonary catheter (Swan-Ganz).

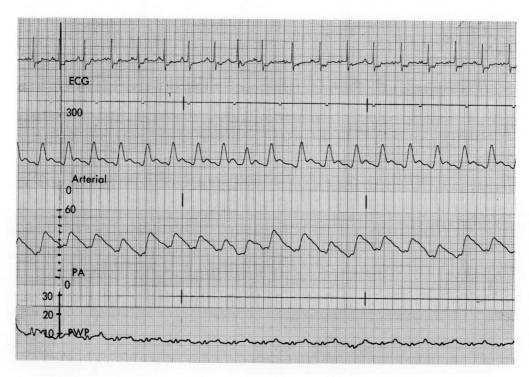

FIGURE 2-43. Pressure waveforms. Electrocardiogram *(ECG)*, arterial pressure, pulmonary artery pressure *(PAP)* and pulmonary capillary wedge pressure *(PCWP)*.

Blood in tubing
Slow blood return from catheter

PRESSURE TRANSDUCER

Air bubbles
Foreign material
   Blood
   Dust particles

DISCONTINUATION

Extravasation of blood
Thrombi formation
Sepsis

Interventions

Check patency of lines, tubings, and connections q4h to 8h
Check pressure in transfer pack q4h to 6h
Flush all lines q1h to 2h
Check calibration of transducer q8h or as indicated by manufacturer; never apply direct pressure to diaphragm of transducer
Relevel transducer as patient position is changed
   Keep level with right atrium
   Record position in which readings are taken
Change pressure line tubing, pressure bag, and manifold q48h
Change dressing qd
Record ECG rhythm strip q6h

Pulmonary artery pressures (PAP, PCWP)

Check that balloon is deflated except when testing PCWP
Record pressure reading q4h to 6h as dictated by patient's condition
Take readings at end-exhalation in presence of respiratory variation
Blood should not be withdrawn routinely from PA line
Parenteral fluids should not be administered routinely through PA line

Cardiac output—thermodilution method

A method of measuring cardiac output using the triple-lumen Swan-Ganz catheter; the proximal lumen is used for injection of an iced or room temperature solution (5 to 10 ml); cardiac output is 5 L/min

Prepare equipment; if using iced injectate, allow 45 to 60 min
Follow manufacturer's manual regarding preparation of computer readout
Calibrate all equipment prior to procedure
Check integrity of catheter before injecting solution
Use aseptic technique in injection of solution
Inject 10 ml rapidly over 4 sec; record amount of injectate on intake and output

Arterial lines

Measure arterial blood pressure directly as ordered
Check connections q2h for tightness
Do not leave patient unattended, especially when restless; use soft restraints as indicated
Record pressure reading q4h as indicated by patient's condition
Check indirect arterial pressure q6h to 8h and record
Check circulation of extremity q2h; observe for changes in color, warmth, pulses, and nail beds
Flush lines before and after withdrawing blood specimens
Measure output of blood samples for replacement in pediatric patients
Change stopcocks qd
Remove dead-space fluid in tubing before removing blood specimens for analysis
Never use force to flush or irrigate a line that is resistant
Notify physician of
   Early signs of inflammation; swelling at insertion site
   Coolness or cyanosis of extremity
   Clotted pressure line
   Absence of pulses

Discontinuation of pressure lines

Maintain direct manual pressure over site for 5 to 10 min following removal of all catheters
Have lidocaine bolus with defibrillator at bedside during removal of pulmonary catheters
Check insertion site and pulses of extremity q2h to 4h for 24 hr
Check and observe for arrhythmias, emboli, and infection for 24 hr following withdrawal of lines

INTRAAORTIC BALLOON COUNTERPULSATION: BALLOON PUMP

A temporary cardiac assistive technique used in management of refractory left ventricular failure, preinfarction angina, MI, and following cardiac surgery

Preinsertion assessment

Observations/findings
PATIENT

Left ventricular failure
   Decreased cardiac output

Elevated LAP and PCWP
Dyspnea
Productive cough
Pulmonary edema
Cardiogenic shock (p. 104)

EQUIPMENT

Clear ECG pattern with upright QRS complex
Patent and functioning hemodynamic monitoring
  (p. 141)
  PAP
  PCWP
  LAP
  Arterial line
Balloon catheter
  Size
  Kinks
  Cracks
  Leaks
Machine console
  Gas level: helium, carbon dioxide
  Mode
    Automatic
    Manual
  Readout
  Alarms (NOTE: Alarms do not function in manual mode)

Required baseline information

Complete physical assessment
ECG
  12-lead
  Rhythm strip
Extremity to be cannulated
  Pulses: quality
  Color
  Temperature
Hemodynamic status
  Arterial pressure
  SVR
  PAP
  PCWP
  Cardiac output

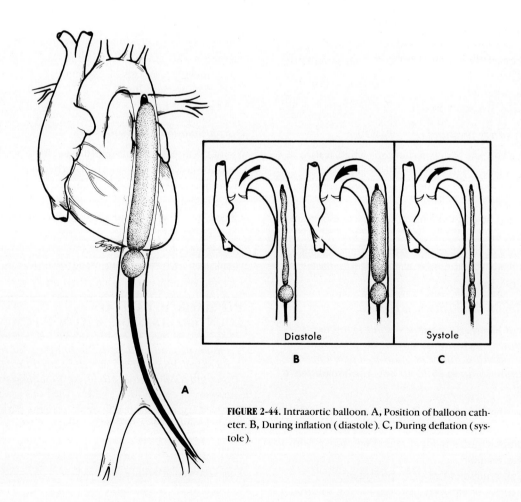

FIGURE 2-44. Intraaortic balloon. **A,** Position of balloon catheter. **B,** During inflation (diastole). **C,** During deflation (systole).

Laboratory/diagnostic studies

Electrolyte profile
CBC
PT
PTT
Type and cross match 1 or 2 units of blood as ordered
Cardiac enzymes
Arterial blood gases

Preprocedure teaching

Reinforce physician's explanation of procedure to patient and/or significant other
Prepare family or significant other for visit at patient's bedside with simple explanation of equipment
Discuss importance of restraining movement of cannulated extremity

Observations during insertion

Dissection or perforation of aorta and/or femoral artery
Clot formation
Hemorrhage
Respiratory failure
Level of consciousness
Hemodynamic status

Assessment during counterpulsation
Observations/findings
GENERAL

Level of consciousness
BP, T, P, and R
Respiratory status
Skin
   Color
   Turgor
   Temperature
Intake and output
Peripheral circulation

SPECIFIC

ECG rhythm disturbances
   Rapid atrial fibrillation
   PVCs
   Ventricular arrhythmias
Heart rate: increase or decrease of greater than 20%
Left ventricular failure
   Increased PAP, PCWP
   Decreased cardiac output
   Oliguria
   Decreased BP
   Rales, rhonchi
Thromboembolism
Volume depletion anemia
Thrombocytopenia
Hemorrhage
Aortic dissection
Atelectasis
Respiratory failure
Balloon pressure waveform
Insertion site
   Infection
   Phlebitis
   Bleeding
Cannulated extremity
   Decreased perfusion
      Pallor
      Coolness
      Decreased capillary filling of nail beds
   Decrease in or absence of pulses
   Ischemia
      Local pain
      Tingling
      Numbness

Laboratory/diagnostic studies

Decreased Hct ratio
Reduced platelet count
Hypoxia
Hypercarbia

Postinsertion care
Patient

Determine parameters of vital signs from physician
Place patient in supine position with head of bed at 45 degrees; never raise head of bed greater than 45 degrees
Do not flex or bend cannulated extremity
Check systolic pressure q6h to 8h using arterial pressure and cuff pressure; report to physician any decrease in systolic/diastolic pressures of greater than 10 mm Hg
Check PAP, PCWP, and CVP with arterial pressure q15 to 30 min until stable, then qh
Check P and R q15 to 30 min until stable, then q1h; check quality and rate of R and P
Check rectal temperature q4h to 6h
Take and record ECG rhythm strips qh, measuring rate and PR and QRS intervals
Check balloon markers q15 to 30 min; balloon inflation marker should be synchronized on T wave during inflation and after P wave during deflation
Check scope pattern q15 to 30 min
Check intraaortic balloon counterpulsation (IABC) augmentation ratio q15 min (i.e., 1:1, 1:2, 1:3, etc.)

Administer oxygen and assisted ventilation as ordered
Measure arterial blood gases as ordered; record if taken on or off pump
Obtain laboratory studies as ordered
  PT
  PTT
  Hct ratio
Record amount of blood removed for laboratory studies
Maintain inspired oxygen concentration as ordered by physician
Auscultate heart sounds q2h to 4h for rhythm and extra heart sounds
Auscultate chest for breath sounds q1h to 2h while on respirator, q4h to 6h while off respirator
Check pulses—femoral, dorsal pedal, posterior tibial, and popliteal—q15 min for 4 hr, then q1h to 2h
  Report any decrease or changes
  Use Doppler sensor if necessary
Obtain and check x-ray film following balloon placement
Connect indwelling catheter to closed urinary drainage
Measure intake and output qh
  Record color and specific gravity of urinary drainage
  Report output of less than 30 ml/hr
Maintain diet as ordered or indicated by physical condition
Maintain parenteral fluids and limit fluid intake as ordered
Administer medications as ordered
  Sedatives
  Diuretics
  Vasopressors
  Heparin
Check dressing q24 hr, noting drainage amount, color, and character
Change dressing q1d to 2d as ordered
Turn and position patient side to side q2h; turn patient with two nurses using logrolling technique
Perform passive ROM exercises of extremities
  Avoid flexing or moving cannulated extemity
  Use footboard for dorsal and plantar flexion
Orient patient to environment as indicated
Plan nursing care to allow maximum rest for patient

Equipment

Check gas level q6h to 8h; fill as necessary
Check ECG leads and electrodes q4h to 8h; if changed, notify IABP technician
NOTE: There should always be spare helium tanks available
Empty cold trap and clear filter qd

Observations during weaning process
BP
  Arterial
  Cuff
Hemodynamic status
Altered level of consciousness
Balloon volume; will be decreased by 50% with pump rate being lowered as ordered
Cardiogenic shock (p. 104)

SHOCK TROUSERS: PNEUMATIC TROUSERS (MAST*)

A pressurized life-support suit designed to correct or counteract hypotension associated with internal or external bleeding situations and hypovolemia

Application

Observations prior to and during application

Level of consciousness change determined by baseline evaluation
Decreased or falling BP: determined by patient's baseline pressure
Respiratory distress
  Dyspnea
  Tachypnea
  Cough
  Pink, frothy sputum
Peripheral pulses
  Dorsal pedal
  Posterior tibial
  Radial
Extremities: feet
  Color
    Pale
    Mottled
  Temperature
Position of trousers (Figure 2-45)
  Abdomen: just below rib cage
  Legs: right, left
Metabolic acidosis
Pulmonary edema
CHF (p. 101)
Hypovolemic shock (p. 104)

Acute care

NOTE: Shock trousers may be contraindicated in patients with pulmonary edema, cardiogenic shock, increased intracranial pressure, or eviscerations

---

*Military antishock trousers.

Cardiovascular System

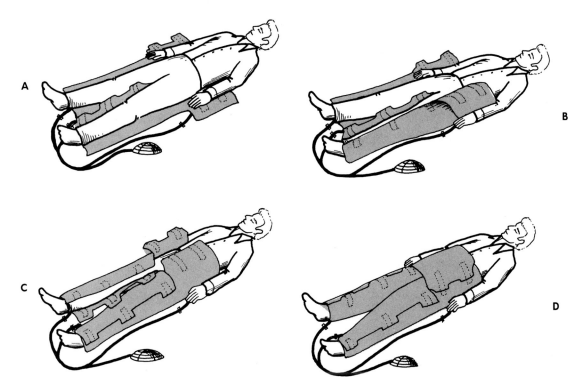

FIGURE 2-45. MAST shock trousers. Application and position of body on trousers.

Equipment

Check trousers with Velcro straps or zippers for tears or leaks prior to application

Secure connecting tubes to pump; remove any kinks or twisting of tubing prior to application

Check valves for proper functioning prior to application

Care during application

Maintain flat, supine position
Check BP, R, and apical pulse q15 min and prn
Record exact time of trouser inflation and sections used
Check inflated sections q15 min
Check peripheral pulses q15 to 30 min
Maintain NPO
Measure intake and output qh
  Maintain parenteral fluids as ordered
  Connect indwelling urethral catheter to closed gravity drainage as ordered
  Notify physician if urinary output is less than 30 ml/hr
Administer whole blood, plasmanate, and other plasma volume expanders as ordered
  Adjust flow rate according to CVP readings as ordered

See standard for specific disease process (e.g., shock, fractured pelvis)
Connect nasogastric tube to intermittent suction as ordered
Monitor arterial blood gases as ordered
Auscultate chest sounds qh
Provide emotional support
  Remain with patient
  Explain purpose of trousers and procedures

Deflation

NOTE: Trousers *must not* be deflated or removed until volume replacement is stable and patient is under care of physician; never deflate all at once

Observations during and following deflation

Level of consciousness
Decreased or falling BP
Respiratory distress
  Dyspnea
  Tachypnea
  Cyanosis
Circulatory collapse
  Hypotension
  Tachycardia
  Oliguria

Cardiac arrhythmias
Pulmonary edema
Cardiac arrest

Acute care

Gradually deflate each section, starting with abdominal section
Check BP, R, and apical pulse q5 to 10 min during deflation; stop deflation process if there is precipitious drop in BP of 4 to 6 mm Hg from ordered BP
Record time deflation started, noting level of consciousness

CARDIOVERSION (SYNCHRONIZED SHOCK)

Delivery of synchronized electrical voltage to the heart to terminate supraventricular tachyarrhythmias via electrodes placed on patient's chest

Preprocedure care

Reinforce physician's explanation of procedure
Obtain signed consent
Withhold diuretics and digitalis preparations 24 to 72 hr prior to procedure as ordered; check digitalis levels if excess is suspected
Maintain NPO 6 to 8 hr prior to procedure
Check serum potassium level for possible hypokalemia as ordered
Obtain 12-lead ECG and rhythm strip
Administer oxygen by mask or cannula as ordered
Have patient void
Remove dentures
Maintain parenteral fluids as ordered
Administer parenteral fluids as ordered
Administer sedation as ordered
Have emergency cart with cardiac drugs, suction, and airway equipment at bedside
Place saline pads or electrode gel on electrode paddles

Observations during and after procedure
Patient

Level of consciousness
ECG
  Return to sinus rhythm
  Atrial fibrillation
  PVCs and/or ventricular tachycardia
  Cardiac standstill
Pulse and respirations
  Quality
  Rate
Skin
  Redness
  Irritation
  Excoriation

Decreased BP
Pulmonary embolus

Equipment

Placement of electrode paddles
  Anterior-posterior: anterior paddle on left precordium; posterior paddle beneath patient
  Standard: one paddle to right of upper sternum and below clavicle; second paddle to left of nipple with center of electrode in midaxillary line
Saline-soaked gauze pads or electrode paste on electrode paddles
Voltage as ordered
  Adults: 50 to 100 joules
  Children: 0.2 to 1 joule/kg
Grounding of equipment surrounding patient
Oxygen via mask or cannula

Postprocedure care

Maintain bed rest: flat, supine position
Check BP, R, and apical pulse q15 min for 1 hr, then q4h as ordered
Monitor cardiac activity; check and obtain rhythm strips immediately after procedure, q4h, and prn
Administer oxygen as ordered
Administer skin care after procedure q4h and prn
  Wash with plain water
  Apply lanolin-based lotion
Maintain diet as ordered
Continue ongoing care for disease process
Check function of equipment on an ongoing basis

DEFIBRILLATION (DIRECT CURRENT COUNTERSHOCK)

NOTE: This is an emergency advanced life support procedure preceded by cardiopulmonary resuscitation until a defibrillator is available

Observations prior to procedure
Patient

Level of consciousness
ECG
  Ventricular tachycardia (unstable)
  Ventricular fibrillation
  Ventricular flutter
Pulse and respirations

Equipment

Placement of electrode paddles
  Anterior-posterior: anterior paddle on left precordium; posterior paddle beneath patient

Standard: one paddle to right of upper sternum (second to fourth intercostal space) and below clavicle; second paddle to left of nipple with center of electrode in midaxillary line
Placement of paddles in patients with permanent pacemakers should not be closer than 5 inches to pacemaker generator
Pulse and respirations
  Quality
  Rate
Skin
  Redness
  Irritation
  Sloughing

Observations following procedure

Level of consciousness
ECG
  Return to sinus rhythm
  Ventricular fibrillation
  Cardiac standstill

Care following defibrillation

Keep defibrillator on standby for immediate use as indicated
Check BP, R, and apical pulse after defibrillation, q5 to 10 min for 4 hr, then q30 to 60 min as ordered
Monitor cardiac activity; check rhythm strips immediately after procedures, then q2h to 4h and prn
Initiate life-support measures with closed-chest compression if no pulse is present
Administer oxygen with assisted ventilation as ordered
Maintain parenteral fluids as ordered
Administer skin care after procedures, q4h, and prn; use lanolin-based lotions
Continue ongoing care for specific disease process
Check function of equipment on an ongoing basis
Obtain laboratory studies as ordered
  Arterial blood gases and pH determinations
  Electrolytes
  Chemistries
  Chest x-ray examination
  Check paddle electrode size
    Infants and children: 4.5 cm in diameter
    Older children: 8 cm in diameter
    Adults: 10 cm in diameter
  Use saline-soaked gauze pads or electrode paste
  Check grounding of equipment surrounding patient
Energy requirements
  Ventricular fibrillation (and pulseless ventricular tachycardia)
    Initial shock: 200 joules
    Second shock: 200 to 300 joules
    Third shock: not to exceed 360 joules
  Ventricular tachycardia (pulse present)
    Initial shock: 50 joules
    Second shock: 100 joules
    Third shock: 200; up to 360 joules
  For children
    Initial dose: 2 watt-seconds (joules)/kg
    Second shock: 4 joules/kg and repeated twice

ANTICOAGULANT THERAPY

anticoagulant *Medication administered to prevent or treat arterial or venous thrombosis; used in treatment of pulmonary embolism, cerebral embolism, valvular heart disease, and with a heart valve prosthesis*

Assessment

Observations/findings

Therapeutic serum levels
  Warfarin: protime—1.5 to 2 × control
  Heparin: partial thromboplastin time—2 to 3 × control
Hematuria
Pain
  Abdominal
  Flank
Tarry stools
Hematemesis
Epistaxis
Bleeding gums
Hemoptysis
Subcutaneous bleeding
Ecchymosis
Hematoma
Joints
  Pain
  Immobility
Site of incision
  Bleeding
  Immobility
Neurologic changes
Increased menstrual flow
Medications
  Potentiate anticoagulation
  Retard anticoagulation

Interventions

Administer parenteral heparin as ordered
  Use heparin lock if ordered
  Give heparin at exact time ordered

Give dosage over a period of 1 min
Never skip doses
Do not remove heparin lock for 2 hr after last dose
Maintain continuous heparin infusion if ordered
Never hang more than 4 hr dose at one time; observe rate q30 min
Administer subcutaneous heparin as ordered rotating sites
Coordinate all laboratory work; avoid multiple punctures
Maintain manual pressure for at least 3 min after venous punctures
Check puncture sites qh
Check BP and P q4h to 8h
Avoid taking rectal temperature
Administer IM medications cautiously; apply manual pressure to injection sites until bleeding stops
Have protamine sulfate or phytonadione (Aqua-Mephyton) available
Administer routine medications cautiously; may potentiate or retard anticoagulation

Warfarin
Patient teaching/discharge outcome

Ensure that patient and/or significant other knows and understands
  Name of medication, dosage, time of administration, purpose, and side effects
  Need to avoid taking over-the-counter medication without checking with physician; to read labels of all medications
    Cold prescriptions with aspirin
    Laxatives
    Vitamins
  Not to take aspirin (acetylsalicylic acid) without physician's order
  Need for diet with moderate to low fat content without abundance of dark, leafy green vegetables; to avoid excessive use of alcohol
  Importance of having laboratory work done as ordered and of contacting physician for possible dosage change
  General side effects: anorexia, nausea, vomiting, abdominal cramps, dermatitis, and uticaria
  Signs of bleeding to report to physician
    Hematuria
    Vomiting
    Elevated temperature
    Pain in joints, swelling
    Epistaxis
    Bleeding gums
    Easy bruisability
    Increased menstrual flow
    Abdominal pain
  Safety precautions to prevent injury
    Avoid vigorous nose-blowing and toothbrushing
    Avoid use of sharp-edged instruments such as razors
    Refrain from water-jet tooth cleaners; use soft-bristled toothbrush
    Refrain from engaging in dangerous hobbies or contact sports
    Wear shoes and slippers at all times
  Importance of avoiding pregnancy while on medication; need to report to physician if pregnancy is suspected
  Need to avoid use of intrauterine device (IUD) for birth control
  Importance of ongoing outpatient care
  Need to carry medical alert or identification care with name of medication
  Need to inform physician when planning to travel in order to
    Obtain extra medications
    Arrange laboratory test

Subcutaneous Heparin Injection
Assessment
Observations/findings

Subcutaneous bleeding
  Hematoma
  Bruises
  Intraabdominal bleeding
    Pain
    Rigid, tender abdomen
  Tarry stools
  Bleeding gums
  Epistaxis
  Hematemesis
  Hemoptysis
  Hematuria
  Injection sites
    Inflammation
    Bruises
    Tenderness
  Increased menstrual flow
Allergic reactions
  Itching
  Urticaria
  Redness
Joints
  Pain
  Immobility

Pain
  Flank
  Abdominal

Patient teaching/discharge outcome
General guidelines

Ensure that patient and/or significant other knows and understands
  Name of medication, dosage, time of administration, purpose, and side effects
  Importance of giving heparin injections at exact time designated
  Importance of not skipping any doses; keep record of all missed doses
  Need to avoid taking over-the-counter medication without checking with physician
    Aspirin
    Salicylates
  Need to avoid drinking alcoholic beverages while on heparin therapy
  Importance of having laboratory work done as ordered
  Signs of bleeding to report to physician
    Bleeding gums
    Joint pain
    Epistaxis
    Hematuria
    Tarry stools
    Increased menstrual flow
    Easy bruisability
  Safety precautions to prevent injury
    Avoid vigorous nose-blowing
    Avoid vigorous toothbrushing
    Avoid use of sharp-edged instruments such as razors
    Refrain from water-jet tooth cleaners; use soft-bristled toothbrush
    Refrain from engaging in dangerous hobbies or contact sports
  Importance of preventing pregnancy while on medication; need to report to physician if pregnancy is suspected
  Need to avoid use of IUD for birth control
  Importance of taking correct dosage at correct time
Demonstrate and explain purpose of each step of heparin therapy
  Preparation for injection
  Rotation of injection sites
  Action of heparin
  Care of equipment
Have patient repeat steps verbally and then perform procedure
Positively reinforce proper performance of procedure and correct errors
Leave equipment at bedside for practice: syringe (1 to 2 ml with needle (25-gauge, ½ to ⅝ inch), vial of sterile water, alcohol swabs, and flat sponge or orange
Arrange to have equipment that will be used at home available
Have patient continue procedure with supervision while in hospital

Preparation of injection

Ensure that patient and/or significant other demonstrates
  Handwashing technique
  Preparation of syringe and needle using sterile technique
  Withdrawal of exact heparin dosage
  Ability to maintain sterile technique throughout procedure

Site of injection

Ensure that patient and/or significant other knows and understands
  Importance of using subcutaneous fatty tissue and avoiding bruised areas, hematomas, incisions, or scarred tissue and the area within 5 cm (2 inches) of umbilicus
  Importance of rotating site of injection with every dose of heparin to prevent bleeding or tissue damage
  Importance of recording site of each injection

Injection

Ensure that patient and/or significant other demonstrates injection technique
  Select injection site (Figure 2-46, A)
  Prepare skin by cleaning with alcohol
  Hold syringe filled with correct heparin dosage like a pencil or a dart
  Pinch up skin, forming a fat roll between fingers (Figure 2-46, B)
  Insert needle at 45-degree angle and quickly push it into subcutaneous tissue up to hub of syringe; may need to guide patient's hand at this point (Figure 2-46, C)
NOTE: Do not pull back on plunger
Inject medication slowly
Withdraw needle; gently release skin as needle is removed
Press area gently; avoid rubbing or massaging area
Record date, time, site, and dosage of each injection on home record

PATIENT CARE STANDARDS

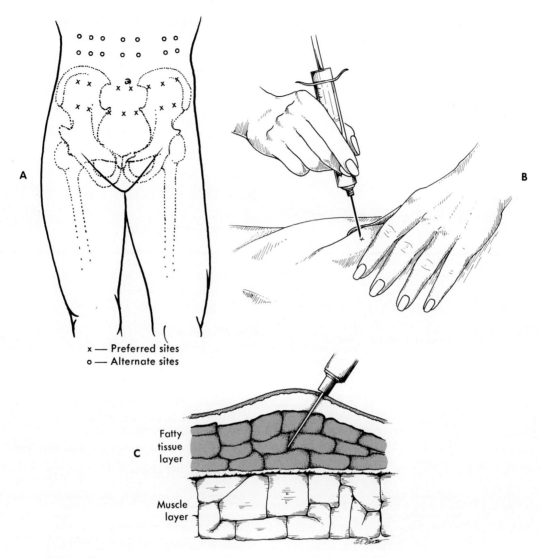

FIGURE 2-46. Subcutaneous heparin injection. A, Sites to be used. B, Pinching skin to form a flat roll between fingers. C, Injection into fatty tissue layer.

Heparin Home Record*

Date	Time	Site	Dosage
1/22/88	6:30 AM	Right upper side	5000 U
	2:30 PM	Left upper side	5000 U
	10:30 PM	Right lower side	5000 U
1/23/88			
1/24/88			

*Physician's order—5000 U heparin injected every 8 hr.

DIGITALIS THERAPY

digitalis Inotropic agent that improves myocardial contractility and efficiency and decreases rapid supraventricular rates

Assessment
Observations/findings
THERAPEUTIC EFFECTS

Increased myocardial contractility
    Increased stroke volume and cardiac output
    Decreased venous pressure
    Diuresis
    Reduced edema
Decreased AV conduction (negative chronotropic effect)

TABLE 2-8. Digitalis Therapy

	Digitoxin	Digoxin (Lanoxin)	Digitalis
Adult dosage (given in divided doses)	Oral: 0.5-1.6 mg over 24 hr IV: 0.5-1.6 mg over 24 hr	1.0-2.5 mg in 24 hr 0.5-1 mg followed by 2-3 additional doses of 0.125-0.25 mg IV or orally in 4-6 hr	1.5 g over 24 hr
Maintenance dose	0.05-0.2 mg	0.125-.25 mg po qd	100 mg po qd
Therapeutic serum levels	10-25 ng/ml	0.5-2.5 ng/ml	15-25 ng/ml
Toxic levels	35 ng/ml	>25 ng/ml	>35 ng/ml
Pediatric dosage			
Digitalization dose	Oral: given in 3 or more doses q6h	Oral Premature neonate: 0.025-0.05 mg/kg	Dose has not been established
	Premature and term neonates: 0.022 mg/kg	Term neonate: 0.04-0.08 mg/kg	
	Infants 2 weeks to 1 yr: 0.045 mg/kg	Infants 2 wk to 2 yr: 0.06-0.08 mg/kg	
	Infants 1 yr to 2 yr: 0.04 mg/kg		
	Children 2 yr and over: 0.03 mg/kg	Children 2 yr to 10 yr: 0.04-0.06 mg/kg IV: calculated at two thirds of oral dose	
Maintenance dose	Oral: one tenth of digitalizing dose once a day	Calculated at one eighth of digitalizing dose given q12h	
Therapeutic serum levels		<1 yr: up to 3.0-3.5 ng/ml >1 yr: 0.6-2.5 ng/ml	

SIDE EFFECTS

Slight hypokalemia
Gynecomastia

TOXIC EFFECTS

Noncardiac
  Anorexia
  Nausea and vomiting
  Diarrhea
  Fatigue
  Muscle weakness
  Headache
  Drowsiness
  Insomnia
  Restlessness
  Irritability
  Vertigo
  Confusion
  Hazy vision; halos around lights
  Visual color disturbance, especially yellow or green
Cardiac
  Regular increase (above 100) or decrease (below 60) in heart rate
  Arrhythmias
    Premature ventricular contractions
    Conduction defects
  Hypotension
  Chest pain
  CHF

Laboratory/diagnostic studies

Decreased potassium levels (below 3.5 mEq/L)
Digoxin level over 2.5 ng/ml
Digitoxin level over 20 ng/ml

ECG
  Prolonged PR interval
  Arrhythmias

Factors predisposing to toxicity

Hypokalemia
Hypercalcemia
Hypomagnesemia
Alkalosis
Renal or liver disease
Hypothyroidism
Rapid digitalization
Advanced heart disease; therapeutic to toxic range narrowed
Cor pulmonale

Medical management

Digitalization (12 to 24 hr; Table 2-8)
Cardiac pacing

Interventions

Check apical and radial pulse rate and rhythm before each dose and q4h
Be certain of correct dosage
Check BP and R q4h
Measure intake and output
Auscultate chest for breath sounds q4h if given for heart failure
Observe for signs of toxicity prn; check after dosages of potassium or diuretics are changed
Monitor serum electrolytes and digitalis levels as indicated

Care for toxicity

  Withhold medication
  Report observations to physician for further orders
  Check apical pulse rate and rhythm qh
  Place patient on cardiac monitor or ECG as ordered; measure rate and PR interval
  Administer medications as ordered
  Prepare for possible placement of pacemaker (p. 134)

Patient teaching/discharge outcome

Ensure that patient and/or significant other knows and understands
  Name and purpose of medication
    Relief of symptoms of heart failure
    Relief of heart rhythm irregularities
  Dosage of medications
    Do not increase or decrease dosage
    Report toxic symptoms to physician (can be caused by extra dose)
  Symptoms of recurrence of disease process to report to physician (can be caused by decreased dosage)
  Frequency of administration
    Take medication at same time each day
    Record dosage on calendar
    Use monthly medication holder
    Take medication exactly as ordered
    Understand that most of drug is excreted within 1 day
    Realize that no addiction is possible
    Do not stop taking drug because feeling better
Ensure that the patient and/or significant other demonstrates
  Pulse taking and recording
    Show location of radial or carotid pulse
    Watch patient find his pulse
    Demonstrate use of watch with second hand
    Tell patient to indicate 1 min by using watch
    Instruct patient to use watch and count pulse for 1 min
    Explain sequence of events
      Rest 2 to 5 min; take and record pulse
      Rest another 10 min and take pulse again if pulse rate is above 100 or below 60 beats/min or as ordered
      Withhold medication and notify physician if pulse is still over 100 or below 60 beats/min
      Take medication when pulse rate is between 60 and 100 beats/min and record on calendar

CHAPTER 3

Hematologic System

HEMATOLOGIC ASSESSMENT

General

Age
Sex
Ethnic background
Cultural background
Appearance
   Stated age equals appearance
   Pallor
   Facial flushing
   Profuse perspiration
   Signs of pain
   Dehydration
   Abnormal body posture, movements, or gait
   Activity level
Vital signs
   T, P, R, or BP changes
   Height and weight changes

Integumentary System

Skin and mucous membranes
   Complaints of
      Pruritus
      Easy bruisability
      Lesions, cuts, infections that do not heal
   Pallor
   Cyanosis
   Plethora
   Erythema
   Jaundice
   Petechiae
   Ecchymosis
   Purpuric lesions
   White patches
   Telangiectasis
   Rashes
   Subcutaneous nodules
   Infiltrates
   Vesicles
   Nonhealing lesions
      Increased skin temperature
      Drainage
      Ulcers
      Diaphoresis
      Turgor
      Note distribution of abnormalities
Nails
   Brittle
   Ridges
   Flattened
   Spoon shaped
   Clubbed
   Loosened
Hair
   Texture
   Growth patterns
Lymph nodes
   Complaints of swelling or tenderness under arms, in neck, or in groin
   Palpate for size, consistency, movement, and pain
   Palpable nodes: note location
      Nodular
      Hard
      Fixed or movable
      Tender
   Skin color over nodes
Eyes
   Edema
   Redness
   Inflammation
   Infection
   Enlarged/engorged vessels
   Vessel tortuosity
   Infiltration
   Hemorrhage
   Cataracts
   Position
   Alignment

Gastrointestinal System

Complaints of
   Nausea
   Vomiting
   Dysphagia

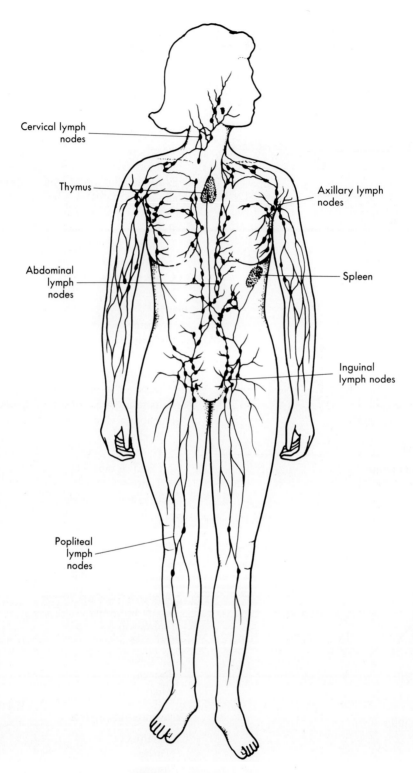

FIGURE 3-1. Lymphatic system.

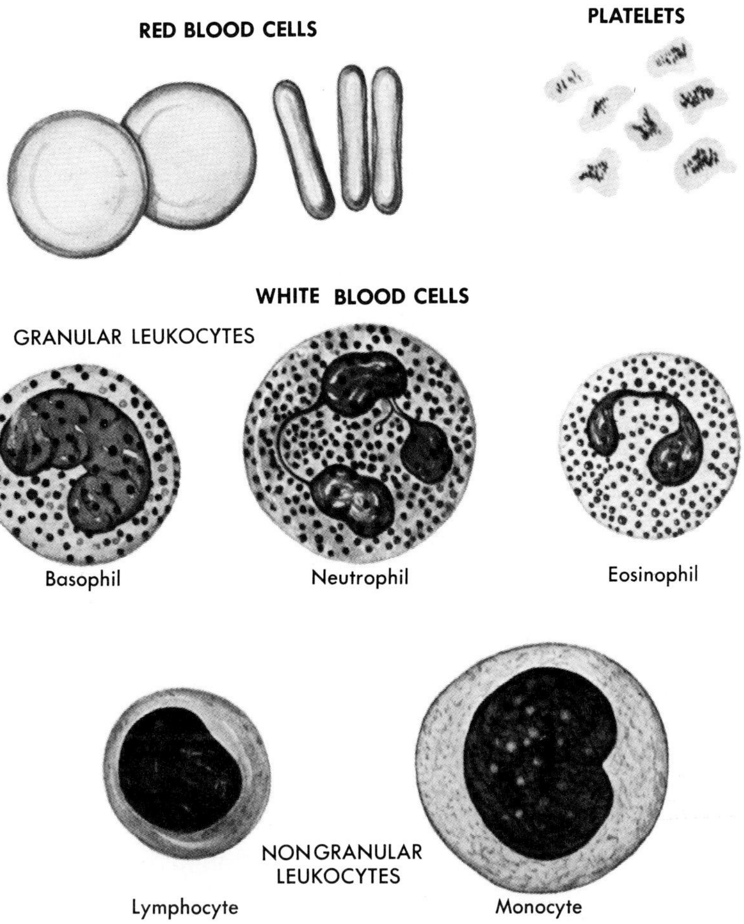

RED BLOOD CELLS

PLATELETS

WHITE BLOOD CELLS

GRANULAR LEUKOCYTES

Basophil Neutrophil Eosinophil

NONGRANULAR LEUKOCYTES

Lymphocyte Monocyte

FIGURE 3-2. Human blood cells. (From Anthony, C.P., and Kolthoff, N.J.: Textbook of anatomy and physiology, ed. 12, St. Louis, 1987, The C.V. Mosby Co.)

Anorexia
Weight loss
Mouth
  Red mucous membranes
  Bleeding of gums and mucosa
  Stomatitis
  Purpura
  Telangiectasis
  Tonsillar hypertrophy
  Gingival hypertrophy
  Ulcers
Tongue
  Complaints of pain
  Appearance
    Beefy
    Swollen
  Texture
    Absence of papillae
    Furrows
  Color: red

Abdomen
  Splenomegaly
  Hepatomegaly
Frank, occult bleeding in stool

Cardiovascular System

Complaints of
  Palpitations
  Shortness of breath
  Fatigue
    After exertion
    All the time
  Angina
Murmurs
Arrythmias
Tachycardia
Extremities
  Color
  Response to temperature changes

Respiratory System

Orthopnea
Tachypnea
Dyspnea
Rhythm
Excursion
Breath sounds change

Musculoskeletal System

Range of motion (ROM)
Joints/bones
    Swelling
    Pain
    Stiffness
Romberg's sign
Soft tissue
    Edema
    Hematoma
    Abscess

Genitourinary System

Hematuria
Incontinence
Impotence
Heavy menses

Neurologic System

Complaints of
    Headache
    Numb, tingling extremities
    Paresthesia
    Weakness
    Frequent napping
    Sleeplessness
Behavior/mood changes
Changes in attention span and responses

Pertinent Background Information
CONCURRENT DISEASES OR CONDITIONS

Frequent illness
Infectious processes
Blood transfusion/component therapy
Multiple allergies
Asthma
Bleeding tendency
Hemorrhage
Renal, cardiovascular, or liver disorders
Cancer

PREVIOUS SURGERY OR ILLNESS

Gastric ulcers
Gastric surgery
Hepatic surgery
Cardiac surgery
Renal surgery
Radioactive exposure and irradiation
Exposure to chemical agents
Recurrent infectious processes: frequent sore throats, etc.

FAMILY HISTORY

Cancer
Blood dyscrasias, anemias
Immune disorders
Allergies
Rh incompatibility

SOCIAL HISTORY

Smoking
Alcohol use
Increased stress
Occupation; exposure to toxic substances
Environmental factors
Diet
    Recent changes
    Cultural or religious restrictions
    Decreased protein intake
    Fad diets

MEDICATION HISTORY

Immunizations
Prescription medications
    Present medications
    Previously taken medications (e.g., chloramphenicol)
Over-the-counter medications
Home remedies
Use of other drugs

Diagnostic Aids
LABORATORY STUDIES

Complete blood cell count (CBC)
White blood cell count (WBC)/differential
Hematocrit (Hct)
Hemoglobin (Hgb)
Reticulocyte count
Platelet count
Mean corpuscular volume (MCV)
Mean corpuscular hemoglobin concentration (MCHC)
Mean corpuscular hemoglobin (MCH)
Bleeding time
Prothrombin time (PT)
Partial thromboplastin time (PTT)
Thrombin time
Activated partial thromboplastin time

Sedimentation rate
Electrophoresis of serum proteins
Immunoelectrophoresis of serum proteins
Total protein
Fibrinogen
Electrolyte values
Bilirubin level
Direct/indirect Coombs' test
Serum iron level
Ferritin titers
Sideroblasts
Hydrochloric acid level
Schilling test
Human lymphocyte antigens (HLA)

OTHER PROCEDURES

Biopsies
   Bone marrow
   Lymph nodes
   Spleen
   Liver
Lymphangiography
Chest and abdominal x-ray examinations
Computed tomography (CT) scans
   Bone
   Liver
Intravenous pyelogram (IVP)

PERNICIOUS ANEMIA (HYPERCHROMIC MACROCYTIC ANEMIA)

Defective red blood cell production caused by lack of the intrinsic factor essential for absorption of vitamin B_{12} (Deficiency of vitamin B_{12} causes gastric, intestinal, and neurologic abnormalities.)

TABLE 3-1. Signs and Symptoms of Blood Loss

Volume lost		Clinical signs
ml	%TBV*	
500	10	None; occasionally vasovagal syncope in blood donors
1000	20	At rest there may be no clinical evidence of volume loss; a slight postural drop in BP may be seen; tachycardia with exercise
1500	30	Resting supine BP and P may be normal; neck veins flat when supine; postural hypotension; exercise tachycardia
2000	40	Central venous pressure, cardiac output, and arterial blood pressure below normal even when supine and at rest; air hunger, rapid thready pulse, cold clammy skin
2500	50	Lactic acidosis, severe shock, death

From Wintrobe, M.M., et al.: Clinical hematology, Philadelphia, 1981, Lea & Febiger.
*Total blood volume.

TABLE 3-2. Approach to Hematologic Disorders; Various Clues That Might Be Found*

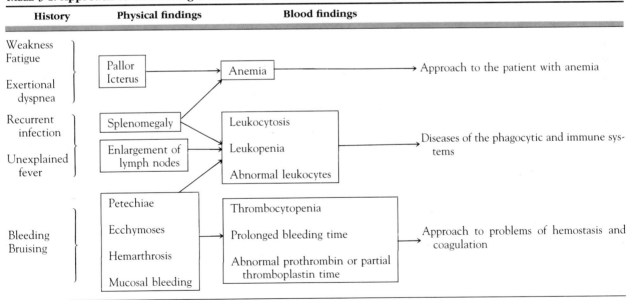

From Wintrobe, M.M., et al.: Clinical hematology, Philadelphia, 1981, Lea & Febiger.
*Features in the history, physical examination, or preliminary blood examination that can guide the examiner toward the solution of a clinical problem.

Assessment

Observations/findings

Central nervous system
  Fatigue
  Weakness
  Paresthesia of hands and feet
  Impaired fine finger movement
  Disturbed coordination and position sense; ataxia
  Positive Romberg's and Babinski's signs
  Disturbances in vision, taste, and hearing
  Irritability
  Poor memory
  Impaired judgment
  Depression
Gastrointestinal
  Tongue: beefy red, smooth, painful
  Flatulence
  Nausea, vomiting
  Anorexia
  Diarrhea
  Constipation
  Weight loss
Cardiovascular
  Palpitations
  Tachycardia
  Wide pulse pressure
  Dyspnea
  Orthopnea
Integumentary
  Skin: waxy, pale to bright lemon-yellow
  Sclera: slight jaundice
  Lips and gums: very pale
Family history of disease
Ethnic background: primarily Northern European
Age: usually between 50 and 60
Previous surgery: gastrectomy

Laboratory/diagnostic studies

Hemoglobin may be reduced to 4 to 5 g/100 ml
Decreased red blood cell count (RBC)
Elevated MCV, MCHC, MCH
RBCs of variable, abnormal size (anisocytosis)
RBCs of variable abnormal shape (poikilocytosis)
Serum $B_{12} < 0.1$ µg/ml
Decreased Schilling test
Bone marrow aspiration: erythroid hyperplasia, increased megaloblasts, and few normally developing RBCs
Gastric analysis: absence of free hydrochloric acid after pengastrin or histamine injection

Potential complications

Cardiomegaly
Congestive heart failure (CHF)
Gastritis
Paranoia
Hallucinations, delusions
Infection, usually genitourinary

Medical management

Vitamin B_{12} replacement therapy
Iron replacement, initially
RBC studies
Vital signs, pulse pressure monitoring

Nursing diagnoses/goals/interventions

ndx: Impaired gas exchange: fatigue and weakness related to impaired oxygen-carrying capacity of blood, with possible compensatory increased cardiac output

GOAL: *Patient will increase activity to desired level and will perform activities of daily living (ADLs) without evidence of fatigue and weakness*

If patient is on bed rest
  Maintain position of comfort
  Perform active or passive ROM exercises qid
  Assist with ADLs and ambulation to conserve energy
Plan undisturbed rest periods to conserve energy and permit performance of activities patient desires
Monitor pulse rate qid and during activities
Assess adverse responses to activities: tachycardia, irregular rhythm, dyspnea, etc.
Set goals with patient to increase activities as symptoms of intolerance decrease
Explain that activity tolerance will increase with therapy

ndx: Alteration in nutrition: less than body requirements related to impaired oral mucosa and fatigue

GOAL: *Patient will increase nutrient intake and increase weight to predisease level if indicated*

Administer oral hygiene q2h and before and after meals
Use dilute mouthwash or normal saline mouth rinse
Avoid irritating, hard-to-chew foods
Assist with meals when necessary to conserve energy
Present food attractively arranged on tray
Provide six small feedings or between-meal nourishment to enhance appetite
Provide foods and fluids of preference
Encourage significant other(s) to remain during mealtime

ndx: Potential for injury related to sensory-motor loss

GOAL: *Patient will not sustain injuries as a result of impaired neurologic or visual disturbance*

Maintain safe environment
Provide safety measures when needed: side rails up, bed in low position if on bed rest
Assess for absence of neurologic deficit before ambulation
Remind patient to call for assistance when needed
Remove obstacles and keep furniture in place when ambulatory
Use support-type slippers or shoes, walkers, canes, or other assistive devices when needed
Orient patient to time, place, or person as necessary
Assess skin integrity bid
Provide warmth through use of extra blankets or layers of clothing; avoid use of heating devices
Keep articles out of bed and prevent wrinkles
Avoid use of restrictive clothing and shoes

ndx: Potential for infection related to increased susceptibility secondary to decrease in WBC

GOAL: *Patient will not exhibit signs of infection*

Assess for signs of infection q8h
Avoid contact with infectious persons
Instruct patient in handwashing technique and when to perform
Teach patient to turn, cough, and deep breathe q4h
Give fluids to 3000 ml/day unless contraindicated
Provide undisturbed rest and sleep periods

ndx: Knowledge deficit regarding medication, disease process, nutrition, and activities

GOAL: *Patient and/or significant other will demonstrate understanding of home care and follow-up instructions through interactive discussion and actual return demonstration*

Medication

Explain need to administer vitamin B_{12} on ongoing basis; teach method for administration, name of medication, dosage, time of administration, purpose, and side effects
Instruct patient to avoid over-the-counter medications without checking with physician

Disease process

Instruct patient to observe and report symptoms of recurrence to physician; explain that symptoms will recede with continuing therapy (check with physician for those symptoms that may be irreversible)
Arrange for visits by public health nurse if needed
Instruct patient to continue follow-up care with physician and laboratory

Nutrition

Explain need to maintain balanced diet and fluid intake as ordered

Activity requirements

Explain need to increase activities gradually to desired level as tolerated
Explain need to avoid fatigue; to maintain planned rest periods
Instruct patient to use safety precautions when needed

Evaluation

Activity level is progressing toward preillness level; patient performs ADLs without evidence of exertional dyspnea or fatigue
Patient takes a balanced diet; weight is increasing toward normal range; skin and mucous membranes show evidence of return to normal
Patient exhibits healing process or no evidence of injuries or impaired skin integrity from falls or other injuries
Patient is free of signs and symptoms of infection in all body systems
Patient and/or significant other verbalizes understanding of home and follow-up care and demonstrates method for medication administration

IRON DEFICIENCY ANEMIA (HYPOCHROMIC, MICROCYTIC ANEMIA)

Defective red blood cell production resulting from depletion of iron stores in the body needed to synthesize hemoglobin

Assessment
Observations/findings

Neuromuscular
  Weakness
  Fatigue
  Vertigo
  Headache
  Inability to concentrate
  Irritability
  Numb, tingling extremities

Gastrointestinal
   Heartburn
   Anorexia
   Pica
   Glossitis
   Stomatitis
   Dysphagia
   Flatulence
   Vague abdominal pains
   Poor skin turgor
   Poor nutrition; inadequate iron intake
   Weight loss
   Chronic diarrhea
   Gastrectomy
   Chronic malabsorption syndrome
Cardiovascular
   Palpitations
   Tachycardia
   Functional systolic murmur
   Tachypnea
   Dyspnea on exertion
   Ankle edema
Integumentary
   Pale skin, mucous membranes
   Blue or pearl-white sclera
   Brittle, spoon-shaped fingernails
Chronic blood loss
   Gastrointestinal (GI) bleeding
   Heavy menses

Laboratory/diagnostic studies

Serum iron <55 mm/100 ml
Iron-binding capacity >350 µg/100 ml
Hgb: 6 to 10 g/100 ml; rings 6.2 to 6.8 µm in diameter
Decreased MCV
Decreased MCHC
Decreased MCH
Poikilocytosis marked
Reduced reticulocytes
Bone marrow studies: depleted or absent iron stores; normoblastic hyperplasia

Potential complications

Chest pain
Cardiomegaly
Hemoglobinuria

Medical management

Iron therapy, orally or parenterally
Diet high in iron-rich foods
Antifungal, anesthetic-type mouth rinse
Ascorbic acid
Stool softeners, laxatives

Nursing diagnoses/goals/interventions

ndx Alteration in nutrition: less than body requirements related to weakness, fatigue, glossitis, stomatitis, and/or anorexia

GOAL: *Patient will return to weight indicated for age, height, and body build within (time frame)*

Maintain balanced diet as ordered, usually high in iron
Provide six small feedings if easily fatigued
Provide foods of patient's preference and according to condition of oral mucosa; be certain that patient receives all nutrients required
Serve food attractively arranged; remove uneaten, undesired trays immediately
Assist with cutting foods, opening containers, and pouring liquids to preserve energy for eating
Have family visit during meals to provide company and assistance when necessary
Administer oral hygiene before and after meals and q2h to 4h; use soft-bristled toothbrush and dilute mouth rinse if glossitis or stomatitis is present
Administer antifungal, anesthetic-type mouth rinses as ordered
Administer iron therapy as ordered
   Oral: use straw if liquid preparation is used, to prevent staining teeth
   Parenteral
     IM
        Avoid staining tissue
        Use second needle after withdrawal from ampule
        Use Z-tract method of injection
        Inject 0.5 cc of air before removing needle from tissue
     IV
        Administer test dose as ordered
        Give cautiously; remain with patient initially
        Use small-gauge needle
        Cover solution with dark plastic
        Observe for symptoms of shock with IV use
Administer ascorbic acid if ordered
Avoid constipation: increase fluids and bulky foods; administer stool softeners or laxatives as ordered
Weigh patient daily at same time with same clothing and scale

ndx Sensory-perceptual alteration related to vertigo, numbness or tingling of extremities, headache, irritability, and/or decreased concentration secondary to decreased oxygen-carrying capacity of the blood

GOAL: *Patient will experience no injury related to neuromotor disturbances (during hospitalization)*

Provide a safe environment free of obstacles

Provide extra bedclothes, warm robes, etc., when needed; avoid added warmth through use of uncontrolled-temperature heating devices

Instruct patient to sit at side of bed and then stand before walking to determine if dizziness is present

Direct patient to call for assistance with ambulation when needed

Assist with hygiene and other care to prevent injury

Avoid very hot liquids at meal or bath time

Plan care with patient to promote consistency and sense of calmness

Encourage verbalization of concerns about concentration ability; assure patient that this will improve with therapy

Inform patient of each step of activity or instruction; do not overload patient with many, varied instructions at one time

Avoid completing sentences for patient; listen with patience

ndx: Activity intolerance related to palpitations, tachycardia, dyspnea on exertion, and/or pallor secondary to decreased oxygen exchange

GOAL: *Patient will increase activity level without evidence of increased pulse rate or pallor and with no complaints of dyspnea*

Monitor vital signs (BP, P, and R) qid, during and after activity

Assess response to activity

Plan with patient so that desired activities can be performed by patient without exertion

Assist with ADLs, when necessary, to preserve energy

Provide uninterrupted rest periods to maintain energy level

Increase activities patient performs in small increments until tolerance level is reached

ndx: Knowledge deficit regarding disease process, medication, nutrition, and activities permitted

GOAL: *Patient and/or significant other will demonstrate understanding of home care and follow-up instructions through interactive discussion and actual demonstration*

Medication

Discuss medications: name, dosage, time of administration, purpose and side effects to report (nausea, vomiting, diarrhea, or constipation)

Explain need to continue iron therapy even though feeling well

Discuss color of stools expected and explain need to avoid constipation

Explain reason for not taking oral iron medication with milk or antacids

Demonstrate method for parenteral administration of iron

Nutrition

Explain importance of maintaining a balanced diet high in iron-rich foods and liquids

Explain importance of monitoring weight weekly

Disease process

Discuss signs and symptoms of recurrence to report to health provider

Activity

Explain importance of increasing exercise and activities to tolerance, alternating with periods of rest

Discuss how to prevent injury through assessment of self-help and ambulation abilities; discuss symptoms that indicate assistance is needed or activities should be decreased

Evaluation

Patient takes a balanced diet; weight is increasing toward normal range; skin, sclera, and mucous membranes show evidence of healing and return to normal color

Patient demonstrates method for and understanding of medication administration

Patient verbalizes precautions to avoid injury and exhibits none

Activity level is progressing toward preillness level; patient performs ADLs without evidence of tachycardia or exertional dyspnea; skin color is no longer pale

Patient and/or significant other verbalizes home care instructions and demonstrates parenteral administration of medication

HEMOLYTIC ANEMIA

A disorder characterized by a rapid rate of erythrocyte destruction; ability of the bone marrow to increase the production of erythrocytes determines the extent of anemia present; may occur with inherited or acquired red blood cell disorders, or in response to toxic agents or drugs, infectious disease, or trauma

Assessment
Observations/findings

Inherited RBC disorder
   Fatigue

Shortness of breath
Jaundice
Urine changes
Trauma/infectious disease
   Chills
   Fever
   Weakness
   Jaundice
   Irritability
   Headache
   Nausea
   Vomiting
   Abdominal pain
   Diarrhea
   Decreased urinary output
Acquired RBC disorder
   Headache
   Fatigue
   Shortness of breath
   Jaundice
   Nocturnal hemoglobinuria
   Abdominal pain
   Splenomegaly
   Venous thrombosis

Laboratory/diagnostic studies

Increased reticulocyte count
Normocytic anemia
Decreased hematocrit
Increased RBC fragility
Shortened erythrocyte life span
Increased bilirubin

Potential complications

Renal failure
Hemogloblinuria

Medical management

Elimination of causative factors
Management of primary condition (trauma, e.g., burns; infectious disease)
Parenteral fluids
Washed PRC transfusions
Whole blood transfusions (for rapid, severe hemolysis)
Osmotic diuretics
Corticosteroids

Nursing diagnoses/goals/interventions

ndx: Fluid volume deficit related to vomiting and/or diarrhea

GOAL: *Patient will maintain balanced intake and output and stable weight*

Monitor intake and output q8h; report imbalances
Weigh patient daily at same time with same clothing and scale; report changes of 2% to 3% of original weight
Monitor vital signs q4h
Assess skin turgor q8h
Administer parenteral fluids, electrolytes, and blood transfusions as ordered
Administer antidiarrheals and antiemetics as ordered
Assess type and amount of foods and liquids tolerated
Provide clear liquid diet to reduce nausea: juices, carbonated beverages, flavored ice pops
Arrange for quiet rest periods prior to meals

ndx: Activity intolerance related to fatigue, weakness, and shortness of breath

GOAL: *Patient will perform activities and self-care procedures*

Plan with patient so that desired activities can be performed by patient without exertion
Assist with ADLs when necessary to preserve energy
Provide uninterrupted rest periods to maintain energy level
Increase activities patient performs in small increments until tolerance level is reached
Assess response to activity; note positive advances
Advise significant others to encourage and assist patient with continuing efforts

ndx: Potential alteration in tissue perfusion: renal related to hemoglobinuria and decreased output; peripheral related to thrombus formation

GOAL: *Patient will maintain urinary output of >500 ml/8 hr with normal color and characteristics (renal) and maintain normal peripheral pulses (peripheral)*

Renal

Monitor intake and output of 8 hr; report output <30 ml/hr and change in color, character, pH, and specific gravity
Force fluids to 3000 ml/day unless contraindicated
Enlist patient's assistance
   Provide fluids of choice and temperature
   Offer small amounts frequently (makes taking fluids less of a chore)
   Serve attractively
Administer parenteral fluids as ordered
Administer osmotic diuretics as ordered
Check T, P, R, and BP q4h; report elevation in BP
Weigh patient daily at same time with same clothing and scale

Avoid chemical oxidants (antimalarials, sulfonamides, phenacetin, chloramphenicol, nitrofurantoin, and fava beans)

Peripheral

Check peripheral pulses q4h; report diminished or absent pulses

Assess color and temperature of extremities q4h; report evidence of thrombosis

Encourage ambulation or ROM exercises q4h

Instruct patient not to cross legs, sit for long periods of time, or wear restrictive clothing

ndx: Alteration in comfort: pain related to headache and abdominal pain

GOAL: *Patient will verbalize feeling of increased comfort*

Maintain environment free of stress

Assess pain: predisposing factors, intensity, frequency, duration, and effective methods of control used by patient

Place patient in position of comfort

Change position qh; assist with ROM exercise if helpful

Consider diversional, relaxation, or imagery measures

Administer pain relief medications as ordered at patient's request; assess effectiveness

ndx: Impairment of skin integrity related to jaundice and/or pruritus

GOAL: *Patient will have intact skin*

Assess condition of skin q8h

Administer daily skin care and as needed
  Soothing baths: sodium bicarbonate or oatmeal
  Avoid skin dryness; apply lotions to slightly moist skin
  Cool sponge baths or tub soaks may be beneficial

Keep clothing light with no constrictions

Elevate bedclothes with bed cradle

Keep bed wrinkle-free

Use linen laundered in nondetergents

Advise patient to avoid scratching; instead, apply pressure or use cool applications

ndx: Knowledge deficit regarding disease process, activity/hygiene, and complications

GOAL: *Patient and/or significant other will verbalize understanding of home care instructions and return-demonstrate method of monitoring fluid balance*

Disease process

Instruct patient about type of hemolytic condition
  Hereditary RBC deficiency: patient is susceptible to hemolysis after ingestion of chemical oxidants; family members should be screened
  Response to trauma or infectious disease
    Explain that primary condition will be treated
    Discuss symptoms of recurrence to report
  Acquired RBC deficiency
    Explain that this may be induced by infection, immunization, iron products, or plasma in whole blood transfusions
    Discuss symptoms of recurrence and thrombus formation to report
    Demonstrate method of inspecting extremities and peripheral pulses

Activity/hygiene

Explain importance of increasing activities daily

Explain need to plan and maintain regular rest and sleep periods

Instruct patient to use assistance from others to conserve energy when needed

Explain need to perform daily skin care; discuss products to use to increase comfort, prevent injury, and decrease itching

Complications

Discuss symptoms of renal failure to report

Demonstrate method of measuring and recording intake and output

Explain importance of taking at least 3000 ml of fluids each day unless contraindicated

Explain importance of eating a balanced diet and using supplements when necessary

Discuss methods of reducing nausea and instruct patient to report persistent vomiting episodes

Evaluation

Patient is taking a balanced diet and at least 3000 ml of fluid daily

Vital signs are stable with balanced intake and output
  Peripheral pulses are present; extremities are warm with good color and turgor

Patient performs self-care procedures

Activity level is increasing daily without evidence of fatigue, weakness, or shortness of breath

Patient verbalizes feelings of increased comfort and reports no headache or abdominal pain

Patient and/or significant other verbalizes understanding of home care and follow-up instructions, and demonstrates methods of taking peripheral pulses and measuring intake and output, and weight

APLASTIC ANEMIA

Anemia, aplastic or hypoplastic, resulting from destruction or injury to the bone marrow stem cells or bone marrow matrix; exposure to toxins, specifically large doses of radiation, benzene, metabolites, alkylating agents, chloramphenicol, or sulfonamides, may cause pancytopenia (bone marrow failure with granulocytopenia, thrombocytopenia, and anemia)

Assessment
Observations/findings

Anemia
    Waxlike pallor
    Fatigue
    Weakness
    Failure to gain energy after rest
    Dyspnea on exertion
    Headache
    Dizziness
    Irritability
    Slowed thought processes
    Confusion
    Unsteady gait
Bleeding tendency
    Petechiae
    Ecchymosis; especially dependent areas, sites of pressure
    Bleeding
        Gums
        Nose
        GI tract
        Urinary tract
        Vagina
Infection
    Elevated temperature
    Cold, flulike symptoms
    Cough
    Nonhealing cuts, lesions
    Burning pain on urination
History of exposure to chemical toxin, or radiation, specific medications

Laboratory/diagnostic studies

Erythrocytes
    <1 million/mm^3
    Normocytic
    Normochromic
Reticulocytes: low
Leukocytes: <2000/mm^3
Granulocytes: reduced
Platelets: <30000/mm^3
Serum iron: elevated
Iron binding capacity: normal if not bleeding
Bone marrow: hypocellular, fatty marrow with few stem cells

Potential complications

Hemorrhage
Cirrhosis
Diabetes
Heart failure
Blood reactions
Overwhelming infections

Medical management

Elimination of identifiable cause
Blood transfusions
    Packed cells
    Platelets
    Leukocytes, HLA matched
Bone marrow transplant
Laboratory studies
Supportive care
    Oxygen therapy
    Corticosteroids
    Antibiotics
    Pain management
    Monitoring of cardiac status

Nursing diagnoses/goals/interventions

ndx: Activity intolerance related to fatigue, weakness, dyspnea, and/or headache

GOAL: *Patient will perform desired activities without evidence of intolerance*

Position patient comfortably
    Position with head elevated 30 degrees or position for maximum chest expansion if respiratory difficulty occurs
    Support with pillows
Administer oxygen therapy as ordered
Take and record vital signs q4h to 8h
Assess respiratory and cardiac status q4h to 8h; report tachycardia, irregular cardiac sounds, dyspnea, wheezes, or rales
Assess neurologic status q8h
Provide adequate periods of sleep and rest
    Plan nursing activities to avoid interrupting sleep
    Provide activity-free periods throughout the day for rest; schedule examinations and tests carefully
Conserve patient's energy for desired activities

Assist with meal preparation
Assist with hygiene measures
Plan activities after rest periods
Maintain activity as tolerated
    Perform passive or assist with active ROM exercises q4h for patient on bed rest
    Assist with ambulation
        Move patient carefully
        Avoid bumps, falls, scratches, or cuts
Determine activity tolerance
    Check pulse rate
    Note posture, respirations, and facial expression
    Allow patient to set own pace
Alternate activity with planned rest periods
Observe safety precautions
    Instruct patient to sit at side of bed before getting up; change position slowly
    Keep needed items close to patient
Keep patient warm
    Encourage use of warm robes, socks, and clothing
    Provide extra blankets; note that cotton sheets are often more comfortable
    Provide nutritious diet high in iron
    Plan rest periods after meals
    Administer blood products when ordered (p. 212)
    Monitor laboratory studies

ndx: Potential alteration in tissue perfusion: cerebral, cardiovascular, gastrointestinal, renal, and/or peripheral related to bleeding

GOAL: *Patient will maintain adequate circulation as evidenced by stable vital signs and no symptoms of bleeding*

Auscultate chest for heart and breath sounds q4h
Monitor cardiac status continuously
Monitor central venous pressure (CVP) q2h to 4h
Check BP, T, R, and apical pulse q4h
Assess sensorium and neurologic status q4h to 8h
Check stools for bleeding
Measure intake and output; check urine for bleeding q4h to 8h
Assess skin and mucous membranes for extension or new sites of ecchymosis, hemorrhage, or hematoma q4h
If bleeding tendency or hemorrhage
    Use smallest-gauge needles possible
    Consolidate laboratory work; use fingersticks when able
    Apply pressure to site of puncture for 5 min and observe q15 min for 1 hr
    Do not disturb clots
    Do not take rectal temperature or administer rectal medications
    Avoid scratching
    Use soft-bristled toothbrush, towels, and nonabrasive soaps
    Assist with walking when necessary to avoid bumps and falls
    Avoid constipation
        Increase fluids to 3000 ml/24 hr if permitted
        Add bulk to diet
        Use stool softeners or laxatives as ordered
Prepare for bone marrow studies when ordered (p. 209)
Administer blood tranfusions as ordered
    If patient is not hemorrhaging, rate of transfusion is not to exceed 1 ml/kg body weight/hr
    The lower the Hgb, the slower the rate of transfusion
Administer platelets as ordered
Observe for blood reactions
Maintain balance sheet
Monitor laboratory studies
Administer corticosteroid therapy as ordered (p. 467)
Prepare for bone marrow transplantation when ordered (p. 181)

ndx: Alteration in nutrition: less than body requirements related to fatigue and possible presence of oral lesions

GOAL: *Patient will maintain optimal weight for disease status as evidenced by decreased weight of not more than 10%*

Assess amount and types of foods and liquids tolerated and desired
Provide diet high in vitamins and proteins; observe patient's preferences
Provide fluids of patient's choice to 3000 ml daily unless contraindicated
Measure intake and output q8h
Notify physician when intake and output are not equivalent and/or weight decreases by 3% to 5%
Weigh patient daily at same time with same clothing and scale
Administer total parenteral nutrition (TPN) when ordered (p. 51)

Fatigue

Arrange for quiet rest periods prior to meals
Eliminate distractions during mealtimes
Provide stress-free, no-hurry environment
Serve tray attractively arranged
Assist with cutting of food and preparation for eating

Position patient and tray to reduce energy expenditure
Assist with meal or ask family or friends to remain during mealtimes to assist as necessary
Small, frequent, high-calorie meals may be preferable

Oral lesions

Teach and assist with routine oral care
  Inspect and palpate lips, gums, and buccal mucosa gently q8h
  Clean teeth and rinse mouth each morning, after meals, and at bedtime
  Increase frequency of oral care to q2h with presence of lesions
Choice of dental equipment will depend on state of oral cavity
  Soft-bristled toothbrush if there are no breaks or lesions
  Gauze or sponge-covered cleaners if there are breaks in skin or gum is bleeding
Rinse mouth q2h to 4h to keep free of particles and reduce bacterial count
  Commercial mouthwash may be irritating
  Peroxide diluted with saline or water, or saline alone may be used
Assess denture fit
  Avoid gumlike grips
  Keep dentures scrupulously clean
  Remove and clean before using mouth rinse
Keep mouth moist
  Provide appealing, tepid liquids for sipping
  Flavored ice pops may be soothing
Keep lips moist; use water-soluble gel
Provide time for patient to prepare for meals
  Perform oral hygiene
  Rinse mouth and gargle 15 to 20 min before meals
  Use local anesthetic or mixture of antihistamine, antacid, and local anesthetic as ordered
  Spray mouth with anesthetic solution in atomizer when ordered
Administer antifungal mouthwash as ordered; diluted frozen antifungal medication may be more appealing and efficacious
If patient is unable to open mouth for oral hygiene
  Prepare irrigating solution; half hydrogen peroxide and half normal saline, or as ordered
  Place solution in irrigating container with tubing (clean, disposable tube feeding bag)
  Hang 12 to 18 inches above patient's chin level
  Place patient in 60- to 90-degree position
  Gently irrigate all surfaces, allowing solution to flow into emesis basin
  Follow with normal saline rinse
  Discard unused solution each time

Provide foods that are nonirritating, easily chewed, and high in nutrition
  Avoid very hot or very cold foods
  Use soft foods often: custards, yogurt, soups, etc.
  Avoid citrus and very sweet foods
  Hot, spicy, or acidic foods are usually intolerable
  Hard fruits and vegetables may be grated to make them palatable
  Puree solid foods or add gravies and sauces to assist with swallowing
  Soft casseroles or soups may be used
Use straws or cups for liquidized foods: utensils, especially forks, may cause more discomfort

ndx: Anxiety related to decreased activity tolerance, slowed thought processes and irritability, and/or threat of dying

GOAL: *Patient will exhibit decreasing signs of irritability and tolerance of limited activities*

Assess level of anxiety and understanding of disease process when appropriate
Visit frequently or have significant other remain with patient
Use touch, reassurance, and positive body language
Be sensitive to needs; listen to nonverbal clues
Plan care with patient to ensure meeting needs and expectations
Be consistent and provide care on time as planned; give explanations if delays are unavoidable
Speak clearly and concisely; allow patient time to complete requests and thoughts; do not anticipate and complete sentences
Provide atmosphere for discussion of fears and consequences of limited ability to carry out ADLs
Provide information about condition, procedures, and diagnostic studies
Encourage questions; answer clearly, consistently, and clarify when necessary
Encourage communication with significant other
Provide diversional activities within limits of patient's energy level
Assess responses to activities and ventilation of feelings
Encourage use of adaptive coping measures
Provide access to others as requested: clergy, social worker, business associates, etc.

ndx: Potential for infection related to increased susceptibility secondary to decreased leukocytes

GOAL: *Patient will not exhibit symptoms of infection*

Place in noninfectious environment
Use physical means to reduce exposure to bacteria
  Instruct and ensure that personnel and visitors follow handwashing procedure with povidone-iodine before entering room
  No one with infectious condition (colds, flu, cold sores, skin rash, etc.) may enter room
  Staff assigned to care for patient must not be assigned to care for patients who have infections
Keep room clean
  Avoid any trash in room and bathroom
  Remove food and examination trays immediately after use
  Maintain furniture, fixtures, floor, and equipment free of dust and spills
Ensure that no plants, flowers, fresh fruits, or vegetables are taken into room
Ensure that allied health personnel (e.g., laboratory technicians) do not bring equipment into patient's room that has been in other areas of hospital
If patient requires transportation, avoid using elevator with potentially infectious passengers present; gown and mask for patient may be required
Assess and record skin condition each shift
Provide mild, antibacterial soaps and soft cloths and towels for skin hygiene, daily and prn
Encourage mobility q2h
Turn and position immobile patient q2h to prevent pressure areas
Initiate and teach perineal care to be performed after each bowel movement; use povidone-iodine wash, ABDs, or very soft cloths; rinse and dry well
Prevent constipation and diarrhea
  Administer medications as ordered
  Avoid use of enemas and suppositories
Maintain skin integrity
  Avoid IM injections
  Observe IV, central line site q4h
    Change dressing daily if nonporous type is used, using aseptic technique
    Change IV tubing and bottles daily
    Avoid infiltrations that necessitate restarting IV
    Position IV site to prevent stress and movement at site of insertion
Consolidate laboratory work; clean skin with povidone-iodine scrub prior to puncture
Assess previous puncture sites each shift
Assess and record condition of oral cavity each shift
  Teach or assist with oral hygiene measures in morning, after food ingestion, at bedtime, and q2h to 4h when patient is awake at night
  Administer antifungal medication as ordered
Assess and record condition of perineum daily

Monitor and record vital signs q4h; take temperature more frequently if trend is beginning
Report temperature elevations immediately
Institute comfort and cooling measures as indicated by condition
  Change linen and clothing to keep patient dry
  Administer antipyretics as ordered
  Prevent chilling; turn q2h
Monitor intake and output; report urinary frequency, burning, or changes in character of urine
Use voiding measures when indicated to avoid catheterization
If catheterization is necessary
  Use strict aseptic technique for insertion
  Perform catheter care each shift
Obtain cultures as ordered and monitor results: blood, urine, sputum, skin, drainage, etc.
Assess and record respiratory status q4h; report changes in breath sounds, cough and sputum, increases in respiratory rate, or presence of sore throat immediately
Assist and teach patient to turn, cough, and deep breathe q2 to 4h
Administer oxygen if ordered
Administer IV antibiotics as ordered
Monitor laboratory data daily; report changes
Administer granulocyte transfusions as ordered (p. 213); monitor migration of transfused granulocytes to site of infection (e.g., complaints of pain at site of infection, such as anal lesion; respiratory complications requiring ventilatory assistance, etc.)

ndx: Knowledge deficit regarding nutrition, activity, and complications

GOAL: *Patient and/or significant other will verbalize understanding of home care and follow-up instructions and return-demonstrate oral and skin care, taking of pulse, management of oxygen therapy, management of minor bleeding, testing of urine and stool for occult blood, and management of TPN*

Nutrition

Explain need to maintain balanced diet of preference and as tolerated: to use frequent, small feedings if preferred; to avoid foods that irritate oral mucous membranes
Explain need to take fluids of preference—at least 3000 ml/day unless contraindicated
Explain need to perform mouth care routinely before and after meals and prn; to report early signs of mouth lesions or those that do not heal; to use special mouth rinses as ordered

Demonstrate method of checking for and explain need to report signs and symptoms of mucositis

Explain need to weigh weekly with same amount of clothing and at same time of day

Demonstrate management of TPN when ordered

Activity

Instruct patient to alternate activities with rest periods to conserve energy

Explain need to increase activity gradually; to not become nonfunctional

Instruct patient on placing personal items at hand and furniture to prevent accidents

Demonstrate use of equipment to assist with ambulation when needed

Explain need to monitor activity tolerance (check pulse rate; if elevated or feeling exhausted, rest, then continue)

Instruct patient to report symptoms to physician if no relief occurs with rest

Demonstrate oxygen therapy administration
  Liters/minute ordered
  Use of equipment: changing tank, cleansing or replacement of cannula
  Mucous membrane observations and care

Bleeding

Discuss signs and symptoms of bleeding to be reported to physician in any of the following areas
  Skin
  Oral
  Nasal
  Rectal
  Stomach
  Cerebral
  Urinary tract

Discuss emergency plan to follow if spontaneous hemorrhage occurs
  Have emergency numbers on hand
  Call paramedics
  Go to nearest emergency area

Explain importance of telling dentist and other medical personnel about disease process and low platelet count

Explain importance of maintaining safe, clutter-free environment

Demonstrate method for applying pressure at blood withdrawal site after laboratory work is completed

Explain importance of avoiding over-the-counter medications, especially those containing acetylsalicylic acid (i.e., aspirin) without checking with physician

Instruct patient to avoid use of sharp objects when possible
  Use electric razor
  Use caution when handling knives or other equipment

Instruct patient to avoid harsh coughing and blowing of nose
  If cough persists, notify physician
  Take cough medication as ordered

Explain need to avoid activities and sports that may cause injury

Explain need to avoid constipation through diet, fluids, and stool softeners

Explain importance of ongoing outpatient care
  Routine laboratory appointments
  Return physician and nurse appointments

Ensure that patient and/or significant other demonstrates
  Method for applying pressure to bleeding site
    Apply dressing or clean material directly over site
    Apply pressure for 5 min
    Apply ice in covered plastic bag over site once bleeding stops
    Check site for further bleeding q15 min for 1 hr
  Method for testing stool and urine for occult blood

Infection

Discuss signs and symptoms of infection to report to physician or nurse

Explain importance of avoiding persons who may be infectious or who may have potentially contagious conditions, as well as persons who have been recently vaccinated and crowds

Explain need to avoid multiple sexual partners

Explain need to wash hands after using bathroom before eating, or before performing any care procedures or food preparation

Discuss importance of preventing injury to skin
  Use electric razors
  Handle knives and sharp objects carefully
  Wear protective gloves when gardening and when using strong household cleaning solutions
  Wear broad-brimmed hat and sun screen when in sun
  Avoid going barefoot
  Wear warm clothing and boots in cold weather
  Avoid cutting cuticles, corns, or calluses
  Wear padded gloves when using oven

Explain need to perform oral hygiene periodically throughout day and importance of daily hygiene, including perineal and rectal care

Explain importance of drinking up to 3000 ml of fluid

each day unless contraindicated; need to avoid using common drinking fountain

Explain need to maintain clean home environment and handle food properly

Explain need to avoid contact with pets or other animals

Demonstrate method for taking and recording temperature

Demonstrate procedure for caring for very small cuts or breaks in skin

Evaluation

Activity level is progressing toward preillness level; patient performs desired activities without evidence of fatigue or weakness

Vital signs remain stable; there is no evidence of bleeding; previous bleeding sites are resolving; skin and mucous membranes are warm and moist with good turgor

Weight is stable and/or increasing toward normal range; patient takes a balanced diet and adequate fluids or maintains TPN therapy; no oral lesions are present, or healing is progressing; bowel elimination has returned to normal pattern

Patient expresses and discusses fears and anxiety regarding prognosis; discusses realistic future plans; seeks out resources and assistance as needed; shows infrequent or no evidence of anxiety

All body systems are free of signs and symptoms of infection, or previous sites are healing; no evidence of lung congestion; urine is clear; oral temperature is 98.6° F (37° C)

Patient and/or significant other verbalizes understanding of home and follow-up care; and demonstrates handwashing, skin, and mouth care, use of oxygen equipment, taking temperature, testing urine and stool for occult blood, and management of TPN

POLYCYTHEMIA

An increase in the number of circulating erythrocytes

polycythemia vera *A chronic disorder in which overproduction of myelocytes, thrombocytes, as well as erythrocytes, occurs with a resulting increase in blood viscosity, blood volume, and hemoglobin concentration*

secondary polycythemia *A compensatory response to hypoxemia, which may result from chronic obstructive pulmonary disease (COPD), congenital heart disease, or prolonged exposure to low oxygen content (high altitude)*

relative polycythemia *A result of decreased plasma volume; erythrocyte level is normal or decreased*

Assessment

Observations/findings

Skin
  Dusky, red-purple (rubor) appearance: face, mucous membranes, and hands
  Pruritus
  Urticaria
Cardiovascular
  Hypertension
  Intermittent claudication
  Chest pain
  Thrombus
  Emboli
  Bleeding
Central nervous system
  Headache
  Dizziness
  Tinnitus
  Lassitude
  Paresthesia
  Bleeding
Respiratory: dyspnea with exertion
Gastrointestinal
  Epigastric distress
  Feeling of fullness
  Thirst
  Flatulence
  Constipation
  Weight loss
  Bleeding
  Hepatosplenomegaly (polycythemia vera)
Eyes
  Blurred vision
  Diplopia
  Engorged veins: fundus, retina
Musculoskeletal: symptoms of gout

Laboratory/diagnostic studies

RBC: 7 to 12 million/mm^3
Hgb: 8 to 25 g/100 ml
Hct: >60%
Myelocytosis ⎫
Thrombocytosis ⎬ polycythemia vera
Hyperuricemia ⎭

Potential complications

Thromboses in any system
  Myocardial infarction (MI)
  Cerebrovascular accident (CVA)
  Gangrene: digits
Hemorrhage in any system
Congestive heart failure (CHF)

Peptic ulcer
Leukemia

Medical management

Phlebotomy, pheresis therapy
Fluid replacement
Myelosuppressive therapy
   Radioisotopes
   Alkylating agents
Secondary, relative polycythemia: treatment of underlying disease or condition; environmental change

Nursing diagnoses/goals/interventions

ndx Alteration in tissue perfusion: cardiopulmonary, cerebral, gastrointestinal, and/or peripheral related to hyperviscosity of blood and potential bleeding

GOAL: *Patient will exhibit stable vital signs and peripheral pulses, absence of dizziness, and paresthesia*

Maintain position of comfort when on bed rest
   No knee gatch
   Active or passive ROM exercises q2h to 4h
   Padded footboard for exercises
   Change position qh
   Avoid restrictive clothing; use bed cradle when necessary
   Keep patient warm and dry
Avoid sitting for long periods; instruct patient not to cross legs when sitting or lock knees when standing; use well-fitting, not tight, slippers or shoes
Monitor BP, T, R, apical pulse, and neurologic status q4h to 6h
Auscultate chest for breath and heart sounds q4h to 6h
Assist and teach patient to turn, cough, and deep breathe q4h
Check peripheral pulses, and color and temperature of extremities q4h to 6h
Auscultate abdomen for bowel sounds q4h to 6h
Assess skin and mucous membranes q4h to 6h
Report early signs or symptoms of thromboses or bleeding to physician
If bleeding tendency
   Avoid invasive procedures when possible.
   Consolidate laboratory procedures; use smallest-gauge needles possible; observe for bleeding at venipuncture sites; apply pressure over site for 5 to 10 min or until bleeding stops
   Avoid trauma
      Provide soft-bristled toothbrush
      Place articles needed by patient within reach
      Arrange furniture and provide good lighting to avoid bumps and falls when ambulating
   Instruct patient to call for assistance if needed
Encourage communication with significant other
Provide information about condition and progress; answer questions consistently; promote other stress-reduction activities
Prepare for phlebotomy or pheresis therapy as ordered
   Explain procedure
   Check vital signs before and after procedure
   Assess for untoward responses during procedure: vertigo; cold, clammy skin; tachycardia; hypotension
   Instruct patient to sit for 10 to 15 min and then stand for 3 to 5 min before attempting ambulation
Administer myelosuppressive agents as ordered

ndx Alteration in nutrition: less than body requirements related to epigastric distress, feelings of fullness, and lassitude

GOAL: *Patient will take balanced meals with fluids to 3000 ml daily (unless contraindicated) to maintain weight at optimal level for age, build, and height*

Assess amount of food or fluids patient can take before feeling full
Provide small feedings of nutritious foods and liquids to patient's tolerance; low-sodium, low-purine diet may be ordered; avoid gas-forming, acidic foods
Have snacks available but out of sight if this contributes to distress
Vary texture of foods and liquids to enhance appetite
Provide time for oral hygiene before and after meals; assist when necessary
Arrange rest periods prior to meals and assist with preparations to conserve energy
Serve meals attractively arranged
Arrange for visitors of patient's preference to enhance social aspect of mealtime
Encourage ROM exercises or ambulation between meals
Weigh patient daily at same time with same clothing and scale
Measure intake and output q8h

ndx Alteration in comfort: pain related to joint discomfort, pruritus, urticaria, or headache

GOAL: *Patient will verbalize feelings of increased comfort*

Joint discomfort

Place patient in position of comfort; support joints anatomically with pillows or pads
Change position qh; assist with ROM exercise
Avoid restrictive clothing; use bed cradle
Use alternate comfort measures: distraction, imagery, etc.
Administer analgesics as ordered; assess effectiveness

Pruritus, urticaria

Assess condition of skin and mucous membranes q4h to 8h
Administer skin care q4h to 6h; provide soothing, cool baths with oil or bicarbonate of soda
Provide unrestrictive clothing that is not rough; clothing laundered with nondetergents may be needed
Keep bedclothes wrinkle-free to prevent irritation
Keep nails short and manicured to prevent scratches
Use distraction and socialization to increase comfort
Administer medications as ordered; assess effectiveness

Headache

Maintain quiet environment
Provide uninterrupted rest periods
Encourage fluid intake
Provide hot or cold compresses of patient's choice
Administer analgesics as ordered; assess response

ndx: Knowledge deficit regarding disease process, complications, activity, nutrition, and medication

GOAL: *Patient and/or significant other will demonstrate understanding of home care and follow-up instructions through interactive discussion and actual return demonstration*

Disease process

Discuss symptoms of recurrence or progression of disease and complications to report to physician
Demonstrate how to check skin and peripheral pulses
Explain importance of regular follow-up care

Complications

Discuss trauma prevention
  Avoid restrictive clothing
  Wear well-fitting shoes
  Keep home and work area free of clutter
  Use assistive devices when needed
  Use caution when performing oral hygiene
  Avoid sports and hobbies that may cause injury
  Handle equipment and sharp objects carefully
  Avoid extremes in environmental temperature

Activity

Instruct patient to balance rest and activity periods
Instruct patient not to cross legs when sitting or lock knees when standing; explain need to change position and exercise extremities q30 min
Explain need to plan regular exercise program

Nutrition

Explain importance of well-balanced diet; low-sodium or low-purine diet may be ordered
Instruct patient to take at least 3000 ml of fluid daily unless contraindicated
Discuss foods to avoid: gas-forming, acidic foods

Medication

Teach name of medication, dosage, time of administration, purpose, and side effects
Instruct patient to avoid taking over-the-counter medications without checking with physician

Evaluation

Vital signs are stable, peripheral pulses are palpable, color and temperature of extremities are within normal limits; no presence of dizziness or paresthesia is verbalized by patient; symptoms of bleeding are not noted
Patient takes a balanced diet with fluids to 2000 to 3000 ml daily; weight is progressing toward or has stabilized at optimal level; bowel and bladder functions are normal (output 1500 to 3000 ml/day)
Patient manages activities without discomfort; there is no evidence of urticaria; skin is clear with good color; patient verbalizes absence of headache

THROMBOCYTOPENIA

A bleeding disorder in which the number of platelets is reduced; defective or diminished production of platelets may be caused by bone marrow infiltration, aplastic anemia, myelosuppressive drugs, radiation, or viral infections; increased peripheral destruction may be caused by immune drug sensitivities, chronic idiopathic thrombocytic purpura (ITP), nonimmune infection, disseminated intravascular coagulation (DIC), or thrombotic thrombocytopenic purpura (TTP)

Assessment
Observations/findings

Mild to excessive bleeding
  Skin: easy bruising, petechiae, ecchymosis
  Epistaxis
  Gum bleeding, blood-filled bullae

"Coffee ground" vomitus or hematemesis
Blood-streaked sputum
Hematuria
Guaiac-positive stool
Heavy menses
Cerebral: headache, slurred speech, malaise
Numb, painful extremities

Laboratory/diagnostic studies

Platelets <100,0000/mm^3
Prolonged bleeding time
Normal coagulation time
Decreased Hgb
Increased capillary fragility
Bone marrow: increased number of megakaryocytes in ITP

Potential complications

Hemorrhage
Loss of consciousness

Medical management

Treatment of underlying cause or removal of precipitating agent
Corticosteroids
Immunosuppressive therapy
Plasmapheresis
Platelet or whole fresh blood transfusions
Splenectomy
Analgesics

Nursing diagnoses/goals/interventions

ndx: Alteration in tissue perfusion: cardiopulmonary, cerebral, and/or renal related to bleeding

GOAL: *Patient will maintain adequate circulation as evidenced by stable vital signs and no evidence of bleeding*

Maintain bed rest when bleeding
  Position patient comfortably
  Support with pillows
  Avoid pressure to any area of body; use foam or gel pads, sheepskin, air mattress, and heel and elbow guards
  Protect from sheet burns; use turn-and-lift sheet to move patient in bed
Check BP, T, P, and R qid
Auscultate chest for breath sounds each shift
Assess neurologic status q2h to 4h when applicable
Check stool and urine for bleeding daily
Assess skin and mucous membranes for bleeding q4h to 8h

Monitor laboratory studies
Administer care to sites of puncture
  Consolidate laboratory work
  Use fingersticks when possible
  Apply pressure at least 5 to 10 min after puncture or until bleeding stops
  Observe site for bleeding or hematoma q15 min for four times
  Clean area with povidone-iodine swab prior to venipuncture
  Place bacteriostatic ointment at site
  Use sterile technique when changing dressings daily
  Observe site q1h to 2h for redness, pain, swelling, or infiltration
Avoid trauma
  Protect patient from falls and bumping into or dropping objects; arrange furniture and equipment conveniently; pad bed rails if necessary; assist with ambulation when necessary
  Avoid use of constrictive clothing; use bed cradle to prevent tight bedclothes
  Use soft towels and cloths for bathing; avoid vigorous skin care
  Advise patient to avoid straining at stool to prevent increasing intracranial pressure; use stool softeners or laxatives as ordered to prevent constipation
  Provide soft-bristled toothbrush; avoid use of nonelectric razors
  Advise patient not to cough to avoid increased intracranial pressure
Administer platelet or whole fresh blood transfusions when ordered; administer platelets quickly through recommended tubing to prevent destruction
Administer corticosteroid therapy and immunosuppressive therapy as ordered (ITP)
Avoid use of antihistamines, phenothiazines, aspirin, and nonsteroidal, antiinflammatory agents in ITP
Prepare for plasmapheresis when ordered (p. 209)
Administer medications (penicillin, sulfinpyrazone, acetylsalicylic acid, dipyridamole, or antihistamines) to inhibit platelet function as ordered in TTP
Prepare for splenectomy if ordered (p. 206)

ndx: Impaired tissue integrity of oral mucous membrane related to blood-filled bullae generally found in the mouth

GOAL: *Patient will tolerate food and fluids as evidenced by not more than a 5% to 10% decrease in weight unless weight reduction is ordered*

Assess integrity of oral mucous membrane q4h
Administer careful oral hygiene before and after meals and q2h to 4h

Use soft-bristled toothbrush; avoid brushing area with bullae

Rinse mouth with dilute mouthwash or irrigate if patient is unable to do so

Maintain diet of preference or as ordered; avoid use of hard, spicy, or difficult-to-chew foods to prevent trauma

Provide fluids of choice to 3000 ml daily unless contraindicated; iced liquids may be more comforting

Measure intake and output q8h

Weigh patient daily at same time with same clothing and scale

ndx: Alteration in comfort: pain related to nerve pressure secondary to bleeding

GOAL: *Patient will verbalize a decrease in or relief from pain*

Assess pain (location, duration, intensity, and predisposing factors) q4h to 6h

Position patient for comfort; use pillows or other support as needed

Provide bed cradle to prevent constriction by bedclothes

Provide warm or cold applications as patient desires

Place articles within patient's reach

Manage visitors according to patient's wishes

Administer analgesics as ordered; assess effectiveness

ndx: Knowledge deficit regarding disease process, nutrition, activity, and medication

GOAL: *Patient and/or significant other will verbalize understanding of home care and follow-up instructions and return-demonstrate methods of checking for bleeding, performing hygiene, and skin care*

Disease process

Demonstrate method to assess for bleeding

Discuss signs and symptoms of recurrence to report to physician: continuous headache, coughing red-streaked sputum, persistent abdominal pain, vomiting frank blood or "coffee ground" material, increased areas of petechiae or ecchymosis, blood-filled bullae in oral cavity, blood in urine or stools

Demonstrate methods of checking for blood in stool and urine

Instruct patient to notify physician when contemplating pregnancy or when pregnancy is first suspected

Caution patient to never donate blood

Explain need to prevent trauma by

Avoiding constipation through diet, fluids, and use of stool softeners or laxatives if needed; avoiding vigorous nose-blowing or coughing; avoiding contact sports or other hazardous hobbies

Careful movements and handling of objects

Use of nonabrasive skin and mouth care products

Explain importance of notifying all health care providers of diagnosis and to keep follow-up appointments

Nutrition

Explain importance of regular oral hygiene; discuss products to use or avoid; demonstrate method for daily inspection

Explain need to maintain balanced diet with adequate hydration; discuss foods to avoid to prevent trauma

Activity

Explain need to balance rest and activity periods; to increase activity as comfort increases; to use assistance when needed to prevent injury

Medication

Teach name of medication, dosage, time of administration, purpose, and side effects

Teach how to read contents of over-the-counter medications, avoiding those that contain acetylsalicylic acid (antihistamines, phenothiazines, or nonsteroidal antiinflammatory agents in ITP)

Evaluation

Vital signs remain stable; there is no evidence of bleeding in new areas, or past areas of bleeding are resolving

Patient is taking a balanced diet with adequate fluids; weight has stabilized; there are no oral lesions, or healing is progressing; bowel and bladder elimination is normal

Patient manages activities without pain or discomfort and uses assistive aids when necessary

Patient and/or significant other verbalizes understanding of home care and follow-up instructions; demonstrates method to detect any bleeding, including checking stool and urine; and demonstrates oral hygiene and skin care measures

ACUTE LEUKEMIA

Uncontrolled proliferation of leukocytes and their precursors in the bone marrow with infiltration of lymph nodes, spleen, liver, and other body organs
acute lymphocytic (lymphoblastic) leukemia (ALL) *Lymphoblasts proliferate in bone marrow*

and lymph nodes and invade other tissues; primarily a disease of childhood

acute myelogenous leukemia (AML) *Proliferation of myeloblasts (immature polymorphonuclear leukocytes); occurs in all age-groups but is more common in adults*

Assessment
Observations/findings

Central nervous system
  Elevated temperature
  Easily fatigued
  Malaise
  Irritability
  Syncope
  Headache
Skin and mucous membranes
  Pallor
  Petechia
  Easy bruising
  Ecchymosis
  Purpura
  Gum bleeding
  Epistaxis
  Infection: may appear red or dark without pus
  Stomatitis
Gastrointestinal
  Abdominal discomfort
  Nausea, vomiting
  Dysphagia
  Esophagitis
  Anorexia
  Weight loss
  Perirectal abscess
  Hepatosplenomegaly
Cardiopulmonary
  Tachycardia
  Palpitations
  Shortness of breath
  Cough
Musculoskeletal
  Bone or joint pain
  Mediastinal mass with tenderness

Laboratory/diagnostic studies

WBC
  May be low or elevated with "shift to the left"
  Excessively elevated (T cell ALL)
  Blasts
  Lymphocytes (ALL)
  Auer rods (AML)
  Phi bodies (AML)
Reticulocytopenia
  Normochromic (AML)
  Normocytic
Anemia
Thrombocytopenia
Elevated serum and urine uric acid
Elevated serum copper
Decreased zinc
Hypergammaglobulinemia (AML)
Bone marrow: proliferation of blast cells

Potential complications

Acute infection
Anemia
Hemorrhage
Organ failure

Medical management

Antineoplastic chemotherapy
Fluid therapy
Antibiotics
Radiation therapy
Transfusions; blood components
Bone marrow transplant
Analgesics, hypnotics, narcotics

Nursing diagnoses/goals/interventions

ndx: Alteration in tissue perfusion: cerebral, cardiopulmonary, gastrointestinal, peripheral, and/or renal related to bleeding or hemorrhage

GOAL: *Patient will exhibit no signs of bleeding; vital signs and peripheral pulses will be within acceptable limits*

Assess for bleeding q4h; more often if bleeding is suspected; report indications of bleeding to physician
  Check BP, P, R, T, and peripheral pulses
  Auscultate chest for breath and heart sounds
  Assess neuro signs
  Assess skin and mucous membranes
  Auscultate abdomen for bowel sounds
  Measure intake and output
  Hematest urine and stool
Initiate and maintain parenteral fluids as ordered
Maintain integrity of central venous line
Administer blood components as ordered
  Platelets
    Observe for changes in bleeding status during and after transfusions
    Usually ordered at fast rate of infusion to ensure therapeutic effectiveness
  Red blood cells: leukocyte-poor; usually ordered

Administer vasopressors and corticosteroids as ordered
  Use mechanical volume/rate controllers to maintain exact rate of infusion required
Monitor laboratory data daily; more often when ordered
  Report changes to physician immediately
  Label requests "bleeding tendency"
  Order fingersticks when possible
  Apply pressure to site for 3 to 5 min after puncture or until bleeding stops; observe for further bleeding
Intubation and mechanical ventilatory assistance may be required during periods of acute sepsis and shock
Place patient in position of comfort; use pillows or pads for support when necessary; provide care for pressure points
Avoid restrictive clothing or bedclothes; use bed cradle or footboard
Use turn-and-lift sheet to move patient
Avoid chilling; provide extra blankets, bed socks, and dry bedding when needed
Teach and assist patient to change position q1h to 2h; perform or assist with ROM exercises
Plan activities to alternate with uninterrupted rest periods
Assist with daily care as needed to conserve energy; assess patient's tolerance level
Encourage ambulation and self-care activities as early as possible
Prevent trauma
  Avoid invasive procedures when possible
  For IM injections use smallest-gauge needle; apply pressure until bleeding stops; recheck
  Monitor invasive procedure sites for bleeding (e.g., IV, catheters, etc.)
  Use soft-bristled toothbrushes or sponge cleaners
  Use electric razors
  Provide safe environment with careful arrangement of furniture and placement of personal items
  Provide good lighting for ambulation
  Advise use of well-fitting slippers or shoes
  Prevent constipation; provide privacy; provide adequate fluids and diet; administer stool softeners or laxatives as ordered
Administer antineoplastic chemotherapeutic agents as ordered; assess for response and reactions (p. 669)
Prepare for radiation therapy (p. 705) or bone marrow transplant (p. 181) when ordered

ndx: Potential for infection related to increased susceptibility secondary to impaired function of white blood cells and myelosuppression

GOAL: *Patient will not exhibit signs of infection*

Place in noninfectious environment
  Private room
  Require handwashing with povidone-iodine scrub for all personnel and visitors prior to entering room
  Remove food, trash, and drainage receptacles from room promptly
  Ensure that no fresh fruits, vegetables, plants, or cut flowers are taken into room
  Screen all personnel and visitors for infection
  Provide support for patient to prevent feelings of isolation and alienation
Plan care with patient
Assist with daily care
  Ensure that skin is dry after bathing
  Assist with oral hygiene before and after meals and q2h
  Handle patient carefully; prevent sheet burns and other injuries to skin integrity
  Assist with and teach perineal care after elimination and daily
Provide adequate, uninterrupted rest periods
Teach patient to turn and deep breathe q2h; avoid vigorous coughing
Assess for infection q4h in all body systems; report early signs to physician immediately
  Temperature of 101° F (38.5° C)
  Sore throat, "cold," "flu," coughing
  Burning on urination
  Small cuts or lesions that do not heal
Cooling measures may be required; avoid chilling; administer antipyretic drugs as ordered
Administer antibiotics on time when ordered
  Obtain necessary cultures quickly to avoid delay in starting antibiotics
  Cultures of throat, blood, urine, stool, and other lesions or areas may be ordered
  Monitor results
Administer granulocytes, HLA-matched, as ordered
  Potential marrow donor will not be used as donor for granulocytes prior to transplant; will use donor's granulocytes after transplant
  Monitor patient for pain at sites of infection or potential infection (e.g., increased respiratory symptoms after infusion)

ndx: Alteration in nutrition: less than body requirements related to nausea, vomiting, anorexia, abdominal discomfort, or impaired oral mucous membrane

GOAL: *Patient will take a balanced diet to maintain or not lose more than 5% to 10% of present weight*

Assess amount and types of foods and liquids tolerated and desired
Administer oral hygiene before and after intake
 Use equipment appropriate to condition of mouth
 Administer oral anesthetic when ordered
Assess predisposing factors, onset, position, frequency, and duration of nausea, vomiting, or discomfort
Eliminate predisposing factors when possible: unpleasant odors, perfume, disturbing sights or sounds
Change eating patterns; provide frequent, light meals; avoid foods and liquids for 2 to 4 hr before meals; and/or change usual place for eating
Serve foods cold or at room temperature to eliminate odors: sandwiches, cereal, cheese, desserts
Provide clear liquid diet to reduce nausea: juices, carbonated beverages, flavored ice pops
Provide high-protein drinks as a supplement
Vary textures and tastes of foods to determine those tolerated: bland, sour, soft, etc.
Sweet, highly seasoned foods are not usually well tolerated
Administer antiemetics when ordered as patient desires
Arrange for quiet or rest periods prior to meals
Assist with preparation to conserve energy
Serve food and liquids attractively
Arrange for visitors, if patient prefers, to enhance social aspect
Weigh patient daily at same time with same clothing and scale
Measure intake and output q8h
Notify physician when intake and output are not equivalent and/or weight decreases by 3% to 5%
Administer TPN as ordered (p. 51)

ndx: Alteration in comfort: pain related to bone or joint discomfort, headache, pressure of bleeding, or lesions

GOAL: *Patient will verbalize feeling of increased comfort or of tolerable level of pain*

Maintain environment free of stress, unexpected sounds, or lighting
Assess pain: predisposing factors, intensity, frequency, duration, and effective methods of control used by patient
Place patient in position of comfort; support joints and extremities with pillows or pads
Change position qh; assist with ROM exercise if helpful
Remove restrictive clothing; use bed cradle or footboard
Provide soothing baths and back care; use warm or cold applications when helpful
Consider diversional, relaxation, or imagery measures
Administer pain relief medications as ordered at patient's request; assess effectiveness

ndx: Fear related to threat of death

GOAL: *Patient will exhibit decreasing symptoms of anxiety/fear and will verbalize feelings about and understanding of condition*

Assess level of anxiety and understanding of disease process when appropriate
Visit frequently or have significant other remain with patient
Use touch, reassurance, and positive body language
Provide an environment conducive to discussion and expression of worries, fears, and loss
Provide information about condition, procedures, and diagnostic studies
Encourage questions; answer clearly, consistently, and clarify when necessary
Be sensitive to needs; listen to nonverbal clues
Maintain and assist with coping strategies
Encourage continuation of relationships
Provide access to others as requested: clergy, social worker, business associates, etc.

ndx: Knowledge deficit regarding disease process, complications, nutrition, activity, anxiety/fear, and medications

GOAL: *Patient and/or significant other will verbalize understanding of home care instructions and return-demonstrate method of checking for complications, hygiene measures, and management of TPN*

Disease process

Discuss symptoms of recurrence or progression of disease to report to physician
Demonstrate how to check skin and peripheral pulses
Explain importance of regular follow-up care: physician, drug administration, laboratory studies

Complications
BLEEDING

Discuss signs and symptoms of bleeding to report to physician
Demonstrate how to check urine and stool for bleeding

Discuss accident/injury prevention
  Avoid restrictive clothing
  Keep home and work area free of clutter
  Use assistive devices for ambulation and work when needed
  Use caution when performing oral hygiene; inspect mouth for breaks or lesions; use special equipment and dentrifices as indicated
  Avoid sports and hobbies that may cause injury
  Handle equipment and sharp objects carefully
  Prevent constipation through adequate fluids and diet, and use of stool softeners or laxatives

INFECTION

Discuss signs and symptoms of infection to report: temperature elevation, sore throat, "cold," "flu," coughing, burning on urination, small cuts, hangnails, lesions that do not heal
Explain need to prevent infection
  Keep environment clean
  Do not handle pets and their equipment
  Avoid persons with infections and large crowds
  Handwashing technique for self and those assisting in the home
  Daily self-care routine including perianal care after elimination

Activity

Instruct patient to balance rest and activity periods
Explain need to plan daily routine, using assistance when necessary
Instruct patient to increase activity or exercise as desired and tolerated

Nutrition

Explain need to have nutritious foods and liquids to 3000 to 4000 ml/day
Emphasize need to continue plan/eating pattern to enhance appetite
Give sources for delivery of prepared meals and high-protein drinks
Demonstrate how to manage TPN therapy (p. 51)

Anxiety/fear

Teach recognition of early symptoms
Explain need to continue open communication to discuss and express feelings
Discuss ways to continue problem solving and decision making
Discuss sources for assistance: psychosocial, financial, spiritual

Medications

Teach name of medication, dosage, time of administration, purpose, and side effects
  Discuss side effects and complications to report to physician
  Demonstrate care and use of volumetric infusion device for medication administration (p. 60)
Explain need to avoid over-the-counter medications without checking with physician

Evaluation

Vital signs remain within acceptable limits; there are no further signs of bleeding; previous bleeding sites are resolving; skin and mucous membranes are warm and moist with good turgor; self-care and activity level are increasing daily
No signs of infection are present; previous sites of infection are healing; there is no evidence of lung congestion; urine is clear; oral temperature is 98.6° F (37° C)
Patient is taking nutritious foods and liquids or maintains TPN therapy; weight has stabilized; oral mucous membranes are intact, or healing is progressing; bowel elimination has returned to normal pattern and consistency
Patient verbalizes feelings of increased comfort; uses alternate pain control methods interspersed with medication; self-care and exercise-activity tolerance are increasing
Patient expresses and discusses feelings about disease, treatment, and prognosis; sets realistic goals; seeks out resources and assistance from others when needed; and shows infrequent or no evidence of symptoms of fear or anxiety
Patient and/or significant other verbalizes home care and follow-up instructions; demonstrates methods for detecting signs of bleeding and infection, including checking urine and stool; and demonstrates oral hygiene and skin care measures, management of TPN therapy, and/or use of volumetric device for medication administration

BONE MARROW TRANSPLANTATION (BMT)

A treatment approach that has resulted in the cure of various neoplastic and hematologic diseases by replenishing depleted bone marrow cell reserves; care is divided into three phases: pretransplant (preparation), conditioning, and transplant

Indications

Several types of leukemia; usually in remission
  Acute lymphocytic leukemia (ALL)

Acute nonlymphocytic leukemia (ANLL)
Chronic myelocytic leukemia (CML)
Aplastic anemia
Severe combined immunodeficiency disease
Thalassemia
Lymphoma
Some solid tumors

Assessment on admission
Observations/findings

May be asymptomatic if in remission
Shortness of breath
Anemia
Bleeding tendency
Easy bruising
Petechiae
Maculopapular rash
Fever
Weakness
Chronic fatigue
Pain in joints and bones

Preparation Phase

Phase during which necessary preparation procedures are performed; these include procedures for decreasing the amount of bacteria on the body surface, as well as inside the body, and diagnostic studies

Assessment
Observations/findings

Response to diagnostic procedures or medications
    Bone marrow biopsy
    Lumbar puncture
    Right atrial catheter insertion
Ability to perform self-care procedures

Laboratory/diagnostic studies

Bone marrow studies
CBC
Platelet count
Fasting blood sugar (FBS)
Serum glutamic oxaloacetic transaminase (SGOT)
Serum glutamic pyruvic transaminase (SGPT)
Bilirubin
Alkaline phosphatase
Blood urea nitrogen (BUN)
Creatinine
Urinalysis
Quantitative immunoglobulin
HAA
HAV

Antigen/antibody titer
EBV
CMV
Type/screen
RBC typing
Chest x-ray examination
ECG

TABLE 3-3. Typical Bone Marrow Transplant Schedule

Day	Scheduled activity
PREPARATION PHASE	

−8	Admission
	  Consents
	  Bone marrow aspiration
	  Lumbar puncture with intrathecal methotrexate instillation (acute leukemia)
	  Administration of nonabsorbable antibiotics
	  Laboratory tests
	  Begin low-bacterial diet

−7	Insertion of double-lumen right atrial catheter Dosimetry Begin teaching self-care procedures and activity requirements
CONDITIONING PHASE	
−6	Insertion of three-way urinary catheter Leukemia: high-dose cytarabine (ARA-C) or cyclophosphamide administered Aplastic anemia: high-dose cyclophosphamide administered Force fluids: 4000 to 4500 ml for adults; 3000 ml/m^2 for children
−5	Continue high-dose chemotherapy and increased fluid intake
−4	Three-way urinary catheter discontinued if no bleeding after completion of high-dose chemotherapy
−3	Total-body irradiation (divided dose) (ordered for leukemia; may be ordered for aplastic anemia)
−2	Total-body irradiation (divided dose) Begin cyclosporine
−1	Total-body irradiation (divided dose)
TRANSPLANT	
0	Marrow, aspirated from donor, is infused to establish graft
POSTTRANSPLANT	
+1 to +30	Observe for engraftment, reactions to total-body irradiation, and complications of transplanted marrow

Medical management

Informed consents
Laboratory and diagnostic studies
Lumbar puncture with intrathecal methotrexate (acute leukemia)
Insertion of double-lumen right atrial catheter
Dosimetry
Low-bacterial diet
Nonabsorbable antibiotics
Allopurinol
Bactrim

Nursing diagnosis/goal/interventions

ndx: Knowledge deficit regarding transplant information and informed consent, central line, dosimetry, self-care procedures, and diet

GOAL: *Patient and/or significant other will verbalize understanding of bone marrow transplant (phases, activities, and procedures) and will return-demonstrate self-care procedures*

BMT procedure

Ensure that patient and/or significant other has read information about BMT, outcome, and possible complications
Encourage questions; give clear, consistent answers; be alert for unspoken questions
Reinforce physician's explanation
Involve other health care workers as necessary to ensure that patient has information required to make decisions
Explain sequence of events for each phase; discuss support systems available to patient and family; introduce all health care providers who will be involved with patient; orient patient to environment: room, unit, radiation therapy department, etc.

Expected care

Explain importance of performing self-care procedures and maintaining exercise and activity levels throughout hospitalization
Teach and have patient demonstrate performance of the following
  Handwashing technique
    Use povidone-iodine solution
    Wash hands prior to self-care activities and meals, and after toileting
  Mouth care
    Must be done at least four times each day
    Never use toothbrush
    May use soft sponge cleaners to clean gums and teeth
    Rinse mouth well with entire amount of one of the following solutions
      Peroxide, 30 mg, in 150 ml of sterile normal saline or sterile water
      Sterile normal saline: 150 to 200 ml
      Sterile water: 150 to 200 ml
    Follow with antifungal rinse and swallow as ordered; usually ordered on day of total-body irradiation (TBI)
  Skin care
    Daily shower with antibacterial soap
    Rinse well
    Dry all body areas thoroughly, especially folds
      Use soft towels
      Avoid vigorous rubbing
  Perineal care
    Must be performed after each voiding or bowel movement
    Wash hands
    Place ordered amount of povidone-iodine peri-wash solution in plastic squeeze bottle
    Add sterile water to solution; never add tap water
    Place solution on sterile pad (ABD)
    Clean perineal area, from front to back for females; avoid use of toilet tissue
    Discard used pad
    Wash hands
  Intake and output
    Give list of measurements
    Discuss measurement tools
    Have patient record amounts on bedside record sheet
  Use of incentive spirometer
Explain and demonstrate assessments that will be done and daily frequency (q8h or more frequently if changes are noted)
  Oral status
  Skin including perianal area
  Respiratory
  Cardiac
  Gastrointestinal
  Neurologic
  Hematest for stool and urine
Discuss activity level that patient will be expected to maintain
  Shower and bathroom activities
  Ambulation and ROM exercises
  Use of exercycle
  Diversionary activities: TV watching, reading, computer/TV games, small handicrafts
Explain procedures, expected effect, and rationale

Bone marrow aspiration
Lumbar puncture
Dosimetry
Insertion of central line
Explain low-bacterial diet
  Diet will be used for 100 days
  Only sterile distilled water and ice cubes will be used; patient should never drink tap water
  Give list of foods permitted (p. 195)
  Food will not be left at bedside
  Food from home must be on the approved list and cooked on the day it is brought to the hospital

Evaluation

Patient and/or significant other verbalizes understanding of BMT procedure, anticipated tests, procedures, medication effects, and self-care expected during hospitalization

Conditioning Phase

First phase of the clinical course; involves treatment of patient with a pretransplant "conditioning regimen"; for patients with leukemia, high-dose cytarabine (ARA-C) or cyclophosphamide and TBI have become standard treatment; for patients with aplastic anemia, high-dose cyclophosphamide is given with or without TBI

Assessment

Observations/findings

Side effects of medications
  Nausea, vomiting
  Stomatitis
  Diarrhea
  Pancytopenia
  Hemorrhagic cystitis
Side effects of TBI
  Nausea, vomiting
  Parotid gland swelling
  Erythema
  Decreased saliva and tears
Psychosocial
  Response to treatments
  Relationships and support systems
  Methods of coping
  Understanding of disease and treatment

Laboratory/diagnostic studies

CBC
Platelet count
FBS
Electrolytes
SGOT
SGPT
Bilirubin
Alkaline phosphatase
BUN
Creatinine
Urinalysis
ECG (weekly)

Potential complications

Pneumonia

Medical management

High-dose cyclophosphamide
Parenteral fluids
Three-way Foley catheter with bladder irrigation
Fractionated TBI for 3 days (total: 1000 rad) or high-dose cytarabine (ARA-C) and fractionated TBI
Cardiac monitoring (during conditioning TBI)
Cyclosporin
Ca-trim
Antiemetics
Antipyretics
Antibiotics
Antidiarrheals
Diuretics
Daily weights
Accurate intake and output
Isolation
TPN
Irradiated blood products

Nursing diagnoses/goals/interventions

ndx: Knowledge deficit regarding medications and TBI procedure

GOAL: *Patient and/or significant other will verbalize understanding of medications and TBI*

Medications

Explain effects of medications and expected care
  Premedication with antiemetics
  Insertion of three-way indwelling catheter with irrigation
  Cardiac monitor use

TBI procedure

Explain TBI procedure
  Patient will be alone in room but will be able to communicate with personnel
  Patient will be visually monitored at all times
  Nurse will remain in department and provide comfort measures as needed

Cardiac status will be monitored throughout procedure
Patient must remain as positioned without moving
Patient must wear mask after completion of TBI while returning to room
Patient will be placed in isolation at completion of procedure

ndx: Alteration in renal (bladder) tissue perfusion related to local effect of cyclophosphamide

GOAL: *Patient will not exhibit signs of hemorrhagic cystitis*

Ensure adequate hydration and diuresis 24 hr prior to, during, and 24 to 48 hr after medication administration (cyclophosphamide)
Force fluids to 4000 to 5000 ml/day unless contraindicated
Enlist patient's assistance
   Provide fluids of choice and at temperature of choice
   Offer small amounts frequently to make taking fluids less of a chore
   Serve attractively
Administer parenteral fluids as ordered: usually dextrose in saline with electrolytes; often ordered at 200 ml/hr for 5 to 6 hr prior to, during, and after chemotherapy infusion
Weigh patient daily at same time with same clothing and scale
Insert indwelling catheter when ordered, using strict aseptic technique
   Connect to closed-gravity drainage system
   Perform catheter care daily
Prepare for bladder irrigation when ordered
   Administer solution as ordered for continuous irrigation
   Maintain irrigation balance sheet; report discrepancies immediately
   Test return flow for occult bleeding q2h to 4h; report positive results and observations to physician
Administer osmotic diuretics when ordered
Check T, P, R, and BP q4h to 8h; report changes

ndx: Potential alteration in cardiac output: decreased output related to effects of cyclophosphamide

GOAL: *Patient will not exhibit symptoms of cardiotoxicity*

Know that ECG changes are *usually* transient and not related to CHF; most ECG changes do not require treatment
Monitor heart function continuously; observe for
   Tachycardia
   Extrasystoles
   ST wave changes
   Transient ECG changes
   30% decrease in limb-lead QRS voltage
Auscultate chest for heart and breath sounds qh during medication administration, then q4h
See Heart Failure (p. 101)

ndx: Alteration in nutrition: less than body requirements related to nausea and vomiting, and/or inability to ingest nutrients

GOAL: *Patient will maintain present weight or lose less than 10% of original body weight*

Nausea and vomiting

Assess amount and types of foods and liquids tolerated and desired
Maintain calorie count
Assess predisposing factors, onset, position, frequency, and duration
Eliminate predisposing factors when possible: unpleasant odors, perfume, disturbing sights or sounds
Administer oral hygiene before and after intake
   Use equipment appropriate to condition of mouth
   Administer oral anesthetic when ordered
Change eating patterns; serve frequent, light meals; avoid food and liquids 2 to 4 hr before meals; and/or change usual place for eating
Provide foods that may be served cold or at room temperature to eliminate odors: cereal, cheese, desserts
Provide clear liquid diet to reduce nausea: juices, carbonated beverages, flavored ice pops
Provide high-protein drinks as a supplement
Vary textures and tastes of foods to determine those tolerated: bland, sour, soft, etc.
Remind patient to eat slowly and chew well
Note that sweet, highly seasoned foods are not usually well tolerated
Administer antiemetics, when ordered, as patient desires
Maintain chart of onset of symptoms, response to varying dosage of medication, and frequency of administration
Arrange for quiet rest periods prior to meals
Assist with preparation to conserve energy
Serve foods and liquids attractively
Arrange for visitors, if patient prefers, to enhance social aspect

Have patient remain in sitting position at least 30 min to 1 hr after meal; avoid rapid position change
Use other methods to prevent onset or reduce severity of symptoms
    Relaxation methods
    Rhythmic breathing exercises
    Imagery experiences
    Self-hypnosis
    Behavior modification techniques
Place patient in well-ventilated room and control odors
    Remove trash frequently
    Empty and remove bedpans and urinals after use
    Remove food trays as soon as patient has eaten
Weigh patient daily at same time with same scale and clothing
Measure intake and output q8h
Notify physician when intake and output are not equivalent and/or weight decreases by 3% to 5%
Explain low-bacterial diet
NOTE: BMT patients require 33 to 38 kcal/kg and 1.5 g protein/kg
Wash hands prior to food preparation
Be certain work area and utensils are clean
Keep foods at proper temperature (p. 196)
Wrap food portions individually
Use only one-serving–size canned or bottled items
Serve only foods and fluids listed on diet (p. 195)
Microwave prepared foods and fluids before serving; never reheat food
Wash thick-skinned fruits or vegetables with alcohol; peel skin off prior to serving
Do not leave warmed food at bedside for longer than mealtime
Cold foods may be left at bedside for 2 hr when placed in container of ice
Remove uneaten foods and liquids from room before disposal
Food from home must be on the low-bacterial food list and cooked on the day it is brought to the hospital
Refrigerate food for not more than 24 hr if not served immediately
Microwave prior to serving

Inability to ingest foods
Administer TPN as ordered (p. 51)

ndx: Potential for infection related to increased susceptibility secondary to TBI and/or chemotherapy
GOAL: *Patient will not exhibit signs of infection*

NOTE: Patient is usually isolated until absolute granulocyte level is >1000 (total WBC × number of granulocytes)
Place patient in isolation after completion of TBI (use of isolation or laminar flow rooms is controversial)
Observe strict isolation precautions
    Wash hands with povidone-iodine solution and put on cap, gown, and mask before entering room
    No infectious personnel or visitors may enter room
    Staff assigned to care for patient must not be assigned to care for patients who have infections
    Be certain that all visitors and personnel entering room know and observe handwashing technique and other protective isolation procedures
    Keep one door to isolation and anteroom closed at all times; never have both doors open at same time
    Provide mask, gown, and gloves if patient must leave room
    Never take flowers or plants into room
    Anything taken into room must be sterilized or washed with bactericidal solution
    Microwave mail or papers before taking into room
    Never use anything that has been dropped on the floor
    Use tap water for bathing only
    Maintain low-bacterial diet using sterile water for drinking
    Be certain that visitors never use patient's equipment or bathroom
    Be certain that room, all equipment, furniture, fixtures, and personal items are cleaned with bactericidal solution daily
    Remove food, trash, and drainage receptacles from room immediately
    Assist with skin, perianal care, and oral hygiene when necessary
Assess and record skin condition q4h
Assist with hygiene as necessary
Maintain skin integrity
    Observe central line site q4h
        Change dressing daily if nonporous type is used, using aseptic technique
        Change tubing daily
Use strict sterile technique for all procedures
Assess and record condition of oral mucous membrane q4h
Remind patient to perform oral hygiene as instructed q2h; assist when necessary
Ensure required nutrient and fluid intake
Administer antifungal medications as ordered
Assess and record condition of perineum q4h

Ensure that perianal care is performed after elimination
Prevent constipation (p. 695) or diarrhea (p. 694); administer medications as ordered
Monitor vital signs q4h
    Take temperature more frequently if trend is beginning
    Report temperature elevations immediately
Institute comfort and cooling measures as indicated
    Change linen and clothing to keep patient dry
    Administer antipyretics as ordered
    Prevent chilling
Monitor intake and output; report urinary frequency, burning, or changes in character of urine
Use voiding measure when indicated
    If catheterization is necessary
        Use strict aseptic technique for insertion
        Perform catheter care q8h
    Obtain and monitor cultures as ordered
Assess and record respiratory status q4h
Report changes in breath sounds, cough and sputum, increases in respiratory rate, or presence of sore throat
Assist or remind patient to turn and deep breathe q2h
Administer oxygen as ordered
Encourage mobility q2h
Turn and position patient q2h if on bed rest
Provide adequate, uninterrupted rest and sleep periods
Administer antibiotics on time as ordered
Administer irradiated granulocytes as ordered; usually ordered with positive cultures and clinical signs of infection after maximal antibiotic therapy

ndx: Anxiety/fear related to severity of responses to conditioning and threat of dying

GOAL: *Patient will exhibit decreasing symptoms of anxiety/fear and will verbalize feelings about and understanding of condition*

Assess level of anxiety and understanding of disease process when appropriate
Visit frequently or have significant other remain with patient
Use touch, reassurance, and positive body language
Provide an environment conducive to discussion and expression of worries, fears, and loss
Continue to provide information about condition and procedures
Encourage questions; answer clearly, consistently, and clarify when necessary
Reassure that patient will not be alone and that care and treatment will be given when needed
Be sensitive to needs; listen to nonverbal clues
Maintain and assist with coping strategies
Encourage continuation of relationships

ndx: Disturbance in self-concept: body image related to sterility, alopecia, and skin and body weight changes

GOAL: *Patient will verbalize feelings about losses and effects on life-style and relationships*

Assess perception of change and its effect on life-style and relationships
Evaluate hygiene and grooming
Provide an atmosphere for expression and discussion of changes that are occurring
Visit frequently and encourage visits by significant other
Be aware of nonverbal clues: patient and nurse
Be sensitive to needs
Provide information about process patient is experiencing
Give correct information about expected positive changes: weight regained, regrowth of hair
Assist patient with decision about temporary measures for hair loss
    Short hair style prior to loss
    Use of wigs, hairpieces, scarves, or caps
Plan with patient to have preferred items available prior to need
Assist with gentle scalp care; use pH-balanced shampoo; expose hair and scalp to air as much as possible
Assist with and encourage routine grooming
Comment on strengths exhibited; value abilities and accomplishments of patient; assist patient with recognizing these also

Evaluation

Patient and/or significant other verbalizes understanding of expected effects and potential complications of medications and TBI
Patient exhibits no signs of hemorrhagic cystitis or cardiotoxicity; vital signs and ECG are within normal limits
NOTE: For further evaluation see p. 194

Transplant Phase

Phase in which histocompatible donor bone marrow is infused to establish a graft and reinstate production of normal blood cellular components

Assessment
Observations/findings

Reaction to marrow infusion
  Anaphylaxis (p. 104)
  Pulmonary emboli (p. 247)
  Transfusion reaction (p. 215)
Skin and mucous membranes
  Petechiae
  Diffuse maculopapular rash; may also be first symptom of graft vs. host disease (GVHD)
  Bruising
  Breaks
  Lesions
  Pruritus
  Hyperpigmentation: usually 2 to 3 weeks after TBI
  Jaundice
  Perianal area
    Erythema
    Excoriation
  Abscess
  Mouth
    Irritation
    Swelling
    Erythema
    Leukoplakia
    Ulcerations
    Secretions
      Consistency
      Amount
      Color
      Taste distortion
      Herpes type 1 viral infection (p. 622)
Lymph nodes: cervical, axillary, groin
  Size
  Tenderness
  Pain
GI system
  Nausea, vomiting
  Anorexia
  Weight loss
  Parotitis: usually 4 to 24 hr after TBI; resolved within 24 to 72 hr
  Diarrhea
    Frequency
    Color
    Consistency
    Occult blood
    Bleeding
Renal system
  Urine
    Color
    Character
    Odor
    Amount
    Bleeding
    Occult blood
    Presence of sugar
Respiratory system
  Breath sounds
    Rales
    Rhonchi
    Diminished
  Rate
  Depth and pattern
  Cough
    Type
    Frequency
  Sputum
    Color
    Character
    Frequency
Cardiovascular system
  Apical rate, rhythm
  Note patient's position and activity prior to taking BP
  Pedal or sacral edema
Eyes
  Photophobia
  Pain
  Abnormal tear secretion

TABLE 3-4. Proposed Clinical Stage of Graft vs. Host Disease According to Organ System

Stage	Skin	Liver	Intestinal tract
+	Maculopapular rash over 25% of body surface	Bilirubin 2-3 mg/dl	Greater than 500 ml diarrhea/day
++	Maculopapular rash over 25%-50% of body surface	Bilirubin 3-6 ml/dl	Greater than 1000 ml diarrhea/day
+++	Generalized erythroderma	Bilirubin 6-15 mg/dl	Greater than 1500 ml diarrhea/day
++++	Generalized erythroderma with bullous formation and desquamation	Bilirubin greater than 15 mg/dl	Severe abdominal pain with or without ileus

From Thomas, E.D. Reprinted, by permission of The New England Journal of Medicine **292**:896, 1975.

Blurred vision
Cataracts: late effect of TBI
Activity level: fatigue associated with activity

Laboratory/diagnostic studies

Same as for conditioning phase with increased frequency

Potential complications

Infections hemorrhage
GVHD (see box)

Nursing diagnoses/goals/interventions*

ndx: Alteration in tissue perfusion: cerebral, cardiovascular, gastrointestinal, and/or peripheral related to thrombocytopenia secondary to TBI

GOAL: *Patient will not exhibit symptoms of bleeding or hemorrhage*

Marrow infusion; cardiovascular alteration

Record baseline vital signs and cardiac rhythm
Administer marrow infusion at rate ordered through central line (must be infused within 4 hr)
  Never infuse through a filter
  Never irradiate marrow
Observe for reactions q15 min
  Anaphylaxis (p. 104)
  Pulmonary emboli (p. 247)
  CHF (p. 101)

---

*See previous nursing diagnoses related to nutrition, infection, anxiety/fear, and body image.

Transfusion reaction (p. 215)
Never stop infusion; slow if reaction occurs and notify physician
Follow orders, continue to observe patient continuously, and monitor vital signs and ECG

Cerebral and peripheral

Monitor platelet count daily
Inspect gums and oral cavity for bleeding q2h to 4h
Inspect skin each shift for increased bruising, petechiae, ecchymosis, and swelling
Inspect and palpate joints each shift for increased size and decreased mobility

TABLE 3-5. Overall Clinical Grading of Severity of Graft vs. Host Disease

Grade	Degree of organ involvement
I	+ to ++ skin rash; no gut involvement; no liver involvement; no decrease in clinical performance
II	+ to +++ skin rash; + gut involvement or + liver involvement (or both); mild decrease in clinical performance
III	++ to +++ skin rash; ++ to +++ gut involvement or ++ to ++++ liver involvement (or both); marked decrease in clinical performance
IV	Similar to grade III with ++ to ++++ organ involvement and extreme decrease in clinical performance

From Thomas, E.D. Reprinted by permission of The New England Journal of Medicine **292**:896, 1975.

GRAFT VS. HOST DISEASE (GVHD)

Condition that occurs when histocompatible differences exist between bone marrow graft and recipient

OBSERVATIONS

Skin
  Maculopapular rash
  Erythroderma
  Exfoliative dermatitis
  Bulbous formation
  Desquamation
  Hair loss
  Jaundice
GI system
  Diarrhea: 500 to 1500 ml/day
  Abdominal pain
    Ileus
  Hepatomegaly
  Splenomegaly
  Muscle wasting
  Emaciation
  Increased susceptibility to infections
  Pneumonitis
  Hemolytic anemia
  Bone marrow aplasia
  Lymphatic depletion
  Death

LABORATORY STUDIES

Bilirubin elevated from 2 mg/100 ml to >15 mg/100 ml
Lymphocytopenia
Thrombocytopenia
Electrolytes
Liver function tests
Coagulation studies

Assess sensorium and neurologic status each shift
Inspect nasal cavity at least once each shift
If epistaxis occurs
   Discourage vigorous nose-blowing
   Stay with patient at first sign of bleeding to decrease anxiety
   Apply pressure and ice at site for 10 min
   Place patient in 90-degree (sitting) position
   Instruct patient to breathe through mouth
   Assist physician with nasal packing if bleeding continues
   Xylocaine/epinephrine packing is usually used initially
   Reassure and encourage patient
   Record estimated blood loss
   Monitor and record vital signs q2h to 4h for 48 hr
Institute safety measures as platelet count decreases below 50,000/mm^3
   Use central line for withdrawal of blood samples and administration of parenteral medications as ordered; avoid skin punctures
   Avoid use of
      Rough towels and washcloths
      Razors
      Restraints
      Tight clothing
   Maintain clutter-free environment
   Provide night-light to prevent bumping into objects or falling
Administer careful oral hygiene
   Use sponge cleaners or gauze pads
   Avoid use of dental floss or toothpicks
   Encourage use of mouth rinse q2h to 4h
      Half saline and half water
      Half saline and half hydrogen peroxide followed by saline rinse
Administer irradiated platelets as ordered; inspect IV or central line site q20 to 30 min for hematoma or oozing

Gastrointestinal

Administer antacids as ordered
Avoid aspirin and aspirin-containing products
Do not take rectal temperatures or administer medications rectally
Test stool for blood after each movement
Administer stool softeners as ordered to prevent bleeding from constipation
Auscultate abdomen for bowel sounds q8h or more frequently if changes occur
Check emesis for frank or occult bleeding; record amount, color, and character; note frequency
Prepare for insertion of nasogastric lavage tube and iced saline lavage
Check and record BP, P, and T q4h
Monitor Hgb, Hct, and electrolytes as ordered
Administer platelets as ordered

ndx: Impaired tissue integrity of oral mucous membrane related to infection or conditioning

GOAL: *Patient will maintain optimal condition of mouth to permit ingestion of food and liquids*

Assess mouth, gums, and teeth on admission; arrange dental care when possible for dental caries, gum disease, or ill-fitting dentures
Teach and assist with routine oral care
   Inspect and palpate lips, gums, and buccal mucosa gently q8h
   Clean teeth and rinse mouth each morning, after meals, and at bedtime
   Increase frequency of oral care and inspection to q2h after beginning conditioning
Choice of dental equipment will depend on state of oral cavity
   Soft toothbrush if no breaks or lesions
   Gauze or sponge-covered cleaners if breaks in skin or gum bleeding
Rinse mouth q2h to 4h to keep free of particles and reduce bacterial count
   Commercial mouthwash may be irritating
   Peroxide diluted with saline or water, or saline alone may be used
Assess denture fit
   Avoid gumlike grips
   Keep dentures scrupulously clean
   Remove and clean before using mouth rinse
Keep mouth moist
   Provide appealing, tepid liquids for sipping
   Flavored ice pops may be soothing
Keep lips moist; use water-soluble gel
Provide time for patient to prepare for meals
   Perform oral hygiene
   Rinse mouth and gargle 15 to 20 min before meals
   Use local anesthetic or mixture of antihistamine, antacid, and local anesthetic as ordered
   Spray mouth with anesthetic solution in atomizer when ordered
Administer antifungal mouthwash as ordered; diluted frozen antifungal medication may be more appealing and efficacious
If patient is unable to open mouth for oral hygiene
   Prepare irrigating solution; half hydrogen peroxide with half normal saline or as ordered

Place solution in irrigating container with tubing (clean, disposable tube feeding bag)
Hang 12 to 18 inches above patient's chin level
Place patient in 60- to 90-degree position
Gently irrigate all surfaces, allowing solution to flow into emesis basin
Follow with normal saline rinse
Discard unused solution each time
Provide foods that are nonirritating, easily chewed, and high in nutrition
　Use soft foods often: custards, yogurt, soups, etc.
　Avoid citrus and very sweet foods
　Hot, spicy, or acidic foods are usually intolerable
　Hard fruits and vegetables may be grated to make them palatable
　Puree solid foods or add gravies and sauces to assist with swallowing
　Soft casseroles or soups may be used
Use straws or cups for liquidized foods; utensils, especially forks, may cause more discomfort
Frequent, small feedings are usually more easily tolerated

ndx: Alteration in skin integrity related to conditioning or GVHD

GOAL: *Patient will have intact skin*

Assess skin condition q4h, especially axillary and breast folds, groin, perirectal area, and dependent extremities
Assist with daily bath prn
　Use antibacterial soaps or povidone-iodine and soft cloths
　Rinse and dry well
　If using lotions, do not leave skin moist; avoid use of perfumes and antiperspirants
Keep linens dry and wrinkle-free; use bed cradle as necessary
Flotation bed may be ordered
Assist patient with turning and repositioning qh; encourage small position change q30 min
Teach and assist with perianal care after each elimination
　Use ABDs, soft towels, or soft cloths
　Wash with povidone-iodine wash
　Ensure that area is kept dry
　Females: wash from front to back
Teach handwashing technique to be used after elimination and prn
Avoid bumps, bruising, cuts, and scratches
　Explain importance of skin care to patient
　Avoid use of sharp objects: razors, cuticle scissors, etc.
　Always wear slippers or shoes when out of bed
　Avoid tight or constrictive clothing
　Avoid use of jewelry: moisture and bacteria collect underneath, and sharp edges can cause scratches or cuts
　Keep nails short
　Instruct patient to avoid scratching
　Use mittens for infant or small child; remove q1h to 2h; inspect skin; keep skin dry; exercise fingers and wrist
Avoid IM injections
Perform daily central line care; withdraw all blood samples for laboratory work via central line using strict aseptic technique

ndx: Alteration in bowel elimination: diarrhea related to GVHD

GOAL: *Patient will not have severe fluid loss and will have regular elimination of soft-formed stool*

Check and record all stools for
　Frequency
　Amount
　Consistency
　Presence of blood, overt or occult
Teach patient to perform perineal care after each stool
　Use povidone-iodine wash and water rinse
　Wash with ABDs or soft cloths; from front to back for women
　Dry by gentle patting with ABDs or soft toweling
　Wash and dry hands well
Perform perineal care if patient is unable to do so
Apply medication to perineum as ordered
Teach patient to test stool for blood after each bowel movement
Assess and record status of perineal area at least each shift (q4h if frequency of stools increases)
Weigh patient daily at same time with same clothing and scale
Monitor intake and output q4h to 8h
Monitor electrolytes daily
Force oral electrolyte-containing fluids to 3000 ml/day unless contraindicated (30 to 60 ml q15 to 30 min)
Administer replacement fluids as ordered
Administer antidiarrheal medications as ordered; observe and report early signs of constipation

ndx: Alteration in comfort: pain related to effects of transplantation or complications

GOAL: *Patient will verbalize feeling of increased comfort or of tolerable level of pain*

Maintain environment free of stress, unexpected sounds, or lighting
Assess pain: predisposing factors, intensity, frequency, duration and effective methods of control used by patient
Place patient in position of comfort; support joints and extremities with pillows or pads
Change position qh; assist with ROM exercise if helpful
Remove constrictive clothing; use bed cradle or footboard
Provide soothing baths and back care; use warm or cold applications when helpful
Consider diversional, relaxation, or imagery measures
Administer pain relief medications as ordered at patient's request; assess effectiveness

ndx: Activity intolerance related to fatigue secondary to anemia, interrupted sleep and rest patterns, or inadequate nutrition (see nursing diagnosis on alteration in nutrition, p. 185)

GOAL: *Patient will perform self-care activities and increase activity and exercise daily*

Provide adequate periods of sleep and rest
   Plan nursing activities to avoid interrupting sleep
   Provide activity-free periods throughout the day for rest
   Schedule examinations and tests carefully
Conserve patient's energy for desired activities
   Assist with meal preparation
   Keep needed items within reach
   Assist with hygiene measures
   Plan activities after rest periods
Keep patient warm
   Encourage use of warm robes, socks, and clothing
   Provide extra blankets; cotton sheets are often more comfortable
Assess neurologic status each shift
Take and record vital signs each shift
Assess respiratory and cardiac status each shift; report tachycardia, irregular cardiac sounds, or presence of wheezes or rales
Place patient at 60-degree angle to facilitate breathing; position with pillows if indicated
Administer oxygen therapy as ordered
Assess extremities, abdomen, and sacrum for presence of edema; report positive findings
Observe safety precautions
   Instruct patient to sit at side of bed before getting up; to change position slowly
   Keep needed items close to patient

Plan rest periods after meals
Monitor laboratory results; report changes
Maintain and increase daily activities as patient's condition improves
   Showering
   Mouth care
   Perineal care
   Use of incentive spirometer
   Walking in room; use of exercycle
   Active participation in all care activities
Assess response to increased activities; change daily plan as needed

ndx: Potential for complication: hepatomegaly related to GVHD*

GOAL: *Patient will not exhibit symptoms of complications*

Assess skin, sclera, and mucous membranes q8h
   Avoid use of artificial light when possible
   Report changes in color, bleeding, and edema to physician
Bathe patient daily; provide soothing baths (i.e., use starch or oil to relieve itching)
Administer skin care as needed to decrease itching
Keep nails short to prevent scratching skin
Encourage fluids to 3000 to 4000 ml/24 hr unless contraindicated; fluids may be limited in presence of edema
Measure intake and output
Report changes in color of urine and stool
If bleeding tendency
   Avoid skin puncture
   Place furniture, equipment, and personal items so as to prevent injuries from falls or bumping into objects
   Administer gentle oral hygiene using sponge cleaners or swabs
   Avoid use of harsh soaps and rough towels and cloths
   Test urine and stool for occult bleeding
Provide diet with amount of calories, carbohydrate, and protein as ordered
Serve meals attractively and at correct temperature; small feedings may be more tempting
Weigh patient daily at same time with same clothing and scale
Measure abdominal girth q8h
Percuss liver and spleen to determine size

---

*Not a NANDA-approved nursing diagnosis.

Report changes in electrolytes, liver function, and coagulation studies
Encourage activity to tolerance
  Assist and teach active ROM exercises q4h
  If patient is on bed rest, position on left side to decrease pressure on liver
Administer methotrexate as ordered, usually days +1, +3, +6, and +11 and then weekly to days +101 and +102
Administer prednisone 0.5 mg/kg to 1 mg/kg as ordered, usually through day +100, then tapered
Administer medications as ordered for itching

ndx: Knowledge deficit regarding self-care procedures, complications, diet, care of home environment, activities, and continuing health care

GOAL: *Patient and/or significant other will verbalize understanding of home care instructions and return-demonstrate self-care procedures, recognizing that precautions are more rigid until day +100*

Self-care procedures

Teach care of central line, heparin flush, administration of TPN (p. 51), and use of volumetric pump
Demonstrate and explain rationale for
  Oral hygiene
  Skin care
  Perianal care
  Handwashing technique
  Use of incentive spirometer
  Measurement of intake and output
  Daily assessment of skin and mucous membranes
  Method for testing urine and stool for blood
  Method for taking and recording temperature

Complications

Instruct patient and/or signficant other how to assess for and report symptoms of
  Anemia
  Bleeding
  Infection
  Stomatitis
  Skin changes
  GVHD
  Nausea, vomiting
  Diarrhea
  Nephrotoxicity
Explain measures to use to avoid complications

ANEMIA

Discuss methods for conserving energy
  Planned rest periods
  Adequate rest
  Activities planned after rest periods
  Assisting with ADLs
  Keeping needed items within reach
Explain need to change position slowly; to use appliances (walker, bars, etc.) for movement if indicated
Emphasize importance of continuing to perform ADLs and other desired activities to tolerance
Explain need to maintain a diet high in iron

BLEEDING

Discuss emergency plan to follow if spontaneous hemorrhage occurs
  Have emergency numbers on hand
  Call paramedics
  Go to nearest emergency area
Explain importance of telling dentist and other medical personnel about chemotherapy and low platelet count
Emphasize importance of maintaining a safe, clutter-free environment
Explain importance of avoiding over-the-counter medications, especially those containing acetylsalicylic acid (aspirin) without checking with physician
Explain need to avoid use of sharp objects when possible
  Use electric razor
  Use caution when handling knives or other equipment
Explain need to avoid harsh coughing and blowing of nose
  If cough persists, notify physician
  Take cough medication as ordered
Ensure that patient and/or significant other demonstrates method for applying pressure to bleeding site
  Apply dressing or clean material directly over site
  Apply pressure for 5 min or until bleeding stops
  Apply ice in covered plastic bag over site once bleeding stops
  Check site for further bleeding q15 min for 1 hr

INFECTION

Explain importance of avoiding persons who may be infectious or who may have potentially contagious conditions, as well as persons who have been recently vaccinated and crowds
Explain need to avoid multiple sexual partners
Explain importance of reporting elevated temperature
Instruct patient to wash hands after using bathroom, before eating, or before performing any procedures
Explain importance of preventing injury to skin
  Use electric razors

Handle knives and sharp objects carefully
Wear protective gloves when gardening and when using strong household cleaning solutions
Wear broad-brimmed hat and sun screen when in sun
Avoid going barefoot
Wear warm clothing and boots in cold weather
Avoid cutting cuticles, corns, or calluses
Wear padded gloves when using oven
Explain need to perform oral hygiene periodically throughout the day
Explain importance of daily hygiene, including perineal and rectal care
Explain importance of drinking up to 3000 ml of fluid each day unless contraindicated; instruct patient to avoid using common drinking fountain

STOMATITIS

Explain importance of routine oral care in the morning, after meals, and at bedtime
Discuss equipment and products to use to avoid irritation
Explain need to avoid commercial mouthwashes containing alcohol
Emphasize need to provide appetizing, high-calorie, high-protein foods in small quantities prepared to the degree of softness tolerated by patient

DIARRHEA

Explain importance of maintaining oral fluid intake at 3000 ml/day unless contraindicated
Explain need to avoid diet high in fiber and roughage
Explain need to take prescribed medication during episodes of diarrhea
Discuss signs and symptoms of constipation to report
Explain need to avoid over-the-counter medications without checking with physician or nurse

Diet

Explain need to maintain low-bacterial diet (Table 3-6)
Discuss methods used during hospitalization to enhance intake of nutrients and liquids
Teach procedures for handling, storing, and cooking foods

Activities

Explain need to perform daily self-care and to increase activity daily to tolerance
Emphasize importance of planning regular rest and sleep periods

Care of home environment, equipment, and supplies

Explain that home environment must be clean and dust-free prior to patient's discharge
All room surfaces and furniture must be washed and/or vacuumed
All plants and flowers should be removed
Pets should be boarded elsewhere until day +100
Daily cleaning and vacuuming is necessary; use of dry dust cloths should be avoided
Equipment and supplies are to be stored in clean area
Towels and wash cloths must be changed daily
Bed linen must be changed at least twice each week
Kitchen equipment must be washed and dried immediately after use
Trash must be taken outside immediately

Continuing health care

Emphasize importance of scheduling and keeping regular appointments with physician, laboratory, and other health care workers
Explain importance of telling dentist and other health care workers about condition
Emphasize need to continue to express and discuss feelings, worries, and fears; to seek assistance as necessary
Provide patient with information concerning community resources, support groups, home care agencies, and equipment suppliers as necessary
Teach name of medication, dosage, time of administration, and side and toxic effects to report to physician
Explain need to avoid use of over-the-counter medications without checking first with physician

Evaluation

No signs of infection are present; any previous sites of infection are healing; there is no evidence of lung congestion; urine is clear; oral temperature is 98.6° F (37° C)
Patient is taking nutritious foods and liquids, or TPN therapy is being maintained; weight has stabilized; oral mucous membrane is intact, or healing is progressing; bowel elimination has returned to normal pattern with elimination of soft-formed stool
Skin is warm and dry with good turgor; color has returned to normal; there is no evidence of breaks, disruptions, or eruptions
Vital signs remain within acceptable limits; there are no signs of bleeding; previous bleeding sites are resolving; skin and mucous membranes are warm and

moist with good turgor; patient is increasing self-care and activity level daily

Urine is clear and yellow; output is equal to intake; there is no evidence of occult bleeding

Patient observes rest periods and maintains sleep pattern when uninterrupted, and performs self-care activities without evidence of fatigue

Patient verbalizes feelings of increased comfort and uses alternate pain control methods interspersed with medication

Patient expresses and discusses feelings about condition, treatment, and prognosis; sets realistic goals; seeks out resources and assistance from others when needed; enhances appearance with use of aids; maintains relationships as before BMT; and has infrequent or no evidence or symptoms of anxiety/fear

TABLE 3-6. Low-Bacterial Diet

Food categories	Foods allowed	Foods to avoid
Beverages	Coffee, decaffeinated coffee, tea, cereal beverages, carbonated beverages, canned or frozen fruit and vegetable juices	Fresh fruit and vegetable juices
Milk (2 or more cups)*	Skim (nonfat), low-fat, or whole milk, buttermilk, commercial milk shakes, and canned eggnog	Milk shakes made with noncommercial ice cream, yogurt, and eggnog made with raw eggs
Meat group (6 to 8 oz cooked)*	Lean meat, fish, fowl, cheese (heated), eggs (cooked), and peanut butter	Cold cuts, stir-fried foods, raw eggs, and cottage cheese
Vegetables (2 to 3 half-cup servings or more)*	All cooked fresh or frozen vegetables and canned vegetables; one serving should be a source of vitamin A (dark green leafy or deep yellow vegetables)	All raw or uncooked vegetables and salads
Fruits (2 to 3 half-cup servings or more)*	All canned or stewed fruits, fresh fruits with thick skin that can be peeled (apple, orange, banana); one serving should be a source of vitamin C (citrus fruits, cantaloupe, or guavas)	All other fresh fruits and dried fruit
Breads and other starches (5 or more servings)*	White enriched, whole wheat, and other breads, rolls, crackers, pretzels, sweet rolls, doughnuts, pancakes, waffles, French toast, all cereals, macaroni, noodles, spaghetti, rice, corn, potatoes, dried beans, and peas	Sweet rolls with custard or cream filling
Fats and oils (2 to 4 tablespoons or more)*	Liquid oil shortenings, margarine, salad dressing, nondairy creamers, nuts, and seeds	Bleu cheese and Roquefort dressing
Soups	Canned, frozen, or dehydrated soups and soups made from "allowed" ingredients	None
Seasonings and miscellaneous	Salt (iodized), spices and herbs (used in the cooking process), condiments, cocoa powder, gravies and sauces made from "allowed" ingredients	Spices, herbs, or seasonings added to food after it has been cooked
Sugars†	Jelly, jam, marmalade, honey, candy, molasses, syrups	None
Desserts†	Individually packaged commercial ice cream, ice milk, sherbert, and individually packaged cakes, cookies, canned or frozen pudding	Noncommercial ice cream, ices, sherbert; custard, gelatin, frozen yogurt

*These foods form the foundation for an adequate diet.
†These foods are not necessary for an adequate diet but add extra calories.

TEMPERATURES (°F) FOR FOOD SAFENESS	
165° to 195°	This temperature kills most harmful bacteria
140° to 150°	Minimum temperature with which to cook foods to kill bacteria
45° to 140°	Danger zone for food safeness; rapid bacterial growth
34° to 45°	Cold or chill food storage; slow bacterial growth
0° to −10°	Frozen food storage

Patient and/or significant other verbalizes understanding of home care and follow-up instructions for avoiding complications, maintenance of home environment, diet, medications, activity management, and continuing health care; and demonstrates methods of checking for signs of complications, oral hygiene and skin/perianal care measures, management of TPN therapy, handwashing technique, use of incentive spirometer, measurement of intake, output, and calories, and procedure for taking and recording temperature

DISSEMINATED INTRAVASCULAR COAGULATION (DIC)

Overstimulation of the normal coagulation process associated with underlying conditions such as snakebite, septicemia, severe hypotension, neoplasms, hemolysis, obstetric emergencies, acidosis, cancer chemotherapy, transplant rejection, and extensive burns, trauma, or surgery; the initial accelerated clotting process consumes large amounts of coagulation factors in the formation of fibrin clots; the fibrinolytic system is then activated to lyse fibrin clots into fibrin degradation products; the activity of these products and the depletion of plasma coagulation factors result in hemorrhage

Assessment
Observations/findings

Abnormal bleeding in all systems and at sites of invasive procedures
  Skin and mucous membranes
    Diffuse oozing of blood or plasma
    Petechiae
    Palpable purpura: initially chest and abdomen
    Hemorrhagic bullae
    Subcutaneous hemorrhage
    Hematoma
    Tape burns
    Acral cyanosis*
  GI system
    Nausea, vomiting
    Guaiac-positive emesis/nasogastric aspiration and stools
    Severe abdominal pain
    Increasing abdominal girth
  Renal system
    Hematuria
    Oliguria
  Respiratory system
    Dyspnea
    Tachypnea
    Blood-tinged sputum
  Cardiovascular system
    Increasing hypotension
    Postural hypotension
    Increasing heart rate
    Absence of peripheral pulses
  Central nervous system
    Changing level of consciousness
    Restlessness
    Vasomotor instability
  Musculoskeletal system
    Pain: muscles, joints, back
Bleeding to hemorrhage
  Surgical incisions
  Postpartum uterus
  Eye fundus: visual changes
  Invasive procedure sites: injection, IV, arterial catheters and chest or nasogastric tubes, etc.

Laboratory/diagnostic studies

Serial studies
  PT >15 sec
  Fibrinogen <160 mg/ml
  Fibrin degradation products (FDP) >1/8
  Platelets <100,000/mm^3
With significant liver disease
  PT >25 sec
  Fibrinogen <125 mg/ml
  FDP >1/64
  Platelets <50,000
Decreased factor assays: V, VII, VIII, X, XIII
PTT >60 to 80 sec
Decreased Hct without clinical bleeding
Schistocytes noted on CBC
Respiratory acidosis

---

*Slightly blue, gray, or dark purple discoloration of the extremities.

Potential complications

Shock
Acute tubular necrosis
Focal gangrene
Pulmonary edema
CHF
Convulsions
Coma
Failure of major organ systems

Medical management

Treatment of underlying disorder
Anticoagulant therapy: heparin IV
Fresh frozen plasma, platelets, clotting factors, other blood products, and parenteral fluids
Thrombolytic therapy
Oxygen therapy

Nursing diagnoses/goals/interventions

ndx: Alteration in tissue perfusion: renal, cardiovascular, and/or cerebral related to bleeding secondary to changes in clotting cycle

GOAL: *Patient will exhibit no evidence of bleeding; vital signs will remain stable*

Maintain venous access using strict aseptic technique
Administer IV heparin and fresh frozen plasma, platelets, and other blood products as ordered (p. 212); assess response and/or reactions
Perform exchange transfusion as ordered for neonates
Observe for bleeding at venipuncture site or clotting at end of catheter; apply pressure dressing if needed
Monitor FDP titers and report to physician for heparin dosage changes
  NOTE: PTT and Lee-White test are prolonged in DIC and are not reliable indicators of heparin therapy
Monitor arterial pressure, ECG, BP, T, P, and R q30 to 60 min; report progressive decrease in BP, increase in heart rate, and elevated temperature
Assess neurologic status q30 to 60 min; report changes
Auscultate chest for heart and breath sounds qh; report abnormal changes immediately
Monitor arterial blood gases; report acidotic states immediately
Administer oxygen therapy as ordered
Assess for increased bleeding and/or new sites of hemorrhage in all body systems; report changes immediately
Measure intake and output qh; report decreasing output or <30 ml/hr; weigh dressings and linen when hemorrhage occurs
Assist patient with turning and deep breathing qh; avoid vigorous coughing
Measure abdominal girth when GI bleeding is suspected
Administer careful skin care as needed; do not disturb clots; use lift sheet to prevent bruising and abrasions; use heel and elbow padding; support joints anatomically
Apply Gelfoam or thrombin dressings to areas with frank bleeding or those that continue to ooze
Provide oral hygiene q2 to 4h; avoid vigorous toothbrushing; use soft-bristled toothbrush, cotton swabs, and dilute mouth rinse or saline
Weigh patient daily at same time with same clothing and scale
Protect from trauma
  Pad side rails if necessary
  Avoid constrictive bedclothes; use bed cradle if needed
  Clip nails to prevent scratching
  Avoid invasive procedures when possible
  Use caution when suctioning or inserting tubes and lines
  Apply pressure to site for 5 to 10 min or until bleeding stops if IM injections are necessary, or when removing IV catheters; observe sites q10 to 15 min; apply pressure dressing if appropriate

ndx: Alteration in comfort: pain related to pressure caused by bleeding

GOAL: *Patient will verbalize increased comfort and/or relief from pain*

Assess location, quality, and intensity of pain
Place patient in position of comfort; provide support with pillows to prevent stress on body parts
Assist with care when patient is actively bleeding or experiencing discomfort
Maintain quiet environment
Provide adequate periods of rest; cluster activities and diagnostic studies, when possible, according to patient's tolerance
Assist patient with alternate comfort measures
Administer analgesics as ordered; assess effectiveness

ndx: Anxiety/fear related to threat of death

GOAL: *Patient will exhibit decreasing symptoms of anxiety/fear and will verbalize feelings about and improvements in condition*

Assess level of patient's fears and understanding of current condition when appropriate

Maintain calm, nonstressful environment
Prepare family/significant other for patient's appearance
Remain with patient or have significant other stay with patient; use touch, reassurance, and positive body language
Provide information about condition, procedures, and diagnostic studies in language understood by patient
Encourage questions; answer clearly and consistently, and clarify when necessary
Note positive progress in physical condition when appropriate
Provide atmosphere conducive to discussion and expression of feelings, worries, fears, and loss
Be sensitive to needs; listen to nonverbal clues
Maintain and assist with coping strategies
Provide access to others to assist patient: clergy, psychologist, social worker, etc.
NOTE: See primary condition for patient teaching and discharge planning

Evaluation

Vital signs remain stable; there is no further evidence of bleeding in any system; past sites of bleeding are resolving
Activity tolerance is increasing with no evidence of pain and little discomfort
There are no signs or symptoms of anxiety; patient verbalizes understanding of condition

MULTIPLE MYELOMA

A malignant disorder in which immature plasma cells proliferate in the bone marrow and form osteolytic tumors of the skeleton; initially, the pelvis, spine, and ribs are involved; other bones, the lymph nodes, spleen, liver, and kidneys are affected later; occurs primarily in males 50 to 70 years of age; diagnosis is often made in late stages, so prognosis is often poor

Assessment
Observations/findings

Medical history: increased susceptibility to infections—upper respiratory infection (URI), pneumonia, urinary tract infection
Musculoskeletal
  Bone pain
    Predominately severe back pain on movement
    Rib
    Extremities
  Fatigue
  Weakness
  Firm, nontender subcutaneous masses over area of skeletal involvement
  Skeletal deformities
  Pathologic fractures
  Shortened stature: 5 inches or more
Hematologic
  Anemia
  Bleeding tendency
Renal: symptoms of calculi

Laboratory/diagnostic studies

Decreased Hgb
Decreased RBC
Elevated sedimentation rate (ESR), calcium level, total protein
Plasma cells: 3%
Lymphocytes: 40% to 50%
Proteinuria: Bence Jones protein
Hypercalciuria
Positive immunoelectrophoresis
Thrombocytopenia
Skeletal survey
  Diffuse osteoporosis
  Osteolytic lesions
IVP: renal involvement
Bone marrow: abnormal increase in immature plasma cells

Potential complications

Vertebral compression
Nephrocalcinosis
Acute renal failure
Bleeding problems
Infections

Medical management

Radiotherapy
Chemotherapy
Pain management
Laminectomy
Intake and output
Vital signs
Parenteral fluids
Treatment of complications

Nursing diagnoses/goals/interventions

ndx: Impaired physical mobility related to osteolytic lesions and/or pathologic fractures

GOAL: *Patient will enhance and reach maximum mobility potential without injury*

Explain importance of maintaining mobility to prevent further bone demineralization

Use pain relief medications prior to ambulation when ordered
Assist with ambulation: patient sits at side of bed, stands, gaining balance, and then walks with assistance
Avoid fast movements and stretching; encourage patient to move at own pace to avoid losing balance
Provide ambulatory aids: walkers, canes, braces, and/or crutches; provide safe environment for learning use of these aids
Arrange furniture, equipment, and personal items within reach to avoid bumping, falls, or the need to reach for items
Provide night-light for safety
Assess ambulatory efforts, stance, gait, and coordination
Assist with and teach patient the use of body mechanics and alignment
Place patient in position of comfort when on bed rest
　Maintain body alignment
　　Support position with pillows or sandbags
Provide trapeze and side rails to assist with position change
Assist with turning and ROM q2h; move smoothly with care; logroll if spine is involved
Remind patient to change position qh
Assess reflexes, motor function, and sensation q8h; report changes and any sudden severe pain or inability to move a body part (may indicate new fracture or spinal cord compression)
Prepare for radiotherapy as ordered; explain rationale, expected results, and side effects
Administer chemotherapy as ordered
Prepare for laminectomy when ordered (p. 487)

ndx: Alteration in comfort: pain related to severe bone pain secondary to fractures or vertebral compression

GOAL: *Patient will verbalize feelings of increased comfort or of tolerable level of pain*

Assess pain: predisposing factors, intensity, frequency, duration, and effective methods of control used by patient; incorporate these methods in plan
Assess neurologic status q8h; report changes (may indicate vertebral compression)
Place patient in position of comfort; support joints and extremities with pillows or pads to maintain body alignment
Change position qh; assist with ROM exercise if helpful
Maintain environment free of stress, unexpected sounds, or lighting
Avoid jarring bed or chair or dropping items
Remove restrictive clothing; use bed cradle or footboard
Provide soothing baths and back care; use warm or cold applications when helpful
Encourage use of diversional, relaxation, or imagery measures
Administer pain relief medications as ordered at patient's request; assess effectiveness

ndx: Potential fluid volume deficit or excess related to renal calculi, nephrocalcinosis, or renal failure

GOAL: *Patient will have balanced intake and output, with urinary output of at least 1500 ml/24 hr, BP within normal limits, and stable weight*

Monitor T, P, R, BP (lying and sitting), central venous pressure (CVP), and breath sounds q4h to 6h; report changes
Observe skin turgor and neck veins q4h to 6h
Measure intake and output q8h
　Note frequency, amount, and color of urine; report difficulty in starting to void, pain, or presence of stones
　Maintain fluids to 3000 to 4000 ml daily or as ordered
　　Space fluids over 24 hr period
　　Avoid dehydration
　Avoid fasting for laboratory work, x-ray studies, etc., without checking with physician
　Maintain urinary output at or >1500 ml/24 hr
Weigh patient daily at same time with same clothing and scale; report changes of more than 3% to 5% daily
Avoid food and liquids with calcium
Ambulate or exercise q4h when possible

ndx: Potential alteration in tissue perfusion: gastrointestinal, peripheral, renal, cerebral, and/or cardiopulmonary related to bleeding secondary to thrombocytopenia

GOAL: *Patient will exhibit no bleeding episodes*

Assess all systems for bleeding q8h; report early symptoms
Administer skin care daily and prn
Maintain skin and mucous membrane integrity
　Avoid invasive procedures when possible
　Change position qh; provide care for pressure areas
　Avoid use of harsh soaps or rough towels, cloths, and bedclothes
　Use soft-bristled toothbrush or foam swabs with evidence of gum bleeding

Assist with and teach deep-breathing exercises; avoid vigorous coughing or nose-blowing

Avoid constipation through diet, stool softeners, or laxatives when ordered

ndx: Potential for infection related to increased susceptibility, possibly secondary to disturbed antibody formation

GOAL: *Patient will not exhibit signs of infection*

Place in noninfectious environment

Ensure that personnel and visitors observe handwashing technique

Screen all personnel and visitors for infection

Assess condition of skin and mucous membranes q8h

Maintain skin integrity; avoid invasive procedures; consolidate laboratory work

Provide mild antibacterial soaps and soft cloths and towels for skin hygiene, daily and prn

Encourage mobility q2h

Turn and position immobile patient q2h

Provide uninterrupted rest and sleep periods

Teach or assist with oral hygiene in morning, after food ingestion at bedtime, and q2h to 4h when awake

Monitor and record vital signs q4h; take temperature more frequently with elevation; report immediately

Institute comfort and cooling measures as indicated by condition
  Change linen and clothing to keep patient dry
  Avoid chilling
  Administer antipyretics as ordered

Monitor intake and output q8h; report urinary frequency, burning, or changes in character of urine

Use voiding measures when indicated to avoid catheterization

Assess and record respiratory status q4h; report changes in breath sounds, cough, and sputum, increases in respiratory rate, or presence of sore throat immediately

Assist and teach patient to turn and deep breathe q2h to 4h

Administer oxygen if ordered

Obtain cultures as ordered: blood, urine, sputum, skin, drainage, etc.

Monitor laboratory data daily; report changes

Administer IV antibiotics as ordered

ndx: Anxiety/fear related to severe pain and/or threat of death

GOAL: *Patient will exhibit infrequent symptoms of anxiety/fear and will verbalize feelings about and understanding of condition*

Assess level of anxiety and understanding of disease process when appropriate

Visit frequently or have significant other remain with patient

Use touch, reassurance, and positive body language

Provide an environment conducive to discussion and expression of worries, fears, and loss

Provide information about condition, procedures, and diagnostic studies

Encourage questions; answer clearly and consistently, and clarify when necessary

Be sensitive to needs; listen to nonverbal clues

Maintain and assist with coping strategies; plan care with patient to enhance decision making and feeling of control

Encourage continuation of relationships

Provide access to others: clergy, social worker, business associates, etc., as requested

ndx: Knowledge deficit regarding disease process and treatment, mobility, pain management, complications, and anxiety/fear

GOAL: *Patient and/or significant other will verbalize understanding of home care instructions and return-demonstrate use of thermometer, ambulatory assistive devices, and hematest materials*

Disease process and treatment

Discuss symptoms of recurrence or progression of disease to report to physician

Demonstrate how to monitor for spinal cord compression

Reinforce rationale, expected outcome, and side effects of radiotherapy and/or chemotherapy

Explain importance of regular follow-up with physician, radiotherapy/chemotherapy appointments, and laboratory studies

Mobility

Explain importance of ambulation and exercise on a regular basis

Discuss methods for preventing accidents and injury; use of assistive devices; arrangement of home environment

Explain use of body mechanics and need to maintain body alignment

Discuss measures to provide support and decrease musculoskeletal strain when on bed rest

Pain management

Instruct patient in alternate pain management methods

Emphasize need to have planned rest and sleep periods

Instruct patient on use of analgesics as ordered for maximal effect

Complications

RENAL DYSFUNCTION

Demonstrate method for recognizing symptoms to report

Demonstrate how to measure and record intake and output, weekly weight, and when to report

Explain importance of taking fluids, especially water, to 3000 to 4000 ml/day

Explain need to decrease calcium intake

BLEEDING

Discuss signs and symptoms to report

Demonstrate how to check urine and stool for bleeding

Explain need to avoid taking over-the-counter medications, especially aspirin or aspirin-containing products, without checking with physician

Instruct patient on how to prevent injury
- Avoid restrictive clothing
- Keep home and work area free of clutter
- Use assistive devices for ambulation and work when needed
- Use caution when performing oral hygiene; inspect mouth for breaks and lesions; use special equipment and dentrifices
- Avoid sports and hobbies that may cause injury
- Handle equipment and sharp objects carefully
- Prevent constipation through adequate fluids and diet, and use of stool softeners or laxatives

INFECTION

Discuss signs and symptoms of infection to report to physician or nurse

Explain importance of avoiding persons who may be infectious or who may have potentially contagious conditions; explain need to avoid crowds

Explain need to avoid persons who have been recently vaccinated

Explain need to avoid multiple sexual partners

Instruct patient to wash hands after using bathroom, before eating, or before performing any procedures

Explain importance of preventing injury to skin
- Use electric razors
- Handle knives and sharp objects carefully
- Wear protective gloves when gardening and when using strong household cleaning solutions
- Wear broad-brimmed hat and sun screen when in sun
- Avoid going barefoot
- Wear warm clothing and boots in cold weather
- Avoid cutting cuticles, corns, or calluses
- Wear padded gloves when using oven

Explain need to perform oral hygiene periodically throughout the day

Explain importance of daily hygiene, including perineal care

Instruct patient to avoid using common drinking fountain

Explain need to maintain clean home environment and handle food properly

Anxiety/fear

Instruct patient on how to recognize early symptoms

Emphasize need to continue open communication to discuss and express feelings

Discuss ways to continue problem solving and decision making

Discuss sources for assistance: psychosocial, financial, spiritual

Evaluation

Patient is increasing periods of ambulation using assistive aids and/or supports as necessary, is aware of surrounding environment, and avoids injury and falls

If on bed rest, patient utilizes trapeze, bedboards, or side rails to change position, keeping body in alignment

Patient uses alternate pain management measures interspersed with analgesics, carries out activities when pain is relieved or diminished, and verbalizes feelings of increased comfort

Vital signs are within normal limits; intake and output are in balance, with output between 1500 to 3000 ml/day

Skin turgor is good; weight is stable; there is no evidence of bleeding, or previous bleeding sites are resolving

No signs of infection are present; lungs are clear; skin is intact, warm, and moist; urine is clear; oral temperature is 98.6° F (37° C)

Patient expresses and discusses feelings about disease, treatment, and prognosis; sets realistic goals; seeks out resources and assistance from others when needed; and has infrequent or no evidence of symptoms of anxiety/fear

Patient and/or significant other verbalizes understanding of home care and follow-up instructions; demonstrates methods for detecting signs of bleeding and infection, including checking urine and stool and taking oral temperature; demonstrates hygiene and skin care measures; and demonstrates use of ambulatory aids and support devices

HODGKIN'S DISEASE

A malignant disorder characterized by painless enlargement of lymphoid tissue; usually one lymph node is affected initially, but other nodes and the spleen become involved throughout the lymphatic system; histiocytes called Reed-Sternberg cells proliferate and replace normal cellular structure; without treatment other organs and structures become involved

Assessment
Observations/findings

Enlarged nodes
    Cervical and supraclavicular nodes are usually involved initially
    Firm, rubbery; become hard with sclerosing
    Vary from nontender without skin changes to tender with skin changes
Skin
    Pruritus: generalized and severe
    Temperature: alternating febrile and afebrile periods
    Night sweats
    Jaundice
    Edema: face and neck
Hematologic
    Fatigue
    Malaise
Gastrointestinal
    Anorexia
    Weight loss

TABLE 3-7. Staging of Hodgkin's Disease

Stage*	Definition
I	Single lymph node region
II	Two or more node regions limited to one side of the diaphragm
III	Disease on both sides of the diaphragm, but limited to the lymph nodes and spleen
IV	Involvement of the bones, bone marrow, lung parenchyma, pleura, liver, skin, gastrointestinal tract, central nervous system, renal, etc.

From Thompson, J.M., et al.: Clinical nursing, St. Louis, 1986, The C.V. Mosby Co.
*All stages are subclassified as A or B to describe the absence (A) or presence (B) of systemic symptoms.

    Splenomegaly
    Hepatomegaly
Musculoskeletal: bone pain

Laboratory/diagnostic studies

Normocytic, normochromic anemia
WBC and differential; any combination of the following
    Neutrophilia
    Monocytosis
    Eosinophilia
    Lymphocytopenia
    Abnormal sedimentation rate
    Increased alkaline phosphatase (indicates bone involvement)
    Lymph node biopsy
        Reed-Sternberg cells
        Nodular fibrosis
        Necrosis

Potential complications

Respiratory distress
Infection
Fractures

Medical management

Staging procedures
    Lymph node biopsy
    Chest x-ray examination
    Bone marrow biopsy
    Liver and spleen biopsy, scans
    Peritoneoscopy
    Laparotomy
    Bone scans
    Lymphangiography
Radiotherapy (usually Stages I, II, and III)
Antineoplastic chemotherapy (usually Stages III and IV)
Treat complications

Nursing diagnoses/goals/interventions

ndx: Impairment of skin integrity related to pruritus, jaundice, and/or immobility

GOAL: *Patient will have intact skin*

Assess condition of skin q8h
Administer daily skin care as needed
    Soothing baths: sodium bicarbonate or oatmeal
    Avoid skin dryness; apply lotions to slightly moist skin
    Cool sponge baths or tub soaks may be beneficial

Apply powders sparingly, avoiding any buildup in tissue folds
Keep clothing light with no constrictions
Check and change q2h during night if patient is experiencing night sweats
Elevate bed clothes with bed cradle
Keep bed wrinkle-free
Use linen laundered in nondetergents
Advise patient to avoid scratching; instead, apply pressure or use cool applications
Use distraction and diversion; keep needed materials within easy reach
Administer medication to relieve severe itching as ordered; assess response
Check temperature q4h to establish pattern; cool sponge baths may be helpful when temperature is elevated

ndx: Alteration in nutrition: less than body requirements related to anorexia and/or abdominal distention secondary to splenomegaly or hepatomegaly

GOAL: *Patient will take a balanced diet to maintain weight at optimal level for age, sex, and body build*

Assess amount and types of foods and liquids tolerated and desired
Provide time for oral hygiene before and after meals
Eliminate unpleasant odors, perfumes, and disturbing sights or sounds
Experiment with various eating patterns: small, light meals; liquids only; change in usual eating place and/or position
Vary textures and tastes of foods to determine those tolerated: bland, sour, sweet, soft, dry, etc.
Add high-protein drinks as a supplement
Serve foods and liquids attractively arranged at temperature desired by patient
Assist with preparation of tray
Arrange for visitors, if patient prefers, to enhance social aspect
Arrange for food-from-home treats
Provide adequate time for meal so patient does not feel rushed
Plan rest periods prior to meals to conserve energy
Weigh patient daily at same time with same clothing and scale
Measure intake and output q8h
Explain that sitting, rather than lying, after a meal may decrease full feeling
Plan periods of exercise (e.g., walking between meals) when possible

ndx: Alteration in comfort: pain related to bone pain or fractures

GOAL: *Patient will verbalize feelings of increased comfort or tolerable level of pain*

Assess pain predisposing factors, intensity, frequency, and duration, and effective methods of control used by patient
Place patient in position of comfort; immobilize or support joints and extremities with pillows or pads; maintain body alignment
Change position qh; assist with ROM exercise if helpful
Remove restrictive clothing; use bed cradle or footboard
Provide soothing baths and back care; use warm or cold applications when helpful
Encourage use of assistive devices when ambulating
Increase activity and self-care to tolerance; note responses; assist patient with being aware of body responses to attain highest level of activity without increasing frequency or intensity of pain
Consider diversional, relaxation, or imagery measures
Administer pain relief medications, as ordered, at patient's request; assess effectiveness

ndx: Anxiety/fear related to unknown outcome of disease

GOAL: *Patient will exhibit infrequent symptoms of anxiety/fear and will verbalize feelings about and understanding of condition*

Assess level of anxiety and understanding of disease process when appropriate
Visit frequently or have significant other remain with patient
Use touch, reassurance, and positive body language
Provide an environment conducive to discussion and expression of worries, fears, and potential loss
Provide information about condition, procedures, and diagnostic studies
Encourage questions; answer clearly and consistently, and clarify when necessary
Reinforce physician's explanation of positive outcome
Be sensitive to needs; listen to nonverbal clues
Maintain and assist with coping strategies; plan care with patient to enhance decision making and feeling of control
Encourage continuation of relationships
Provide access to others as requested: clergy, social worker, business associates, etc.

ndx: Potential for ineffective airway clearance related to airway edema and/or enlarged mediastinal lymph nodes

GOAL: *Patient will exhibit no respiratory difficulty*

Assess respiratory effort, breathing pattern, and breath sounds q4h to 8h (more frequently if abnormalities are noted)

Place patient in position of comfort; usually sitting position will decrease respiratory effort

Assist and teach patient to turn and deep breathe q2h

Administer oxygen as ordered

Note patient's response to activities; assist as necessary to avoid respiratory distress

Keep emergency airway maintenance equipment available

ndx: Potential for infection related to increased susceptibility secondary to changes in WBC

GOAL: *Patient will not exhibit signs of infection*

Place in noninfectious environment

Ensure that personnel and visitors observe handwashing technique

Screen all personnel and visitors for infection

Assess condition of skin and mucous membranes q8h

Maintain skin integrity; avoid invasive procedures; consolidate laboratory work

Provide mild antibacterial soaps, and soft cloths and towels for skin hygiene, daily and prn

Encourage mobility q2h

Turn and position immobile patient q2h

Provide uninterrupted rest and sleep periods

Teach or assist with oral hygiene in morning, after food ingestion, at bedtime, and q2h to 4h when awake

Monitor and record vital signs q4h; take temperature more frequently with elevation; report immediately

Institute comfort and cooling measures as indicated by condition
   Change linen and clothing to keep patient dry
   Avoid chilling
   Administer antipyretics as ordered

Monitor intake and output; report urinary frequency, burning, or changes in character of urine

Use voiding measures when indicated to avoid catheterization

Assess and record respiratory status q4h; report changes in breath sounds, cough, and sputum, or increases in respiratory rate, or presence of sore throat immediately

Assist and teach patient to turn and deep breathe q2h to 4h

Administer oxygen if ordered

Obtain cultures as ordered: blood, urine, sputum, skin, drainage, etc.

Monitor laboratory data daily; report changes

Administer IV antibiotics as ordered

ndx: Knowledge deficit regarding disease process, treatment, complications, nutrition, activities, comfort, and anxiety/fear

GOAL: *Patient and/or significant other will verbalize understanding of home care instructions and return-demonstrate use of thermometer, breathing exercises, and ambulatory devices*

Disease process and treatment

Discuss symptoms of recurrence or progression of disease to report to physician

Explain expected outcome and responses to radiation and/or chemotherapy

Explain importance of regular follow-up care: physician, radiation therapy/chemotherapy, laboratory studies

Reinforce physician's explanation of need to delay pregnancy (for patients of childbearing age) until patient is in remission for a period of time

Complications

INFECTION

Discuss how to check for and report signs and symptoms of infection: elevated temperature, sore throat, "cold," "flu," coughing, burning on urination, and small cuts, hangnails, and lesions that do not heal

Explain need to prevent infection
   Maintain skin integrity: avoid scratching; observe careful skin care; observe for skin changes
   Maintain adequate rest and sleep periods
   Keep environment clean
   Avoid persons with infection and crowds
   Use handwashing technique for self and those assisting

RESPIRATORY DISTRESS

Discuss signs and symptoms of early respiratory distress to report: increasing cough, hoarse voice, decreased activity tolerance, any change in breathing pattern

Teach deep-breathing exercises and explain need to pace activities to avoid acute distress

Emphasize need to have emergency plan and phone numbers available for acute distress

Nutrition

Explain need to maintain balanced diet and liquids of choice to 3000 ml/day

Emphasize need to continue meal plan and eating pattern to enhance appetite

Instruct patient to weigh weekly and to report more than 10% loss

Activities and comfort

Explain importance of returning to normal life-style as soon as possible

Explain need to balance rest and activity periods

Instruct patient to plan daily routine; to use assistance when necessary

Instruct patient to increase activities and self-care as condition improves

Explain need to continue skin care measures to decrease pruritus

Instruct patient to continue alternate pain relief measures that are successful; to use assistive devices when ambulating to prevent injury; teach body alignment if patient is on bed rest, with ROM exercises and methods for preventing injury

Anxiety/fear

Instruct patient on how to recognize symptoms

Emphasize need to continue open communication to express and discuss feelings

Discuss ways to continue problem solving and decision making

Discuss sources for assistance if needed: psychosocial, spiritual, financial

Evaluation

No signs of infection are present: skin is intact and warm, with good turgor; breathing pattern is normal; lungs are clear; respiratory excursion is normal; urine is clear; oral temperature is 98.6° F (37° C)

Patient is taking a balanced diet and liquids to 3000 ml daily; weight is stabilized

Patient verbalizes feelings of increased comfort and uses alternate pain control methods interspersed with medication; self-care and exercise/activity tolerance are increasing

Respiratory rate, excursion, and breath sounds are normal; there is no evidence of cough, stridor, or hoarseness

Patient expresses and discusses feelings about disease, treatment, and prognosis; sets realistic goals; and seeks out resources and assistance from others when needed

There is infrequent or no evidence of symptoms of anxiety/fear

Patient and/or significant other verbalizes understanding of home care and follow-up instructions, plan to increase self-care and other activities with adequate rest and sleep periods, signs and symptoms of disease or complications to report, methods for avoiding complications, diet and eating plan, plan for emergency assistance, and plan for unexpected results or side effects of radiation and/or chemotherapy; and demonstrates methods to detect complications, general hygiene care (including specific care for skin), breathing exercises, use of thermometer, and use of any needed ambulatory devices

MALIGNANT LYMPHOMA

Refers to a grouping of neoplasms originating in lymphoid tissue, which are classified by degree and differentiation of cellular content; grouping includes non-Hodgkin's lymphomas and lymphosarcoma; etiology is unknown, but a viral source is suspected; it can occur in all age-groups and is more common in males, Caucasians, and people of Jewish ancestry

Assessment
Observations/findings

Enlarged lymph nodes
   Cervical and supraclavicular initially
   Nontender, movable, rubbery
   Size fluctuations
   Enlarged tonsils and adenoids
   Oropharyngeal and mediastinal mass
Fatigue
Malaise
Weight loss
Elevated temperature
Susceptibility for infections
Pressure symptoms in areas of involvement
   GI system
      Dysphagia
      Anorexia
      Nausea, vomiting
      Constipation
   Retroperitoneal: abdominal and low back pain
   Central nervous system
      Paresthesia, weakness
      Nerve pain

Laboratory/diagnostic studies

EARLY

Abnormal-appearing lymphocytes
Lymphocytes with monoclonal surface immunoglobulin (Ig)
Bone marrow infiltration
Hypercalcemia
Elevated copper
Elevated lactic dehydrogenase
Positive antiglobulin (Coombs') test

LATE

Hypoalbuminemia or hypergammaglobulinemia
Monoclonal Ig spikes

Potential complications

Pleural effusions
Bone fractures
Paralysis

Medical management

Staging procedures
    Biopsies for histologic evaluation
        Lymph nodes
        Tonsils
        Liver
        Bone marrow
        Bowel
        Tissue removed during laparotomy
    Lumbar puncture
    Chest x-ray examination
    CT scans
        Spleen
        Liver
        Abdomen
        Bone
    Lymphangiography
Radiotherapy
Chemotherapy

Nursing diagnoses/goals/interventions

See Hodgkin's Disease (p. 202)

SPLENECTOMY

Surgical removal of the spleen to treat traumatic injuries or blood dyscrasias in which hypersplenism occurs (The spleen produces leukocytes, lymphocytes, monocytes, and plasma cells. It also destroys nonfunctional red blood cells and platelets, stores blood, and assists in maintaining hemopoiesis. The spleen indiscriminantly sequesters normal red blood cells and platelets, thereby removing them from the circulation when hypersplenism occurs.)

Assessment

Postoperative observations/findings

Cardiovascular
    Bleeding
    Tachycardia
    Thrombosis
Respiratory
    Splinting with respiration
    Decreased breath sounds
    Tachypnea
    Atelectasis
    Subdiaphragmatic abscess
Gastrointestinal
    Character and amount of gastric drainage
    Nausea, vomiting
    Dehydration
    Abdominal distention
Infection
    Elevated temperature
    Site of incision
        Redness
        Swelling
        Draining
        Dehiscence

Laboratory/diagnostic studies

Elevated thrombocyte level
Bleeding and clotting times: normal
Electrolytes

Potential complications

Hemorrhage
Infection
Paralytic ileus
Shock

Medical management

Nasogastric tube
Parenteral therapy
Pain management
Management of complications

Nursing diagnoses/goals/interventions*

ndx: Potential for ineffective airway clearance related to anesthetics and/or site of incision

GOAL: *Patient will have normal respiratory rate, excursion, and breath sounds*

---

*See also standard for primary condition, General Preoperative Care/Teaching (p. 29), and Care of Patient in Recovery Room (p. 30).

Assess respiratory effort, breath sounds, and rate q4h for 48 hr, then q8h

Position patient to decrease respiratory effort

Assist and teach patient to turn, cough, and deep breathe q2h to 4h; support incision

Teach patient to use incentive spirometer q4h or as ordered

Assist with ambulation as soon as possible

ndx: Alteration in comfort: pain related to surgical incision

GOAL: *Patient will verbalize feelings of increased comfort and will perform activities without discomfort*

Assess pain location, frequency, intensity, and duration

Assist patient with assuming position of comfort; support as necessary

Administer analgesics as ordered and needed for pain (usually required q3h to 4h during immediate postoperative period); assess effectiveness of ordered medication

Administer pain medication prior to performing activities to increase comfort, thereby increasing compliance
 Coughing and deep breathing
 ROM exercises
 Early periods of ambulation and self-care activities pain increases, assess for other factors (e.g., complications, exacerbation of primary condition)

ndx: Potential fluid volume deficit related to nasogastric drainage, abdominal distention, and/or paralytic ileus

GOAL: *Patient will have balanced intake and output; weight will not change more than 5%*

Maintain NPO as ordered

Connect nasogastric sump tube to low, intermittent suction apparatus as ordered
 Do not change position of tube
 Maintain tube patency
 Check drainage q2h to 4h; report excessive bleeding

Administer parenteral fluids with electrolytes as ordered

Measure intake and output q8h; report imbalance

Weigh patient daily at same time with same clothing and scale

Observe voiding: frequency, amount, color, odor, discomfort, distention

Institute voiding measures as needed

Insert catheter when ordered for retention or overflow voiding; perform daily catheter care

Auscultate abdomen for bowel sounds q8h; report return of bowel sounds

Begin oral liquids, progressing to regular diet when ordered after return of bowel sounds; note tolerance

Encourage fluids to 3000 ml/day unless contraindicated

Administer Harris flush q6h prn for distention if ordered

Monitor for first bowel movement after surgery; give stool softeners or enemas as ordered

ndx: Potential alteration in tissue perfusion: cardiopulmonary, renal, gastrointestinal, and/or peripheral related to bleeding or thrombosis

GOAL: *Patient will exhibit no symptoms of bleeding or signs of thrombosis*

Monitor BP, P, R, CVP, and T q4h for 48 hr, then q8h

Assess for signs of bleeding or thrombosis q4h to 8h

Check dressing for bleeding q2h to 4h for 48 hr
 Reinforce as necessary
 Report excessive bleeding to physician

Change dressing daily and prn; observe healing process

Position patient comfortably; assist with turning q2h; avoid knee gatch or pillows under knees

Assist with and teach active or perform passive ROM exercises q4h

Provide correct-size antiembolic stockings when ordered

Plan uninterrupted rest and sleep periods to avoid fatigue

Assist with ambulation as necessary
 Avoid sitting for long periods
 Walk in place when standing

Administer skin care and oral hygiene q4h

Encourage patient to participate in self-care activities

ndx: Potential for infection related to increased susceptibility secondary to surgical procedure

GOAL: *Patient will exhibit no signs of infection, with good wound healing*

Monitor T, P, R, and breath sounds q4h for 48 hr, then q8h; report changes indicative of infection

Observe incision for swelling, redness, drainage, odor, or dehiscence
 Report immediately
 Change dressing daily using sterile technique
 Remove sutures when ordered and when incision is healing

Assess for urinary frequency or burning sensation; report findings

Force fluids to 3000 to 4000 ml/day unless contraindicated

Assist patient with turning, coughing, and deep breathing and ambulate to prevent pulmonary infections

ndx: Knowledge deficit regarding self-care, activities, and nutrition

GOAL: *Patient and/or significant other will verbalize understanding of home care instructions and return-demonstrate incision care, breathing, and ROM exercises*

Self-care

Instruct patient to shower daily; to dry incision well
Teach patient to observe for and report increased pain, swelling, redness, or drainage
Emphasize importance of not applying creams, lotions, or powders to incision
Instruct patient to support incision if needed, when deep breathing and coughing
Emphasize need for follow-up care

Activities

Explain need to increase ambulation and activities each day and to plan regular, uninterrupted rest periods
Explain need to exercise extremities routinely; demonstrate ROM and breathing exercises
Instruct patient to avoid sitting for long periods; explain importance of not crossing legs
Instruct patient to avoid heavy lifting and contact sports for 6 to 8 weeks or as directed by physician

Nutrition

Instruct patient to maintain well-balanced diet, taking 3000 ml of liquids daily
Instruct patient to report inability to tolerate food or liquids, nausea, any vomiting, diarrhea, or constipation

Evaluation

Vital signs are within normal limits; lungs are clear; respiratory excursion is adequate; all peripheral pulses are palpable; color and temperature of extremities are normal
Patient verbalizes feelings of increased comfort; performs self-care, exercise, and ambulation without limitations; and no longer requires analgesics
Patient takes regular diet and fluids to 3000 ml/day; intake equals output; mucous membranes are moist; skin turgor is good; patient is voiding without difficulty and has had soft-formed bowel movement
Incision is dry and healing, with no evidence of bleeding or infection; sutures have been removed
Patient and/or significant other verbalizes understanding of home care and follow-up instructions and demonstrates incision care, breathing, and ROM exercises

LYMPHANGIOGRAPHY

Injection of opaque dye into the lymphatic system for x-ray visualization

Observations

Allergic reaction to dye
　Dyspnea
　Nausea, vomiting
　Numbness of extremities
　Diaphoresis
　Tachycardia
Site of injection
　Irritation
　Redness
　Swelling
　Drainage
　Thrombus

Preprocedure care

Explain procedure
　Local injection of dye into hands or feet
　Small surgical incision to locate lymph ducts
　Some discomfort is to be expected while lymph ducts are being located
　Injection of dye into lymphatic system
　Patient must lie still for long period of time
　Feeling of warmth is normal response to dye
　X-ray examinations of body immediately after injection, 24 hr later, and prn thereafter
　Bluish cast to skin will disappear within 1 month
Start ordered IV in extremity that is expected to be injected during procedure

Postprocedure care

Increase fluids to 3000 ml unless contraindicated
Administer back care q2h to 4h until discomfort is gone
Check T, P, and R q2h for four times or as ordered
Check extremities for numbness q2h for four times
Check site of incision q2h to 4h; warm compresses may be ordered if local tissues are infiltrated

BONE MARROW STUDY

Bone marrow is obtained by aspiration or biopsy to examine types and numbers of cells, maturation level, and composition of supporting tissue; used for diagnosis and treatment response

Observations

Site of puncture
    Redness
    Pain
    Drainage
    Hematoma
Tachycardia
Apprehension
Pericardial puncture
Bone marrow histologic results
Indications for aspiration: symptoms of decreased production or increased destruction of cells, including
    Megaloblastic anemia
    Sideroblastic anemia
    Hypochromic, microcytic anemia
    Neutropenia
    Leukemia
    Thrombocytopenia
    Immunoglobulin disorders
Indications for biopsy
    Failure to obtain material by aspiration
    Pancytopenia
    Myelofibrosis
    Tumor, lymphoma, or granulomatous disease of marrow

Preprocedure care

Explain procedure to patient and assess understanding
    Local anesthetic will be administered
    Pressure will be felt on insertion of needle
    Pain will be felt as marrow is aspirated, but it lasts only a few minutes
    Pressure will be applied at site
Provide time for expression of anxiety
Notify laboratory technologist if appropriate

Care during and after procedure

Ensure privacy
Position patient on back with small pillow under thoracic spine if sternal puncture is planned
Position for good visualization and patient comfort if puncture of other areas (iliac crest) is planned
Assist with sterile procedure as necessary
    Shave skin area if appropriate
Prep skin with povidone-iodine solution
Remain with patient during procedure
Provide emotional support
Make slides if appropriate and if laboratory technologist is not available
Send biopsy specimen for histologic studies
Check BP and R q30 min for three times
Apply pressure dressing if needed
Report excessive drainage to physician
Manage pain as indicated
Assess effectiveness of pain relief measure(s)

PHERESIS

Selective removal of blood or blood components for therapeutic goals; also used to provide cell-specific support therapy; types of pheresis—procedures are named depending on the blood component to be removed

Plasmapheresis

Removal of multiple liters of plasma containing abnormal substances with replacement of equal volumes of a plasmalike solution

Indications

Hemolytic anemia (AIHA), ITP (acute)
Myasthenia gravis
Renal transplant rejection syndrome
Goodpasture's syndrome
Systemic lupus
Rheumatoid arthritis
Multiple myeloma
Macroglobulinemia (Waldenström's)
Biliary cirrhosis
Hyperlipidemia
Hypercholesterolemia
Cancer conditions in which plasma substances interfere with patient's immune system

Assessment

Observations/findings

See primary condition
Bleeding
    Venipuncture sites
    All body systems (e.g., bleeding gums, tarry stools—rare; if this happens, it is a reaction to citrate)
Pyrogenic reactions
    Elevated temperature
    Urticaria
    Pruritus

Electrolyte imbalance
    Citrate toxicity: hypocalcemia
        Perioral or periorbital paresthesia
        Numbness
        Tingling
        Twitching
        Positive Chvostek's/Trousseau's sign
        Arrhythmia
    Hypokalemia
        Leg cramps
        Malaise
        Dizziness
        Mental confusion
        Lengthened QT interval on ECG
Hypothermia
    Chilling
    Hypertension (very rare; related to anxiety)
Hypovolemia
    Increasing heart rate
    Decreasing BP
    Decreasing urinary output
Fluid overload
    Tachypnea
    Tachycardia
    Increased urinary output
    Shortness of breath
    Edema
    Hypoxia
Vasovagal reaction
    Sudden bradycardia
    Sudden hypotension
Thrombus or air embolus formation
    Venipuncture site
    Extremities
        Color change
        Decreased sensation
        Decreased temperature
    Behavioral changes
    Numbness (in body part)
    Paralysis
Hypotension
Chest pain
ECG changes compatible with ischemia or infarction
Tachypnea
Abnormal breath sounds not present before pheresis therapy
Decreased or absent urinary output
Shock

Prepheresis laboratory/diagnostic studies

Total albumin and protein
Potassium
Magnesium
Calcium
CBC
Hgb
Hct
Platelet count
PT
Activated PTT
Hepatitis-associated antigen/VDRL
Cold agglutinins
Liver and renal function tests

Prepheresis care

Reinforce physician's explanation of procedure; include significant other
Obtain written consent after physician has explained procedure
Assess patient's existing condition and note routine and special nursing care requirements for primary condition
Check prepheresis laboratory values
Take and record vital signs, and standing and lying BP
Assess patient's heart and lung sounds
Administer medications and fluids as ordered
NOTE: Wear protective gloves when handling blood components, needles, and centrifuge equipment to protect against hepatitis

General care during procedure

Explain each step of procedure prior to initiation
Use strict aseptic technique in performing venipunctures and maintaining sites
Monitor ECG as ordered; check rhythm strip qh
Check BP, P, R, and T q30 min to 60 min and prn (for each 500 ml of plasma removed)
Auscultate chest for breath sounds qh
Measure intake and output qh
Monitor volume of blood component removed and fluid replaced to maintain balance or as ordered
Monitor infusions and rates q15 to 30 min
With every 500 ml removed, observe for signs and symptoms of RBC agglutination and hemolysis (e.g., restlessness, skin discoloration, increased potassium, decreased Hct)
Give heparin, protamine, and Ringer's lactate solution as ordered
Observe bottles and tubings for breaks, leaks, and clots
Assist and teach patient to turn, cough, and deep breathe q1h to 2h
Administer skin care q2h

Administer routine medications, sedatives, and pain medications as ordered and indicated

Offer diet and fluids of preference or as ordered; assist patient as needed

Provide atmosphere for discussion of feelings about condition and therapies

Encourage visiting with significant other

Provide diversions such as television and radio

Draw sample for postpheresis blood work as ordered

Apply pressure to venipuncture sites after removal of needles until clotted

Apply bandage strip over puncture site when clotted

Postpheresis care
Immediate care

Continue with same care as during procedure and decrease frequency of nursing functions as vital signs and intake and output stabilize

Instruct patient to report signs of bleeding or cramping

Maintain fluid intake and limit activities as ordered

Ongoing care

If antecubital veins are used for access
  Never use for other venipunctures
  Apply warm soaks qid
  Have patient do arm-strengthening exercises qid

Relate to patient that treatment is usually done every other day but can be done daily if indicated by physician

Relate to patient that there will be a replacement solution as ordered by physician

If fresh frozen plasma is ordered (Table 3-8), understand that Ig and coagulation factors will be replaced but that there is an increased risk for hypersensitivity and hepatitis

If normal saline and albumin are ordered, understand that volume is replaced without risk of hepatitis or hypersensitivity; however, Ig and coagulation factors will not be replaced; understand that there are usually six treatments, with each one lasting 1 to 2 hr, depending on blood flow and vascular access, as well as volume that needs to be removed (usually 2 to 4 hr)

All Pheresis Treatments
Laboratory/diagnostic studies

NOTE: The following laboratory studies are required to be drawn at initial treatment and prn per physician's order: CBC, Hgb, Hct, platelet count, PT, activated PTT, HAA, VDRL, cold agglutinins, liver and renal function tests

Plateletpheresis

Removal of abnormal or excessive platelets for thrombocytopenia; removal of donor platelets for infusion

Assessment
Observations/findings

See primary condition

Prepheresis laboratory/diagnostic studies

Platelet count
CBC

Ongoing care

Understand that length of pheresis therapy varies with underlying condition

Relate to patient that treatment usually lasts from 2 to 4 hr, until platelet count is at desired level

Relate to patient that since only 200 to 300 ml is removed, it is not necessary to replace this volume (for donors only); for therapeutic treatment, usually 1000 ml is removed, depending on platelet count

Leukapheresis

Removal of excessive or abnormal white blood cells for chronic lymphatic leukemia, rheumatoid arthritis, and multiple sclerosis: lymphocytes for multiple sclerosis; removal of donor granulocytes for infusion for chronic myelogenous and granulocytic leukemia

Assessment
Observations/findings

See primary condition

Prepheresis laboratory/diagnostic studies

CBC
Differential

Ongoing care

Understand that there may be 18 to 20 treatments, depending on disease; rate of mobilization and rate of cell proliferation dictate frequency of leukapheresis procedures necessary to achieve sustained reduction in leukocyte count

Relate to patient that each treatment usually lasts 3 to 4 hr

Relate to patient that treatments are usually scheduled three times first week, two times second week, and one time each remaining week until total ordered is completed

Relate to patient that no replacement solution is given, since volume removed is only 200 to 300 ml (donor only)

TABLE 3-8. Blood and Blood Components

Product	Description	Indication(s)	Action	Administration
Red blood cells, packed (PRC)	Concentrated red blood cells that remain after plasma is separated	To improve oxygen-carrying capacity of the blood (hemolytic anemia in aplastic crisis, chronic hypoplastic anemia, leukemia, lymphoma, and other malignant diseases with bone marrow failure); exchange transfusions; surgery; shock; conditions in which sudden changes in blood volume are not tolerated	Increases oxygen-carrying capacity; elevates Hct (3% if unit of PRC has Hct of 70%-80%)	See blood administration standard; administer through a filter; regulate flow to 25 ml/hr for 15 min; remain with patient; observe for reaction; if no reaction, regulate flow to 100-200 ml/hr in adult with no cardiac failure or elevated CVP and in infants and children regulate flow to 2-6 ml/kg/hr; add sodium chloride to PRC prior to administration when ordered; *no other solution or medication may be added to red cells*
Red blood cells, leukocyte poor	Concentrated red cells with leukocytes removed, usually by continuous flow centrifuge or washing	See PRC; severe febrile transfusion reactions due to anti-leukocyte or anti-platelet antibodies; candidates for transplantation	See PRC	See PRC
Red blood cells, frozen	Glycerol added to red cells to protect cell from hemolysis while suspended in hypertonic solution when frozen; glycerol is removed before administration	See PRC; hypersensitivity reactions to plasma components such as IgA	See PRC	See PRC
Whole blood	Plasma and red blood cells; may or may not contain other cells and factors; dependent on length of time transpired after collection; unit usually contains 520 ± 45 ml of anticoagulated blood with Hct of about 40%	Restoration of blood volume due to hemorrhage or trauma	Restores blood volume and increases oxygen-carrying capacity	Administer through a filter; remain with patient until 25-50 m transfused, usually 15-30 min; observe for transfusion reactions; if no reaction, adjust flow rate to administer complete unit within 4 hr; warm unit no higher than 37° C using special coils when refrigerated blood needs to be administered quickly
Whole blood with platelets and cryoprecipitate removed	Platelets and certain labile components removed	Hypovolemic shock	Increases oxygen-carrying capacity and provides volume without adding platelets, which release serotonin (a vasoconstrictor)	See whole blood

TABLE 3-8. Blood and Blood Components—cont'd

Product	Description	Indication(s)	Action	Administration
Whole blood with antihemophilic factor (factor VIII) removed	Prepared by removing factor VIII, using heparin in initial collection, or converting a previously collected unit of blood containing a citrate anticoagulant	Exchange tranfusion in the adult; priming pump oxygenator	Provides volume without contributing to coagulation ability	See whole blood
Plasma	Plasma prepared from single donor unit of fresh blood	Volume expansion; burns; traumatic shock; replacement of certain coagulation factors	Provides plasma proteins for volume expansion, oncotic pressure and coagulation factors	Administer unit in less than 1 hr in hypovolemic patient; in normovolemic patient, administer at rate of 5-20 ml/kg
Plasma, fresh-frozen or freeze-dried	Plasma prepared from single donor unit of fresh blood; it is frozen within 6 hr of collection	Volume replacement; hypoproteinemia in selected patients; source of fibrinogen and factors V and VIII	See plasma; 1 U usually contains approximately 400 mg fibrinogen, 200 U factors VIII and IX, and other stable and labile coagulation factors	Thaw frozen plasma in 37° C water bath with gentle agitation; *do not warm*; administer through a filter; *never add* medications or fluids
Plasma, frozen	Plasma prepared from single donor unit within 26 days after collection; stored frozen	Factor VII, IX, X, XI, and XIII deficiencies or abnormalities	Replacement of factors VII, IX, X, XI, or XIII	See plasma, fresh-frozen or freeze-dried
Cryoprecipitate	Precipitate derived from pooled fresh-frozen plasma is refrozen, then thawed prior to administration	Hemophilia A; von Willebrand's disease (factor VIII deficiency)	Provides high concentrations of factor VIII and fibrinogen	Administer at flow rate of 10 ml/min or as ordered
Cryoprecipitated antihemophilic factor (factor VIII)	Preparation containing factor VIII is obtained from a single unit of blood; contains approximately 80 U factor VIII, and 200 mg fibrinogen in 15 ml of plasma	Hemophilia A; von Willebrand's disease (factor VIII deficiency)	Provides high concentrations of factor VIII and fibrinogen	Thaw in warm water bath at 37° C with gentle agitation; administer through filter rapidly within 6 hr after thawing if container not entered; 2 hr after thawing if container entered
Leukocyte concentrate	Leukocytes, platelets, and erythrocytes in varying amounts in 200-500 ml of plasma collected by pheresis; a compatible HLA donor is usually preferred (not identical donor whose use as a tissue donor is anticipated)	Bacterial sepsis not responsive to antibiotic therapy in presence of neutropenia; chronic granulomatous disease	Provides granulocytes to more effectively control infection	Administer irradiated leukocytes to prevent engraphment and possible GVHD; regulate rate of flow to give 250-850 granulocytes/μl/M^2; usually 1 U/day is ordered; slow rate of transfusion at appearance of elevated T wave, chills, and urticaria; stop transfusion when symptoms of transient pulmonary infiltrate appear

Continued.

TABLE 3-8. Blood and Blood Components—cont'd

Product	Description	Indication(s)	Action	Administration
Platelet concentrate	Platelets separated from whole blood suspended in plasma; collection from single donor preferred	Hemorrhage due to thrombocytopenia; prevention of potential hemorrhage in bone marrow suppression due to chemotherapy; abnormalities in platelet function	Corrects hemostatic deficit in thrombocytopenia and abnormally functioning platelets; I U usually increases platelet count 5000/ml in 70 kg adult	Administer through a filter (*never* a microaggregate filter); regulate flow rate to assure administration of total unit in less than 20 min; must be infused by 6 hr after collection
Normal serum albumin, USP 25% solution	Derived from pooled venous plasma; contains 25 g normal serum albumin/100 ml	Hypoproteinemia; burns; shock due to trauma, hemorrhage	Increases oncotic pressure; increases circulating volume by drawing 3½ times the infused volume of albumin into circulation unless patient is dehydrated; reduces hemoconcentration and blood viscosity	Administer at flow rate <2-3 ml/min to prevent rapid rise in BP, circulatory embarrassment, or pulmonary edema
Hespan, Hetastarch	An *artificial* colloid derived from a waxy starch composed of amylopectin; it has a molecular weight suitable for use as a plasma expander; Hespan is 6% Hetastarch in 0.9% sodium chloride injection	An adjunct in treatment of hemorrhagic shock, burns, and septic shock Leukapheresis	Volume expansion due to albumin-like properties Increases ESR when added to whole blood, thereby improving efficacy of granulocyte collection	For hemorrhagic shock, administer at 20 ml/kg/hr, slower rate usually ordered for other indications; contraindications: severe bleeding disorders, severe CHF, renal failure

Red Cell Pheresis

Removal of excessive or abnormal red blood cells for polycythemia vera and sickle cell anemia

Assessment
Observations/findings

See primary condition
During the procedure, watch for signs and symptoms of hypovolemia and red cell alloimmunization

Prepheresis laboratory/diagnostic studies
CBC

Ongoing care

Understand that treatment schedule varies with disease
Relate to patient that no replacement solution is given when excess cells are removed
Relate to patient that an equal amount of red blood cells will be replaced if treatment is for removal of abnormal cells

General principles of care for hemapheresis patient

If arteriovenous fistula is used for access
    Check patency daily
    Never use for venipunctures
    Never take BP in that extremity; no IM injections in same extremity
See standard of care for primary condition

Patient teaching/discharge outcome

Ensure that patient and/or significant other demonstrates
    Care of venous or arteriovenous fistula care
    Extremity exercises to perform daily
Ensure that patient and/or significant other knows and understands

TABLE 3-9. Reactions to Transfusion of Blood and Blood Components

Product	Type of reaction	Onset	Observations	Nursing actions
Red blood cells, all preparations	Febrile	Initiation of transfusion to 24 hr post-transfusion	Chills, elevated temperature, headache, nausea, vomiting	Check and record baseline T, P, R, and BP; slow infusion; notify physician; administer antipyretic or antihistamines as ordered; check and record T, P, and R q15 min; saline-washed RBCs: frozen, thawed, washed RBCs or leukocyte filter may be ordered to decrease reaction
Whole blood	Allergic plasma sensitivity	Within 30 min after initiating transfusion Immediately to 30 min after initiation of transfusion	Mild reaction: chills, elevated temperature, backache, pain in legs Moderate to severe reaction: erythematous rash, urticaria, dyspnea, wheezing, hypotension, intestinal hyperperistalsis, anaphylactic shock	Check and record baseline T, P, R, and BP; stop infusion; initiate slow (4-6 ml/hr) infusion of saline using new sterile IV tubing; notify physician and blood bank; monitor T, P, R, and BP q10 to 15 min; ensure that blood specimen is drawn for testing; return remainder of blood product, tubing, and transfusion record to blood bank; indicate observations on transfusion record; usually red cells without IgA will be ordered for administration; oxygen, steroids, vasopressors, or epinephrine may be ordered for anaphylactic shock; prepare for resuscitation
	Other allergic reactions	During transfusion to several days after	Urticaria, swelling of lymph nodes, sore throat	Slow transfusion rate; report observations to physician; administer antihistamines as ordered; blood obtained from a fasting donor may be ordered if reaction is severe
	Circulatory overload	During transfusion to 24 hr after	Sharp cough, precordial pain, back pain, dyspnea, cyanosis, increased venous pressure, distended neck veins, productive cough, frothy sputum, pleural rales	Slow transfusion rate; report observations to physician; continue rate of flow as ordered; usually 2 ml/kg/hr; monitor T, P, R, BP, and CVP q15-30 min; see CHF (p. 101)
	Hemolytic	Immediately to 30 min after initiation of transfusion or when 25-50 ml infused	Restlessness, anxiety, precordial oppression, elevated T to 105° F (40.6° C), tachycardia, tachypnea, flushed face, back and thigh pain, generalized tingling, chills, nausea, vomiting, shock, disseminated intravascular coagulation (DIC), renal failure, oliguria, hematuria, anuria	Stop transfusion immediately; change IV tubing; initiate normal saline at 4-6 ml/hr; cap blood tubing with sterile needle or cap; report symptoms to physician and blood bank; recheck identifying blood numbers with patient's numbers; monitor and record T, R, and cardiac rate and rhythm q10-15 min; measure and record urine output with each voiding or q½h; send first

Continued.

TABLE 3-9. Reactions to Transfusion of Blood and Blood Components—cont'd.

Product	Type of reaction	Onset	Observations	Nursing actions
				specimen to lab for testing; report output less than 15 ml/30 min or presence of bleeding; ensure that blood samples are drawn for testing; the following are usually ordered: Hgb, haptoglobin level, methemalbumin, bilirubin, differential agglutination, serologic studies, renal function tests, and aerobic and anaerobic cultures; complete transfusion record, send discontinued blood, tubing, and record to lab for testing; administer medications and fluids IV as ordered; diuretics, oxygen, electrolytes, and heparin may be ordered; prepare for dialysis
Massive transfusions of red blood cells or whole blood	Metabolic hyperkalemia and citrate toxicity with acid citrate dextrose (ACD) anticoagulant	Citric acid elevations of 100 mg/100 ml	Tremors, prolonged QT segment on ECG, hypocalcemia, acidosis then alkalosis, cardiac arrest if citric acid levels higher	When massive transfusions required, transfusion products with citrate-phosphate dextrose (CPD) anticoagulant usually ordered; monitor and record T, R, and cardiac function q10-15 min; ensure that blood samples are drawn for electrolytes, calcium, pH, CO_2, bicarbonate levels; administer calcium gluconate IV as ordered; administer oral or rectal cation exchange resins as ordered for hyperkalemia
	Pulmonary infiltrates	During transfusion	Chills, elevated temperature, tachycardia, nonproductive cough, dyspnea, respiratory distress syndrome (p. 263)	Stop blood immediately; change tubing; institute normal saline IV at 4-6 ml/hr; monitor and record T, P, R, and BP; auscultate chest for breath and heart sounds; report observations to physician; see respiratory distress syndrome (p. 263)
	Bleeding tendency due to dilutional effect	Transfusion volume equal to blood volume of patient	Bleeding in any body system, thrombocytopenia, coagulation abnormalities	Report observations to physician immediately; check and record T, P, R, and BP q10-15 min; monitor cardiac function continuously; auscultate chest for heart and breath sounds q15-30 min; administer platelet concentrate, fluids, and medications as ordered; manage hemorrhage as indicated and ordered

TABLE 3-9. Reactions to Transfusion of Blood and Blood Components—cont'd.

Product	Type of reaction	Onset	Observations	Nursing actions
	Pulmonary air embolus	During transfusion	SOB, chest pain, cyanosis, syncope, hypotension, shock	Stop transfusion immediately; place patient on left side; administer oxygen as ordered; monitor vital signs, CUP q15 min; see pulmonary embolus (p. 247)
Leukocyte concentrate	Acute reaction	Immediately	Elevated temperature, chills	Slow transfusion; monitor and record T, P, R, and BP q15-30 min; auscultate chest for breath and heart sounds q15-30 min; report observations to physician; see respiratory distress syndrome (p. 263)
	Transient pulmonary infiltrate		Retrosternal constriction, pallor, cyanosis, tachycardia, cough	
	GVHD			Usually only irradiated leukocytes are administered for prevention
Platelets	Febrile; usually due to infusion of incompatible leukocytes contaminating platelet preparations	Immediately to 12-24 hr posttransfusion	Chills, hives, flushing	Check and record T, P, R, and BP q15-30 min; administer medications when ordered; reaction usually self-limiting; patient may develop antibodies and destroy platelets in subsequent transfusions
Plasma	Similar to whole blood	Similar to whole blood	Similar to whole blood	Similar to whole blood
Whole blood with factor VIII removed	Bleeding due to heparin used as anticoagulant; reactions as in whole blood	During and after transfusion when large volumes administered; see whole blood	Bleeding in any body system See whole blood	Report observations to physician immediately, check and record T, P, R, and BP; monitor cardiac status continuously; administer protamine sulfate as ordered; measure and record urinary output See whole blood
Normal serum albumin	Reactions are rare	During administration	Chills, elevated temperature, nausea	Slow transfusion rate; report observations to physician; check and record T, P, R, and BP q15-30 min
	Circulatory overload/bleeding during rapid infusion	During transfusion	Rising or elevated BP, circulatory overload, pulmonary edema; new areas of bleeding appear in hemorrhagic shock	Monitor rate of infusion carefully; slow rate of transfusion; report observations to physician; check and record T, P, R, and BP q10-15 min; monitor cardiac status continuously; auscultate chest for heart and breath sounds q15-30 min; observe closely for new sites of bleeding

Signs and symptoms of bleeding and infection to report to physician
To avoid exposure to persons with infections, especially URIs
See standard of care for primary condition

BLOOD TRANSFUSIONS

Assessment
Observations/findings

Venipuncture site
  Pain
  Warmth
  Redness
  Swelling
  Leakage at insertion site
Position of extremity
Blood
  Type and Rh factor
  Flow rate
  Amount

Potential reactions (Table 3-9)

Hemolysis
  Elevated temperature
  Decreased BP
  Hemoglobinuria
  Hematuria
  Chills
  Pain
Circulatory overload
  Shortness of breath
  Lung congestion: rales, rhonchi
  Frothy sputum
Pyrogenic reaction
  Sudden chilling
  Elevated temperature
  Headache
Allergic reaction
  Urticaria
  Laryngeal edema
  Asthmatic wheezing
Hepatitis

Pretransfusion care

Select equipment needed for venipuncture according to hospital policy, procedure, and physician's order
Prepare venipuncture site
Prepare equipment and normal saline solution
Obtain blood no more than 30 min prior to administration; check blood according to hospital policy

Care during transfusion

Flush blood tubing with normal saline solution prior to starting blood
Remain with patient for at least 15 min (or 50 ml) after starting blood
Discontinue blood immediately if transfusion reaction occurs, call physician, and follow hospital procedure
Change blood tubing after transfusion

Posttransfusion care

Apply pressure to venipuncture site
Apply adhesive bandage and/or dressing as indicated
Observe for reaction 1 hr after infusion of blood
Record whether or not a reaction occurred

Patient teaching

Ensure that patient and/or significant other knows and understands
  Importance of maintaining position of extremity
  Importance of reporting symptoms of reaction
  Rash
  Flushed feeling
  Chills
  Shortness of breath
Importance of not regulating flow rate

CHAPTER 4

Respiratory System

RESPIRATORY ASSESSMENT

Subjective Data

Cough
Pain
  Chest
  Abdomen
Wheeze
Shortness of breath
Use of how many pillows
Amount of exercise tolerated
Fever
Chills
Rapid breathing
Tiring easily
Change in voice
Dizziness
Sweating
Swelling of feet and hands

Objective Data

Anxious facies
Flaring nostrils
Red, swollen nose
Nasal discharge
Color
  Cyanosis
    Lips
      Circumoral area
      Nail beds
      Gums
      Earlobes
      Soles of feet
      Palms of hands
  Pallor
  Ashen
  Gray
  Cherry red
  Red
  Reddish blue
Confusion, restlessness
Hallucinations
Cough
  Nonproductive
  Productive
    Amount of sputum
    Color, characteristics of sputum
Stridor
Wheeze
Assuming upright position: orthopnea
Clubbing of extremities: nail beds
Use of accessory muscles of respiration
Telegraphic speech pattern
Eyes
  Engorged veins
  Papilledema
Elevated temperature
Diaphoresis
Anorexia
Weight
  Obese
  Gain
  Loss
Ascites
Rash
Respirations (Table 4-1)
  Bradypnea
  Tachypnea
  Long expiratory phase
  Irregular
  Asymmetric
  Periods of apnea
  Cheyne-Stokes
  Shallow
  Pursed lip breathing
  Biot's
  Kussmaul's
  Apneustic
  Hyperventilation
Retractions
  Suprasternal
  Supraclavicular
  Substernal
  Intercostal

TABLE 4-1. Patterns of Respiration

Type		Characteristics
Normal respirations	⋎⋎⋎⋎⋎⋎⋎⋎⋎⋎	Rate Rhythm, regular
Cheyne-Stokes respiration	⋎⋎⋀⋀⋀⋁⋁	Periods of apnea alternating with series of respiratory cycles Rate and amplitude of successive respiratory cycles increase to a maximum and then decrease until terminated by period of apnea
Biot's respiration	⋎⋎ ⋀ ⋀	Variation of Cheyne-Stokes respiration in which periods of apnea alternate irregularly with periods of breaths of equal depth
Sighing respiration	⋀⋀⋀⋀⋀⋀⋀⋀	Deep audible sighs that interrupt normal respiratory rhythm
Painful respiration	⋎⋎⋀⋀⋀⋀⋎⋎	Interruption of normal respiratory rhythm due to pain; breathing frequently becomes shallow during interruption
Ataxic respiration	⋎⋀⋀⋀⋀⋎⋀⋎	Gross irregularity in rate, rhythm, and depth of respiration; also referred to as meningitic respirations

Modified from Abels, L.F.: Mosby's manual of critical care, St. Louis, 1979, The C.V. Mosby Co.

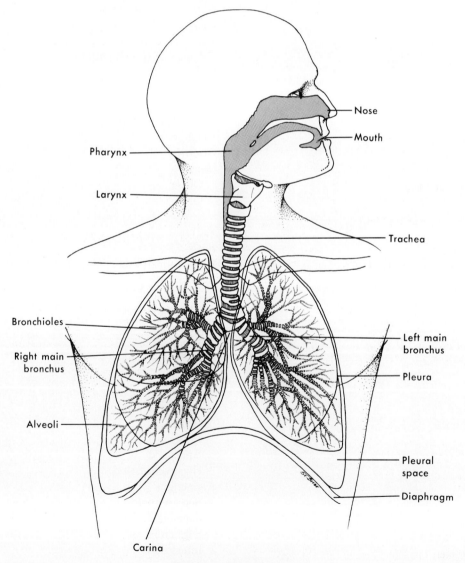

FIGURE 4-1. Respiratory system.

TABLE 4-2. Normal Respiratory Findings

Area of concern	Normal adult findings	Variations in child	Variations in older adult
General appearance	Appears relaxed Breathing is quiet and easy without apparent effort Facial expressions and limb movements are relaxed		
Breathing pattern	Diaphragmatic-thoracic pattern is smooth and regular May have occasional sighing respirations Breathing is quiet and passive	Abdominal and nasal breathing during childhood until 6 to 7 years of age, then change to adult pattern Newborns may demonstrate Cheyne-Stokes breathing until 3 to 4 weeks of age	Pattern is same as for adults, but calcification at rib articulation points may decrease chest expansion
Respiratory rate	12-20 resp/min Ratio of pulse to respirations is 4:1	Newborn: 30-50 resp/min 1 yr: 20-40 resp/min 3 yr: 20-30 resp/min 6 yr: 16-22 resp/min 10 yr: 16-20 resp/min 17 yr: 14-20 resp/min	
Skin	Appears well oxygenated; no cyanosis or pallor present Palpation of skin and chest wall reveals smooth skin and a stable chest wall; there are no crepitations, bulging, or painful spots	Babies may become mottled if left uncovered	
Nail bed, nail configuration	Minimal angulation between base of nail and finger No thickening of distal finger width		
Chest wall configuration	Symmetric, bilateral muscle development A:P to transverse ratio is 1:2 to 5:7; larger than these ratios is considered to be barrel chest Straight spinal processes Downward and equal slope of ribs; costal angle 90 degrees or less	Newborns have rounded chest wall configuration; by 6 years of age, A:P ratio should be 1:2	Kyphosis is a common finding in elderly persons; there is dorsal scoliosis with slight tracheal deviation; this may also cause a slight increase in A:P to transverse ratio
Tracheal position	Midline and straight directly above the suprasternal notch		May be slightly deviated if kyphosis is present

From Thompson, J.M., et al.: Clinical nursing, St. Louis, 1986, The C.V. Mosby Co.

Cardiac status
  Elevated BP
  Tachycardia
  Bradycardia
  Sinus arrhythmia
  Congestive heart failure (CHF)
    Crackles
    Rhonchi
    Jugular venous distention
    Edema
    Abdominal distention and pain
    Hepatosplenomegaly

Thoracic examination
  Scoliosis
  Kyphosis
  Kyphoscoliosis
  Pectus excavatum (funnel chest)
  Pectus carinatum (pigeon chest)
  Barrel chest
  Unequal shoulder height
Palpation
  Thoracic expansion
  Fremitus (vocal/tactile)
  Tracheal deviation

TABLE 4-3. Breath and Voice Sounds: Normal and Abnormal

Breath and voice sounds	Characteristics	Findings
NORMAL		
Vesicular	Heard over most of lung fields; low pitch; soft and short expirations	Low pitch, soft expirations
Bronchovesicular	Heard over main bronchus area and over upper right posterior lung field; medium pitch; expiration equals inspiration	Medium pitch, medium expirations
Bronchial	Heard only over trachea; high pitch; loud and long expirations	High pitch, loud expirations
ABNORMAL		
Bronchial when heard over peripheral lung fields	High pitch; loud and long expirations	
Bronchovesicular sounds when heard over peripheral lung fields	Medium pitch with inspirations equal to expirations	
Adventitious	Crackles: discrete, noncontinuous sounds	
	Fine crackles (rales): high-pitched, discrete, noncontinuous crackling sounds heard during the end of inspiration (indicates inflammation or congestion)	
	Medium crackles (rales): lower, more moist sound heard during the midstage of inspiration; not cleared by a cough	
	Coarse crackles (rales): loud, bubbly noise heard during inspiration; not cleared by a cough	
	Wheezes: continuous musical sounds; if low pitched, may be called rhonchi	
	Sibilant wheeze: musical noise sounding like a squeak; may be heard during inspiration or expiration; usually louder during expiration	
	Sonorous wheeze (rhonchi): loud, low, coarse sound like a snore heard at any point of inspiration or expiration; coughing may clear sound (usually means mucus accumulation in trachea or large bronchi)	
	Pleural friction rub: dry, rubbing, or grating sound, usually due to the inflammation of pleural surfaces; heard during inspiration or expiration; loudest over lower lateral anterior surface	

From Thompson, J.M., et al.: Clinical nursing, St. Louis, 1986, The C.V. Mosby Co.

TABLE 4-3. Breath and Voice Sounds: Normal and Abnormal—cont'd

Breath and voice sounds	Characteristics	Findings
RESONANCE OF SPOKEN VOICE		
	Bronchophony: using diaphragm of stethoscope, listen to posterior chest as patient says "ninety-nine"	Negative response: muffled "nin-nin" sound heard
		Positive response: clear, loud "ninety-nine" response heard because the lung tissue is consolidated
	Whispered pectoriloquy: listen to posterior chest as patient whispers "one, two, three"	Negative response: muffled sounds heard
		Positive response: clear "one, two, three" is heard because of lung consolidation
	Egophony: listen to posterior chest as the patient says "e-e-e"	Negative response: muffled "e-e-e" sound heard
		Positive response: sound of *e* changes to an a-a-a sound because of consolidation

    Crepitations
Percussion
    Resonance
    Hyperresonance
    Tympany
    Dullness
    Flatness
Auscultation
    Decreased or absent breath sounds
    Crackles
    Rhonchi
    Wheezing
    Friction rubs
    Pectoriloquy
    Bronchophony
    Egophony

Pertinent Background Information

Concurrent diseases or conditions
    Cancer
    Heart disease
    Renal disease
    Liver disease
    Ascites
    Polycythemia
    Obesity
    Hypertension
    Guillian-Barré syndrome
    Myasthenia gravis or other neurologic disease affecting respiratory function
Psychologic responses
    Response to stress
    Methods of coping
    Response to pain
    Relationships with others

Previous respiratory condition/medical history
    Asthma
    Bronchitis
    Emphysema
    Tuberculosis
    Fibrocystic disease
    Premature birth
    Previous operations
Family history
    Heart disease
    Hypertension
    Diabetes
    Obesity
    Pulmonary disorders
Social history
    Smoking: packs per day times how many years
    Alcohol use
    Exercise and activity levels
    Occupation
    Sleep patterns
    Environmental factors: exposure to dust, fumes, asbestos, or chemicals
    Recent exposure to infections
    Travel out of country
Medication history
    Prescription medications
    Over-the-counter medications

Diagnostic Aids

Chest x-ray examination
Complete blood cell count (CBC)
Arterial blood gases (ABGs)
Serum electrolytes
Electrocardiogram (ECG)
Sputum culture

Throat or nasopharyngeal culture
Pulmonary function tests
Gastric washings
Skin tests
Bronchoscopy
Bronchograms
Lung biopsy
Lung scans
Scalene node biopsy
Aortography
Pulmonary angiography
Tomography
Fluoroscopy
Barium swallow
Computed tomography (CT) scan
Pulmonary echograms

THERAPEUTIC BRONCHOSCOPY

Direct visual examination of the trachea and tracheobronchial tree by means of a bronchoscope; the flexible fiberoptic bronchoscope is commonly used because it is better tolerated by the patient and allows better visualization of distal airways

Purpose

Collect secretions for laboratory examinations
Obtain tissue for biopsies
Locate and biopsy tumors
Diagnose hemoptysis, lesions, or masses
Remove foreign bodies or mucous plug secretions
Treat lung abscesses, pneumonia, or aspiration

Preparation

Explain procedure to patient
Maintain NPO for 6 hr before procedure
Manage pain with sedation as indicated; assess effectiveness of pain relief measures
Provide emotional support (patient may be fearful of discomfort and/or possible findings)
Remove dentures
Place patient in sitting or supine position as directed
Instruct patient to breathe in and out of nose with mouth open during procedure:
  Fiberoptic bronchoscope is inserted through nose or mouth
Rigid bronchoscope is inserted through mouth

Postbronchoscopic assessment
Observations/findings

Difficulty in breathing
Stridor
Nasal flaring
Suprasternal and/or supraclavicular retractions
Hemoptysis
Hypotension
Tachycardia
Tachypnea
Cyanosis
Nausea, vomiting
Absence of gag and cough reflex
Hoarseness
Throat pain
Chest pain

Potential complications

Crepitus and/or subcutaneous emphysema
Absence of breath sounds

Immediate postbronchoscopic care

Check BP, P, and R q15 min for four times, then q2h to 4h and prn
Assist and teach patient to
  Not eat or drink until gag reflex returns
  Maintain bed rest; elevate head of bed 45 degrees
  Dispose of tissue after coughing
  Understand importance of not smoking
  Manage pain as indicated; assess effectiveness of pain relief measure(s)
  Establish means of communication
    Call bell within reach
    Pad and pencil or Magic Slate*
Auscultate chest for breath sounds q2h to 4h and prn
Report absent or diminished breath sounds to physician
Perform postural drainage as ordered
Perform oropharyngeal suctioning prn
Administer oxygen as ordered

Convalescent care

Check BP, T, P, and R q8h and prn
Assist and teach patient to
  Gargle with warm saline solution q2h to 4h as indicated
  Maintain position of comfort
  Progress from liquids to diet as tolerated; avoid extremely hot foods

Patient teaching/discharge outcome

Ensure that patient and/or significant other knows and understands
Importance of not driving self home if procedure is done on an outpatient basis

---

*Registered trademark of Western Publishing Co., Inc., Racine, Wis.

Importance of maintaining liquid or soft diet as ordered until throat pain disappears
Importance of forcing fluids to 3000 ml daily unless contraindicated by patient's condition
Need to avoid extremely hot foods and liquids
Need to avoid smoking
Symptoms to report to physician
  Chest pain
  Difficulty in breathing
  Inability to swallow
Importance of ongoing outpatient care
Name of medication, dosage, time of administration, purpose, and side effects
Need to avoid taking over-the-counter medications without checking with physician
Importance of avoiding persons with upper respiratory infections (URIs)

THORACENTESIS

Puncture of the chest wall with a large-gauge needle in order to remove air or fluid from the pleural space

Preparation

Auscultate chest for breath sounds
Obtain chest x-ray examination as ordered by physician
Obtain baseline BP, T, P, and R
Administer sedation as ordered
Prepare local anesthetic as ordered
Position patient on edge of bed with feet supported; head and arms should be resting on overbed table; if patient is unable to sit on edge of bed, have him lie on unaffected side with head of bed elevated and arm raised over head
Provide emotional support
Obtain signed consent form

Preprocedure teaching

Ensure that patient and/or significant other knows and understands
  Procedure to be performed
  Importance of remaining immobile during procedure
  Importance of not coughing during procedure
  That sensations of pain and/or pressure are to be expected

Assessment during and after thoracentesis
Observations/findings
DURING PROCEDURE

Chest tightness
Difficulty in breathing
Tachypnea
Tachycardia
Vertigo
Hypotension
Cyanosis
Diaphoresis
Pallor
Anxiety

POSTPROCEDURE

Difficulty in breathing
Chest pain
Uncontrollable cough
Hemoptysis
Decreased BP
Tachycardia
Tachypnea
Absent or diminished breath sounds
Crepitus
Hyperresonance
Diminished chest wall movement on affected side
Distended neck veins
Cyanosis
Elevated temperature
Deviation of larynx and trachea

Potential complications

Mediastinal shift
Pneumothorax
Pulmonary edema

Immediate postprocedure care

Check BP, P, and R q15 min for four times, then q2h to 4h and prn
Check temperature q4h for 24 hr
Apply adhesive bandage or dressing to site of puncture
Check dressing q15 to 30 min
Turn patient on unaffected side for 1 hr, then to position of comfort
Manage pain as indicated; assess effectiveness of pain relief measure(s)
Administer oxygen as ordered
Measure and record total amount of fluid removed; note color and character
Auscultate chest for breath sounds q2h for two times; then q4h for 24 hr
  Report diminished or absent breath sounds and/or audible rales to physician
  Obtain chest x-ray examination as ordered by physician

Ongoing care

Continue with immediate postprocedure care and decrease frequency of nursing functions as patient's condition improves

Change dressing prn
Assist and teach patient to
  Turn and deep breathe q2h to 4h
  Ambulate as tolerated
  Maintain diet as ordered

Patient teaching/discharge outcome

Ensure that patient and/or significant other knows and understands
  Importance of deep breathing q2h to 4h
  Importance of maintaining a well-balanced diet
  Importance of forcing fluids to limit allotted for patient's condition
  Importance of not smoking
  Importance of avoiding persons with URIs
  Name of medication, dosage, time of administration, purpose, and side effects
  Need to avoid taking over-the-counter medications without checking with physician
  Symptoms to report to physician
    Difficulty in breathing
    Chest pain
    Vertigo
    Elevated temperature
    Diaphoresis
    Uncontrollable cough
    Hemoptysis
  Importance of ongoing outpatient care

ASPIRATION OF SECRETIONS

Preprocedure assessment
Observations/findings

Restlessness
Wheezing
Crowing (ineffective cough)
Inability to expectorate
Difficulty in breathing
Tachycardia
Crackles
Rhonchi over large airways
Decreased breath sounds
Cyanosis

Preprocedure teaching

Explain procedure to patient
Discuss what is expected of patient during procedure
Demonstrate suction equipment
Assist and teach patient to cough and deep breathe prior to procedure

Assessment during procedure
Observations/findings

Tachycardia
Hypoxemia
Trauma to airway; bloody aspirate
Bronchospasm
Aspirate
  Color
  Consistency
  Amount
Cyanosis
Tachypnea
Dyspnea
Nausea

Potential complications

Hypotension
Sudden hypertension
Bradycardia
Cardiac arrhythmias
  Atrioventricular (AV) heart block
  Premature ventricular contractions (PVCs)
  Cardiac arrest

Care during procedure

Auscultate chest for breath sounds
Maintain sterile technique
Use vented or Y catheter
Choose correct catheter to prevent airway occlusion and/or trauma; should be half diameter of airway
  General guide
    Adult: 12 to 18 French
    Child: 6 to 12 French
    Infant: 5 to 6 French
Hyperoxygenate and hyperinflate patient's lungs for four to five breaths
Avoid use of force when inserting catheter
Apply suction only while removing catheter; do not exceed 10 sec
Rotate catheter while removing; avoid moving catheter up and down while suctioning
Suction pressure must not exceed
  Adult: 120 to 150 mm Hg
  Child: 100 to 120 mm Hg
  Infant: 60 to 100 mm Hg
Release suction every 10 sec; ventilate patient for four or five breaths or longer if necessary as soon as suction has been released
Use separate sterile catheter for tracheal suctioning if catheter has already been used for oral suctioning
Observe patient for

Adequate chest expansion
Changes in color
Increased restlessness
Increased pulse rate
Cardiac arrhythmias
Bronchospasm

If bronchospasm, bradycardia, PVCs, or AV block occurs, stop suctioning immediately and ventilate and hyperoxygenate patient

Observe aspirate: if purulent or colored, obtain specimen for culture

Postprocedure assessment
Observations/findings

Breath sounds
  Crackles
    Decreased
    Increased
  Rhonchi over large airways
    Decreased
    Increased
Arterial blood gases: decreased PaO_2
Elevated temperature
Bronchospasm
Tachycardia
Cyanosis

Immediate postprocedure care
General

Auscultate chest for breath sounds; prepare to repeat suctioning procedure if crackles and rhonchi are present

Return oxygen concentration to setting ordered by physician

Check apical pulse and/or record ECG rhythm strip

Assist and teach patient to deep breathe following suctioning procedure

Specific

Oropharyngeal and nasopharyngeal suction

Avoid nasopharyngeal suctioning if patient has a spinal fluid leak or epistaxis

Elevate head of bed 45 degrees

Suction mouth and throat and discard catheter

Lubricate sterile catheter with water-soluble lubricant or water and insert into nares for suctioning

NASOTRACHEAL SUCTION

Avoid nasotracheal suction if patient has a spinal fluid leak or epistaxis

Elevate head of bed 60 to 90 degrees

Hyperoxygenate and hyperinflate patient's lungs for four to five breaths prior to suctioning

Lubricate sterile catheter with water-soluble lubricant or water and insert through nostril to pharynx

Have patient cough or deep breathe and pass catheter into trachea

Suction no more than 10 sec at a time

Hyperoxygenate and hyperinflate patient's lungs for four or five breaths after suctioning

Return oxygen to setting ordered by physician

ENDOTRACHEAL OR TRACHEOSTOMY SUCTION

Be aware that a coudé (curved-tip) catheter may be used in an attempt to suction left mainstem bronchus in certain disease states

Hyperoxygenate and hyperinflate patient's lungs for four or five breaths prior to suctioning

Suction oropharynx and discard catheter

Suction endotracheal tube or tracheostomy tube with a sterile catheter

Suction no more than 10 sec at a time

Hyperoxygenate and hyperinflate patient's lungs for four or five breaths after suctioning

Return oxygen to setting ordered by physician

OXYGEN THERAPY

Use of oxygen to relieve hypoxemia and avoid hypoxia; oxygen flow rate and concentration should be regulated to maintain PaO_2 between 60 mm Hg and 100 mm Hg

Preprocedure assessment
Observations/findings

Hypoxemia
  Hypotension
  Sudden hypertension
  Bradycardia
  Tachycardia
  Cardiac arrhythmias
  Cyanosis
  Tachypnea
  Dyspnea
  Drowsiness
  Disorientation
  Headache
  Excitement
  Decreased attention span
  Poor judgment
  Decreased long- and short-term memory
  Nausea

Nasal flaring
Muscle weakness
Retractions

Potential complications

Atelectasis
Pulmonary edema
Pneumonia
Emphysema
Airway obstruction
Central nervous system (CNS) depression
Decreased PaO_2

Preprocedure teaching

Explain procedure to patient
Demonstrate equipment to be used

Assessment during procedure
Observations/findings

Respiratory depression
Somnolence
Substernal pain with deep inspiration
Arterial blood gases
  PaO_2
  $PaCO_2$
  pH
Tidal volume
Vital capacity (VC)
Elevated temperature
Tachycardia
Psychosocial problems
  Anxiety
  Depression
  Dependence

Potential complications

Oxygen toxicity: time and dose related
  Decreased lung compliance
  Reduced VC
  Sore throat
  Cough
  Diminished breath sounds
  Crackles
  Visual impairment
    Tearing eyes
    Papilledema
Substernal pain with deep inspiration
Circulatory depression: falling central venous pressure (CVP)

Care during procedure
General

Maintain patent airway
Assist and teach patient to maintain position best suited for optimal lung expansion; head of bed usually elevated 45 to 90 degrees
Initiate and maintain oxygen flow rate and concentration with humidification as ordered; have portable oxygen tank and/or extension tubing available if oxygen is to be used continuously and patient is ambulatory or needs to be transported
Check BP, T, R, and apical pulse q15 min for 4 hr, then q2h to 4h if stable
Check level of consciousness q15 min for 4 hr, then q2h to 4h if no change
Auscultate chest for breath sounds q2h to 4h; report diminished or absent breath sounds or audible crackles to physician
Administer oral and nasal hygiene q2h to 4h
Assist and teach patient to turn, cough, and deep breathe q2h to 4h
Provide emotional support; remain with patient while acutely anxious
Continue other nursing functions required for primary disease process
Avoid high-flow rate and concentration of oxygen for patients who require some degree of hypoxemia to maintain respirations
Monitor arterial blood gases as ordered
NOTE: Oxygen toxicity can occur with oxygen concentrations of 50% or higher administered for 24 to 48 hr; symptoms include tachypnea, substernal pain, and dizziness; physiologic effects include atelectasis, ciliary dysfunction, and nitrogen washout; in carbon dioxide retainers, hypoventilation, somnolence, and apnea may occur with minimal elevations in PaO_2

General precautions

Provide humidification with oxygen administration
Always use sterile equipment when administering oxygen; change connecting tubing, humidification equipment, masks, and nasal cannulas q24h
Do not allow smoking while oxygen is in use
Do not permit oil, grease, or other combustible material to come in contact with cylinders, regulators, gauges, valves, or fittings
Administer oxygen only with a safely functioning and properly fitting regulating device
Cylinders

Secure safely to prevent from falling
Transport only in proper carrier
Maintain valve in closed position when not in use
Open valve slowly to full open position when using

Care with use of various devices
NASAL CATHETER

Check catheter patency before insertion
Lubricate catheter with water-soluble lubricant
Position catheter so it cannot be seen when patient's tongue is depressed
Tape securely to nose
Remove catheter q6h to 8h
Reinsert new catheter in opposite nostril if possible
Observe patient for abdominal distention

NASAL CANNULA (PRONGS)

Useful for providing approximately 24% to 44% oxygen at flow rates of 1 to 6 L/min (rate above 6 L/min does not deliver more oxygen)
Ensure proper positioning; avoid kinking or twisting, which impedes oxygen flow
Apply water-soluble lubricant to nares
Observe patient for sinus area pain or nasopharyngeal irritation
Reposition q2h

SIMPLE OXYGEN MASK

Can deliver 40% to 60% oxygen at flow rates of 6 to 10 L/min (rate lower then 5 L/min with face mask can lead to carbon dioxide retention in dead space of mask)
Choose correct size for patient
Remove mask periodically for a few seconds
   Dry patient's face
   Observe for pressure areas
Use face mask only with artificial airway in unconscious patient
Have nasal cannula available for patient to use while eating

PARTIAL REBREATHING MASK

Used for higher oxygen concentrations (40% to 60%) at flow rates of 8 to 12 L/min
Choose correct size for patient
Ensure proper positioning of mask
Apply mask as patient exhales
Avoid twisting or kinking bag
Avoid letting bag totally deflate when patient is inhaling; increase oxygen flow rate if necessary

Remove mask periodically for a few seconds
   Dry patient's face
   Observe for pressure areas
   Apply water-soluble lubricant to lips
Have nasal cannula available for patient to use while eating
Observe for signs of oxygen toxicity

NONREBREATHING MASK

Provides 60% to 90% oxygen at flow rates of 6 to 15 L/min
Choose correct size for patient
Ensure proper positioning of mask
Avoid letting bag totally deflate
Avoid twisting bag
Ensure that all rubber flaps stay in place
Remove mask periodically for a few seconds
   Dry patient's face
   Observe for pressure areas
   Apply water-soluble lubricant to lips
Observe patient for signs of oxygen toxicity; monitor arterial blood gases as ordered
Have a nasal cannula available for patient to use while eating

VENTURI MASK

Provides 24% to 50% oxygen at 3 to 8 L/min flow rate
Choose correct size for patient
Ensure proper positioning; avoid kinking of tubing and blockage of oxygen intake parts that alters FlO_2
Maintain oxygen flow rate as ordered by physician
Remove mask periodically for a few seconds
   Dry patient's face
   Observe for pressure areas
   Apply water-soluble lubricant to lips
Rid tubing of excessive moisture prn
Have nasal cannula available for patient to use while eating

HUMIDITY AND AEROSOL THERAPY

Valuable in loosening up thick secretions and in the delivery of medications; aerosol and humidity devices used to provide humidity when artificial airways are being used are as follows
jet nebulizers   Hand-held nebulizers commonly used to provide medicated aerosol treatment; these are large-reservoir nebulizers for continuous aerosol treatment with or without supplemental oxygen
ultrasonic nebulizers   Can be given to patients

breathing on their own or installed into ventilator circuits; treatments generally last 20 to 30 min

humidifiers Used to prevent humidity deficit when artificial airways are in use; the most commonly used are the bubble humidifiers in conjunction with low-flow oxygen devices

Assessment
Observations/findings
PATIENT

Respirations
  Quality
  Rate
  Depth
Breath sounds
  Crackles
  Diminished or absent
Secretions
  Amount
  Color
  Character
Fluid overload

EQUIPMENT

Oxygen concentration ordered
Oxygen concentration delivered
Heat control
Connecting tubing patent; free from excess moisture

Ongoing care
Patient

Maintain patent airway
Check patient as frequently as indicated by disease or patient's condition during treatment
Suction as indicated
Auscultate chest for breath sounds q2h to 4h; report absent or diminished breath sounds to physician
Position patient comfortably
Dry face of moisture as indicated
Assist and teach patient to turn, cough, and deep breathe q2h to 4h

Equipment

Use sterile distilled water in nebulizer; check water level in reservoir q4h—when adding water, empty reservoir, then refill to correct level
Free tubing of excess moisture q2h to 3h and prn
Check heat control q2h to 4h
Maintain temperature between 95° and 97.8° F (35° and 36.6° C)
Change mask, adaptors, and tubing q24h
Secure and allow sufficient tubing for turning

CHRONIC OBSTRUCTIVE PULMONARY DISEASE (COPD), CHRONIC OBSTRUCTIVE LUNG DISEASE (COLD)

Chronic condition associated with a history of emphysema, asthma, chronic bronchitis, bronchiectasis, cigarette smoking, or exposure to air pollution; there is persistent airway obstruction that progessively increases

Assessment
Observations/findings

Audible expiratory wheeze
Prolonged expirations with considerable effort
Pursed lip breathing
Use of accessory muscles of respiration
Increased anteroposterior diameter of chest (barrel chest)
Distant breath sounds
Crackles
Rhonchi
Bronchospasm
Restlessness
Anorexia
Type of cough
Amount and character of sputum
Malaise
Pulsus paradoxus
Dependent edema
Carbon dioxide retention
  Decreased pH
  Elevated PCO_2
  Confusion
  Somnolence
  Loss of memory

Laboratory/diagnostic studies

ABG studies
Chest x-ray
Pulmonary function studies
White blood cell count (WBC) and sputum specimen analysis
ECG

Potential complications

Arrhythmias
Respiratory failure
Cardiac failure
Gastric ulcer
Cor pulmonale
Polycythemia
Psychosocial problems

Apprehension
Fear of death
Fear of suffocation
Pleural effusion
Ascites

Medical management

Oxygen therapy
Artificial airway/mechanical ventilation if required
Chest physiotherapy
Serial ABG assessment
Medications
  Bronchodilators
  Antibiotics
  Corticosteroids
  Diuretics
  Cardiotonics
Parenteral fluids
Restriction of smoking

Nursing diagnoses/goals/interventions

ndx: Impaired gas exchange related to alveolar-capillary membrane changes

GOAL: *Patient will demonstrate optimal gas exchange for condition*

Maintain bed rest in quiet environment during exacerbation of symptoms
Check respirations qh; note quality and rate
Auscultate chest for breath sounds q1h to 2h; note area of abnormal sounds
Elevate head of bed 45 to 90 degrees
  Allow patient to assume position of comfort
  Padded overbed table may be helpful for patient's comfort
Administer humidified oxygen per nasal catheter or cannula at low flow as ordered
Observe for signs of cyanosis
Be aware that patient may require continuous mechanical ventilation (p. 277)
Administer intermittent positive pressure breathing (IPPB) or aerosol with bronchodilators as ordered
Check BP, T, and apical pulse q2h to 4h and prn
Monitor ABGs
Assist and teach patient to turn, cough, and deep breathe q2h; note type of cough and color and character of sputum
Collect sputum for culture as ordered
Allow absolutely no smoking
Administer medications as ordered
  Bronchodilators
  Antibiotics
  Adrenal corticosteroids
  Avoid respiratory depressant medications
Observe level of consciousness q2h; report confusion, somnolence, or restlessness to physician

ndx: Ineffective airway clearance related to tracheobronchial obstruction and/or secretions

GOAL: *Patient will maintain a patent airway*

Be aware that an endotracheal tube or tracheostomy may be required
Auscultate lung q1h to 2h and prn
Encourage incentive breathing with large tidal volumes
Have patient turn and cough q2h; teach effective coughing technique
Assist and teach patient to perform postural drainage as needed
Administer chest physiotherapy
Suction prn; see Aspiration of Secretions (p. 226)
Administer bronchodilators as ordered

ndx: Alteration in nutrition: less than body requirements related to decreased oral intake associated with dyspnea, anorexia, and fatigure

GOAL: *Patient will maintain an adequate nutritional status*

Maintain liquid to soft, high-protein diet
  Administer supplementary feedings
  Provide attractive meals
Reassess nutritional status on a regular basis; consult with dietitian
Monitor percent of meals eaten
Implement measures to relieve dyspnea
Place in high-Fowler's position at meals to reduce dyspnea
Encourage rest periods prior to meals to reduce fatigue
Provide small, frequent meals to decrease abdominal pressure on diaphragm
Encourage significant others to bring in patient's favorite foods
Administer stool softeners, laxatives, and enemas as ordered
Weigh patient daily at same time with same clothing and scale

ndx: Alteration in tissue integrity of oral mucous membrane: dryness related to prolonged O_2 therapy

GOAL: *Patient will maintain a moist, intact oral mucous membrane*

Assess for dryness of oral mucosa
Administer oral hygiene q2h to 4h and prn
Lubricate lips with petroleum jelly or mineral oil
Encourage fluid intake to 2000 to 3000 ml/day

ndx: Anxiety/fear related to change in health status

GOAL: *Patient will experience a reduction in anxiety/fear*

Provide quiet, nonstressful environment
Provide emotional support
   Remain with patient during anxious periods
   Be aware of subjective statements of patient
   Encourage communication with significant other
   Limit visitors as necessary
   Plan care to provide frequent rest periods
   Avoid "you brought it on yourself" attitude
   Encourage patient; condition can stabilize if a plan of care is followed
   Assess usual coping skills
   Encourage verbalization of fear and anxiety
   Explain all procedures and treatment
   Introduce support groups available to patient and family

ndx: Activity intolerance related to imbalance between oxygen supply and demand

GOAL: *Patient will demonstrate an increased tolerance for activity*

Plan care to provide optimum rest
Assist and teach patient to perform active or passive ROM exercises q4h
Instruct patient on energy conservation measures
Teach pursed lip breathing
Provide O_2 therapy as ordered
Monitor vital signs during time of increased activity
Monitor for signs of extreme fatigue, chest pain, or diaphoresis
Encourage participation in pulmonary rehabilitation program (p. 242)

ndx: Knowledge deficit regarding disease process and home care management

GOAL: *Patient and/or significant other will demonstrate understanding of home care and follow-up instructions through interactive discussion and actual return demonstration*

Explain importance of maintaining respiratory function
Explain importance of not smoking and of avoiding those who smoke
Explain need to avoid respiratory irritants
   Dust
   Fumes
   Smoke
   Perfumes
   Aerosol sprays
   Cold temperatures
Explain need to avoid persons with infections, especially URIs
Explain importance of ongoing outpatient care
Discuss symptoms to report to physician immediately
   Elevated temperature
   Sore throat
   Increase in sputum production
   Change in color of sputum
   URI
   Increased difficulty in breathing
   Decreased activity tolerance
   Decreased appetite
   Increased use of IPPB and oxygen
Explain need to keep warm and avoid chilling
Explain importance of influenza immunization if ordered
Explain importance of environmental control
   Avoid dry air by using humidifier
   Be aware that some patients tolerate high humidity poorly
   Keep free of irritating factors
   Avoid emotional stress; teach stress reduction techniques
   Provide warm house (75° to 80° F [23.8° to 26.6° C])
Explain importance of activity and rest
   Exercise to tolerance
   Need to limit activity on days of high air pollution
   Plan rest periods during day
   Rest before and after meals if shortness of breath increases at mealtimes
   Breathe deeply and slowly during periods of activity
   Understand own life-style and avoid waste of energy
Discuss medications: name, dosage, time of administration, purpose, and side effects
Explain need to avoid taking over-the-counter medications without checking with physician
Demonstrate use of bronchodilator nebulizers if ordered
   Use tid or qid

Take one or two deep inhalations
Release medication only one or two times with each use
Watch for side effects such as tachycardia
Avoid overuse

Explain need to wear medical alert band re chronic obstructive lung disease

Explain need to maintain high-calorie diet as indicated; to force fluids to 2000 to 3000 ml daily unless contraindicated

Explain need to avoid constipation and straining

Ensure that patient and/or significant other demonstrates
  Deep-breathing exercises: pursed lip breathing
  Positions for postural drainage if needed
  Use of ventilator if applicable
  Use of oxygen equipment if applicable

Evaluation

Patient
  Maintains adequate gas exchange as evidenced by
    Usual mental status
    Usual skin color
    Blood gases within acceptable levels for patient
  Maintains a patent airway as evidenced by
    Improved breath sounds
    Normal rate and depth of respirations
    Absence of dyspnea and cyanosis
    Blood gases within acceptable levels
  Maintains an adequate nutritional status as evidenced by weight remaining stable and within or moving toward normal range for patient's height, age, and build
  Has moist, intact oral mucosa as evidenced by
    No verbalization of pain
    No evidence of dryness or cracking of lips and oral mucosa
  Experiences a decrease in fear and anxiety as evidenced by
    Relaxed facial expression
    Verbalization of feeling less anxious
    Verbalization of understanding hospital routines, procedures, and disease process
  Demonstrates an increased tolerance for activity as evidenced by ability to resume activities of daily living (ADLs) without extremes in fatigue or dyspnea
  Demonstrates understanding of home care management of disease process as evidenced by
    Regular attendance at doctor's appointment
    Increased activity tolerance
    Decreased admissions to hospital

ASTHMA

A reversible obstructive disease characterized by increased reactivity of the trachea and bronchi to stimuli, manifested by wheezing and dyspnea; narrowing is due to a combination of bronchospasm, mucosal swelling and increased secretions

Assessment
Observations/findings

Sudden onset of respiratory distress
  Prolonged expiratory wheeze
  Short inspiratory period
  Intercostal and sternal retraction
  Use of accessory muscles of respiration
  Air hunger
  Crackles
Breath sounds
  Decreased
  Absent
Assumes upright sitting position; leans forward
Diaphoresis
Tachycardia
Distended neck veins
Cyanosis
  Circumoral area
  Nail beds
Hard, dry cough; productive cough is difficult
Altered level of consciousness
Hypoxemia
Hypotension
Pulsus paradoxus
Dehydration
Increased anxiety
  Fear of suffocation
  Fear of death

Laboratory/diagnostic studies

Arterial blood gases
  Mild decrease in PaO_2 and $PaCO_2$: common between attacks
  Decreased PaO_2, increased PaO_2 with severe attacks
Chest x-ray examination
  Normal between attacks
  Hyperinflation with attacks
Skin testing (extrinsic asthma)
Pulmonary function tests
  Normal or increased lung volumes
  Decreased flow rates; improvement with bronchodilators
WBC and sputum examination
  Sputum and blood eosinophilia are common
  Serum IgE levels are elevated in extrinsic asthma

Potential complications

Pulmonary edema
Respiratory failure
Status asthmaticus
Pneumonia

Medical management

Oxygen therapy
Fluid management
Artificial airway and ventilatory support if necessary
Medications
Sympathomimetics
Theophylline
Steroids
Cromolyn sodium
Antibiotics

Nursing diagnoses/goals/interventions

ndx: Anxiety related to difficulty in breathing, fear of suffocation, and/or fear of recurrent attacks

GOAL: *Patient will experience a reduction in anxiety/fear*

Provide emotional support
   Remain with patient when anxious
   Anticipate patient's needs
   Provide quiet reassurance
   Maintain bed rest in quiet environment
Remain with patient during coughing episodes
   Encourage sips of water
   Give hard candy if it helps control coughing
Evaluate patient coping skills
Teach relaxation techniques
Explain procedures
Reassure patient that oxygen and medical therapy usually can control attacks
Implement measures to promote airway clearance; encourage patient to change position q1h to 2h and prn
Administer oral hygiene q2h to 4h and prn
Maintain planned rest periods
   Pace and plan ADLs
   Discourage talking if extremely dyspneic
   Limit visitors as necessary
   Encourage frequent rest periods
Perform active or passive range-of-motion (ROM) exercises q4h if on bed rest
Keep environment free from flowers, smoke, and dust

ndx: Ineffective airway clearance related to excessive mucous production and bronchospasm

GOAL: *Patient will maintain a patent airway*

Check BP, R, and apical pulse q2h
Check rectal temperature q4h
Auscultate chest for breath sounds q1h to 2h
Observe skin color and temperature q2h
Check arterial blood gases as ordered
Check level of consciousness q1h to 2h; report decrease to physician
   Elevate head of bed 60 to 90 degrees
   Support back with pillows
   Provide well-padded overbed table to lean over
   Place side rails up for safety and support
   Place humidifier or steam vaporizer at bedside as ordered
   Administer low flow of oxygen by nasal catheter as ordered
   Avoid oxygen mask (it increases sensation of suffocation)
   Administer IPPB as ordered
Administer medications as ordered
   Epinephrine preparations
   Aminophylline
   Sympathomimetics
   Antihistamines
   Expectorants
   Adrenal corticosteroids
   Sedatives; avoid respiratory depressants
   Antibiotics
   Isoproterenol or cromolyn nebulization; avoid using isoproterenol and aminophylline together (can cause arrest)
Force fluids as ordered to keep secretions thin
Assess sputum for color, tenacity, and amount
Collect sputum for culture as ordered
Suction prn

ndx: Ineffective breathing pattern related to decreased lung expansion during acute attack

GOAL: *Patient will resume an effective breathing pattern*

Monitor for signs and symptoms of ineffective breathing: shallow respirations, diaphoresis, dyspnea, use of accessory muscles
Monitor vital signs and arterial blood gases
Place patient in high-Fowler's position for maximal chest expansion
Administer oxygen therapy if ordered
Maintain patent airway
Suction prn
Remain with patient during acute attack to decrease fear and anxiety
Administer medications as ordered

TABLE 4-4. Broncholidators

Generic name	Brand names	Availability	Adult dosage range
SYMPATHOMIMETICS			
Albuterol	Proventil, Ventolin	Tablets: 2, 4 mg Aerosol: 90 mcg	PO: 2-4 mg 3-4 times daily Inhale: 2 inhalations every 4-6 hours
Ephedrine	Ephedrine	Tablets: 25 mg Capsules: 25, 50 mg Syrup: 11, 20 mg/5 ml Injection: 25, 50 mg/ml	PO: 25-50 mg every 3-4 hours SC, IM, IV: 25-50 mg
Epinephrine	Primatene, Vaponefrin, Bronkaid Mist	Nebulization: 1:100 Aerosol: 0.2, 0.25, 0.3 mg Injection: 1:200, 1:100	See manufacturer's recommendations
Ethylnorepinephrine	Bronkephrine	2 mg/ml	SC or IM: 0.5-ml
Isoetharine	Bronkosol, Beta-2, Bronkometer	Nebulization: 0.125, 0.2, 0.5, 1% Aerosol: 0.61%	See manufacturer's recommendations
Isoproterenol	Isuprel, Aerolone, Norisodrine	Nebulization: 0.25, 0.5, 1% Aerosol: 0.2, 0.25% Injection: 0.2 mg/ml SL: 10, 15 mg tabs	See manufacturer's recommendations
Metaproterenol	Alupent, Metaprel	Tablets: 10, 20 mg Syrup: 10 mg/5 ml Aerosol: 225 mg Nebulization: 5%	See manufacturer's recommendations
Terbutaline	Brethine, Bricanyl	Tablets: 2.5, 5 mg Injection: 1 mg/ml	PO: 5 mg every 6 hours SC: 0.25 mg; repeat, if needed, in 30 minutes
XANTHINE DERIVATIVES			
Aminophylline		Tablets: 100, 200 mg Elixir: 250 mg/15 ml Liquid: 105 mg/5 ml Suppositories: 250, 500 mg Injection: 250, 500 ml Others	See manufacturer's recommendations
Dyphylline	Dilor, Dyflex, Lufyllin	Tablets: 200, 400 mg Liquid: 100 mg/5 ml Elixir: 100, 160 mg/15 ml Injection: 250 mg/ml	PO: 15 mg/kg, 5 times daily IM: 250-500 mg slowly
Oxtriphylline	Choledyl	Tablets: 100, 200 mg Elixir: 100 mg/5 ml Syrup: 50 mg/5 ml	200 mg 4 times daily
Theophylline	Bronkodyl, Elixophyllin, Theolair, others	Tablets: 125, 200, 225, 300 mg Capsules: 50, 100, 200, 250 mg Elixir: 80 mg/15 ml Liquid: 80 mg/15 ml Syrup: 80 mg/15 ml Suspension: 300 mg/15 ml Others	9-20 mg/kg/24 hours in 4 divided doses

From Clayton, B., Stock, Y., and Squire, J.: Squire's basic pharmacology for nurses, St. Louis, 1985, The C.V. Mosby Co.

ndx: Fluid volume deficit potentially related to increased respiratory distress and diaphoresis

GOAL: *Hydration will be maintained*

Encourage oral intake as tolerated
Provide liquid to soft diet
Provide high-calorie, high-protein diet
Assist with feeding if extremely weak
Administer parenteral fluids as ordered
Measure intake and output
Monitor weight daily

ndx: Knowledge deficit regarding self-care management

GOAL: *Patient and/or significant other will demonstrate understanding of home care and follow-up instructions through interactive discussion and actual return demonstration*

Explain importance of preventing future attacks
    Avoid known irritants
    Avoid stressful situations
    Express anxieties and fears
    Encourage communication with significant other and/or family
    Provide adequate humidity
        Nonflowering plants can increase humidity 5% to 10%
        Humidifiers are helpful (provide instructions on use of humidifiers and need to keep clean)
    Avoid persons with infections, especially URIs
    Do not smoke; avoid persons who smoke
Explain importance of breathing exercises
Explain importance of exercise to tolerance
    Avoid fatigue
    Plan rest periods
Explain importance of diet and fluids
    Eat balanced, nutritious meals
    Force fluids to 2000 to 3000 ml daily unless contraindicated
    Avoid gaining weight
Explain importance of ongoing outpatient care
Discuss symptoms to report to physician
    URI
    Flu
    Elevated temperature
Discuss medications: name, dosage, time of administration, purpose, and side effects
Demonstrate proper use of inhalers and maintenance of containers
Explain that tachycardia may occur
Explain need to wear medical alert band re asthma
Explain importance of taking medications as ordered

Evaluation

Patient
    Demonstrates a reduction in fear and anxiety as evidenced by
        Relaxed facial expression
        Verbalization of feeling less anxious
        Vital signs within normal parameters
    Maintains a patent airway as evidenced by
        Improved breath sounds
        Normal rate and depth of respirations
        Absence of dyspnea
        Absence of cyanosis
        Blood gases within normal range
    Maintains an effective breathing pattern as evidenced by
        Normal rate, rhythm, and depth of respirations
        Absence or reduction of dyspnea
        Blood gases within acceptable range for patient
    Maintains hydration as evidenced by
        Skin turgor, mucous membranes, and specific gravity within normal limits
        Bronchial secretion liquified and easily coughed up
    Demonstrates knowledge in health care management as evidenced by verbalization of principles of health care management of the disease

BRONCHITIS

Acute or chronic inflammation of the bronchial mucous membrane (Chronic bronchitis is the most common respiratory disease.)

Assessment
Observations/findings

Elevated temperature
Chills
Cough (morning)
    Nonproductive
    Mucopurulent sputum
Breath sounds
    Crackles
    Rhonchi
    Decreased
    Absent
Hemoptysis
Malaise
Wheezing respirations
Bronchospasm
Atelectasis
Hypoxemia
Anorexia
Dyspnea

Laboratory/diagnostic studies

Arterial blood gases
    Hypoxemia (decreased PaO_2)
    Hypercapnea (increased PaO_2)
    Respiratory acidosis
Sputum culture: eosinophils
Chest x-ray examination
    Increased peribronchial markings at both bases
    Normal-size heart
Pulmonary function tests
    Normal lung volumes
    Decreased flow rates
CBC: polycythemia in chronic hypoxemia

Potential complications

Infections of respiratory tract
Respiratory insufficiency
Respiratory failure

Medical management

O_2 therapy
Chest physiotherapy
Fluid management
Medications
    Bronchodilators
    Antibiotics
    Diuretics
    Steroids

Nursing diagnoses/goals/interventions

ndx: Ineffective airway clearance related to increased tracheobronchial secretions

GOAL: *Patient will maintain a patent airway*

Position patient comfortably: usually with head of bed elevated 45 to 60 degrees
Provide humidified air
Force fluids to 2000 to 3000 ml daily unless contraindicated
Assist and teach patient to turn, cough, and deep breathe q2h; postural drainage may be ordered
Auscultate chest for breath sounds q8h
Administer oral hygiene after productive coughing
Check T, P, and R q4h
Administer antibiotics as ordered
Administer bronchodilators as ordered
Administer IPPB as ordered
Suction prn

ndx: Ineffective breathing pattern related to decreased lung expansion secondary to increased mucous production blocking airways

GOAL: *Patient will resume an effective breathing pattern*

Monitor for signs and symptoms of ineffective breathing: shallow respirations, diaphoresis, dyspnea, use of accessory muscles
Oxygen therapy if ordered
Monitor vital signs and arterial blood gases
Encourage fluids to keep secretions thin if not medically contraindicated
Suction prn
Place patient in high-Fowler's position to maximize chest expansion when possible
Administer medications as ordered

ndx: Knowledge deficit regarding home care management

GOAL: *Patient and/or significant other will demonstrate understanding of home care and follow-up instructions through interactive discussion and actual return demonstration*

Explain importance of not smoking; need to avoid persons who smoke
Explain need to reduce exposure to air pollution and occupational respiratory hazards
Explain importance of maintaining diet as ordered; need to force fluids to 2000 to 3000 ml daily unless contraindicated
Explain importance of maintaining weight within normal limits for age, sex, and height
Explain need to exercise to tolerance; to avoid fatigue and plan rest periods
Explain need to avoid persons with URIs
    Avoid crowds
    Sleep in a cool, not cold, room
    Use vaporizer prn
    Keep warm
    Avoid chilling
Discuss medications: name, dosage, time of administration, purpose, and side effects
Explain need to avoid taking over-the-counter medications without checking with physician
Explain importance of ongoing outpatient care
Discuss symptoms to report to physician
    Elevated temperature
    Cough
    Respiratory distress
    Flu or cold
Ensure that patient and/or significant other demonstrates
    Diaphragmatic breathing
    Coughing techniques

Evaluation

Patient
- Maintains a patent airway as evidenced by
  - Improved breath sounds
  - Normal rate and depth of respirations
  - Absence or improvement of dyspnea
  - Absence of cyanosis
  - Blood gases within acceptable range
- Maintains an effective breathing pattern as evidenced by
  - Normal rate, rhythm, and depth of respirations
  - Absence or reduction of dyspnea
  - Blood gases within acceptable range for patient
- Demonstrates increased knowledge regarding self-care management as evidenced by verbalization of self-care management principles pertaining to diagnosis

BRONCHIECTASIS

Chronic dilation of a bronchus or bronchi, secreting large amounts of purulent sputum

Assessment

Observations/findings

Cough: paroxysms in early morning
Sputum
  Profuse
  Purulent
  Foul odor
  Hemoptysis
Breath sounds
  Crackles
  Rhonchi
  Decreased
  Absent
Weight loss
Chronic fatigue
Anorexia
Recurrent pneumonia
Elevated temperature
Chronic sinusitis
Clubbing of fingers and toes

Laboratory/diagnostic studies

Chest x-ray examination
  Usually normal
  Air fluid levels and infiltrates may be seen in advanced diffuse disease
Bronchography
Sputum examination: staphylococci, streptococci, and pseudomonas commonly seen on sputum smears and cultures
Pulmonary function tests
  Normal or slightly decreased lung volumes
  Decreased flow rates
Arterial blood gases: mild decrease in PaO_2 and $PaCO_2$ are common

Potential complications

Respiratory failure

Medical management

O_2 therapy with humidity
Postural drainage
Medications
  Bronchodilators
  Antibiotics
Surgical resection of lung

Nursing diagnoses/goals/interventions

ndx: Ineffective airway clearance related to tracheobronchial secretions and decreased ciliary function

GOAL: *Patient will maintain a patent airway*

Auscultate chest for breath sounds q4h to 8h
Perform postural drainage as indicated by patient's condition; avoid mealtimes
Assist and teach patient to turn and deep breathe; encourage incentive breathing
Avoid vigorous coughing (could spread infection)
Check T, P, and R q4h
Assist and teach patient to perform diaphragmatic breathing
Administer oral hygiene after sputum production
Force fluids to 2000 to 3000 ml daily unless contraindicated
Observe closely during coughing paroxysms for dyspnea and cyanosis
Administer antibiotics as ordered
Administer IPPB as ordered
Prepare for bronchoscopy as ordered (p. 224)
Suction prn

ndx: Disturbance in sleep pattern: sleep deprivation related to frequent coughing and chronic increased work of breathing

GOAL: *Patient will attain adequate amounts of sleep within parameters of treatment regimen*

Plan frequent rest periods
Avoid fatigue
Teach energy conservation techniques
Exercise to tolerance
Utilize techniques to maintain patent airway during rest/sleep periods

Deep breathing and coughing prior to rest period
Postural drainage to clear airways 1 to 2 hr before bedtime
Medication regimen utilized to enhance sleep at night

ndx: Knowledge deficit regarding disease process

GOAL: *Patient and/or significant other will demonstrate understanding of home care and follow-up*

Instructions through interactive discussion and actual return demonstration
Explain need to maintain high-protein, high-calorie diet through small, frequent feedings
Explain need to force fluids to 2000 to 3000 ml daily unless contraindicated
Explain importance of not smoking; need to avoid persons who smoke
Explain need to reduce exposure to air pollution and occupational respiratory hazards
Explain need to exercise to tolerance; to avoid fatigue and plan rest periods
Explain need to avoid persons with respiratory infections
   Avoid crowds
   Keep warm
   Avoid chilling
Discuss medications: name, dosage, time of administration, purpose, and side effects
Explain need to avoid taking over-the-counter medications without checking with physician
Explain importance of ongoing outpatient care
Discuss symptoms to report to physician
   Chest pain
   Difficulty in breathing
   Hemoptysis
   Elevated temperature
   Flu or cold

Evaluation

Patient
   Maintains a patent airway as evidenced by
      Improved breath sounds
      Normal rate and depth of respirations
      Absence of dyspnea
      Absence of cyanosis
      Blood gases within acceptable range
   Attains adequate amounts of sleep as evidenced by
      Statements of feeling rested
      Absence of frequent yawning, dozing during the day, and fatigue
   Demonstrates an increased understanding of disease process as evidenced by verbalization of self-care management principles

EMPHYSEMA

Destruction of elastic tissues of the alveolar walls, causing a reduced expiratory flow rate and overinflated alveoli; a progressive disease that is irreversible

Assessment

Observations/findings

Shortness of breath
Difficulty in breathing
Use of accessory muscles of respiration
Cough: may be productive
Pursed lip–breathing
Cyanosis
Orthopnea
Unequal chest expansion
Increased AP chest diameter
Tachypnea
Tachycardia
Elevated temperature
Anxiety
Carbon dioxide retention; decreased pH
Elevated $PaCO_2$
   Restlessness
   Confusion
Hypoxemia
Breath sounds
   Distant
   Crackles
   Wheezing
Hyperresonance
Weakness
Fatigue
Anorexia
Weight loss
Peripheral edema if cardiac involvement
Clubbed fingers

Laboratory/diagnostic studies

Arterial blood gases
   Decreased PaO_2; increased $PaCO_2$
   pH within normal limits if compensation has occurred
Chest x-ray examination
   Hyperlucent lung fields; small, narrow heart; increased AP diameter; low, flat diaphragm
   Apical bullae are common
Pulmonary function tests
   Increased total lung capacity
   Increased residual volume
CBC: polycythemia if chronically hypoxic
ECG: low-voltage, right axis deviation is common in moderately advanced disease
Sputum culture

Potential complications

Respiratory failure
Cor pulmonale
Heart failure
Arrhythmias

Medical management

O_2 therapy
Fluid management
Medications
    Bronchodilators
    Antibiotics
    Steroids
Artificial airway/mechanical ventilation

Nursing diagnoses/goals/interventions

ndx: Impaired gas exchange related to decreased lung capacity secondary to tissue destruction

GOAL: *Patient will maintain optimal gas exchange within limits of disease process*

Administer oxygen with humidification as ordered
Be aware that patient may be placed on continuous mechanical ventilation (p. 277)
Administer IPPB with nebulization as ordered
Administer medications as ordered
    Bronchodilators
    Antibiotics
    Expectorants
    Steroids
    Pain management
    Avoid sedation
Check BP, P, and R q2h to 4h
Check quality and rate of respirations
Check rectal temperature q4h to 6h
Auscultate chest for breath sounds q2h to 4h and prn
Maintain bed rest, if necessary, during exacerbation of symptoms
Maintain good body alignment; elevate head of bed 45 to 60 degrees
Assist and teach patient to turn, cough, and deep breathe q2h to 4h; splint chest when coughing
Assist and teach patient to perform breathing exercises as ordered
    Pursed lip breathing
    Diaphragmatic breathing
Check arterial blood gases as ordered

ndx: Ineffective airway clearance related to excessive mucous, impaired cough effort

GOAL: *Patient will maintain a patent airway*

Auscultate lung q1h to 2h and prn
Encourage incentive breathing
Have patient turn and cough q2h
Administer chest physiotherapy or assist and teach patient postural drainage following aerosol treatments as needed
See Aspiration of Secretions (p. 226); if this is necessary obtain sputum for culture and sensitivity as ordered
Administer bronchodilators as ordered
Assist and teach patient to ambulate to tolerance as ordered
    Avoid overtiring
    Encourage self-care
    Teach energy conservation techniques
    Maintain planned rest periods

ndx: Ineffective breathing pattern related to decreased lung expansion

GOAL: *Patient will resume an effective breathing pattern*

Monitor for signs and symptoms of ineffective breathing: shallow respirations, diaphoresis, dyspnea, use of excessory muscles
Monitor vital signs and arterial blood gases
Administer oxygen therapy if ordered
Place patient in positions to maximize chest wall expansion
Maintain patent airway
Suction prn
Administer medications as ordered

ndx: Alteration in nutrition: less than body requirements related to decreased oral intake associated with dyspnea, anorexia, and fatigue

GOAL: *Patient will maintain an adequate nutritional status*

Maintain liquid to soft, high-protein diet
    Administer supplementary feedings
    Provide attractive meals
Reassess nutritional status on a regular basis; consult with dietitian
Monitor percent of meals eaten
Place in high-Fowler's position at meals to reduce dyspnea
Encourage rest periods prior to meals to reduce fatigue
Encourage significant others to bring in patient's favorite foods
Administer stool softeners, laxatives, and enemas as ordered

ndx: Activity intolerance related to dyspnea and fatigue

GOAL: *Patient will demonstrate an increased tolerance for activity*

Plan care to provide optimum rest
Assist and teach patient to perform active or passive ROM exercises q4h
Instruct patient on energy conservation measures
Teach pursed lip breathing
Provide O_2 therapy as ordered
Monitor vital signs during time of increased activity
Monitor for signs of extreme fatigue, chest pain, and diaphoresis
Encourage admission to pulmonary rehabilitation program

ndx: Knowledge deficit regarding health care management of disease process

GOAL: *Patient and/or significant other will demonstrate understanding of home care and follow-up instructions through interactive discussion and actual return demonstration*

Explain nature of disease and importance of treatment and management
Explain need to exercise to tolerance
   Avoid excessive fatigue
   Rest before and after meals if shortness of breath is increased during mealtime
   Plan ADLs carefully to allow maximum functioning with minimum energy expenditure
Discuss medications: name, dosage, time of administration, purpose, and side effects
Explain need to avoid taking over-the-counter medications without checking with physician
Explain importance of avoiding persons with URIs
Explain importance of influenza vaccination if ordered
Explain importance of ongoing outpatient care
Discuss first signs of a cold or flu to report to physician
   Fever
   Increased difficulty in breathing
   Sore throat
Explain need to avoid respiratory irritants
   Smoke
   Fumes
   Dust
   Perfumes
   Aerosol sprays
   Cold temperatures
Explain need to limit physical activities during days of high air pollution concentration
Discuss symptoms to report to physician
   Change in color or character of sputum
   Decreased activity tolerance
   Increased use of IPPB and oxygen
   Decreased appetite
Explain importance of maintaining high-protein, high-carbohydrate diet if indicated; need to force fluids to 2000 to 3000 ml daily unless contraindicated
Explain importance of environmental control
   Avoid decreasing humidity by using humidifier or nonflowering house plants
   Maintain comfortable temperature in house to avoid extremes; prevent chilling
Explain need to avoid constipation and straining
Explain need to wear medical alert band re emphysema
Ensure that patient and/or significant other demonstrates
   Breathing exercises
      Diaphragmatic breathing
      Pursed lip breathing
      Inhaling and exhaling slowly
   Postural drainage as needed
   Use of ventilator if ordered
   Use of oxygen equipment if ordered

Evaluation

Patient
   Maintains adequate gas exchange as evidenced by
      Usual mental status
      Usual skin color
      Blood gases within acceptable range
   Maintains a patent airway as evidenced by
      Improved breath sounds
      Normal rate and depth of respirations
      Absence of dyspnea
      Absence of cyanosis
      Blood gases within acceptable range
   Maintains an effective breathing pattern as evidenced by
      Normal rate, rhythm, and depth of respirations
      Absence or reduction of dyspnea
      Blood gases within acceptable range for patient
   Maintains an adequate nutritional status as evidenced by weight remaining stable and within normal range for patient's height, age, and build
   Demonstrates an increased tolerance for activity as evidenced by ability to resume ADLs without extremes in fatigue or dyspnea
   Demonstrates an increased understanding of home care management as evidenced by

Regular attendance at doctor's appointments
Decreased admissions to hospital
Increasing activity tolerance

PULMONARY REHABILITATION

An inpatient or outpatient program designed to increase exercise tolerance in COPD patients while educating them to understand and assist in the management of their disease; components generally include physical therapy, respiratory therapy, exercise conditioning, medications, and education

Admission criteria

Symptomatic pulmonary disease
    Dyspnea (see dyspnea classification)
    Cough
    Wheezing
    Sputum production
    Chest pain
Patient motivation
Restricted ADLs (see COPD Disability Scale, Table 4-5)
No underlying condition that would interfere with the program (psychosis, alcoholism, drug abuse)
Medically stable: no signs of CHF, uncontrolled arrhythmias, or myocardial infarction (MI) in previous 6 months
Adequate financial/insurance status
Family support system

TABLE 4-5. COPD Disability Scale

Class I	No significant restriction of normal activities, but dyspnea on strenuous exertion.
Class II	No dyspnea with essential activities of daily living; dyspnea on climbing stairs and in other climbs but not on level walking. Employability limited to sedentary occupations.
Class III	Dyspnea with some activities of daily living (e.g., showering, dressing), but can perform all such activities without assistance. Able to walk at own pace for a city block, but cannot keep up while walking with normal others of the same age.
Class IV	Dependent on others in some activity of daily living; not dyspneic at rest, but dyspneic with minimal exertion.
Class V	Dyspneic at rest; dependent on assistance from others for most activities of daily living.

From Hodgkin, J., Zorn, E., and Connors, G., editors: Pulmonary rehabilitation: guidelines to success, Stoneham, Mass., 1984, Butterworth Publishers. Adapted from Moser, K.M., et al.: Results of a comprehensive rehabilitation program, Arch. Intern. Med. **140**:1596, 1980.

Exclusion criteria

Terminal cancer
Heart failure
Stroke
Alcoholism, active
Drug abuse
Organic brain disease
End-stage COPD

Inpatient Program

Assessment

Observations/findings

Heart rate
    Increase of 30 beats/min above resting rate with activity
    Heart rate less than 50 during activity
    Consistent drop in heart rate of more than 10 beats/min during activity
ECG rhythm: presence of irregular rhythm
Blood pressure
    Increase of 20 mm Hg above normal
    Diastolic increase of more than 10 to 15 mm Hg
    Systolic drop to below 90 at rest; diastolic below 40

Symptoms during activity

Dyspnea
Dizziness
Fatigue
Pain
Palpitations
Diaphoresis

Indicators of energy expenditure during activity

Arterial oxygen saturation values
PaO_2
Oxygen consumption rate

Indicators of ventilatory response during activity

Minute ventilation
Respiratory rate
Carbon dioxide production

Ongoing care

Activity progression program
    Follow physician activity prescription
    Initiate exercise program
Evaluate daily progress and plan activity levels
Maintain progressive increase in activities until discharge
Monitor ECG and respiratory parameters
Record and report any signs or symptoms of shortness of breath (SOB), fatigue, or nausea during or following exercise

> **PULMONARY REHABILITATION PROGRAM: SUGGESTED CLASS CONTENT**
>
> Orientation to rehabilitation program
> Anatomy and physiology of pulmonary system
> Nutrition
> Effects of stress and emotions on lung disease
> Coping with chronic lung disease
> COPD, specific diseases
> Medications
> Impact of COPD on family and friends
> Oxygen, IPPB treatments
> Principles of exercise
> Relaxation techniques
> Breathing exercises: pursed lip breathing and diaphragmatic breathing
> Energy conservation techniques
> Postural drainage
> Prevention of Infection
> Stop smoking sessions
> Discussions on sexuality

Assist patient in performing ADLs and monitor HR, R, and BP 1 min and 4 min after activity (response to activity should return to preactivity level within 5 min; if it does not, monitor every 2 min until pretest levels are reached)
Observe, record and report patient's tolerance

Discharge evaluation

Self-care/ADL skills
Equipment needs for the home
Weekly schedule of exercise and rest
Assessment of level of knowledge
Knowledge of agency referral sources

Benefits of Pulmonary Rehabilitation Program

Reduced symptoms
Decreased anxiety and depression
Improved ability to perform ADLs
Increased exercise tolerance
Reduced hospital admissions/days/cost of care
Improved quality of life

PNEUMONIA

Inflammation of the alveolar spaces of the lung caused by bacteria, viruses, chemicals, dust, and allergens; lung tissue is consolidated as alveoli fill with exudate

Assessment

Observations/findings

Difficult and painful respirations
    Pleuritic pain
    Shortness of breath and grunting
    Tachypnea
    Diminished, progressing to absent, breath sounds
    Crackles
    Rhonchi
    Asymmetric chest movements
Chills and fever (102° to 106° F [38.8° to 41.1° C]); delirium
Anorexia
Malaise
Abdominal distention
Productive, tenacious cough
    Incessant, painful
    Copious amounts of green-yellow sputum progressing to pink or rusty
Restlessness
Cyanosis
    Circumoral area
    Nail beds
Tachycardia
Pleural effusion
Lung abscess
Bacteremia
Atelectasis
Paralytic ileus
Herpes simplex
Psychosocial problems
    Disorientation
    Anxiety
    Fear of death

Laboratory/diagnostic studies

Chest x-ray examination: patchy or diffuse infiltrates
Sputum culture
WBC count
Blood culture
Arterial blood gases

Potential complications

Respiratory failure
Superinfection
Pleural effusion

Medical management

Fluid management
Parenteral therapy
Oxygen therapy
Bed rest

Chest physiotherapy
Artificial airway or ventilator support if necessary
Medications
    Antipyretics
    Antibiotics
    Antimicrobials

Nursing diagnoses/goals/interventions

ndx: Impaired gas exchange related to tracheobronchial secretions and lung consolidation with decrease in effective lung surface

GOAL: *Patient will have adequate gas exchange*

Elevate head of bed 45 to 60 degrees; isolation precautions may be necessary
Provide humidified oxygen per mask or nasal catheter as ordered
Maintain continuous vaporizer at bedside
Provide croup tent if helpful
Administer IPPB as ordered
Assist during coughing episodes
    Have patient sit upright
    Splint chest with pillows
Assist and teach patient to turn and deep breathe q2h to 4h
Auscultate chest for breath sounds q2h to 4h
Prepare for chest x-ray examination and laboratory work
Administer medications as ordered
    Antibiotics
    Analgesics
    Antipyretics
    Sedatives; avoid respiratory depressants
    Expectorants
Pace activities to patient's tolerance

ndx: Ineffective airway clearance related to increased tracheobronchial secretions secondary to infectious process

GOAL: *Patient will maintain a patent airway*

Encourage turning and deep breathing q2h to 4h
Incentive spirometry
Suction prn
Force fluids as ordered to help liquify secretions
Auscultate chest for breath sounds q2h to 4h
Assist and teach patient postural drainage as soon as tolerated

ndx: Alteration in comfort: pain related to respiratory distress and coughing

GOAL: *Patient will experience diminished pain*

Encourage patient to verbalize any pain
Administer medications to treat cough
Administer analgesics as ordered
    Be aware of potential for depression of respiratory function
    Evaluate effectiveness
Keep patient warm and dry
Maintain planned rest periods
    Avoid unnecessary talking if necessary
    Limit visitors as necessary
Provide emotional support
    Remain with patient as much as possible
    Explain all equipment and procedures
    Anticipate needs
Discourage smoking
Encourage communication with significant other
Administer oral hygiene q2h to 4h ac, and prn; assess for lesions and dry mouth (ice chips at bedside are helpful)

ndx: Potential alteration in body temperature regulation related to bacterial or viral infection

GOAL: *Temperature will be within normal range*

Collect blood cultures as ordered
Collect sputum cultures as ordered
Check T, P, and R q4h; check T, P, and R during periods of chilling
Administer prescribed antimicrobials and/or antipyretics
Encourage oral fluids as ordered
Administer cooling procedures as ordered
Isolate patient if required

ndx: Knowledge deficit regarding self-care management

GOAL: *Patient and/or significant other will demonstrate understanding of home care and follow-up instructions through interactive discussion and actual return demonstration*

Explain importance of avoiding transmission of disease
    Turn head away when coughing and cover mouth with tissue
    Use tissue only once
    Dispose of tissue in waste container
Explain importance of gradual convalescence
    Limit exercise and activity to tolerance
    Plan two or three rest periods during day
    Avoid fatigue

Explain importance of postural drainage and deep-breathing exercises; continue deep-breathing exercises qid for 6 to 8 weeks
Explain importance of maintaining diet as tolerated
    Avoid high-calorie diet if overweight
    Force liquids to 3000 ml daily unless contraindicated
Explain need to avoid recurrence of disease
    Keep warm
    Avoid chilling
    Avoid persons with infections, especially URIs
    Receive influenza vaccine as ordered
Explain need to use vaporizer or humidifier at home
Explain importance of ongoing outpatient care
Discuss symptoms to report to physician
    Elevated temperature
    Diaphoresis
    Difficulty in breathing
    Persistent cough
    Cold or flu
Discuss medications: name, dosage, time of administration, purpose, and side effects
Explain need to avoid taking over-the-counter medications without checking with physician
Ensure that patient and/or significant other demonstrates methods of postural drainage

Evaluation

Patient maintains adequate gas exchange as evidenced by
    Usual mental status
    Usual skin color
    Blood gases within acceptable range
Patient maintains an effective breathing pattern as evidenced by
    Normal rate, rhythm, and depth of respirations
    Clear lungs
    Decreased dyspnea
    Blood gases within normal range
Patient experiences decreased pain as evidenced by
    Verbalization of pain relief
    Relaxed facial expression and body movements
    Improved breathing pattern
    Effective cough
Infection is minimized as evidenced by
    Normal temperature
    Negative culture following medication regimen
Patient demonstrates knowledge of self-care management principles as evidenced by verbalization of those principles indicating understanding of disease process, compliance with treatment regimen, and isolation procedures as necessary

PULMONARY EDEMA

Abnormal accumulation of fluid in the alveoli due to an increase in pulmonary microvascular pressure, usually a result of abnormal cardiac function

Assessment

Observations/findings

Bounding pulse
Engorged peripheral veins
Hoarseness
Apprehension
Restlessness
Respiratory distress
    Orthopnea
    Tachypnea: shallow, moist respirations
    Crackles: in dependent parts of lung initially, extending progressively upward
Cough: pink, frothy sputum
Tachycardia: thready pulse
Elevated BP
Jugular venous distention
Pallor
Cyanosis
Diaphoresis
Edema of extremities
Acid-base disorder
    Decreased pH
    Elevated $PaCO_2$
See Cardiovascular Assessment (p. 67)

Laboratory/diagnostic studies

Arterial blood gases: hypoxemia and hypocapnea
Chest x-ray examination
    Bilateral interstitial and alveolar infiltrates
    Kerley's lines are common
ECG
Pulmonary capillary pressure
    Left atrial pressure (LAP):
        14 to 20 mm Hg—mild
        25 to 30 mm Hg—moderate to severe
Protein concentration of edema fluid

Potential complications

Arrhythmias
Heart failure
Respiratory/cardiac arrest

Medical management

O_2 therapy
Parenteral therapy
Intake and output

Hemodynamic monitoring
Cardiac monitor
Rotating tourniquets and/or phlebotomy may be used
Medications
    Morphine
    Diuretics
    Cardiotonics
    Bronchodilators
Mechanical ventilatory support

Nursing diagnoses/goals/interventions

ndx: Impaired gas exchange related to alveolar-capillary membrane changes

GOAL: *Patient will have adequate gas exchange*

Elevate head of bed 60 to 90 degrees with lower extremities dependent
Administer medications as ordered
Administer oxygen therapy as ordered
Administer IPPB as ordered (p. 280)
Check BP, R, and apical pulse qh and prn
Check rectal temperature q4h
Assist and teach patient to cough and deep breathe qh and prn
Auscultate chest for breath sounds qh
Maintain bed rest during acute phase

ndx: Alteration in comfort related to pain and effort of breathing

GOAL: *Patient will verbalize relief of pain*

Manage pain with morphine sulfate as ordered; assess effectiveness of pain relief measure(s)
Monitor for potential effect of pain medications on respiratory function
Assist and teach patient energy conservation techniques as tolerated
Encourage use of incentive spirometer and other breathing exercises

ndx: Anxiety related to difficulty in breathing

GOAL: *Patient will demonstrate reduced anxiety*

Provide emotional support
    Remain with patient
    Create a nonstressful environment
    Explain procedures and treatments thoroughly
    Use short, simple sentences
    Use calm, reassuring voice
    Ensure quiet environment
Plan rest periods

ndx: Knowledge deficit regarding disease process

GOAL: *Patient and/or significant other will demonstrate understanding of home care and follow-up instructions through interactive discussion and actual return demonstration*

Explain need to exercise to tolerance
    Avoid strenuous exercise
    Plan frequent rest periods
Explain need to maintain a low-sodium diet as ordered
Explain importance of avoiding constipation
Explain importance of not smoking
Explain need to avoid persons with URIs
Explain importance of ongoing outpatient care
Discuss symptoms to report to physician
    Sudden weight increase
    Decreased urinary output
    Swollen feet and ankles
    Chest pain
    Difficulty in breathing
    Persistent cough
    Discuss medications: name, dosage, time of administration, purpose, and side effects

Evaluation

Patient
    Has adequate gas exchange as evidenced by
        Demonstrated effortless breathing
        Usual mental status
        Usual skin color
        Blood gases within normal range
        Ability to perform self-care activities without signs of SOB
        Increased activities
        Frequent use of incentive spirometer without evidence of discomfort
    Demonstrates decreased anxiety as evidenced by
        Verbalized reduced anxiety
        Demonstrated understanding of treatment
        Decreased use of tranquilizers and/or pain medication
        Vital signs within normal limits
    Demonstrates knowledge of self-care management as evidenced by
        Verbalized principles of home management
        Demonstrated understanding of disease process
        Stated symptoms to report to physician
        Ability to name medications with purpose, dose, and times
    Demonstrates relief from pain as evidenced by
        Effortless breathing
        Decreased use of pain medication

PULMONARY EMBOLISM

Occurs when the pulmonary artery or one of its branches is partially or completely occluded; damage to the lung depends on the number of clots and the extent of obstruction to pulmonary circulation

Assessment

Observations/findings

Sudden, severe substernal pain
Shortness of breath
Diaphoresis
Cyanosis, pallor
Faintness
Tachypnea
Tachycardia
Elevated temperature
Hypotension
Anxiety, sense of doom
Hemoptysis (rare)
Cough
Distended neck veins
Breath sounds
   Decreased
   Wheezing
   Crackles
Weakness

Laboratory/diagnostic studies

Chest x-ray examination
   Elevated diaphragms
   Atelectasis
   Hyperlucent lung fields
   Small pleural effusion
   Interstitual infiltrates
Arterial blood gases
   Decreased PaO_2
   Decreased $PaCO_2$
ECG
   Right axis deviation
   Incomplete right bundle branch block (BBB)
Ventilation/perfusion scan
Pulmonary angiogram
Elevated LDH, elevated bilirubin
Fibrin split products/fibrin degradation tests
Prothrombin time (PT), partial thromoplastin time (PTT)

Potential complications

Extended/recurrent pulmonary embolism
Arrhythmias
   Atrial fibrillation
   PVCs
CHF
Shock (p. 104)
Cardiopulmonary arrest

Medical management

Bed rest
Oxygen therapy
Cardiac monitor
Medication
   Heparin
   Coumadin
   Streptokinase
   Vasopressors
   Analgesics/sedatives
Parenteral fluids
Nutritional support

Nursing diagnoses/goals/interventions

ndx: Impaired gas exchange related to ventilation/perfusion abnormalities

GOAL: *Patient will experience adequate gas exchange*

Monitor for and report signs of impaired gas exchange
Administer oxygen as ordered; intubation and assisted ventilation may be indicated
   Turn and deep breathe q2h to 4h
   Check BP, R, and apical pulse q1h to 2h and prn
   Check quality and rate of P and R q2h to 4h and prn
   Auscultate chest for breath sounds q2h to 4h
   Check arterial blood gases as ordered
   Use cardiac monitor as ordered
   Check sputum for amount, color, and character

ndx: Potential for injury: bleeding related to increased risk of bleeding from anticoagulant therapy

GOAL: *Patient will not exhibit signs of bleeding*

Check PT and clotting functions or coagulation factors daily as ordered
Observe for bleeding
   Stools
   Urine
   Sputum
Do not administer aspirin-containing products
Maintain bed rest; elevate head of bed 45 to 60 degrees as tolerated
Never gatch knee; avoid back rubs
Provide antiembolic stockings as ordered
Avoid constipation and straining; use stool softeners or mild laxatives

Administer anticoagulants as ordered
Prepare for lung scan, pulmonary angiography, and possible surgery

ndx: Anxiety related to fear of perceived and/or actual threat to biologic integrity

GOAL: *Patient will experience a reduction in anxiety/fear*

Assess verbal and nonverbal signs and symptoms of anxiety/fear
Assess usual coping skills
Provide emotional support; maintain quiet environment
Continue with acute care and decrease frequency of nursing functions as patient's condition improves

ndx: Knowledge deficit regarding health care management

GOAL: *Patient and/or significant other will demonstrate understanding of home care and follow-up instructions through interactive discussion and actual return demonstration*

Discuss methods of prevention
　Avoid sitting or standing for long periods of time
　Elevate legs while sitting
　Do not cross legs
　Use antiembolic stockings if ordered
　Perform regular exercise such as walking
Explain need to exercise to tolerance with planned rest periods
Explain need to avoid constipation and straining
Explain importance of ongoing outpatient care
Discuss symptoms to report to physician
　Sudden, sharp chest pain
　Bloody sputum
　Elevated temperature
Discuss medications: name, dosage, time of administration, purpose, and side effects
Explain need to avoid taking over-the-counter medications without checking with physician
Explain need to check for bleeding in urine, stools, and sputum if sent home on anticoagulants
Explain need to avoid persons with URIs
Explain importance of not smoking
Explain need to wear medical alert band re anticoagulants

Evaluation

Patient
　Experiences adeqaute O_2/CO_2 exchange as evidenced by
　　Usual mental status
　　Usual skin color
　　Blood gases within normal range
　Experiences no bleeding or extension of embolism as evidenced by
　　Normal clotting parameters
　　Absence of blood in stool, urine, sputum, or other sites
　　No evidence of pain
　Experiences a reduction in anxiety as evidenced by
　　Relaxed facial expression
　　Verbalization of feeling less anxious
　　Decreased use of sedatives and/or tranquilizers
　　Verbalization of an understanding of routines and treatments
　Demonstrates an understanding of home care management principles as evidenced by verbalization of management principles of the disease process

PULMONARY TUBERCULOSIS

A chronic acute or subacute infectious disease caused by the tubercle bacillus, Mycobacterium tuberculosis, most commonly affecting the alveolar structure of the lung; clinical presentation varies from asymptomatic with only a positive skin test to extensive pulmonary and systemic involvement

Assessment

Observations/findings

Elevated temperature, night sweats
Tachycardia
Anorexia
Weight loss
Malaise
Fatigue
Cough: usually mild
　Blood-streaked sputum
　Hemoptyisis
　Mucoid or mucopurulent sputum
Lymph nodes
　Inflamed
　Painful
Crackles over apex of lung
Pleuritic chest pain
Irregular menses

Laboratory/diagnostic studies

Skin testing
　PPD (5 units of purified protein derivative)
　Mantoux test: PPD or OT (old tuberculin) injected with pressure gun

Tine test: OT pressed into skin with tine unit
Gastric washings
Sputum cultures: positive for *M. tuberculosis* within 2 to 3 weeks if active
Chest x-ray examination
    Calcification, enlarged lymph nodes, and infiltrates if extension of original site has occurred
    Pleural effusion or cavitation
    CAUTION: Other lung abnormalities (pneumonia, tumors) can look like TB
Fiberoptic bronchoscopy
Needle biopsy of pleura

Potential complications

Atelectasis
Hemoptysis
Pneumothorax
Recurrence
Tuberculosis pericarditis, peritonitis, meningitis, lymphadenitis

Medical management

Chemotherapy treatment
    Isoniazid (INH)
    Ethambutal
    Rifampin
    Streptomycin
    Para-aminosalicylic acid (PAS)
    Pyrazinamide
Analgesics
High-protein, high-carbohydrate diet
Respiratory isolation as necessary
Report to Board of Health for follow-up on family and contacts

Nursing diagnoses/goals/interventions

ndx Ineffective breathing pattern related to decreased total lung capacity

GOAL: *Patient will achieve full lung expansion with adequate ventilation within limits of the disease*

Check quality and depth of respirations and record any changes
Auscultate chest for breath sounds q4h
Assist and teach patient to turn, cough, and deep breathe q2h to 4h
Provide frequent rest periods, avoid fatigue, and exercise to tolerance
Check T, P, and R q4h
Administer chemotherapy as ordered

ndx Potential for infection transmission related to noncompliance with medical regimen

GOAL: *Potential for infection transmission will be decreased*

Maintain respiratory isolation; avoid direct contact with sputum
Teach patient to cough into tissues
    To turn head with coughing
    How to dispose of tissues
    Use of mask if unable to follow directions
Collect and care for sputum cultures as ordered
Teach patient importance of not stopping antituberculosis medications until directed to do so by physician

ndx Alteration in nutrition: less than body requirements related to chronic infection

GOAL: *Optimal nutritional status will be maintained*

Obtain admission weight and monitor daily
Maintain high-protein, high-carbohydrate diet with small, frequent feedings
Administer stool softeners, laxatives, or enemas as ordered
Assess for additional causes of malnutrition (e.g., alcoholism)
Reassess nutritional status on a regular basis; consult with dietitian
Monitor percent of meals eaten
Implement measures to relieve dyspnea
Place in high-Fowler's position at meals to reduce dyspnea
Encourage rest periods prior to meals to reduce fatigue
Encourage significant others to bring in patient's favorite food
Measure intake and output

ndx Potential for noncompliance with treatment regimen related to alteration in perception and/or lack of motivation

GOAL: *Patient will follow recommended diet and medication regimen as ordered*

Evaluate patient's health belief system, including spiritual and cultural factors
Assess for evidence of noncompliant behavior (weight, alcohol, or drug abuse)
Arrange for visiting nurses or social service referral
Reeducate patient to importance of following prescribed medical regimen
    Utilize patient/nurse contract if helpful

Discuss with family or significant others possible reasons for noncompliant behavior

ndx: Knowledge deficit regarding disease process and home care management

GOAL: *Patient and/or significant other will demonstrate understanding of home care and follow-up instructions through interactive discussion and actual return demonstration*

Explain nature of disease and purpose of treatment and procedures
Explain importance of good hygiene and handwashing (coughing into tissues, use of mask if unable to follow directions, how to dispose of tissues, to turn head if coughing, and to avoid direct contact with sputum)
Explain importance of maintaining high-protein, high-carbohydrate diet; need to force fluids to 2000 to 3000 ml unless otherwise contraindicated
Explain importance of maintaining respiratory isolation until necessary medication levels are obtained
Explain importance of exercise, frequent rest periods, and avoiding fatigue
Explain importance of avoiding close contact with others until advised by physician
Explain need to avoid crowds and persons with URIs
Explain importance of ongoing outpatient care
Discuss symptoms to report to physician
  Hemoptysis
  Chest pain
  Difficulty in breathing
  Hearing loss
  Vertigo
Discuss medications: name, dosage, time of administration, purpose, and side effects
Explain need to avoid taking over-the-counter medications without checking with physician
Discuss importance of not stopping medication without physician's approval

Evaluation

Patient
  Maintains an effective breathing pattern as evidenced by
    Normal rate, rhythm, and depth of respirations
    Decreased dyspnea
    Blood gases within normal range
  Has decreased potential for transmission of disease as evidenced by failure of patient contacts to convert to positive skin test
  Maintains an adequate nutritional status as evidenced by weight remaining stable and within normal range for patient's height, age, and build
  Follows medical regimen as evidenced by
    No active infection
    Laboratory values within normal limits
    Patient's being free of infection
  Demonstrates increased level of knowledge regarding health care as evidenced by verbalization of those principles indicating understanding of health care management

SARCOIDOSIS

A multisystem disease of unknown etiology; any organ system may be involved, but pulmonary manifestations are most common; in most cases process is benign and self-limiting without residual; 10% become chronic conditions; staged according to international standards, based on chest x-ray findings; fatal in 5% of cases; most common in young adults and among blacks

Assessment
Observations/findings

Weight loss
Anorexia
Fever, night sweats
Arthralgias
Fatigue
Respiratory
  Pulmonary hypertension
  Pulmonary fibrosis
  Cor pulmonale
  Clubbing of fingers
  Dyspnea
  Cough: usually unproductive but may be incapacitating and occur in paroxysms that lead to vomiting
  Hypoxemia
  Hypercapnia
  Crackles: diffuse or just at bases
Ocular
  Uveitis (common)
  Iritis
  Glaucoma
  Cataracts
  Blindness (rare)
Cardiovascular
  Mild to severe chest pain (rare)

Palpitations
Fatigue
Arrhythmias: PVCs, bundle branch or complete heart block
Cardiomyopathy (rare)
Cutaneous
Erythema nodosum
Bone cysts in hands and feet
Nasal mucosal lesions
Alopecia
Lymphatic
Parotid and cervical lymphadenopathy
Splenomegaly

Laboratory/diagnostic studies

Kveim skin test: positive in 3 to 6 weeks
Blood work
CBC
Serum protein levels
Erythrocyte sedimentation rate (ESR): elevated
Angiotensins converting enzyme level: may be elevated
Skin and lymph node biopsy
Transbronchial biopsy via bronchoscopy
Open-lung biopsy
Bronchoalveolar lavage
Galium-67 scan
Chest x-ray examination
Abnormal in 90% of patients during course of illness
Varies from hilar lymphadenopathy to diffuse infiltrates and pulmonary fibrosis
Pulmonary function tests: spirometry may be normal or show decreased vital capacity and expiratory flow rates, as well as decreased lung compliance

Potential complications

Restrictive lung disease (pulmonary fibrosis, progressive lung disability)
Complications of steroid therapy (diabetes mellitus, fluid retention, electrolyte imbalances, infection)

Medical management

No treatment if symptoms are mild
Medications
Systemic or topical steroids
Azathioprine (Imuran) if steroids are contraindicated
Optic agents
Antiarrhythmic agents
Calcium-chelating medication if needed
Routine chest x-ray and pulmonary function monitoring
Low-calcium, low-salt, low-potassium diet
Vitamin D supplements

Nursing diagnoses/goals/interventions

ndx Impaired gas-exchange related to pulmonary fibrosis or parenchymal lesions

GOALS *Patient will maintain adequate oxygenation and ventilation status*

Assess respiratory status, observing for cough, adventitious sounds, dyspnea, and abnormal rate, rhythm, or quality
Obtain sputum specimens as ordered
Instruct patient on energy conservation techniques and breathing exercises (slow, deep breaths; pursed lip breathing)
Monitor pulmonary function results
Administer medications and oxygen as ordered

ndx Potential alteration in cardiac output related to arrhythmias

GOAL *Patient will have normal cardiac output without signs of cardiac arrhythmias*

Maintain bed rest
Monitor cardiac activity as indicated
Monitor vital signs q2h to 4h and prn
Monitor signs and symptoms of decreased cardiac output, including edema, dyspnea, hypotension, crackles, jugular venous distention, decreased urine output, increased heart rate, cool, clammy skin, and fatigue
Administer oxygen as ordered
Report abnormal ECG, hemodynamic, and laboratory findings
Assess heart and breath sounds q2h to 4h
Administer medications as ordered

ndx Alteration in comfort: pain related to disease-induced arthralgias and ocular discomfort

GOAL: *Patient will verbalize absence of pain*

Assess pain, location, onset, duration, and precipitating and alleviating factors
Administer analgesics as ordered
Provide comfort measures as needed
Positioning
Warm compresses
Rest

ndx: Knowledge deficit regarding home care needs

GOAL: *Patient and/or significant other will demonstrate understanding of home care and follow-up instructions through interactive discussion*

Explain the nature of disease: even if symptoms are mild, will require ongoing evaluation and care
   Routine chest x-ray examinations
   Pulmonary function tests
   Yearly eye examination
Explain need to avoid
   Strenuous exercise
   Lengthy exposure to sun
   Smoking: recommend support group prn
   Persons who smoke
Explain need to restrict salt, foods high in potassium, and vitamin D supplements; to restrict calcium intake if necessary
Discuss symptoms to report to physician
   Shortness of breath
   Red, watery eyes
   Dizziness
   Chest pain
   Swollen joints
   Unusual fatigue
Discuss medications: name, dosage, time of administration, purpose, and side effects of corticosteroid therapy
Take antacid with dose
Watch for signs of infection
Be aware of mood swings
Avoid taking over-the-counter medications without checking with physician

Evaluation
Patient
   Maintains adequate gas exchange as evidenced by
     Usual mental status
     Usual skin color
     Blood gases within normal range
   Maintains normal cardiac output as evidenced by
     Blood pressure within normal range
     Unlabored respiration
     Usual mental status
     Usual skin color
     Normal urine output
   Experiences decreased pain as evidenced by
     Verbalization of pain relief
     Relaxed facial expression and body positioning
     Improved breathing pattern
     Increased activity
   Demonstrates knowledge of home care activities as evidenced by verbalization of principles of self-care management

PNEUMOTHORAX

Collection of air or gas in the pleural space, causing the lung to collapse; may be partial or total collapse; can be the result of an open chest wound that permits entry of air, or from the rupture of a bleb or bullae on the surface of the lung; or it may occur spontaneously without obvious cause

Assessment
Observations/findings

Sudden, sharp chest pain
Anxiety
Dyspnea
Tachypnea
Absent or decreased breath sounds on affected side
Hyperresonance over affected thoracic space
Asymmetric chest movements
Pleural pain
Diaphoresis
Elevated temperature
Tachycardia with weak pulse
Vertigo
Pallor
Cyanosis
Hypotension
Mediastinal shift

Laboratory/diagnostic studies

Chest x-ray examination
   Unequal lung expansion
   Mediastinal shift to affected side
Arterial blood gases
   Decreased PaO_2

Potential complications

Respiratory failure
Infection
Cardiac arrest

Medical management
Oxygen therapy
Analgesics
Chest tube insertion

Nursing diagnoses/goals/interventions
ndx: Ineffective breathing pattern related to inadequate chest expansion

GOAL: *Patient will demonstrate an effective breathing pattern*

Remain with patient and have another person notify physician
Reassure and try to calm patient
Teach patient to suppress cough
Place patient in a sitting position, with head of bed elevated 60 to 90 degrees
Administer oxygen per nasal cannula at 2 to 6 L/min as ordered unless contraindicated
Assist with insertion of chest tube
See Chest Tubes (p. 271)
Administer oxygen and IPPB as ordered
Check BP, T, R, and apical pulse q2h to 4h
Auscultate chest for breath sounds q2h to 4h
Assist and teach patient to
   Turn and deep breathe q2h to 4h: diaphragmatic, segmental breathing
   Encourage use of incentive spirometer (p. 281)
   Perform passive and active ROM exercises to extremities q4h
   Avoid stretching, reaching, or sudden movements
Continue with acute care and decrease frequency of nursing functions as patient's condition improves
Care for chest puncture site as needed after removal of chest tube
Assist and teach patient to ambulate when ordered
Increase activity as tolerated
Maintain planned rest periods to avoid fatigue

ndx: Impaired gas exchange related to decreased lung capacity

GOAL: *Patient will maintain arterial blood gas values within an acceptable range*

Monitor ABG results
Observe for signs of increased work of breathing
Observe for unequal lung expansion
Observe for signs and symptoms of hypoxemia
Administer supplemental oxygen as ordered
Monitor function of chest tube

ndx: Alteration in comfort related to biologic, (tissue trauma) and physical factors (chest tube insertion)

GOAL: *Patient will verbalize relief from pain*

Assess for presence of pain (verbal and nonverbal)
Administer analgesic as prescribed
Assess effectiveness of pain relief measures
Premedicate patient prior to breathing/coughing exercises
Instruct patient on splinting techniques
Secure chest tubes to limit movement and resulting irritation

ndx: Knowledge deficit regarding self-care management

GOAL: *Patient and/or significant other will demonstrate understanding of home care and follow-up instructions through interactive discussion and actual return demonstration*

Explain importance of maintaining diet as ordered; need to force fluids to 2000 to 3000 ml daily unless contraindicated
Explain need to exercise to tolerance; to avoid fatigue and plan rest periods
Explain importance of avoiding strenuous activity or exercise, especially contact sports
Explain importance of not smoking
Explain need to avoid persons with infections, especially URIs
Explain importance of ongoing outpatient care
Discuss symptoms to report to physician
   Cold
   Sore throat
   Flu
   Elevated temperature
   Cough
   Sudden, sharp chest pain
   Difficulty in breathing
   Any redness, pain, swelling, or tenderness of puncture wound
Discuss medications: name, dosage, time of administration, purpose, and side effects
Explain need to avoid taking over-the-counter medications without checking with physician
Ensure that patient and/or significant other demonstrates care of chest puncture wound

Evaluation

Patient
   Maintains an effective breathing pattern as evidenced by
      Normal rate, rhythm, and depth of respirations
      Decreased dyspnea
      Blood gases within normal range
   Maintains adequate gas exchange as evidenced by
      Usual mental status
      Usual skin color
      Blood gases within normal range
   Experiences decreased pain as evidenced by
      Verbalization of pain relief

Relaxed facial expression and body positioning
Improved breathing pattern
Increased activity
Demonstrates increased level of knowledge regarding health care as evidenced by verbalization of those principles indicating understanding of health care management

TENSION PNEUMOTHORAX

An opening through the pleura that allows air to pass into the pleura but not out; this produces a shift in the affected lung and mediastinum toward the unaffected side (Tension pneumothorax is a medical emergency.)

Assessment
Observations/findings

Respiratory distress
   Increases
   Sudden
   Severe
Use of accessory muscles of respiration
Tachypnea
Chest pain
Anxiety
Tachycardia
Cyanosis
Bulging sternum
Tracheal shift: toward unaffected side
Breath sounds
   Absent (affected side)
   Diminished (unaffected side)
   Crepitus

Laboratory/diagnostic studies

Chest x-ray examination: mediastinal or tracheal shift to unaffected side
Arterial blood gases
   Decreased PaO_2

Potential complications

Respiratory or cardiac arrest
Infection

Medical management

Chest tube insertion
Oxygen therapy
Analgesics

Nursing diagnoses/goals/interventions

ndx: Impaired gas exchange related to decrease lung capacity

GOAL: *Patient will maintain adequate gas exchange*

Notify physician immediately
Remain with patient
Maintain patent airway
Use mechanical ventilation as necessary
Administer oxygen, 2 to 6 L/min, as ordered
Initiate IV: maintain patent vein
Have emergency equipment available
   Emergency cart
   Intubation tray
   Chest tubes and water seal drainage system
Check BP, R, and apical pulse q5 to 10 min
Place patient on cardiac monitor
Prepare for insertion of chest tubes
Assist physician with insertion of chest tubes (p. 271)
Initiate resuscitative measures if necessary

ndx: Alteration in comfort related to biologic (tissue trauma) and physical factors (chest tube insertion)

GOAL: *Patient will verbalize relief from pain*

Assess for presence of pain (verbal and nonverbal)
Administer analgesic as prescribed
Assess effectiveness of pain relief measures
Premedicate patient prior to breathing/coughing exercises
Instruct patient on splinting techniques
Secure chest tubes to limit movement and resulting irritation

ndx: Knowledge deficit regarding self-care management

GOAL: *Patient and/or significant other will demonstrate understanding of home care and follow-up instructions through interactive discussion and actual return demonstration*

Explain importance of maintaining diet as ordered; need to force fluids to 2000 to 3000 ml daily unless contraindicated
Explain need to exercise to tolerance; to avoid fatigue and plan rest periods
Explain importance of avoiding strenuous activity or exercise, especially contact sports
Explain importance of not smoking
Explain need to avoid persons with infections, especially URIs
Explain importance of ongoing outpatient care
Discuss symptoms to report to physician
   Cold
   Sore throat
   Flu

Elevated temperature
Cough
Sudden, sharp chest pain
Difficulty in breathing
Any redness, pain, swelling, or tenderness of puncture wound

Discuss medications: name, dosage, time of administration, purpose, and side effects

Explain need to avoid taking over-the-counter medications without checking with physician

Ensure that patient and/or significant other demonstrates care of chest puncture wound

Evaluation

Patient
- Maintains adequate gas exchange as evidenced by
  - Usual mental status
  - Usual skin color
  - Blood gases within normal range
- Experiences decreased pain as evidenced by
  - Verbalization of pain relief
  - Relaxed facial expression and body positioning
  - Improved breathing pattern
  - Increased activity
- Demonstrates increased level of knowledge regarding health care as evidenced by verbalization of those principles indicating understanding of health care management

HEMOTHORAX

Accumulation of blood in the pleural space, causing the lung to partially or totally collapse; often a complication of chest trauma and can occur after chest surgery

Assessment

Observations/findings

Difficulty in breathing
Hyperresonance on percussion
Distant to absent breath sounds on affected side
Asymmetric chest movements
Elevated temperature
Tachypnea
Tachycardia
Anxiety
Restlessness
Pain
Shock if blood loss is significant

Laboratory/diagnostic studies

Chest x-ray examination
Arterial blood gases
CBC

Potential complications

Respiratory failure
Shock from hemorrhage
Infection
Hypotension
Tension pneumothorax

Medical management

Thoracentesis
Chest tube
Analgesics
IV replacement of fluid/blood
Oxygen therapy

Nursing diagnoses/goals/interventions

ndx: Ineffective breathing pattern related to inadequate chest expansion

GOAL: *Patient will demonstrate an effective breathing pattern*

Check BP, T, P, and R q2h to 4h
Auscultate chest for breath sounds q2h to 4h
Assist and teach patient to
  Turn, cough, and deep breathe q2h to 4h
  Perform active ROM exercises to extremities q4h
  Avoid stretching, reaching, or sudden movements
Administer oxygen or IPPB as ordered
Position patient comfortably; elevate head of bed 45 to 60 degrees
Assist with chest tube insertion (p. 271)
Continue with acute care and decreased frequency of nursing functions as patient's condition improves
Assist and teach patient to ambulate as tolerated
Maintain planned rest periods to avoid fatigue
Care for chest puncture site as needed after removal of chest tube

ndx: Impaired gas exchange related to decreased lung capacity

GOAL: *Patient will maintain arterial blood gas values within an acceptable range*

Monitor ABG results
Observe for signs of increased work of breathing
Observe for unequal lung expansion
Observe for signs and symptoms of hypoxemia
Administer supplemental oxygen as ordered
Monitor function of chest tube

ndx: Alteration in comfort related to biologic (tissue trauma) and physical (chest tube insertion) factors

GOAL: *Patient will verbalize relief from pain*

Assess for presence of pain
Premedicate patient prior to increased activity (coughing exercises)
Instruct patient on splinting techniques
Secure chest tubes to limit movement and subsequent irritation
Manage pain as indicated; avoid use of respiratory depressants; assess effectiveness of pain relief measure(s)

ndx: Knowledge deficit regarding self-care maintenance

GOAL: *Patient and/or significant other will demonstrate understanding of home care and follow-up instructions through interactive discussion and actual return demonstration*

Explain importance of maintaining diet as ordered; need to force fluids to 2000 to 3000 ml daily unless contraindicated
Explain need to exercise to tolerance; to avoid fatigue and plan rest periods
Explain importance of not smoking
Explain need to avoid persons with infections, especially URIs
Explain importance of ongoing outpatient care
Discuss symptoms to report to physician
  Elevated temperature
  Cold
  Flu
  Cough
  Sudden, sharp chest pain
  Difficulty in breathing
  Any redness, pain, swelling, or drainage from chest puncture wound
Discuss medications: name, dosage, time of administration, purpose, and side effects
Explain need to avoid taking over-the-counter medications without checking with physician
Ensure that patient and/or significant other demonstrates care of chest puncture wound

Evaluation

Patient
  Demonstrates effective breathing pattern as evidenced by
    Normal respiratory rate and depth
    Arterial blood gas measurements within acceptable range
    Bilateral chest expansion
  Maintains adequate gas exchange as evidenced by
    Usual mental status
    Usual skin color
    Blood gases within normal range
  Demonstrates relief from pain as evidenced by
    Verbalization of less pain
    Decreased use of analgesics
    Increased ambulation and movement
  Demonstrates knowledge and skills of self-care management as evidenced by verbalization of principles of self-care management

THORACIC EMPYEMA

Pus in the pleural cavity due to underlying infections of the lung such as pneumonia or lung abscess, following thoracic surgery, or from penetrating chest wounds

Assessment
Observations/findings

Difficulty in breathing
Orthopnea: mild to severe
Localized chest pain
  Constant
  Only during inspiration
Asymmetric chest expansion
Decreased or absent breath sounds over affected area
Productive cough
Malaise
Fatigue
Elevated temperature
Tachycardia
Tachypnea
Weight loss
Anorexia

Laboratory/diagnostic studies

Chest x-ray examination
Thoracentesis
Fluid cell count/differential
Cytologic examination of fluid

Potential complications

Pneumothorax
Pneumonia
Bronchopleural fistula

Medical management

Chest tube insertion
Thoracentesis
Thoracotomy if necessary
High-protein, high-carbohydrate diet
O_2 therapy as necessary

Medications
   Antibiotics
   Antipyretics
   Analgesics
Fluid management

Nursing diagnoses/goals/interventions

ndx: Ineffective breathing pattern related to decreased lung expansion secondary to pus in the pleural space

GOAL: *Patient will demonstrate an effective breathing pattern*

Reassure and try to calm patient
Place patient in a sitting position, with head of bed elevated 60 to 90 degrees
Administer oxygen per nasal cannula at 2 to 6 L/min as ordered unless contraindicated
Assist with insertion of chest tube (p. 271)
Administer oxygen and IPPB as ordered
Check BP, T, R, and apical pulse q2h to 4h
Auscultate chest for breath sounds q2h to 4h
Assist and teach patient to
   Turn and deep breathe q2h to 4h: diaphragmatic, segmental breathing
   Encourage use of incentive spirometer (p. 281)
   Perform passive and active ROM exercises to extremities q4h
   Avoid stretching, reaching, or sudden movements
   Order chest x-ray examination as indicated by physician

ndx: Alteration in comfort related to biologic (tissue trauma) and physical (chest tube insertion) factors

GOAL: *Patient will verbalize relief from pain*

Assess for presence of pain (verbal and nonverbal)
Administer analgesic as prescribed
Assess effectiveness of pain relief measures
Premedicate patient prior to breathing/coughing exercises
Instruct patient on splinting techniques
Secure chest tubes to limit movement and resulting irritation

ndx: Knowledge deficit regarding disease process and self-care management

GOAL: *Patient and/or significant other will demonstrate understanding of home care and follow-up instructions through interactive discussion and actual return demonstration*

Explain need to exercise to tolerance
   Plan rest periods
   Avoid fatigue
Explain importance of ongoing outpatient care
Discuss symptoms to report to physician
   Difficulty in breathing
   Chest pain
   Elevated temperature
   Persistent cough
Explain importance of avoiding persons with URIs
Discuss symptoms of a cold or flu to report to physician
Explain importance of influenza vaccination as ordered
Discuss medications: name, dosage, time of administration, purpose, and side effects
Explain need to avoid taking over-the-counter medications without checking with physician

Evaluation

Patient
   Maintains an effective breathing pattern as evidenced by
      Normal rate, rhythm, and depth of respirations
      Decreased dyspnea
      Blood gases within normal range
   Experiences decreased pain as evidenced by
      Verbalization of pain relief
      Relaxed facial expression and body positioning
      Improved breathing pattern
      Increased activity
   Demonstrates increased level of knowledge regarding health care as evidenced by verbalization of those principles indicating understanding of health care management

ATELECTASIS

Collapse of alveoli or airless condition of the lung caused by mucous plugs, excessive secretions, compression, or shallow breathing

Assessment

Observations/findings

Elevated temperature
Absent or decreased breath sounds over affected area
Tachypnea
Tachycardia
Shortness of breath
Anxiety
Restlessness
Pleuritic pain
Cyanosis

Egophony and bronchophony with auscultation
Asymmetric chest movement on inspiration

Laboratory/diagnostic studies

Arterial blood gases
    Decreased PaO_2
    Elevated PCO_2
Chest x-ray examination
    Elevated diaphragm on affected side
    Shift of trachea to affected side if large area is atelectatic

Potential complications

Pneumonia
Pneumothorax

Medical management

Oxygen therapy as needed
Chest physiotherapy
IPPB/incentive spirometry
Bronchoscopy
Nutritional support
Fluid management

Nursing diagnoses/goals/interventions

ndx: Ineffective breathing pattern related to inactivity and/or failure of deep breathing instructions

GOAL: *Patient will maintain an effective breathing pattern*

Assist and teach patient to turn, cough, and deep breathe q1h to 2h and prn
Ambulate patient as soon as possible
Auscultate chest for breath sounds q2h to 4h
    Check quality and rate of respirations
    Note area of lung without breath sounds
Assist and teach patient to perform postural drainage qid and prn; clapping may be ordered
Perform nasotracheal suction as ordered
Administer nebulization as ordered
Administer oxygen and/or IPPB as ordered
Assist and teach patient to use incentive spirometer as ordered
Check BP, T, and apical pulse q4h
Check arterial blood gases as ordered
Administer medications as ordered
    Antibiotics
    Antipyretics
    Analgesics
    Avoid respiratory depressants

Prepare for chest x-ray examination and/or bronchoscopy

ndx: Knowledge deficit regarding disease process and health care management

GOAL: *Patient and/or significant other will demonstrate understanding of home care and follow up instructions through interactive discussion and actual return demonstration*

Explain need to avoid persons with infections, especially URIs
Explain importance of not smoking
Explain importance of ongoing outpatient care
Discuss symptoms to report to physician
    URI
    Flu
    Difficulty in breathing
    Persistent cough
    Elevated temperature
Explain importance of exercising to tolerance; need to avoid fatigue and plan rest periods
Discuss medications: name, dosage, time of administration, purpose, and side effects
Explain need to avoid taking over-the-counter medications without checking with physician

Evaluation

Patient
    Maintains an effective breathing pattern as evidenced by
        Normal rate, rhythm, and depth of respirations
        Blood gases within acceptable range
    Demonstrates understanding of health care management of disease process as evidenced by
        Use of incentive spirometer as ordered
        Ambulation as directed by health team
        Verbalization of principles of health care management

PLEURAL EFFUSION

Abnormal amount of fluid in the pleural space; may be caused by numerous conditions such as congestive heart failure, pneumonia, pulmonary embolism, carcinoma of the breast, and renal diseases

Assessment

Observations/findings

Related to underlying disease and may be asymptomatic if effusion is small

Shortness of breath
Respiratory difficulty
Diminished or absent breath sounds over affected area
Pleural friction rub
Localized chest pain
Asymmetric chest expansion
Elevated temperature
Fatigue
Cough

Laboratory/diagnostic studies

Chest x-ray examination
    Blunting of costophrenic angle
    Partially obscured diaphragm
    Complete "white out" of involved side in large effusions
    Thoracentesis
    Pleural biopsy
    Cytologic examination of fluid

Potential complications

Pneumothorax
Pneumonia

Medical management

Bed rest
Chest tube insertion (p. 271)
Medications
    Antibiotics
    Antipyretics
    Analgesics
High-protein, high-carbohydrate diet
Fluid management
Oxygen therapy as needed
Nitrogen mustard installation or tetracycline via chest tube

Nursing diagnoses/goals/interventions

***ndx*:** Ineffective breathing pattern related to decreased lung expansion secondary to fluid accumulation in the pleural space

GOAL: *Patient will maintain an effective breathing pattern*

Provide oxygen therapy as ordered
Maintain bed rest; assist patient in assuming position of comfort
See Thoracentesis (p. 225) and/or Chest Tubes (p. 271) if ordered
Check BP, T, P, and R q4h and prn
Auscultate chest for breath sounds q2h to 4h
Administer medications as ordered
    Antibiotics
    Antipyretics
    Analgesics
Manage pain as indicated; assess effectiveness of pain relief measure(s)
Assist and teach patient to
    Turn, cough, and deep breathe q2h to 4h
    Encourage incentive breathing
    Splint chest when coughing
    Perform active ROM exercise to all extremities q2h to 4h
    Increase activity as tolerated
    Prepare patient for x-ray examination

***ndx*:** Knowledge deficit regarding disease process

GOAL: *Patient and/or significant other will demonstrate understanding of home care and follow-up instructions through interactive discussion and actual return demonstration*

Explain need to exercise to tolerance
    Plan rest periods
    Avoid fatigue
Explain importance of ongoing outpatient care
Discuss symptoms to report to physician
    Difficulty in breathing
    Chest pain
    Elevated temperature
    Persistent cough
Explain importance of avoiding persons with URIs
Discuss symptoms of a cold or flu to report to physician
Explain importance of influenza vaccination as ordered
Discuss medications: name, dosage, time of administration, purpose, and side effects
Explain need to avoid taking over-the-counter medications without checking with physician

Evaluation

Patient
    Maintains an effective breathing pattern as evidenced by
        Normal rate, rhythm, and depth of respirations
        Decreased dyspnea
        Blood gases within normal range
        Afebrile
    Demonstrates understanding of disease process and principles of self-care management as evidenced by verbalization of those principles that indicate understanding of self-care management

FLAIL CHEST

Chest cage abnormality usually due to crushing chest injury where multiple fractures of ribs have occurred

Assessment

Observations/findings

Sharp chest pain
Difficulty in breathing
Respirations
    Shallow
    Paradoxical chest wall movement
    Splinting
Tachypnea
Tachycardia
Cyanosis
Decreased breath sounds
Mediastinal and tracheal shift
Sputum
    Copious
    Blood tinged
Pain

Laboratory/diagnostic studies

Chest x-ray examination
    Atelectasis
    Pneumothorax
    Evidence of fractured ribs
Arterial blood gases
    Decreased PaO_2
    Increased $PaCO_2$
Pulmonary function tests: decreased lung volumes

Potential complications

Tension pneumothorax
Hemothorax
Pulmonary edema
Cardiac tamponade
Respiratory arrest
Shock

Medical management

O_2 therapy
Chest tube insertion
Intubation and mechanical ventilation
Medications
    Pavulon
    Curare
    Antibiotics
    Pain management

Nursing diagnoses/goals/interventions

ndx: Potential for ineffective breathing pattern related to unstable chest wall movement

GOAL: *Patient will maintain an effective breathing pattern*

Maintain bed rest; assist patient in assuming position of comfort; do not turn patient onto flailed side
Understand that endotracheal tube (p. 273) or tracheostomy (p. 275) may be ordered
Place on continuous mechanical ventilation (p. 277) as ordered
    Positive pressure ventilator
    Volume-cycled ventilator
    Respirations may be controlled by ventilator
Understand that chest tubes may be ordered (p. 271)
Check BP, P, and R q1h to 2h and prn
Auscultate chest for breath sounds q1h to 2h and prn
Report decreased or absent breath sounds to physician
Perform oropharyngeal suctioning prn
Check arterial blood gases as ordered
Turn and reposition patient q2h and 4h and prn
Maintain body alignment
Assist and teach patient to deep breathe q2h and 4h and prn in absence of tracheostomy or endotracheal tube; do not splint chest manually when deep breathing
Continue acute care management but decrease frequency of nursing functions as patient's condition improves
Administer IPPB with humidification as ordered
Assist and teach patient to use incentive spirometer as ordered

ndx: Alterations in comfort related to chest trauma and presence of chest tubes and ventilator

GOAL: *Patient will experience decreased pain*

Assess for verbal and nonverbal signs of pain
Manage pain as indicated; assess effectiveness of pain relief measure(s)
Prepare for possible intercostal nerve block
Establish means of communication of pain
    Call bell within reach
    Pad and pencil or Magic Slate
Explain all procedures thoroughly, using calm, reassuring voice

ndx: Knowledge deficit regarding health care management

GOAL: *Patient and/or significant other will demonstrate understanding of home care and follow-up instructions through interactive discussion and actual return demonstration*

Explain importance of exercising to tolerance; avoid fatigue periods
Explain need to avoid persons with infections, especially URIs
Explain importance of ongoing outpatient care
Discuss symptoms to report to physician
    URI
    Shortness of breath
    Persistent cough
    Persistent chest pain
Discuss medications: name, dosage, times of administration, purpose, and side effects
Explain need to avoid taking over-the-counter medications without checking with physician

Evaluation

Patient
    Maintains an effective breathing pattern as evidenced by
        Normal rate, rhythm, and depth of respirations
        Decreased dyspnea
        Blood gases within normal range
    Experiences decreased pain as evidenced by
        Verbalization of pain relief
        Relaxed facial expression and body positioning
        Improved breathing pattern
        Increased activity
    Demonstrates knowledge and skill in self-care management as evidenced by verbalization of principles required for self-care management

RESPIRATORY FAILURE

Inability of the respiratory system to maintain normal oxygenation of blood (hypoxic failure) and/or elimination of carbon dioxide (hypoventilatory failure) due to problems with ventilation, diffusion, and/or perfusion; may be chronic or acute

Assessment

Observations/findings

Respiratory distress
    Nasal flaring
    Tachypnea or bradypnea
    Retractions
    Use of accessory muscles of respiration
    Diminishing chest wall movement
    Labored breathing
    Air hunger
    Diaphoresis
Altered level of consciousness
    Anxiety
    Restlessness
    Confusion
Headache
Pallor
Cyanosis
Diaphoresis
Anorexia
Impaired motor function; asterixis
Hypotension
Tachycardia or bradycardia
Anorexia
Breath sounds
    Crackles
    Rhonchi
    Wheeze
    Decreased
Respiratory secretions
    Increased
    Purulent
Bronchospasm
Arrhythmias
    Atrial
    Ventricular
CHF (p. 101)
Decreased cardiac output
    Restlessness
    Lethargy
    Tachycardia
    Decreased urinary output
    Shock (p. 104)
    Respiratory arrest
    See Cardiovascular Assessment (p. 67)

Laboratory/diagnostic studies

Arterial blood gases
    Hypoxemia
    Acidosis
    Increased or decreased CO_2, depending on stage of failure
Pulmonary function
    Decreased VC
    Decreased tidal volume
    Decreased minute volume
Hemodynamic findings: increased pulmonary artery/wedge pressures

Chest x-ray examination: depends on underlying cause of failure
ECG
  May show evidence of right-sided heart strain
  Arrhythmias

Potential complications

Cardiac failure
Infection
  Bronchopulmonary
  Systemic
Barotrauma

Medical management

Oxygen therapy
Mechanical ventilatory support/IPPB treatment
Chest physiotherapy
Hemodynamic/cardiac monitoring
Parenteral therapy
Medications
  Antibiotics
  Bronchodilators
  Steroids
  Cardiotonics
Nutritional support as needed

Nursing diagnoses/goals/interventions

ndx: Ineffective breathing pattern related to decreased lung expansion

GOAL: *Patient will demonstrate an effective breathing pattern*

Be aware that endotracheal tube (p. 273) or tracheostomy (p. 275) may be inserted if $PaCO_2$ is over 50 mm Hg or PaO_2 is less than 60 mm Hg
Administer oxygen with assisted ventilation and humidification as ordered
Monitor arterial blood gases as ordered
  Record on flow sheet
  Report $PaCO_2$ of 50 mm Hg or above or PaO_2 of 60 mm Hg or below to physician
Prepare mechanical ventilator as ordered
Be aware that continuous mechanical ventilation (p. 277) may be necessary if pH is 7.25 or less, $PaCO_2$ is over 60 mm Hg, $PaCO_2$ increases at a rate of 5 mm Hg or more per hour, $PaCO_2$ cannot be maintained at 60 mm Hg or higher, or if patient is unable to cooperate with treatment regimen
Check BP, P, apical pulse, and level of consciousness qh and prn
  Report changes in level of consciousness to physician

Auscultate chest for breath sounds qh
Maintain bed rest with head of bed elevated 30 to 45 degrees
Remain with patient if respiratory distress is acute
Initiate resuscitative measures if necessary

ndx: Ineffective airway clearance related to obstructed airway and poor ventilation secondary to retention of secretions

GOAL: *Patient will achieve airway patency*

Assist and teach patient to turn, cough, and deep breathe if crackles or rhonchi are auscultated
Encourage use of incentive spirometry (p. 281)
Instruct patient in effective coughing techniques
Assist and teach patient to perform postural drainage as ordered
Provide humidity as ordered
Maintain adequate fluid intake
Suction (p. 225) patient if necessary
  Use sterile technique
  Hyperoxygenate and/or hyperinflate patient's lungs for four or five breaths prior to and following procedure
  Observe cardiac monitor for arrhythmias during procedure
Report diminished or absent breath sounds to physician
Monitor and record amount, consistency, and color of sputum
Administer medications as ordered
  Antibiotics
  Bronchodilators
  Mucolytic agents
  Steroids

ndx: Impaired gas exchange related to chronic tissue hypoxia

GOAL: *Patient will demonstrate arterial blood gas values within acceptable parameters*

Observe for signs and symptoms of hypoxia and hypercapnia
Monitor arterial blood gases as ordered
Record on flow sheet
Report $PaCO_2$ of 50 mm Hg or above or PaO_2 of 60 mm Hg or below to physician
Administer oxygen with assisted ventilation and humidification as ordered
Check BP, P, apical pulse, and level of consciousness qh and prn; report changes in level of consciousness to physician

Auscultate chest for breath sounds qh
Maintain adequate ventilation
Monitor cardiac rhythm
Monitor hemodynamics, pulmonary artery pressure (PAP), and pulmonary capillary wedge pressure (PCWP)
Suction airways as needed (p. 225)
Administer parenteral fluids as ordered
Administer drugs as ordered
- Bronchodilator
- Antibiotics
- Steroids
- Cardiotonics

Evaluate ADLs in relation to decreased oxygen demands
Prepare to assist with intubation and mechanical ventilation when indicated

ndx: Anxiety/fear related to inability to breathe effectively

GOAL: *Patient will demonstrate reduced anxiety*

Provide emotional support
Allow patient and family to verbalize questions and concerns
Explain procedures and treatments
Instruct patient on energy conservation techniques
- Pursed lip breathing
- Diaphragmatic breathing

Use calm, reassuring manner
Monitor vital signs

ndx: Knowledge deficit regarding disease process, procedures, and treatment

GOAL: *Patient and/or significant other will demonstrate understanding of home care and follow-up instructions through interactive discussion and actual return demonstration*

Encourage patient and/or family to verbalize feelings and questions
Explain disease process and discuss need for necessary equipment (oxygen, ventilators, incentive spirometers, suctioning material)
Explain all tests and procedures
Identify agencies available to assist patient
Demonstrate use of respirator if required
Emphasize importance of periodic turning, coughing, and deep breathing
Demonstrate postural drainage procedure if necessary
See standard of care for primary condition

Evaluation

Patient
- Maintains an effective breathing pattern as evidenced by
  - Normal rate, rhythm, and depth of respirations
  - Decreased dyspnea
  - Blood gases within normal range
- Maintains a patent airway as evidenced by
  - Improved breath sounds
  - Normal rate and depth of respirations
  - Absence of dyspnea
  - Absence of cyanosis
  - Blood gases within normal range
- Maintains adequate gas exchange as evidenced by
  - Usual mental status
  - Usual skin color
  - Blood gases within normal range
- Experiences a reduction in anxiety/fear as evidenced by
  - Relaxed facial expression
  - Verbalization of feeling less anxious
- Demonstrates knowledge of disease process and self-care management as evidenced by verbalization of principles of self-care management

ADULT RESPIRATORY DISTRESS SYNDROME (ARDS)

Nonspecific result of acute injury to the lung characterized by a group of symptoms that include decreased compliance of the lung, noncardiac pulmonary edema, and refractory hypoxemia (Figure 4-2); etiology is diverse and includes shock, chest trauma, aspiration, fat embolism, and massive viral pneumonia; end result is a uniform hyaline membrane development that leads to gas exchange abnormalities; mortality is 50% to 60%

Assessment
Observations/findings

Anxiety
Dyspnea
Tachypnea
Restlessness
Cough
Grunting respirations
Use of accessory muscles of respiration
Color
- Pallor
- Cyanosis

Decreased pulmonary compliance

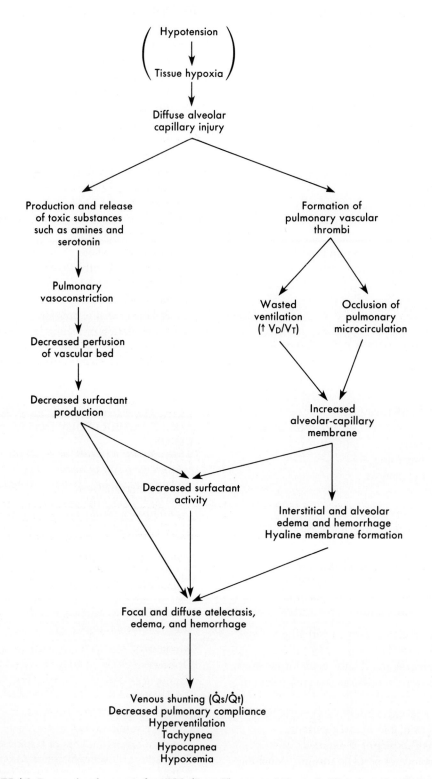

FIGURE 4-2. Proposed pathogenesis for ARDS. (From Thompson, J.M., et al.: Clinical nursing, St. Louis, 1986, The C.V. Mosby Co.)

Increased peak inspiratory pressures necessary to deliver tidal volume
Breath sounds
　Crackles
　Rhonchi
Pulmonary edema
Oxygen toxicity
CVP
　Normal
　Decreased

Laboratory/diagnostic studies

Arterial blood gases
　Decreased PaO_2
　Decreased $PaCO_2$ initially; then elevated $PaCO_2$ in later stages
CBC
Chest x-ray examination
　Diffuse pulmonary infiltrates
　"White out" on x-ray film, giving ground glass appearance
Pulmonary artery pressures (PAP, PCWP)
　Early stages: normal
　Late stage: elevated

Potential complications

Arrhythmias
Renal failure
Cardiac/respiratory arrest
Infection
Barotrauma

Medical management

Oxygen therapy
Ventilator support, intubation
Parenteral therapy
Nutritional support
Medications
　Antibiotics
　Steroids
　Heparin
　Cardiotonics
Cardiac monitor
Hemodynamic monitoring

Nursing diagnoses/goals/interventions

ndx Impaired gas exchange related to ventilation/perfusion abnormalities

GOAL: *Patient will demonstrate arterial blood gas values within an acceptable range*

See Respiratory Failure (p. 261)
See standard of care for primary condition

Place patient on volume-cycled ventilator with positive end-expiratory pressure (PEEP) or continuous positive airway pressure (CPAP) as ordered (p. 279); PEEP is contraindicated in patients with chronic obstructive pulmonary disease (COPD)
Administer oxygen as ordered by physician
Monitor arterial blood gases; report increases or decreases of PaO_2 and $PaCO_2$ to physician
Administer parenteral fluids and electrolytes as ordered by physician
Check BP, P, and R qh; assess level of consciousness qh and prn; report changes to physician
Auscultate chest for breath sounds qh and prn
　Suction patient if crackles or rhonchi are present
　Notify physician if pulmonary edema is present
　Administer corticosteroids as ordered by physician
　Administer diuretics as ordered by physician
　Measure PAP and PCWP qh
　Measure and record urinary output qh
　Turn from side to side q1h to 2h
　Maintain bed rest with head of bed elevated 30 to 45 degrees
Monitor hemodynamics (PAP, PCWP, arterial pressure) as indicated

ndx Ineffective breathing pattern related to decreased lung compliance

GOAL: *Patient will exhibit an effective breathing pattern*

Prepare mechanial ventilator as ordered
Be aware that continuous mechanical ventilation may be necessary if pH is 7.25 or less, $PaCO_2$ is over 60 mm Hg, $PaCO_2$ increases at a rate of 5 mm Hg or more per hour, $PaCO_2$ cannot be maintained at 60 mm Hg or higher, or if patient is unable to cooperate with treatment regimen
Report changes in level of consciousness to physician
Auscultate chest for breath sounds qh
　Assist and teach patient to turn, cough, and deep breathe if crackles or rhonchi are auscultated
　Suction (p. 225) patient if necessary
Limit fluid intake as ordered; titrate by CVP, PAP, or PCWP readings
　Hyperoxygenate and hyperinflate patient's lung for four or five breaths prior to and following procedure
　Observe cardiac monitor for arrhythmias during procedure
　Report diminished or absent breath sounds to physician
　Assist and teach patient to perform postural drainage as ordered

Administer medications as ordered
  Antibiotics
  Cardiotonics
  Steroids
  Sodium bicarbonate
  Bronchodilators
  Mucolytic agents
Provide emotional support
  Remain with patient as much as possible
  Provide means of communicating
  Have call bell or tap bell within reach

ndx: Knowledge deficit regarding disease process and medical management

GOAL: *Patient will demonstrate understanding of home care and follow-up instructions through interactive discussion and actual return demonstration*

See standard of care for primary condition
See Volume-Cycled Positive Pressure Ventilators (p. 279)
See Respiratory Failure (p. 261)

Evaluation

Patient
  Maintains adequate gas exchange as evidenced by
    Return to baseline: level of consciousness, skin color
    Blood gases within acceptable range
  Maintains an effective breathing pattern as evidenced by
    Normal rate, rhythm, and depth of respirations
    Decreased dyspnea
    Blood gases within acceptable range
  Demonstrates increased knowledge of disease process and management regimen as evidenced by verbalization of principles indicating understanding of the disease and its management

LARYNGECTOMY: RADICAL NECK DISSECTION

Removal of the larynx and surrounding neck tissue to treat a cancerous condition; a permanent stoma is formed

Preoperative assessment
Observations/findings

Tachypnea
Dysphagia
Hemoptysis
Stridor
Hoarseness
Enlarged cervical nodes
Pain in Adam's apple; radiates to ears
Cough
Fear of surgery
Body image change
Panic
Denial
Disbelief
Anger

Preparation

Prepare patient for operation
  See General Preoperative Care/Teaching (p. 29)
  Demonstrate
    Laryngectomy tube
    Cleaning equipment
    Suctioning equipment
  Explain that nasogastric tube will be in place for feeding
  Explain that IV will be in place for 24 to 48 hr
  Determine if patient can write English or other language
  Determine if patient can hear
  Explain that patient will not be able to talk postoperatively
  Have pad and pencil or Magic Slate available
  Have picture cards available if patient is unable to write
Explain that patient may be in critical care area for 24 to 48 hr; tour critical care area with patient and family
Have family purchase a mirror with a stand
Have speech therapist visit patient preoperatively if possible

Postoperative assessment
Observations/findings

Hemorrhage
Airway obstruction
  Restlessness
  Tachycardia
  Use of accessory muscles of respiration
  Tachypnea
  Noisy respirations
  Wheezing
  Stridor
  Pallor
  Cyanosis
Atelectasis
Pneumonia
Tracheoesophageal fistula
Dehydration

Sensory deprivation
Fear of suffocation
Behavioral response
   Helplessness
   Fear
   Anger
Sputum
   Amount
   Character
Site of incision
   Discoloration
   Pain
   Swelling
   Drainage
   Sloughing of tissue
   Stoma
Wound drains
   Sump drains
   Hemovac
Infection
   Elevated temperature
   Purulent aspirate

Laboratory/diagnostic studies

Chest x-ray examination
Arterial blood gases
Baseline pulmonary function tests
ECG
Electrolytes
Fiberoptic endoscopy
Biopsy of suspect lesions
Skull and neck radiographic studies
Bone scan
Anti-Epstein-Barr virus antibody titers

Potential complications

Pneumonia
Respiratory failure
Metastasis
Carotid erosion
Pneumothorax
Hypovolemic shock
Tracheoesophageal fistula

Medical management

Radiation therapy
Artificial airway and mechanical ventilation if required
Nasogastric tube
Oxygen therapy with hydration
Parenteral therapy
Nutritional support

Nursing diagnoses/goals/interventions

ndx: Anxiety/fear related to perceived and/or actual threat to biologic function

GOAL: *Patient will experience a reduction in anxiety/fear*

Provide emotional support (p. 14)
   Encourage verbalization of fears
   Answer all questions honestly
   Encourage communication with significant other
   Arrange for visit by someone who has had laryngectomy as indicated

ndx: Potential for ineffective breathing pattern related to effect of anesthesia and presence of artificial airways

GOAL: *Patient will maintain an effective breathing pattern*

Maintain patent airway
   Apply humidification to laryngectomy
   Suction prn: need for suction determined by auscultation of chest for breath sounds qh
      Suction if crackles or rhonchi over large airways are heard
      Use sterile technique when suctioning patient
      Hyperoxygenate and/or hyperinflate patient's lungs prior to suctioning for four to five breaths
   Clean inner cannula q2h to 4h and prn
   Avoid occluding airway with bed linen or when turning patient
   Have hand-held resuscitator with adaptor at bedside
Have standby laryngectomy tube available: same size and type
Assist and teach patient to turn, cough, and deep breathe q2h
Auscultate chest for breath sounds q2h to 4h

ndx: Impairment of skin integrity related to surgical incision, tracheostomy, and impaired wound healing secondary to preoperative radiation

GOAL: *Patient will experience normal healing of surgical wounds*

Clean skin around stoma q4h and prn
   Wash with hydrogen peroxide
   Rinse with saline solution
Administer oral hygiene q2h to 4h
Elevate head of bed 45 to 60 degrees; prevent forward flexion of neck
   Remove pillows if necessary
   Place small towel under shoulders
Record drainage q8h if Hemovac or sump drains for continuous suction are in place

Pat dry
Change laryngectomy ties prn; make sure ties are loose enough not to cause pressure on neck
Place 4 × 4 inch gauze under laryngectomy tube
Change dressing as ordered
    Report excessive drainage to physician
    Clean area around drains with hydrogen peroxide
Observe for signs of infection; check temperature q4h for 48 hr, then qid

ndx: Impaired verbal communication related to surgical removal of larynx

GOAL: *Patient will use an effective communication system*

Present calm, reassuring manner
Maintain open communication
    Have call light at bedside
    Have pad and pencil or Magic Slate available
    Avoid asking questions that require "yes" or "no" answers
    Wait for patient to write answer
    Do not anticipate end of sentence
    Read statements aloud; encourage patient to communicate feelings
Provide emotional support
    Encourage communication with significant other
    Deal with fear of suffocation, helplessness, and anger
    Prepare visitors for patient's appearance
    Help visitors and staff not to exclude patient from conversations or talk exclusively to one another
Assist patient with operation of artificial larynx if available

ndx: Knowledge deficit regarding disease process and self-care management

GOAL: *Patient and/or significant other will demonstrate understanding of home care and follow-up instructions through interactive discussion and actual return demonstration*

Explain importance of maintaining diet as ordered; need to eat, even though food will taste dull because of loss of senses of smell and taste
Explain need to shower
    Wear shield over stoma
    Use shower hose to direct spray below neck
    Avoid getting soap into stoma
Explain that male patients may shave with electric razor or safety razor; need to avoid getting lather into stoma
Explain need to exercise to tolerance but no swimming; to plan rest periods
Explain need to keep stoma covered at all times; to wear clothing with high necklines, scarves, and jewelry
Explain importance of covering stoma when coughing; to report persistent cough to physician
Explain need to avoid smoking; to avoid persons who smoke
Explain need to avoid persons with URIs
Explain need to wear medical alert band re neck breather
Explain that bowel movements will be controlled with diet and suppositories
Explain importance of ongoing outpatient care
Explain importance of not using aerosol sprays around patient
Discuss symptoms of respiratory distress to report to physician
    Increasing dyspnea
    Increased respiratory rate and pulse
    Increased temperature
    Mental status changes
Discuss medications: name, dosage, time of administration, purpose, and side effects
Explain need to avoid taking over-the-counter medications without checking wih physician
Ensure that patient and/or significant other demonstrates
    Administration of tube feeding if ordered
    Care of incision
    Symptoms to report to physician
        Swelling
        Pain
        Drainage
Ensure that patient and/or significant other demonstrates care of laryngectomy and stoma; provide mirror
    Handwashing procedure
    Taking four or five deep breaths before suctioning
    Suctioning: clean procedure, not sterile
    Caring for inner cannula: clean procedure, not sterile
    Removing and replacing outer cannula
    Changing laryngectomy ties
    Cleansing skin around stoma bid
        Use hydrogen peroxide
        Rinse with water
        Pat dry

Evaluation

Patient
- Experiences a reduction in anxiety/fear as evidenced by
  - Relaxed facial expression
  - Verbalization of feeling less anxious
  - Increased understanding of treatment regimen
- Maintains an effective breathing pattern as evidenced by
  - Normal rate, rhythm, and depth of respirations
  - Decreased dyspnea
  - Blood gases within normal range
- Experiences normal healing of surgical wounds as evidenced by
  - Gradual reduction of redness and swelling
  - Presence of granulation tissue
  - No sign of elevated temperature
- Develops and uses an effective communication system as evidenced by
  - Ability to make needs known to medical and nursing staff
  - Increasing use of Magic Slate or voice box
- Demonstrates knowledge of disease process and home care management as evidenced by verbalization of principles of home management

THORACOTOMY, LOBECTOMY, PNEUMONECTOMY

thoracotomy *Surgical excision of the chest wall*
lobectomy *Removal of one or more lobes of the lung*
pneumonectomy *Removal of an entire lung*

Preoperative care

See General Preoperative Care/Teaching (p. 29)

Postoperative assessment

Observations/findings

Patent airway
Labored breathing
Use of accessory muscles of respiration
Dyspnea
Tachycardia
Breath sounds
- Present
- Absent

Chest expansion
Elevated temperature
Hemoptysis
Crepitus
Amount
Location
Cyanosis
Mediastinal shift
Chest tubes and water seal drainage if applicable
Incision
- Redness
- Pain
- Swelling
- Drainage

Arm contracture: operative side

Laboratory/diagnostic studies

Chest x-ray examination
Arterial blood gases
ECG

Potential complications

Pulmonary embolism
Pulmonary edema
Hemorrhage
Shock
Atelectasis
Tension pneumothorax
Infection

Medical management

O_2 therapy
Intubation and ventilator support
NPO until stable
Parenteral therapy
Medications
- Antibiotics
- Diuretics
- Cardiotonics

Chest tube insertion

Nursing diagnoses/goals/interventions

ndx: Potential for ineffective breathing pattern related to pain secondary to surgical incision

GOAL: *Patient will maintain an effective breathing pattern*

Administer oxygen as ordered
Elevate head of bed 60 to 90 degrees
Assist and teach patient to turn, cough, and deep breath qh
- *Do not turn to unaffected side when pneumonectomy is done*
- Pad area around chest tube when turned to operative side

Splint chest to assist with coughing
Administer IPPB as ordered
Assist and teach patient to use incentive spirometer as ordered
Observe for creptitation
Note amount and location
Report extension of or excessive crepitation to physician
Provide emotional support
Auscultate chest for breath sounds q2h; report diminished or absent breath sounds on unaffected side to physician
Check BP, T, P, and R q2h; report elevated temperature or tachycardia to physician
Check chest tube q1h to 2h
Administer pain medications as indicated
Report to physician
Sudden, sharp chest pain
Asymmetry of chest
Tracheal deviation
Continue with immediate postoperative care and decrease frequency of nursing functions as patient's condition improves
Assist and teach patient to exercise to tolerance
Ambulate as ordered
Plan rest periods q1h to 2h
Assist physician with removal of chest tubes
Apply sterile dressing to wound
Change dressing as ordered and prn
Report redness, swelling, pain, or drainage to physician

ndx: Ineffective airway clearance related to incisional pain and presence of chest tubes

GOAL: *Patient will maintain a patent airway*

Maintain patent airway; suction when necessary
Assist and teach patient to turn, cough, and deep breathe qh
Splint chest when coughing
Assist and teach patient to use incentive spirometer
Auscultate chest q2h; report any abnormalities
Medicate for pain as ordered; assess for effectiveness of pain relief measures

ndx: Impaired physical mobility (arm on affected side) related to incisional pain and edema

GOAL: *Patient will regain full range of motion of affected extremity*

Consult with physical therapy department to obtain ROM exercises
Encourage patient to rotate arm 360 degrees as ordered
Document progress
Medicate for pain as needed

ndx: Knowledge deficit regarding self-care management

GOAL: *Patient and/or significant other will demonstrate understanding of home care and follow-up instructions through interactive discussion and actual return demonstration*

Explain need to continue coughing and deep breathing qid at home
Explain need to avoid smoking
Explain importance of exercising to tolerance
Increase amount of exercise gradually
Adjust activities according to degree of fatigue experienced
Plan rest periods
Explain that some numbness, pain, or heaviness in operative area is expected; it is caused by interruption of intercostal nerves and is usually temporary
Explain need to avoid persons with URIs
Explain importance of ongoing outpatient care
Discuss symptoms to report to physician
Persistent dyspnea
Cough
Elevated temperature
URI
Redness
Pain
Swelling
Drainage from incision
Explain importance of maintaining diet as ordered
Discuss medications: name, dosage, time of administration, purpose, and side effects
Explain need to avoid taking over-the-counter medications without checking with physician
Ensure that patient and/or significant other demonstrates care of incision

Evaluation

Patient
Maintains an effective breathing pattern as evidenced by
Normal rate, rhythm, and depth of respirations
Decreased dyspnea
Blood gases within acceptable range
Maintains a patent airway as evidenced by
Improved breath sounds
Normal rate and depth of respirations

Absence of dyspnea
Absence of cyanosis
Blood gases within acceptable range
Has full range of motion of affected side as evidenced by ability to rotate full 360-degree arm circles by discharge
Demonstrates understanding of home care management as evidenced by verbalization of principles of health management

CHEST TUBES

Drainage tubes placed in the pleural cavity and attached to a water seal drainage system and/or suction to remove air and/or fluid and allow expansion of the affected lung

Assessment
Observations/findings
PATIENT

Chest drainage
  Amount
  Character
Dyspnea
Labored breathing
Tachypnea
Cyanosis
Tachycardia
Elevated temperature
Chest expansion
Breath sounds
  Crackles
  Rhonchi
  Diminished
  Absent
Atelectasis
Crepitus
Hemorrhage
Tension pneumothorax
Mediastinal shift
Shock

EQUIPMENT

Patency of tube(s) and water seal drainage system
Continuous fluctuation of water in water seal drainage system
Water level in water seal drainage system
Stability and security of water seal drainage system
Amount of added suction applied to water seal drainage system

Ongoing care
Patient

Position patient on affected side with head of bed elevated 45 to 60 degrees after insertion of chest tube
Explain purpose of chest tube(s)
Check and record BP, T, P, and R q4h and prn
Check and record amount, color, and character of drainage q2h to 4h; report drainage in excess of 100 ml/hr to physician
Manage pain as indicated (p. 8); assess effectiveness of pain control measure(s)
Check chest tube site and surrounding area q2h to 4h for crepitus and air leaks
Assist and teach patient to turn, cough, and deep breathe q2h
  Splint chest when coughing
  Pad area around chest tube(s) when patient is turned to operative side
Assist and teach patient to perform active or passive ROM exercises to extremities q2h to 4h
Ambulate patient as ordered
Auscultate chest for breath sounds q2h to 4h; report diminished breath sounds in unaffected lung to physician
Change dressing as ordered
Encourage fluids as ordered

Equipment

Tape connecting tubing securely
Maintain pressure if patient is on added suction as ordered
Avoid kinking and obstruction of chest tubing
Keep water seal drainage system lower than patient's chest at all times
Secure connecting tubing and chest tube(s) to avoid tension and allow freedom of movement
Check fluctuation of water in water seal drainage system; if absent, report to physician
Change water seal drainage system as indicated; never allow drainage to fill collection unit
Have petroleum jelly gauze at bedside for emergency use
Keep two rubber-tipped hemostats at bedside at all times
Clamp chest tube(s) only under the following circumstances
  If ordered to do so by physician
  When disconnecting closed water seal drainage system to change collection unit
  If closed water seal drainage system breaks or integrity is disrupted for any reason

Patient teaching

See standard of care for primary condition
Ensure that patient and/or significant other knows and understands
- Purpose of chest tube(s)
- Importance of turning, coughing, and deep breathing
- Importance of keeping closed water seal drainage system below level of patient's chest when sitting or ambulating
- Importance of not placing tension on chest tube(s)
- Need to report difficulty in breathing and chest pain to nurse and/or physician

Ensure that patient demonstrates coughing and deep breathing

Removal of Chest Tube
Interventions

Place patient in a sitting position
Instruct patient to take a deep breath and hold it until chest tube(s) is (are) removed by physician
Assist physician in applying pressure dressing to chest tube site
Instruct patient to breathe normally
Auscultate chest for breath sounds q4h for 24 hr; report diminished or absent breath sounds to physician

Patient teaching/discharge outcome

See standard of care for primary condition
Ensure that patient and/or significant other knows and understands
- Importance of reporting any sudden, sharp chest pain or difficult breathing to nurse and/or physician
- Importance of coughing and deep breathing
- Importance of exercising to tolerance
- Need to avoid having contact with any person with URI
- Need to avoid crowds
- Importance of not smoking

ARTIFICIAL AIRWAYS

Oropharyngeal Airway

An artificial airway that extends from the lips to the pharynx, displacing the tongue anteriorly

Assessment
Observations/findings

Level of consciousness
Difficulty in breathing
Airway obstruction
- Restlessness
- Stridor
- Labored breathing
- Retractions
  - Intercostal
  - Suprasternal
  - Supraclavicular
  - Nasal flaring
- Cyanosis or pallor
- Tachycardia
- Gagging
- Breath sounds
  - Crackles
  - Rhonchi
  - Decreased
- Position of tongue
- Position of head and neck

Ongoing care

Check airway for patency and proper size
Ensure that tongue is not between teeth and airway
Assist and teach patient to maintain supine position; if gagging or vomiting occurs, turn head to side
Suction oropharynx or nasopharynx as indicated
Administer oxygen as ordered
Change airway q8h and prn
Administer oral hygiene q8h and prn
Auscultate chest for breath sounds q2h and prn

Removal of airway

Note level of consciousness
Instruct patient to push airway out with tongue when possible
Do not remove airway until gag and swallow reflexes are present
Remain with patient until normal respirations are maintained without airway

Patient teaching

Explain purpose of airway
Establish method of communication
- Call light within reach
- Pad and pencil or Magic Slate at bedside

Nasopharyngeal Airway (Figure 4-3)

An artificial airway that extends from the naris to the pharynx

Assessment
Observations/findings

Level of consciousness
Difficulty in breathing

Airway obstruction
  Restlessness
  Stridor
  Shortness of breath
  Retractions
    Intercostal
    Suprasternal
    Supraclavicular
Tachycardia
Cyanosis or pallor
Mouth breathing
Pressure sores on naris
Breath sounds
  Crackles
  Rhonchi
  Decreased
Position of head and neck

Ongoing care

Suction oropharynx and nasopharynx q2h to 4h and prn
Administer oxygen as ordered
Check P and R q4h and prn; note quality of respirations
Auscultate chest for breath sounds q2h and prn
Administer oral hygiene q4h and prn
Change airway q72h and alternate nares if possible
Clean nares q8h and prn
  Use cotton-tipped applicator with saline solution
  Apply water-soluble lubricant to nares
Use soft restraints if indicated
Establish means of communication when necessary
  Call light within reach
  Pad and pencil or Magic Slate at bedside

Removal of airway

Suction prior to removal
Administer oxygen when ordered
Remain with patient for 15 min after removal; report any signs of respiratory distress to physician
Check P and R q10 min for three times, noting quality and rate, then as ordered
Auscultate chest for breath sounds q15 to 30 min for three times, then q2h to 4h as ordered

Patient teaching

Explain purpose of airway as indicated
Explain need to avoid mouth breathing

Endotracheal Tube

An artificial airway that extends from the nose (Figure 4-4) or mouth into the trachea

Assessment

Observations/findings

Correct position of tube
  Taped securely
  Patency
Decreased or absent breath sounds
Crackles
Rhonchi over large airways
Respiratory distress
  Cyanosis or pallor
  Tachypnea
  Asymmetric chest movement
  Retraction of chest muscles
  Contraction of cervical muscles
  Presence of secretions

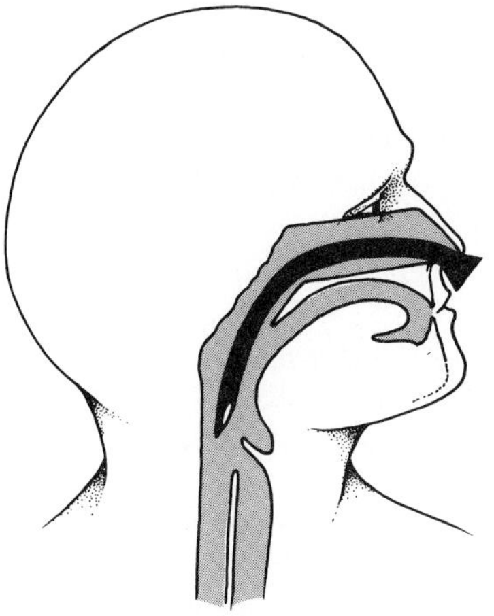

FIGURE 4-3. Nasopharygeal airway.

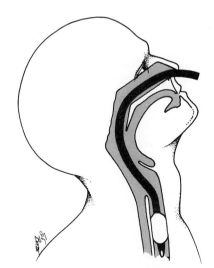

FIGURE 4-4. Nasotracheal tube.

Wheezing
　　Restlessness
　　Biting on tube
Level of consciousness
Gag reflex
Tachycardia
Bradycardia
Pressure sores on nares
Infection
　　Elevated temperature
　　Purulent aspirate
　　Colored aspirate
Inflated cuff
　　Minimal leak technique
　　Minimal occlusion volume technique
Deflated cuff
Humidification with room air or oxygen
Psychosocial problems
　　Anxiety
　　Fear of unknown

Ongoing care

Maintain patent airway
　　Auscultate chest for breath sounds qh; report decreased or absent breath sounds to physician
　　Suction patient when crackles and/or rhonchi over large airways are heard
　　　　Observe color of aspirate: if purulent or colored, obtain specimen for culture
　　　　Irrigate with normal saline solution if ordered
　　Check position of tube q½h to 1h to prevent slippage into right or left mainstem bronchus
　　Obtain chest x-ray examination after insertion in order to ascertain position of tube
　　Keep hand-held resuscitator with adaptor at bedside
Check respirations for quality and rate qh
Be aware that respirations are usually maintained on a continuous mechanical ventilator (p. 277)
Use air or oxygen blow-by if indicated
Be certain cuff is inflated while patient is on ventilator
　　Maintain inflated cuff with either a minimal leak or minimal occlusion volume technique
　　Test pressure in inflated cuff q2h to 4h: cuff pressure should remain below 20 mm Hg
Deflate cuff when patient is off ventilator for long periods of time; suction mouth and trachea prior to deflating cuff
Check rectal temperature q4h
Check BP and P q2h to 4h
Turn patient q1h to 2h
Maintain NPO

Administer parenteral fluids as ordered
Measure and record intake and output
Check level of consciousness qh; establish means of communication if patient is conscious
　　Call bell within reach
　　Pad and pencil or Magic Slate at bedside
Provide emotional support
Administer oral hygiene q1h to 2h
Clean naris gently around endotracheal tube q8h and prn; use cotton-tipped applicator with saline solution—apply water-soluble lubricant to naris
Provide oropharyngeal airway or bite-block if patient bites on endotracheal tube
Apply soft restraints as necessary if patient is restless
Provide humidification to endotracheal tube when patient is off ventilator

CARE DURING/AFTER REMOVAL OF ENDOTRACHEAL TUBE
Assessment
Observations/findings

Level of consciousness
Gag reflex
Able to maintain spontaneous respirations without assistance
BP and P
Breath sounds
Arterial blood gases
Laryngospasm

Ongoing care

Auscultate chest for breath sounds
Assess level of consciousness
Ascertain if patient is able to maintain spontaneous respirations at a rate sufficient to maintain normal arterial blood gases
Elevate head of bed 45 to 90 degrees
Hyperoxygenate and hyperinflate patient's lungs for four or five breaths
Suction oropharynx and/or nasopharynx
Suction endotracheal tube
Deflate cuff
Assist and teach patient to take deep breaths as tube is removed
Remove tube, using a smooth, slightly downward motion
Provide emesis basin and tissues
Administer humidified oxygen
Assist and teach patient to cough and deep breathe qh
Auscultate chest for breath sounds q15 min for four times, then q1h to 2h; report absent or diminished breath sounds to physician

Check BP, R, and apical pulse q15 min for four times, then q1h to 2h
Monitor arterial blood gases as ordered
Prepare for reinsertion of endotracheal tube if laryngospasm occurs or if patient is unable to maintain adequate respiratory rate
Administer oral hygiene
Provide emotional support
  Remain with patient as much as possible
  Explain that throat will be sore
  Encourage patient to minimize talking for a few hours
  Provide a pad and pencil or Magic Slate
  Have call light within reach

Patient teaching

Explain all procedures whether patient appears conscious or not; orient patient to date, time, and place
Explain why patient is unable to talk and that it is only a temporary condition
Establish means of communication
  Call bell within reach
  Pad and pencil or Magic Slate at bedside
Emphasize importance of turning and coughing up secretions

TRACHEOSTOMY (Figure 4-5)

Insertion of a tube into the trachea through an incision

Preoperative care

See General Preoperative Care/Teaching (p. 29)
Teach as much of the following as possible
  Provide emotional support
    Explain purpose of tracheostomy
    Remain with patient as much as possible
    Speak calmly and act unhurried
    Involve family or significant other in care and instructions
  Demonstrate
    Tracheostomy tube
    Cleaning equipment
    Suctioning equipment; explain suctioning procedure
  Determine if patient can write English or other language
  Determine if patient can hear
  Explain that patient will not be able to talk postoperatively
    Have pad and pencil or Magic Slate at bedside
    Have picture cards available if patient is unable to write
  Explain that patient may be in critical care area after operation; tour critical care area with patient and family
  Establish means of contacting nurse
    Call light
    Tap bell

Postoperative assessment

Observations/findings

Hemorrhage
Airway obstruction
  Restlessness
  Tachycardia
  Tachypnea
  Noisy respirations
  Wheezing
  Stridor
  Pallor
  Cyanosis
Position of tracheostomy
Cuff
  Present
  Inflated
  Deflated
Bilateral expansion of chest
Atelectasis (p. 257)
Pneumonia (p. 243)
Tracheoesophageal fistula
Dehydration
Infection
  Elevated temperature
  Purulent aspirate
Sputum
  Amount
  Character

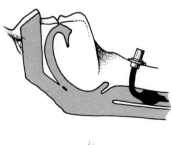
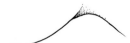

FIGURE 4-5. Tracheostomy tube with cuff.

Stoma
   Pain
   Swelling
   Drainage
Anxiety
Sensory deprivation
Fear of suffocation
Helplessness

Immediate postoperative care

See Care of Patient in Recovery Room (p. 30)
Maintain patent airway
   Administer humidification to tracheostomy
   Suction prn; need for suctioning is determined by auscultation of chest for breath sounds qh
      Suction when crackles and rhonchi over large airways are heard
      Use sterile technique when suctioning patient
      Hyperoxygenate and hyperinflate patient's lungs for four or five breaths before suctioning
   Clean inner cannula (if present) q2h to 4h and prn
   Avoid occluding airway with bed linen or when turning patient
   Tape tracheostomy obturator to head of bed
   Have standby tracheostomy tube available: same size and type
   Have hand-held resuscitator with adaptor at bedside
Elevate head of bed 45 to 60 degrees; prevent forward flexion of neck
   Remove pillow if necessary
   Place small towel under shoulder area
Administer oxygen or mechanical ventilation as ordered; see appropriate standard
If a cuffed tracheostomy tube is used, have cuff deflated whenever possible
   Maintain inflated cuff with either minimal leak or minimal occlusive volume technique; test pressure in inflated cuff q2h to 4h—cuff pressure should remain below 20 mm Hg
   Use a low-pressure–cuffed tube
Cleanse skin around stoma q4h and prn
   Wash with hydrogen peroxide
   Rinse with saline solution
   Pat dry
   Change and secure tracheostomy ties prn
   Place 4 × 4 inch gauze under tracheostomy tube
Manage pain as indicated (p. 8); assess effectiveness of pain relief measure(s)
Check BP, P, R, and rectal temperature q4h for 48 hr, then qid
Assist and teach patient to turn, cough, and deep breathe q2h
Auscultate chest for breath sounds q2h to 4h; report diminished or absent breath sounds to physician
Administer oral hygiene q2h to 4h and prn
Administer parenteral fluids as ordered
Measure and record intake and output
Assist and teach patient to perform active or passive ROM exercises to extremities
Establish means of communication
   Have pad and pencil or Magic Slate available
   Avoid asking questions that require "yes" or "no" answers
   Wait for patient to write answer; do not anticipate end of sentence
   Read statements aloud
   Encourage patient to communicate feelings
Provide emotional support
   Encourage communication with significant other; help visitors and staff not to exclude patient from conversation or talk exclusively to one another
   Remain with patient as much as possible
   Answer call light promptly
   Deal with fear of suffocation and helplessness
Give laxatives, stool softeners, or enemas as ordered

Ongoing care

Continue with immediate postoperative care and decrease frequency of nursing functions as patient's condition improves
Maintain diet as ordered
   Force fluids to 3000 ml daily unless contraindicated
   Inflate cuff prior to feedings and leave inflated for 30 min after each feeding
   Test swallowing reflex with gelatin; have suctioning equipment available
   Observe for signs of aspiration and tracheoesophageal fistula
Decannulate tracheostomy as ordered
   Be aware that a fenestrated tube may be used for decannulation process
   Partially cork tracheostomy tube
      Make sure cuff is deflated throughout procedure
      Observe patient for respiratory obstruction
      Progressively increase size of cork until tracheostomy is completely occluded; notify physician when patient is able to tolerate complete occlusion of tracheostomy for 24 hr
Be aware that physician may change tracheostomy tube daily using progressively smaller sizes
Involve patient in care if tracheostomy is permanent; demonstrate tracheostomy care while patient watches in mirror
Ensure that patient and/or significant other knows and

understands importance of establishing a means of communication
    Pad and pencil
    Magic Slate
    Call light within reach
    Tap bell
Ensure that patient and/or significant other demonstrates
    Care of tracheostomy and stoma; provide mirror
    Handwashing procedure
    Taking four to five deep breaths prior to suctioning procedure: clean procedure, not sterile
    Care of inner cannula: clean procedure, not sterile
    Changing tracheostomy ties
    Cleansing skin around stoma bid
        Use hydrogen peroxide
        Rinse with water
        Pat dry
Understand that patient may not be motivated to participate initially
Assist and teach patient to ambulate as ordered
Have patient shower daily
    Direct spray below neck
    Cover tracheostomy with waterproof material
Refer to Visiting Nurses Association or other home health agency or patient help groups in area

Patient teaching/discharge outcome

Ensure that patient and/or significant other knows and understands
    Importance of maintaining diet as ordered
        Eat, even though food tastes dull because of loss of sense of smell
        Force fluids to 3000 ml daily unless contraindicated
    Need to shower daily
        Wear shield over stoma
        Use shower hose
        Direct spray below neck
        Avoid getting soap into stoma
    Need for male patients to shave with electric razor or safety razor; avoid getting lather into stoma
    Need to exercise to tolerance but no swimming; to plan rest periods
    Need to keep stoma covered at all times; to wear clothing with high neckline, scarves, and jewelry
    Importance of covering stoma when coughing; need to report persistent cough to physician
    Importance of not smoking
    Need to wear medical alert band re neck breather
    Need to control bowel movements with diet and suppositories
    Importance of not using aerosol sprays around patient
    Need to use commercial humidifier or pan of water on stove to add to comfort
    Importance of ongoing outpatient care
    Need to avoid persons with URIs
    Need to report any respiratory distress to physician
    Name of medication, dosage, time of administration, purpose, and side effects
    Need to avoid taking over-the-counter medications without checking with physician
Ensure that patient and/or significant other demonstrates
    Administration of tube feeding if ordered
    Care of tracheostomy and stoma

CONTINUOUS MECHANICAL VENTILATION

A method of providing ventilatory support for those patients whose respiratory apparatus fails to maintain adequate oxygenation of the blood, with or without carbon dioxide retention; two types of ventilators can be used, pressure limited and volume limited; examples of a pressure-limited ventilator are the Bird Mark 7 and Bennett PR2; Bennett MA-1, Emerson, Bourns Bear 1, Ohio 560, and Engstrom are volume-limited ventilators

Care of Patient on Continuous Mechanical Ventilation
Assessment
Observations/findings

Position of airway
    Endotracheal tube
    Tracheostomy
Patency of airway
Respiratory distress
    Tachypnea
    Restlessness
    Apprehension
    Pallor
    Cyanosis
Breath sounds
    Crackles
    Rhonchi
    Diminished
    Absent
Respiratory acidosis (acidemia)
    Decreased pH: below 7.4
    Elevated $PaCO_2$: above 40 mm Hg
Respiratory alkalosis (alkalemia)
    Increased pH: above 7.4
    Decreased $PaCO_2$: below 40 mm Hg

Hypoxemia
Sputum
  Amount
  Color
  Consistency
Infection
  Elevated temperature
  Purulent sputum
Tachycardia
Diaphoresis
Oxygen toxicity (time and dose related)
  Diminished breath sounds
  Crackles
  Decreased lung compliance
  Decreased VC
  Decreased $PaCO_2$ while using same oxygen concentration
  Changes on chest x-ray examination
  Visual impairment
  Papilledema
Fluid and electrolyte imbalance
  Dehydration
  Positive water balance
Decreased cardiac output
Atelectasis
Psychosocial problems
  Anxiety
  Dependence on ventilator

Potential complications

Disconnection from ventilator
Acid-base imbalance
Infection
Oxygen toxicity
Fluid and electrolyte imbalance
Pneumothorax
GI bleeding

Acute care

Maintain patent airway
  Suction prn; determine need for suctioning by auscultating chest for breath sounds qh—suction when crackles or rhonchi are present
    Hyperoxygenate and hyperinflate lungs for four or five breaths prior to suctioning patient
    Use sterile technique when suctioning patient
    Place respirator attachment on sterile towel while suctioning patient
  Keep hand-held resuscitator with adaptor at bedside
Maintain visual contact with patient
Avoid placing tension on airway
Avoid obstructing airway when turning patient

See Tracheostomy (p. 275)
See Endotracheal tube (p. 273)
Provide controlled ventilation if necessary
Administer sedative as ordered
Administer morphine sulfate as ordered
Administer neuromuscular blocking agents as ordered
Attach arterial line to monitor if ordered
Check arterial blood gases as ordered; report acidemia, alkalemia, or abnormal PaO_2 to physician
Check BP, R, and apical pulse q1h to 2h
Check rectal temperature q4h
Monitor CVP if ordered
Auscultate chest for breath sounds q1h to 2h; report diminished or absent breath sounds to physician
Maintain position of optimal ventilation; turn q1h to 2h and prn, alternating postural drainage positions
Have patient sigh q15 min or as ordered
Check exhaled tidal volume q8h and prn
Maintain oxygen concentration as ordered
Check FIO_2 qh and immediately after suctioning patient
Check delivered oxygen concentration q8h and prn
Avoid turning alarm systems off
Maintain temperature in inspiratory tubing between 89.6° and 95° F (32° and 35° C)
Administer parenteral fluids as ordered
Measure and record intake and output
Administer oral fluids as ordered; tube feedings may be ordered
Administer oral and nasal care q2h to 4h and prn
Administer skin care q2h and prn; use air mattress or sheepskin prn
Assist and teach patient to perform active or passive ROM exercises to extremities
Provide emotional support
  Remain with patient as much as possible
  Answer call light promptly
  Establish means of communication: pad and pencil or Magic Slate
  Allow patient sufficient time to communicate thoughts and feelings
  Maintain nonstressful environment
  Be calm, confident, and unhurried when caring for patient
  Encourage communication with significant other

Ongoing care: subacute

Continue with acute care and decrease frequency of nursing functions as patient's condition improves
Wean patient off respirator as ordered
  Obtain baseline respiratory rate, VC, and tidal volume

Explain weaning process thoroughly
Remain with patient during weaning process
Check R and apical pulse q5 to 15 min
Place on ventilator immediately if respiratory distress occurs
Be prepared to repeat weaning process several times if necessary

Convalescent care

See standard of care for primary condition

Patient teaching

Ensure that patient and/or significant other knows and understands
- Purpose of ventilator
- Importance of breathing with ventilator
- Importance of coughing up secretions
- Importance of artificial airway
- Need to avoid placing any tension on airway; to never touch airway with hands
- Need to communicate in writing

Pressure-Limited Positive Pressure Ventilator

Delivers a volume of air until a preset pressure is reached; used primarily for IPPB treatments in the adult population

Assessment/care of equipment

Attached to gas source
Connecting tubing
  Patent
  Free of excessive moisture
Air leaks
  Cuff of endotracheal tube
  Cuff of tracheostomy
Patent airway
Adequate humidification
  Nebulizer
  Heated humidification
Temperature of inspired gas
Settings as ordered
  Respiratory rate: should not be less than 12/min
  Oxygen concentration: air mix control
  Inspiratory pressure control
  Apnea control
  Sensitivity control

Ongoing care

Maintain inspiratory rate and respiratory pressure as ordered
  Patent airway
  System free of leaks
  Connective tubing patent and free of excessive moisture
Be aware that inspiratory positive pressure ventilators may not have alarm systems
Remain with patient as much as possible
Determine respiratory rate, oxygen concentration, and inspiratory pressure setting by arterial blood gases
Establish flow sheet
  Record ventilator settings
  Record laboratory values
Maintain oxygen concentration as ordered; measure FIO_2 q8h and prn
Maintain respiratory rate as ordered
  Measure tidal volume q8h and prn
  Auscultate chest for breath sounds qh
Provide humidification
Make sure that equipment continues to cycle when cuff is deflated
Have patient sigh q15 min or as ordered; use hand-held resuscitator
Change connecting tubing, nebulizer, and humidification system q24h; replace with sterile equipment

Volume-Cycled Positive Pressure Ventilator

Delivers breathing gas at a predetermined volume; once the desired volume has been delivered, the ventilator will cycle and patient will passively exhale

Assessment/care of equipment

Electrical system
  Plugged in
  Alarms on
Connecting tubing
  Patent
  Free of excessive moisture
Air leaks
  Cuff of endotracheal tube
  Cuff of tracheostomy
Patent airway
Adequate humidification
  Heated humidification
  Nebulizer
Temperature of inspired gas
Settings as ordered
  Flow rate
  Inspiratory pressure
  Tidal volume
  Positive end-expiratory pressure (PEEP)
  Ventilator rate: should not be less than 12/min
  Oxygen concentration
  Sigh pressure
  Sigh volume
  Number of sighs per hour

Ongoing care

Maintain tidal volume as ordered
    Patent airway
    System free of leaks
    Connective tubing patent and free of excessive moisture
Determine ventilator settings by arterial blood gases
Establish flow sheet
    Record ventilator settings
    Record laboratory values
Maintain oxygen concentration as ordered (determined by PaO_2; measure FIO_2 q8h and prn
Maintain respiratory rate as ordered
Provide heated humidification
Have patient sigh q15 min or as ordered; sigh pressure and volume as ordered
Avoid turning alarm system off
Measure tidal volume q8h and prn
Test alarm system q8h
Change connecting tubing, nebulizer, and humidification q24h; replace with sterile equipment

INTERMITTENT POSITIVE PRESSURE BREATHING (IPPB)

intermittent positive pressure ventilator *A ventilator that delivers breathing gas until equilibrium is established between the patient's lungs and the ventilator; depends on pressure buildup in the patient's lungs rather than on time or volume; a valve mechanism shuts off the gas flow when the pressure has been reached and patient exhales passively; should be used only after less expensive modalities have been tried*

Pretreatment assessment
Observations/findings

BP
Pulse
Color
Respiratory effort
Breath sounds

Preparation

Check BP and apical pulse prior to treatment
Auscultate chest for breath sounds
Place patient in sitting position
Prepare machine
    Secure all tubing connections
    Place medication or saline solution in nebulizer
    Set pressure and oxygen concentration as ordered
    Control nebulizer to produce fine mist

Preprocedure teaching

Explain procedure and what is expected of patient
    Concentrate on using diaphragm
    Breathe at normal rate through mouth
    Allow machine to fill lungs to desired volume
    Prolong expiration
    Purse lips around mouthpiece

Assessment during treatment
Observations/findings

Respiratory rate
Chest expansion
Sudden respiratory distress
Hyperventilation
    Circumoral numbness
    Tingling of fingers
    Dizziness
Fatigue
Nervousness
Tachycardia
Chest pain
Function of equipment

Ongoing care

Check pulse one or two times during treatment
Remain with patient during initial treatment
Stop treatment if sudden respiratory distress or chest pain occurs
Have patient deep breathe slowly one or two times during treatment
Have patient cough one or two times during and after treatment
Check pressure gauge and adjust flow to avoid negative inspiratory pressure
Administer oral hygiene after treatment

Patient teaching/discharge outcome

Ensure that patient and/or significant other knows and understands
    Need to follow physician's instructions regarding use of IPPB
    Need to cough during treatment and immediately following treatment
    Importance of using saline solution or medication in nebulizer
    Symptoms of respiratory distress to report to physician
    Need to stop treatment if dizziness, nervousness, chest pain, rapid pulse, or sudden respiratory distress occurs during treatment
    Importance of avoiding persons with URIs
    Symptoms of URI to report to physician

Importance of ongoing outpatient care
Name of medication, dosage, time of administration, purpose, and side effects
Need to avoid taking over-the-counter medications without checking with physician
Ensure that patient and/or significant other demonstrates
  Preparation of machine for treatment
  Use of machine during treatment
  IPPB procedure
  Coughing techniques
  Care of equipment

INCENTIVE SPIROMETER

A mechanical device that assists patient in maintaining maximal inspiratory effort; effective when used by postoperative patients in order to prevent development of atelectasis and pneumonia; more physiologic and less hazardous than IPPB

Assessment

Observations/findings

PATIENT

Presence or absence of pain
Motivation
Weakness
Hyperventilation
  Dizziness
  Lightheadedness
  Numbness around mouth and nose
  Tingling in fingers and toes
Cough
  Productive
  Nonproductive
Breath sounds
  Crackles
  Rhonchi over large airways
  Diminished
  Absent

EQUIPMENT

Type of device
Tidal volume

Ongoing care

Patient must be alert and cooperative
Assess degree of pain present
  Administer analgesics as ordered
  Assess effectiveness of pain relief measure(s)
Elevate head of bed 60 to 90 degrees or have patient sit in chair
Assist and teach patient to use incentive spirometer
  Exhale slowly
  Place mouthpiece in mouth between teeth
  Close lips tightly around mouthpiece
  Inhale through mouth only, taking a slow, deep breath
  Hold breath for 3 to 5 sec
  Remove mouthpiece from mouth
  Exhale slowly
Repeat procedure 10 to 20 times qh
Caution patient not to breathe too rapidly
Observe for signs of hyperventilation; stop use of incentive spirometer if dizziness or lightheadedness occurs
Assist and teach patient to cough after using incentive spirometer
Auscultate chest for breath sounds q4h
  Assist and teach patient to cough if crackles or rhonchi are heard
  Report diminished or absent breath sounds to physician
Monitor patient's progress q4h
Increase tidal volume as patient tolerates it

Patient teaching

Ensure that patient and/or significant other knows and understands
  Purpose of incentive spirometer
  Importance of using it 10 to 20 times qh
  Importance of holding breath for 3 to 5 sec
  Need to inhale through mouth
  Importance of not exhaling into apparatus
  Importance of reaching desired tidal volume
  Importance of coughing after using apparatus
Ensure that patient demonstrates
  Use of incentive spirometer
  Coughing productively

Chapter 5

Neurologic System

NEUROLOGIC ASSESSMENT

Subjective Data

Loss of consciousness
Dizziness, vertigo
Weakness
Headaches
Numbness
Paralysis
Bowel and/or bladder dysfunction
Pain
Memory loss
Tremors, tics
Nervousness
Seizures
Irritability
Drowsiness
Hallucination
Confusion
Disturbances in
  Smell
  Taste
  Vision

Objective Data

Mental status
Level of consciousness
  See Glascow Coma Scale (GSC, p. 288)
  Awake, alert, and oriented; able to maintain conversation
  Responds to verbal and/or painful stimuli
  Drowsy, lethargic, sleeplike
  Able to follow commands
  Disoriented and stuporous
  Unable to respond to verbal or painful stimulus
  Comatose
Behavior
  General appearance
  Mood, affect
  Personal grooming
  Verbal and nonverbal expression
  Facial expression
  Ability to concentrate
  Attention span
Intellectual or cognitive performance
Memory: immediate, recent, and past
Abstract reasoning; insight
Emotional status
Level of dependence vs. independence in activities of daily living (ADLs)
Sensory dysfunctions
  Visual agnosia
  Tactile agnosia
Language dysfunction
  Dysarthria
  Motor, expressive aphasia: Broca's aphasia
    Aphemia (pure word mutism)
    Sensory, receptive aphasia (Wernicke's aphasia)
    Auditory verbal agnosia (pure word deafness)
    Apraxia
Meningeal signs
  Brudzinski's sign: to assess meningeal irritation—patient in supine position bends knees to avoid pain when neck is flexed
  Kernig's sign: to assess meningeal irritation—patient in supine position with hips flexed is unable to extend knees without pain
  Nuchal rigidity: stiff neck
    High-pitched cry
    Severe retraction of head
    Arm and leg extension
Abnormal findings of particular gaits and postures
General appearance
  Skin
    Temperature
    Color, discolored areas
    Turgor
    Rashes
    Angiomatous lesions
    Moles
Vital signs
  BP
    Both arms, standing, sitting
    Increased
    Decreased
    Widening pulse pressure
  Arterial pulses
  Respirations (Table 5-1)

TABLE 5-1. Patterns of Respiration in Neurologic Dysfunction

Terms	Description	Selected neurologic causes
Eupnea	Normal breathing	
Cheyne-Stokes respirations	Breathing characterized by regular, alternating periods of hyperpnea and apnea; breathing builds from respiration to respiration in a smooth crescendo and, as peak is reached, declines in an equally smooth decrescendo; ordinarily, hyperpneic phase endures longer than apneic phase	Deep bilateral diencephalic lesions, hypertensive encephalopathy, uremia, anoxia, or imminent transtentorial herniation
Central neurogenic hyperventilation	Sustained regular, rapid hypocapnic hyperpnea	Brain dysfunction
Biot's respirations	Regular periods of hyperventilation and irregular periods of apnea	
Apneustic respirations	Ataxic, gasping, shallow breathing	Infarction at mid- or caudal pontine level, usually as a result of basilar artery occlusion; *not* characteristically observed with progressive rostral-caudal brainstem dysfunction
Posthyperventilation apnea	Respirations interrupted for up to 30 seconds after five voluntary breaths in wakeful patients	Diffuse metabolic or structural forebrain disease
Cluster breathing	Breaths follow each other in disorderly sequence with irregular pauses between them	Low pons or high medulla lesion; may be result of expanding lesion in posterior fossa (cerebellar hemorrhage)
Ataxic breathing	Completely chaotic pattern with deep and shallow breaths occurring randomly; progressively leads to apnea	Dorsomedial medulla dysfunction; may appear in relation to meningitis or acute parainfectious demyelination

From Barber, J.M., Stokes, L.G., and Billings, D.M.: Adult and child care: a client approach to nursing, ed. 2, St. Louis, 1977, The C.V. Mosby Co.

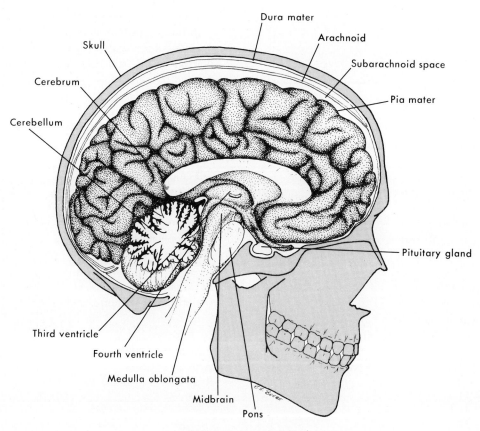

FIGURE 5-1. Nervous system.

Rate
Rhythm
Quality
Type of breathing
Chest movements
Breath sounds
Eyes (Figure 5-3)
  Pupils
    Equality
    Size
    Pinpoint
    Dilation
    Reaction to light
  Ptosis
  Nystagmus
  "Doll's eyes"
  Diplopia
  Visual acuity
  Visual fields
  Ophthalmoscopic assessment
Motor function
  Balance
  Coordination of body movements
  Posture
  Gait
  Strength
    Hands, arms
    Lips, legs, ankles
  Muscle mass
    Tone
    Strength
    Abnormal movement
      Tremors
      Tics
  Seizures
  Reflex responses

Classification		Description
0	(0)	Absent
1	(+)	Sluggish or diminished
2	(++)	Active or normal
3	(+++)	Slightly hyperactive or increased response
4	(++++)	Brisk with intermittent or transient clonus
5	(+++++)	Very brisk with sustained clonus

Autonomic functions
  Bowel and/or bladder dysfunctions
  Sexual dysfunction
Cranial nerve abnormalities (Table 5-2)

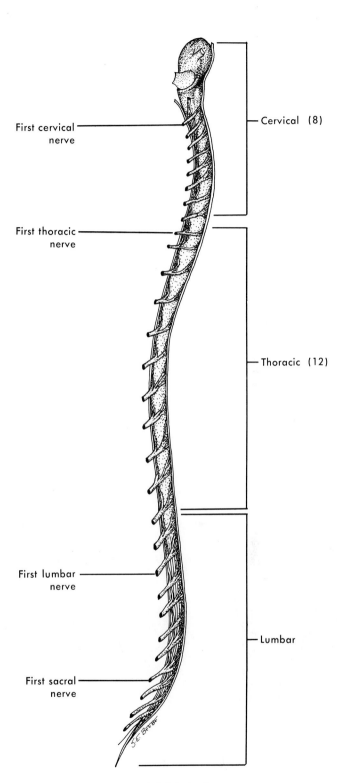

FIGURE 5-2. Spinal column.

TABLE 5-2. Cranial Nerve Function

Nerve	Findings
I. Olfactory	Smell
II. Optic	Visual acuity, visual fields; examination of fundi
III. Oculomotor	Pupillary reflex, external ocular muscles inducing upward, downward, and medial movements; involvement will cause ptosis, dilation of pupils
IV. Trochlear	Ocular movements; involvement will cause inability to look downward and laterally; nystagmus
V. Trigeminal	Sensory function: corneal reflex, skin of face and forehead, mucosa of nose and mouth; motor function; maxillary "jaw" reflex
VI. Abducens	Ocular movements; involvement will cause inability to look downward and laterally; nystagmus
VII. Facial	Motor function of upper and lower face; involvement will cause asymmetry of face and paresis; sensory function is tested by taste
VIII. Acoustic	Cochlear nerve test: hearing, lateralization, air and bone conduction; involvement will cause tinnitus, decreased hearing, or deafness
IX. Glossopharyngeal	Motor function: pharyngeal gag reflex, swallowing; vocal cord assessment: speak clearly without hoarseness
X. Vagus	
XI. Accessory	Strength of trapezius and sternocleidomastoid muscle; involvement will cause inability to elevate shoulder
XII. Hypoglossal	Motor function of tongue; involvement will cause lateral deviation, atrophy, tremor, inability to extend or move tongue from side to side

INFANTS

Fontanel evaluation
   Bulging
   Flat
   Pulsating
Cry quality: high pitched
Reflexes
   Moro's
   Grasping
   Rooting
   Sucking
Muscle tone
   Jitteriness
   Tremors
   Seizures

Pertinent Background Information
HISTORY OF PRESENT ILLNESS

Description of past or concurrent condition
Hypertension
Cancer
Coronary artery disease
Hyperlipidemia
Pernicious anemia
Obesity
Diabetes
Coarctation of aorta
Epilepsy
Loss of consciousness
Headaches
Allergies
Seizure disorders
Infections
Neurologic medical-surgical procedures
Motor and/or sensory disturbances
Behavioral or emotional changes
Head trauma
Drug abuse
Alcohol use

FAMILY HISTORY

Hypertension
Seizure disorders
Neurologic disorders
Cancer
Tumors
Strokes
Mental retardation
Alcoholism
Mental illness
Sudden death

SOCIAL HISTORY

Sleep patterns
Exercise and activity level
Occupation; work patterns
Leisure activities
Eating habits
Smoking
Alcohol use

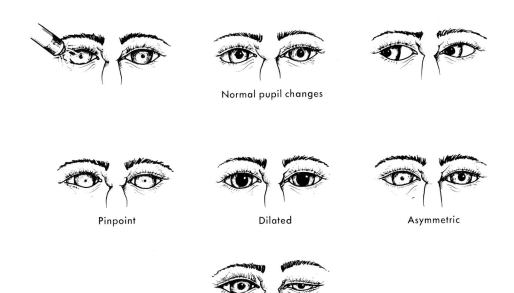

FIGURE 5-3. Variations in pupil response.

Psychosocial patterns
   Personality changes
      Relationships with family and friends
School history; learning disorders

MEDICATION HISTORY

Prescription medications
Over-the-counter medications

Diagnostic Aids
LABORATORY STUDIES

Cerebrospinal fluid (CSF) analysis
Complete blood cell count (CBC)
Erythrocyte sedimentation rate (ESR)
Gastric analysis with histamine
Blood chemistries
Arterial blood gases
Blood glucose and pH
Fluid and electrolyte levels
Enzyme studies

DIAGNOSTIC PROCEDURES

Skull x-ray examinations
Electroencephalogram (EEG)
Myelogram
Lumbar puncture
Cisternal puncture
Ventricular puncture

Tomography
Echoencephalography
Pneumoencephalography
Ventriculography
Brain scan
Computed tomography (CT) scan
Positron emission tomography (PET) scan
Nuclear magnetic resonance (NMR)
Cerebral angiography
Doppler scan
Cerebral blood flow (CBF)
Biopsy
   Brain
   Nerve
   Muscle
Pulmonary function
   Vital capacity (VC)
   Minute ventilation
   Tidal volume

SURGICAL PROCEDURES

Craniotomy; burr holes
Cranioplasty
Craniectomy
Cordotomy
Sympathectomy
Laminectomy
Ventriculostomy

DIAGNOSTIC PROCEDURES

Numerous procedures, both invasive and noninvasive, performed for neurologic diagnostics; general guidelines for preprocedure preparation and postprocedure observations/interventions are listed

Preprocedure preparation

For all tests or procedures patient and family or significant others should be fully informed of the nature of the procedure, its rationale, and risks involved
Reinforce physician's explanation
Explain procedure and any sensations or discomforts that will be experienced during and after procedure
Reinforce importance of cooperation and immobility of patient for appropriate procedures
Determine patient's allergies to iodine or procaine, or kidney function when indicated
Whenever possible, be present to provide physical and emotional support during procedure

Postprocedure observations/interventions

Changes in level of consciousness or orientation
Changes in any neurologic functions: speech, range of motion (ROM), visual acuity, sensory function
For vascular procedures: observe for hemorrhage, bleeding, and stability in vital signs
Maintain positioning postprocedurally as indicated
Restrict fluids and/or foods as ordered
Maintain bed rest as ordered
Measure intake and output
Control pain as indicated

GLASGOW COMA SCALE (GCS)

Assessment scale designed to quickly and quantitatively relate level of consciousness to eye opening, motor response, and verbal responses
Scores of 9 or greater (14: normal) not indicative of coma; may be assigned to responses indicating increased arousal states; scores of 7 or less qualify as coma; lowest score of 3 is compatible with but not indicative of brain death

EYE OPENING

a.	Open spontaneously	4
b.	Open to voice	3
c.	Open to pain or noxious stimuli	2
d.	No response	1
	Unable to open eyes due to bandages or edema	

MOTOR RESPONSE

a.	Obeys simple commands	6
b.	Localizes pain	5
c.	Flexion withdrawal (pain)	4
d.	Abnormal flexion (pain); decorticate rigidity	3
e.	Abnormal extension (pain); decerebrate rigidity	2
f.	No motor response	0

VERBAL RESPONSE

a.	Oriented	5
b.	Confused	4
c.	Verbalizes; inappropriate word	3
d.	Vocalizes; incomprehensive words, sounds	2
e.	No verbal response	1

CARE OF PATIENT WITH ALTERED CONSCIOUSNESS

altered consciousness (lowered) *The state where alteration in the interaction of the cerebral hemisphere and the reticular activating system (RAS) results in an inability of the individual to relate to himself and his environment*

Assessment
Observations/findings

Level of consciousness
   GSC (see box): motor, verbal, eye opening
   Reflex eye movements
   Occulovestibular
   (See level of consciousness under Neurologic Assessment, p. 283)
Seizure activity
Cranial nerve assessment
Pulmonary
   Airway patency
      Secretions
      Artificial airway placement
      Positioning
   Respirations
      Quality
      Rate
      Character
   Breath sounds: equal or decreased
      Dullness
      Crackles
Cardiovascular
   Heart rate, rhythm, quality
   Peripheral pulses
   BP
Skin
   Color
   Temperature
   Turgor

Laboratory/diagnostic studies

Electrolytes, chemistry profile
    Fasting blood sugar (FBS)
    Sodium
    Potassium
    Calcium
    Phosphorus
    Magnesium
Serum ETOH (alcohol)
CSF
Arterial blood gas (ABG) studies
Intracranial pressure (ICP) may be elevated
Skull x-ray examination
Brain scan
NMR
Urine
    Toxicology screening
    Creatinine clearance

Potential complications

Aspiration, atelectasis
Pneumonia
Decubitus, constipation, contractures malnutrition
Respiratory failure/arrest
Increased ICP

Medical management

Oxygen/ventilatory support
Respiratory therapy
Fluids and electrolytes
ICP monitoring (Figure 5-4)
Nutritional support
Medications
    Diuretics
    Antihypertensives
    Antibiotics

Nursing diagnoses/goals/interventions

ndx: Potential for ineffective breathing pattern related to neuromuscular impairment

GOAL: *Patient will demonstrate an effective breathing pattern*

Maintain patent airway; avoid flexion of neck
Administer oxygen and humidification as indicated
Administer assisted ventilation as indicated
Check level of consciousness q15 min until respiratory status is sufficiently stable
Inspect, auscultate, and percuss chest frequently
Check rectal temperature q2h to 4h; cooling measures may be indicated
Provide oral nasopharyngeal airway as indicated for managing secretions; suction naso-oropharynx prn
Elevate head of bed to 30 degrees to maximize breathing potential
    Maintain in prone or semiprone position
    Turn side to side and prone q2h to optimize alveolar expansion

ndx: Self-care deficit: hygiene, nutrition, toileting, mobility, and/or self-protection related to alteration in cognitive process

GOAL: *Patient's self-care needs will be met*

Maintain nutritional balance
    Assess daily caloric and fluid requirements
    Administer high-calorie, high-protein tube feedings q2h to 3h as ordered
    Initiate hyperalimentation or intralipid therapy as indicated
Administer skin care q2h
    Use air mattress or egg crate mattress
    Rub back and pressure points with lanolin-based lotions
    Use cottonseed oil over feet and hands to prevent loss of cutaneous oil
    Keep linen taut, dry, and wrinkle-free
    Comb hair on daily basis; shampoo every week as indicated
    Keep nails clipped and clean
Perform passive ROM exercise to all extremities q2h to 4h and prn; involve large (arms, legs) and small (fingers, toes) muscle groups
Maintain safety for restless patient
    Maintain side rails up when patient is unattended
    Use padded side rails if patient is restless or if seizures occur
    Provide hand mittens as indicated; remove q8h for hand care
    Provide soft restraints; contraindicated if seizures occur
Administer oral hygiene q2h to 4h and prn
    Remove dentures
    Brush teeth three times a day
    Clean mucous membranes with water and/or alkaline mouthwash
    Keep lips moist with cold creams or glycerin-type lipsticks
    Initiate oral lavages as indicated
    Inspect tongue daily for cuts or crusting
Perform eye inspection and care q4h
    Observe for signs of corneal ulcerations, keratitis, inflammation, or irritation
    Remove any formed crusts
    Cleanse with lubricating eye drops
    Close eyes and apply eye shield as necessary

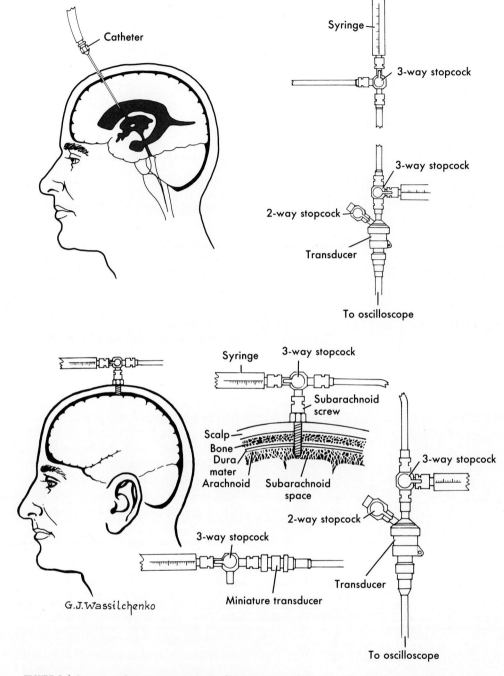

FIGURE 5-4. Intracranial pressure monitoring. (Modified from Rudy, E.B.: Advanced neurological and neurosurgical nursing, St. Louis, 1984, The C.V. Mosby Co.)

Apply topical ointments as indicated
Avoid positioning patient on side with eyes open
Administer nose care q4h to 5h
    Remove any formed crusts
    Apply ointment to nares
    Change nasal tube q72h as ordered; alternate nares

Inspect ears q4h to 6h for signs of dry or fresh drainage
    Report any fresh drainage to physician
    Remove crusts as ordered
Ensure elimination
    Connect indwelling catheter to closed gravity drainage as ordered

Use external catheters as ordered
Care for catheter q8h and prn
Check for bowel movement daily; if none, check for impaction q2d to 3d
Initiate bowel program
    Give mild cathartics q2d to 3d
    Give enemas as ordered

ndx: Ineffective family coping related to situational crisis

GOAL: *Family will maintain family process within limitations imposed by illness*

Provide emotional support for family or significant other
    Encourage verbalization of feelings of death, dying, and loss
    Encourage participation in patient care as desired
    Allow family to do small tasks for patient: combing hair, applying lotion, etc.
Call for spiritual counselor if requested

Patient teaching/discharge outcome

See standard of care for primary condition

Evaluation

Patient has a patent airway
Patient has a normal rate, rhythm, and pattern of breathing
Patient's needs for hygiene, elimination, and toileting are met
Patient is free of injury
Patient experiences normal ROM and joint mobility
Patient and family show adaptation to and coping with the illness

SEIZURES

Involuntary motor movements characteristic of an underlying disease process, neurologic impairment, trauma, or chronic disorder such as epilepsy; generally, are transitory and often involve disturbances in consciousness as well as motor-sensory and/or autonomic function

Assessment
Observations/findings

Assess patient for characteristics before, during, and after seizure activity
Document time, length, and body parts involved
Loss of consciousness or alteration in consciousness
Motor activity

GENERALLY RECOGNIZED SEIZURE CLASSIFICATIONS

GENERALIZED
Tonic clonic (grand mal)
Absence (petit mal)
Myoclonic
Akinetic

PARTIAL
Motor: focal motor (Jacksonian), simple partial
Sensory
Psychomotor: temporal lobe, complex partial

Tonic, clonic
Jerking, patting, rubbing movements
Sudden, brief contractions of muscle groups
Fluttering of eyelids
Facial jerking
Lip smacking
Movements may be confined to one area or may spread from one side to the other
Head and eyes deviate to the side
Respiratory function
    Tachypnea
    Apnea
    Difficulty in breathing
    Occluded airway

Laboratory/diagnostic studies

EEG
Echoencephalogram
Cerebral angiography
CT brain scan/magnetic resonance imaging (MRI)
Urine screening
FBS
Blood urea nitrogen (BUN)
Serum ETOH
Chemistries
    Magnesium levels
    Ammonia

Potential complications

Physical trauma, self-inflicted injury
Aspiration pneumonia
Respiratory function impairment
Status epilepticus

Medical management

Oxygen therapy
Medications (Table 5-3)

TABLE 5-3. Drugs Used in Seizure Disorders

Drug	Plasma therapeutic levels	Average daily dose	Side and toxic effects
Acetazolamide (Diamox)		1-3 g 750 mg	Drowsiness; aplastic anemia; headache; paresthesia
Carbamazepine (Tegretol)	4-10 µg/ml	450-700 mg (maximum dose 1200 mg); children: 20-30 mg/kg	Skin rash; blurred vision; ataxia; bone marrow depression
Clonazepam (Clonopin)	40-100 µg/ml	1.5-20 mg; children: 100-200 µg/kg/day	Drowsiness; ataxia; anorexia; behavior changes
Diazepam (Valium)		8-30 mg	Drowsiness; ataxia
Ethosuximide (Zarontin)	40-90 µg/ml	500-1500 mg; children: 20-40 mg/kg	Drowsiness; aplastic anemia; headache; lethargy
Mephenytoin (Mesantoin)		200-600 mg; children: 100-400 mg	Nystagmus; ataxia; skin rashes; serious toxicity common; pancytopenia
Methsuximide (Celontin)		300-600 mg	Drowsiness; ataxia; anorexia aplastic anemia
Paramethadione (Paradione)		300-900 mg	Nephrotoxicity; neutropenia
Phenobarbital (Luminal)	20-40 µg/ml	80-120 mg; adults: 60-250 mg; children: 3-6 mg/kg	Drowsiness; ataxia; nystagmus
Phenytoin, sodium diphenylhydantoin (Dilantin)	10-20 µg/ml	300 mg or 4-7 mg/kg/day	Drowsiness; ataxia; nausea; rash; gingival hyperplasia; nystagmus; anemia
Primidone (Mysoline)	7-15 µg/ml	750-1500 mg; children: 10-25 mg/kg	Drowsiness; ataxia
Timethadione (Tridione)		900-1200 mg/day; children: 900 mg/day	Bone marrow depression; dermatitis; photophobia; irritability
Valproic acid (Depakene)	50-100 µg/ml	1000-3000 mg; children: 15-60 mg/kg	Nausea hepatotoxicity

    Anticonvulsants
    Sedatives
    Barbiturates

Nursing diagnoses/goals/interventions

ndx: Potential for ineffective breathing pattern related to neurogenic impairment

GOAL: *Patient will demonstrate an effective breathing pattern*

Preseizure

Keep oral airway at bedside
Have suction equipment readily available
Administer oxygen if ordered

Postseizure

Maintain airway
Suction oropharynx as indicated prn
Administer oxygen as ordered

Check BP, P, and R and do neuro check immediately after seizure and prn
Continue with preconvulsive care as indicated
Note frequency, time, level of consciousness, body parts involved, and length of seizure activity
Be prepared for administration of diazepam, intubation IV therapy, and nasogastric suction for status epilepticus
Administer medications as ordered (Table 5-3)
    Anticonvulsants
    Sedatives

ndx: Potential for injury related to rapid onset of altered state of consciousness and seizure activity

GOAL: *Patient will be free of injury*

When patient is on bed rest, pad side rails
If out of bed during seizure activity, assist patient to floor and remove objects of potential harm

Observe patient carefully after seizure
Maintain effective respiratory pattern and patent airway
Assess patient for injury carefully, noting oral cavity
Assess in postictal phase for
  Altered level of consciousness
  Headache
  Malaise
  Nausea, vomiting
  Muscular soreness, backache, or back weakness
  Aspiration
    Choking, difficulty in breathing, cyanosis
    Decreased or absent breath sounds
    Tachycardia
    Tachypnea
    Pneumonia
Check pulse and pupils immediately after seizure activity
Provide emotional support
Inform patient of seizure and reorient if necessary
Resume routine activity

ndx: Knowledge deficit regarding disease process

GOAL: *Patient and/or significant other will demonstrate understanding of home care and follow-up instructions through interactive discussion and actual return demonstration*

Teach patient and family to recognize seizure activity and course of action to take
  Avoid restraining or interrupting behavior
  Observe and record behaviors exhibited during preictal and convulsive phases
Teach patient and family nature of disorder and need to attempt to adopt positive attitude toward patient's life and treatment
Dispel and clarify common fears and myths about convulsive disorders
  Epilepsy is not a form of insanity
  It does not get progressively worse
Emphasize importance of communication between patient and family regarding feelings of shame and humiliation associated with epilepsy
Explain importance of identifying aura and course of action to take
Explain need to identify and avoid stimuli that can stimulate onset of seizure activity
  Flickering lights
  Certain sounds
  Certain types of food
  Full bladder
Discuss medications: name, dosage, frequency of administration, purpose, and toxic or side effects
Explain need to avoid taking over-the-counter medications without checking with physician

Explain importance of maintaining regularity of diet, exercise, and all activity
Explain importance of well-balanced diet; avoid excessive use of alcohol
Explain to family
  Need to encourage patient to continue with normal routines, such as work, recreation, and other outside interests
  Need to avoid being overprotective; assure patient and family that activity often inhibits seizure activity
Explain need to avoid excessive physical and emotional excitement or stress; need to avoid stimulants and alcohol
Explain need to wear or carry medical alert band or card re epileptic
Discuss available agencies for use as references, such as Epilepsy Foundation of America*
Educate patient regarding possible limitations or restrictions of driving privileges

Children

Discuss child's needs with parents
  To have an understanding about condition
  To participate actively in care and treatment
  To avoid rigid restrictions and overprotection
Emphasize importance of allowing child to attend regular school and engage in normal activities with other children
Stress need to inform school nurse and/or teacher of
  Patient's epileptic status
  Child's understanding of the disorder
  Treatment to implement should seizure occur while child is at school

Evaluation

Patient demonstrates a patent airway
Patient has clear breath sounds
Patient is free of injury
Patient and/or significant other demonstrates knowledge and understanding of home care and disease management

CEREBROVASCULAR DISRUPTIONS

Alterations in cerebrovascular circulation; causes— ruptured cerebral aneurysm, hypertensive intracerebral hemorrhage, ruptured arteriovenous malformation, or cerebral infarction; may be classified as ischemic and hemorrhagic and may be

---

*Epilepsy Foundation of America, 4351 Garden City Dr., Landover, Md. 20785.

commonly termed stroke or cerebrovascular accident (CVA); assessment and intervention depend on location and timing (before or after rupture or leak)

Assessment

Observations/findings

ISCHEMIC

Altered level of consciousness
- Vertigo
- Drowsiness
- Stupor
- Mental confusion
- Disorientation
- Irritability
- Coma

Visual disturbances
- Diplopia
- Ptosis
- Monocular blindness
- Photophobia

Sensory disturbances
- Tingling
- Numbness
- Tinnitus

Motor disturbances
- Paresis
- Weakened reflexes
- Hemiplegia

Dysphasia
Aphasia
Nausea, vomiting
Elevated T and BP
Tachycardia
Tachypnea
Positive Kernig's and Brudzinski's signs

HEMORRHAGIC

Symptoms generally abrupt in onset
Altered level of consciousness
- Headaches (may be severe)
- Vertigo
- Mental confusion
- Irritability
- Stupor
- Drowsiness
- Coma

Altered visual, auditory, and/or sensory disturbances
Ocular disturbances
Hemiplegia
Nausea, vomiting
Sweating and/or chills
Fever
Nuchal rigidity

Laboratory/diagnostic studies

CSF evaluation (may not be performed because of elevated ICP)
Elevated pressure
Xanthochromic to grossly bloody
Clotting studies
CT scan
Cerebral angiography
X-ray examinations
Brain scan
NMR
Cerebral blood flow studies
Carotid Doppler flow studies

Potential complications

Neuromuscular deficit: mild to severe
- Paresis
- Paralysis

Major cognitive deficit
Respiratory failure
Increased ICP

Medical management

Ischemic

Parenteral therapy
Medications
- Anticonvulsants
- Antiplatelet aggregation
- Antihypertensives
- Corticosteroids
- Diuretics
- Antihistimines
- Narcotic analgesic

Ventilatory support when indicated
Cardiac monitoring
Seizure precautions
Intracranial pressure monitoring
Nutritional support

Hemorrhagic

Ventilatory/oxygen support
Complete activity restriction
Control of ICP
Fluid restrictions
Medications
- Osmotic diuretics
- Aminocaproic acid therapy
- Codeine

Hyperventilation
Hypothermia

Nursing diagnoses/goals/interventions

ndx Alteration in cerebral tissue perfusion related to ischemic or hemorrhagic injury

GOAL: *Patient will maintain or regain optimal cerebral tissue perfusion within physiologic limitations*

Maintain bed rest with head of bed elevated 15 to 60 degrees
Check BP, P, and R and do neuro check q15 to 30 min to assess alterations in circulatory status
Report any sudden changes in BP, pupillary, or neurologic status immediately
Check rectal temperature q2h to 4h; hypothermia or cooling measures may be indicated
Maintain parenteral fluids as ordered

ndx: Self-care deficit: toileting, hygiene, and/or mobility related to altered neurologic functioning

GOAL: *Patient's self-care needs will be met*

Limit activities and perform nursing functions as indicated
Perform passive ROM exercises to all extremities if allowed within activity restrictions
Turn patient gently q2h to 4h
Avoid straining and constipation
Provide nutritional support as ordered
    Assess chewing and swallowing abilities; monitor for aspiration
    Maintain adequate hydration
Provide for physical hygiene
    Promote self-care as indicated
    Maintain skin, eye, oral, and perineal care
Maintain elimination needs
    Check time and amount of voiding
    Initiate voiding measures as needed
    Assess bowel sounds
    Keep stools soft; avoid straining and constipation

ndx: Sensory-perceptual alterations related to altered cerebral vascular perfusion

GOAL: *Patient will demonstrate minimal sensory-perceptual alterations*

Maintain method of communication
Provide for social interaction
Maintain safe environment
Provide orientation and appropriate level of stimuli

ndx: Potential for alteration in airway clearance related to perceptual or cognitive impairment

GOAL: *Patient will maintain a patent airway*

Position patient to maximize airway patency and ventilatory exchange
Provide oral or nasopharyngeal airway if indicated
Suction prn
Assess rate and rhythm of respirations
Auscultate lungs
Assess for restlessness and confusion as indicators of hypoxia
Monitor ABG
Administer oxygenation/ventilatory support as indicated
Hyperventilate, cough, and deep breathe q1h to 2h

ndx: Knowledge deficit regarding disease process and home management

GOAL: *Patient and/or significant other will understand the diagnosis, medical and surgical management, and will demonstrate understanding of physical care management*

Discuss medications: name, dosage, frequency of administration, purpose, and toxic or side effects
Explain need to avoid taking over-the-counter medications without checking with physician
Encourage verbalization; help patient understand nature of disorder
Explain need to increase activities as ordered
Explain importance of physical activity as tolerated
Explain need for planned rest periods
Discuss need for speech therapy when appropriate
Discuss symptoms of progression of condition to report to physician
Explain importance of ongoing outpatient care

Evaluation

Patient demonstrates effective cerebral perfusion
    Is oriented to time, person, and place
    There is no alteration in consciousness
    Vital signs are normal
Patient demonstrates effective sensory perceptual function
    Has effective hearing, speech, and ROM
    Has an effective communication method
Patient's self-care needs are met
    Fluid and nutritional needs are met
    Elimination needs are met
    Skin, oral, and eye hygiene needs are met
    Passive or active ROM is performed
Patient's ventilatory status is maintained
    Airway is patent
    Breath sounds remain clear
    Breathing rate and pattern are normal
Patient and/or significant other demonstrates knowledge and understanding of home care management
    Demonstrates passive or active ROM exercises
    States all relevant information regarding medications, time of dose, side effects, and purpose

Identifies high-calorie, high-protein food and states understanding of need for maintenance of diet
States understanding of fluid intake maintenance to avoid infection risk and constipation

CEREBROVASCULAR ACCIDENT (CVA)

Decreased blood flow to part of the brain due to occlusion or stenosis of the blood vessels from embolism, thrombosis, or hemorrhage (NOTE: Symptoms depend on location and size of lesion)

Assessment
Observations/findings

Altered level of consciousness
Presence or absence of movement of extremities; may be of sudden onset or gradual
Loss of sensation and reflexes
    Usually unilateral
    May be temporary or permanent
Generalized weakness
Noisy respirations: Cheyne-Stokes (see Table 5-1)
Pupil inequality
Ptosis of eyelid
Visual loss
Drooping mouth
Elevated temperature
Elevated BP
Paralysis: may be unilateral or bilateral
Language and communication dysfunction
    Aphasia
    Apraxia
    Agnosia
Dysphagia
Aspiration
Dehydration
Bladder and bowel incontinence
Nausea and vomiting
Nuchal rigidity
Bruits on auscultation

Laboratory/diagnostic studies

CSF (perform with caution)
    Elevated pressure
    Elevated protein level
    Serum electrolytes
    ABG
    ESR
CT scan
MRI
Cerebral arteriography
EEG
Brain scan
Digital subtraction angiography
B-mode ultrasound
Skull x-ray examination
Echoencephalography
Doppler ultrasonography

Potential complications

Herniation
Aspiration, atelectasis
Increased ICP
Respiratory failure
Seizure activity
Cardiac arrhythmia
Neurologic deficit: mild to severe
    Paresis
    Paralysis
Malnutrition
Contractures, ankylosis

Medical management

Airway patency support
    Oxygen/assisted ventilation
    Tracheostomy
Bed rest
Nutritional and fluid management
Medications
    Antihypertensives
    Antifibrinolytics
    Antispasmodics
    Anticonvulsants
    Anticoagulants
    Analgesics
    Antipyretics
    Corticosteriods
Electrocardiogram (ECG) and cardiac monitoring
Hypothermia
ICP monitor

Nursing diagnoses/goals/interventions

ndx: Ineffective airway clearance related to inability to maintain secretions

GOAL: *Patient will have airway patency*

Position body and head to avoid obstruction of airway and provide optimal secretion removal
Suction secretions prn
Provide oral or nasopharyngeal airway to maintain airway patency
Auscultation chest for breath sounds q2h to 4h
See Care of Patient with Altered Consciousness (p. 288)

Neurologic System

Administer oxygen/humidification as ordered
Provide mechanical ventilation as ordered
Monitor arterial blood gases and hemoglobin

ndx: Impaired physical mobility related to impaired neurophysiologic function

GOAL: *Patient will maintain or regain maximal neuromuscular function of affected limbs*

Maintain body alignment; use bedboard, air mattress, or footboard as indicated (Figure 5-5)
Assist and teach patient to turn, cough, and deep breathe q2h to 4h; pull sheet may be indicated
When patient is on side, support with pillows; may use hand rolls and arm splints as ordered (Figure 5-5)
Perform active and/or passive ROM exercise to all extremities q2h to 4h and prn
Perform quadriceps setting and gluteal exercises q4h
Perform hand, finger, and foot exercises
  Squeeze rubber sponge ball
  Perform extension and flexion
  Perform extension of fingers, legs, and feet
Assist patient with using supportive devices as indicated: overhead trapeze, braces, wheelchair, canes, walker
Explain need to avoid use of slings
Encourage use of involved side when possible

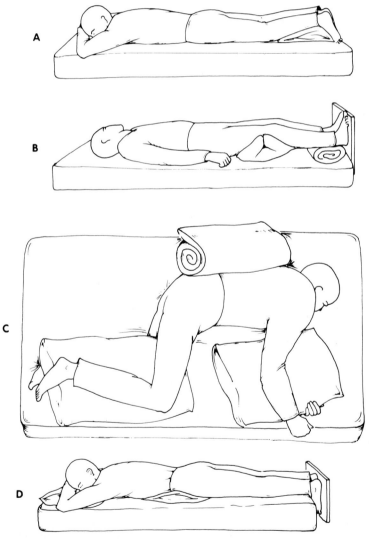

FIGURE 5-5. Various body positions to maintain correct alignment. **A,** Prone position. **B,** Supine position. **C,** Side-lying position. **D,** Prone position with support of feet.

Instruct patient to use good extremity to support weaker side (e.g., lift involved left leg with good right leg or lift involved left arm with good right arm)
Encourage patient to perform basic ADLs as soon as possible using unaffected side
  Bathing
  Brushing teeth
  Combing hair
  Eating
Begin progressive ambulation as ordered; assist to sitting position—begin with transfer procedure from bed to chair to regain position sense

ndx: Self-care deficit: hygiene, feeding, and/or toileting related to impaired physical mobility and alteration in cognitive process

GOAL: *Patient will manage own self-care needs*

Administer skin care q4h to 5h
  Use oil-based lotions
  Inspect area over bony prominences daily for any breakdown
Maintain bed rest; assist patient in assuming position of comfort
  Maintain body alignment
  Avoid neck flexion
  Use footboard (Figure 5-5)
Provide for total physical hygiene as indicated
Elevate affected limbs on pillow
Assist and teach patient to turn q2h; maintain on side as much as possible; avoid positioning on affected side for periods longer than 30 min
Administer tube feeding as ordered
Maintain oral feedings as ordered
  Progress from clear liquids
  Assist with feedings as necessary
  Observe for difficulty in swallowing
  Position on side with head of bed elevated if feeding patient in bed
Encourage fluid intake to 2000 ml daily unless contraindicated; apply antiembolic stockings, avoid leg massage

ndx: Sensory-perceptual alterations related to impaired transmission and/or integration secondary to neurologic deficit

GOAL: *Patient's physical and emotional needs related to sensory-perceptual impairment will be met*

Provide emotional support; explain all procedures and treatments as they occur
Orient patient frequently to time and place
Be positive and reassuring in approach
Anticipate needs of patient
Recognize and accept behavioral changes: depression, frustration, crying
Establish means of communication
  Call bell within reach
  Pad and pencil or Magic Slate
  Word board
  Symbols and gestures
  One-word commands
Maintain safe environment
  Use side rails
  Use protective vest restraints
Explain importance of beginning activity as soon as it is safe
Explain need for regular exercise program to maintain joint mobility: ROM exercises to all body joints q2h to 4h (Figures 5-6 and 5-7)

ndx: Knowledge deficit regarding disease process

GOAL: *Patient and significant other will demonstrate understanding of home care and follow-up instructions through interactive discussion and actual return demonstration*

Explain to family
  Need to encourage as many independent activities as possible; be alert to limitations
  Need to set realistic, achievable goals
  Need to avoid being overprotective
  Need to praise any tasks accomplished
  Importance of dealing with body image changes and behavioral changes
  Need to allow patient to be expressive
Encourage diversional activities
  Reading to patient
  Watching television
  Listening to radio
Plan regular rest periods; avoid fatigue
Encourage verbalization and communication between patient and family
Be sympathetic to emotional upsets, but be firm in carrying out regimen
Reinforce physician's explanation of medical management
Stress importance of ongoing outpatient care and follow-up visits
Stress importance of continuation of exercise program
Instruct patient and significant other in proper dietary and fluid needs
Stress importance of safety measures: side rails, ramps, flat shoes, removal of scatter rugs

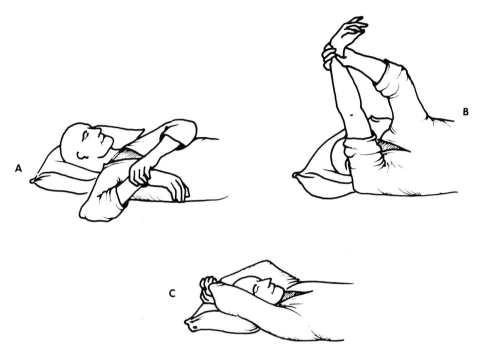

FIGURE 5-6. Range of motion of affected shoulder and elbow.

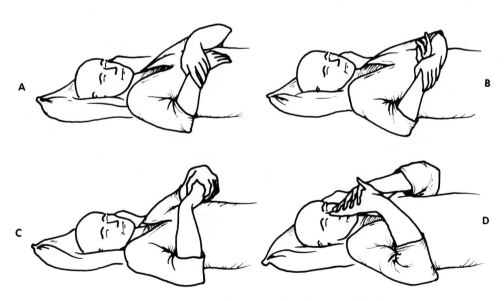

FIGURE 5-7. Range of motion of affected wrist and hand.

Evaluation

Patient demonstrates a patent airway
   Chest expansion is symmetric
   Breath sounds are clear to auscultation
   ABGs and vital signs are within normal limits
   There are no signs of respiratory distress
Patient demonstrates maximal physical mobility within physiologic limitations
Patient functions at an optimal level of orientation
Patient remains free of injury
Patient demonstrates skin integrity
Patient's self-care deficits are minimal
Patient's sensory-perceptual needs are met appropriately to accommodate physiologic status
Patient and/or significant other demonstrates knowledge and understanding of home care management
   Demonstrates passive and/or active ROM exercises
   States all relevant information regarding medications, time of dose, side effects, and purpose
   Identifies high-calorie, high-protein food and states understanding of need for maintenance of diet
   States understanding of fluid intake maintenance to avoid infection risk and constipation

BRAIN TUMORS

Abnormal growths of primary, metastatic, or developmental origin occurring within the brain or supporting structures

Assessment

Observations/findings

Headache: localized or general; may increase with activity
Dizziness occurring with position change; vertigo
Altered level of consciousness
Decreased response to verbal and painful stimuli
Inability to follow commands
Mental or personality changes
   Irritability
   Forgetfulness
   Loss of memory
   Impaired judgment
   Depression
Pupils: unequal response to light
Diplopia
Blurring or decreased vision
Ptosis
Tinnitus
Loss of hearing
Weakness or paralysis of face and/or extremities
Discoordination of extremities
Paresthesia
Gait
   Staggering
   Uncoordinated
   Wide-based walking
Difficulty in chewing with dysphagia
Vomiting with or without nausea
Aphasia
Agraphia (inability to express oneself in writing)
Obesity

ACCORDING TO LOCATION

FRONTAL LOBE

Inappropriate affective responses; memory loss
Lack of concern; moral laxity
Facetiousness
Impaired sphincter control
Focal seizures
Headaches

TEMPORAL LOBE

Visual phenomenon: "deju vu"
Auditory disturbances: "auditory agnosia"
Psychomotor seizure
Olfactory or gustatory hallucinations
Sensory aphagia
Dysphagia

OCCIPITAL LOBE

Visual disturbances
   Hemianopsia (blindness of one half of visual field)
   Central blindness
   Cortical blindness and anosognosia
   Visual hallucinations

CEREBELLUM

Uncoordination: ataxia
Loss of equilibrium

PARIETAL LOBE

Sensory loss
Apraxia
Body perceptional disorders

ACCORDING TO TYPE

GLIOMAS (ASTROCYTOMAS)

Occurring in cerebral hemispheres
Headache
Vomiting
Personality changes; irritable, apathetic

ACOUSTIC NEUROMAS

Vertigo
Ataxia
Parasthesia and weakness of face (cranial nerves V, VII)
Loss of corneal reflex
Decreased sensitivity to touch or pain (cranial nerves V, XI)
Unilateral hearing loss
Vertigo

MENINGIOMAS

Seizures
Unilateral exophthalmos
Extraocular muscle palsy
Visual disturbances
Olfactory disturbances
Paresis

PITUITARY ADENOMAS

Acromegaly
Hypopituitarism: decreased thyroid, pancreatic, and gonadal function
Cushing's syndrome
Female: amenorrhea, sterilization
Male: loss of libido, impotence
Visual disturbances
Diabetes mellitus
Hypothyroidism
Hypoadrenalism
Diabetes insipidus
Inappropriate antidiuretic hormone (IADH)

Laboratory/diagnostic studies

Physical and neurologic examination
Visual fields examination
NMR
Skull x-ray examination
Lumbar puncture
EEG
Echoencephalography
CT scan
Cerebral angiography
Hyperglycemia
CSF: elevated protein

Potential complications

Herniation
Elevated BP
Seizure activity
Neurologic deficit: mild to severe

Increased ICP
Alteration in respiratory function
Alteration in consciousness
Personality change

Medical management

Surgical excision
Medications
    Antineoplastic agents
    Corticosteroids
    Anticonvulsants
    Antibiotics
Radiation therapy
Fluid/electrolyte therapy
Oxygenation/ventilatory support
Nutritional support
ICP monitoring
Cardiac monitoring
Neurologic rehabilitation

Nursing diagnoses/goals/interventions

ndx: Potential for injury related to changes in ICP and sensory-perceptual function

GOAL: *Patient will remain free of injury*

Obtain baseline history of signs and symptoms to observe for progression
Note level of consciousness q4h to 5h and prn
Utilize Glasgow Coma Scale for rapid assessment (p. 288)
Note quality and strength of facial muscles and extremities q4h to 5h
Check BP, P, and R, and do neuro check q2h to 4h and prn
Maintain seizure precautions
Maintain safe environment
    Use side rails with padding as indicated
    Use soft restraints
Maintain quiet environment
Check rectal temperature q2h to 4h; hypothermia or cooling measures may be indicated
Maintain parenteral fluids as ordered
Control pain
Establish means of communication as necessary
    Call bell within reach
    Pad and pencil or Magic Slate
Deal with mental and personality changes
    Allow patient time to eat and to complete all activities: walking, dressing, bathing
    Orient patient to surroundings as necessary
Provide emotional support

Explain all procedures and treatments, using vocabulary understood by patient
Allow patient and family to assist in planning and implementing care
Explain that changes in behavior and speech may be uncontrollable and part of disease process
Explain and prepare for diagnostic tests when ordered
Prepare for treatment as ordered
  Radiation therapy
  Surgery
  Neurologic rehabilitation

ndx: Self-care deficit: hygiene, feeding, toileting, and/or mobility related to perceptual, cognitive, and/or neurologic impairment

GOAL: *Patient's self-care needs will be met*

Administer oral hygiene prn
Administer skin care
Administer eye care
  Remove any formed crusts
  Apply water-based eye drops as ordered
Familiarize patient with surroundings if eyesight and/or visual fields are impaired
Ensure elimination
  Use external or indwelling catheter as indicated
  Initiate voiding measures as necessary
  Avoid constipation and straining through use of stool softeners or mild laxatives
Maintain diet as ordered
Feed and assist with nutritional intake as needed
Ambulate as tolerated; assist as necessary with wheelchair, walker, or cane
If patient is unable to ambulate, assist and teach patient to turn, cough, and deep breathe q2h and prn
Elevate head of bed to 30 to 45 degrees
Perform active and passive ROM exercises to all extremities q4h to 5h

ndx: Knowledge deficit regarding disease process and home management

GOAL: *Patient and/or significant other will demonstrate understanding of home care and follow-up instructions through interactive discussion and actual return demonstration*

Reinforce physician's explanation of the disease and its causes, symptoms, and treatment
Discuss medications: name, dosage, frequency of administration, purpose, and toxic or side effects
Explain need to avoid taking over-the-counter medications without checking with physician
Explain need for well-balanced diet
Explain need for ongoing rehabilitation therapy
Explain importance of physical exercise program

Evaluation

Patient remains free of injury
  Respiratory function is adequate
  Patient is free of symptoms of increased intracranial pressure
Patient's self-care needs are met
  Nutritional status is adequate
  Elimination needs are met
  Skin integrity is maintained
Patient and/or significant other demonstrates knowledge and understanding of home care management and disease process
  Demonstrates passive or active ROM exercises
  States all relevant information regarding medications, time of dose, side effects, and purpose
  Identifies high-calorie, high-protein food; states understanding of need for maintenance of diet
  States understanding of fluid intake maintenance to avoid infection risk and constipation

CRANIOCEREBRAL TRAUMA

Any sudden impact or blow to the head with or without loss of consciousness; the following are types of head injuries

linear fracture *A break in the continuity of bone without displacing bone tissue*
comminuted fracture *Multiple breaks leading to fragmentation of bone*
depressed fracture *Bone fragments displaced below the surface of the skull*
compound fracture *A fracture complicated by laceration of surrounding scalp or membranes*
concussion *Shock of brain soft tissue without bruising or lacerations; accompanied by temporary memory loss and amnesia lasting approximately 48 hr*
contusion *Shock of brain soft tissue with bruising and laceration; accompanied by loss of consciousness and amnesia; patient may exhibit varying degrees of consciousness: stupor, agitation, disorientation, coma*
coup-contracoup phenomenon *Brain injury due to acceleration type of injury causing contusion and laceration in areas remote or opposite from the site of impact*
subdural hematoma *An accumulation of blood between the arachnoid and dura mater due to contusion or laceration of subdural blood vessels; symptoms (headaches, increasing drowsiness, seizures, unilateral pupil dilation) may not occur for weeks or months*

epidural hematoma *Bleeding in the epidural space between the skull and dura mater; usually involves a temporoaparietal fracture, which causes a lacerated middle meningeal artery; transient loss of consciousness occurs and is followed by lucid periods; patient then lapses into unconsciousness again with signs of rapidly developing increased ICP; this is usually a surgical emergency*

Assessment
Observations/findings

Altered level of consciousness; periods of consciousness followed by unconsciousness
Headache
Dizziness, vertigo
Posturing
  Decorticate rigidity
  Decerebrate rigidity
  Motor and/or sensory movement of extremities: unilateral, bilateral
  Weakness, paresis, paralysis, stimulus, response
Mental changes
  Irritability
  Restlessness
  Confusion
  Delirium
  Stupor
  Coma
Pupillary response
  Size, equality, response to light
  Corneal reflex
Brainstem integrity
  EOM (extraoccular movement), gag or swallow reflex
Airway patency
  Rate and rhythm of respirations
  Breathing pattern
  Secretion management
Unequal pupils and uncoordinated eye movement
Periocular edema
Seizure activity
Hematemesis
Projectile vomiting
Lacerations and abrasions around head and face
Drainage from ears and nose
Elevated temperature
Elevated or decreased BP
Increased weakness
Paresis or paralysis
Facial asymmetry
Aphasia
Nuchal rigidity
Dehydration
Polyuria

Laboratory/diagnostic studies

Skull x-ray examinations
Cervical x-ray examinations
CT scan
CSF sampling (may be contraindicated)
ABGs
Serum electrolytes
CBC
EEG
Echoencephalogram

Potential complications

Increased ICP
Hemorrhage
Herniation
Respiratory failure
Neurologic deficit: mild to severe
  Paresis
  Paralysis

Medical management

Respiratory management
Oxygenation/mechanical ventilation with volume ventilation
Surgical repair
  Craniotomy
  Ventriculostomy
  Cranioplasty
  Shunting procedures
  Tracheostomy
Medications
  Anticonvulsants
  Diuretics
  Corticosterods
  Antibiotics
  Analgesics
ICP monitoring
Hypothermia
Cardiac monitoring
Fluid and electrolyte management
Nutritional support
Physical therapy
Rehabilitation

Nursing diagnoses/goals/interventions

ndx: Ineffective airway clearance related to impaired neurologic function

GOAL: *Patent airway will be maintained*

Maintain patent airway: endotracheal tube or tracheostomy as ordered; suction prn
Administer oxygen, humidification, or mechanical ventilation as ordered

Assess respiratory exchange by auscultation and inspection prn

Maintain $PaCO_2$ and PaO_2 as ordered to prevent hypoxia and hypercapnia

Assist patient in coughing and deep breathing when conscious

Maintain head of bed elevated to 30 degrees if patient is unconscious unless contraindicated to maximize airway patency and control secretions

Check BP, P, and R and GSC q15 to 30 min; report any pupillary or mental changes immediately, since changes may signal respiratory embarrassment

ndx: Self-care deficit: bathing, feeding, toileting, and/or mobility related to neurologic impairment

GOAL: *Patient's self-care needs will be provided for*

Administer oral hygiene q2h to 4h

Administer skin care q2h to prn

Provide for all hygiene needs as indicated

Maintain NPO for first 24 hr, progressing to clear liquids as ordered

Assess nutritional status
  Assess daily caloric intake
  Initiate intralipid or hyperalimentation as indicated
Maintain diet as tolerated; assist with feeding as indicated

Encourage fluids to 3000 ml daily unless contraindicated

Provide for patient's elimination needs

Initiate voiding measures as indicated

Instruct patient and family in exercise activities

Encourage early ambulation as ordered
  Structure day's activities, allowing for periods of rest
  Initiate progressive activity levels
Perform active or passive ROM exercises to all extremities

ndx: Potential for alteration in self-concept related to actual or perceived changes in physical and personal self-image

GOAL: *Patient's self-care needs will be met*

Provide emotional support; allow patient to verbalize needs and to participate in planning care

Encourage verbalization of feelings about body image and function changes

Provide for alternative communication methods if vocalization is impaired: Magic Slate, pencil and paper

ndx: Knowledge deficit regarding disease process and home management

GOAL: *Patient and/or significant other will demonstrate understanding of home care and follow-up instructions through interactive discussion and actual return demonstration*

Discuss nature of disorder, treatment, and procedures; explain as they occur

Explain to family need to encourage verbalization about any body image change or limitations

Explain need to ambulate as tolerated

Explain importance of planned rest periods

Discuss possible residual effects such as dizziness, headache, and memory loss, which may persist for 3 to 4 months after trauma

Discuss medications: name, dosage, frequency of administration, purpose, and toxic or side effects

Explain need to avoid taking over-the-counter medications without checking with physician

Discuss symptoms of progression of condition to report to physician

Explain importance of ongoing outpatient care
  Physician's visits
  Physical therapy
Explain importance of diet as ordered; need to chew and swallow slowly

Discuss care of abrasions or lacerations as indicated

Evaluation

Patient demonstrates an effective breathing pattern
  Chest expansion is symmetric
  Breath sounds are clear to auscultation
  ABGs and vital signs are within normal limits
  There are no signs of respiratory distress
Patient's self-care needs are met
  Medications are administered as ordered
  Fluid and nutritional needs are met
  Elimination needs are met
  Skin, oral, and eye hygiene needs are met
  Passive or active ROM is performed
  Planned rest periods are maintained
Patient accepts changes in self-concept, and body image

Patient and/or significant other demonstrates knowledge and ability needed for self-care and home management

SPINAL CORD INJURIES

cord injuries *Injuries in which the spinal cord is compressed by fracture or displaced vertebrae, bleeding, or edema*

cervical cord injuries *Level of injury is located in the cervial spine C_2 to C_6*

thoracic cord injuries *Level of injury is located in the thoracic spine T_1 to T_{12}*
lumbar cord injuries *Level of injury is located in the lumbar spine L_1 to L_2*

NOTE: Clinical descriptions of spinal cord injuries generally refer to deficits in terms of upper motor neuron (UMN) and lower motor neuron (LMN): UMN lesions involve injury above L_1 to L_2 and result in muscle spasticity and increased tendon reflexes; LMN injuries involve anterior horn cells or nerve fibers after their exit from the spinal cord and result in muscle flaccidity, loss of reflexes, loss of tone, and muscle atrophy (Table 5-4)

Assessment
Observations/findings
CORD INJURIES

Loss of power, movement, and sensation of extremities below level of injury
Pain at level of injury
Urinary retention
Priapism
Absence of vasomotor tone and perspiration in cervical and upper thoracic cord injuries

CERVICAL CORD INJURIES

Paralysis of all extremities and trunk
Respiratory failure: hypoxemia
Bladder and bowel disturbances
    Bladder retention, spasticity
    Bowel incontinence
Autonomic dysreflexia
    Bradycardia
    Sweating
    Elevated temperature
    Paroxysmal hypertension
    Headache

THORACIC CORD INJURIES

Paralysis of lower extremities; initially muscles are flaccid—later become spastic
Paralysis of bladder, bowel, and sphincters
Pain to chest or back
Abdominal distention
Loss of sexual function

LUMBAR CORD INJURIES

Paralysis of lower extremities, bladder, and rectum
    Flaccid muscles during spinal shock phase
    Spastic muscular activity
Loss of sexual function

Laboratory/diagnostic studies
Arterial blood gases
CBC with differential
Coagulation studies
Electrolytes
X-ray examination
Myelography
CT scan

Potential complications
Respiratory arrest
Spinal shock
    Decreased BP
    Tachycardia
    Loss of reflex activity below level of cord injury
    Urinary retention
    Paralytic ileus
    Fecal retention
Hemorrhage
Urinary tract infection
Paralytic ileus
Autonomic dysreflexia
Pneumonia, atelectasis

TABLE 5-4. Clinical Manifestations of Upper and Lower Motor Neuron Lesions

Upper motor neuron	Lower motor neuron
Muscle spasticity, possible contractures	Muscle flaccidity
Little or no muscle atrophy	Muscle atrophy
Hyperreflexia	Loss of muscle tone
Damage above level of brainstem will affect opposite side of the body	Hypoflexia or areflexia
	Fasciculations
	Muscle changes will be in muscles supplied by that nerve—usually muscle on same side as lesion

From Rudy, E.B.: Advanced neurological and neurosurgical nursing, St. Louis, 1984, The C.V. Mosby Co.

Malnutrition: acute or chronic
Decubitus
Contractures, ankylosis
Spasms
Foot-drop, wrist-drop
Behavioral changes
    Anxiety
    Grief reaction
    Acute depression

Medical management

Surgical decompression, stabilization
    Skull tongs (Crutchfield, Vinke, Gardner-Wells)
    Halo
    Traction
Ventilatory support
Medication
    Analgesics
    Antibiotics
    Steroids
Cardiac monitoring
Fluid/electrolyte management
Intake and output

Nursing diagnoses/goals/interventions

ndx: Ineffective breathing pattern related to neurogenic or traumatic injury

GOAL: *Patient will have a patent airway*

Maintain patent airway
Auscultate breath sounds
Administer assisted ventilation and oxygenation as ordered; measure vital capacity and minute ventilation to ensure adequate ventilation
Be aware that tracheostomy may be indicated
Provide nasal or oropharyngeal airway and suction as needed
Monitor vital signs and consciousness q1h to 2h as indicators of impaired ventilatory status
Assess motor-sensory function to ensure adequate rhythm or pattern of respiration

ndx: Self-care deficit: hygiene, feeding, toileting, and/or mobility related to neurophysiologic impairment

GOAL: *Patient's self-care needs will be met*

Maintain parenteral fluids as ordered
Maintain NPO until chewing, swallowing, and gastrointestinal (GI) function is established
Provide nutritional support as ordered
Connect indwelling catheter to closed gravity drainage as ordered
Check urine for presence of calculi
Administer catheter care bid
Give colon lavage or enemas q3d as ordered
Perform passive ROM exercises to extremities; check with physician before starting exercises
Administer oral hygiene q2h to 4h
Administer skin care q2h to 4h
    Give back rubs
    Use sheepskin
    Use footboard
    Use heel and/or elbow guards
Explain importance of daily exercises and planned rest periods
Explain importance of skin care
Teach muscle-building exercises
    Squeeze toys
    Rubber balls
    Clay
Use trapezes and pulleys

ndx: Potential for ineffective individual coping related to actual or perceived body self-image changes

GOAL: *Patient will utilize positive coping strategies*

Involve family or significant other in care and instructions
Explain nature of disorder and its limitations and allowances
Deal with body image changes, as well as fears and grief over loss of body function
Encourage communication between patient and family or significant other
Encourage socialization and visiting privileges
Encourage independence when possible; be aware of limitations
Provide emotional support
    Explain all treatments and procedures as they occur
    Be reassuring and positive in approach
    Encourage verbalization

ndx: Knowledge deficit regarding diagnosis and potential home management

GOAL: *Patient and significant other will demonstrate understanding of home care and follow-up instructions through interactive discussion and actual return demonstration*

Ensure that patient and significant other are informed about disease and prognosis
Prepare for chronicity and duration of rehabilitative process
Discuss medications: name, dosage, route, side effects, and purpose

Refer to appropriate rehabilitative and counseling resources

Evaluation

Patient demonstrates an effective breathing pattern
    Chest expansion is symmetric
    Breath sounds are clear to auscultation
    ABGs and vital signs are within normal limits
    There are no signs of respiratory distress
Patient's self-care needs are met
    Medications are administered as ordered
    Fluid and nutritional needs are met
    Elimination needs are met
    Skin, oral, and eye hygiene needs are met
    Passive or active range of motion is performed
    Planned rest periods are maintained
Patient and/or significant other demonstrates knowledge and understanding of home care management
    Demonstrates passive or active ROM exercises
    States all relevant information regarding medications, time of dose, side effects, and purpose
    Identifies high-calorie, high-protein foods and states understanding of need for maintenance of diet
    States understanding of fluid intake maintenance to avoid infection risk and constipation
Patient demonstrates effective coping
    States realistic goals and plans for the future
    Discusses feelings about physical limitations
    Identifies fears and concerns, and describes methods and resources for resolution

SURGICAL INTERVENTION OF CENTRAL NERVOUS SYSTEM

Surgical repair of conditions involving the brain, spinal cord, cranial nerves, and cerebral vasculature
craniotomy *Surgical revision, resection, or removal of growths or abnormalities within the cranium; consists of removing and replacing bones of the skull to provide access to intracranial structures*
craniectomy *Removal of a portion of the skull; includes burr hole performance*

Assessment

Postoperative observations/findings*

Level of consciousness
    See Glasgow Coma Scale for rapid assessment (p. 288)
    Pupillary response
    Visual disturbances

Motor-sensory
    Paresthesia
    Paralysis
Speech
Swallowing
Pulmonary
    Respirations
        Quality
        Rate
        Character
    Breath sounds: equal or decreased
        Dullness
        Rales
        Rhonchi
Cardiovascular: hemodynamic parameters
    Arterial BP
    HR, rhythm
Restlessness
Seizure activity
Peripheral vascular
    Peripheral pulses
    Skin temperature
    Color
    Pressure
Genitourinary, gastrointestinal
    Bowel sounds, distention
    Time and amount of voiding

Potential complications

Increased ICP
Hemorrhage
Shock
Aspiration
Respiratory failure
Paralysis

Medical management

Oxygenation/ventilatory support
Medications
    Corticosteroids
    Analgesics
    Diuretics
    Antibiotics
Parenteral therapy
Enteral therapy
ICP monitoring
Cardiac monitoring

Nursing diagnoses/goals/interventions

ndx: Potential for ineffective breathing pattern related to postanesthesia recovery and possible neurologic depression

---

*Generalized observations indicated are for the entirety of the nervous system; some procedures may require only partial assessments.

GOAL: *Patient will demonstrate an effective breathing pattern*

See Care of Patient in Recovery Room (p. 30)
Maintain patent airway
Report any change in vital signs, level of consciousness, or restlessness immediately
Administer oxygen with assisted ventilation as ordered
Monitor arterial blood gases
Maintain parenteral therapy as indicated
Assess ventilatory status
  Auscultate chest for breath sounds q1h to 2h and prn
  Maintain optimal positioning to promote ventilatory status and enhance CSF outflow
  Assist and teach patient to turn and deep breathe q2h

ndx: Alteration in cerebral/peripheral tissue perfusion related to interruption of arterial flow

GOAL: *Patient will maintain adequate cerebral/peripheral tissue perfusion*

Maintain bed rest with head of bed elevated 15 to 30 degrees or as ordered
Check BP, P, and R and do neuro check q15 to 30 min
Monitor ICP and report sustained or trends in elevations immediately
Report any sudden changes in BP, pupillary or neurologic status, numbness, tingling, or weakness or loss of pulses immediately
Assess for restlessness and seizure activity
Check rectal temperature q2h to 4h; hypothermia or cooling measures may be indicated
Maintain parenteral fluids as ordered
Maintain bed rest; use firm mattress or bedboard
Provide cervical collar or cervical traction as ordered
Keep head in neutral or slightly flexed position

ndx: Self-care deficit: feeding, hygiene, toileting, and/or mobility related to physical postoperative limitations

GOAL: *Patient's self-care needs will be met*

Maintain proper positioning as indicated by surgical restrictions
Limit activities and perform nursing functions as indicated
Maintain quiet environment
Administer skin care q4h to 5h
  Give back rubs
  Use air mattress (for patient in traction)
  Use sheepskin
  Check for redness, irritation, and pressure areas q2h to 4h when patient is in traction
  Provide additional padding and pressure reduction if indicated
  Keep skin dry
Provide passive or active ROM to nonoperative extremities
Maintain patient NPO until otherwise ordered
Provide fluid and/or diet within restrictions as ordered; assess for swallowing and chewing ability
Maintain adequate elimination
  Initiate voiding measures as appropriate
  Monitor time and amount

ndx: Knowledge deficit regarding disease process and potential home management

GOAL: *Patient and/or significant other will demonstrate understanding of home care and follow-up instructions through interactive discussion and actual return demonstration*

Explain nature of disorder, symptoms, and importance of maintaining traction, corset, or braces at home
Explain to family need to encourage verbalization; to deal with body image changes and anxieties over disability and loss of work
Teach principles of body mechanics
  Avoid bending from waist: keep back straight, bend knees, and lower body to pick up objects
  Use straight, flat chairs; avoid soft-cushioned chairs
  Avoid crossing knees
  Avoid lifting while back is flexed or twisted
Explain need to avoid constipation through use of stool softeners, mild laxatives, and/or fruit juices and roughage in diet
Explain need to avoid extremes of hot and cold to lower extremities because of possible sensory nerve loss
Explain need to avoid hyperextension of spine while sleeping; to avoid sleeping in prone position or straight supine position
Explain need to sleep on side with knees and hips in flexion
Explain need to wear corset or brace support as ordered
Explain need for exercise as ordered; instruct patient to stop exercises if pain is unrelieved or worsens
Explain importance of maintaining diet as ordered
Discuss medications: name, dosage, time of administration, purpose, and side effects
Explain need to avoid taking over-the-counter medications without checking with physician

Explain importance of ongoing outpatient care
    Physician's visits
    Physical therapy
Ensure that patient and/or significant other demonstrates proper use and maintenance of traction and corsets

Evaluation

Patient demonstrates an effective breathing pattern
    Chest expansion is symmetric
    Breath sounds are clear to auscultation
    ABGs and vital signs are within normal limits
    There are no signs of respiratory distress
Patient demonstrates no alteration in cerebral/peripheral tissue perfusion
    Is alert and oriented
    Cognitive processes are intact
    There is sensory-perceptual integrity
    Speech is normal; ROM is intact
Patient's self-care needs are met
    Medications are administered as ordered
    Fluid and nutritional needs are met
    Elimination needs are met
    Skin, oral, and eye hygiene needs are met
    Passive or active ROM is performed
    Planned rest periods are maintained
Patient and/or significant other demonstrates knowledge and understanding of home care management
    Demonstrates passive or active ROM exercises
    States all relevant information regarding medications, time of dose, side effects, and purpose
    Identifies high-calorie, high-protein food and states understanding of need for maintenance of diet
    States understanding of fluid intake maintenance to avoid infection risk and constipation

ALZHEIMER'S DISEASE

Progressive deterioration of intellect, memory, personality, and self-care, leading to severe dementia from degeneration of nerve cells in the cerebral cortex

Assessment

Observations/findings
MILD TO MODERATE

Memory loss
    Loss of orientation to time and location
    Inability to recognize close family and friends
    Lack of recent memories but can recall early life events
Personality changes
    Anxiety, fear, belligerence, stubbornness
    Suspicion progressing to paranoia
    Loss of sense of humor
    Insensitivity to others
Intellectual changes
    Difficulty in making decisions or plans
    Inability to calculate (e.g., money transactions)
    Loss of train of thought during conversations
    Requires repetitive directions
Conversation changes: slow speech, loss of words, use of cliches
Mood
    Reactive depression
    Crying spells
    Fatigues easily
    Lethargic
    Neglect of self-care
    Nocturnal wandering

ADVANCED

Apathetic, mute
Inability to recall recent or remote events
Disorientation
Inability to perform ADLs
Incontinence

Potential complications

Physical and/or psychologic dependence
Social isolation
Injury

Medical management

Supportive management
Physiologic and psychologic support measures for patient and family to enhance coping with progressive deterioration

Nursing diagnoses/goals/interventions*

ndx: Potential for injury related to physiologic deterioration of cognitive function

GOAL: *Patient will remain free of injury*

Maintain safety precautions
    Have attendant with patient during any treatment or procedure
    Remove or disconnect door locks
    Avoid use of razors without assistance
    Avoid potentially dangerous tasks (e.g., smoking, cooking)

---

*Care and teaching are combined to provide nurse and family with consistent approach.

Assist with ADLs prn
Maintain regular exercise/activity level with help
  Daily walks
  Use of rocking chair
Explain to patient and family the nature of this disorder; that this is progressive
Assist with reality orientation
  Introduce all care givers by name each time; repeat on regular basis
  Writing instructions and directions may be helpful
  Provide large-face clock and current calendar
  Orient patient to day, hour, and location frequently
Speak in quiet tones
Maintain calm atmosphere; avoid rushing
Use consistency and repetition with patient
Give singular, simple instructions

ndx: Self-care deficit: hygiene, nutrition, and/or toileting related to physiologic and/or psychologic dependence

GOAL: *Patient's self-care needs will be met*

Provide for physical hygiene needs
Provide properly balanced diet
Administer diet as ordered; present one course at a time (e.g., salad first, then entree)
Assist patient in cutting food as needed
Establish regular bowel habits
  Determine patient's normal patterns
  Instruct patient to go to bathroom at scheduled times
  Recognize signs of impaction
    No formed stool for 3 days
    Semiliquid stools
    Restlessness
  Discuss treatment for impaction: laxative, suppository, enema
Establish routine voiding measures
  Remind patient to go to bathroom q2h
  Avoid fluids before bedtime
  Use disposable diapers prn
Administer medications as ordered

ndx: Potential for ineffective family coping related to long-term deteriorating effects of disease process

GOAL: *Family and/or significant others will demonstrate ability to cope with disease process*

Provide emotional support
Refer family to support groups
Refer to social services for financial concerns and potential placement
Refer to home care services for potential in-home assistance for home maintenance and management problems
Ensure that family and/or significant others are informed about disease process and physician's instructions for supportive care

Evaluation

Patient is free of injury; has no physical injury resulting from trauma
Patient has intact skin
Patient's self-care needs are met
Patient has adequate nutritional intake
Patient's elimination needs are met
Family and/or significant others are coping effectively with home management
Proper resources are being utilized for patient care needs, counseling, and financial assistance

PARKINSON'S DISEASE

A progressive, degenerative disease of the brain's dopamine neuronal system, most commonly idiopathic in nature

Assessment
Observations/findings

Rigidity of limbs: arms lose natural swing and remain at side of body
Tremors
  Exaggerated by stress and anxiety
  Most severe when limb is resting; absent during sleep
  Fingers: pill-rolling movement
  Head: to-and-fro tremor
Movements
  Voluntary body movements become slower (bradykinesia)
  Starting activities become difficult (akinesia)
Posture
  Bent forward
  Walks with slow, short, shuffling steps
  May break into run if pushed
Uncoordinated and/or loss of muscular activity: impaired writing (micrographia)
See Musculoskeletal Assessment (p. 470)
Stiffness and diffuse pain in legs and shoulders
Blank facial expression (masked facies)
  Wide-eyed
  Infrequent blinking of eyes
Speech
  Slowed, monotonous

Dysarthric
Slurred
Soft spoken, decreased volume
Dysphagia
Excessive salivation and drooling
Emotional changes
- Depression
- Nervousness
- Mood swings
- Hallucinations
- Paranoia
- Dementia

Side effects of drugs
- Levodopa
  - Anorexia
  - Nausea, vomiting
  - Postural hypotension
  - Mental confusion
  - Memory loss
  - Behavioral changes
  - Cardiac arrhythmias
- Trihexyphenidyl (Artane)
  - Blurred vision
  - Vertigo
  - Tachycardia
  - Dizziness
  - Dry mouth

Laboratory/diagnostic studies

CSF
- Usually within normal limits
- May show slight increase in protein level

Mild microcytic anemia

GI studies
- Hypomotility
- Delayed emptying of stomach
- Varying degrees of bowel distention

EEG
- Normal with minimal slowing
- Marked or moderate slowing and/or disorganization (with marked dementia and bradykinesia)

Medical management

Surgical stereotactic thalamotomy to relieve contralateral tremor and rigidity*

Chemotherapeutic agents
- Levodopa
- Dopamine
- Anticholinergics

Tricyclic antidepressants (may decrease effectiveness of levodopa)
Sedatives
Antihistamines
Fluid and electrolyte management
Physical therapy
Occupational therapy
Speech therapy

Nursing diagnoses/goals/interventions

ndx: Impaired physical mobility related to neuromuscular deterioration

GOAL: *Patient will demonstrate optimal level of mobility*

Encourage ambulation to tolerance
Assist to chair
Perform active or passive ROM exercises q4h to all extremities
- Neck
- Hands and fingers
- Wrists
- Elbows
- Knees

Provide physical therapy as ordered: massage and stretching exercises
Have patient practice lifting legs while walking rather than shuffling; try to maintain erect posture
Maintain planned rest periods
Conduct occupational therapy as indicated by amount of tremors
Administer skin care q4h to 5h and prn; avoid oil-based lotions
Assist patient with turning q2h to 4h if unable to move self

ndx: Alteration in self-care ability: feeding, hygiene, toileting

GOAL: *Patient's self-care needs will be met*

Assist and teach patient to cough and deep breathe q4h to 6h and prn
Maintain well-balanced soft diet
Avoid foods and medications that contain pyridoxine HCl (vitamin B_6)
Maintain frequent small feedings as indicated
Maintain fluid intake to 2000 ml daily unless contraindicated
Maintain supplemental high-calorie fluids such as eggnog, milk shakes, and malts
Use bibs and straws as indicated; place food and drinks within easy reach of patient

---

*May be considered somewhat controversial.

Initiate voiding measures as necessary
Institute bladder control program as indicated
Avoid constipation through use of high-residue foods, stool softeners, and/or enemas
Provide or assist with general hygiene as indicated
Administer oral hygiene q4h to 6h and prn
Encourage self-care as tolerated: bathing, mouth care
Promote adequate pulmonary toilet by encouraging coughing and deep-breathing exercises

ndx: Potential for alteration in self-concept related to actual or perceived changes in physical and personal self-image

GOAL: *Patient will adapt to perceived or actual physical changes*

Provide emotional support; allow patient to verbalize needs and to participate in planning care
Encourage verbalization of feelings about body image and function changes
Provide for alternative communication methods if vocalization is impaired: Magic Slate, pencil and paper

ndx: Knowledge deficit regarding diagnosis and home maintenance

GOAL: *Patient and/or significant other will demonstrate understanding of home care and follow-up instructions through interactive discussion and actual return demonstration*

Reinforce physician's explanation of disease and its causes, symptoms, and treatment
Discuss importance of verbalization about loss of body function, self-esteem, and sexuality
Explain that behavioral changes may be part of disease process or may be due to medications
Emphasize need to discuss feelings about symptoms
  Tremors
  Drooling
  Slurred speech
Explain to family
  Need to provide psychologic support
  Need to emphasize capabilities rather than limitations
  Need to encourage active participation in family activities
  Need to encourage socialization
  That although patient may be physically disabled, he is intellectually normal
    Discuss need for family to show security, love, a need for patient, and patience with and understanding of patient's slowness and clumsiness
  Explain that frustration over tremors and dependence may be source of patient's irritability and loss of self-interest
  Need to encourage independence; avoid overprotection
  Need to permit patient to do things for himself
    Self-care
    Feedings
    Dressing
    Ambulation
Discuss available agencies for use as resources, such as the American Parkinson Disease Association*
Explain importance of daily exercise to delay progression of disease
Explain importance of performing any physical task that is difficult 5 to 10 times a day
Explain importance of ongoing outpatient care
  Physician's visits
  Physical therapy
Discuss medications: name, dosage, frequency of administration, purpose, and toxic or side effects
Explain need to avoid taking over-the-counter medications without checking with physician
Explain need for well-balanced, soft diet; limit high-protein foods, which may block effects of drugs
  Cut foods for patient
  Place all utensils within easy reach
  Use blender for thick foods
  Use braces for severe tremors occurring during meals
  Maintain fluid intake to 2000 ml daily unless contraindicated
  Serve frequent, small feedings
  Serve supplemental high-calorie fluids such as eggnog and milk shakes
  Use straws and bibs for excessive drooling
  Avoid food high in vitamin B_6 (reverses effects of levodopa)
  Instruct patient to swallow slowly and to take small bites of food
Explain need for activity
  Plan rest periods
  Perform passive or active ROM exercises to all extremities
  Encourage family or significant other to participate in physical therapy exercise of stretching and massaging muscles
  Give warm baths

---

*American Parkinson Disease Association, 116 John St., New York, N.Y., 10038; National Parkinson's Foundation Hotline: 1-800-327-4545.

Encourage daily ambulation outdoors, but avoid extremely hot or cold weather
Encourage patient to practice lifting feet while walking, using heel-toe gait, and swinging arms deliberately while walking
Place head of bed or back of chair on blocks to facilitate getting out of bed or chair; use pulleys such as sheets tied to end of bed
Avoid sitting for long periods of time
Encourage patient to dress daily
Avoid clothing with buttons; use zippers instead
Avoid shoes with laces or snaps
Provide diversional activities depending on extent of tremors and disability
  Reading
  Watching television
  Listening to radio
  Engaging in hobbies
  Painting
Prevent falls by clearing walkways of furniture and scatter rugs; build side rails on stairs and in tub or shower
Provide supports when ambulating with walker or cane as indicated
Provide speech therapy
  Instruct patient to speak slowly and practice reading aloud slowly in an exaggerated manner
  Provide electronic amplifiers as ordered for weak voice
Explain need for oral hygiene q2h to 4h and prn; need to control drooling
  Have tissues easily accessible to patient (e.g., in pockets)
  Use bib while eating
  Clean corners of mouth after eating and prn
  Apply ointment if necessary
Explain importance of proper elimination
  Conduct voiding measures as necessary
  Conduct bladder control program as necessary
  Provide raised toilet seat with side rails in home to facilitate sitting and standing

Evaluation

Patient demonstrates optimal mobility appropriate to physical limitations
Patient's self-care needs are met
Patient demonstrates optimal nutritional intake
Patient demonstrates skin integrity
Patient has optimal respiratory function
Patient and/or significant other demonstrates optimal knowledge concerning Parkinson's disease and related home maintenance

MULTIPLE SCLEROSIS (DISSEMINATED SCLEROSIS)

A chronic, progressive disease characterized by scattering of demyelinating lesions in the central nervous system (CNS), which affect the white matter of the brain and spinal cord

Assessment
Observations/findings

Fatigue; may be enhanced by hot bath or shower
Sensory impairment
  Numbness
  Tingling
Weakness of extremities
  Facial palsy
  Exaggerated reflexes
Dizziness, vertigo
Visual disturbances
  Diplopia
  Blurred vision or loss of vision
  Nystagmus
  Optic neuritis
Speech impairment: scanning speech
Muscular spasms
Babinski's sign
Poor coordination
  Ataxia
  Spasticity of extremities
  Tremors
  Staggering gait
Weakness of throat muscles: difficulty in chewing and swallowing
Loss of position sense: staggering gait
Fecal and/or urinary incontinence or retention
Mental changes
  Mood swings
  Depression
  Euphoria
  Irritability
  Apathy
  Inattention
  Lack of judgment
  Weeping

Laboratory/diagnostic studies

CSF
  Usually normal
  Increased white blood cell count (WBC)
  Increased gamma globulin level
MRI
Myleography
CT scan

Potential complications

Neurologic deficit; paralysis
Sexual dysfunction
Spastic bladder, urinary retention
Respiratory failure

Medical management

Medications
    Antiinflammatory agents
    Corticosteroids
    Muscle relaxants
    Immunosuppressive agents
    Vitamin B
    Antianxiety drugs/tranquilizers
    Beta-adrenergic blocking agents
Physical therapy
Psychotherapy/counseling
Nutritional therapy

Nursing diagnoses/goals/interventions

ndx: Self-care deficit: mobility, hygiene, feeding, and/or toiletry related to limitations in physical mobility imposed by disease process

GOAL: *Patient's self-care needs will be met*

Maintain quiet and relaxing environment
Institute activity
    Massage and stretch muscles
    Perform resistive exercises to all extremities and joints
    Perform active or passive ROM exercises q4h to 5h and prn
    Encourage ambulation to tolerance
    Encourage self-care
    Avoid use of heating pad; measure bathwater temperature (heat diminishes muscle strength)
    Plan all activities to avoid fatigue
    Plan rest periods
    Encourage diversional activities
        Reading
        Watching television
        Listening to radio and/or talking books
If patient is confined to bed rest
    Position comfortably
    Turn q2h to 4h and prn
    Perform active or passive ROM exericises q2h to 4h
    Perform dorsiflexion of ankles and quadriceps q2h to 4h
    Help out of bed and into chair two or three times daily
    Feed as necessary; hand braces may be indicated
Catheterize intermittently as indicated
Teach self-catheterization whenever possible
Plan bladder dysfunction program as appropriate for spasticity or flaccidity
Institute bowel control program
    Establish regular bowel routines
    Avoid constipation
Maintain high-calorie, high-vitamin, high-protein diet
Encourage fluids to 3000 ml daily unless contraindicated
Administer oral hygiene q4h to 5h and prn
Assist with or provide physical hygiene as indicated by physical ability
Maintain appropriate bathing temperatures
Administer eye care q4h to 5h as indicated

ndx: Potential for disturbance in self-concept: body image and self-esteem related to altered perception of self

GOAL: *Patient will accept changes in body image and self-esteem*

Establish means of communication
    Call bell within reach
    Pad and pencil, Magic Slate, word board
Acknowledge concerns about body image
Be supportive of patient's emotional changes and needs for improving image and esteem; encourage verbalization of feelings

ndx: Potential for ineffective airway clearance related to motor weakness and/or immobility

GOAL: *Patient will maintain a patent airway*

Suction oral pharynx as needed
Assist and teach patient to cough and deep breathe q2h to 4h and prn
Maintain patent airway and avoid flexion of patient's neck if immobile
Auscultate breath sounds q2h to 4h and prn
Position patient for maximal respiratory expansion and control of respiratory secretions

ndx: Knowledge deficit regarding disease process

GOAL: *Patient and/or significant other will demonstrate understanding of home care and follow-up instructions through interactive discussion and actual return demonstration*

Explain nature of disease, emphasizing that this is not a hereditary disease
Explain that warm weather and hot baths may increase weakness

Explain importance of avoiding fatigue and becoming overworked or emotionally stressed, since these may be precipitating factors in exacerbation
Explain importance of exercising regularly; need to maintain rest periods
Explain need to do muscle stretching exercises daily
Explain need for ROM exercises for patient with spasticity
Explain importance of daily routines for activities and rest periods
Discuss need for patient support when ambulating with walker, cane, or braces as indicated
Instruct patient to walk with a wide base, keeping feet apart
Emphasize importance of speech therapy; instruct patient to speak slowly and practice reading aloud
Emphasize need for diversional activities
   Reading
   Watching television
   Listening to radio
   Knitting
   Playing quiet games
Explain importance of decubitus care if patient is confined to bed rest or wheelchair
Explain importance of regulating bathwater temperature; need to avoid extremes of hot and cold due to loss of temperature change sense
Discuss symptoms of disease progression to report to physician
Explain importance of avoiding persons with infections, especially URIs
Discuss symptoms of cold or flu to report to physician
   Elevated temperature
   Chills
   Cough
   Extreme fatigue
Encourage activity as long as patient is able
   Recreational activities
   Work
   Household chores
Encourage verbalization
Allow time for patient to complete all activities and deal with any body image changes and loss of self-esteem
Encourage socialization with friends and family
Encourage independence and self-care to point of tolerance

Evaluation

Patient's self-care needs are met
   Medications are administered as ordered
   Fluid and nutritional needs are met
   Elimination needs are met
   Skin, oral, and eye hygiene needs are met
   Passive or active ROM is performed
   Planned rest periods are maintained
Patient demonstrates an effective breathing pattern
   Chest expansion is symmetric
   Breath sounds are clear to auscultation
   ABGs and vital signs are within normal limits
   There are no signs of respiratory distress
Patient demonstrates adaptation to actual or perceived changes in body image and self-esteem
Patient and/or significant other demonstrates knowledge necessary for home maintenance management

MYASTHENIA GRAVIS

A neuromuscular disorder characterized by muscular weakness and fatigue due to a defect in transmission of motor impulses at the neuromuscular junction; probably a result of an autoimmune response

Assessment
Observations/findings

Fatigue
Expressionless facies
Generalized weakness
   Increases with exercise
   May be confined to one area
   Weakness of face, jaw, neck, arms, hands, and/or legs
Difficulty in raising arms above head or extending fingers outward
Dysphagia
Difficulty in chewing
Weak voice
Ptosis of one or both eyelids
Diplopia
Inability to walk on heels; may walk on toes
Strength decreases as day progresses
Stress incontinence
Anal sphincter weakness
Respirations
   Shallow
   Decreased VC
   Use of accessory muscles
   Muffled cough

Laboratory/diagnostic studies

CT scan of chest or chest x-ray examination indicating thymoma
Tensilon test

Single-fiber electromyogram
Nerve conduction studies
Anti–acetylcholine receptor (ACLR) antibody test

Potential complications

Neuromuscular deficit: mild to severe
Pneumonia
Aspiration, atelectasis
Respiratory failure

Medical management

Plasmapheresis
Thymectomy
Tracheostomy
Mechanical ventilation/oxygen therapy
Physical therapy
Occupational therapy
Medications
    Anticholinesterase
    Corticosteroids
    Pituitary hormones
Nutritional support
Ventilatory management

Nursing diagnoses/goals/interventions

ndx: Ineffective breathing pattern related to neuromuscular impairment

GOAL: *Patient will demonstrate maximal respiratory function within physiologic limits*

Inspect, auscultate, and percuss chest q2h to 4h and prn
Assist and teach patient to cough and deep breathe q2h to 4h
Position patient to maximize breathing pattern effectiveness
Suction excessive oral secretions as indicated
Keep tracheostomy tray at bedside at all times
Provide oxygenation/ventilatory support as ordered
Monitor muscular strength by tidal volume and VC, since deterioration may severely impact on breathing pattern

ndx: Self-care deficit: feeding, hygiene, and/or toileting related to decreased motor function

GOAL: *Patient's self-care needs will be met*

Maintain regular diet as tolerated; with persistent dysphagia, tube feeding may be indicated; small, frequent feedings may be indicated
Administer oral hygiene q2h to 4h, after meals, and prn
Administer skin care q4h to 6h
    Turn patient q2h to 4h if patient is unable to ambulate
    Apply sheepskin
    Rub back
Administer eye care q4h to 5h
    Remove any formed crusts
    Place eye patch over affected eye
    Administer eye drops as ordered

ndx: Alteration in mobility related to neuromuscular weakness

GOAL: *Patient will experience optimal mobility*

Increase activity to tolerance; plan treatments and major activities early in day or 30 min after medication is taken
Perform passive or active ROM exercises q4h to 5h and prn
Maintain planned rest periods
Administer medication as ordered
    Anticholinesterase: to be given 20 to 30 min prior to meals; note increase in muscular strength within 30 min of taking medication
    Medication should always be taken at scheduled time; never miss a dose (rationale: anticholinesterase maximizes physical mobility)

ndx: Potential for alteration in self-concept related to actual or perceived changes in physical and personal self-image

GOAL: *Patient will accept changes in body image and function*

Provide emotional support; allow patient to verbalize needs and to participate in planning care
Encourage verbalization of feelings about body image and function changes
Provide for alternative communication methods if vocalization is impaired
    Magic Slate
    Pencil and paper

ndx: Knowledge deficit regarding disease process and home management

GOAL: *Patient and/or significant other will demonstrate understanding of home care and follow-up instructions through interactive discussion and actual return demonstration*

Explain to family
    Need to encourage patient to deal with body image

changes and fears of permanent disability, dying, or loss of body function
Need to encourage verbalization
Need to encourage independence and continued socialization
Discuss medications: name, dosage, time of administration, purpose, and side effects
Anticholinesterase
Importance of dosage
Take at scheduled times
Do not miss doses
Take with milk, crackers, or bread
Avoid taking with coffee, or fruit or tomato juice
Avoid taking with sedatives or tranquilizers
Toxic side effects: muscular weakness, abdominal cramps, diarrhea
Discuss symptoms and first signs of drug toxicity to report to physician
Explain need to avoid taking over-the-counter medications without checking with physician
Explain need to wear medical alert band
Discuss symptoms of recurrence or progression of disease or of any complications, such as respiratory failure, to report to physician
Explain importance of avoiding persons with infections, especially URIs
Discuss symptoms of URI to report to physician
Increased weakness
Low-grade fever
Chills
Cough
Explain need to avoid use of tobacco and alcohol and prolonged exposure to hot or cold weather
Explain importance of ongoing outpatient care
Explain need to maintain regular diet according to patient's status
Serve soft or solid food as tolerated
Arrange foods and utensils so as to be easily managed by patient
Instruct patient to chew small pieces of food well and to eat slowly
Explain need for exercise to tolerance; to avoid strenuous activity
Plan activities when maximum effect of medication is seen; patient will usually exhibit most strength in morning or after nap
Assist in planning ADLs in a manner in which patient will accomplish tasks without too many motions
Explain need for active or passive ROM exercises to all extremities

Explain need for planned rest periods and at least 8 hr of sleep at night
Emphasize need for diversional activities
Reading
Watching television
Listening to radio
Knitting
Working puzzles
Emphasize importance of avoiding physical and emotional stress
Discuss need for speech therapy; instruct patient to speak slowly and practice reading aloud
Explain need to use eye patch over affected eye or frosted lens to increase clear vision if diplopia persists
Explain importance of avoiding constipation; may need to use stool softeners or mild laxatives
Explain need for adequate fluid intake: up to 2000 ml daily unless contraindicated
Discuss available agencies for use as references, such as Myasthenia Gravis Foundation*
Refer patient and/or significant other to Visiting Nurses Association or social service worker for obtaining any necessary equipment for home use, such as suctioning equipment

Evaluation

Patient demonstrates an effective breathing pattern as evidenced by
Clear breath sounds
Maximum VC physiologically possible
Patency of airway at all times
Patient's self-care needs are met as evidenced by
Optimal nutritional status
Skin integrity
Optimal ROM and physical mobility
Patient demonstrates positive coping strategies to deal with body image and function changes
Patient and/or significant other demonstrates knowledge of the disease process and home management needs

MYASTHENIA GRAVIS CRISIS, CHOLINERGIC CRISIS

myasthemia gravis crisis Acute exacerbation of myasthenic process resulting in increased signs of weakness; usually a result of infection, surgery, or emotional upset

---

*Myasthenia Gravis Foundation, 7-11 South Broadway, Suite 304, White Plains, N.Y. 10601.

cholinergic crisis *Acute exacerbation of myasthenic process resulting from an overdose of anticholinesterase*

Assessment

Observations/findings

MYASTHENIA GRAVIS CRISIS

Respiratory distress progressing to periods of apnea and respiratory failure
Tachypnea
Increased muscular weakness
Extreme fatigue
Restlessness
Anxiety
Irritability
Difficulty in handling secretions
Dysphagia
Inability to chew or move jaws
Facial weakness
Speech impairment
Elevated temperature
Ptosis of one or both eyelids

CHOLINERGIC CRISIS

Respiratory distress progressing to periods of apnea and respiratory failure
Dyspnea and wheezing
Vertigo
Blurred vision
Sweating
Lacrimation
Salivation
Anorexia
Abdominal cramping
Nausea and vomiting
Dysarthria
Dysphagia
Muscular cramps and spasms (fasiculations)
General weakness
Toxic effects of anticholinesterase
    Anorexia
    Abdominal cramps
    Nausea, vomiting
    Excessive salivation
    Sweating
    Diarrhea

Potential complications

Aspiration
Respiratory failure
Respiratory arrest

Medical management

Oxygenation/assisted ventilation
Tracheostomy
Bronchoscopy
Fluid and electrolyte support
Intake and output
Medication therapy; reduce or withdraw anticholinergic drugs
NPO as indicated

Nursing diagnosis/goal/interventions

ndx: Ineffective breathing pattern related to neuromuscular (respiratory) impairment

GOAL: *Patient will maintain an effective breathing pattern*

Maintain patent airway
Administer oxygen with assisted ventilation as ordered if tracheostomy is performed
Inspect and auscultate chest frequently to monitor adequate ventilation
Monitor VC q2h to 4h as ordered
Assist and teach patient to turn, cough, and deep breathe q2h as possible
Suction q1h to 2h and prn
Monitor consciousness until breathing pattern is stabilized
Check rectal temperature q2h to 4h; cooling measures may be ordered to decrease work of breathing
Maintain bed rest to maximize effective breathing
    Elevate head of bed 30 degrees as tolerated
    Maintain body alignment
Administer medication to optimize ventilatory muscular activity
    Reduce or withdraw anticholinergic drugs as ordered; may be given to differentiate type of crisis
        Myasthenia gravis crisis: patient worsens
        Cholinergic crisis: patient improves
    Keep atropine at bedside; *avoid use of morphine*
Maintain ventilatory support until crisis is resolved, then resume noncrisis management

Evaluation

Patient demonstrates an effective breathing pattern without ventilatory support
Respiratory rate, rhythm, and pattern are within normal limits without mechanical support

AMYOTROPHIC LATERAL SCLEROSIS (ALS)

A progressive lower motor neuron disorder of unknown etiology that results in muscular wasting and atrophy; commonly referred to as "Lou Gehrig's disease"

Assessment
Observations/findings

Irregular muscular fasciculations
Cramping
Incoordination of movement of hands and fingers
Muscle stiffness and wasting involving hands, arms, and shoulders
Spastic gait
Progressive weakness, flaccidity, and atrophy of legs
Dysarthria
Dysphagia
Dyspnea
Excessive drooling
Loss of reflexes

Laboratory/diagnostic studies

Elevated creatinine phosphokinase (CPK)
CSF: elevated protein
Myelography
CT scan
Muscle biopsy
Electromyelogram
Nerve conduction studies

Potential complications

Neuromuscular deficit: mild to severe
Respiratory infection
Aspiration, atelectasis
Injury
Respiratory failure

Medical management

Cricopharyngeal myotomy to alleviate dysphagia
Cervical esophagostomy
Medications
    Anticholinesterase
    Steroids
    Antibiotics
    Muscle relaxants
Oxygenation/ventilatory support
Cardiac monitoring
Parenteral fluids/nutritional support
Physical therapy

Nursing diagnoses/goals/interventions

ndx: Ineffective airway clearance related to progressive neuromuscular impairment

GOAL: *Patient will demonstrate a patent airway*

Maintain patent airway through
    Proper body and head positioning
    Suction q2h to 4h as indicated
    Encourage coughing and deep breathing as patient's condition permits
    Auscultate chest for adventitious sounds
    Observe for alterations in respiratory pattern
Administer oxygen, humidification, and ventilatory support as ordered
Perform chest percussion and vibration to loosen secretions
Test muscular strength for respiratory effort by tidal volume and VC
Auscultate chest for breath sounds q6h to 8h

ndx: Potential for self-care deficit: feeding, bathing, and/or toileting related to progressive neuromuscular deterioration

GOAL: *Patient's self-care needs will be met*

Encourage self-care as long as possible
    Bathing
    Feeding
Direct nursing care to promote self-care and prevention of complications according to severity of symptoms
Initiate and teach gentle oral suction as indicated
Administer oral hygiene q4h to 5h
Check gag reflex
Modify eating patterns as gag reflex diminishes
Maintain high-calorie, high-protein soft diet as tolerated
Initiate parenteral fluids as ordered
Administer skin care q4h and prn
    Use air mattress
    Use sheepskin
    Use footboard
    Rub back
Anticipate and manage elimination needs
Avoid constipation
    Encourage drinking fluids
    Use daily suppositories or stool softeners

ndx: Alteration in mobility related to neuromuscular deterioration

GOAL: *Patient will maintain optimal mobility*

Perform active or passive ROM exercises q4h to all extremities
Utilize braces or splints to support ankles and hands
Turn q2h to 4h if patient is confined to bed
Encourage ambulation to tolerance
Avoid strenuous exercise
Provide physical therapy as ordered: massage and stretching exercises
Maintain planned rest periods
Test muscular strength of extremities q4h and prn

ndx: Anticipatory grieving related to perceived or actual loss of body function

GOAL: *Patient and family will feel supported in grieving process*

Provide emotional support; be aware that there is no cure
    Deal with body image changes
    Encourage communication with family and/or significant other
Deal with feelings of frustration, helplessness, and powerlessness associated with progressive weakness
Assist family and patient with accepting reality of loss as they progress through phases of grief process
Be supportive; encourage active listening and expression of feelings by patient and family members

ndx: Knowledge deficit regarding disease process and home management

GOAL: *Patient and significant other will demonstrate understanding of home care and follow-up instructions through interactive discussion and actual return demonstration*

Reinforce physician's explanation of disease, symptoms, progression of disease, and management
Emphasize that while activity is impaired, cognitive processes are not affected
Emphasize importance of verbalization about progressive muscular wasting and weakness
Emphasize need to discuss feelings about
    Excessive salivation
    Weakening voice, hoarseness
    Dysphagia
Emphasize need by family to encourage active participation in family activities
Demonstrate use of electrolarynx to facilitate vocalization as tolerated
Discuss need to develop alternative methods of communication when voice becomes nonfunctional: use of eyes and eyelid blinking
Explain importance of ongoing outpatient care and physician's visits
Explain need for high-calorie, high-protein soft diet as tolerated
Assist patient with dealing with problems of swallowing
    Place pureed foods on posterior aspect of tongue
    Cut foods for patient
    Use wrist and hand braces
    May need to consider nasogastric or gastrostomy feedings
Explain need for oral suctioning as disease progresses
Instruct patient to swallow slowly to avoid danger of aspiration
Explain need for oral hygiene q2h to 4h and prn
    Have tissues easily accessible to patient
    Use bib while eating
    Clean corners of mouth after eating and prn
Discuss use of braces, splints, and/or cervical collars for support of hands, ankles, and neck
Explain need to avoid strenuous exercise/activity
Explain need to perform ROM activities as tolerated
Discuss available agencies for use as resources
Explain need to provide skin care frequently, turning patient q2h to 4h to alternate potential pressure areas
Explain need to provide for and anticipate elimination needs

Evaluation

Patient demonstrates an effective breathing pattern
    Chest expansion is symmetric
    Breath sounds are clear to auscultation
    ABGs and vital signs are within normal limits
    There are no signs of respiratory distress
Patient's self-care needs are met
    Fluid and nutritional needs are met
    Elimination needs are met
    Skin, oral, and eye hygiene needs are met
Patient's needs for mobility are met
    Passive or active ROM is performed
    Planned rest periods are maintained
Patient and family utilize supports/resources to deal with anticipated or actual loss
Patient and/or significant other demonstrates knowledge and understanding of home care management
    Demonstrates passive or active ROM exercises
    States all relevant information regarding medications, time of dose, side effects, and purpose
    Identifies high-calorie, high-protein foods and states understanding of need for maintenance of diet

States understanding of fluid intake maintenance to avoid infection risk and constipation
Demonstrates abilities in physical hygiene care
States principles important in maintaining skin integrity

GUILLAIN-BARRÉ SYNDROME (ACUTE INFECTIOUS POLYNEURITIS; POLYRADICULITIS)

A neurologic syndrome of increasing weakness, numbness, pain, and paralysis; etiology is unknown, but syndrome generally follows a recent infection; onset is rapid, and symptoms are generally reversible

Assessment
Observations/findings

Muscular weakness of lower extremities, progressive to arms, trunk, head, and face
See Musculoskeletal Assessment (p. 470)
Paresthesia, pain, often "stocking-glove" distribution
Paralysis of upper extremities may be partial, or complete quadriplegia may develop
See Respiratory Assessment (p. 219)
Unstable BP
Choking, difficulty in breathing, tachypnea, tachycardia
Decreased or absent breath sounds
Dysphagia, difficulty in swallowing
Speech impairment
Low back and muscle pain
Low-grade fever
Weight loss
Anorexia
Urinary retention or infection
Personality changes

Laboratory/diagnostic studies

CSF
  Increased protein
  Normal WBC
Lumbar puncture
Electromyography
Nerve conduction studies

Potential complications

Aspiration, atelectasis
Respiratory failure
  Decreased tidal volume
  Hypercapnea
Respiratory arrest
Neuromuscular deficit

Medical management

Tracheostomy
Oxygen or mechanical ventilation
Arterial blood gases
Chest physiotherapy
Physical and/or occupational therapy
Medications
  Antibiotics
  Analgesics (not opiates)
  Steroids
  Pituitary hormones
Bed rest; monitoring of muscular strength
Parenteral therapy
Enteral or oral nutrition with high-protein, high-calorie diet
Cardiac monitor
Plasmapheresis

Nursing diagnoses/goals/interventions

ndx: Potential for ineffective breathing pattern related to neuromuscular impairment (ascending paralysis)

GOAL: *Patient will demonstrate an effective breathing pattern*

Maintain patent airway
Administer oxygen, humidification, and assisted ventilation as ordered
Provide tracheostomy care if indicated (p. 275)
Monitor closely for signs of impending respiratory failure; do not leave patient unattended during periods of respiratory distress
Auscultate chest q2h to 4h
Elevate head of bed 30 degrees
Maintain body alignment and position
Check BP, P, and R with neuro signs q1h to 2h and prn for change
Test muscular strength q4h to 6h
Suction prn
Assist and teach coughing and deep breathing as appropriate
Keep intubation equipment and mechanical ventilator on standby in acute phase

ndx: Self-care deficit related to neuromuscular paralysis

GOAL: *Patient's self-care needs will be met*

Administer oral hygiene q2h, after meals, and prn
Administer skin care and eye care q2h to 4h; remove crusts, apply eye shields, and administer artificial tears
Turn patient q2h

Observe carefully for pressure points
Use positioning devices and alternating pressure mattresses as needed
Observe for sensory alteration to heat and cold
Perform passive ROM to all extremities
Increase frequency of nursing functions as patient's condition requires
Encourage ambulation as tolerated
  Begin by sitting on bedside with support, progressing to chair two to three times daily
  Later walk in room or hall for 15 min four times daily
Maintain planned rest periods
Administer diet as tolerated; progress from soft to solid foods as tolerated
Supplement feedings with high-calorie, high-protein fluids such as eggnog and milk shakes
Administer enteral feedings as indicated
Encourage fluids to 2000 ml daily unless contraindicated
Maintain parenteral fluids
Indicate voiding measures as necessary
Monitor elimination and catheter care, as well as intake and output
Avoid constipation through use of daily suppositories or stool softeners

ndx: Potential for powerlessness related to physical limitations imposed by progressive physical deterioration, loss of body control, and/or threat to physical integrity

GOAL: *Patient will feel in control or participate in as many routine activities as possible*

Establish and maintain means of communication
  Call bell within reach
  Magic Slate, pad and pencil, or word board at bedside
Provide emotional support, thorough explanations, and reassurance
Be alert to emotional changes and mood swings
Encourage patient's participation and expression of needs and feelings
Maintain planned rest periods
Encourage self-care (eating, dressing, shaving) as indicated
Provide physical care as indicated
Provide physical, occupational, and psychosocial diversity

ndx: Knowledge deficit regarding disease process

GOAL: *Patient and/or significant other will demonstrate understanding of home care and follow-up instructions through interactive discussion and actual return demonstration*

Ensure that patient and/or significant other understands that recovery may take up to 1 year or more
Stress importance of dealing with body image changes and fears of permanent disability, loss of function, and dying
Explain to family
  Need to encourage verbalization
  Need to encourage independence and socialization
  Need to encourage self-care as a strategy for health maintainence
  Importance of allowing patient to take meals with family
Discuss medications: name, dosage, frequency of administration, purpose, and side effects
Explain need to avoid over-the-counter medications without checking with physician
Stress need to avoid individuals with infections, especially URIs
Encourage diversional activities: TV, reading, radio
Stress importance of high-calorie, high-protein diet
Reinforce need to arrange utensils and foods for easy patient management
Stress need to maintain fluid intake of 2000 ml per day
Teach patient to avoid constipation by drinking fluids
Explain importance of ongoing outpatient care, including physical and/or occupational therapy
Encourage need to exercise to tolerance
Explain use of warm baths to alleviate stiffness and pain
Ensure that patient and/or significant other demonstrates
  Active and passive ROM exercise with massage to all extremities
  Strengthening and mobility exercises to fingers
  Exercises that increase mobility and strength of fingers; use of rubber squeeze toys, balls, or clay

Evaluation

Patient demonstrates an effective breathing pattern
  Chest expansion is symmetric
  Breath sounds are clear to auscultation
  ABGs and vital signs are within normal limits
  There are no signs of respiratory distress
Patient's self-care needs are met
  Fluid and nutritional needs are met
  Elimination needs are met
  Skin, oral, and eye hygiene needs are met
  Passive or active ROM is performed

Planned rest periods are maintained
Patient participates in decision making and activities related to his care
  Identifies his need areas
  Participates in self-care
  Optimal communication is established
  Participates in diversional activities
Patient and/or significant other demonstrates knowledge and understanding of home care management
  Demonstrates passive/active ROM exercises
  States all relevant information regarding medications, time of dose, side effects, and purpose
  Identifies high-calorie, high-protein foods and states understanding of need for maintenance of diet
  States understanding of fluid intake maintenance to avoid infection risk and constipation
  Demonstrates abilities in physical hygiene care
  States principles important in maintaining skin integrity

NEUROLOGIC INFECTIONS

Those conditions in which a microorganism has gained entry into the body, producing a reaction, brain abscess, or meningitis

brain abscess Secondary to systemic infections or may be introduced through trauma; results in space-occupying lesions causing a potential for increased ICP

meningitis Infection of the meninges causing inflammatory reaction in the pia-arachnoid membrane

encephalitis Infection of the brain parenchyma

myelitis Infection of the spinal cord parenchyma

Assessment
Observations/findings

History of recent URI, sinus or ear infection, penetrating trauma, or basal skull fracture
Headache
Positive Kernig's sign

TABLE 5-5. Antibiotic Therapy in Meningitis

Causative organisms	Antibiotic	Method of administration	Monitor
Meningococci	Aqueous penicillin G Ampicillin Choramphenicol (for allergic persons)	IV for 7-10 days	Skin for rash Tongue for glossitis CBC Platelet count
	For exposed persons prophylactic: Rifampin Minocycline	Orally for 14 days	
Pneumococci	Aqueous benzyl penicillin	IV for 7-10 days	
Streptococci	Ampicillin	IV for 12-15 days	
Staphylococci	Methicillin Nafcillin	IV for 2-4 weeks	
Haemophilus influenzae	Moxalactam	IV for 10-14 days Loading dose for children: 100 mg/kg, then 50 mg/kg q5h Never exceed 200 mg/day	Hematuria Vertigo Tinnitis Hearing loss CBC Protrombin time
E. coli, Pseudomonas	Gentamicin or Moxalactam	IV for 14 days, then 3 times weekly for 2 years (children: 20-30 mg/kg)	
Tuberculosis bacillus	Streptomycin Isoniazid daily	Adults: 1 g daily IM, 400 mg orally for 10-14 days	Hearing loss
Coccidioides immitis	Amphotericin B	IV, 0.25-1 mg/kg	BUN
Cryptococcus		Mix well in 500 ml dextrose (5%) in water Administer every other day over 6 hr period for 6 weeks	Serum creatinine CBC Headache Vomiting

From Vogt, G., Miller, M., and Esluer, M.: Mosby's manual of neurological care, St. Louis, 1985, The C.V. Mosby Co.

Positive Brudzinski's sign
Meningeal irritability; nuchal rigidity
Disorientation
Altered level of consciousness: irritability to coma
Diplopia
Photophobia
Seizures
Malaise
Increased ICP
Elevated temperature
Tachycardia
Dyspnea
Tachypnea
Nausea, vomiting
Petechial rash
Dehydration

Laboratory/diagnostic studies

CSF
   Elevated protein level and pressure
   Elevated glucose level
Serum blood cultures
EEG
CT scan
Chest x-ray examination
Skull x-ray examination
Brain scan

Potential complications

Herniation
Increased ICP
Neurologic deficit
Respiratory failure
Shock

Medical management

Institution protocol for infection control as indicated by organism (identified)
Medications
   Antibiotic therapy
   Analgesics
   Anticonvulsants
Ventilatory/oxygenation support
Hypothermia
ICP monitoring
Fluid/electrolyte therapy

Nursing diagnoses/goals/interventions

ndx: Potential for ineffective airway patency related to increased intracranial pressure or depressed cerebral functioning

GOAL: *Patient will demonstrate a patent airway*

Maintain respiratory function
   Assess respiratory status q1h to 2h
   Auscultate breath sounds
   Administer oxygen ventilatory support as ordered
   Position patient for optimal ventilation
   Maintain artificial airway as indicated
   Suction prn
Check BP, P, R, and consciousness prn as indications of neurologic and respiratory stability
Check rectal temperature q2h to 4h
Administer cooling measures as ordered

ndx: Self-care deficit: hygiene, feeding, toileting, and/or mobility related to alteration in neurophysiologic function

GOAL: *Patient's self-care needs will be met*

Maintain quiet environment; darken room if photophobia occurs
Maintain bed rest; assist patient in assuming position of comfort
Maintain parenteral fluids as ordered
Maintain high-calorie, high-protein diet as tolerated
Force fluids unless contraindicated
Control pain as ordered
Assist and teach patient to turn, cough, and deep breathe q2h to 4h
Perform active or passive ROM exercises q4h to 6h
Administer skin care q2h to 4h
   Use air mattress
   Give back rubs
Administer comfort measures
   Tepid sponges
   Ice cap to head
Administer oral hygiene q2h to 4h
Provide for all hygiene measures as indicated
Initiate voiding measures as necessary
Ensure elimination through use of stool softeners, daily suppositories, and/or enemas as necessary

ndx: Knowledge deficit regarding disease process and eventual home management

GOAL: *Patient and significant other will demonstrate understanding of home care and follow-up instructions through interactive discussion and actual return demonstration*

Discuss medications: name, dosage, frequency of administration, purpose, and toxic or side effects
Explain need to avoid taking over-the-counter medications without checking with physician
Explain to family need to encourage verbalization; help patient understand nature of disorder

Explain need to increase activities as ordered
Explain importance of physical activity as tolerated
Explain need for planned rest periods
Explain need for balanced nutritional diet
Discuss symptoms of progression of condition to report to physician
Explain importance of ongoing outpatient care

Evaluation

Patient demonstrates an effective breathing pattern
   Chest expansion is symmetric
   Breath sounds are clear to auscultation
   ABGs and vital signs are within normal limits
   There are no signs of respiratory distress
Patient's self-care needs are met
   Medications are administered as ordered
   Fluid and nutritional needs are met
   Elimination needs are met
   Skin, oral, and eye hygiene needs are met
   Passive or active ROM is performed
   Planned rest periods are maintained
Patient and/or significant other demonstrates knowledge and understanding of home care management
   Demonstrates passive or active ROM exercises
   States all relevant information regarding medications, time of dose, side effects, and purpose
   Identifies high-calorie, high protein foods, and states understanding of need for maintenance of diet

SUBSTANCE ABUSE (DRUG ABUSE AND INTOXICATION)

NOTE: Care of the intoxicated patient will depend on the amount and type of drug ingested; for severe drug overdose or intoxication refer to Care of Patient with Altered Consciousness (p. 288), Shock Syndrome (p. 104), Respiratory Failure (p. 261), Respiratory Assessment (p. 219), and Seizures (p. 291).

Alcohol Intoxication

Assessment

Observations/findings

Acute intoxication
   Confusion
   Slurred speech
   Ataxia
   Depressed deep tendon reflexes
   Nystagmus
   Anxiety, restlessness
   Dilated pupils
   Stupor

DRUGS COMMONLY ABUSED

NARCOTICS
   Opium
   Heroin (horse, smack)
   Oxycodone
   Codeine
   Methadone
   Hydromorphone (Dilaudid)
   Meperidine (Demerol)

HALLUCINOGENS
   LSD (acid)
   Mescaline
   DMT
   Scopolamine
   Atropine
   Phencyclidine: PCP (angel dust, crystal, dust mist, peace pill, superweed)
   Psilocybin

ORGANIC SOLVENTS
   Glue
   Cleaning fluid

DEPRESSANTS
   Alcohol
   Barbiturates
   Meprobamate
   Chloral hydrate
   Glutethimide (Doriden)

STIMULANTS
   Cocaine (coke)
   Amphetamines
   Methylphenidate (Ritalin)

CANNABIS
   Marijuana (grass, weed, joints)
   Hashish (weed oil, hash)

   Coma
   Gastric irritation: vomiting
Withdrawal
   Anxiety
   Tremors
   Diaphoresis
   Nausea, vomiting
   Anorexia
   Confusion
   Moroseness
   Confabulation
   Delirium tremens
   Seizure activity
   Uncontrolled rage
   Hallucination
   Toxic psychosis
Chronic intoxication
   Mental confusion
   Cerebellar degeneration
      Ataxic gait
      Nystagmus
      Dysarthric speech
   Nutritional deficiencies
   Myopathy
   Hepatic coma
   Seizure disorders

Marchiafava-Bignami syndrome (progressive organic dementia)
Wernicke's syndrome
   Ophthalmoplegia
   Apathy, apprehension
   Confusion
   Coma
Korsakoff's syndrome
   Disorientation to time and place
   Peripheral neuropathy
   Confabulation

Laboratory/diagnostic studies

Serum ETOH (Table 5-6)
Serum chemistries

Potential complications

Aspiration
Severe stages
   Hypoventilation
   Hypotension
   Hypothermia
   GI hemorrhage

Medical management

Acute

Airway support and management: oxygenation/ventilatory
Fluid/electrolyte therapy

Medications during withdrawal

Phenothiazines
Tranquilizers
Barbiturates
Anticonvulsants
Thiamin

Nursing diagnosis/goals/interventions

ndx: Potential for ineffective airway clearance or breathing pattern

GOAL: *Patient will demonstrate a patent airway*

Maintain patent airway: assisted ventilation as indicated
See Care of Patient with Altered Consciousness (p. 288) and Respiratory Failure (p. 261)
Position to optimize respiratory excursion, airway patency, and secretion removal
Check BP, P, and R q2h to 4h and prn
Provide oral or nasopharyngeal airway as indicated
Suction prn
Auscultate breath sounds prn
Provide oxygenation/respiratory therapy
Avoid use of sedatives; may potentiate effects of alcohol
Provide soft restraints as indicated
   Keep restraints loose
   Position patient on side or stomach

ndx: Ineffective individual coping related to inadequate coping methods

GOAL: *Patient will demonstrate use of positive coping behaviors*

Maintain quiet, supportive environment; avoid punitive approach
Maintain safety precautions for anxious and restless patients
Administer high-calorie, high-protein diet as ordered
Assist with or provide self-care hygiene as needed
Provide supportive counseling services to patient when receptive
Ensure that patient and/or significant other is knowledgeable about effects of alcohol abuse

Evaluation

Patient
   Demonstrates an effective breathing pattern
      Chest expansion is symmetric
      Breath sounds are clear to auscultation
      ABGs and vital signs are within normal limits
      There are no signs of respiratory distress
   Demonstrates effective coping strategies
      Discusses effects of alcohol abuses
      Attends counseling/educational support groups

Chemical Substance Abuse

Intermittent or chronic use of stimulants or depressants resulting in alterations in mental and physiologic function

Assessment

Observations/findings

DEPRESSANTS: NARCOTICS, OPIATES*

Level of consciousness
   Apathy
   Withdrawal
   Euphoria
   Coma
Airway obstruction
Stridor
Decreased BP

---

*Refers to all drugs that possess some morphinelike activity.

TABLE 5-6. Serum Alcohol Levels

Serum alcohol levels	Effects
Mild: 0.5 to 1.5 mg/ml	Muscular incoordination, personality changes; talkative, morose, noisy
Moderate: 1.5 to 3 mg/ml	Marked ataxia, mental impairment, incoordination, prolonged reaction time, nausea, vomiting, diplopia
Severe: 3 to 5 mg/ml	Dysarthria, amnesia, hypothermia, hypoventilation, coma

Tachycardia or bradycardia
Pupillary changes
   Pinpoint (opiates)
   Dilated (barbiturates)
Depressed gag and swallow reflexes
Respiratory distress, respiratory rate < 8/min or > 30/min
Seizure activity
Hypothermia
Method of administration
   Oral
   Subcutaneous: "skin popping"
   Nasal insufflation: "snorting"
   Intravenous
   Signs of withdrawal
      Abdominal and muscular pain
      Severe cramping

HALLUCINOGENS, STIMULANTS
GENERAL

Anxiety progressing to pain
Paranoid reaction
Combativeness progressing to violence
Insomnia
Hallucinations
   Auditory
   Visual
Confusion
Ataxia
Depression: mild to severe
Suicidal tendencies
Anorexia
Nausea
Headache
Elevated BP
Elevated temperature
Tachycardia palpitations
Hypertension progressing to crisis
Pupillary changes: dilated
Photophobia
Diplopia
Horizontal and vertical nystagmus
Hot flashes
ECG disturbances
Decreased urine output

LSD, MESCALINE

Hyperactivity
Pupil dilation
Increased vital signs
Low doses: euphoria
High doses: hallucinatory psychosis

PCP: "ANGEL DUST"

Low to moderate doses: effect begins within 5 min and peaks within 30 to 60 min
   Elevated systolic and diastolic pressures
   Tachycardia
   Increased deep tendon reflexes
   Small pupils
   Nystagmus: horizontal and vertical (persists for 4 days)
   Tremors, clonus
   Euphoria
   Amnesia
   Agitation
   Image distortion
   Increased urine output
High doses
   Slurred speech
   Drowsiness
   Depressed deep tendon reflexes
   Seizures
   Opisthotonos
   Bradypnea
   Decreased BP
   Disordered thought processes, hallucinations

Laboratory/diagnostic studies

Serum chemical screening
Urinalysis
Arterial blood gases

Potential complications

Aspiration
Respiratory failure
Shock
Acute psychosis

Medical management
Depressants

Respiratory support with oxygenation or ventilation
Fluid/electrolyte therapy

Emetics
Gastric lavage
Activated charcoal for ingested opiates
Naloxone for opioid overdose
Peritoneal dialysis

Stimulants

Decreased external stimuli
Medications
  General
    Barbiturates, phenothiazines
    Sedatives, anticonvulsants
  For LSD, mescaline
    Diazepam (oral)
    Avoid phenothiazine; may potentiate psychotic reaction
  For PCP
    Haloperidol
    Diazepam
    Activated charcoal (high doses)
  Parenteral fluids
  Gastric suction for PCP
  Psychiatric liason

Nursing diagnoses/goals/interventions

ndx: Potential for ineffective breathing pattern

GOAL: *Patient will demonstrate an effective breathing pattern*

Refer to p. 288 if patient arrives in coma or in respiratory failure
Check respirations q2h to 4h, noting rate, quality, and depth
Check level of consciousness q2h to 4h
Report any changes in consciousness or vital signs to physician
Administer parenteral fluids as ordered
Understand that peritoneal dialysis may be indicated for long-acting barbiturates
Obtain accurate and detailed history regarding drug ingested: type, amount, time of ingestion, method of administration
Administer emetics as ordered; contraindicated in presence of depressed gag reflex, seizures, or coma
Administer gastric lavage as ordered (within 2 hr of ingestion); endotracheal tube is usually inserted prior to lavage in comatose patient
Keep patient physically active and stimulated
Provide patient with positive reassurance about condition; avoid punitive approach
Be firm, patient, and understanding

Administer medication as ordered: naloxone (Narcan) for opiate overdose; effects can be noted within 1 to 2 min for IV
Give activated charcoal orally for ingested opiates
Check BP and P on admission and q4h as indicated by condition
Monitor cardiac status for dysrhythmias
Provide self-care needs as indicated

ndx: Potential for violence

GOAL: *Patient will demonstrate calm and nondestructive behavior*

Admit to private room when possible
Decrease external stimuli
  Use low lighting
  Avoid loud voices and rapid movements
Allow friend or family member to remain in room during all procedures to assist in "talking down"
Provide patient with support, reassurance, and reality-defining information
Instruct patient to avoid trying to differentiate between real perceptions and effects of drug; remind patient that effects of drug will end
Avoid mechanical restraints
Approach cautiously; avoid whispering to others
Explain all procedures; allow same person to care for patient at all times
Administer medications as ordered
Avoid phenothiazine (may potentiate effect or produce anticholinergic crisis)
NOTE: Administration of the following care may heighten patient's paranoid state and cause increased agitation; approach patient quietly, utilizing friend to assist if required
Administer parenteral fluids as ordered
Check BP, P, and R q2h to 4h or as indicated by level of consciousness

ndx: Knowledge deficit regarding potential side effects of drug abuse and dependence

GOAL: *Patient and/or significant other will demonstrate understanding of home care and follow-up instructions through interactive discussion*

Explore patient's willingness to participate in self-help and support group experiences
Provide supportive, nonjudgmental approach to patient
Provide opportunity for participation in counseling and group support

Evaluation

Patient
Has an effective breathing pattern
Exhibits nondestructive behavior
Understands effects of drug abuse and dependence

LUMBAR PUNCTURE (SPINAL TAP)

Puncture usually made at the junction of the third and fourth lumbar vertebrae to obtain CSF for purposes of measuring CSF pressure and laboratory examination

Preprocedure preparation

Explain procedure
Have patient empty bowel and bladder
Position patient on side with spine close to edge of bed; support soft mattress with bedboards
Maintain aseptic technique throughout procedure
   Handle specimen with care
     Ensure specimen delivery to lab within 30 min to ensure diagnostic accuracy
Instruct patient that procedure may be uncomfortable
Explain importance of immobilization during procedure
Instruct patient to breathe normally; to not hold breath
Provide patient with physical and emotional support during procedure

Postprocedure assessment

Observations/findings

Altered level of consciousness
Headache: mild to severe
Nuchal rigidity
Hypotension
Tachycardia
Tachypnea
Bleeding from site of puncture
Elevated temperature

Laboratory/diagnostic studies

Normal adult CSF
   Pressure: 70 to 200 mm of water
   Color: colorless, clear
   Glucose level: 45 to 75 mg/100 ml
   Protein level (total): 20 to 45 mg/100 ml
   Red blood cells: none
   White blood cells: 0 to 5 cells/mm^3
   Microorganisms: none
Normal child CSF (above 6 months)
   Pressure: 70 to 200 mm of water
   Color: colorless, clear
   Glucose level: > 40 mg/100 ml
   Protein level (total): < 40 mg mg/100 ml
   Red blood cells: none
   White blood cells: 0 to 4
   Microorganisms: none

Potential complications

Increased ICP
Infection

Immediate postprocedure care

Maintain bed rest; place patient in supine position, keeping head of bed flat for 4 to 8 hr as ordered; if headache occurs, elevate feet 10 to 15 degrees above head
Assist and teach patient to turn and deep breathe q2h to 4h
Check BP, P, and R q15 min for four times, then qh for four times, then as ordered
Control pain as ordered
Observe site of puncture for redness, swelling, or drainage and report any symptoms to physician
Maintain diet as ordered
Force fluids unless contraindicated
Explain importance of keeping head and body position flat in bed

Ongoing care

Resume activities as ordered
Ambulate to tolerance

HYPOTHERMIA: CARE OF PATIENT

Controlled reduction and maintenance of body temperature to decrease the metabolic rate

Assessment

Observations/findings
PATIENT

Shivering
Decreased BP
Bradycardia
Bradypnea
Altered level of consciousness
Medication reactions
Pupil inequality

EQUIPMENT

Cooling solution; amount in unit
Patency of connections
Pads

Potential complications

Arrhythmias
Increased ICP
Respiratory failure
Decreased urinary output
Intestinal ileus
Frostbite and burns

Immediate care

Take and record temperature before starting treatment and q5 min until desired temperature is reached, then q15 min
Check BP, P, and R and do neuro check q5 min to 10 min while temperature is stabilizing
Observe for any change in skin color or for presence of edema and induration; report any changes to physician immediately
Assist and teach patient to turn, cough, and deep breathe q1h to 2h
Measure intake and output; measure output qh; report output less than 30 ml/hr to physician; specific gravity test may be ordered
Connect indwelling catheter to closed gravity drainage as ordered
Auscultate chest for breath sounds q1h to 2h
Administer medication for shivering as ordered
Test gag reflex prior to administering any oral fluids or food to patients with temperatures of less than 90° F (32.2° C)
Perform naso-oral suction as indicated
Administer skin care q1h to 2h
  Lubricate skin before and during procedure with oil or lotion
  Place bath blankets over thermal blankets
Maintain good body alignment
Perform passive or active ROM exercises q4h
Administer oral hygiene q1h to 2h; keep lips well lubricated
Administer nose care q1h to 2h
Provide emotional support
  Remain with patient when anxious
  Anticipate needs

Ongoing care

Patient

Check BP, T, P, and R and do neuro check q30 min for four times, then q4h for 24 hr, then as ordered
Check any dressing and all skin surfaces q1h to 2h until patient's temperature is stable
Measure intake and output
Assist and teach patient to turn, cough, and deep breathe q2h
Resume care of disease as ordered

Equipment

Check for leaks or punctures in pads prior to applying to patient

INTRACRANIAL PRESSURE (ICP) MONITORING

Insertion of a catheter for purposes of monitoring ICP and/or removing CSF

intraventricular (ventriculostomy) *Placement of catheter into lateral ventricle; CSF may be removed for control of ICP or diagnostic evaluation*

subarachnoid method *Screw or commercial bolt with stopcock that can be rapidly passed into subarachnoid space*

epidural method *Placement of sensor through a burr hole between the skull and dura*

Assessment
Observations/findings
PATIENT

Normal levels: 1 to 15 mm Hg
Moderate elevation: 15 to 40 mm Hg
High levels: > 40 mm Hg
Cerebral perfusion pressure (CPP): 50 to 85 mm Hg
  Calculation of formula:

  CPP = MABP (mean arterial blood pressure) − ICP

  CPP < 50 mm Hg: ischemia
  CPP < 20 to 30 mm Hg: irreversible ischemia
Wave forms
  A waves: large plateau formations characterized by varying increases and decreases of ICP ranging from 50 to 90 mm Hg and lasting 5 to 20 min; related to cerebral dysfunction
  B waves: occur more regularly—1½ to 1/min, ranging from 10 to 50 mm Hg
  C waves: rapid rhythmic oscillations at amplitudes to 20 mm Hg
Hemodynamic measurements
  Intraarterial pressure
  Pulmonary capillary wedge pressure (PCWP)
  Pulmonary artery diastolic pressure
  Cardiac output (CO)
Level of consciousness
Decreased BP
Increased ICP: changes determined by baselines pressure
CSF
  Clear
  Cloudy
  Blood tinged
  Xanothochromic
Elevated temperature

EQUIPMENT

Flush solution
    Ringer's lactated injection
    Normal saline solution
Pressure line tubing
Transducer
Pressure monitor

Potential complications

Meningitis
Hemorrhage: catheter insertion site
Infection
    Swelling
    Inflammation
    Redness
    Leaking of CSF

Preparation
Patient

Reinforce physician's explanation of procedure, duration, and equipment that will be used
Record baseline observations of patient and ICP at time of insertion

Equipment

Calibrate all equipment prior to insertion
    Transducer
    Recording display unit
Position transducer to eye of patient for ventriculostomy or at level of both for subarachnoid screw
Be aware that insertion must be done under sterile conditions

Ongoing care
Patient

Maintain head of bed elevated at 30 degrees with patient in supine position; avoid neck flexion, prone position, or extreme hip flexion
Record pressures qh, prn, and following changes in body position or condition
Notify physician if plateau wave forms begin to increase steadily
Calculate CPP qh
Check BP, P, and R and do neuro check q1h to 2h
Check rectal temperature q2h to 4h
Report any changes in level of consciousness or pressures to physician
Check dressing q1h to 2h
Change dressing qd
Never flush or irrigate ventricular cannula
Administer stool softeners as ordered; avoid straining
See Increased Intracranial Pressure (ICP)
NOTE: The following items may change pressure readings

    Obstructed airway
    Suctioning
    Body position
    Valsalva maneuver
Report any changes in patient's condition to physician
Observe monitor during removal of CSF for precipitous drop in pressure
Remove CSF slowly and by gravity; never aspirate

Equipment

Level transducer to eye of patient for ventriculostomy; to bolt for subarachnoid screw
Flush pressure tubings with 10 ml of fluid at a time
Check patency of pressure lines q4h; remove air bubbles
Prevent kinking, compression, or tension on tubing
Calibrate transducer q4h to 6h or as indicated by manufacturer; never apply direct pressure to diaphragm of transducer
Change pressure tubing q24h

INCREASED INTRACRANIAL PRESSURE (ICP)

Slow or sudden elevation in CSF pressure due to edema, hemorrhage, or trauma; caused by increase in CSF or obstruction to outflow

Assessment
Observations/findings

Altered level of consciousness
Restlessness
Instability
Anxiety
Variability in concentration
Purposeless movements
Paresis
Dysphasia
Decreased level of response
Headache: location, duration, severity
Pupil inequality (dilation on side of hemorrhage)
Progressive weakness or paralysis of extremitites
Decreasing respiratory rate progressing to periods of apnea; Biot's or Cheyne-Stokes respirations (p. 220)
Elevated BP (systolic); widened pulse pressure
Pulse rate decreased to 50 beats/min or below
Cerebral perfusion pressure (CPP)
Hemodynamic pressure
    Cardiac output (CO)
    Pulmonary capillary wedge pressure (PCWP)
    Pulmonary artery pressure (PAP)
Nausea, vomiting (projectile)
Elevated temperature

Visual disturbances
    Diplopia
    Blurred vision
Seizure activity
After cranial surgery
    Swelling around surgical site
    Elevation of bone flap

Laboratory/diagnostic studies

CT scan
MRI
Ventriculostomy
ICP monitoring
Arterial blood gases
Electrolytes
BUN, creatinine, glucose
CBC
Coagulation

Potential complications

Deterioration of neurologic function
Impaired respiratory function
Brainstem herniation

Medical management

Management of ventilatory status
    Oxygenation
    Ventilatory support
    Hyperventilation
Medications
    Osmotic diuretics
    Fluid restriction
    Steroids
    Anticonvulsants
    Barbiturate coma
    Antiinfectives
    Antacids
Cardiac monitoring
Surgical intervention
Shunting

Nursing diagnosis/goal/interventions

ndx: Potential for injury related to physiologic effects of sustained elevations in intracranial pressure

GOAL: *Patient will be free of injury from increased intracranial pressure*

Maintain airway patency
Elevate head of bed to 30 degrees
Maintain body position
    Avoid semiprone or prone position
    Avoid flexion of neck
    Avoid compression of neck veins
    Avoid extreme hip flexion
Check BP, P, and R q30 min; if possible take BP on same arm each time
Perform neuro check q30 min using Glasgow Coma Scale; report scores of 8 or less or any significant changes
Check rectal temperature q2h to 4h and prn; perform cooling measures as needed
Report any changes in vital signs or level of consciousness to physician immediately
Maintain parenteral fluids as ordered; hypertonic solutions may be ordered
Initiate specific medical management as indicated
Avoid Valsalve-type maneuvers: vomiting, retching, straining
Avoid isometric muscular contractions; instruct patient to avoid pushing feet against bedboard
Perform passive ROM activities as ordered
Avoid stress-producing procedures during rapid eye movement (REM) stages of sleep
Explain and prepare for diagnostic tests and/or return to surgery as ordered
See standard of care for primary condition

Evaluation

Patient
    Remains free of injury
    Demonstrates appropriate orientation and level of consciousness
    Demonstrates an effective breathing pattern
    Demonstrates normal intracranial pressure
    Demonstrates normal ROM

BOWEL TRAINING

Method of bowel evacuation by reflex conditioning

Assessment

Observations/findings

Impaction
Diarrhea
Bowel incontinence
Autonomic hyperreflexia (dysreflexia)
    Restlessness
    Chills
    Hypertension
    Diaphoresis
    Headache
    Elevated temperature
    Bradycardia

Patient teaching/discharge planning

Explain purpose and necessity of developing bowel regulation
Encourage patient's participation in developing his program
Evaluate previous bowel habits
Establish regular bowel habits
    Time of day that will be convenient for patient once discharged: after breakfast
    Development of program to have bowel evacuation at same time each day or q3d
Teach exercises that will help develop abdominal muscles and tone
    Pushing up
    Bearing down
    Contracting abdominal muscles
Ensure privacy
Provide bedside commode rather than bedpan when possible; encourage sitting position rather than lying
Keep equipment easily available at bedside
Teach patient to recognize signals or "cues" that may indicate full bowel
    Goose pimples
    Perspiration
    Raising of hair on arms or legs
    Sense of fullness

SKULL TONGS (HALO TRACTION)

Method of immobilizing the neck and stabilizing the spine

Assessment

Observations/findings

Site of insertion of tongs
    Redness
    Swelling
    Drainage
Skin condition: decubiti of scapula, coccyx, and heels
Alignment of head, pulleys, and weights: avoid head touching head of bed
Weights
    Pounds ordered
    Off floor, hanging freely
Position of bed

Ongoing care

Inspect and clean site of insertion q1h to 2h; remove *any* formed crusts with hydrogen peroxide q6h to 8h and prn
Administer skin and scalp care q2h to 4h
    Use air mattress
    Use sheepskin
    Give back rubs
    Keep linen dry and wrinkle-free
    Avoid powders
Perform passive ROM exercises to all extremities q4h
Check alignment of pulleys and weights q4h to 6h; sandbags may be indicated for restlessness as ordered
Turn patient q2h as ordered
Assist and teach patient to deep breathe q2h
Establish means of communication and keep within easy reach of patient: call bell

Patient teaching

Explain purpose of tongs
Explain methods of turning when possible
Explain importance of keeping head straight

CARE OF PATIENT ON A CIRCLE BED

Assessment

Observations/findings

PATIENT

Body alignment
Pressure areas
Numbness of any area
Dizziness or nausea related to turning
Foot-drop

BED

Position, condition, and proper functioning of
    Canvas supports
    Anterior and posterior frame
    Locks
    Side rails
    Armrests
    Wheel brakes
    Footboard
    Electrical outlets

Ongoing care

Check position, condition, and proper functioning of bed parts prior to use and daily; report breakage, missing parts, or malfunction to appropriate person
Turn and reposition patient as ordered
    Free drainage tubing and call light prior to turning and reaffix after turning
    Maintain any traction during turning
    Turn slowly; ask patient to describe how he feels during turning
Use footboard at all times
Place armrests in desired position

Provide some method to increase field of vision when possible

STRYKER FRAME

Metal frame bed used to facilitate administration of nursing care to patient with spinal cord injuries

Assessment

Observations/findings

PATIENT

Body position
- Straight body alignment
- Place in center of frame
- Body parts not resting on metal frame

Skin
- Temperature
- Color

Pressure areas
Pulse
Respirations
Lightheadedness
Numbness

EQUIPMENT

Canvas supports
Arm and foot supports
Locks
Frame
- Anterior
- Posterior

Preparation of unit

Check unit for security of bolts, locks, and frame before placing patient on Stryker frame
Prepare bed with linens, foam mattress, arm rests, and footboards prior to receiving patient

Ongoing care

Turn patient q2h during day
Turn patient q4h during night
Check P and R before and after turning
Free all excess tubing before turning
Secure all bolts tightly before turning
Reassure patient when turning
Administer skin care q2h and 4h and prn
Inspect pressure points q2h to 4h

GENERAL REHABILITATIVE CARE OF NEUROLOGIC PATIENT

May involve minimal to long-term chronic rehabilitative care; specialized settings have programs designed to meet special need areas; the following describe general guidelines for observation and intervention of the neurologically impaired patient

Conditions requiring rehabilitative approach

Cognitive impairment
Sensory-perceptual impairment
Alteration in memory, speech, auditory or visual function
Paralysis
Behavioral changes
Spinal cord injuries (see p. 305 for assessment)
Alteration in elimination function
Alteration in physical mobility
Self-care deficit
Ineffective individual coping

Rehabilitative approach

Reinforce physician's explanation of disorder and its limitations and allowances
Deal with behavioral changes
- Allow patient to go through stages of grief over loss of body function
- Be supportive but firm in dealing with patient

Encourage verbalization of feelings and fears
Use positive and reassuring approach to patient
Encourage independence when possible; be alert to limitations
Involve family or significant other in care and instructions
Establish program for ADLs
Encourage patient's participation in developing his program
Establish daily routines of activity and rest periods
Sample
- 7:00 to 7:30 Morning care
- 7:30 to 8:30 Breakfast
- 9:00 to 9:30 Commode (bowel training)
- 9:30 to 10:30 Bath
- 10:30 to 11:00 Chair, stretcher
- 11:00 to 12:00 Bed rest; turn and position
- 12:00 to 12:30 Lunch
- 12:30 to 2:30 Bed rest; turn and position
- 2:30 to 3:00 Exercises
- 3:00 to 5:00 Bed rest
- 5:00 to 6:00 Chair, stretcher
            Dinner
- 6:00 to 9:00 Bed rest
- 9:00 to 9:30 Exercises
- 9:30 to 10:00 Evening care
- 10:00 PM to 7:00 AM Bed rest

Turn and reposition to
- Right side

Left side
Prone position
Supine position

Attempt to avoid sensory deprivation by providing
Calendars
Clocks
Pictures
Include in schedule favorite television or radio programs, hobbies, and visiting hours

Explain all treatments and procedures as they occur

Alert staff to emotional changes and mood swings

Allow patient time to express needs

Refer to social service, Visiting Nurses Association, and/or local rehabilitation centers as ordered

Report symptoms of urinary tract infection to physician
Foul odor of urine
Sedimentation, pus, or blood in urine
Decreased output
Low-grade fever
Chills

Encourage participation in bowel and bladder training

Avoid constipation

Cleanse perineal region; wipe from front to back after urination

Cleanse perineal region with soap and water after each bowel movement

Give high-calorie, high-protein diet as ordered; avoid high-calcium foods

Activities

Explain importance of exercise programs
Exercise to tolerance; avoid fatigue
Plan rest periods

Nutrition

Assess daily caloric needs
Maintain high-calorie, high-protein, low-residue diet as ordered
Limit high-calcium and gas-producing foods

Elimination

Encourage fluids to 3000 ml daily unless contraindicated
Avoid constipation through use of stool softeners, mild cathartics, suppositories, and/or enemas
Check for bowel movement q3d
Institute bowel and bladder programs
Avoid overdistention of bladder and bowel
Initiate intermittent catheterization as indicated

Patient teaching

Ensure patient and/or significant other knows and understands
  Importance of exercise programs
  Need to exercise to tolerance; to avoid fatigue
  Importance of fluid intake; measure intake and output
  Importance of turning q2h to 4h while in bed
  Need to inspect skin and bony prominences for detection of breakdown
  Importance of skin care q2h to 4h while in bed
  Need to avoid constrictive clothing below level of lesion (e.g., garters, belts)
  Need to avoid urinary tract infections
  Avoid overdistention of bladder; empty on regular basis
  Encourage fluid to 3000 ml daily
Need to ensure daily bowel evacuation to avoid fecal impaction; encourage participation in bowel training (p. 332)
Need for ongoing support and counseling services
  Sexual counseling: patients can engage in some form of satisfying sexual activity
  Limitations depend on site of injury; incomplete injuries and high cord injuries allow for varying amounts of sensation and sexual function—even if spinal reflexes are absent, sensation of genital organs may endure
  Female reproductive system usually remains intact; patient can bear children—refer for family planning counseling

PARAPLEGIA

Paralysis of the lower extremities resulting from injury to the spinal cord

Assessment
Observations/findings

Atrophy of nonfunctioning body parts
See Musculoskeletal Assessment (p. 470)
Bladder distention
Dysuria
Bowel
Incontinence
Impaction

Rehabilitation

Give praise for tasks completed
Avoid tasks that patient cannot complete
Provide diversional activities as indicated
  Reading
  Watching television
  Listening to radio
  Working puzzles
  Listening to tape cassettes

Establish means of communication
  Call bell within reach
  Calling out to nurse

Bed activities

Perform weight-bearing exercises
  Begin elevating head of bed, progressing to high-Fowler's position as tolerated when condition stabilizes
  Use tilt or circle bed as ordered
    Begin elevating patient's head at 10 degrees for 10 to 15 min three times daily, progressing to 15 degrees for 1 hr two or three times daily
    Keep legs wrapped with elastic stockings as ordered
    Take BP before tilting patient and q5 min at 10 degrees; in absence of hypotension or dizziness, progress to 15 degrees as tolerated
    Gradually progress to 90-degree elevation as tolerated
Change position qh: maintain body alignment
  Prone position
  Supine position
  Rolling to side
  Sitting up
  Moving forward and backward
Check placement of lower extremities with each movement
Administer skin care q2h to 4h
  Use air mattresses
  Use sheepskin
  Give back rubs with lanolin-based lotions
  Put foam rubber pads on chairs
  Keep linen dry and wrinkle-free
  Place rubber sheet under bath blanket
  Use body corset as ordered
See p. 619 if decubitus develops
Perform muscle-building exercises
  Active ROM exercise to support extremities
  Dumbbells: extending and flexing of arms
  Overhead trapezes
  Push-ups
  Sit-ups
  Hand-finger exercises
    Rubber sponge balls
    Extension and flexion
Teach method of turning self and pulling up in bed

Wheelchair activities

Get patient out of bed two or three times daily
Demonstrate method of transferring from bed to wheelchair, and from wheelchair to toilet or shower
Demonstrate management of wheelchair: moving forward, backward, turning, stopping, and locking

Self-care activities

Allow self-care as tolerated
  Bathing
  Dressing
  Combing hair
  Shaving
  Oral hygiene
Encourage patient to wear own clothing: pajamas, slippers, or shoes

Motion activities

Use long leg braces as ordered
Perform physical therapy as ordered
  Weight-bearing exercises
  Parallel bar exercises
  Balancing exercises
  Crutch-walking exercises
To relieve spasticity
  Perform active or passive ROM exercises
  Wear long leg braces
  Give medications as ordered

Elimination

Perform urinalysis weekly as indicated
Check urine output for sedimentation or presence of renal calculi
Perform intermittent catheterization as ordered
Initiate bowel and bladder programs
Teach self-catheterization when appropriate

QUADRIPLEGIA

Paralysis of the upper and lower extremities resulting from injury to the spinal cord (thoracic and cervical regions)

Assessment

Observations/findings

Loss of sweating reflex
Bladder distention and incontinence
Mass reflex of bladder
  Muscular spasms
  Diaphoresis
  Elevated BP
  Headache

Rehabilitation

Encourage staff to allow time for patient care; do not rush patient

Provide diversional activities as indicated
  Reading
  Socializing with nursing staff
Provide means of communication
  Calling out to nurse
  Whistling

Bed activities

Maintain good body alignment
Use circle bed as indicated
Turn and position patient q1h to 2h
  Use supports: sandbags and pillows
  Avoid external rotation of lower extremities
  Position patient: supine, prone, and on side
Cough and deep breathe q1h to 2h
Administer skin care q1h to 2h
  Use air mattress
  Use footboard
  Use sheepskin
  Keep bed linen dry and wrinkle-free
  Rub back and heels with lanolin-based lotions
  Change bed clothing prn
  Place rubber sheet under bath blanket to be used as draw sheet
  Assist with or provide perineal care after each voiding or bowel movement
  Begin elevating head of bed as condition stabilizes, progressing to high-Fowler's position as tolerated
Tilt table or circle bed as ordered
  Begin raising head to 10 degrees for 10 to 15 min three times daily, progressing to 20 degrees for 1 hr two or three times daily, on to 90 degrees for 1 hr two or three times daily, on to 90 degrees as tolerated
  Take BP before tilting patient and at 5 to 10 min intervals as head is being raised; in absence of hypotension or dizziness progress to 90 degrees
  Apply elastic bandages or stockings as ordered

Wheelchair activities

Use three or four persons to transfer patient to stretcher chair or stretcher for 15 to 30 min two to three times daily as ordered
Encourage wheelchair activity as ordered as condition stabilizes
Provide braces, splints, and other supports as ordered
Take safety measures
  Soft jacket restraints
  Soft abdominal binders
  Side rails when indicated

Self-care activities

Encourage patient to wear clothing from home and to make selections

Motion activities

To relieve spasticity
  Perform gentle passive ROM exercises
  Wear braces
  Give medications as ordered
  Prepare for rhizotomy or chordotomy as ordered

Nutrition

Give tube feedings as indicated
Position patient with head of bed at 30 to 45 degrees
Feed patient
  Allow 30 to 45 min for feeding time
  Give small bites of food
Perform oral hygiene q4h and after meals
  Clean with hydrogen peroxide and water
  Gargle and mouthwash
  Brush teeth

Elimination

Provide indwelling or external catheter to closed gravity drainage as ordered
Instruct patient to develop exercise or signals that may help to stimulate urge to defecate
  Smoking
  Pressure on inner thigh
  Stroking anus
  Digital rectal stimulation
  Drinking coffee
  Massaging abdomen downward or right to left
Instruct patient to respond to "cues" promptly
Discuss importance of established well-balanced diet that includes bulk and roughage
Discuss foods to avoid
  Bananas
  Beans
  Cabbage
  Foods that have been previously constipating
Encourage fluids to 3000 ml daily unless contraindicated
Include prune and orange juice and coffee in daily diet as preferred
Discuss possible programs to develop
  Instruct patient to take 8 to 10 oz of prune juice 12 hr prior to time set for defecating; insert glycerin suppository high in rectum 15 to 20 min before set time, then place patient on bedpan, toilet, or commode

Insert lubricated glycerin suppository 2 hr before set time and position patient in sitting position or transfer to bedpan or commode

Instruct patient to drink 4 to 8 oz of prune juice each night

Instruct patient to drink a warm drink 30 min before set time
- Water
- Coffee
- Milk

Insert laxative suppository for 2 to 4 days, then glycerin suppository for 2 to 4 days; note length of time between insertion and defecation; place patient on bedside commode at appropriate time; if no bowel movement, give small tap water enema

Instruct patient to recognize signs of impaction
- No formed stool for 3 days
- Semiliquid stools
- Restlessness and increased feeling of discomfort

Discuss treatment for impaction
- Laxative suppository
- Tap water or oil-retention enemas
- Manual clearing of bowel followed by enema

CHAPTER 6

Digestive System

GASTROINTESTINAL ASSESSMENT

Subjective Data

Mouth, gums, tongue, lips
  Painful
  Tender
Dysphagia
Eructation
Anorexia, loss of weight
Indigestion
Pyrosis (heartburn)
Fullness after eating
Nausea, vomiting; regurgitation without vomiting
Abdomen
  Painful
  Tender
  Cramping
Easily fatigued
Change in eating or bowel habits
Change in color, character, or frequency of stools or urine
Constipation
Diarrhea
Hemorrhoids
Painful defecation
Use of laxatives or enemas
Change in skin color or texture; rash or itching
Edema of extremities

Objective Data

General appearance
Vital signs
  BP, P, and R
    Lying
    Sitting
    Standing
Temperature
Weight
Urinary output, color, amount
Allergies
Mouth
  Stomatitis
  Condition and color of tongue, gums, mucous membrane, and teeth
  Halitosis
  Saliva production: increased or decreased
Abdomen
  Distention, rigidity, ascites
  Symmetry
  Hepatomegaly
  Keloid tissue, scars
  Visible peristalsis
  Bowel sounds
    Present
    Absent
  Visible palpable masses; hernia(s)
  Presence of ostomies
Perianal area
  Hemorrhoids
  Color and condition of area
  Odor
  Color, consistency, and frequency of stools
Sclera: jaundice
Skin
  Jaundice
  Turgor
  Pruritus
  Spider angioma
  Purpura
  Palmar erythema
  Peripheral edema
  Distended, tortuous blood vessels
  Abdominal striae

Pertinent Background Information
CONCURRENT DISEASES OR CONDITIONS

Carcinoma
Cardiovascular disease (hypertension)
Alcoholism
Endocrine disorders
Severe burns
Psychologic problems
Drug abuse
Neurologic conditions
Epistaxis

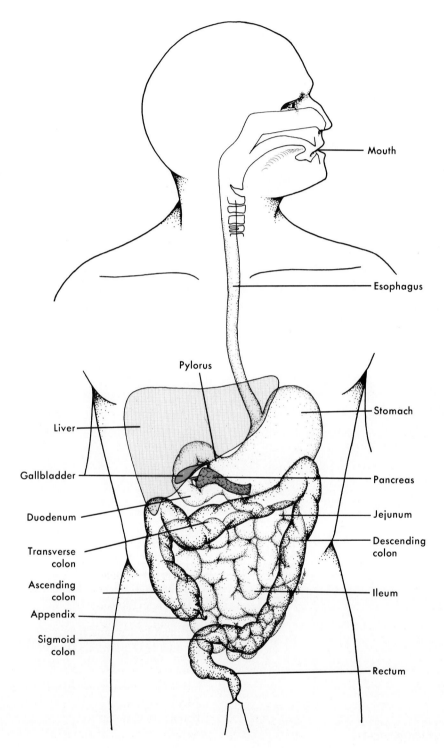

FIGURE 6-1. Digestive system.

PREVIOUS SURGERY OR ILLNESS

Inflammatory bowel disease
Carcinoma
Gastrointestinal (GI) surgery
   Cholecystectomy
   Gastric surgery
   Ostomies
   Other abdominal, pelvic, or rectal surgeries
Hepatitis
Cirrhosis
Pancreatitis
Diabetes mellitus

FAMILY HISTORY

Carcinoma
GI-related disease
Diabetes mellitus

SOCIAL HISTORY

Alcohol, tobacco use
Cultural food use; eating habits
Personality type: tense, stressful
View of life's work

MEDICATION HISTORY

Antacids
Laxatives, cathartics
Anticholinergics
Steroids
Antidiarrheals
Antiemetics
Tranquilizers
Sedatives
Antihypertensives
Barbiturates
Antibiotics
Acetylsalicylic acid

Diagnostic Aids

LABORATORY STUDIES

Complete blood cell count (CBC)
Alkaline phosphatase level
Bilirubin level
   Serum
   Urine
   Fecal
Serum glutamic oxaloacetic transaminase (SGOT)
Serum glutamic pyruvic transaminase (SGPT)
5-Nucleotidase
Lactic acid dehydrogenase (LDH)
Prothrombin time (PT)
Amylase level
   Serum
   Urine
Blood urea nitrogen (BUN)
Stool examination
   Occult blood
   Fat
   Protein
   Parasite ova
Secretin stimulation test
Serum lipase, cholinesterase levels
Serum calcium level
Serum ammonia level
Serum gastrin level
Serum alpha-fetoprotein
Sulkowitch's urine test
Serum albumin level
Total protein level
Serum glucose level
Serum electrolyte profile
Serum carotene test
D-Xylose tolerance test
Schilling's test
Albumin-globulin (A/G) ratio
Urobilinogen level
Galactose tolerance test
Insulin tolerance test
Hollander test
Carcinoembryonic antigen (CEA)

PROCEDURES

Endoscopy and biopsy
   Esophageal
   Gastric
   Duodenal
Cine-esophagogram
Basal secretion
Gastric acid stimulation test
Esophageal manometry
Contrast radiography
Hypotonic duodenography
Radionuclide imaging
Computed tomography (CT) scan
Ultrasonography
Upper GI series
Small bowel series
Barium enema or swallow gastrography
Cholecystography
Intravenous cholangiography
T tube cholangiography
Biopsy
   Liver
   Rectum

Colon
    Small bowel
Sigmoidoscopy
Colonoscopy
Fluoroscopy
Complete abdominal x-ray examination
Bernstein test
Gastric cytology
Percutaneous transhepatic cholangiography
Celiac and mesenteric arteriography
Superior and inferior mesenteric angiogram
Scans
    Liver, spleen
    Pancreas
Splenoportography
Endoscopic retrograde cholangiopancreatography (ERCP)

Esophagus

ESOPHAGEAL TRAUMA

Major traumatic conditions affecting the esophagus (e.g., chemical burns, foreign bodies, and injuries from external forces)

Assessment

Observations/findings

Type and cause of injury: internal or external
Patent airway
Amount of bleeding and source
Level of consciousness
Vital signs
Respiratory distress
Cyanosis
Dysphagia
Nausea, vomiting
Restlessness
Amount, type, and location of pain

Laboratory/diagnostic studies

Endoscopy
Radiography
CBC
Urinalysis

Potential complications

Esophageal perforation
Aspiration pneumonia
Hemorrhage
Shock

Medical management

Specific poison antidote
Oxygen therapy
NPO
Nasogastric tube with intermittent suction
Gastrostomy (if applicable)
Analgesics, antibiotics
Oropharyngeal suctioning
Gastric lavage

Nursing diagnoses/goals/interventions

ndx: Impaired gas exchange related to airway obstruction and/or lung aspiration

GOAL: *Patient's airway will be maintained, and gas exchange will be adequate*

Internal injuries
CAUSTIC SUBSTANCES

Maintain patent airway
Perform oropharyngeal suctioning prn
Administer specific antidote as ordered
Administer oxygen therapy as ordered
Do not induce vomiting
Elevate head 30 to 40 degrees
Turn and deep breathe q2h

FOREIGN BODIES

Maintain patent airway
Perform oropharyngeal suctioning prn
Determine type of object ingested
Keep patient as quiet as possible
Elevate head 30 to 40 degrees
Turn and deep breathe q2h

External injuries

Maintain patent airway
Perform oropharyngeal suctioning prn
Administer oxygen therapy as ordered
Turn and deep breathe q2h

ndx: Alteration in nutrition: less than body requirements related to esophageal trauma

GOAL: *Patient's nutrition will be maintained*

Administer parenteral therapy with electrolytes as ordered
Maintain NPO
Assist with insertion and connect nasogastric tube to intermittent suction apparatus as ordered
Check color, consistency, and amount of gastric drainage q4h
Measure intake and output q8h
Administer oral hygiene q4h

If patient is not NPO and nasogastric tube is not in place
    Force fluids to 3000 ml daily, unless contraindicated, or according to weight in a child
    Provide diet as ordered when allowed
Monitor vital signs 4h; take rectal temperature if nasogastric tube is in place
For gastrostomy insertion, see p. 367
For esophageal surgery, see p. 349

ndx: Alteration in comfort: pain related to trauma

GOAL: *Patient will state pain is minimal or controlled*

Administer analgesics as ordered
Perform passive or teach active range-of-motion (ROM) exercises q4h
Change position q2h
Administer back rubs prn
Offer diversional activities

ndx: Anxiety/fear related to traumatic experience and hospitalization

GOAL: *Patient will demonstrate adaptive responses when anxiety/fear is understood*

Encourage and allow time for verbalization
Explain all procedures and treatments
Involve patient in planning care
Reinforce physician's explanation of course of therapy and possible surgery
Provide quiet, nonstressful environment

ndx: Knowledge deficit regarding home care

GOAL: *Patient and/or significant other will demonstrate understanding of home care and follow-up instructions through interactive discussion*

Discuss dietary management following foreign object removal
    Provide soft, bland diet until soreness disappears
    Avoid hot liquids, spicy foods, alcohol, and caffeine
    Force fluids to 3000 ml/24 hr or, if child, according to weight unless contraindicated
Discuss ways of preventing further ingestion of foreign objects or caustic substances
Discuss signs of perforation to report to physician
    Increased pain or dysphagia
    Edema of neck or respiratory distress
    Excessive bleeding
Following gastrostomy insertion, see p. 367
Following esophageal surgery, see p. 349
Explain importance of follow-up appointments with physician

Evaluation

There are no complications
Patient is well hydrated and comfortable
There is no respiratory distress
Patient demonstrates knowledge of home care and follow-up instructions

ESOPHAGEAL STRICTURE, ESOPHAGITIS, ACHALASIA, DIVERTICULOSIS

stricture *Narrowing of the wall of the esophagus (usually lower two thirds); most commonly due to reflux esophagitis, chemical ingestion, sliding hiatal hernia, or neoplastic infiltration*

esophagitis *Acute or chronic inflammation caused by gastroesophageal reflux, trauma, bacteria, chemical ingestion, hiatal hernia, or overindulgence in alcohol and/or spices*

achalasia *Disruption or absence of peristaltic action in the lower two thirds of the esophagus and failure of the cardiac sphincter to relax on swallowing*

diverticulosis *Saclike protrusion in the esophageal wall, usually of a congenital nature*

Assessment

Observations/findings

Midsternal or substernal pain; may radiate to back, neck, and arms
Discomfort after eating, when bending, or when in supine position
Sore throat
Nocturnal choking
Pyrosis (heartburn)
Regurgitation without vomiting
Weight loss
Eructation
Dysphagia
Hematemesis

Laboratory/diagnostic studies

Endoscopy with biopsy, cytology, and/or dilation
Barium swallow esophagram
Splash down time
Chest radiologic study
Manometry
CBC and electrolytes
Bernstein test

Potential complications

Aspiration pneumonia
Esophageal obstruction
Malnutrition
Esophageal perforation

Medical management

High-calorie diet according to tolerance
Antacids
Topical liquid anesthetics
Stool softeners
Antibiotics

Nursing diagnoses/goals/interventions

ndx: Alteration in nutrition: less than body requirements related to dysphagia

GOAL: *Patient will maintain intake to meet metabolic requirements*

Provide small, frequent meals
Teach patient to chew food well and to eat slowly
Encourage fluids with meals
Avoid extremes in food temperatures
Measure intake and output
Administer liquid topical anesthetic prior to meals as ordered
Administer antacids between meals and at bedtime as ordered
Provide high-fiber foods if tolerated and/or administer stool softeners as ordered
Monitor CBC, electrolytes
Weigh patient daily at same time with same clothing and scale
Discourage smoking

ndx: Ineffective airway clearance related to inability to clear oral secretions

GOAL: *Patient will demonstrate ability to free airway of secretions and/or food*

Assist and teach patient to cough and deep breathe q4h
Monitor breath sounds q4h
Elevate head of bed 30 to 45 degrees after meals and at bedtime
Avoid supine position
Provide planned rest periods
Encourage fluid intake to 2500 ml/24 hr if not contraindicated
Assist with and teach active or perform passive ROM exercises qid if patient is not ambulatory
Administer oral hygiene qid

ndx: Anxiety related to hospitalization and disease process

GOAL: *Patient will verbalize increasing freedom from stress*

Provide calm, nonstressful environment
Reinforce physician's explanation of disease process
Explain all procedures, treatments, and plans of care
Encourage verbalization of fears; assist patient with identifying stressors and positive coping behaviors

ndx: Knowledge deficit regarding home and follow-up care

GOAL: *Patient and/or significant other will demonstrate understanding of home care and follow-up instructions through interactive discussion*

Discuss with patient and/or significant other the importance of diet and diet restrictions
  Explain need to avoid foods that cause dysphagia
  Provide high-calorie, high-protein diet instruction sheet if applicable
  Encourage increased fluid intake
Explain need to avoid tobacco, aspirin, and phenylbutazone
Explain need to elevate head while sleeping
Explain need for nonstressful environment
Explain need to avoid bending and stooping
Discuss methods of avoiding constipation
  High-fiber foods if tolerated
  Natural laxatives
Explain need to increase activities to tolerance
Discuss medications: name, dosage, time of administration, purpose, and side effects
Explain importance of follow-up care with physician
Discuss symptoms of recurrence or progression of disease to report to physician

Evaluation

There are no complications
Optimal caloric and fluid intake is maintained
Patient demonstrates understanding of correct breathing and coughing techniques
Patient demonstrates decreased feelings of anxiety
Patient demonstrates understanding of principles of home and follow-up care

BLEEDING ESOPHAGEAL VARICES

A condition usually associated with cirrhosis and portal hypertension in which the small esophageal veins become distended and rupture as a result of the increased pressure in the portal system; may be controlled medically, but surgery (portacaval shunt) is often required

Assessment
Observations/findings

Character, frequency, and amount of hematemesis
Respiratory distress

Aspiration of emesis
Disorientation
Confusion
Dehydration
Electrolyte imbalance
Abdominal distention
Anxiety
Melena
Jaundice

Laboratory/diagnostic studies

Esophagoscopy
Esophageal arteriogram
CBC, platelets, PT, arterial blood gases, electrolytes
Blood alcohol
SGOT, SGPT, LDH, alkaline phosphatase
Liver function tests
Guaiac stools for blood

Potential complications

Aspiration pneumonia
Hemorrhage
Shock
Hepatic coma
Death

Medical management

NPO
Esophagogastric tube with suction and pressures to be maintained
Iced saline lavages
Parenteral fluids with electrolytes
Fresh whole blood
Indwelling urinary catheter with hourly measurements
Orotracheal suctioning
Oxygen therapy
Central venous pressure (CVP) line or Swan-Ganz catheter
Arterial blood gases
Saline enemas
Vasopressin (Pitressin), antibiotics, vitamin K
Analgesics, usually phenobarbital
Esophageal sclerotherapy
Surgical intervention (portacaval shunt, p. 407)

Nursing diagnoses/goals/interventions

ndx: Ineffective airway clearance related to inability to clear oral secretions

GOAL: *Patient's airway will be maintained*

Maintain bed rest in quiet environment
    Position on side during vomiting episodes
    Elevate head of bed 30 degrees
Perform orotracheal suctioning prn
Auscultate chest for breath sounds q1h to 2h
Administer oxygen therapy by mask or catheter
Assist and teach patient to turn and deep breathe qh; instruct not to cough
Administer oral hygiene q1h to 2h; keep mouth and nares well lubricated

ndx: Alteration in tissue perfusion related to abnormal fluid loss and hemorrhage

GOAL: *Patient's fluid volume and electrolyte balance will be maintained, and hemorrhage will be managed*

Assist with insertion of esophagogastric tube
    Sengstaken-Blakemore tube (p. 352)
    Linton tube (p. 352)
Check character and amount of gastric drainage q1h to 2h
Administer iced saline lavages as ordered
Maintain NPO
Administer parenteral fluids with electrolytes as ordered
Administer fresh whole blood as ordered
Monitor hemoglobin (Hgb), hematocrit (Hct), serum electrolytes, and PT
Monitor CVP line or Swan-Ganz catheter
Draw arterial blood gases as ordered
Monitor BP, R, and apical pulse q15 min to 30 min
Take rectal temperature q2h
Connect indwelling urinary catheter to gravity drainage as ordered
Measure intake and output qh; if urine output is less than 30 to 50 ml/hr, report to physician
Observe for signs of coma or ascites
Measure abdominal girth q1h to 2h; report increase to physician
Observe character, amount, and color of stools; give saline enemas as ordered
Administer medications as ordered
    Antibiotics
    Vitamin K
    Vasopressin
    Antacids
Prepare for surgery if ordered
After esophagogastric tube is removed
    Initiate clear liquids q1h to 2h, 30 to 60 ml at a time
    Keep liquids at room temperature or below
    Progress from nonroughage soft to regular diet as tolerated and ordered
    Provide meals in six small feedings
    Consult with dietitian (RD), since amounts of car-

bohydrate, fat, and protein depend on liver function
Administer mild laxative as ordered to clear bowel of old blood
Monitor stools for melena
Continue to monitor intake and output

ndx: Alteration in comfort: pain related to procedures and position restriction

GOAL: *Patient will verbalize that pain is minimized or relieved*

Maintain position of comfort within limits of ongoing treatments
Administer skin care and back rubs q2h to 4h
Keep patient warm and dry
Perform passive (ROM) exercises q4h
Manage pain as indicated
    Administer phenobarbital as ordered
    Avoid morphine and meperidine
    Assess effectiveness of pain relief measures
Increase activity as tolerated

ndx: Alteration in sensory perception related to sensory overload

GOAL: *Patient will express feelings of decreased sensory overload*

Remain with patient at onset of bleeding as much as possible
    Use restraints if applicable
    Keep side rails up
Plan care to provide rest periods
Orient patient to place, date, and time frequently
Explain each procedure as much as time allows
Reinforce physician's explanation of disease process
Maintain nonstressful environment
    Dim lights when possible
    Discourage loud talking and noises
Encourage verbalization of fears and anxieties

ndx: Knowledge deficit regarding home and follow-up care

GOAL: *Patient and/or significant other will demonstrate understanding of home care and follow-up instructions through interactive discussion*

Explain diet restrictions of carbohydrate, fat, and protein
Consult dietitian (RD) for low-roughage diet plan
Discuss importance of avoiding alcohol
Explain about available counseling
    Alcoholics Anonymous
    Al-Anon, Al-Ateen
    Chemical dependency agencies
Instruct patient in a mild exercise to tolerance program with planned rest periods
Reinforce physician's explanation of effects of alcohol on disease process
Discuss medications: name, purpose, dosage, time of administration, and side effects; caution patient not to take over-the-counter medications without checking with physician
Explain symptoms of recurrence or progression to report to physician
Discuss importance of follow-up care with physician

Evaluation

There are no complications
Patent airway is maintained
Diet is sufficient to meet metabolic needs
Patient demonstrates freedom from pain
Patient expresses feeling of decreased stress due to sensory overload
Patient demonstrates understanding of principles of home and follow-up care

HIATAL HERNIA WITH ESOPHAGEAL REFLUX

Protrusion of part of the stomach through the diaphragm, causing gastric juices to reflux into the esophagus, in turn causing irritation, scar tissue, and possible stricture

Assessment

Observations/findings

Gradual onset of symptoms
Burning sensation in throat after eating; increases in supine position
Regurgitation without vomiting
Dull substernal, epigastric pain; may radiate to shoulder
Dysphagia, except for water
Abdominal distention after eating
Nausea
Belching
Borborygmus
Tachypnea
Pyrosis (heartburn)
Fear and anxiety: symptoms similar to myocardial infarction and peptic ulcer

Laboratory/diagnostic studies

CBC, urinalysis, electrolytes
Thyroid studies

Electrocardiogram (ECG)
Upper GI series
Barium swallow
Chest radiologic study
Endoscopy with biopsy and cytology
Stool for occult blood
Bernstein test

Potential complications

Esophageal stricture
Malnutrition
Electrolyte imbalance
Aspiration pneumonia
Hemorrhage

Medical management

Antacids
Histamine receptor antagonists: cimetidine (Tagamet), Zantac
Antiemetic agent: metoclopramide (Reglan)
Autonomic agent: bethanechol chloride (Urecholine)
Stool softeners
Surgical repair

Nursing diagnoses/goals/interventions

ndx: Alteration in comfort: pain related to disease process

GOAL: *Patient will express reduced or minimized discomfort or pain*

Maintain bed rest
    Place patient in sitting position
    Avoid supine position
Measure intake and output
Monitor vital signs q8h
Assist with and teach patient to turn and deep breathe qid
Provide bland diet as ordered; small, frequent feedings are beneficial
Encourage water with meals unless contraindicated
Maintain sitting position after meals
Manage pain as indicated; change in position is beneficial
Discourage smoking
Avoid constipation
Ambulate when ordered; caution against bending from waist
Explain and prepare for GI series, endoscopy, or dilation if ordered
Discuss stress management and ways of handling stress
Encourage and allow time for verbalization of fears and anxieties
Reinforce physician's explanation of disease process

ndx: Knowledge deficit regarding home and follow-up care

GOAL: *Patient and/or significant other will demonstrate understanding of home care and follow-up instructions through interactive discussion*

Instruct patient to elevate head of bed on 4-inch blocks and to avoid using pillows under head
Discuss dietary plan and restrictions
Encourage patient to eat slowly, chew foods well, take small bites, and have small, frequent meals
Stress importance of exercise and weight reduction if applicable; some modification of activities may be needed
Explain disease process and symptoms to report to physician
Discuss stool softeners and natural laxatives as alternatives to cathartics/laxatives
Outline medication management as to name, dosage, purpose, time of administration, and side effects
Stress importance of continuing follow-up care

Evaluation

There are no complications
Nutritional intake is adequate within limits of dietary restrictions
Pain is controlled with diet and medications
Principles of follow-up care are understood

ESOPHAGEAL CARCINOMA

Carcinoma developing in the middle or lower one third of the esophagus; usually fatal because the condition is advanced before symptoms appear

Assessment
Observations/findings

Increasing dysphagia
Painful swallowing
Substernal pain
Feeling of fullness
Pyrosis (heartburn)
Fear and anxiety
Weight loss
Generalized malaise
Dehydration
Regurgitation after eating
Increased salivation and mucus formation
Foul breath
Singultus (hiccups)
Eructation

Hoarseness and coughing
Hepatomegaly
Diaphragmatic paralysis (phrenic nerve involvement)

Laboratory/diagnostic studies

Endoscopy with biopsy and cytology
CBC and electrolytes
Chest radiologic study
Barium studies
Bronchoscopy
CT scan: liver and chest
Liver function tests

Potential complications

Malnutrition, anemia
Electrolyte imbalance
Fluid volume depletion
Aspiration pneumonia
Infection
Metastasis to other organs
Hemorrhage

Medical management

Analgesics
Chemotherapeutic agents
Radiation therapy
Insertion of plastic tubes (Celestin tube) to maintain nutrition
Esophageal surgery (esophagogastrectomy)
Gastrostomy tube insertion

Nursing diagnoses/goals/interventions*

ndx: Ineffective airway clearance related to esophageal obstruction

GOAL: *Patient will demonstrate ability to maintain a clear airway*

Maintain bed rest if condition warrants
  Elevate head of bed 30 to 45 degrees
  Avoid supine position
  Do not gatch knees
Assess patient's ability to swallow and teach coughing techniques
Perform orotracheal suction as needed
Provide emesis basin and tissues for expectorating
Assist and teach patient to turn and deep breathe q2h to 4h
Administer oral hygiene q2h to 4h and prn
Monitor vital signs q4h

ndx: Alteration in nutrition: less than body requirements related to anorexia and dysphagia

GOAL: *Patient's caloric intake will be maintained*

Assess patient's ability to swallow liquids and solid foods
Provide high-calorie, high-protein diet as ordered
Encourage patient to chew foods well, to take small bites, and to eat slowly
Assist with feedings prn
Force fluids to 3000 ml/24 hr unless contraindicated
Measure intake and output
Weight patient daily at same time with same clothing and scale
Initiate parenteral therapy with vitamins and electrolytes as ordered
Total parenteral nutrition (TPN) may be ordered (p. 51)
Assist with insertion of nasogastric tube if ordered; connect to low, intermittent suction or closed gravity drainage as ordered
Provide gastrostomy or Celestin tube feedings if appropriate (p. 367)

ndx: Alteration in comfort: pain related to disease process

GOAL: *Patient will express that pain is minimal or absent*

Administer analgesics as ordered
Assess effectiveness of medication
Change position q2h to 4h
Provide planned rest periods
Assist with and teach active or perform passive ROM exercises q4h

ndx: Anxiety/fear related to poor disease prognosis

GOAL: *Patient and/or significant other will verbalize fears and anxieties and utilize effective coping mechanisms*

Assess patient and/or significant other's ability to communicate feelings
Assist in dealing with emotional reactions to disease process
Recommend outside supportive groups (visiting nurses, American Cancer Society) for home care assistance
Encourage and provide time for verbalization of concerns
Involve dietitian (RD) for assistance in planning specific types of meals
Develop means of communication if patient has speaking difficulties

---

*Patient's condition dictates amount of care required; modify accordingly.

ndx: Knowledge deficit regarding home care

GOAL: *Patient and/or significant other will demonstrate understanding of home care and follow-up instructions through interactive discussion and actual return demonstration*

Instruct patient and/or significant other on type of diet required
   For gastrostomy tube (p. 367)
      Method for ascertaining correct placement and amount of residual contents
   For Celestin tube (p. 350)
      Elevating head at all times
      Swallowing only small amounts
      Method for clearing obstructions
Discuss and teach pain management and injection administration if ordered
Enlist support of dietitian (RD), home health agencies, etc.
Discuss schedule of radiation or chemotherapy treatments as ordered
Explain need to maintain physician's follow-up appointments

Evaluation

Nutritional status is maintained within limits of disease process
Pain is managed adequately
Appropriate coping mechanisms are observed
There are no complications

ESOPHAGEAL SURGERY

Surgery performed when medical management of esophageal disorders such as diverticulitis, perforation, and hiatal hernia has been unsuccessful; for carcinoma of the esophagus, an esophagogastrectomy is usually performed—approach may be thoracic or abdominal

Assessment

Observations/findings

Decreased breath sounds
Splinting with respirations
Tachypnea
Bradypnea
Function of chest tubes (thoracic approach)
Character and amount of gastric drainage and urine output
Location and character of pain

Laboratory/diagnostic studies

CBC and electrolytes
Chest radiologic study

Potential complications

Respiratory distress
Electrolyte imbalance
Gastroesophageal anastomosis leak
Hemorrhage
Shock
Tracheoesophageal fistula
Suture line infection
Pheumothorax (thoracic approach)
Pneumonia

Medical management

Analgesics
NPO
Parenteral fluids with electrolytes
Whole blood
Nasogastric tube and urinary catheter
Orotracheal suction
Oxygen per mask or catheter
Chest tubes (thoracic approach)
Intermittent positive pressure breathing (IPPB)
Gastrostomy tube if appropriate

Nursing diagnoses/goals/interventions

ndx: Ineffective airway clearance related to anesthesia

GOAL: *Patient's airway will remain patent and free of secretions*

Auscultate chest for breath sounds q2h to 4h
Elevate head of bed 35 to 45 degrees
Do not gatch knees
Teach and assist patient to turn, cough, and deep breathe q2h to 4h; splint chest as needed
Administer oxygen or IPPB as ordered
Connect chest tubes to underwater seal if appropriate (p. 271)
Following immediate postoperative care ambulate with assistance as ordered

ndx: Fluid volume deficit related to abnormal fluid loss

GOAL: *Patient's intake of fluids and electrolytes will be maintained*

Maintain NPO
Administer parenteral fluids with electrolytes as ordered
Administer whole blood as ordered
Measure intake and output
Monitor vital signs q4h
Connect nasogastric tube or gastrostomy tube to intermittent suction or gravity drainage as ordered
Check placement of nasogastric tube and do not change its position; tape in place

Check character and amount of gastric drainage q8h
Administer oral hygiene q2h to 4h; keep nares clean and moist
Assist with and teach active or perform passive ROM exercises q4h
Following nasogastric tube removal
    Initiate oral fluids in small amounts
    Observe for signs of fistula
    Progress to soft, bland diet as tolerated
    Report pain, retching, or vomiting to physician
For gastrostomy tube: administer tube feedings as ordered (p. 367)

ndx: Alteration in comfort: pain related to surgical intervention

GOAL: *Patient will express minimal discomfort or freedom from pain*

Assess type and location of pain
Administer analgesics as ordered and assess effectiveness of pain relief measures
Turn and change position q2h to 4h
Provide back rubs and skin care
Maintain planned rest periods

ndx: Actual impairment of skin integrity due to surgical incision

GOAL: *Patient's skin will remain clean, dry, and intact*

Check incision and surgical dressings q4h
Reinforce dressings as needed
Report increased drainage or bleeding to physician
Maintain skin integrity around gastrostomy tube site if applicable
Observe for signs of wound infection

ndx: Potential for ineffective coping related to surgical procedure and possible changes in life-style

GOAL: *Patient will verbalize knowledge concerning surgical procedure and demonstrate progress toward positive behavioral attitudes toward coping with expected changes*

Reinforce physician's explanation of surgical procedure and expected outcome
Encourage and allow time for verbalization of concerns; involve significant others
Explain nursing care plan and all procedures
Assess present coping patterns; assist patient with identifying alternative and positive ways of coping

ndx: Knowledge deficit regarding home care needs

GOAL: *Patient and/or significant other will demonstrate understanding of home care and follow-up instructions through interactive discussion and actual return demonstration*

Discuss diet and dietary restrictions
    Need for small, frequent meals
    Need to chew foods well and eat slowly
    Need to drink water with meals
    Need to elevate head of bed at night
    Procedure for gastrostomy feedings
Discuss need to avoid smoking and stress
Explain importance of activity and rest
Discuss need to avoid constipation with natural laxatives
Demonstrate wound and dressing care
Explain signs of wound infection and fistula formation
Discuss importance of follow-up care with physician

Evaluation

There are no complications
Nutritional status is adequate for weight
Patient demonstrates positive coping patterns related to changes in life-style
Patient demonstrates understanding of home and follow-up care

CARE OF PATIENT WITH CELESTIN TUBE

Celestin tube *A semirigid prosthesis inserted through the obstructing esophageal tumor to form a passage for food and fluids; used when disabling dysphagia and aspiration are present and surgical intervention is not possible*

Postinsertion assessment
Observations/findings

Level of consciousness
Swallowing reflex
Placement of nasogastric tube
Location and character of pain
Head of bed elevated

Laboratory/diagnostic studies

Electrolytes, CBC
Chest radiologic study

Potential complications

Aspiration pneumonia
Prolapse of mucosa into tube
Esophageal hemorrhage from perforation
Tube slippage

Medical management

Analgesics
Nasogastric aspiration
Intake and output
Oxygen therapy
Oropharyngeal suctioning
NPO
Parenteral fluids with electrolytes and vitamins
TPN
Diet when tolerated

Nursing diagnoses/goals/interventions

ndx Ineffective airway clearance related to inability to manage secretions

GOAL: *Patient's airway will remain patent and free from secretions*

Keep head of bed elevated at all times, even at night
Observe for respiratory distress
Perform oropharyngeal suctioning prn
Assess ability to swallow
Administer oxygen therapy as ordered
Assist and teach patient how to manage saliva
Assist and teach patient to turn, cough, and deep breathe q2h to 4h
Monitor vital signs q4h

ndx Alteration in nutrition related to swallowing difficulties

GOAL: *Patient's nutritional intake will be maintained*

Maintain NPO
Connect nasogastric tube to intermittent suction apparatus as ordered; observe character and amount of gastric drainage q8h
Administer parenteral fluids with electrolytes and vitamins as ordered
Administer TPN if ordered (p. 51)
Measure intake and output
Monitor Hgb, Hct, and electrolytes
Administer oral hygiene q2h to 4h; keep nares clean and moist
On fourth or fifth postoperative day initiate small amounts of water: 5 ml q15 to 30 min
Assist and teach patient to take only small amounts at one time and assess ability to swallow
Increase fluids to 10 to 15 ml by seventh postoperative day; add tea to fluid intake
As swallowing ability increases, remove nasogastric tube as ordered
Increase intake to blended and soft foods as tolerated
Instruct patient to always keep head elevated, since peristaltic action is absent
Observe for signs of tube obstruction; report to physician immediately

ndx Alteration in comfort related to surgical implant of prosthesis and/or disease

GOAL: *Patient will express that discomfort is minimal or absent*

Administer analgesics as ordered; assess effectiveness of pain relief measures
Assess location and character of pain; observe for signs of perforation
Change position frequently and administer skin care and back rubs prn
Perform passive or assist with and teach active ROM exercises q4h

ndx Ineffective or compromised family coping related to possible poor prognosis

GOAL: *Patient and/or significant other will demonstrate positive coping behaviors through interactive discussions of feelings*

Assess present coping abilities
Encourage and allow time for verbalization of feelings
Support patient's coping strengths and discuss alternative coping measures
Involve patient and/or significant other in nursing care and procedures
Reinforce physician's explanation of disease process and prognosis
Explain all treatments and procedures

ndx Knowledge deficit regarding home care needs

GOAL: *Patient and/or significant other will demonstrate understanding of home care and follow-up instructions through interactive discussion and actual return demonstration*

Discuss and demonstrate preparation of diet; involve dietitian (RD)
Reinforce procedure for eating
   Take and swallow small amounts
   Keep head elevated at all times
   Chew semisolid foods well before swallowing
Explain signs of obstruction of tube
   Food cannot be swallowed
   Regurgitation will occur
   Instruct patient and/or significant other to report obstruction to physician; sips of meat tenderizer or hydrogen peroxide may be used to open tube
Discuss and demonstrate administration of analgesics: liquid or IM injections

Explain availability of home health care agencies to assist in activities of daily living (ADLs)
Provide information on available support groups (I Can Cope, American Cancer Society, etc.)
Stress importance of follow-up care with physician

Evaluation

There are no complications
Nutrition is adequate
Patient demonstrates ability to clear airway of secretions
Pain is managed with analgesics and comfort measures
Patient demonstrates positive coping behaviors
Patient demonstrates knowledge of home care needs

ENDOSCOPY: ESOPHAGEAL, GASTRIC, DUODENAL

Insertion of a fiberoptic scope into the esophagus, stomach, or duodenum to determine pathologic conditions and/or obtain tissue specimens for diagnostic studies; also used to remove foreign bodies

Preendoscopy care

Encourage and allow time for verbalization of fears and concerns
Reinforce physician's explanation of procedure
Maintain NPO
Remove dentures and partial plates
Administer oral hygiene
Administer premedications as ordered

Postendoscopy assessment

Observations/findings

Level of consciousness and vital signs
Swallow and gag reflexes present
Respiratory rate and depth
Hoarseness
Sore throat

Potential complications

Respiratory distress
Esophageal, gastric, or duodenal perforation
  Dysphagia
  Subcutaneous crepitus in neck
  Extreme pain: increases with respirations or neck or shoulder movement
  Hematemesis

Medical management

NPO until reactive
Warm saline gargles for discomfort

Nursing diagnoses/goals/interventions

ndx: Alteration in comfort related to procedure

GOAL: *Patient will verbalize minimal discomfort or relief from pain*

Assist and teach patient to turn and deep breathe q2h
Administer warm saline gargles as ordered
Provide warm liquids until patient is able to swallow, then diet as tolerated
Administer oral hygiene prn

ndx: Knowledge deficit regarding self-care at home

GOAL: *Patient and/or significant other will demonstrate knowledge of home and follow-up care*

Explain importance of liquid diet until soreness disappears
Discuss deep-breathing exercises and oral hygiene
Explain safety precautions; keep small items and caustic substances away from children
Encourage ongoing outpatient care

Evaluation

There are no complications
Discomfort is minimal
Patient demonstrates knowledge of home care

CARE OF PATIENT WITH SENGSTAKEN-BLAKEMORE TUBE OR LINTON TUBE

Sengstaken-Blakemore tube *Nasoesophagogastric tube with three lumens and two pressure balloons: two lumens are used to inflate the balloons, and the third is for gastric drainage; used to control esophageal hemorrhage (Figure 6-2, A)*
Linton tube *Three-lumen nasogastric tube for control of gastric hemorrhage: two lumens suction esophageal and gastric contents and the third lumen inflates the gastric balloon (Figure 6-2, B)*

Preinsertion assessment and care

Assess patient's ability to swallow and mouth breathe; maintain patent airway
Explain purpose of tube and procedure
Observe amount and color of emesis after stomach contents have been aspirated
Check tube for patency of each lumen and strength of balloon(s)
  Tube should not be over 1 year old
  Use sphygmomanometer for balloon inflation of Sengstaken-Blakemore tube
  Use 50 cc syringe for balloon inflation of Linton tube
  Lubricate and chill tube according to instructions

Postinsertion assessment

Observations/findings

SENGSTAKEN-BLAKEMORE TUBE

Tube is inserted through nose into stomach
Balloons are inflated to 20 to 40 mm Hg each or as ordered (Figure 6-2, A)
Lumens are securely clamped and labeled from each balloon
Gastric suction tube is labeled and attached to intermittent suction apparatus
Traction (¼ to 1 lb) is applied to gastric balloon as ordered
Tube is securely taped to nose or traction sponge

LINTON TUBE

Tube is inserted through nose into stomach
Gastric tube and esophageal tube are labeled and connected to separate intermittent suction apparatuses
Balloon is inflated with 100 to 200 cc of air or as ordered, and lumen is securely clamped and labeled
If helmet is used (Figure 6-2, B), tube is taped to face mask and traction applied
If helmet is not used, tube is taped to traction sponge and traction applied (see Figure 6-2, A, for Sengstaken-Blakemore tube)

Laboratory/diagnostic studies

Chest radiologic study for correct placement of Sengstaken-Blakemore tube
Electrolytes

Potential complications

Respiratory distress
Aspiration pneumonia
Chest pain
Abdominal distention

Medical management

Amount of pressure in balloons
Amount of traction on tube
Length of time pressure and traction are maintained
Iced saline lavage of tube
Oropharyngeal suctioning
Type of gastroesophageal aspiration
NPO
Parenteral fluids with electrolytes and vitamin K
Whole blood transfusions
Analgesics

Nursing diagnoses/goals/interventions

ndx: Ineffective airway clearance related to inability to manage secretions

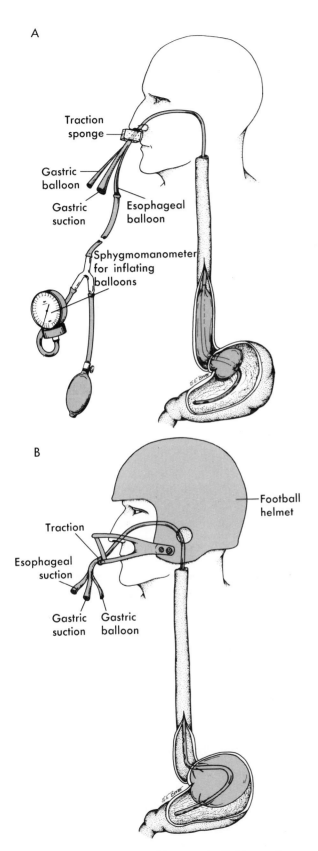

FIGURE 6-2. A, Sengstaken-Blakemore tube. **B,** Linton tube.

GOAL: *Patient's airway will remain patent and free of secretions*

Assist and teach patient to manage saliva and other oral secretions
Elevate head of bed 30 to 45 degrees unless patient is in shock
Auscultate chest for breath sounds q2h
Observe for respiratory distress: stridor, retraction, cyanosis; *notify physician immediately and remove clamps, deflate balloons, and remove tube*
Suction oropharynx qh and prn
Assist and teach patient to deep breathe qh; avoid coughing and gagging
Maintain ordered balloon pressure; check amount of pressure qh and prn
Release traction and deflate balloon q8h to 12h to avoid necrosis of tissues

ndx: Potential fluid volume deficit related to abnormal fluid and blood loss

GOAL: *Patient's fluid and electrolyte intake will be maintained at normal levels and blood loss replaced*

Observe for signs of shock
Maintain NPO
Administer parenteral fluids with electrolytes and vitamin K as ordered
Administer fresh whole blood as ordered
Measure intake and output
Irrigate only gastric lumen of Linton tube with measured amounts of saline prn; iced saline lavage may be ordered
Irrigate gastric lumen of Sengstaken-Blakemore tube with measured amounts of saline as ordered
  Irrigate continuously until bleeding subsides or as ordered
  Note consistency, color, and amount of return flow
Observe for abdominal distention or chest pain
Check and measure gastric drainage qh
Monitor electrolytes, Hgb, and Hct

ndx: Alteration in comfort related to pain and discomfort of gastric tube

GOAL: *Patient will express minimal discomfort or absence of pain*

Administer analgesics as ordered
  Observe for respiratory distress
  Assess effectiveness of pain relief measures
Provide skin care and back rubs when patient can be turned
Place sheepskin under patient
Perform passive ROM exercises q2h to 4h

ndx: Impairment of tissue integrity related to inadequate oral hygiene and/or oronasal tube

GOAL: *Patient's oral and nasal mucosa will be maintained*

Administer oral and nasal hygiene q2h to 4h and prn
Apply lip balm or lubricant to nares and mouth prn
Assess areas frequently for signs of necrosis

ndx: Anxiety/fear related to emergent situation

GOAL: *Patient will demonstrate understanding of needed procedure*

Provide quiet reassurance; avoid showing own anxiety
Stay with patient as much as possible and explain procedures as they occur
Reinforce physician's explanation of disease process and possible surgical treatment
Assess patient's coping abilities and support positive behaviors
Promote adaptive coping styles
Allow time for and encourage verbalization of fears and anxieties

Evaluation

Fluid volume is maintained
Discomfort is controlled
Skin integrity is maintained
There are no complications, nor is surgery performed

Stomach

PEPTIC ULCER DISEASE (GASTRIC AND DUODENAL)

gastric ulcer *Ulceration of gastric mucosa due to a break in the mucosal barrier, allowing backwash of hydrochloric acid; causative factors include medications (aspirin, indomethacin), chemicals (tobacco, alcohol), stress, and heredity*

duodenal ulcer *Ulceration of duodenal mucosa due to increased amounts of hydrochloric acid in the duodenum; causative factors include heredity, psychosocial stressors, and medications*

Assessment
Observations/findings
GASTRIC ULCER

Left to midepigastric pain; may radiate to back
Pain experienced 60 to 90 min after eating

DUODENAL ULCER

Right epigastric pain; may radiate to back or thorax; pain occurs 2 to 4 hr after eating

Pyrosis (heartburn)
Fullness after eating
Eructation
Nausea
Abdominal tenderness

Laboratory/diagnostic studies

Endoscopy with biopsy and cytology
Barium studies
Abdominal radiologic studies
Gastric analysis
Hgb, Hct, blood pepsinogen
Stool for melena

Potential complications

Electrolyte imbalance
Gastric, duodenal hemorrhage, perforation
Hemorrhage
Shock

Medical management

Aluminum-magnesium antacids: Delcid, Mylanta-II
Cimetidine (Tagamet)
Ranitidine (Zantac)
Sucralfate (Carafate)
Diet

Nursing diagnoses/goals/interventions

ndx: Alteration in nutrition: less than body requirements related to discomfort after eating

GOAL: *Patient will understand nutritional concepts and maintain adequate caloric intake*

Assess patient's nutritional status: present diet, eating patterns, foods precipitating pain
Assess patient's medication history: aspirin, steroids, vasopressors
Maintain nonstressful environment
Provide diet as ordered in small, frequent meals
Administer antacids, cimetidine or ranitidine as ordered

ndx: Knowledge deficit regarding home care and nutritional status

GOAL: *Patient and/or significant other will demonstrate understanding of home care, nutritional regimen, and follow-up instructions through interactive discussion*

Discuss relationship of causative agents to peptic ulcer disease
Provide written instructions concerning medications, including name, purpose, dosage, time of administration, and side effects; instruct patient to take only antacids prescribed by physician
Discuss dietary plan: importance of eating meals at regular times, necessity of not missing a meal, and benefits of small, frequent meals
Explain signs and symptoms of perforation: extreme epigastric pain and hematemesis
Describe importance of nonstressful environment, especially at mealtime
Encourage follow-up care with physician

Evaluation

There are no complications
Patient demonstrates understanding of dietary regimen, medication use, and home care plan

GASTRIC BLEEDING

Condition in which ulceration of the mucosa has progressed to the vasculature of the stomach or duodenum; may be insidious or acute

Assessment

Observations/findings

Abdominal distention
Nausea, vomiting
Hematemesis
Melena
Hyperperistalsis
Abdominal tenderness, pain
Increased bowel sounds
Dehydration
Chills, fever
Anxiety/fear

Laboratory/diagnostic studies

Endoscopy
GI series
Stools for occult blood
CBC, electrolytes, BUN

Potential complications

Electrolyte imbalance
Gastric perforation
Hemorrhage
Shock

Medical management

Analgesics
NPO
Nasogastric tube or Linton tube, depending on bleeding site
Parenteral fluids with electrolytes and vitamins

Cimetidine intravenously
Antacids via nasogastric tube
Iced saline lavage (Norepinephrine bitartrate [Levophed] may be added to produce vasoconstriction)
Endoscopy: endoscope electrocoagulation
Vasopressin arterially
Surgical intervention: repair or resection

Nursing diagnoses/goals/interventions

ndx: Alteration in tissue perfusion related to bleeding and fluid loss

GOAL: *Patient's circulating blood and fluid volume will be maintained*

Maintain bed rest with head elevated 30 degrees
Assess acuteness of bleeding and for signs of hypovolemia
Monitor vital signs q15 to 30 min until stable; take apical pulse
Maintain NPO
Administer parenteral therapy as ordered: electrolytes, volume expanders, whole blood, packed cells
Monitor CVP line or Swan-Ganz line if appropriate
Insert nasogastric tube and connect to intermittent suction apparatus as ordered; measure gastric output q4h to 8h
　Irrigate with iced saline solution as ordered
　Initiate gastric hypothermia if ordered
Measure intake and output
Monitor electrolytes, Hgb, Hct, and BUN
Insert indwelling urethral catheter if ordered; attach to closed gravity drainage system; monitor hourly output as ordered
Auscultate abdomen for bowel sounds and distention q4h: increased bowel sounds may indicate increased bleeding
Measure abdominal girth q4h
Check stools for melena
Administer vasopressin via infusion pump as ordered; observe for side effects: hypertension, bradycardia, fibrillation, hyponatremia
Prepare for endoscopic electrocoagulation or surgery as ordered
When bleeding subsides and nasogastric tube is removed, initiate fluids in small amounts as tolerated
　Progress to blended or soft foods in small, frequent meals
　Continue monitoring intake and output and stools for melena
　Administer saline enemas to clear bowel of old blood as ordered
　Avoid constipation
　Administer iron, vitamin K, antacids, and cimetidine as ordered
When indwelling urethral catheter is removed, initiate voiding measures as needed

ndx: Alteration is comfort: pain related to disease process

GOAL: *Patient will verbalize minimal discomfort or absence of pain*

Administer analgesics as ordered (e.g., morphine); meperidine is usually avoided because it can cause nausea and vomiting
Assist and teach patient to turn and deep breathe q2h to 4h
Administer back care and oral hygiene when turning patient
Assist with and teach active or perform passive ROM exercises q4h
Keep patient warm and dry
Provide planned rest periods
Ambulate with assistance when allowed

ndx: Anxiety/fear related to emergent situation and hospitalization

GOAL: *Patient will verbalize anxieties and fears and demonstrate progress toward positive coping behaviors*

Maintain quiet environment
Explain all procedures and treatments
Encourage and allow time for verbalization of concerns
Assess level of anxiety/fear and present coping styles
Discuss alternative coping behaviors and listen carefully
Encourage communication with significant other(s)

ndx: Knowledge deficit regarding home care needs

GOAL: *Patient and/or significant other will demonstrate understanding of home care and follow-up instructions through interactive discussion*

Discuss nutritional plan, stressing importance of
　Small, frequent meals at regular intervals
　Chewing food well and eating slowly
　Avoiding caffeine, alcohol, tobacco, stressful situations, and aspirin
Reinforce physician's explanation of relationship of causative factors to disease process
Provide medication instructions as to name, dose, purpose, time of administration, and side effects; instruct patient to take only antacids prescribed by physician

Explain signs and symptoms of further bleeding: hematemesis, abdominal distention, tarry stools, fainting, dyspnea
Discuss importance of exercise to tolerance and planned rest periods
Encourage follow-up visits with physician

Evaluation

There are no complications
Nutritional intake is adequate, and Hgb, Hct, and electrolytes are within normal limits
Pain is decreased or absent
Anxieties are identified, and adaptive behaviors are demonstrated
Home care needs and follow-up care are understood

GASTRIC SURGERY

Surgery performed for medical emergencies such as gastric hemorrhage, perforation, obstruction, and carcinomas or for ulcers that have not responded to medical management

Assessment

Observations/findings

Splinting with respirations
Decreased breath sounds
Tachypnea
Bradypnea
Character and amount of gastric drainage
Nausea, vomiting
Urinary output
Abdominal distention

Laboratory/diagnostic studies

Hgb, Hct, electrolytes

Potential complications

Dehydration, anemia
Electrolyte imbalance
Atelectasis
Hemorrhage
Shock
Thrombophlebitis (p. 74)
Dumping syndrome (p. 358)
Paralytic ileus (p. 377)
Wound evisceration, infection
Postprandial hypoglycemia
Gastrojejunocolic fistula

Medical management

NPO until bowel sounds return
Parenteral fluids with electrolytes until diet is allowed
Nasogastric aspiration
Analgesics
Antiembolic stockings

Nursing diagnoses/goals/interventions

ndx: Alteration in nutrition: less than body requirements related to preoperative and postoperative food and fluid restrictions

GOAL: *Patient's nutritional status will be maintained adequately*

Maintain NPO
Connect nasogastric tube to intermittent suction apparatus
   Note color and amount of gastric output q4h
   Do not reposition tube
   Maintain patency of tube by irrigation with measured amounts of saline *only* if ordered
   Note that following gastrectomy, drainage will be minimal
   Report excessive bleeding to physician
Monitor electrolytes, Hgb, and Hct
Administer parenteral fluids with electrolytes as ordered
Measure intake and output
Administer oral hygiene q2h to 4h
Auscultate bowel sounds and passage of flatus q8h
When bowel sounds return, administer small amounts of water via nasogastric tube as ordered
   Aspirate stomach 2 hr after last feeding of the day; contents should be <100 ml and no pain, distention, or nausea should be present
   Report to physician if amount is >100 ml and/or the above symptoms occur
Initiate oral fluids when nasogastric tube is removed
   Offer 5 to 10 ml of warm water or tea with sugar qh as ordered
   Increase amounts until 90 to 120 ml is tolerated qh
Progress to small, frequent meals of soft foods as ordered; avoid milk, since it may cause dumping syndrome
Discontinue feedings if pain, nausea, distention, or vomiting occur and notify physician
Continue measuring intake

ndx: Ineffective breathing pattern related to location of surgical incision

GOAL: *Patient's breathing will be maintained to meet body requirements*

Assess respirations, observing for signs of distress
Maintain bed rest with head elevated 30 degrees

Auscultate chest for breath sounds q4h

Assist and teach patient to turn, cough, and deep breathe q2h to 4h; provide support to incision

Administer incentive spirometer and/or IPPB as ordered

ndx: Alteration in peripheral tissue perfusion secondary to surgical intervention and postoperative restrictions

GOAL: *Patient's peripheral circulation will be maintained*

Monitor vital signs q4h; check extremities for temperature, color, and sensation

Check pedal pulses q4h

Do not gatch knees

Assist with and teach active or perform passive ROM exercises q4h

Apply antiembolic stockings as ordered

Assist with ambulation when allowed

ndx: Impairment of skin integrity related to surgical incision

GOAL: *Patient's incision will remain clean, dry, and intact without signs of inflammation*

Check dressings and incision for drainage q4h; reinforce as needed

When allowed, change dressings prn and observe healing process

Observe for signs of wound infection

ndx: Alteration in comfort: pain related to surgical intervention

GOAL: *Patient will express minimal discomfort or absence of pain*

Administer analgesics as ordered

Change position often and support with pillows to decrease discomfort

Administer skin care and back rubs q4h

Maintain quiet environment

Schedule rest periods between treatments

ndx: Anxiety/fear related to surgery and hospitalization

GOAL: *Patient will express and identify anxieties and fears and progress toward adaptive responses and behavior*

Explain all procedures and treatments

Reinforce physician's explanation of surgical procedure and treatment

Encourage and allow time for verbalization of feelings; listen carefully

Assess present coping behaviors and support positive responses

Encourage communication with significant others

ndx: Knowledge deficit regarding home care needs and follow-up instructions

GOAL: *Patient and/or significant other will demonstrate understanding of home care and follow-up instructions through interactive discussion and actual return demonstration*

Discuss and explain dietary plan and restrictions
 Eat small, frequent meals at regular intervals; avoid high-fiber foods, sugar, salt, caffeine, alcohol, milk, and tobacco
 Take fluids between meals, not with meals
 Eat slowly and chew foods well
 Measure weight q2d to 4d

Provide instructions and demonstrate wound care; identify signs of wound infection

Reinforce importance of avoiding stressful situations, especially at mealtimes

Explain symptoms of dumping syndrome: epigastric pain, weakness, nausea, vomiting after eating

Discuss medications: name, dosage, time of administration, purpose, and side effects; instruct patient to avoid over-the-counter medications

Discuss importance of adequate rest and exercise with planned rest periods

Encourage follow-up care with physician

Evaluation

There are no complications

Wound is clean, dry, and intact

Dietary regimen is understood

Pain or discomfort is minimal

Knowledge of home care needs is demonstrated

DUMPING SYNDROME

Postgastrectomy syndrome due to loss of the pyloric valve allowing food and fluid to pass too rapidly into the small bowel; appears 1 to 3 weeks after surgery

Assessment
Observations/findings

Time of onset of symptoms: usually during or immediately after meal

Epigastric fullness
Nausea, vomiting
Abdominal distention
Malaise
Profuse diaphoresis
Palpitations
Vertigo
Tachypnea
Decreased BP
Increased bowel sounds
Urge to defecate

Potential complications

Syndrome becomes chronic
ECG changes

Medical management

Anticholinergics, pectin powder
Surgery to alter dumping rate

Nursing diagnoses/goals/interventions

ndx: Potential alteration in nutrition: less than body requirements related to inability to absorb nutrients

GOAL: *Patient's nutritional status will be maintained to adequately meet body needs*

Provide diet as ordered
  Provide six small meals a day
  Avoid milk and milk dishes
  Do not give liquids with meals
  Provide dry foods such as toast, crackers, and cereals
  Provide diet low in carbohydrates and salt, moderate in fat, and high in protein
  Include foods containing pectin: citrus fruits, yellow vegetables, bananas, apples, apricots, cherries, beans
  Avoid extreme temperatures in foods
Administer pectin powder as ordered; thoroughly mix with water, since patient may experience a sense of dryness if mixture is not liquid enough
Provide liquids between meals as allowed
Administer anticholinergics 30 min before meals as ordered
Monitor vital signs q4h
Measure intake and output q8h
Position patient in recumbent position after meals to allow food to pass more slowly into intestine
Assess perianal area for excoriation; promote correct hygiene; provide perianal care and apply protective ointments

ndx: Knowledge deficit regarding disease process and management

GOAL: *Patient and/or significant other demonstrates understanding of syndrome and its management through interactive discussion*

Discuss importance of dietary plan, stressing small, frequent meals, foods to avoid, and foods to eat
Explain that syndrome is usually only temporary, but to report its continuance to physician after 2 to 3 weeks
Instruct patient to lie down after meals and to avoid stressful situations, especially at mealtimes
Encourage follow-up visits with physician

Evaluation

There are no complications
Symptoms of syndrome have decreased or are absent
Patient demonstrates knowledge of disease process and dietary management

SURGICAL INTERVENTION FOR OBESITY

Insertion of two rows of staples across upper one tenth of the stomach to reduce capacity and ensure early satiety; performed for patients highly motivated to lose weight and where medical management of obesity has been unsuccessful; there are three types performed:

gastric bypass Anastomosis of jejunum to upper one tenth of the stomach, bypassing the remaining stomach (Figure 6-3, A)

gastroplasty/partitioning Small opening left in rows of staples, allowing small amounts of food to pass into stomach (Figure 6-3, B)

jejunoileal bypass End-to-end or end-to-side anastomosis of 10 to 14 inches of jejunum to terminal ileum; distal end of ileum is closed, and proximal end is either anastomosed to transverse colon (Figure 6-3, C) or to shortened jejunum (Figure 6-3, D)

Preoperative Care
Assessment
Observations/findings

Nutritional history
  Previous eating patterns and types of foods eaten
  Present weight greater than 100 lb over ideal body weight
Medical history
  Absence of renal, cardiac, bowel, or liver disease
  No history of hypertension, diabetes, or arthritis
  No signs of upper respiratory infection (URI) or anemia
Psychologic adjustment to procedure
  Motivation to lose weight
  Weight loss minimal or absent after many attempts
  Presence of positive coping behaviors

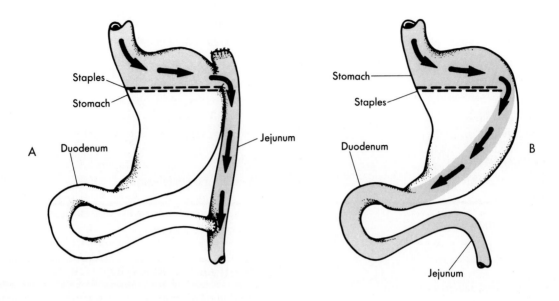
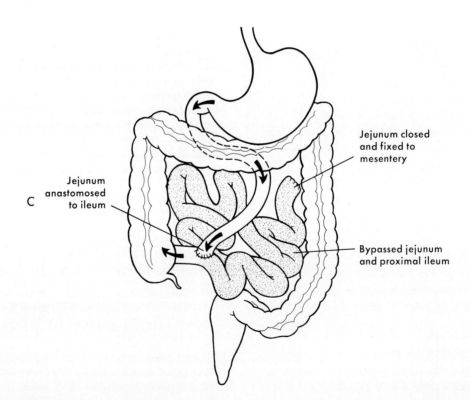

FIGURE 6-3. **A,** Gastric bypass. **B,** Gastroplasty/partitioning. **C,** End-to-end jejunoileal anastomosis (type 1).

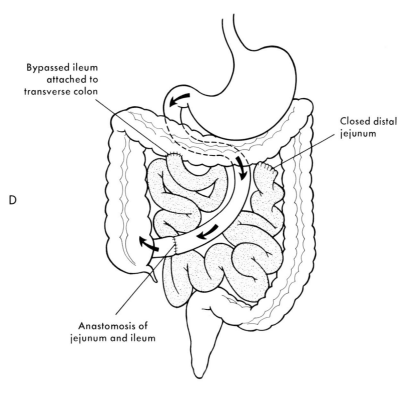

FIGURE 6-3, cont'd. **D,** End-to-end jejunoileal anastomosis (type 2). (C and D from Given, B.A., and Simmons, S.J.: Gastroenterology in clinical nursing, ed. 4, St. Louis, 1984, The C.V. Mosby Co.)

Laboratory/diagnostic studies

Renal and liver function studies
Abdominal and chest radiologic studies
Upper GI series
Cholecystogram
Intravenous pyelogram
Barium enema
Pulmonary function test
Serum glucose, insulin, cholesterol, triglycerides, creatinine, protein, iron, CBC, urinalysis
Baseline arterial blood gases

Medical management

Preoperative medication
Parenteral fluids with heparin
Nasogastric tube and/or indwelling urethral catheter

Nursing diagnoses/goals/interventions

ndx: Anxiety/fear related to hospitalization, procedures, and surgery

GOAL: *Patient will express concerns and display a more calm, relaxed appearance*

Attempt to maintain nonstressful environment
Orient patient to surroundings and provide comfortable armless chair
Encourage and allow time for verbalization of concerns; listen carefully
Reinforce physician's explanation of preoperative and postoperative care and surgical procedure
Perform activities in an unhurried manner, explaining each as it occurs
Encourage verbalization with significant other

ndx: Knowledge deficit regarding preoperative and postoperative care

GOAL: *Patient will indicate understanding of nursing care, procedures, and activities through interactive discussion and actual return demonstration*

Discuss with patient and teach
  Use of trapeze bar and getting in and out of bed
  Method for turning, coughing, and deep breathing with incisional support
  Use of inspirational spirometer and diaphragmatic breathing procedure

Procedure for sipping from a cup, 30 ml in 5 min
Active ROM exercises
Explain that early ambulation (2 to 4 hr after surgery) will be required and trapeze bars will be in place
Explain that preoperatively a nasogastric tube and indwelling urethral catheter will be inserted
Discuss postoperative dietary management; small sips of water increasing to 30 to 60 ml as tolerated
Explain that IV line will be in place preoperatively and an anticoagulant will be administered
Discuss need for bowel preparation for jejunoileal bypass surgery

Postoperative Care

Assessment

Observations/findings

Location and character of pain
Splinting with respirations
Decreased breath sounds
Hypoventilation
Tachypnea
Character, color, and amount of
    Gastric drainage
    Urine output
    Wound drainage
Placement and patency of nasogastric tube
Pressure delivered by suction machine
Nausea, vomiting
Abdominal distention

Laboratory/diagnostic studies

Hgb, Hct, electrolytes
Chest radiologic study

Potential complications

Dehydration
Electrolyte imbalance
Thrombophlebitis (p. 74)
Atelectasis
Anastomotic leak
    Tachycardia
    Referred abdominal pain to left shoulder
Peritonitis
Hemorrhage
Shock
Wound infection
Liver dysfunction, malabsorption syndrome (jejunoileal bypass)

Medical management

Analgesics, heparin, antidiarrheals
Ambulation q2h to 3h
Parenteral fluids with electrolytes
Connection of nasogastric tube to intermittent suction and indwelling urethral catheter to gravity drainage
IPPB and/or incentive spirometer
Arterial blood gases
Diet, activity, rest

Nursing diagnoses/goals/interventions

ndx: Ineffective breathing pattern related to surgical incision and decreased lung expansion

GOAL: *Patient's breathing will be optimal, and oxygenation will be maintained*

Maintain bed rest with head elevated 30 degrees
Monitor respirations q1h to 2h; observe for shallow breathing, splinting, hypoventilation, and respiratory distress
Auscultate chest for breath sounds q2h
Provide incentive spirometer q2h
Place pads on side rails and encourage patient to use as arm rests (aids in lung expansion)
Encourage diaphragmatic breathing
Assist patient to turn, cough, and deep breathe q2h; support incision
Avoid abdominal binders

ndx: Potential alteration in tissue perfusion: cardiopulmonary, GI, renal, and peripheral systems related to interruption of blood flow

GOAL: *Patient's circulation will be maintained*

Monitor vital signs q4h; take rectal temperatures
Monitor arterial blood gases and CVP or Swan-Ganz catheter
Monitor Hgb and Hct
Administer heparin as ordered
Assist with active ROM exercises q2h to 4h
Avoid elevating knee gatch and antiembolic stockings
Check calves of legs for pain on dorsiflexion
Avoid sitting with legs in dependent position
Ambulate with assistance as ordered

ndx: Potential fluid volume deficit related to decrease intake, gastric suction, and/or electrolyte loss

GOAL: *Patient's fluid intake will be adequate for body requirements, and electrolyte balance will be maintained*

Maintain NPO
Administer parenteral fluids with electrolytes as ordered
Monitor serum electrolytes, magnesium, and calcium
Measure intake and output
Connect nasogastric tube to intermittent suction apparatus

Note color, consistency, and amount of drainage
Label tube: "Do not reposition"
Mark tube where it enters nose and avoid placing tension on tube
Irrigate gently with 20 to 30 ml of normal saline q2h to 4h or as ordered
Administer oral hygiene q2h to 4h
Connect indwelling catheter to closed gravity drainage system as ordered; measure hourly urine output; if output is less than 50 ml, notify physician
Auscultate abdomen for bowel sounds q4h
Weigh patient daily at same time with same clothing and scale

ndx: Potential for infection related to surgical incision

GOAL: *Patient's wound will be clean, dry, and intact with no evidence of infection*

Observe incision and dressings q2h to 4h; reinforce or change dressings prn
Monitor incision for signs of wound infection
Maintain dressings securely; avoid taping too tightly
Keep skin clean and dry, especially in skin folds

ndx: Alteration in comfort: pain related to surgical intervention

GOAL: *Patient will express minimal discomfort or absence of pain*

Assess location, type, and character of pain
Administer analgesics as ordered; assess effectiveness of relief measure(s)
Assess patency of nasogastric tube, since obstruction of tube may cause pain
Medicate 20 to 30 min prior to procedures when possible
Monitor type of pain closely and observe for abdominal distention, tenderness, and fever
Change position slightly at frequent intervals to alleviate discomfort

ndx: Alteration in nutrition: less than body requirements related to decreased size of stomach and desired weight loss

GOAL: *Patient's nutritional intake will be adequate to maintain body requirements and provide weight loss*

Remove nasogastric tube when ordered (third to fourth day postoperatively)
Provide 1 oz medication cup and assist patient with sipping 30 ml of water per hour (adequate hydration demands almost constant fluid intake)
Progress to clear liquids, using 1 oz cup, until soft, high-protein, low-fat diet is tolerated
Instruct patient to heed feeling of satiety to avoid nausea or vomiting

ndx: Alteration in bowel elimination: diarrhea due to induced malabsorption

GOAL: *Patient will adapt to new bowel pattern and express understanding of dietary restrictions*

Provide diet high in bulk with moderate fluid intake
Observe for signs of dumping syndrome
Provide perianal care following bowel movement; apply protective ointments as needed
Observe frequency, color, amount, and consistency of stools
Administer antidiarrheals as ordered

ndx: Alteration in urinary elimination pattern related to urethral catheter and decreased output

GOAL: *Patient will manage altered urinary pattern, and complications will be minimal*

Remove urethral catheter when ordered; assist with voiding measures as needed
Observe for retention or frequency
Monitor intake and output until stable

ndx: Knowledge deficit regarding home care needs

GOAL: *Patient and/or significant other will demonstrate understanding of home care and follow-up instructions through interactive discussion and actual return demonstration*

Discuss importance of following eating regimen
  Eat and drink slowly and chew foods well
  Always sit up while eating or drinking
  Do not overeat: stomach will expand and void surgical procedure
  Eat small amounts of all food and heed satiety feeling
  Avoid drinking 30 min before and after meals
  Eat with family in nonstressful environment
  Use small plate and glass to make portions appear larger
  Do not snack between meals
  Avoid carbonated beverages
  Eat only two meals a day
Explain importance of diet management
  Avoid high-calorie, high-carbohydrate foods and drinks
  Maintain well-balanced, high-protein diet, 300 to 500 calories/day or as ordered

Be accurate in measuring all food allowances
Use 30 ml medication cup or 1½ tablespoon measuring scoop
Maintain 1500 ml/day fluid intake
Add new foods to diet one at a time as intolerances occur, especially with meat and chicken
    Discuss methods of blenderizing foods for gastroplasty patients
    Discuss availability of high-protein liquid supplements
Measure urine output daily
Keep accurate record of daily intake
Take chewable multivitamin daily
Weigh weekly since weight loss is more noticeable
Instruct patient regarding rest and exercise
    Avoid heavy lifting and strenuous exercise
    Walk daily with goal of 1 to 2 miles/day in 4 weeks
    Maintain rest periods
Demonstrate incisional and perianal care
Explain symptoms to report to physician
    Elevated temperature
    Wound drainage
    Persistent nausea and/or vomiting
    Hematemesis
    Abdominal tenderness and/or pain
    Abdominal distention
    Urine output of less than 750 ml/day for 3 consecutive days
    Constipation or continuing diarrhea
Discuss availability of support groups to assist in ADLs
    Public health nurses
    Dietitians (RDs) and nutritionists
    "Reflections" group
Explain importance of not taking over-the-counter medications without physician's permission
Encourage follow-up visits with physician, including laboratory testing as ordered

Evaluation

There are no complications
Incision is clean, dry, and intact
Nutritional intake is adequate to produce desired weight loss
Patient demonstrates understanding of home care and follow-up instructions

GASTRIC CARCINOMA

Carcinoma most commonly occurring in the pyloric segment and along the lesser curvature of the stomach; there are no early definitive signs of the disease process

Assessment

Observations/findings

Feeling of fullness after eating
Indigestion
Eructation
Epigastric pain or discomfort after eating
Dysphagia
Anorexia
Malaise, fatigue
Generalized weakness
Weight loss
Pallor
Vertigo/syncope
Nausea, vomiting
Occult blood in stool

Laboratory/diagnostic studies

Endoscopy with biopsy and cytology
Upper GI series
CBC, Hct (below normal), albumin (decreased)
Gastric analysis
Tomography
Stool for occult blood (positive)
Chest radiologic examination

Potential complications

Malnutrition
Dehydration
Electrolyte imbalance
Hematemesis
Pyloric obstruction
Epigastric mass
Enlarged axillary and/or supraclavicular lymph nodes
Recurrent phlebitis
Metastasis to liver

Medical management

Analgesics
Parenteral fluids, diet, fluid intake
Chemotherapeutic agents
Radiation therapy
Surgery (gastric resection, gastrectomy)

Nursing diagnoses/goals/interventions*

ndx Alteration in nutrition: less than body requirements related to dysphagia and/or nausea and vomiting

GOAL: *Patient's nutritional status will be maintained to meet body requirements*

---

*Patient's condition dictates type and amount of care required; modify accordingly.

Provide light, well-balanced, high-calorie, high-protein diet or parenteral therapy with electrolytes and vitamins as ordered
Assess and identify foods that cause discomfort
Measure intake and output
Weigh patient daily at same time with same clothing and scale
Monitor stools for occult blood
Provide adequate fluid intake, 2500 ml/24 hr, unless contraindicated

ndx: Alteration in comfort: pain related to progressive disease process

GOAL: *Patient will express minimal discomfort or absence of pain*

Administer analgesics as ordered; assess effectiveness of pain relief measures
Coordinate care to provide planned rest periods between procedures
Assist and teach patient to turn and deep breathe q4h
Change position frequently to relieve pressure
Provide diversional activities

ndx: Ineffective individual coping or responses related to disease process and prognosis

GOAL: *Patient will express concerns and learn to manage stress with positive coping behaviors*

Provide quiet environment
Encourage and allow time for verbalization of feelings
Support positive coping behaviors and assist patient with managing stress
Encourage communication with significant other
Reinforce physician's explanation of disease process and plan of treatment
Involve patient and/or significant other in care and explain procedures and treatments

ndx: Anticipatory grieving related to poor prognosis

GOAL: *Patient and/or significant other will verbalize feelings of grief and be provided opportunities to discuss them in a supportive atmosphere*

Assess present coping styles and interdependence in relationship with others
Provide caring and accepting environment
　Listen carefully
　Encourage and allow time for communication with significant other
　Encourage verbalization of feelings

Provide reassurance as needed
Offer hope realistically

ndx: Knowledge deficit regarding home care needs

GOAL: *Patient and/or significant other will demonstrate understanding of home care and follow-up instructions through interactive discussion*

Explain dietary and nutrition care plan according to patient's condition; provide written instructions as needed
Discuss performing ADLs with assistance from home health care agencies as needed
Identify appropriate support groups for assistance
Explain grieving process and ways of working through it: denial, anger, bargaining, and accepting (p. 18)
Demonstrate methods of pain management
Encourage follow-up physician care

Evaluation

There are no new complications
Pain is managed with minimal discomfort
Nutrition is maintained
Patient demonstrates ability to cope with disease and prognosis
Patient understands importance of follow-up care

CARE OF PATIENT WITH NASOGASTRIC TUBE

nasogastric tube *A tube that is used for gastric decompression, such as Levine or Salem sump (Figure 6-4), or for administration of food, fluid, or medication; a Levine tube must always be connected to intermittent suction; a Salem sump tube is most usually connected to low, continuous suction (since it is air vented), but can also be connected to intermittent suction*

Preinsertion assessment and care

Assess patient's ability to swallow and mouth breathe
Check tube for patency
Lubricate and chill tube according to instructions
Explain purpose of tube and procedure

Postinsertion assessment
Observations/findings

Character and consistency of gastric output
Patency of tube
Patency of sump if Salem tube is used
Placement for optimal drainage
Tube taped securely and comfortably to nose

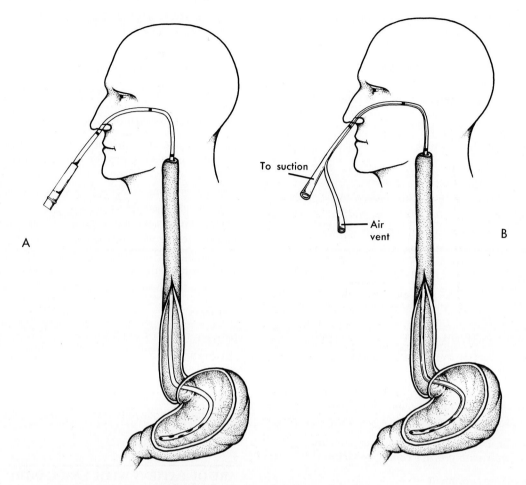

FIGURE 6-4. **A,** Levine tube. **B,** Salem sump tube.

Pressure of suction apparatus
Nasal irritation
Dry lips and mouth
Dysphagia
Sore throat

Laboratory/diagnostic studies

Electrolytes
Gastric analysis

Potential complications

Dehydration
Electrolyte imbalance
Aspiration pneumonia

Medical management

Parenteral fluids with electrolytes
Type of nasogastric aspiration
Irrigation of tube
Intake and output
NPO with ice chips
pH of gastric contents

Nursing diagnoses/goals/interventions

ndx: Potential fluid volume deficit related to abnormal fluid loss via tube

GOAL: *Patient's fluid and electrolyte balance will be maintained to meet body requirements*

Maintain NPO
Administer parenteral fluids with electrolytes as ordered
Measure intake and output
Check character, amount, and consistency of gastric contents q4h; monitor gastric pH; if pH is less than 3.5, notify physician

Auscultate stomach for placement of tube prn
Connect tube to low, intermittent suction apparatus as ordered; irrigate with measured amounts of normal saline solution as ordered
Salem sump tube
　Maintain patency of sump (air vent): keep opening higher than gastric tube and do not plug
　Sump tube may be irrigated, but instill 20 to 30 cc of air following irrigation to maintain patency
Avoid dislodgment: tape securely to nose and allow enough tube for freedom of movement

ndx Ineffective airway clearance related to oral secretion collection

GOAL: *Patient's airway will remain patent and free of secretions*

Assist and teach patient to manage saliva and other oral secretions
Elevate head of bed 40 to 60 degrees
Assist and teach patient to turn and deep breathe q2h to 4h
Assist with and teach active or perform passive ROM exercises q4h

ndx Impairment of tissue integrity related to inadequate oral hygiene and presence of tube

GOAL: *Patient's oral and nasal mucosa will be maintained*

Administer oral hygiene q2h to 4h and prn
Provide ice chips if ordered; avoid indiscriminate use; chewing gum may help dryness also
Apply lip balm or lubricant to nares and mouth prn
Check tape holding tube prn; observe for reddened area

Evaluation

There are no complications
Fluid balance is maintained
Oral hygiene is adequate
Understanding of purpose of tube is demonstrated
Oral secretions are managed safely

CARE OF PATIENT WITH UPPER GI OSTOMY, TUBE, OR PROSTHETIC VALVE

esophagostomy *A surgically constructed stoma used to drain saliva and other secretions in patients with esophageal carcinoma, stricture, dysphagia, or atresia; may be used to administer tube feedings for the above conditions; this procedure is similar to gastrostomy except a longer tube is used (e.g., Levin); the stoma may be permanent or temporary (Figure 6-5)*

gastrostomy *A surgically constructed stoma or opening for a tube or prosthetic valve in patients with esophageal carcinoma, stricture, trauma, atresia, and dysphagia; used for tube feedings or decompression and drainage; the ostomy and valve are usually permanent, whereas the tube is either temporary or permanent (Figure 6-5)*

duodenostomy-jejunostomy *Surgical incision for placement of a catheter (tube) for tube feedings or decompression and drainage in patients where oral intake is prohibited or following gastrointestinal-esophageal surgery; may be permanent or temporary (Figure 6-5)*

Assessment

Observations/findings

Type and patency of GI stoma, tube, or valve present
Placement of dressing or stoma appliances
Length of catheter (tube) from incision to distal end
Taping of catheter or tube
Pressure delivered by low, intermittent suction apparatus
Placement of closed gravity drainage system, clamp, or other collecting device
Character, color, and amount of gastric drainage
Skin integrity around catheter, stoma, or valve
Condition of lips and mouth
Weight
Urinary output and specific gravity
Abdominal distention
Diminished bowel sounds
Character and color of stool

Laboratory/diagnostic studies

Electrolytes
Abdominal radiologic study for tube placement

Potential complications

Dehydration
Nausea, vomiting
Electrolyte imbalance
Aspiration pneumonia
Wound infection
Hemorrhage/shock

Medical management

Analgesics
Intermittent gastric suction or gravity drainage
Tube feedings, amount, and caloric content
Parenteral therapy with electrolytes and vitamins
Intake and output

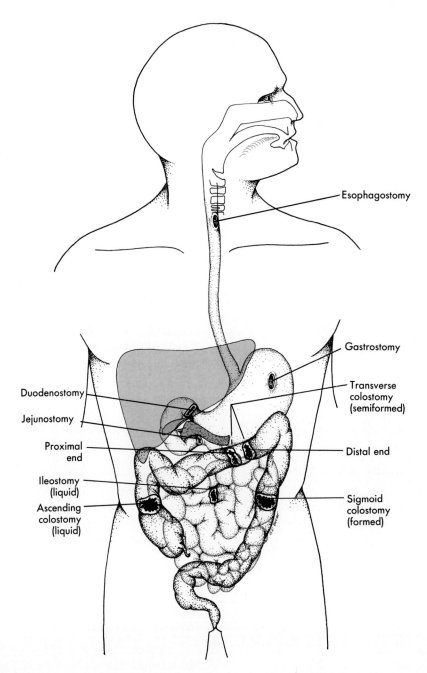

FIGURE 6-5. Types of ostomies and viscosity of fecal material from ileostomy and large intestine ostomies.

Nursing diagnoses/goals/interventions

ndx: Potential fluid volume deficit related to abnormal loss of body fluids, electrolytes, or blood

GOAL: *Patient's fluid volume and electrolytes will be maintained*

Maintain NPO

Administer parenteral fluids with electrolytes and vitamins as ordered

Measure intake and output q8h

For catheters (tubes)

    Check color and consistency of drainage q4h; measure amount q8h

    Connect catheter (tube) to suction apparatus or gravity drainage as ordered

Measure length of catheter (tube) q8h
    Tape securely to abdomen or neck; allow sufficient tubing for freedom of movement
For prosthetic valve or ostomy
    Check dressings and place valve cap in safe place
    Place stoma appliance over ostomy
Auscultate abdomen for bowel sounds q8h; report return to physician
Check operative site for bleeding q2h to 4h
When bowel sounds return or drainage is less than 300 to 500 ml/24 hr
    Clamp catheter, cap valve, or cover ostomy as ordered
    Instruct patient in signs of retention and bowel obstruction
        Nausea
        Abdominal distention
        Abdominal pain
    If these symptoms occur, notify physician immediately and unclamp tube or uncap valve and connect to gravity drainage system
Initiate tube feedings when ordered
Weigh patient daily at same time with same clothing and scale
Maintain fluid intake as ordered after parenteral therapy is discontinued: usually 2000 ml/24 hr unless contraindicated

ndx: Ineffective airway clearance related to oral secretion management

GOAL: *Patient's airway will be maintained and free of secretions*

Maintain bed rest with head elevated 30 to 45 degrees; do not gatch knees
Assist and teach patient to turn, cough, and deep breathe q4h
Assist and teach patient to expectorate saliva rather than swallow it
Perform passive or assist with and teach active ROM exercises q4h

ndx: Potential impairment of skin integrity related to surgical procedure

GOAL: *Patient's skin around catheter, ostomy, or valve will be clean, dry, and intact*

Provide skin care around surgical site q4h to 8h
    Wash area gently with soap and water
    Rinse and pat dry
    Apply skin barrier as needed (p. 391)
    Reapply dressings and appliance prn

ndx: Alteration in comfort: pain related to surgical intervention

GOAL: *Patient will express minimal discomfort or absence of pain*

Administer analgesics as ordered; assess effectiveness of pain relief measures
Change position to position of comfort prn
Provide planned rest periods between procedures
Maintain clean, comfortable bed in safe environment

ndx: Ineffective coping by individual related to disease process, surgical procedure, and/or prognosis

GOAL: *Patient will express feelings and concerns and be given opportunities to adjust in a supportive environment*

Assess patient's present coping patterns and identify strengths
Encourage and allow time for verbalization; listen carefully
Assess past coping methods based on previous experiences
Involve patient in all care, explaining treatments and procedures
Encourage communication with significant other
Encourage diversional activities

ndx: Knowledge deficit regarding home care needs

GOAL: *Patient and/or significant other will demonstrate understanding of home care and follow-up instructions through interactive discussion and actual return demonstration*

Discuss with and demonstrate to patient procedure of tube feeding and tube feeding preparation, as well as amount and times of feeding
Discuss and demonstrate ostomy care (p. 391) and skin care around tube sites
Demonstrate dressing change procedure and care of prosthetic valve and cap
Explain importance of weighing q2d to 3d
Provide information on symptoms of bowel obstruction and wound infection
Demonstrate medication preparation via tube feeding; discuss name, dose, purpose, time of administration, and side effects
Encourage follow-up appointments with physician

Evaluation

There are no complications
Fluid and nutrition intake are adequate to meet body requirements

Pain is managed adequately
Adaptive responses are demonstrated as related to coping behavior
Home and follow-up care are demonstrated adequately

Intestines

IRRITABLE BOWEL SYNDROME: REGIONAL ENTERITIS (CROHN'S DISEASE) AND ULCERATIVE COLITIS

regional enteritis *Chronic, recurrent nonspecific inflammation of the entire intestine, usually the terminal ileum, involving the mucosa and surrounding musculature and leading to deep fissure formation*

ulcerative colitis *Inflammatory intestinal disease of unknown cause, usually affecting the mucosal lining of the colon; may be mild, chronic, or acute*

Assessment

Observations/findings

Regional enteritis: cramplike abdominal pain; often in right lower quadrant with frequent diarrhea containing melena and/or steatorrhea
Ulcerative colitis: colicky abdominal cramps; pain is usually minimal; diarrheal stools are frequent and contain mucus, melena, and pus
Anorexia
Weight loss
Fever
Nausea, vomiting
Generalized malaise
Increased peristalsis
Emotional instability

Laboratory/diagnostic studies

Barium studies of intestine
Sigmoidoscopy, colonoscopy
Biopsy
Radiologic study of abdomen
Serum electrolytes, albumin
Liver function tests
Hematologic studies
Stools for melena

Potential complications

Electrolyte imbalance
Dehydration, malnutrition, anemia
Intestinal obstruction, perforation
Hemorrhage, shock
Fistula, peritonitis
Perianal abscess, fistula, fissure

Medical management

Corticosteroids
Antibiotics
Antidiarrheals
Sedatives, analgesics
Parenteral fluids, elemental diet, TPN (depending on severity of disease)
Nasogastric aspiration
Activity, rest
Surgical interventions: ileostomy, colostomy, resection

Nursing diagnoses/goals/interventions

ndx Potential fluid volume deficit related to abnormal fluid loss (diarrhea)

GOAL: *Patient's fluid balance and electrolytes will be maintained to meet body requirements*

Maintain NPO as ordered
Administer parenteral fluids with electrolytes and vitamins as ordered
Measure intake and output q8h
Monitor electrolytes
Weigh patient daily at same time with same clothing and scale
Monitor vital signs q4h; avoid rectal temperature

ndx Alteration in bowel elimination related to diarrhea

GOAL: *Patient's bowel elimination will be less frequent and less painful*

Assess and monitor stools for amount, frequency, consistency, and color
Monitor stools for occult blood
Auscultate abdomen for bowel sounds q8h
Measure abdominal girth q8h
Administer antidiarrheal, antibiotic, and steroid therapy as ordered
Provide rest and activity as ordered
Provide odor-free environment; keep covered bedpan within easy reach and empty and return promptly

ndx Alteration in nutrition: less than body requirements related to diarrhea

GOAL: *Patient's nutritional status will be maintained within parameters of disease process*

Assess nutritional status and assist patient with identifying irritating foods
Provide diet as ordered: usually high in calories, protein, and minerals; low in residue, fat, and fiber

Prepared elemental diets are available
TPN as ordered
Six small meals are beneficial
Encourage patient to eat slowly, chew well, and take small bites
Monitor Hgb and Hct

ndx: Potential impairment of skin integrity related to malnourished state and/or diarrhea

GOAL: *Patient's skin integrity will be maintained and symptoms of inflammatory process will be relieved*

Assess perirectal area for inflammation, abscess, or fistula
Administer perirectal skin care following each bowel movement
   Wash gently with soap and water
   Pat dry and apply soothing protective ointments as ordered
Administer sitz baths as ordered
Provide other skin care to bony prominences as needed

ndx: Alteration in comfort: pain related to disease process

GOAL: *Patient will verbalize minimal discomfort or absence of pain*

Administer sedatives, analgesics, and rectal suppositories and ointments as ordered
Change position frequently and administer back rubs
Provide diversional activities and frequent rest periods
Ambulate with assistance as allowed

ndx: Family coping: potential for growth related to disease process and prognosis

GOAL: *Patient and/or significant other will express feelings and concerns, identify strengths, and demonstrate adaptive behaviors in managing changes in life-style*

Assess present and past coping patterns
Provide time for and encourage communication with significant other
Establish a supportive relationship with patient and/or significant other
   Explain all procedures and treatments
   Involve patient and/or significant other in plan of care and realistically reinforce physician's explanation of disease process
   Maintain quiet and nonstressful environment

Accept patient's dependency and encourage independent activities as strength returns
Provide information about outside support groups: United Foundation for Ileitis and Colitis, United Ostomy Association, etc.

ndx: Sexual dysfunction related to chronicity of disease and inflammation of perineal area

GOAL: *Patient will express concerns and feelings and demonstrate knowledge of needed sexual activity limitations*

Explain to patient and/or significant other that sexual activity only needs to be curtailed while perineal area is inflamed or there are fistulas or abscesses present
Explain that following surgery with ostomy, sexual activity can be normal after incision is healed; explain need to avoid excessive pressure on ostomy site
Encourage patient to read about alternative positions and techniques
Explain that odor may be controlled by changing ostomy appliance prior to sexual activity and/or using light scent of perfume or aftershave lotion
Provide supportive environment

ndx: Knowledge deficit regarding home care needs

GOAL: *Patient and/or significant other will demonstrate understanding of home care and follow-up instructions through interactive discussion and actual return demonstration*

Provide instructions in diet management, stressing foods to avoid: raw fruits and vegetables, alcohol, chocolate, and gas-producing foods
Discuss importance of avoiding stress during meals; need to chew food well and eat slowly
Demonstrate procedure for perineal care for inflammation, abscess, and/or fistula and for washing and drying area after each bowel movement
Explain causal relationship of stress on disease process and symptoms of recurrence or progression of disease to report to physician
Provide information about medications, including name, dosage, purpose, time of administration, side effects, and interactions; explain need to avoid over-the-counter medications
Encourage follow-up appointments with physician

Evaluation

There are no complications
Nutrition is adequate, and fluid balance is maintained

Skin integrity is maintained
Adaptive behaviors are demonstrated
Pain and diarrhea are diminished
Home care needs are demonstrated accurately

PERITONITIS

Inflammation of the peritoneal cavity due to infiltration of intestinal contents from such conditions as a ruptured appendix, gastric or intestinal perforation or trauma, and anastomotic leaks

Assessment

Observations/findings

Abdominal pain and rigidity over area of inflammation
  Rebound tenderness
  May refer to shoulder
Abdominal distention
Anorexia
Nausea, vomiting
Decreased to absent bowel sounds
Failure to pass flatus or stool rectally
Chills, fever
Tachycardia
Hypotension
Leukocytosis
Anxiety
Thoracic breathing: rapid, shallow
Fecal emesis

Laboratory/diagnostic studies

CBC, electrolytes
Radiologic examination of abdomen
Peritoneal aspiration

Potential complications

Electrolyte imbalance
Dehydration
Metabolic acidosis
Respiratory alkalosis
Shock

Medical management

Parenteral fluids with electrolytes, antibiotics, and vitamins
Nasogastric aspiration
Arterial blood gases
Central venous lines
Oxygen therapy
Peritoneal lavage with antibiotics
Surgical intervention

Nursing diagnoses/goals/interventions

ndx: Alteration in tissue perfusion, actual or potential, secondary to increased blood flow to peritoneum

GOAL: *Patient's tissue perfusion will be maintained*

Maintain NPO
Monitor vital signs and CVP qh or prn; observe for signs of shock
Administer parenteral fluids with electrolytes, antibiotics, and vitamins as ordered
Measure intake and output q8h; measure urine output hourly
Assist with peritoneal aspiration
Monitor electrolytes, blood gases, Hgb, and Hct
Perform passive or assist with and teach active ROM exercises q4h

ndx: Ineffective breathing pattern secondary to thoracic breathing

GOAL: *Patient's breathing will be maintained adequately to meet body requirements*

Maintain bed rest in quiet environment with head elevated 35 to 45 degrees
Administer oxygen therapy or incentive spirometer as ordered
Assist and teach patient to turn and cough q4h and deep breath q½h
Auscultate chest for breath sounds q4h

ndx: Alteration in nutrition: less than body requirements

GOAL: *Patient's nutritional intake will be reestablished to preperitonitis status*

Insert nasogastric tube or assist with insertion of naso-oral intestinal tube; connect to low, intermittent suction apparatus as ordered
  Observe character, amount, color, and odor of drainage
  Provide frequent oral and nasal hygiene
Measure abdominal girth q4h
Observe for passing of flatus
Auscultate abdomen for bowel sounds q8h
Administer TPN as ordered
When bowel sounds return and nasogastric-intestinal tube is removed, provide clear liquid diet as tolerated
If surgery is performed, see Intestinal Surgery (p. 380)

ndx: Alteration in comfort: pain related to inflammatory process

GOAL: *Patient will express minimal discomfort or absence of pain*

Assess type, location, and severity of pain
Administer analgesics only after diagnosis has been made
Maintain position of comfort to minimize stress on abdomen and change frequently
Provide planned rest periods

ndx: Anxiety/fear related to severity of illness

GOAL: *Patient will express concerns, feelings, and demonstrate positive coping behaviors*

Assess present coping patterns
Encourage and allow time for verbalization of feelings
Explain all treatments and procedures
Reinforce physician's explanation of illness and treatment
Assist with and teach relaxation techniques

Evaluation

There are no complications
Nutritional and fluid intake is adequate
Fluid volume has been restored

SHORT BOWEL SYNDROME

Malabsorption that follows small bowel resection; severity depends on the amount and portion of small bowel removed

Assessment

Observations/findings

Frequent, watery diarrhea; may be steatorrheic
Rapid dehydration from malabsorption
Rapid weight loss
Weakness
Purpura, generalized bleeding
Anemia
Malabsorption of fat and fat-soluble vitamins (A, E, D, K)

Laboratory/diagnostic studies

Barium enema
Serum studies: iron, vitamins B_{12} and A, calcium, folate, magnesium, electrolytes, CBC, carotene, cholesterol
PT (increased)
Stool for steatorrhea and culture
Lactose tolerance, D-lactate level, xylose tolerance

Potential complications

Malnutrition
Electrolyte imbalance
Osteoporosis, osteomalacia
Night blindness
Tetany
Confusion, stupor

Medical management

Antidiarrheals
Anticholinergics
Antibiotics
Antacids
Vitamins
Histamine receptor antagonists (cimetidine)
TPN, parenteral fluids
Elemental diet progressing to low-lactose, high-calorie diet

Nursing diagnoses/goals/interventions

ndx: Actual fluid volume deficit related to profuse diarrhea and electrolyte loss

GOAL: *Patient's fluid intake will be sufficient to meet body requirements*

Administer parenteral fluids with electrolytes and vitamins as ordered
Assess for signs of dehydration and shock; check level of consciousness q2h
Monitor vital signs q2h to 4h
Measure intake and output q8h
Weigh patient daily at same time with same clothing and scale
Monitor serum electrolytes, Hgb, and Hct

ndx: Alteration in bowel elimination: diarrhea

GOAL: *Patient's stools will be increasingly normal in consistency, amount, and frequency*

Administer antidiarrheals, antacids, and cimetidine as ordered
Monitor stools for color, consistency, amount, and frequency
Provide perineal care following each bowel movement; keep environment free from odor
Auscultate abdomen for bowel sounds q4h

ndx: Alteration in nutrition: less than body requirements related to diarrhea

GOAL: *Patient's nutritional status will be sufficient to meet body needs and provide weight gain*

Administer TPN as ordered
Monitor urine for sugar and acetone qid
Observe site of catheter for infection
Institute elemental diet (Vivonex, Precision LR) when ordered, usually when weight gain is apparent and diarrhea is less frequent
    Administer diet through nasogastric tube or orally, depending on patient's appetite: 300 to 350 ml/q2h
    When given orally, provide a straw because the taste may be unpalatable to some patients
    Discuss with and assist patient with accepting nutritional plan, since it may be necessary for a long period of time
Administer antacids and anticholinergics as ordered

ndx: Knowledge deficit regarding home care needs

GOAL: *Patient and/or significant other will demonstrate knowledge of home care and follow-up instructions through interactive discussion and actual return demonstration*

Provide written information about nutritional plan, usually low-lactose, high-calorie; introduce milk slowly and observe tolerance
Instruct patient and/or significant other concerning signs and symptoms to report to physician: nausea, vomiting, diarrhea, or other intestinal problems
Provide written instructions for home TPN if applicable; arrange for home health care visits (p. 51)
Discuss medication: name, dosage, purpose, time of administration, and side effects
Encourage follow-up visits with physician

Evaluation

There are no complications
Nutritional status is improving or normal
Fluid balance is maintained
Diarrhea has diminished
Home care instructions are understood

INTESTINAL OBSTRUCTION

Blockage of the intestinal tract, which inhibits the passage of fluids, flatus, and food; may be mechanical or functional

Causes
Mechanical

Strangulated hernia
Abscess
Adhesions
Carcinoma
Volvulus
Intussusception
Obstipation

Functional

Paralytic ileus
Spinal cord lesions
Regional enteritis
Electrolyte imbalance
Uremia

Assessment
Observations/findings
SPECIFIC

Small bowel
    Severe, cramplike abdominal pain
    Mild distention
    Nausea, vomiting
    Rapid dehydration: acidosis
Large bowel
    Mild abdominal discomfort
    Severe distention
    Latent fecal vomiting
    Latent dehydration: rare acidosis

COMMON

Anorexia and malaise
Fever
Tachycardia
Diaphoresis
Pallor
Abdominal rigidity
Failure to pass stool or flatus rectally or per ostomy
Increased bowel sounds
Urinary retention
Leukocytosis

Laboratory/diagnostic studies

Serum electrolytes, CBC, amylase
Barium enema
Radiologic studies of abdomen

Potential complications

Dehydration
Electrolyte imbalance
Metabolic acidosis
Perforation
Shock

Medical management

NPO
Nasointestinal aspiration

Surgical intervention: see Intestinal Surgery (p. 380)
Parenteral fluids with electrolytes, antibiotics, and vitamins
Analgesics

Nursing diagnoses/goals/interventions

ndx: Actual fluid volume deficit secondary to nausea and vomiting, fever, and/or diaphoresis

GOAL: *Patient's fluid volume will be maintained to meet body requirements*

Monitor vital signs and observe level of consciousness and for symptoms of shock
Maintain NPO
Administer parenteral fluids with electrolytes, antibiotics, and vitamins as ordered
Assist with insertion of nasointestinal tube and connect to low, intermittent suction as ordered (p. 365) if no surgery is to be performed
Position patient on right side, then left side to facilitate passage into intestine; do not tape nasointestinal tube to nose
Monitor tube for advancement qh and note character and amount of drainage
Insert nasogastric tube if surgery is to be performed; connect to low, intermittent suction apparatus as ordered (p. 365)
Administer oral and nasal hygiene frequently
Measure intake and output; indwelling urethral catheter may be ordered; report output of less than 500 ml/24hr to physician
Auscultate abdomen for bowel sounds q4h and note increased rigidity or pain; gentle enema may be ordered
Measure abdominal girth q4h
Monitor electrolytes, Hgb, and Hct
Initiate oral fluids when ordered, either by clamping intestinal tube for 1 hr and giving measured amounts of water or tea or giving these fluids after intestinal tube is removed
Open tube, if in place, at specified times as ordered, to estimate amount of absorption
Observe abdomen for discomfort, distention, pain, or rigidity and report to physician
Auscultate bowel sounds tid, 1 hr after meals
Force fluids to 2500 ml daily unless contraindicated
Measure intake and output until adequate
Observe initial stool for color, consistency, and amount; avoid constipation
Administer supplementary vitamins as ordered

ndx: Alteration in comfort: pain related to disease process

GOAL: *Patient will verbalize minimal discomfort or absence of pain*

Maintain bed rest in position of comfort; do not gatch knees
Administer analgesics as ordered; avoid morphine
Provide planned rest periods
Assist with and teach active or perform passive ROM exercises q4h
Change position frequently and administer back rubs and skin care

ndx: Ineffective breathing pattern related to abdominal distention and/or rigidity

GOAL: *Patient's respirations will be adequate to meet body requirements*

Assess respiratory status; observe for shallow, rapid breathing
Elevate head of bed 40 to 60 degrees
Administer oxygen therapy or incentive spirometer as ordered
Assist and teach patient to turn and cough q4h and deep breathe qh
Auscultate chest for breath sounds q4h

ndx: Anxiety/fear related to hospitalization and emergent situation

GOAL: *Patient will verbalize concerns and demonstrate understanding of disease process and treatment*

Assess present coping behaviors
Encourage and allow time for verbalization of anxieties and fears
Explain procedures and treatments and reinforce physician's explanation of illness, treatment, and prognosis
Maintain quiet, nonstressful environment

ndx: Knowledge deficit regarding home care needs

GOAL: *Patient and/or significant other will demonstrate understanding of home care and follow-up instructions through interactive discussion*

Discuss dietary management, stressing importance of eating slowly, chewing foods well, and eating at regular intervals
Explain need to avoid constipation
  Use natural laxatives or stool softeners

Maintain fluid intake of 2500 ml/day
Increase activity as tolerated
Provide instructions on symptoms to report to physician: abdominal pain, cramps, distention, and/or nausea and vomiting
Encourage follow-up care with physician
See Intestinal Surgery (p. 380) if surgery was performed

Evaluation

There are no complications
Nutritional status is adequate
Home care needs and follow-up instructions are understood

INTESTINAL CARCINOMA

carcinoma of small intestine Malignancy most frequently found in the lower duodenum and lower ileum; mortality is high; early signs and symptoms are usually absent

carcinoma of large intestine Slow-growing malignancy most frequently found in the cecum, lower ascending, and sigmoid colon; prognosis is optimistic; early signs and symptoms are usually absent

Assessment

Observations/findings

SPECIFIC

Small intestine
    Nausea, vomiting
    Anorexia
    Upper abdominal pain
Large intestine
    Alteration in bowel habits and function
    Rectal bleeding, tarry stool
    Abdominal cramps, pain, distention

COMMON

Generalized weakness
Weight loss

Laboratory/diagnostic studies

Upper GI series
Duodenoscopy with biopsy
Radiologic abdominal series
Barium enema
Sigmoidoscopy and colonoscopy with biopsy
CBC, electrolytes

Potential complications

Electrolyte imbalance
Dehydration
Anemia
Intestinal obstruction
Bowel abscess: fistula
Metastatic involvement: lungs, kidneys, bone

Medical management

Diet or parenteral fluids with electrolytes and vitamins
Nasogastric/intestinal aspiration
Bed rest, ambulation
Analgesics
Chemotherapeutic agents
Radiotherapy, immunotherapy
Surgical intervention (resection, ostomy, abdominal-perineal resection)

Nursing diagnoses/goals/interventions*

ndx: Alteration in nutrition: less than body requirements related to vomiting and/or anorexia

GOAL: *Patient's nutritional status will be maintained to meet body needs*

Maintain NPO
Administer parenteral fluids with electrolytes and vitamins C and K as ordered
Insert nasogastric, nasointestinal tube as ordered; connect to low, intermittent suction; observe color and amount of drainage
Measure intake and output
Monitor serum electrolytes, Hgb, and Hct
Monitor vital signs
Provide high-protein, high-carbohydrate, high-calorie, low-residue diet if diet is allowed; note foods that cause irritation and anorexia

ndx: Alteration in comfort: pain related to disease process

GOAL: *Patient will express minimal discomfort or absence of pain*

Maintain bed rest in position of comfort; do not gatch knees
Plan all care to provide rest periods
Administer analgesics as ordered: large doses are sometimes needed in terminally ill patients; assess effectiveness of pain relief measures
Perform passive or assist and teach active ROM exercises q2h to 4h
Assist and teach patient to cough and deep breathe q4h
Change position frequently; provide back rubs prn
Ambulate with assistance as ordered and tolerated

---

*Patient's condition dictates type and amount of care required; modify accordingly.

ndx: Alteration in bowel elimination related to altered bowel function and/or bleeding

GOAL: *Patient's elimination will be maintained within parameters of disease process*

Auscultate abdomen for bowel sounds and measure abdominal girth q4h
Monitor stools for color, consistency, frequency, and amount

ndx: Ineffective individual coping related to illness and prognosis

GOAL: *Patient will express concerns and feelings and be allowed to form adaptive behaviors in a supportive environment*

Encourage and allow time for verbalization of concerns and feelings; listen carefully
Involve significant other and encourage communication with patient
Reinforce physician's explanation of disease process and prognosis
Explain all procedures and treatments and involve patient in plan of care
Assess present coping patterns and identify strengths and provide supportive environment

ndx: Anticipatory grieving related to poor prognosis

GOAL: *Patient and/or significant other will be allowed time to express grief and participate in decision making for the future*

Encourage and allow time for verbalization of feelings; assist patient in identifying steps in grieving process
Assess present patterns of coping; identify strengths
Promote family cohesiveness and communication
Provide a supportive environment in which hope is presented realistically
Provide information on outside support groups (American Cancer Society)

ndx: Knowledge deficit regarding home care needs and chemotherapy and/or radiotherapy

GOAL: *Patient and/or significant other will demonstrate understanding of home care and follow-up instructions through interactive discussion and actual return demonstration*

Provide patient and/or significant other with information about diet management, activity, and rest; refer to dietitian (RD)
Discuss medications: name, dosage, purpose, time of administration, and side effects
Explain side effects of chemotherapy and/or radiotherapy and ways of managing them
Refer to outside health care agencies for assistance with home care
Encourage follow-up visits with physician

Evaluation

There are no complications
Pain is managed adequately
Nutritional status is maintained within confines of disease process
Patient is working through grieving process or has accepted prognosis, and coping behaviors are adaptive
Demonstration of home care is adequate

PARALYTIC ILEUS

Decrease in or absence of intestinal motility following intestinal or abdominal surgery or in connection with any severe metabolic disease; cause may be neuromuscular, resulting from lack of potassium, or gastrointestinal, resulting from gastric inactivity and air swallowing

Assessment
Observations/findings

Abdominal tenderness and distention
Absent or diminished bowel sounds
Nausea, vomiting
Lack of flatus
Decreased urinary output
Fever

Laboratory/diagnostic studies

Electrolytes (decreased potassium)
Abdominal radiography series

Potential complications

Dehydration
Electrolyte imbalance
Shock
Perforation of ileum
Peritonitis (p. 372)
Circulatory failure
Respiratory distress

Medical management

Parenteral fluids with electrolytes
Nasointestinal, nasogastric aspiration
Oxygen therapy
Medications to promote peristalsis: dexpanthenol (Ilopan), vasopressin (Pitressin), bethanechol (Urecholine) and neostigmine (Prostigmin)

Nursing diagnoses/goals/interventions

ndx: Ineffective breathing pattern related to abdominal distention

GOAL: *Patient's oxygen–carbon dioxide exchange and effective breathing pattern will be maintained*

Maintain bed rest in position to facilitate respirations; do not gatch knees
Assess respiratory status
Administer oxygen therapy as ordered
Assist and teach patient to turn and cough q4h and deep breathe q1h
Provide planned rest periods
Assist patient with active or perform passive ROM exercises q4h
Monitor vital signs q4h
Ambulate as ordered

ndx: Actual fluid volume deficit related to vomiting and distention

GOAL: *Patient will be adequately hydrated*

Maintain NPO
Administer parenteral fluids with electrolytes as ordered
Insert nasointestinal tube and attach to low, intermittent suction apparatus as ordered (p. 365)
  Do not tape tube to nose; position patient to facilitate passage into intestine
  Monitor advancement qh
Check character, amount, and color of intestinal drainage q4h; report any change in the above to physician
Nasogastric tube may be inserted in lieu of intestinal tube; connect to low, intermittent suction apparatus
  Irrigate with measured amounts of normal saline
  Observe color and amount of drainage
Measure intake and output; report urine output of less than 30 ml/hr to physician
Administer oral and nasal hygiene q2h to 4h
As intestinal or gastric output decreases and bowel sounds return
  Clamp tube as ordered
  Administer liquids (warm tea, carbonated beverages) in measured amounts as ordered
  Observe for pain, distention, and cramps; unclamp tube if these signs occur
  Remove tube when ordered and progress to previous diet
  Continue measuring intake and output until adequate

ndx: Alteration in bowel elimination: constipation related to decreased intake and electrolyte loss

GOAL: *Patient's normal bowel elimination pattern will return*

Administer medication to increase peristalsis as ordered
Auscultate abdomen for bowel sounds q4h; observe for return of flatus and normal bowel elimination
Measure abdominal girth q4h
Administer rectal tube, Harris flush, or enemas as ordered

ndx: Knowledge deficit regarding illness and its outcome

GOAL: *Patient will demonstrate understanding of disease process, needed treatments, and procedures through interactive discussion and actual return demonstration*

Reinforce physician's explanation of cause of paralytic ileus and that it is a temporary condition
Explain all procedures and treatments
Demonstrate swallowing technique so as not to ingest air

Evaluation

There are no complications
Fluid and nutritional intake are adequate
Bowel elimination is normal for patient
Treatments and procedures are understood

DIVERTICULAR DISEASE OF COLON

Herniation (pocket formation) along the mucosa of the large intestine caused by low-fiber diets (diverticulosis); an inflammatory process may take place when a diverticulum ruptures or feces becomes impacted in the diverticulum (diverticulitis)

Acute Diverticulitis
Assessment
Observations/findings

Cramplike pain and tenderness in left lower quadrant
Anorexia
Nausea
Low-grade fever
Irregular bowel function
  Constipation
  Diarrhea
  Mucus, blood in stool
  Increased flatulence

Abdominal distention
Decreased bowel sounds

Laboratory/diagnostic studies

Barium enema
Sigmoidoscopy, colonoscopy with biopsy
Ultrasonography
WBC, ESR (increased)
Urinalysis
Examination of surrounding organs (kidney, bladder) for possible involvement

Potential complications

Leukocytosis
Dehydration
Intestinal obstruction, perforation
Peritonitis
Fistula, abscess
Hemorrhage

Medical management

Parenteral fluids with electrolytes and antibiotics
Nasogastric aspiration (severe vomiting, distention)
Analgesics, anticholinergics
NPO increasing to high-fiber diet
Vasopressin for severe bleeding
Surgical intervention (resection, colostomy)

Nursing diagnoses/goals/interventions

ndx: Potential fluid volume deficit related to vomiting, diarrhea, and/or anorexia

GOAL: *Patient's fluid intake will be maintained to meet body requirements*

Maintain NPO
Administer parenteral fluids with antibiotics and electrolytes as ordered
As pain and fever subside, provide clear liquid diet and progress to soft diet until high-fiber diet can be tolerated as ordered
Force fluids to 2500 ml daily unless contraindicated

ndx: Alteration in tissue perfusion: cerebral, cardiopulmonary, renal, gastrointestinal, and/or peripheral secondary to intestinal bleeding

GOAL: *Patient's circulation will be maintained*

Assess and monitor amount of bleeding; check stools for occult blood
Monitor vital signs q4h and Hgb, Hct
Administer blood transfusions as ordered
Assist with active or perform passive ROM exercises q4h

ndx: Alteration in bowel elimination: constipation related to anorexia, low-fiber diet, and/or bleeding

GOAL: *Patient's bowel elimination will be normal*

Insert nasogastric tube and connect to low, intermittent suction apparatus as ordered
   Maintain tube patency
   Measure gastric output q8h
Auscultate abdomen for bowel sounds q4h
Measure abdominal girth q4h
Observe stools for consistency, color, amount, and frequency
Administer anticholinergics as ordered
Measure intake and output; report urinary output of less than 30 ml/hr to physician
Administer oral and nasal hygiene q4h

ndx: Alteration in comfort: pain related to disease process

GOAL: *Patient will express minimal discomfort or absence of pain*

Maintain bed rest in position of comfort
Administer analgesics as ordered; avoid morphine; assess effectiveness of pain relief measures
Assist and teach patient to turn and deep breathe q2h; administer back rubs
Maintain planned rest periods
Change position frequently to prevent pressure and fatigue

ndx: Knowledge deficit regarding dietary management and home care needs

GOAL: *Patient and/or significant other will demonstrate understanding of home care and follow-up instructions through interactive discussion*

Provide written dietary instructions and discuss relationship of diet to disease process
Include listing of high-fiber foods: bran, fruits, vegetables, nuts
Explain importance of regular meals, eating slowly, and chewing well
   Avoid large meals, extremely cold foods, and alcohol
   Increase fluid intake to eight glasses/day unless contraindicated
Discuss importance of elimination
   Establish regular bowel habits
   Avoid constipation, straining, enemas, and harsh laxatives
   Take psyllium (Metamucil) or high-fiber wafers or powder

Explain signs and symptoms of recurrence to report to physician
Encourage regular visits to physician

Evaluation

There are no complications
Nutritional status is adequate
Bowel elimination is normal
Home care and dietary management is understood

INTESTINAL SURGERY

Any surgery performed on the intestine from the jejunum to the colon for such conditions as carcinoma, obstruction, acute enteritis or colitis, benign tumors, trauma, appendicitis, incarcerated hernia, or diverticulitis

Preoperative assessment and care

Assess respiratory status
Bowel preparation
    Low-residue, clear liquid diet
    Magnesia preparations, antibiotics po
    Enemas until clear; avoid depleting debilitated or elderly patients with multiple enemas at one time
    Nasogastric/nasointestinal tube insertion
Provide patient with information regarding drains, tubes, etc., that may be present postoperatively
Teach patient to turn, cough, and deep breathe and methods for incisional support

Postoperative assessment

Observations/findings

Character and amount
    Gastric or intestinal drainage
    Urinary output
    Ostomy drainage, if ostomy performed
    Wound drainage
Nausea, vomiting
Abdominal distention
Placement of nasogastric tube
Location and type of pain
Decreased, shallow respirations
Decreased breath sounds

Laboratory/diagnostic studies

Electrolytes, Hgb, Hct
Urine culture after indwelling catheter is removed
Wound culture; suspected infection

Potential complications

Dehydration
Electrolyte imbalance
Atelectasis
Shock
Hemorrhage
Peritonitis
Paralytic ileus
Pulmonary embolus
Thrombophlebitis
Wound evisceration
Wound infection

Medical management

Parenteral fluids with electrolytes
Nasogastric aspiration
NPO progressing to prescribed diet
Analgesics, antibiotics, vitamins
Oxygen therapy
Activity

Nursing diagnoses/goals/interventions

ndx Potential alteration in tissue perfusion: cardiopulmonary, renal, gastrointestinal, and/or peripheral related to surgical intervention/anesthesia

GOAL: *Patient's circulation will be maintained to meet body requirements*

Monitor vital signs q4h
Check peripheral pulses, color, and temperature q4h
Apply antiembolic stockings as ordered
Assist and teach active or perform passive ROM exercises q4h
Ambulate with assistance bid

ndx Ineffective breathing pattern related to placement of incision and/or pain

GOAL: *Patient's respirations will be maintained to meet body needs*

Assess respiratory status: type, frequency, and character of respirations
Elevate head of bed 35 to 45 degrees; do not gatch knees
Auscultate lungs for breath sounds q2h
Assist and teach patient to turn, cough q2h, and deep breathe q1h; support incision
Provide incentive spirometer q2h

ndx Potential fluid volume deficit related to gastric aspiration, anesthesia, and/or surgical procedure

GOAL: *Patient's hydration will be adequate*

Maintain NPO
Administer parenteral fluids with electrolytes, vitamins, and antibiotics as ordered

Connect nasogastric/intestinal tube to low, intermittent suction as ordered
   Check color and consistency of drainage
   Irrigate with measured amounts of normal saline as ordered
Measure intake and output q8h
Monitor serum electrolytes
Connect indwelling urethral catheter to closed gravity drainage system as ordered
   Measure output hourly; if less than 30 to 50 ml/hr, report to physician
   Initiate voiding measures prn after catheter is removed
Observe for abdominal distention and monitor bowel sounds 2 to 3 days postoperatively

ndx: Potential for infection related to bacterial invasion of surgical incision

GOAL: *Patient's wound will remain clean, dry, and intact without signs of inflammation*

Observe incision for drainage, inflammation, or wound separation
Reinforce dressings or change prn
Observe ostomy site, if present, for correct appliance (p. 391) and skin integrity
Assess healing process

ndx: Alteration in comfort: pain related to surgical intervention

GOAL: *Patient will verbalize reduction or absence of pain*

Maintain bed rest in quiet environment
Administer analgesics as ordered; assess effectiveness of pain relief measures and note location and character of pain
Encourage patient to take pain medication as prescribed for 48 hr; addiction will not result
Coordinate care to allow for planned rest periods
Change position frequently; administer back rubs

ndx: Potential impairment of skin/mucous membrane integrity related to wound drainage, nasogastric tube, and/or urethral catheter

GOAL: *Patient's skin and mucous membranes will remain clean and dry with no signs of inflammation or irritation*

Administer nasal and oral hygiene frequently and keep nares and mouth moist
Change dressings as needed; use nonallergenic tape or Montgomery straps
Maintain permanency of tubes and catheters by taping comfortably and securely
Initiate a wound pouching system if drainage is profuse
Assess color and condition of stoma and peristomal skin integrity if present

ndx: Alteration in bowel elimination related to constipation or diarrhea

GOAL: *Patient's bowel elimination will be normal within confines of surgical procedure*

Assess preoperative bowel habits and auscultate abdomen for bowel sounds
Observe for first postoperative bowel movement; assess color, consistency, amount, and frequency
Keep perineal area clean and dry
Assess rectal dressing and incision if abdominal-perineal resection was performed

ndx: Self-care deficit: bathing/hygiene related to fatigue and limited movement

GOAL: *Patient will demonstrate self-care abilities by time of discharge or express acceptance of limitations*

Assist with hygienic needs as needed
Encourage patient to participate and take responsibility for care as tolerated

ndx: Alteration in nutrition: less than body requirements related to NPO status/parenteral fluids

GOAL: *Patient's nutritional status will be adequate to meet body requirements*

After bowel sounds return and nasogastric/intestinal tube is removed or clamped, initiate clear liquids in measured amounts; observe for tolerance and discomfort or distention
Progress to soft or regular diet as ordered and tolerated
Observe for malabsorption syndrome in surgery of small intestine: steatorrhea, diarrhea, weight loss
Weigh patient daily at same time with same clothing and scale

ndx: Knowledge deficit regarding home and follow-up care

GOAL: *Patient and/or significant other will demonstrate understanding of home care and follow-up instructions through interactive discussion and actual return demonstration*

Provide written dietary instructions and restrictions
Demonstrate dressing changes, wound care, aseptic technique, and signs of infection

Explain importance of avoiding constipation and to use natural laxatives or those prescribed

Discuss activities allowed, need for rest and mild exercise, and necessity of not lifting heavy objects for 6 to 8 weeks

Reinforce physician's explanation of surgical procedure and outcome expected

Discuss medications: name, dosage, purpose, time of administration, and side effects

Encourage follow-up visits with physician

Evaluation

There are no complications
Nutritional status and fluid intake are adequate
Pain is minimal or absent
ADLs can be performed by patient or with assistance
Home care instructions are understood

CONTINENT ILEOSTOMY (KOCK'S POUCH)

Surgical removal of the rectum and colon (proctocolectomy) with construction of an internal ileal reservoir, nipple valve, and stoma, allowing intermittent drainage of ileal contents; performed for patients with ulcerative colitis, familial polyposis, or existing ileostomy diversion (Figure 6-6)

Preoperative care

Administer bowel preparation as ordered
    Oral antibiotics
    Mild laxatives
    Colonic irrigations
    Ileostomy irrigation

Bowel preparation will depend on
    Age and nutritional status
    Extent of disease process in colon
    Presence of existing ileostomy

Insert nasogastric tube and indwelling urethral catheter as ordered
Involve enterostomal therapist in preoperative education
Reinforce physician's explanation of surgical procedure and postoperative care

Postoperative assessment

Observations/findings

Patency and placement of plastic ileal reservoir catheter
Placement of suture holding catheter in place
Color and amount of
    Ileal reservoir drainage
    Gastric drainage
    Urine output
    Wound drainage
Patency of nasogastric tube
Color of stoma
Nausea, vomiting
Abdominal distention
Abdominal cramps
Diminished breath sounds

Laboratory/diagnostic studies

Electrolytes, Hgb, Hct

Potential complications

Electrolyte imbalance
Atelectasis
Intestinal obstruction, perforation
Peritonitis
Wound infection: stoma and rectum
Valve prolapse, leakage
Pouch perforation

Medical management

Parenteral fluids with electrolytes
Nasogastric/ileal reservoir aspiration
Analgesics
Diet management
Activity

Nursing diagnoses/goals/interventions

ndx: Potential for ineffective breathing pattern related to pain and location of incision

GOAL: *Patient's respirations will be adequate to meet body requirements*

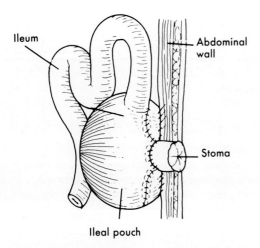

FIGURE 6-6. Continent ileostomy (Kock's pouch).

Assess respiratory status and respiratory rate q2h to 4h
Assist and teach patient to turn and cough q2h to 4h and deep breathe q1h; support incision
Auscultate chest for breath sounds q4h
Elevate head of bed 30 to 45 degrees; do not gatch knees

ndx: Potential fluid volume deficit related to increased ileal output

GOAL: *Patient's fluid intake will be adequate to maintain hydration*

Maintain NPO
Administer parenteral fluids with electrolytes as ordered
Measure intake and output q8h
Monitor vital signs q4h
Connect nasogastric tube to low, intermittent suction apparatus as ordered; irrigate gently with measured amounts of normal saline q2h to 4h
Connect indwelling urethral catheter to closed gravity drainage system as ordered; report output of less than 30 to 50 ml/hr to physician
Monitor serum electrolytes, Hgb, and Hct

ndx: Potential impairment of skin integrity related to acidity of ileostomy drainage and surgical procedure

GOAL: *Patient's skin around ostomy and incisions will remain clean, dry, and intact*

Check dressings q1h to 2h for 24 hr; then q4h for 48 hr
  Change dressings as needed; include rectal dressing
  Place dressing around reservoir catheter to avoid tension and absorb drainage from stoma
  Report excessive bleeding to physician
  Check color of stoma (pink-red); report any change to physician
  Administer wound and stomal care prn
    Wash around stoma and wound with clear water, pat dry, and allow to air dry for 30 min
    Apply lanolin-based ointment or pectin wafer if skin is irritated
  Reapply dressings prn
Administer sitz baths tid as ordered

ndx: Alteration in bowel elimination: diarrhea related to ileostomy and ileal pouch reservoir

GOAL: *Patient's bowel elimination will be managed within confines of disease process and surgical intervention*

Connect ileal reservoir catheter to closed gravity drainage system as ordered
  Avoid placing tension on suture and catheter
  Irrigate gently with 20 to 30 ml of normal saline q2h and prn as ordered
  Observe return flow: should equal amount of instilled plus ileal contents
  Check color and consistency of drainage
Auscultate abdomen for bowel sounds q4h
Observe and monitor for signs of reservoir catheter obstruction
  Feeling of fullness in lower abdomen or around catheter
  Nausea, vomiting
  Increased pain or cramps
If these symptoms occur, notify physician and perform the following procedure if ordered
  Gently irrigate catheter with 20 to 30 ml of normal saline
  If there is no outflow, carefully remove skin suture
  Retain suture around catheter, since it marks length of insertion
  Gently irrigate with 20 ml of normal saline and rotate catheter clockwise until outflow begins
  If no results occur, notify physician immediately

ndx: Alteration in nutrition: less than body requirements related to nasogastric aspiration and increased ileal output

GOAL: *Patient's nutritional status will be maintained to meet body needs*

Clamp or remove nasogastric tube as ordered when bowel sounds return or bubbles appear in ileal catheter
Provide water and clear liquids as tolerated
Avoid carbonated beverages
Progress to soft, low-residue, low-fiber diet to prevent catheter plugging
Avoid gas-producing foods
Teach patient to chew foods well with mouth closed, to eat slowly, and to avoid talking while eating
Avoid drinking with straw
Consider patient's food preferences when possible
Ileal catheter will remain in place 14 to 21 days to allow reservoir healing
  Continue irrigations q2h to 3h with 30 to 40 ml of normal saline; contents will thicken as diet increases
Measure instillation and outflow amounts
Increase fluid intake to 3000 ml/day unless contraindicated

Provide grape and prune juice to keep ileal contents thin

If plugging occurs, gentle milking of catheter and rotation clockwise while irrigating may help; having patient cough and apply light pressure to lower abdomen may also help

Catheter may be removed, rinsed, and reinserted as ordered

ndx: Alteration in comfort: pain related to surgical intervention

GOAL: *Patient will express minimal discomfort or absence of pain*

Maintain bed rest in quiet environment

Assess location and character of pain; severe gas pains are usually present

Administer analgesics and monitor effectiveness of pain relief measures

Assist with and teach active or perform passive ROM exercises q4h

Coordinate care to provide planned rest periods

Provide diversional activities

Ambulate with assistance as ordered

ndx: Disturbance in self-concept related to body image change

GOAL: *Patient will verbalize concerns and demonstrate adaptive responses and coping patterns toward stoma, intubation, and loss of rectum*

Encourage and allow time for verbalization of feelings and concerns; listen carefully

Encourage communication with significant other

Assess present coping behaviors and strengths and assist in promoting self-confidence

Encourage patient to view stoma and catheter and discuss their positive aspects

Reinforce physician's explanation of procedure and treatment; clarify misconceptions

ndx: Knowledge deficit regarding care of continent ileostomy, home care needs, and follow-up instructions

GOAL: *Patient and/or significant other will demonstrate understanding of ileostomy care, home care, and follow-up instructions through interactive discussion and actual return demonstration*

Assist and teach patient to care for ileal reservoir catheter when physical and psychologic status warrants

Involve patient and significant other in plan of care

Set and explain daily goals, with ultimate goal being total patient management

Phase I

Familiarize patient with anatomy and physiology of ileal reservoir

Explain that type of drainage will depend on food ingested and importance of high-liquid intake

Teach patient to irrigate catheter; use 50 ml syringe, normal saline, and 500 ml graduate

Instill 30 to 50 ml of normal saline

Measure outflow

Make certain all irrigating fluid is returned

Reconnect catheter to closed gravity drainage system

Phase II

When ordered, clamp catheter for 1 hr, then release for 30 min and reclamp

Irrigate prn with normal saline if outflow is thick

Teach patient procedure in small segments until mastered

Explain that clamping procedure is to gradually increase reservoir capacity

Explain that clamping time will increase by 15 to 30 min daily until 3 to 4 hr time is reached, usually in 5 to 6 days

Continue to connect catheter to closed gravity drainage system at night

See box on p. 385

Phase III

When ordered, remove catheter and teach patient reinsertion procedure using the following equipment and guidelines

Equipment
  No. 28 plastic catheter with insertion tube
  50 ml graduate
  50 ml syringe
  Normal saline
  Water-soluble lubricant
  Tissues
  4 × 4 dressing
  Nonallergic tape

Guidelines
  Have patient sit on side of bed
  Remove dressings and catheter; disconnect catheter from drainage system
  Rinse catheter with water and lubricate tip; place open end into graduate
  Place graduate below stoma

TWO METHODS FOR INCREASING ILEAL RESERVOIR CAPACITY

EXAMPLE 1

1. Leave catheter in pouch with continuous drainage for 2 to 3 weeks from day of surgery.
2. Week 3 and/or 4:
   a. During daytime hours, clamp catheter for 2 hours, then open and drain.
   b. Connect to straight drainage at bedtime.
   c. Irrigate catheter with 1 ounce of tap water when drainage is thick. This may be repeated several times.
   d. Catheter may be removed for 15 minutes every 24 hours for showering.
3. At the end of the fourth week, remove catheter and begin intubation schedule.
4. Week 5: Intubate every 3 hours.
5. Week 6: Intubate every 4 hours.
6. Week 7: Intubate every 5 hours.
7. Week 8: Intubate every 6 hours.
8. Week 9: Intubate three to four times in 24-hour period. Maintain this schedule.

EXAMPLE 2

1. Leave catheter in pouch with continuous drainage for 2 to 3 weeks from day of surgery.
2. Week 3:
   a. During daytime hours, clamp catheter for 2 hours, then open and drain.
   b. Connect to straight drainage at bedtime.
   c. Irrigate catheter with 1 ounce of tap water when drainage is thick. This may be repeated several times.
   d. Catheter may be removed for 15 minutes every 24 hours for showering.
3. Week 4: During daytime hours, clamp catheter for 3 hours, then open and drain. Follow steps b, c, and d.
4. Week 5: During daytime hours, clamp catheter for 4 hours, then open and drain. Open and drain one time during the night. Follow steps c and d.
5. Week 6: During daytime hours, clamp catheter for 5 hours, then open and drain. Open and drain at night if necessary. Follow steps c and d.
6. Week 7: During daytime hours, clamp catheter for 6 hours, then open and drain. Open and drain at night if necessary. Follow steps c and d.
7. Week 8: Remove catheter and begin intubation schedule. Intubate three to four times in 24-hour period. Maintain this schedule.

From Broadwell, D.C., and Jackson, B.S.: Principles of ostomy care, St. Louis, 1982, The C.V. Mosby Co.

Gently intubate stoma until resistance of nipple valve is felt (2 inches [5 cm])
Slide catheter through valve with gentle pressure to insertion line
  If catheter meets resistance, do not force
    Have patient lie down, relax, and take deep breaths
    Insert catheter through valve during exhalation
Drainage time is about 5 to 10 min unless fecal material is thick; irrigating with 30 ml of normal saline will help
Air bubbles in catheter are normal
When drainage is complete, remove catheter and wash with soap and water; rinse well and dry; store in plastic bag
Cleanse stoma and skin with warm water; pat dry and apply 4 × 4 dressing; secure with tape
Discuss importance of maintaining drainage schedule
Time between will increase as reservoir capacity increases
Provide written schedule (see box above)
Provide needed equipment and information concerning where it may be purchased
Explain importance of well-balanced diet and foods to avoid
  Avoid gas-producing foods: cabbage, cauliflower, carbonated beverages
  Avoid foods that clog catheter: corn, nuts, mushrooms, lettuce, fruit peels
  Eat at regular times, chew food well, eat slowly, and avoid straws
  Maintain fluid intake of 3000 ml/24 hr; drink prune and grape juice to help liquidize drainage
Discuss signs and symptoms to report to physician
  Inability to intubate stoma
  Abdominal distention
  Nausea, vomiting

Increased abdominal pain
Elevated temperature
Incontinence of stool and/or flatus (nipple valve dysfunction)
Explain need to wear nonirritating clothes until wound heals
Demonstrate care of surgical incisions
Encourage follow-up visits with physician

Evaluation

There are no complications
Nutritional status is maintained
Care of ileal pouch and wounds is demonstrated
Self-care activities are performed
Follow-up physician care is understood

ILEOANAL RESERVOIR

A two-stage surgical procedure anastamosing the ileum to an ileal reservoir constructed at the anus, allowing normal bowel elimination without an ileostomy

Stage I: Colectomy, Temporary Ileostomy, and Construction of Ileal Reservoir at Anus

Preoperative assessment and care

Reinforce physician's explanation of surgical procedure and expected outcome; clarify misconceptions
Contact enterostomal therapist for preoperative assessment
Monitor baseline vital signs
Prepare bowel as ordered: tap water enemas, oral antibiotics
Encourage and allow time for expression of concerns and feelings; promote positive aspects of surgical procedure
Explain possibility of nasogastric tube, indwelling urethral catheter, and presacral drainage tube exiting from abdomen postoperatively

Postoperative assessment

Observations/findings

Location of ileostomy and presacral drain
Color, character, and amount of drainage
  Incision (abdominal and rectal)
  Gastric
  Ileostomy
  Presacral drain
Skin integrity of ileostomy and rectal area
Urine output
Location and character of pain

Laboratory/diagnostic studies

Electrolytes, CBC, urinalysis

Potential complications

Skin erosion from ileostomy
Reservoir abscess, ischemia, fistula
Intestinal obstruction
Wound infection: pouchitis (inflammation of reservoir)
Cystitis, retention
Phlebitis

Medical management

Analgesics, antibiotics, dermatologic creams
Parenteral fluids with electrolytes and vitamins
Nasogastric aspiration
Diet, rest, ambulation, exercise

Nursing diagnoses/goals/interventions

ndx: Actual fluid volume deficit related to abnormal body fluid loss from ileostomy, gastric aspiration, and NPO status

GOAL: *Patient will remain adequately hydrated to meet body requirements*

Maintain NPO
Administer parenteral fluids with electrolytes and vitamins as ordered
Connect indwelling urethral catheter to closed drainage system; monitor hourly output for 12 hr
Connect nasogastric tube to low, intermittent suction apparatus as ordered; irrigate with measured amounts of normal saline to keep patent
Monitor and measure ileostomy output; 800 to 1000 ml/24 hr is not uncommon
Connect presacral catheter to closed gravity drainage system or as ordered; monitor output q2h for 12 hr, then q4h
Measure intake and output q8h; observe for urinary retention
Monitor vital signs q2h until stable; then q4h
Weigh patient daily at same time with same clothing and scale
Monitor electrolytes, Hgb, and Hct
When nasogastric tube is removed, initiate liquids as ordered; progress to well-balanced diet as tolerated; monitor stools for tolerance of food
Initiate voiding measures as needed after indwelling catheter is removed

ndx: Actual impairment of skin integrity related to ileostomy and rectal/anal drainage

GOAL: *Patient's skin will return to normal integrity and be clean, dry, and intact*

Monitor perianal area for drainage and mucus; may be copious and odorous
    Change dressings prn and clean area well; dry with hair dryer and apply skin sealants and creams as ordered
    Irrigate reservoir daily as ordered to remove mucus and other drainage and prevent pouchitis
    Provide absorbent pads to wear while ambulating or at night
Assist with and teach patient ileostomy and skin care (p. 391)
    Apply suitable appliance as soon as possible
    Maintain skin integrity with use of skin barriers
    Demonstrate ileostomy care as soon as tolerated physically and emotionally

ndx: Knowledge deficit regarding home care management

GOAL: *Patient and/or significant other will demonstrate understanding of home care and follow-up instructions through interactive discussion and actual return demonstration*

Reiterate ileostomy care and appliance change; observe return demonstration
Stress importance of and demonstrate skin care of perianal area and ileostomy site
Demonstrate daily reservoir irrigation as ordered
Discuss and teach patient Kegel exercises (squeezing and relaxing perineal muscles) to increase anal sphincter tone
Reinforce physician explanation of Stage II procedure and clarify misconceptions
Explain that Gastrografin film of reservoir will be taken in about 6 to 12 weeks to assess reservoir capacity and anatomic location
Explain that manometric studies of anal sphincter tone will also be performed
Stress importance of well-balanced diet, rest, and exercise
Instruct patient on signs and symptoms to report to physician: increasing diarrhea, drainage, foul odor from anus, abdominal distention, absence of feces
Promote follow-up visits with physician

Stage II: Ileostomy Closure and Anastomosis of Ileum to Anal Reservoir

Preoperative assessment and care

See Stage I (p. 386)
Presacral drainage tube is not usually in place, and enemas are not given
Irrigation of reservoir is usually ordered

Postoperative assessment
Observations/findings

Location and character of pain
Color, character, and amount of drainage
    From abdominal incision
    Gastric drainage
    Rectal drainage
Urine output
Skin integrity (perianal area)

Laboratory/diagnostic studies

Electrolytes, CBC, urinalysis

Potential complications

Reservoir abscess, ischemia, fistula
Skin erosion (perianal area)
Intestinal obstruction
Wound or reservoir infection
Cystitis, retention
Phlebitis

Medical management

Analgesics, antibiotics, antidiarrheals, dermatologic creams, ointments
Parenteral fluids with electrolytes and vitamins
Nasogastric aspiration
Diet, rest, ambulation, exercise
Sitz baths

Nursing diagnoses/goals/interventions

ndx: Potential fluid volume deficit related to abnormal body fluid loss from NPO status and nasogastric aspiration

GOAL: *Patient will remain adequately hydrated to meet body requirements*

Maintain NPO
Administer parenteral fluids with electrolytes and vitamins as ordered
Connect nasogastric tube to low, intermittent suction apparatus as ordered; irrigate with measured amounts of normal saline to keep patent
Connect indwelling urethral catheter to closed gravity drainage system as ordered; monitor hourly output
Measure intake and output q8h
Monitor vital signs q4h
Weigh patient daily at same time with same clothing and scale
Monitor electrolytes, Hgb, and Hct
Initiate voiding measures as needed following urethral

catheter removal; observe for retention and signs of infection

ndx: Potential impairment of perianal skin integrity related to diarrhea

GOAL: *Patient's perianal area will become clean, dry, and remain in good condition as stools diminish*

Cleanse perianal area as needed with water or aluminum acetate (Domeboro solution) and soft cloth or cotton balls; dry thoroughly with hair dryer
Cover with skin barrier prn and use Tuck's pads
Administer sitz baths as ordered
Irrigate ileal reservoir daily if ordered

ndx: Alteration in bowel elimination: diarrhea related to ileal output and lack of sphincter control

GOAL: *Patient will progress toward fewer and more formed bowel movements*

Monitor bowel movements for frequency and consistency; will be frequent, initially (10 to 20/day)
Provide well-balanced diet when allowed, avoiding fresh fruits, spices, and dairy products on a trial-and-error basis
Administer psyllium (Metamucil), diphenoxalate (Lomotil) as ordered to control diarrhea
Promote Kegel exercises qh to increase sphincter tone

ndx: Knowledge deficit regarding home care management

GOAL: *Patient and/or significant other will demonstrate understanding of home care and follow-up instructions through interactive discussion and actual return demonstration*

Stress importance of protecting perineal area
   Cleanse area after urinating or defecating with water and dry with hair dryer; take sitz baths prn
   Apply skin sealants, lotions, and dermatologic creams prn
   Avoid harsh, perfumed soaps and nylon underwear
   Daily reservoir irrigation may be needed to prevent infection
Discuss bowel elimination; frequency will become less (6 to 10/day) and eventually drop to 3 to 4/day
   Some incontinence may be noted at night; pads may be worn as protection
   Psyllium (Metamucil) and loperamide (Imodium) will help avoid diarrhea
Provide information on diet and foods that cause diarrhea (spices, fresh fruit, and dairy products)

Instruct patient on signs and symptoms to report to physician: increasing diarrhea, drainage or foul odor from rectum, abdominal distention, absence of feces
Promote follow-up visits with physician

Evaluation

There are no complications
Ileoanal reservoir is functioning properly
Skin integrity is maintained
Home care management is understood

CARE OF PATIENT WITH NASO-ORAL INTESTINAL TUBE (CANTOR OR MILLER-ABBOTT TUBE)

Cantor or Miller-Abbott tube *An intestinal tube, 6 to 10 ft (2 to 3.3 m) in length, that is passed through the nose or mouth into the stomach and intestine; a balloon for mercury is attached to the distal end; used for decompression and drainage in patients with bowel obstruction or paralytic ileus; tube is advanced manually, by peristaltic action, by gravity and weight of mercury (Figure 6-7)*

Preinsertion assessment and care

Reinforce physician's explanation of procedure and its purpose
Assess patient's ability to swallow and willingness to cooperate
Assess abdomen for
   Size, shape, softness
   Presence or absence of bowel sounds
Assess patient for presence of nausea, vomiting, and pain
Elevate head of bed 60 to 70 degrees; tilt head slightly forward to facilitate tube passage
Check tube for patency
Check that balloon is securely attached and test for leakage by inserting water into balloon with syringe
Prepare syringe with correct amount of mercury
   Cantor tube: mercury is injected into balloon prior to insertion
   Miller-Abbott tube: mercury is inserted into balloon after insertion
Ice tube according to procedure and lubricate with water-soluble jelly prior to insertion

Insertion assessment

Heart rate and rhythm: arrhythmias may occur as a result of vagal stimulation
Respiratory distress
Vomiting

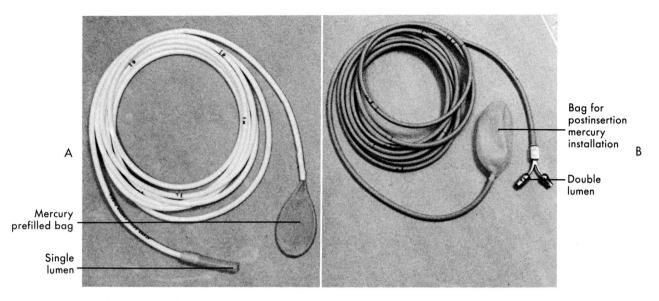

FIGURE 6-7. A, Cantor tube. **B,** Miller-Abbott tube.

Postinsertion assessment
Observations/findings
Nausea, vomiting
Character and amount of drainage
Accurate placement of tube in stomach
Pressure delivered by intermittent suction apparatus
Patency of tube
Position of patient and tube to facilitate passage of tube
Dysphagia
Sore throat
Abdominal distention, pain, or cramps
Increasing bowel sounds
Erosion of nares
Condition of mouth
Blockage of eustachian tube on insertion side

Laboratory/diagnostic studies
Electrolytes
Abdominal radiologic series

Potential complications
Dehydration
Electrolyte imbalance
Oliguria

Medical management
NPO
Parenteral fluids with electrolytes
Nasointestinal aspiration with suction pressure
Analgesics

Nursing diagnoses/goals/interventions
ndx: Potential fluid volume deficit related to vomiting and loss of gastric contents via aspiration

GOAL: *Patient's fluid intake will be adequate to maintain hydration*

Maintain NPO
Administer parenteral fluids with electrolytes as ordered
Insert prescribed amount of mercury into correct lumen of Miller-Abbott tube and label "mercury"
Connect nasointestinal tube to low, intermittent suction apparatus as ordered
Coil tube and pin to patient's gown; do not tape to nose and avoid placing tension on tube
Measure intake and output q8h; if urinary output is less than 30 to 40 ml/hr, notify physician
Monitor color and consistency of intestinal drainage q4h
Irrigate tube gently with measured amounts of normal saline as ordered; if no return flow is obtained, include amount as intake
Measure abdominal girth and auscultate abdomen, for bowel sounds q4h
Turn patient to right side, to back, to left side until tube passes into intestine

Advance tube as ordered, usually 3 to 4 inches at specified times
Monitor vital signs and electrolytes

ndx: Potential alteration in nutrition: less than body requirements secondary to required NPO status

GOAL: *Patient's nutritional status will return to normal when causative disease process is eliminated*

When bowel sounds return and/or flatus or stool is passed
   Clamp tube for 2 to 4 hr as ordered
   Measure abdominal girth and observe for signs of distention, cramps, or nausea
   If these symptoms occur, unclamp tube and notify physician
If patient tolerates clamping procedure, administer small, frequent, measured amounts of water and observe tolerance
If patient tolerates fluids, tube is removed slowly, 2 to 3 inches at a time, or allowed to pass out through rectum
Provide clear liquid diet as ordered and progress to diet as tolerated
If bowel sounds do not return, prepare patient for surgical release of bowel obstruction as ordered (p. 374)

ndx: Alteration in comfort: pain related to tube insertion and placement

GOAL: *Patient will express minimal discomfort or absence of pain*

Maintain bed rest in position of comfort: usually head elevated 30 to 40 degrees
Maintain quiet environment and coordinate care to allow frequent rest periods
Assess character and location of pain
Administer analgesics as ordered and assess effectiveness of pain relief measures
Assist and teach patient to turn and cough q4h and deep breathe q1h; administer back rubs
Perform passive or assist with and teach active ROM exercises q4h

ndx: Potential impairment of tissue integrity secondary to nasointestinal tube insertion

GOAL: *Patient's oronasal tissues will be maintained and free from irritation or discomfort*

Administer oral hygiene q2h; provide lozenges or hard candy if allowed to stimulate salivation
Assess nares for irritation or dryness q2h; gently clean and apply lubricant as needed

Administer topical anesthetic spray to throat as ordered
Lubricate intestinal tube well before advancing it

ndx: Knowledge deficit regarding understanding of nasointestinal tube and its purpose

GOAL: *Patient and/or significant other will demonstrate understanding of procedure following interactive discussion*

Explain purpose of tube and appropriate anatomy and physiology
Discuss advancement of tube and how to avoid dislodgment
Discuss signs and symptoms to report
   Ear pain or fullness on side of insertion
   Nausea, or vomiting
   Increased abdominal pain or cramps
   Feeling of abdominal fullness or pressure

Evaluation

There are no complications
Nutritional and fluid intake is adequate
Tube is removed or surgery is performed

ABDOMINAL HERNIORRHAPHY

Surgical repair of a herniation of the intestine through a weakened portion of the abdominal wall

Assessment
Observations/findings

Site of incision for bleeding
Abdominal distention
Urinary retention
Scrotal edema and pain

Potential complications

Evisceration
Wound infection

Medical management

Analgesics, antibiotics (epididymitis)
Scrotal support, ice bags
Catheterization if unable to void
Stool softeners
Activity, diet
Intake and output

Nursing diagnoses/goals/interventions

ndx: Potential alteration in urinary elimination related to discomfort

GOAL: *Patient will void and will not develop retention*

Encourage and assist patient with voiding
   Avoid retention
   Assist male patients with standing and voiding
   Assist females with ambulation to bathroom
Observe males for scrotal edema; apply scrotal support and/or ice bags as ordered

ndx: Knowledge deficit regarding home care needs

GOAL: *Patient and/or significant other will demonstrate understanding of home care and follow-up instructions through interactive discussion*

Discuss activity restrictions: no strenuous exercise or heavy lifting until allowed, increase activities as tolerated
Explain importance of diet and elimination
   Eat well-balanced diet
   Drink six to eight glasses of water daily
   Avoid straining and constipation by using natural laxatives or stool softeners
Demonstrate incisional care and discuss signs of wound infection
Encourage follow-up visits with physician

Evaluation

There are no complications
Wound healing is adequate
Home care is understood

OSTOMY MANAGEMENT AND CARE

ostomy *Surgical opening into the intestine to provide temporary or permanent passage of feces; necessitated by carcinoma, inflammation, trauma, or obstruction below the site of the incision*

Assessment

Observations/findings

Type of ostomy (see Figure 6-5)
   Ileostomy: usually permanent
   Colostomy: ascending, transverse, descending; may be temporary or permanent
Level of patient's understanding of surgical procedure
Emotional status
   Acceptance of ostomy
   Understanding of ostomy function
   Ability to verbalize feelings
   Acceptance of body image change
Character, frequency, and amount of feces
Size, location, and color of stoma (see Figure 6-5)
Condition of skin around stoma
Correct placement and size of appliance
Hydration

Laboratory/diagnostic studies

Electrolytes, Hbg, Hct

Potential complications

Leakage under appliance
Signs of wound infection
Electrolyte imbalance
Dehydration
Obstruction
Prolapse
Hemorrhage
Stricture
Retraction
Necrosis

Medical management

Diet management
Corticosteroid aerosol spray, hystatin powder
Odor-control preparation

Nursing diagnoses/goals/interventions

ndx: Potential impairment of skin integrity (peristomal) secondary to ostomy drainage

GOAL: *Patient's peristomal skin will remain clean, dry, and intact without signs of inflammation*

Initiate peristomal care and apply ostomy appliance as soon postoperatively as possible
Measure stoma for correct appliance size at each appliance change; size should be 1/8 inch larger than stoma measurement
Change appliance prn and observe color, amount, and consistency of feces, and color of stoma
Maintain peristomal skin integrity
   Wash with mild soap and water and rinse thoroughly with each appliance change; to avoid skin irritation, start with appliance that can be emptied, cleaned, and deodorized
   Pat skin dry with towel and apply effective skin barrier (Skin Prep, Stomahesive, Releaseal)
NOTE: *Never place appliance directly on irritated skin*
Apply only clear appliance directly to facilitate monitoring stoma
Maintain a tight seal around stoma
Involve enterostomal therapist if available
Control odor with deodorant drops or bismuth/chlorophyll preparations

ndx: Disturbance in self-concept secondary to body image change

GOAL: *Patient will express feelings and concerns and be assisted in developing adaptive behaviors in a supportive environment*

Assist patient and significant other in accepting ostomy
   Allow time for and encourage verbalization
   Answer all questions and explain treatments and procedures
   Provide care in positive manner; avoid facial expressions connoting distaste
   Observe for signs of denial, grief, or anger
   Provide privacy and a safe environment
Assess present coping patterns and explore strengths and resources
Encourage self-care and independence

ndx: Sexual dysfunction related to change in self-image due to ostomy

GOAL: *Patient and/or siginificant other will demonstrate understanding of any sexual restrictions and will explore alternate methods of attaining satisfaction*

Assess stage of adaptation of patient to ostomy and explain its normalcy
Encourage communication with significant other and explain the need to share feelings
Explain that near-normal sexual activity can be resumed when allowed except to avoid pressure on ostomy site and rectal area
Discuss methods of controlling odor
Provide information about alternative sexual techniques and positions
Encourage counseling if impotency is a problem

ndx: Alteration in bowel elimination: constipation (colostomy) or diarrhea (ileostomy) secondary to shortened bowel and/or change in life-style

GOAL: *Patient will establish an elimination pattern that will sustain body needs and promote life-style acceptance*

Assess patient's previous bowel habits and life-style
Reinforce physician's explanation of surgical procedure and anatomy and physiology of ostomy
   Colostomy feces will be more solid, whereas ileostomy will be liquid to pasty
   Colostomy may be irrigated to establish near-normal elimination; ileostomy should not be irrigated
     Involve significant other where appropriate
     Demonstrate procedure and have patient return demonstration until patient can perform it alone
   Provide information on where to purchase equipment and symptoms of obstruction or prolapse to report to physician
Consult dietitian (RD) for diet instructions, since each patient will differ in foods tolerated
   Most ostomy patients are discharged on a general diet and given a list of foods that may cause gas or diarrhea
   Follow this general rule of thumb
     Ileostomates should have foods high in sodium and potassium: bananas, bouillon, citrus juices, tea, cola, rye flour, molasses
     Ileostomates should avoid gas-producing foods, fried foods, highly seasoned foods, nuts, raisins, rich foods, pineapple, and all raw fruits except bananas if they cause a problem
     Colostomates should avoid gas-producing foods such as cabbage, beans, corn, broccoli, and cauliflower if gas is uncomfortable or embarrassing
   Each patient will have to use a trial-and-error method to establish which foods can be tolerated
   Introduce new foods one at a time
   Stress adequate nutritional and fluid intake
   Stress eating slowly, chewing food well, and eating regular meals
   Avoid extremes in temperature of foods and carbonated beverages
   Involve patient and/or significant other in meal planning
Auscultate abdomen for bowel sounds q8h; report absent sounds to physician
Discuss signs and symptoms of obstruction or stricture
   Decreased drainage, constipation
   Diarrhea
   Cramps, abdominal distention
   Nausea, vomiting

ndx: Knowledge deficit regarding ostomy and diet management and home care needs

GOAL: *Patient and/or significant other will demonstrate understanding of home care and follow-up instructions through interactive discussion and actual return demonstration*

Explain and demonstrate stomal care step-by-step and have patient return demonstration
Discuss equipment used and where to purchase it; provide enough supplies to last a few days after discharge
Explain and provide written information on diet management

Provide information on outside support groups available (United Ostomy Association) and refer to home health care as needed
Discuss signs of wound infection, obstruction, prolapse, etc.
Encourage follow-up visits with physician

Evaluation

There are no complications
Correct ostomy management is demonstrated
Nutrition is adequate
Home care instructions are understood

COLOSTOMY IRRIGATION

A procedure used by some colostomates to clear the bowel of fecal matter and to help establish an evacuation schedule; may not be applicable for all patients

Assessment

Observations/findings

Patient's emotional status
    State of acceptance
    Knowledge and understanding of procedure
    Ability to comprehend
    Tolerance of procedure
Size and color of stoma
Location of stoma(s)
    Single
    Double, with proximal and distal stomas—which stoma to irrigate
Hydration of patient
Temperature and amount of irrigating solution
Retention of irrigating solution; dehydrated patients may retain some fluid
Amount and character of return flow
Constipation
Diarrhea
Pain
Distention

Potential complications

Stoma constriction
Obstruction
Prolapse

Irrigating procedure

When irrigations are ordered (7 to 10 days after surgery)
    Explain procedure and equipment
    Use equipment that will be used at home
    Demonstrate step-by-step
    Assess patient's normal bowel habits
    Involve patient in assisting with procedure as soon as physically and emotionally able
    Use commode as soon as possible for irrigations to provide psychologic support
    Provide diversional activities after instillation of irrigating solution
During procedure observe these precautions
    Have patient sit on commode when possible; elevate head of bed 50 to 80 degrees if in bed
    Prepare 500 to 750 ml of warm tap water
        Remove all air in tubing
        Hold bag at shoulder level or 12 to 18 inches above stoma
    Apply irrigation sleeve over stoma; place end in commode or bedpan
    Insert lubricated cone tip gently into stoma; avoid using catheter, since it may cause intestinal perforation
    Allow solution to run in slowly
    Allow 45 min to 1 hr for return flow
        Position change and/or abdominal massage will help if return is slow
        Irrigation sleeve may be folded and clipped, and patient allowed to ambulate
    Stoma dilation may be ordered
        Using glove, lubricate finger closest to size of stoma
        Insert finger gently into stoma, *never* force
        Rotate finger gently for 1 min to dilate
    Involve significant other where appropriate
    Demonstrate procedure and have patient return demonstration until patient can perform it alone
    Provide information on where to purchase equipment and symptoms of obstruction or prolapse to report to physician

RECTAL SURGERY

Any surgery performed on the rectum, such as for prolapse, polyps, thrombosed hemorrhoids, tumors, fistulas, or fissures

Assessment

Observations/findings

Character and amount of rectal drainage
Placement of drain
Character and location of pain
Urinary output

Potential complications

Abdominal distention
Urinary retention

Hemorrhage
Infection

Medical management

Analgesics, topical anesthetic ointment
Ice packs, sitz baths, warm compresses
Stool softeners
Diet progression

Nursing diagnoses/goals/interventions

ndx: Alteration in comfort: pain related to surgical intervention

GOAL: *Patient will verbalize minimal discomfort or decreased pain*

Maintain bed rest in prone position as ordered; turn side to side q2h
Administer analgesics as ordered; if ointments are ordered, test first for allergic reaction; assess effectiveness of pain relief measures
Avoid supine position if possible; place pillows between knees while on side
Apply warm, wet compresses or ice bag as ordered
Ambulate with assistance; encourage small steps at first; provide Gelfoam or flotation pads for sitting; avoid rubber rings
Provide planned rest periods; avoid sitting in chair for long periods of time
Administer analgesic prior to removing packing

ndx: Alteration in bowel elimination: constipation related to NPO status and painful defecation

GOAL: *Patient will pass soft, formed stool with minimum discomfort*

Maintain NPO until nausea subsides
Provide low-residue, soft diet as ordered
Force fluids to 2500 to 3000 ml/day unless contraindicated
Administer stool softeners as ordered; encourage defecation as soon as urge occurs
Encourage activity and ambulation as soon as possible

ndx: Potential alteration in urinary elimination pattern related to proximity of surgical procedure to bladder

GOAL: *Patient will urinate adequately with minimal discomfort*

Measure intake and output for 24 hr; observe for signs of retention
Assist patient with voiding: males stand and void; females elevate head or use commode
Encourage patient to void during sitz bath

ndx: Potential for infection related to break in suture line or bacterial invasion

GOAL: *Patient's wound will be clean, dry, and intact with no evidence of inflammation or bleeding*

Monitor vital signs q4h
Observe dressings q2h to 4h; check for bleeding, drainage, and packing
Change dressings prn; apply petroleum gauze
Cleanse perianal area after each bowel movement

ndx: Knowledge deficit regarding home care

GOAL: *Patient and/or significant other will demonstrate understanding of home care and follow-up instructions through interactive discussion and actual return demonstration*

Discuss importance of diet management
   Maintain low-residue diet for 1 week
   Increase roughage as tolerated
   Include fresh fruits
   Force fluids to 2500 ml daily unless contraindicated
Demonstrate care of incision and perirectal area
   Take sitz baths as ordered
   Use warm compresses
   Use petroleum gauze pads
   Maintain care of perineal area after each bowel movement
   Apply dressing
Discuss symptoms of wound infection and anal stricture to report to physician
Discuss maintaining soft bowel movements with use of stool softeners and natural laxative foods
Explain importance of avoiding heavy lifting and straining
Encourage follow-up visits with physician

Evaluation

There are no complications
Bowel elimination is returning to normal
Pain is minimal or absent
Home care management is understood

Gallbladder

BILIARY OBSTRUCTION (STONES, INFECTION)

Obstruction of the common and/or cystic bile ducts due to stones, which inhibits the drainage of bile and causes an acute inflammatory process to occur

Assessment

Observations/findings

Midepigastric colicky pain
Pain may radiate to shoulder
Nausea, vomiting
Chills
Fever
Dark, concentrated urine
Clay-colored feces
Weight loss
Tachycardia
Tachypnea
Abdominal distention

Laboratory/diagnostic studies

WBC (elevated)
Serum bilirubin (elevated)
Serum amylase (elevated)
Ultrasound/radiologic abdominal series
Biliary scintigraphy
Cholecystogram (for chronic cholecystitis only)
Chest radiologic study (to rule out pneumonitis)
PT

Potential complications

Jaundice
  Skin
  Sclera
Dehydration
Electrolyte imbalance
Bleeding tendencies (vitamin K deficiency)
Peritonitis if rupture occurs

Medical management

Analgesics, antibiotics, antiemetics, anticholinergics
NPO
Nasogastric aspiration
Parenteral fluids with electrolytes
Surgical intervention: cholecystectomy with exploration of common bile duct or cholecystotomy

Nursing diagnoses/goals/interventions

ndx: Potential fluid volume deficit related to abnormal loss of body fluids

GOAL: *Patient's hydration and electrolyte balance will be maintained*

Maintain NPO
Monitor vital signs q4h prn
Administer parenteral fluids with electrolytes and antibiotics as ordered
Connect nasogastric tube to low, intermittent suction apparatus as ordered; irrigate to maintain patency (p. 365)
Measure intake and output q8h; note color and consistency of urine, stools, and gastric contents
Monitor serum electrolytes, PT
Observe stools for clay color or return of bile

ndx: Alteration in comfort: pain related to disease process

GOAL: *Patient will express minimal discomfort or absence of pain*

Assess character, location, and severity of pain
Administer analgesics (avoid morphine) and anticholinergics; assess effectiveness of pain relief measures
Maintain bed rest in position of comfort: usually head elevated 30 to 45 degrees; do not gatch knees
Assist and teach patient to turn and deep breathe q2h
Perform passive or assist with active ROM exercises q4h

ndx: Alteration in nutrition: less than body requirements related to vomiting and decreased nutritional intake

GOAL: *Patient will gain or maintain optimal weight, and vomiting will cease*

Following removal of nasogastric tube, initiate clear liquid diet and progress to low-fat, soft diet as tolerated
Force fluids to 2500 ml/day unless contraindicated
Observe for food intolerances
Provide quiet, nonstressful environment at mealtimes
Encourage activity and ambulation
Weigh patient daily at same time with same clothing and scale

ndx: Knowledge deficit regarding surgical procedure or home care needs

GOAL: *Patient and/or significant other will demonstrate understanding of surgical procedure or home care and follow-up instructions through interactive discussion*

If cholecystectomy (p. 396) is to be performed, reinforce physician's explanation of needed tests and procedure and provide preoperative instructions
On discharge, provide written dietary instructions on low-fat diet
Advise patient and/or significant other to increase fat in diet slowly
Discuss importance of rest and activity
Encourage follow-up visits with physician

Evaluation

There are no complications
Nutrition is adequate, and pain is absent

Urine and feces are normal in color and consistency
Home care instructions are understood

BILIARY SURGERY

Any surgery of the gallbladder, such as cholecystectomy (removal of gallbladder), choledocholithotomy (removal of stones in common bile duct), or choledochojejunostomy (anastomosis of the common bile duct to the jejunum)

Assessment
Observations/findings

Respiratory distress
Diminished breath sounds
Splinting with respirations
Tachypnea
Bradypnea
Character and amount
   Gastric drainage
   Bile drainage (T tube)
   Drainage from incision
   Urinary output
Location and character of pain

Laboratory/diagnostic studies

Electrolytes, Hbg, Hct

Potential complications

Dehydration
Electrolyte imbalance
Hemorrhage
Shock
Peritonitis (p. 372)
Jaundice (3 to 4 days postoperatively)
Signs of wound infection
Thrombophlebitis (p. 74)
Atelectasis
Pulmonary embolus (p. 247)

Medical management

Analgesics, antibiotics, vitamin K
Nasogastric aspiration
Parenteral fluids with electrolytes
Oxygen therapy, incentive spirometer
Oral replacement of bile salts
T tube drainage and clamping
Diet, activity, rest

Nursing diagnoses/goals/interventions

ndx Ineffective breathing pattern related to placement of incision and pain

GOAL: *Patient's respirations will remain adequate to meet body requirements*

Assess respiratory status; observe for splinting and shallow, rapid breathing
Auscultate lungs for breath sounds q2h
Administer incentive spirometer q2h to 4h
Assist and teach patient to turn and cough q2h and deep breathe q1h; support incision
Elevate head 20 to 30 degrees; do not gatch knees

ndx Potential fluid volume deficit related to NPO status and increased body fluid loss

GOAL: *Patient will remain adequately hydrated to meet body requirements*

Maintain NPO
Administer parenteral fluids with electrolytes and vitamin K as ordered
Connect nasogastric tube to low, intermittent suction apparatus as ordered; irrigate prn to maintain patency with measured amounts of normal saline
Monitor intake and output q8h; observe for urinary retention
Connect T tube to closed gravity drainage system as ordered; observe color and amount of drainage
   Measure bile drainage q8h; report drainage greater than 500 ml/24 hr to physician
   Replace bile salts as ordered
Monitor serum electrolytes
Monitor stools for clay-colored feces and urine for presence of bile
Provide diet as ordered; monitor for fat tolerance

ndx Alteration in tissue perfusion: bleeding related to decreased resistance and vitamin K deficiency

GOAL: *Patient's incision will remain clean, dry, and intact without signs of bleeding*

Observe incision q2h for 8 hr, then q4h
Reinforce dressing prn
Report excess drainage or bleeding to physician
Cover "stab wound" drain with ostomy appliance or sterile dressing; change prn
Monitor vital signs q4h; monitor Hgb and Hct
Discourage visitors with upper respiratory infections (URIs) or other infections
Administer injections with small-gauge needle and apply more pressure longer
Provide swabs for oral hygiene if bleeding gums are noted
Administer antibiotics as ordered

ndx: Potential impairment of skin integrity related to bile drainage from T tube

GOAL: *Patient's skin around T tube will remain clean and dry with no signs of inflammation*

Assess patency of T tube q2h; observe for kinks in tubing

Anchor tubing to allow for freedom of movement

Assess skin around T tube q2h to 4h; clean prn with soap and water; rinse and pat dry
- Apply petroleum jelly gauze or Skin Prep as needed for irritation
- Apply Montgomery straps as indicated

Observe skin and sclera for jaundice or pruritus

Clamp T tube as ordered after meals; observe for distention, cramps, and pain; unclamp T tube if symptoms occur and notify physician

ndx: Alteration in comfort: pain related to surgical intervention

GOAL: *Patient will express minimal discomfort or absence of pain*

Assess location, type, and severity of pain

Administer analgesics as ordered; assess effectiveness of pain relief measures

Maintain bed rest in quiet environment

Change position frequently; administer back rubs

Perform passive or assist with and teach active ROM exercises q4h

Ambulate with assistance as ordered; abdominal binder may be required for obese patient

ndx: Knowledge deficit regarding home care needs

GOAL: *Patient and/or significant other will demonstrate understanding of home care and follow-up instructions through interactive discussion and actual return demonstration*

Provide written diet instructions and restrictions; fats may be added as tolerated

Demonstrate care of incision and T tube (if applicable)

Explain signs of wound infection to report to physician

Discuss importance of increasing activity to tolerance and planned rest periods

Explain that bowel movements may be loose for a while because of increased amount of bile

Encourage regular visits with physician

Evaluation

There are no complications
Pain is minimal or controlled
Nutrition is adequate
Skin integrity around T tube is maintained
Home care instructions are understood

CARE OF PATIENT WITH T TUBE

T *tube* *A tube placed in the duct to carry off excessive bile, decrease the amount of bile flowing into the intestine, and prevent backflow of bile into the liver when the common bile duct has been explored*

Assessment

Observations/findings

Character, color, and amount of bile drainage; less than 500 ml/24 hr is within normal limits
Patency of tube
Leakage around tube
Tube taped securely to skin
Skin integrity around tube
Color, consistency, and frequency of stools

Laboratory/diagnostic studies

Electrolytes
T tube cholangiogram

Potential complications

Jaundice: sclera, skin
Electrolyte imbalance
Abdominal distention
Fat-soluble vitamin (A, D, E, K) deficiency

Medical management

T tube drainage collection
T tube clamping schedule

Nursing diagnoses/goals/interventions

ndx: Potential impairment of skin integrity secondary to bile secretion problems

GOAL: *Patient's skin integrity will be maintained with no signs of inflammation or irritation*

Connect T tube tubing to closed gravity drainage system placed well below incision or cover with ostomy pouch

Secure connections with tape and allow enough tubing to allow for freedom of movement

Place rolled 4 × 4 pads under T tube at exit site and tape to skin to prevent tension

Monitor skin around T tube exit site; keep clean and dry; use Stomahesive wafer or Skin Prep to prevent irritation

Measure bile output q8h; report output of greater than 500 ml/24 hr to physician

Monitor electrolytes and signs of sodium or potassium deficiency

Replace bile salts orally or administer florantyrone (Zanchol) or dehydrocholic acid (Decholin) as ordered

Administer bile salts chilled in orange juice; patients do not need to know what mixture contains

ndx: Alteration in bowel elimination: diarrhea related to increased amount of bile in intestine

GOAL: *Patient will adapt to new bowel pattern and understand it is usually only temporary*

Auscultate abdomen for bowel sounds q8h; report return to physician

Observe first stool for color, consistency, and amount; should be dark—clay color may indicate bile duct blockage

Clamp tube as ordered and observe for abdominal pain, distention, chills, fever, and nausea; if these occur, unclamp tube and notify physician

Increase time tube is clamped as ordered: usually before and after meals to facilitate digestion

Prepare for T tube cholangiogram (7 to 10 days postoperatively); T tube is removed after 24 hr if bile duct is patent

ndx: Knowledge deficit regarding home care of T tube

GOAL: *Patient and/or significant other will demonstrate home management of T tube through interactive discussion and return demonstration*

Demonstrate care of skin, drainage system, and incision
Discuss measuring and clamping procedure
Discuss symptoms to report to physician
Provide instructions for medications, including name, dosage, purpose, time of administration, and side effects
Encourage follow-up visits with physician

Evaluation

There are no complications
Skin integrity is maintained
Bowel elimination is manageable
Home care instructions are understood

TRANSHEPATIC BILIARY DECOMPRESSION CATHETER

A multivented catheter inserted through the abdominal wall, liver, common bile duct, and into the duodenum to allow bile to drain past the obstructed bile duct into the intestine; performed for hepatic dysfunction, biliary obstruction (jaundice), and inoperable malignancy of the biliary system

Assessment

Observations/findings

Location of catheter, type of drainage system
Character, color, and amount of drainage
Presence of stabilizing device or sutures
Decreasing jaundice and serum bilirubin
Color, frequency, and amount of stool and urine

Laboratory/diagnostic studies

Catheter usually inserted in radiology department
Postinsertion x-ray examination, cholangiography
Serum bilirubin, electrolytes
Stool for occult blood
Urine for bilirubin

Potential complications

Biliary sepsis
Bleeding or increased retrograde flow of bile
Catheter obstruction
Hyponatremia, electrolyte imbalance

Medical management

Parenteral fluids with electrolytes
Type of catheter drainage system and length of time to remain open
Irrigating procedure: solution, amount of irrigant, frequency
Diet, activity, rest

Nursing diagnoses/goals/interventions

ndx: Potential fluid volume deficit related to abnormal body fluid loss

GOAL: *Patient will remain adequately hydrated*

Connect catheter to closed gravity drainage system as ordered; place stopcock between catheter and tubing; keep open

Monitor and measure amount of drainage q2h for 8 hr, then q4h; observe for increased amount of drainage; if more than 1500 ml/24 hr, notify physician immediately

Administer parenteral fluids with electrolytes as ordered

Monitor catheter site for drainage, type of sutures, and dressing q2h to 4h; change dressing prn and apply antibacterial ointment as ordered

Monitor vital signs q4h; elevated temperature and hypotension may be signs of sepsis

Irrigate catheter as ordered through external port of stopcock, closing off drainage bag
  Aspirate a few milliliters to ascertain patency
  Irrigate gently with prescribed amount of solution; this may be painful for patient—explain prior to procedure
  Do not force irrigation if resistance is met; notify physician, since catheter may be obstructed
  Following instillation open stopcock to allow irrigant to drain into drainage bag
  Assess patient's tolerance and observe for increasing, continuous pain, cramping, or abdominal distention (peritonitis, catheter slippage)
Clamp catheter as ordered; observe patient for decreasing jaundice
  Monitor stools, urine, skin, and sclera for more normal appearance
  Monitor serum bilirubin
  Tape catheter comfortably to abdomen; cover with sterile dressing
Monitor electrolytes, especially for hyponatremia; observe for lethargy or altered mental status

ndx: Disturbance in self-concept related to body image change

GOAL: *Patient will express feelings and progress toward adaptive behaviors and coping patterns*

Encourage and allow time for verbalization of feelings; promote communication with significant other
Explain all procedures and treatments; involve patient in planning care
Assess present coping patterns and strengths; assist patient with identifying past behaviors that have been successful
Focus on positive aspect of procedure and begin self-care activities and teaching when patient is physically and emotionally able

ndx: Knowledge deficit regarding managing catheter at home

GOAL: *Patient and/or significant other will demonstrate understanding of catheter care, home care, and follow-up instructions through interactive discussion and actual return demonstration*

Demonstrate and observe return demonstration for catheter irrigation and care
Provide written instructions for irrigating procedure
Discuss signs and symptoms of malfunction to report to physician
  Fever, chills, weakness
  Bleeding, increased bile output
  Increasing jaundice, abdominal pain, distention
  Dislodgment of catheter
  Food particles in catheter drainage
Refer to home health care agency
Explain need for frequent visits to radiology department for evaluation of catheter position and function
Promote follow-up visits with physician

Evaluation

There are no complications
Catheter functions properly
Jaundice is decreasing
Patient is more comfortable
Home care management of catheter is understood

Liver

CIRRHOSIS: PORTAL, POSTNECROTIC, BILIARY

Liver disease characterized by the destruction of cells, progressive fibrosis, and eventual nodular formation that results from excessive alcohol intake (70% to 80%), hepatitis, drug toxicity, biliary obstruction, metabolic disease, or congestive heart failure (CHF)

Assessment
Observations/findings

Anorexia
Nausea, vomiting
Weight loss or gain
Abdominal distention
Irregular bowel function
  Clay-colored stools
  Flatulence
  Melena
Right upper quadrant pain
Elevated temperature
Pruritus
Decreased urinary output
Generalized malaise/weakness
Foul breath
History of substance abuse
History of hepatitis or biliary obstruction
Spider angiomas
Jaundice
Edema of extremities
Gynecomastia
Clubbing of fingers
Dehydration
Abnormal liver function tests, PT, clotting time, serum albumin, SGOT, and SGPT
Altered mental status

Laboratory/diagnostic studies

Electrolytes
Serum bilirubin (elevated, jaundice)
SGOT, SGPT, LDH (elevated)
Serum albumin (decreased), ammonia (elevated)
CBC, prothrombin time (prolonged), urinalysis
Endoscopic retrograde cholangiopancreatography (ERCP) (common bile duct obstruction)
Esophagoscopy (varices) with barium esophagraphy
Liver biopsy, scans
Ultrasonography
Percutaneous transhepatic porotography (visualizes portal venous system)
Paracentesis (ascites)

Potential complications

Electrolyte imbalance
Malnutrition
Ascites
Oliguria
GI bleeding
Portal hypertension, esophageal varices, caput medusae (umbilical venous distention)
Hepatomegaly, splenomegaly
Coma

Medical management

Diuretics, analgesics, antibiotics
Digestants, vitamins K and C, iron, thiamin, folic acid
Stool softeners
Parenteral fluids with electrolytes
Fresh whole blood, fresh frozen plasma, or platelets
Nasogastric aspiration
Diet management according to disease process
Sodium and/or fluid restriction
Oxygen therapy

Nursing diagnoses/goals/interventions

ndx: Alteration in nutrition: less than body requirements related to inadequate diet, vomiting, and/or anorexia

GOAL: *Patient's nutritional intake will be maintained to meet body needs*

Maintain bed rest in quiet environment
Provide small, frequent feedings of prescribed diet; amount of fat, carbohydrate, and protein will depend on patient's ability to metabolize these nutrients; salt may be restricted
Assist and encourage patient to eat, and consider preferences in food choices

ndx: Potential fluid volume deficit related to loss of body fluids

GOAL: *Patient will remain hydrated, and electrolytes will be within normal limits*

Maintain NPO; administer parenteral fluids with electrolytes and vitamins; restrict fluid intake as ordered
Measure intake and output and abdominal girth q8h
Note consistency, color, and frequency of stools and urine
Monitor serum and urine electrolytes; observe for signs of sodium and/or potassium imbalance
Monitor vital signs q4h; observe for elevated temperature
Weigh patient daily at same time with same clothing and scale
Administer diuretics as ordered
Provide oral hygiene and ice chips prn

ndx: Potential impairment of skin integrity related to edema, dehydration, and/or jaundice

GOAL: *Patient's skin will remain intact, clean, and dry with no signs of inflammation*

Assess skin for breaks, reddened areas, and pruritus
Provide sheepskin with alternating pressure or egg crate mattress
Administer skin care frequently; provide clean linen prn; use lanolin-based lotion and clip nails as needed; administer cholestyramine for pruritus
Provide perineal care following urination and bowel movement; apply lotions to prevent breakdown
Turn patient q2h and administer back care; change position slightly prn to promote comfort
Monitor for signs of jaundice and pruritus
Perform passive or assist with active ROM exercises q4h

ndx: Ineffective breathing pattern related to debilitated state and ascites

GOAL: *Patient's respirations will be adequate to meet body requirements; pneumonia will not develop*

Elevate head of bed 45 to 60 degrees or as needed to maintain ventilation
Assist and teach patient to turn and cough q4h; deep breath q½h
Auscultate lungs for breath sounds q4h
Assist and teach patient to use incentive spirometer q2h
Prepare for paracentesis as ordered (p. 405)

ndx: Alteration in tissue perfusion related to renal dysfunction and decreased urine formation

GOAL: *Patient's urinary output will be maintained*

Measure urine output q1h until stable
Monitor urine for potassium and sodium
Administer corticosteroids and salt-poor albumin as ordered

ndx: Alteration in tissue perfusion related to impaired blood coagulation or hemorrhage from portal hypertension

GOAL: *Patient will experience minimal bleeding, or it will not occur*

Monitor mucous membranes for signs of bleeding; avoid hard-bristled toothbrushes
Observe injection sites for prolonged bleeding; apply extra pressure and pressure bandage; use small-gauge needles
Monitor patient's use of razors and glass bottles and jars
Avoid straining during bowel movement and forceful nose-blowing
Monitor PT and platelet count
Administer vitamin K and antifibrinolytic agents as ordered
Observe for signs of bleeding; decreasing BP, increasing P, hematemesis, melena
Monitor vital signs, Hgb, and Hct
Prepare for endoscopy if bleeding occurs
Insert nasogastric tube and connect to low, intermittent suction apparatus as ordered
Measure gastric output qh and note color and consistency; irrigate, if ordered, to maintain patency
Administer parenteral fluids and/or transfusions as ordered
Administer vitamin K, vasopressin, and neomycin as ordered
Refer to Bleeding Esophageal Varices (p. 344)

ndx: Alteration in thought process related to potential increase of serum ammonia and hepatic coma

GOAL: *Patient's mental status will be maximized, and mental deterioration minimized*

Observe frequently for changes in mental status, lethargy, drowsiness, and confusion
Monitor neurologic status for decreased motor ability
Avoid use of sedatives, tranquilizers, and narcotics
Provide safe environment: side rails up and bed in low position; restraints if necessary
Provide high-calorie, low-protein diet if mental deterioration occurs, as ordered

ndx: Knowledge deficit regarding home care management

GOAL: *Patient and/or significant other will demonstrate understanding of home care and follow-up instructions through interactive discussion*

Provide written dietary instructions from dietitian (RD), listing amount of protein, carbohydrate, fat, and salt allowed
Discuss with patient importance of avoiding stress during meals and need to eat small, frequent meals
Provide information on community resources available for alcohol rehabilitation and assistance
Reinforce physician's explanation of relationship between alcohol and cirrhosis
Provide information on medications, including name, purpose, dosage, time of administration, and side effects; caution against using any medicine not prescribed by physician
Explain importance of rest and exercise, avoiding exposure to infection
Discuss skin care if pruritus persists
Discuss signs of progression of disease: hematuria, melena, abdominal distention, edema, fever, bleeding that does not subside, mental deterioration, personality changes
Encourage follow-up visits with physician

Evaluation

There are no complications
Nutritional intake is adequate
Skin integrity is maintained
Laboratory values are within normal limits
Thought processes are stable
Home care management is understood

VIRAL HEPATITIS

infectious Virus A (HAV); *rapid onset of symptoms and destruction of liver cells caused by contaminated water or food; usually affects young adults*

serum Virus B (HBV); *slow onset of symptoms and destruction of liver cells caused by contaminated serum from needles and instruments; affects all age-groups*

non-A, non-B *Little is known about these two viruses, but they manifest symptoms similar to HBV*

Assessment

Observations/findings

Anorexia
Malaise
Headache
Tenderness and pain in right upper quadrant
Arthritic pain (HBV)
Elevated temperature (HAV)
Jaundice
    Pruritus
    Urticaria
    Sclera
    Clay-colored stools
    Dark urine
Nausea, vomiting
Diarrhea

Laboratory/diagnostic studies

Serum SGOT, SGPT, bilirubin (elevated)
Alkaline phosphatase, lactic dehydrogenase (elevated)
PT (elevated in severe hepatitis)
Stool and serology for HAV
Serum antigen/antibody tests for HBV
CBC, urinalysis, electrolytes
Liver biopsy

Potential complications

Decreased urinary output
Dehydration and electrolyte imbalance
Altered mental status
Hyperglycemia or hypoglycemia
Hepatic coma

Medical management

Sedatives, antiemetics, antacids, vitamin K
Diet according to tolerance of protein, carbohydrates, and fat
Parenteral therapy with electrolytes and vitamins for vomiting or GI bleeding
Nasogastric aspiration
Antihistamines for pruritus

Nursing diagnoses/goals/interventions

ndx: Activity intolerance related to weakness or fatigue secondary to infection

GOAL: *Patient will progress toward maximum activities as energy returns*

Maintain bed rest in quiet environment; assist patient in assuming position of comfort; bathroom privileges may be allowed
Assist and teach patient to turn q2h and deep breathe q½h
Change position frequently to promote comfort
Administer sedatives as ordered
Discuss with patient and institute isolation precautions
    HAV: gown plus gloves when handling excretions
    HBV and non-A, non-B: gloves when handling serum
Assist with and teach active or perform passive ROM exercises q4h while in bed
Coordinate care to provide planned rest periods
Ambulate with assistance when allowed

ndx: Alteration in nutrition: less than body requirements secondary to anorexia and/or vomiting

GOAL: *Patient's nutritional status will improve and be maintained as evidenced by weight gain*

Provide diet as ordered, monitoring intake of protein, fat, and carbohydrates
Offer small, frequent meals, attractively prepared
Force fluids to 3000 ml/24 hr unless contraindicated; include fruit juices and carbonated beverages, since they are easily digested
Administer antacids and antiemetics as ordered; avoid Compazine and Thorazine
Weigh patient daily at same time with same clothing and scale

ndx: Potential fluid volume deficit related to excessive loss of body fluids

GOAL: *Patient will remain adequately hydrated, and electrolytes will be normal*

Maintain NPO if vomiting and/or anorexia
Administer parenteral fluids with electrolytes and vitamins as ordered
Measure intake and output q8h
Monitor stool and urine for color, consistency, and frequency
Observe for ascites, increasing jaundice, and mental deterioration
Monitor vital signs, electrolytes, Hgb, and Hct
Observe for signs of bleeding: mucous membranes, injection sites, emesis, stool

ndx: Potential impairment of skin integrity related to jaundice and ensuing pruritus

GOAL: *Patient will express minimal discomfort, and skin integrity will be maintained*

Administer frequent skin care; avoid soap
Provide shower or bath with baking soda or starch; apply lotions; use cholestyramine as ordered
Offer frequent back rubs and changes in position
Encourage short fingernails or use of gloves
Provide diversional activities

ndx: Disturbance in self-concept related to disease process, hospitalization, and isolation

GOAL: *Patient's self-esteem will be restored, and positive coping patterns will be demonstrated*

Encourage and allow time for communication of fears and concerns
Reinforce physician's explanation of disease process and treatment rationale
Explain purpose of isolation procedure to patient and/or significant other
Assess present coping patterns, and be supportive and understanding
Encourage communication with significant other

ndx: Knowledge deficit regarding disease process and home care management

GOAL: *Patient and/or significant other will demonstrate understanding of disease process, home care, and follow-up instructions through interactive discussion*

Provide written diet instructions on amounts of protein, carbohydrate, and fat allowed; no alcohol for 1 year
Explain importance of rest and exercise
  Avoid heavy lifting, strenuous exercise, and contact sports
  Exercise to tolerance and get plenty of rest and sleep
Discuss importance of personal hygiene
  HAV: perineal care and handwashing after toileting and disinfection of soiled articles of clothing
  HBV-NANB: caution not to share razors or toothbrushes and to avoid serum or secretion contact with others
Explain infectious nature of HAV, HBV, and non-B and need to avoid infecting others until laboratory values are normal; importance of not donating blood; need to avoid others with infections, especially URIs
Stress importance of follow-up medical care for 1 year
  Regular laboratory tests as ordered
  Routine follow-up care with physician
Encourage family members and friends to seek injection of gamma globulin for HAV

Discuss symptoms of recurrence to report to physician
Provide instructions on medication, including name, purpose, dosage, time of administration, and side effects; explain need to avoid medicines not prescribed by physician

Evaluation

There are no complications
Nutritional status is adequate
Liver function studies are near normal or normal
Skin integrity is maintained
Home care instructions are understood

CONTINUOUS PERITONEAL-JUGULAR SHUNT FOR ASCITES (LeVEEN SHUNT)

Subcutaneous shunt with one-way pressure valve to continuously reinfuse ascitic fluid subcutaneously from peritoneal cavity to jugular vein and superior vena cava; procedure reduces ascites and overcomes fluid and electrolyte imbalance

Preoperative assessment

Assess patient's understanding of surgical procedure; reinforce and clarify as needed
Assess respiratory and neurologic status
Assess and measure abdominal girth; mark measuring point on abdomen

Postoperative assessment
Observations/findings

Increased or decreased abdominal distention
Dyspnea
Diminished breath sounds
Tachypnea
Tachycardia
Right upper quadrant pain
Neck edema on shunt side
Increased or decreased urinary output
Level of consciousness

Laboratory/diagnostic studies

Electrolytes, especially potassium
Hgb, Hct, urine for potassium

Potential complications

Leakage of fluid from incision site
Electrolyte imbalance
Increased clotting time
Elevated bilirubin
Intravascular coagulation
Peritonitis (p. 372)

GI bleeding
Hepatic coma
Wound infection

Medical management

Furosemide and spironolactone diuretics
Sedatives
Parenteral fluids with electrolytes
Fluid restriction first 2 to 4 days
Abdominal binder

Nursing diagnoses/goals/interventions

ndx Ineffective breathing pattern secondary to ascites and placement of shunt

GOAL: *Patient's respirations will be maintained to meet body requirements*

Assess respiratory status q2h to 4h; observe for signs of edema over superior vena cava
Auscultate chest for breath sounds q4h and listen for diminished breath sounds
Encourage patient to breathe normally, since respirations control mechanical operation of valve
Assist with and teach patient Valsalva maneuver, and to exhale against closed glottis to close valve and inhale through tube connected to closed bottle to open valve; perform three to four times daily to check patency of shunt
Assist and teach patient to turn and deep breathe q4h
Elevate head of bed to 45 to 90 degrees or as ordered

ndx Potential fluid volume deficit related to abnormal loss of body fluids (diuresis) secondary to hemodilution caused by shunt

GOAL: *Patient's fluid volume and electrolytes will be maintained*

Maintain NPO as ordered
Administer parenteral fluids with electrolytes as ordered; usually restricted to less than 1 L/day for 3 to 4 days
Measure intake and output q8h; urine output will be increased
Monitor vital signs q2h to 4h
Monitor electrolytes
Weigh patient daily at same time with same clothing and scale
Administer diuretics as ordered
Apply abdominal binder when ordered, usually after first postoperative day
Measure abdominal girth q4h

Monitor mental status for signs of deterioration
Observe dressing for drainage or bleeding; reinforce prn

ndx Alteration in nutrition: less than body requirements related to disease process and NPO status

GOAL: *Patient's nutritional intake will be maintained*

Provide diet according to allowed amounts of fat, carbohydrates, and protein when oral intake is allowed
Encourage small, frequent meals and provide a quiet environment
Restrict fluid intake as ordered

ndx Alteration in comfort: pain related to surgical intervention

GOAL: *Patient will express minimal discomfort or absence of pain*

Maintain bed rest in quiet environment
Assess location and character of pain
Administer sedatives and/or analgesics as ordered; assess effectiveness of pain relief measures
Change position frequently and keep linen clean and dry
Perform passive or assist with and teach active ROM exercises q4h while in bed
Provide diversional activities
Ambulate with assistance when allowed

ndx Knowledge deficit regarding home care and management of shunt

GOAL: *Patient and/or significant other will demonstrate understanding of home care and follow-up instructions through interactive discussion and actual return demonstration*

Provide written dietary instructions and fluid restriction if applicable
Demonstrate incisional care and explain signs of wound infection
Discuss management of shunt and signs to report to physician
  Demonstrate measuring abdominal girth (to be done daily)
  Redemonstrate methods of ensuring shunt patency
Weigh patient three times a week
Report weight gain, increased abdominal girth, neck edema, pain, decreased urine output, respiratory distress, or change in mental status to physician
Promote follow-up care with physician

Evaluation

There are no complications
Incision is clean, dry, and intact
Nutritional intake is adequate
Home care instructions are understood

CARE OF PATIENT UNDERGOING PARACENTESIS FOR ASCITES

paracentesis *Needle aspiration of small amounts of ascitic fluid from peritoneal cavity for increasing, disabling abdominal distention or for laboratory analysis; provides only palliative action and is performed only when alternate measures have been unsuccessful*

Preinsertion assessment and care

Reinforce physician's explanation of purpose and procedure
Be aware that rapid removal and/or removal of large amounts of fluid can be life-threatening
Monitor baseline vital signs and measure abdominal girth
    Check BP, P, and R q5 min during procedure
    Notify physician of any change
Check for allergy to local anesthetic
Elevate head of bed 60 to 90 degrees or have patient sit on side of bed
    Support feet with footstool
    Support back with pillows
Have patient void just prior to procedure or check indwelling catheter for patency
Be certain all equipment is in readiness and remain with patient during procedure
Provide continuous emotional support
Assess neurologic, cardiovascular, and respiratory status during procedure; report any changes to physician

Postinsertion assessment

Observations/findings

Total amount of aspirate removed
Color and consistency of aspirate
Leakage of ascitic fluid
Respiratory distress
Hyperventilation
Fetor hepaticus
Cyanosis of lips, skin, and nail beds
Tachycardia
Tachypnea
Hypotension
Vertigo
Syncope
Level of consciousness

Laboratory/diagnostic studies

Electrolytes
Culture/sensitivity of aspirate

Potential complications

Flapping tremors
Hypovolemia
Electrolyte imbalance
Nausea, vomiting
Shock
Hepatic coma

Medical management

Diet and activity management
Disbursement of aspirate
Sedatives

Nursing diagnoses/goals/interventions

ndx: Potential fluid volume deficit related to abnormal body fluid loss secondary to paracentesis

GOAL: *Patient will remain adequately hydrated to meet body requirements*

Monitor vital signs q15 min until stable, then q4h for 24 hr
Assist patient in assuming position of comfort, usually head elevated 30 to 45 degrees unless patient is hypotensive
Maintain parenteral fluids with electrolytes as ordered
Measure intake and output
Apply pressure dressing to insertion site and cleanse area with povidone-iodine solution; observe for signs of bleeding or drainage qh for 4 hr, then q4h for 24 hr
Continue with diuretics as ordered

ndx: Alteration in tissue perfusion: cerebral, cardiopulmonary, renal, gastrointestinal, and/or peripheral related to sudden loss of ascites fluid

GOAL: *Patient's vital signs, urinary output, and peripheral pulses will be maintained*

Monitor level of consciousness q15 min until vital signs are stable; observe for syncope and vertigo
Observe and monitor color and temperature of lips, skin, and nail beds, and check peripheral pulses q15 min until vital signs stabilize

Monitor urine output; observe color and amount q4h
Perform passive or assist with and teach active ROM exercises q4h
Ambulate with assistance when allowed
Continue care for cirrhosis (p. 399)

Evaluation

There are no complications
Vital signs are normal for patient
Adequate hydration is maintained

HEPATIC SURGERY

Surgical removal or repair of portions of the liver due to trauma or carcinoma

Preoperative assessment and care

Assess cardiovascular, respiratory, cerebral, and renal status; obtain baseline vital signs; observe for jaundice
Prepare bowel as ordered: enemas, oral antibiotics, magnesium preparations
Insert nasogastric tube and/or indwelling urethral catheter as ordered; monitor aspirate and urine for color and consistency
Administer vitamin K and/or blood transfusions as ordered
Reinforce physician's explanation of surgical procedure and postoperative care; explain that chest tubes may be present
Provide emotional support to patient and/or significant others

Postoperative assessment

Observations/findings

Placement of chest tubes and drainage apparatus if applicable
Character and amount of
 Chest drainage if applicable
 Gastric drainage
 Urinary output
 Wound drainage
Nausea, vomiting
Abdominal distention
Tachycardia
Tachypnea
Splinting of respirations
Decreased breath sounds
Elevated temperature

Laboratory/diagnostic studies

Serum electrolytes, albumin, liver function studies
Electrolytes, CBC, glucose, PT

Potential complications

Electrolyte imbalance
Decreased serum albumin levels
Hypoglycemia
Atelectasis (p. 257)
Pneumonia (p. 243)
Paralytic ileus (p. 377)
Hemorrhage
Shock
Subdiaphragmatic abscess
Jaundice
Ascites
Hepatic coma
Wound infection

Medical management

Analgesics
Nasogastric aspiration
Parenteral fluids with electrolytes and vitamin K
Antibiotics, albumin, transfusions
Connection of chest tubes to underwater seal
Oxygen therapy
Urethral catheter drainage

Nursing diagnoses/goals/interventions

***ndx**:* Ineffective breathing pattern related to surgical intervention, chest tube placement, and/or pain

GOAL: *Patient's respirations will be maintained to meet body requirements*

Elevate head of bed 30 to 45 degrees; do not gatch knees
Connect chest tubes and underwater seal to low, intermittent suction or as ordered; monitor amount and color of aspirate
Auscultate chest for breath sounds q2h; observe respiratory rate and for splinting
Assist and teach patient to turn and cough q2h and deep breathe q½h; support incision
Provide incentive spirometer as ordered

***ndx**:* Potential fluid volume deficit related to NPO status and/or nasogastric aspiration

GOAL: *Patient will remain hydrated, and electrolytes will remain within normal range*

Maintain NPO
Administer parenteral fluids with electrolytes and/or antibiotics as ordered
Connect nasogastric tube to low, intermittent suction apparatus as ordered; irrigate gently with measured amounts of normal saline
Connect urethral catheter to closed gravity drainage

system; monitor output q1h; report output of less than 30 to 50 ml/hr to physician
Measure intake and output q8h
Monitor vital signs q½h until stable, then q4h
Monitor serum electrolytes, albumin, and glucose
Auscultate abdomen for bowel sounds q8h
Observe for signs of hypoglycemia: nausea, shakiness, lethargy
Monitor mental acuity q4h

ndx: Alteration in tissue perfusion: hemorrhage related to surgical procedure and/or vascular nature of liver

GOAL: *Patient's incision will remain clean, dry, and intact and without signs of bleeding*

Observe dressings and incision q2h for drainage or bleeding; reinforce prn and change when allowed
Monitor incision for signs of healing
Monitor Hgb, Hct, and vital signs
Observe for jaundice
Administer antibiotics and/or vitamin K as ordered
Assist with removal of chest tubes when ordered; place petroleum jelly gauze over wound and apply dressing; observe for signs of healing or infection

ndx: Alteration in comfort: pain related to surgical intervention

GOAL: *Patient will express minimal discomfort or absence of pain*

Maintain bed rest in quiet environment
Assess type and location of pain
Administer analgesics as ordered; assess effectiveness of pain relief measures
Change position frequently; administer back rubs; observe bony prominences for reddened areas or breakdown
Provide naso-oral hygiene q2h to 3h prn; keep areas moist
Perform passive or teach active ROM exercises q4h while patient is in bed
Ambulate with assistance when ordered

ndx: Alteration in nutrition: less than body requirements related to surgery and NPO status

GOAL: *Patient's nutritional status will be maintained to meet body requirements*

Remove or clamp nasogastric tube when bowel sounds return and as ordered
  Provide small amounts of water or clear liquids and monitor tolerance
  Progress to soft diet as tolerated; amounts of fat, carbohydrate, and protein will depend on ability of liver to metabolize
  Measure intake
Remove urethral catheter as ordered; initiate voiding measures as needed; measure output
Force fluids to 3000 ml daily unless contraindicated
Administer stool softeners to prevent constipation and straining
Weigh patient daily at same time with same clothing and scale

ndx: Knowledge deficit regarding home care management

GOAL: *Patient and/or significant other will demonstrate understanding of home care and follow-up instructions through interactive discussion and actual return demonstration*

Provide written diet instructions with amounts of fat, carbohydrate, and protein allowed
Demonstrate care of incision and discuss signs of wound infection
Provide information on signs and symptoms to report to physician
  Decreased mental acuity, lethargy
  Abdominal distention, pain
  Jaundice, dyspnea, fever
Discuss medications: name, dosage, purpose, times of administration, side effects, and importance of taking only medicines prescribed by physician
Promote follow-up visits with physician

Evaluation

There are no complications
Nutritional status and hydration are maintained
Pain is managed adequately
Home care management is understood

PORTACAVAL-SPLENORENAL SHUNTS FOR PORTAL HYPERTENSION

Procedures for correction of portal hypertension, which develops in patients with cirrhosis of the liver; subsequent bleeding esophageal varices and ascites are a result of obstruction of blood flow within the portal system

portacaval shunt *Blood flow is diverted from the liver by anastomosing the portal vein to the inferior vena cava; performed when obstruction is intrahepatic*

splenorenal shunt *Blood flow is diverted from the liver by anastomosing the splenic vein to the renal vein; performed when the portal vein is obstructed*

Preoperative assessment and care

Be aware that
   Shunts are usually not performed on patients with active varices because of increased surgical risk
   Extensive preparation time may be required to physically and emotionally prepare patients for surgery
Assess respiratory, cardiovascular, and neurologic status
Assess nutritional and integumentary status
Measure abdominal girth to assess presence or absence of ascites; assist with paracentesis as ordered
Monitor liver function studies, serum electrolytes, Hgb, Hct, and PT results
Administer medications as ordered
   Antibiotics
   Multivitamins
   Vitamin K
Provide diet with regulated amounts of protein, carbohydrates, salt, fat, and calories as ordered until NPO is required
Administer parenteral fluids with electrolytes as ordered
   TPN may be required
   Whole blood may be ordered
   Observe puncture site for bleeding
Insert nasogastric tube and indwelling urethral catheter as ordered; be aware that nasogastric tube may be inserted in operating room, since insertion may activate variceal bleeding
Discuss with and teach patient
   ROM exercises to extremities
   Method of turning, deep breathing, and coughing, and use of incentive spirometer
   That chest tubes may be in place postoperatively
   That a regional heparinization catheter may be in place
Provide supportive environment
Reinforce physician's explanation of surgical procedure
Encourage and deal with verbalization of fears and anxieties
Encourage communication with significant other

Postoperative assessment

Observations/findings

Placement of chest tubes and drainage apparatus
Placement of regional heparinization catheter if applicable
Character and amount of
   Chest drainage
   Gastric drainage
   Urinary output
   Wound drainage
Splinting of respirations
   Decreased breath sounds
   Tachypnea
   Difficulty in breathing
Mental alertness and acuity
Nausea, vomiting

Laboratory/diagnostic studies

Serum electrolytes, albumin, bilirubin, PT
Arterial blood gases
Chest radiography

Potential complications

Dehydration
Electrolyte imbalance
Atelectasis
Decreased serum albumin
Prolonged PT
Jaundice
Ascites
Peripheral edema
Hemorrhage
Shock
Hepatic coma
Wound infection

Medical management

Analgesics, antibiotics, albumin, vitamin K, lactulose, antacids
Parenteral fluids with electrolytes or TPN
Nasogastric aspiration
Chest tube aspiration
Arterial blood gases
Oxygen therapy
Regional heparinization catheter
Diet, activity

Nursing diagnoses/goals/interventions

ndx: Ineffective breathing pattern related to surgical incision, chest tube placement, and/or pain

GOAL: *Patient's respiratory status will be maintained to meet body requirements*

Elevate head of bed 30 to 45 degrees; do not gatch knees
Connect chest tubes and underwater seal to low, intermittent suction or as ordered (p. 271); monitor amount and color of aspirate
Auscultate chest for breath sounds q2h; observe respiratory rate and for splinting
Monitor arterial blood gases
Provide incentive spirometer as ordered

Assist and teach patient to turn and cough q2h and deep breathe q½h; support incision

ndx: Potential fluid volume deficit related to NPO status and/or nasogastric aspiration

GOAL: *Patient will remain hydrated and electrolytes will remain within normal limits*

Maintain NPO
Administer parenteral fluids with electrolytes, vitamins, antibiotics, and/or salt-poor albumin as ordered
Connect nasogastric tube to low, intermittent suction apparatus as ordered; irrigate with measured amounts of normal saline as ordered
Connect urethral catheter to closed gravity drainage system as ordered; monitor hourly output; report output of less than 30 to 50 ml/hr to physician; assist with voiding measures when removed
Measure intake and output q8h
Monitor vital signs q½h until stable, then q4h
Monitor serum electrolytes, albumin, and PT
Auscultate abdomen for bowel sounds and measure abdominal girth q4h (some ascites may be normal)
Monitor ankles for edema (some edema is normal for 2 to 3 days)
Monitor skin and sclera for jaundice
Connect regional heparinization catheter to flow rate controller as ordered; avoid tension and obstruction

ndx: Alteration in tissue perfusion: hemorrhage related to surgical procedure and/or portal hypertension

GOAL: *Patient's incision will remain intact without signs of hemorrhage; there will be no GI bleeding*

Observe incision and dressings for drainage or bleeding q2h; reinforce prn and change when allowed
Monitor nasogastric aspirate for bleeding; report any bleeding immediately to physician
Monitor Hgb, Hct, PT, and vital signs
Administer antibiotics and vitamin K as ordered
Administer injections with small-gauge needle; observe for bleeding
Observe mucous membranes for bleeding
Assist with removal of chest tubes as ordered; place petroleum jelly gauze over wound and observe for signs of healing

ndx: Potential for infection related to bacterial invasion of incision

GOAL: *Patient's incision will be clean, dry, and intact*

Change dressings as ordered; observe for signs of infection and healing process
Monitor temperature carefully
Administer antibiotics and antipyretics as ordered
Collect urine specimen for culture/sensitivity when indwelling catheter is removed; initiate voiding measures

ndx: Alteration in thought processes related to anesthesia, shunting of venous blood away from liver, and/or surgical blood loss

GOAL: *Patient will remain oriented to time and place, and BUN and ammonia levels will be within normal limits*

Monitor mental acuity q4h; observe for confusion, lethargy, or inappropriate behavior
Monitor serum BUN, ammonia, and albumin levels
Orient patient frequently to time and place and explain all procedures and treatments
Avoid analgesics that require liver metabolism: morphine, sedatives
Administer lactulose and antacids as ordered

ndx: Alteration in comfort: pain related to surgical intervention

GOAL: *Patient will verbalize minimal discomfort or absence of pain*

Maintain bed rest in quiet environment
Assess type and location of pain
Administer analgesics as ordered; avoid morphine and sedatives; phenobarbital or chloral hydrate is usually drug of choice
Assess effectiveness of pain relief measures
Change position frequently; administer back rubs; observe bony prominences for redness or breakdown
Provide naso-oral hygiene q2h and prn; keep areas clean and moist
Perform passive or assist with and teach active ROM exercises q4h
Ambulate with assistance when allowed

ndx: Alteration in nutrition: less than body requirements related to presurgical nutritional status, NPO status, and negative nitrogen balance

GOAL: *Patient's nutritional status will improve as evidenced by normal weight gain*

Continue with TPN as ordered; monitor urine for sugar and acetone q4h

Remove or clamp nasogastric tube when bowel sounds return as ordered

Provide small amounts of water and/or clear liquids and monitor tolerance

Progress to soft diet as tolerated; amount of fat, carbohydrate, and protein will be regulated by liver metabolism

Measure intake

Force or restrict fluids as ordered

Weigh patient daily at same time with same clothing and scale; measure abdominal girth to ensure that weight gain is not ascites

Administer stool softeners to prevent constipation and straining; test each stool for occult blood

ndx: Knowledge deficit regarding disease process and home care management

GOAL: *Patient and/or significant other will demonstrate understanding of disease process, home care, and follow-up instructions through interactive discussion and actual return demonstration*

Reinforce physician's explanation of disease process and treatments; discuss and clarify any misconceptions

Provide written diet instructions with amount of fat, carbohydrate, salt, and protein allowed; avoid alcohol and spicy foods
  Maintain prescribed fluid intake
  Eat slowly; chew foods well

Demonstrate incisional care, measuring abdominal girth, daily weights, method of record keeping, and stool testing with Hemastix

Discuss prescribed activities and rest; explain need to avoid heavy lifting and straining

Discuss signs and symptoms to report to physician
  Decreased mental acuity
  Increased girth and weight
  Peripheral edema, jaundice
  Fever, nausea, vomiting
  Tarry stools, hematuria

Provide instructions about medications, including name, purpose, dosage, time of administration, and side effects; explain importance of taking only medications prescribed by physician

Encourage follow-up care with physician

Evaluation

There are no complications
Nutrition and hydration are adequate
Mental acuity is normal for patient
Pain is managed adequately
Home care management is understood

HEPATIC CARCINOMA

Malignant tumor most commonly due to metastatic lesions in other organs; primary lesions are rare and may be asymptomatic

Assessment
Observations/findings

Slow onset of symptoms
Anorexia
Weakness, general fatigue
Progressive weight loss
Nausea, vomiting
Increased flatulence
Light-colored, bulky stools containing fat
Diarrhea
Abdominal fullness or discomfort
Abdominal pain when coughing or deep breathing
Referred pain to subscapular area
Low-grade fever
Dehydration
Melena
Anemia
Electrolyte imbalance
Abnormal liver function studies
Leukocytosis

Laboratory/diagnostic studies

Increased PT, ESR, bleeding/clotting time
CBC, urinalysis, fasting blood sugar (FBS)
Liver function studies
Alkaline phosphatase: elevated
Decreased serum albumin
Immunoserologic assay
Stools for steatorrhea
Chest radiologic study
Hepatic scintiscanning/scan, arteriography
Liver biopsy
Paracentesis cytology

Potential complications

Hypoglycemia
Hepatomegaly
Splenomegaly
Hematemesis, GI bleeding
Portal hypertension
Respiratory distress
Change in mental status
Jaundice
Ascites
Peripheral edema
Hepatic coma

Medical management

Analgesics, antiemetics, diuretics, antacids, corticosteroids
Diet, activity
Parenteral fluids with electrolytes, vitamins, and/or salt-poor albumin
TPN
Nasogastric aspiration, urethral catheter
Percutaneous transhepatic catheter, chemotherapeutic agents
Hepatic lobectomy

Nursing diagnoses/goals/interventions*

ndx: Potential fluid volume deficit related to dehydration, electrolyte imbalance, NPO status, and/or nasogastric aspiration

GOAL: *Patient will remain hydrated, and electrolytes will be within normal limits*

Maintain NPO if ordered; discriminate use of ice chips may be beneficial
Administer parenteral fluids with electrolytes, vitamins, and salt-poor albumin as ordered
Insert nasogastric tube and connect to low, intermittent suction apparatus as ordered; irrigate gently with measured amounts of normal saline; monitor aspirate for color and amount
Insert indwelling urethral catheter as ordered; connect to closed gravity drainage system and monitor color and amount of urine
Measure intake and output q8h
Monitor ankles for edema and measure abdominal girth q8h
Monitor vital signs q4h; provide cooling measures for temperature above 102° F (38.9° C) as ordered; take rectal temperature if nasogastric tube is in place; observe for venous distention around rectum
Monitor electrolytes, FBS, and liver function studies
Administer medications as ordered: diuretics, antacids, corticosteroids, chemotherapeutic agents

ndx: Alteration in tissue perfusion: hemorrhage and/or jaundice related to liver dysfunction and/or prolonged bleeding/clotting time

GOAL: *Patient will exhibit no signs of GI bleeding, bleeding from mucous membranes, or jaundice*

Monitor gastric aspirate and stools for bleeding; check each for occult blood with Hemastix

---

*Patient's condition dictates amount of care required; modify accordingly.

Observe for signs of vitamin K deficiency
   Bleeding gums, purpura
   Bleeding after injections; use small-gauge needle and apply pressure
   Monitor PT and clotting time
Monitor skin, sclera, and urine for jaundice
Administer vitamin K as ordered

ndx: Alteration in thought processes related to liver dysfunction and/or potential negative nitrogen balance

GOAL: *Patient will remain oriented to time and place, and blood ammonia levels will be within normal limits*

Monitor mental acuity frequently; observe for signs of disorientation, lethargy, personality changes, or depressed motor skills
Monitor serum albumin and BUN levels

ndx: Alteration in comfort: pain related to disease process

GOAL: *Patient will verbalize minimal discomfort or absence of pain*

Assess type and location of pain
Administer analgesics as ordered; avoid morphine and sedatives; assess effectiveness of pain relief measures
Maintain bed rest in quiet environment in position of comfort; no knee gatch
Assist and teach patient to turn q2h and deep breathe q1h
Change position frequently and administer back rubs
Administer skin care and oronasal hygiene prn
Perform passive or assist with and teach active ROM exercises q4h
Ambulate with assistance when allowed

ndx: Alteration in nutrition: less than body requirements related to anorexia, malnutrition, and/or fatigue

GOAL: *Patient's nutritional status will be maintained within parameters of disease process*

Administer TPN as ordered; monitor urine for sugar and acetone q4h
Provide diet, when allowed, with amounts of protein, fat, and carbohydrate regulated
   Avoid stress during meals
   Present meal trays attractively
   Encourage small, frequent meals
   Assist with meals as needed
   Sodium may be restricted if ankle edema/ascites is present

Weigh patient daily at same time with same clothing and scale

Monitor intake and output; institute voiding measures as needed when urethral catheter is removed

ndx Ineffective family coping related to poor prognosis of disease

GOAL: *Patient and/or significant other will verbalize concerns and feelings and be allowed to adopt positive coping behaviors in a supportive environment*

Reinforce physician's explanation of prognosis and clarify misconceptions

Encourage and allow time for verbalization of feelings and concerns; listen carefully

Assess present coping patterns and be supportive of those strengths that assisted in past experience

Encourage communication with significant other and assist in identifying problems

Promote feelings of self-worth and self-esteem

ndx Grieving related to anticipated loss

GOAL: *Patient will express grief and be allowed to work through grieving process in supportive environment*

Encourage expression of feelings about death with patient and/or significant other

Provide hope in small ways, but be realistic (short-term goals)

Provide supportive environment for patient and/or significant other to begin grieving process and assess and understand stages as they occur

ndx Knowledge deficit regarding home care management

GOAL: *Patient and/or significant other will demonstrate understanding of home care and follow-up instructions through interactive discussion and actual return demonstration*

Explain chemotherapy schedule, where to come, length of procedure, and possible side effects

Provide written diet instructions regarding amounts of nutrients allowed

Demonstrate care of percutaneous transhepatic catheter if applicable

Discuss signs and symptoms to report to physician
 Decreased mental acuity
 Increased abdominal girth: weight gain
 Jaundice
 Hematemesis, tarry stool
 Mucosal bleeding
 Peripheral edema, dyspnea

Discuss medications: name, dosage, purpose, time of administration, and side effects; explain importance of taking only medicines prescribed by physician; demonstrate injection administration if applicable

Encourage follow-up visits with physician

Evaluation

Nutritional status is maintained within confines of disease process

Pain is managed adequately

Appropriate coping behaviors are demonstrated

Home care management is understood

There are no complications

LIVER BIOPSY

Introduction of a special needle into the liver to obtain a specimen for pathologic examination

Prebiopsy care

Be certain unit of whole blood is available

Monitor baseline vital signs

Assess mental alertness and ability to cooperate

Explain procedure and follow-up care

Administer analgesics or sedatives as ordered

Check for allergy to local anesthetic

Teach patient how to inhale and hold breath during needle insertion

Monitor bleeding, clotting, and PT results; report abnormal results to physician

Postbiopsy observations

Intraperitoneal hemorrhage

Shock

Pneumothorax

Peritonitis

Interventions

Apply pressure to biopsy site for first 15 min following procedure

Maintain bed rest in supine position for 24 hr

Position patient on right side for first 12 hr

Monitor vital signs q15 min for four times, then q30 min for four times, then q4h or as ordered

Observe biopsy site q30 min for bleeding, swelling, or increased pain

Manage pain as indicated; epigastric pain or referred shoulder pain may occur

Report prolonged pain to physician: pain lasting over 24 to 48 hr

Administer vitamin K as ordered

Assist patient with eating and other activities as needed for 24 hr

Pancreas

ACUTE AND CHRONIC PANCREATITIS

acute pancreatitis *Acute inflammatory disease in which autodigestion of the organ occurs as a result of obstruction of the pancreatic duct; exact cause is unknown, but various causative factors are thought to be excessive use of alcohol, stones, tumors, and trauma*

chronic pancreatitis *Chronic, progressive disease that may or may not follow acute pancreatitis; causative factors include gallbladder disease, carcinoma, and excessive use of alcohol; pancreas becomes fibrotic and necrotic, and enzyme action is markedly decreased or nonexistent*

Assessment

Observations/findings

ACUTE PANCREATITIS

Pain in upper left quadrant: dull, unrelenting, boring
  Increases in supine position
  May radiate to shoulder and thoracic vertebrae
Mild abdominal distention, ascites
Nausea, vomiting
Fever, chills
Tachycardia, hypovolemia, hypotension
Respiratory impairment, dyspnea, splinting; adult respiratory distress syndrome (ARDS) may develop
Decreased urine output
Discoloration of abdomen and/or flanks
Jaundice
Hyperglycemia

CHRONIC PANCREATITIS

Intermittent epigastric pain: steady, boring, dull, or sharp
  Radiates to back
  Relieved when leaning forward
Nausea, vomiting
Weight loss
Diarrhea, steatorrhea
Malnutrition
Minimal jaundice
Fat-soluble vitamin deficiencies
Symptoms of diabetes mellitus

Laboratory/diagnostic studies

ACUTE PANCREATITIS

CBC, BUN, urinalysis, FBS
Arterial PO_2 less than 60 mm Hg
Serum calcium, albumin (decreased)
Serum LDH, SGOT, SGPT (increased)
Amylase: serum, urine, lipase (elevated)

CHRONIC PANCREATITIS

CBC, urinalysis
Alkaline phosphatase: elevated
Serum amylase, lipase: normal

ACUTE AND CHRONIC PANCREATITIS

Serum glucose: elevated
Radiologic abdominal films
Ultrasonography/CT scan
Upper GI series/cholangiography
Stool for steatorrhea

Potential complications

Electrolyte imbalance, hypocalcemia
Respiratory, circulatory, renal failure
Paralytic ileus
Jaundice
Shock, hemorrhage

Medical management

Analgesics, antacids, cimetidine, antibiotics, anticholinergics
Hemodynamic monitoring
Parenteral fluids with electrolytes, vitamins, serum albumin, and/or dextran
Nasogastric aspiration
Diet, activity, TPN
Digestants (pancreatic enzymes) for chronic pancreatitis
Insulin for hyperglycemia
Paravertebral block

Nursing diagnoses/goals/interventions

ndx: Potential fluid volume deficit related to vomiting, fever, and/or gastric aspiration

GOAL: *Patient will remain adequately hydrated, and electrolytes will be within normal limits*

Maintain NPO
Administer parenteral fluids with electrolytes, vitamins, albumin, and antibiotics as ordered or initiate TPN as ordered
Connect nasogastric tube to low, intermittent suction apparatus as ordered; irrigate with measured amounts of normal saline as ordered
Monitor vital signs q2h to 4h; check apical pulse; take rectal temperature
Monitor CVP or Swan-Ganz catheter; check arterial blood gases as ordered
Measure intake and output; check urine output qh; report output of less than 30 to 50 ml/hr to physician

Monitor electrolytes, glucose, liver function studies, PT, and calcium
Auscultate abdomen for bowel sounds and measure abdominal girth q4h
Administer medications as ordered

ndx: Potential for complications related to pancreatitis: abscess, cyst, ileus, decreased mental acuity, infection*

GOAL: *Patient will be afebrile with minimal complications*

Monitor respiratory status: breath sounds, cough, and sputum
Assist and teach patient to turn and cough q2h and deep breathe q½h
Administer skin care and oral hygiene q2h to 4h; observe for reddened areas or breakdown
Observe for signs of jaundice: skin, sclera, urine
Monitor temperature for elevation; initiate cooling measures for temperature greater than 101° F (38.2° C) as ordered
Test urine for sugar q4h
Monitor stools for fat, clay color, or odor
Observe for signs of hypocalcemia (tetany)
Observe for mental/emotional changes due to alcohol withdrawal, anxiety, and/or electrolyte imbalance
Monitor PT and observe mucous membranes and injection sites for bleeding

ndx: Alteration in comfort: pain related to disease process

GOAL: *Patient will express minimal discomfort or absence of pain*

Maintain bed rest in quiet environment in position of comfort; no knee gatch
Assess type and location of pain; provide analgesics as ordered
  Avoid morphine; small, frequent doses of meperidine are beneficial
  Medicate before pain becomes severe
  Assist with paravertebral block if ordered
  Observe for signs of addiction
Change position frequently; administer back rubs
Perform passive or assist with and teach active ROM q4h
Coordinate care to provide for rest periods

---

*Not a NANDA-approved nursing diagnosis.

Ambulate with assistance when allowed
Promote diversional activities

ndx: Alteration in nutrition: less than body requirements related to anorexia, vomiting, and/or decreased digestive enzymes

GOAL: *Patient's nutritional status will be maintained*

Initiate liquid to soft diet when tolerated and allowed
  Provide high-protein, high-carbohydrate, low-fat, or diabetic diet in small, frequent meals
  Avoid coffee, tea, stimulants, and gas-producing foods
Administer antacids, insulin, and anticholinergics as ordered
Weigh patient daily at same time with same clothing and scale
Monitor stools for diarrhea and steatorrhea

ndx: Knowledge deficit regarding home care management

GOAL: *Patient and/or significant other will demonstrate understanding of home care and follow-up instructions through interactive discussion*

Provide written dietary instructions
Reinforce causal relationships of pancreatitis and alcohol use; promote outside counseling with rehabilitation centers
Explain and teach about diabetes, urine testing, insulin therapy, and symptoms to report to physician
Discuss medications: name, schedule, dosage, purpose, and side effects; explain importance of taking only medicines prescribed by physician; promote discriminate use of narcotics
Encourage follow-up visits with physician

Evaluation

Complications are minimal
Nutrition is adequate
Pain is manageable
Home care management is understood

PANCREATIC SURGERY

Surgery of the pancreas, including total pancreatectomy with or without islet cell autotransplant for chronic pancreatitis and carcinoma, subtotal pancreatectomy for islet cell tumor and carcinoma; and pancreatoduodenectomy (Whipple procedure) for carcinoma

Preoperative assessment and care

Assess respiratory, circulatory, and neurologic status; take baseline vital signs; observe for abdominal distention and peripheral edema

Assess nutritional status and substance abuse history of alcohol and/or narcotics

Provide nourishing diet as ordered and tolerated

Administer parenteral fluids, TPN, and/or blood transfusions as ordered

Insert nasogastric tube and/or indwelling urethral catheter as ordered

Provide emotional support and reinforce physician's explanation of surgical procedure; clarify misconceptions

Administer vitamin K, salt-poor albumin, and antibiotics as ordered

Explain and teach about possibility of insulin and pancreatic enzyme therapy postoperatively

Postoperative assessment

Observations/findings

Hypotension
Patency of nasogastric tube
Character and amount of
    Gastric drainage
    Wound drainage
    Urine output
    Bile drainage if T tube is in place
Location and character of pain
Type of parenteral therapy equipment
    CVP line
    TPN line
Tachycardia
Splinting of respirations
Decreased breath sounds
Nausea, vomiting
Abdominal distention

Laboratory/diagnostic studies

Electrolytes, PT, FBS, Hgb, Hct
Arterial blood gases, pH, serum albumin
Serum and urine osmolalities

Potential complications

Oliguria
Dehydration
Electrolyte imbalance
Decreased serum albumin levels
Increased PT
Hyperglycemia
Hypoglycemia
Atelectasis
Pneumonia
Elevated temperature
Jaundice
Subdiaphragmatic abscess, intraperitoneal infection
Paralytic ileus
Gastric/wound hemorrhage
Shock
Wound infection

Medical management

Analgesics, antibiotics, vasopressors, diuretics
Parenteral fluids with electrolytes, vitamins, and/or albumin
Nasogastric aspiration, urine monitoring, T tube
Oxygen therapy
TPN
Stool softeners
Diet, activity

Nursing diagnoses/goals/interventions

ndx: Ineffective breathing pattern related to surgical incision, pain, and anesthesia

GOAL: *Patient's respirations will be adequate to meet body requirements*

Elevate head of bed 30 to 45 degrees; no knee gatch
Monitor respiratory status q1h to 2h; observe for dyspnea and splinting
Auscultate chest for breath sounds q4h
Provide incentive spirometer as ordered
Monitor CVP, Swan-Ganz catheter, and check arterial blood gases and pH
Assist and teach patient to turn and cough q2h and deep breathe q½h; support incision

ndx: Potential fluid volume deficit related to abnormal body fluid loss

GOAL: *Patient will remain hydrated, and electrolytes will be within normal limits*

Maintain NPO
Administer parenteral fluids with electrolytes, vitamins, and insulin as ordered
Connect nasogastric tube to low, intermittent suction apparatus as ordered; irrigate with measured amounts of normal saline
Connect indwelling catheter and/or T tube to closed gravity drainage system as ordered
Measure intake and output; observe urine output qh;

report output of less than 30 to 50 ml/hr to physician; check for sugar and acetone q4h
Monitor vital signs qh until stable; report hypotension to physician; administer vasopressors as ordered
Monitor electrolytes, glucose, and albumin levels
Auscultate abdomen for bowel sounds and measure girth q4h
Administer diuretics as ordered

ndx: Alteration in tissue perfusion related to hemorrhage and/or jaundice

GOAL: *Patient will remain afebrile; incision will remain clean, dry, and intact; and complications will be minimized*

Monitor incision and dressings q2h for bleeding or drainage; reinforce prn
Observe character and color of gastric aspirate and bile drainage for bleeding
Observe skin, sclera, and urine for jaundice
Monitor PT and liver function levels
Administer transfusions and salt-poor albumin
Monitor Hgb and Hct

ndx: Potential for infection related to bacterial invasion of incision and lowered resistance

GOAL: *Patient's incision will remain clean, dry, and intact*

Change dressings as ordered; observe for signs of infection and healing process
Monitor temperature carefully
Administer antibiotics and antipyretics as ordered
Collect urine specimen for culture/sensitivity when indwelling catheter is removed; initiate voiding measures

ndx: Alteration in comfort: pain, related to surgical intervention

GOAL: *Patient will express minimal discomfort or absence of pain*

Assess type and location of pain
Administer analgesics as ordered; provide prior to pain becoming severe and before treatments
Change position frequently; administer back rubs and observe for reddened areas or breakdown
Provide skin care and oral hygiene q4h
Perform passive or assist with and teach active ROM exercises q4h
Ambulate with assistance when allowed

ndx: Alteration in nutrition: less than body requirements related to malnutrition preoperatively, NPO status, and/or anorexia

GOAL: *Patient's nutritional status will be maintained as evidenced by normal weight gain*

Continue with TPN as ordered
Provide water and other clear liquids in small amounts following removal of nasogastric tube; observe for tolerance
Progress to soft diet or diabetic diet as tolerated; provide small, frequent meals; measure intake
Administer insulin and pancreatic enzymes as ordered
Continue monitoring urine for sugar and acetone
Clamp T tube as ordered and observe for signs of pain, distention, and nausea
Avoid constipation with stool softeners; discourage straining

ndx: Knowledge deficit regarding diabetes and home care management

GOAL: *Patient and/or significant other will demonstrate understanding of diabetes, home care, and follow-up instructions through interactive discussion and actual return demonstration*

Provide written dietary instructions for regular or diabetic diet as needed
Demonstrate insulin administration and urine testing procedures
Demonstrate care of T tube if applicable
Discuss medications: name, schedule, dosage, purpose, and side effects; explain importance of taking only medicines prescribed by physician and need to use narcotics discriminately
Explain incisional care and signs of wound infection
Provide information about outside sources available for substance abuse rehabilitation
Demonstrate management of TPN if applicable
Discuss symptoms to report to physician
  Increased abdominal pain, distention
  Fever, jaundice
  Nausea, vomiting
  Gastric bleeding, tarry stools
  Mucosal bleeding
Encourage follow-up visits with physician

Evaluation

There are no complications
Nutrition and hydration are adequate
Pain is manageable
Respirations are normal
Home care management is understood

PANCREATIC CARCINOMA

Malignancy in the pancreas with high mortality due to the lack of early symptoms, symptoms similar to those of other diseases, and rapid metastasis to other organs; 50% occur in the head of the pancreas; 50% occur in the body and tail

Assessment
Observations/findings

Midepigastric pain, varying in severity
    May radiate to lower back and subscapular area
    May be related to eating, activity, or supine position
Signs of biliary obstruction
    Jaundice
    Dark, concentrated urine
    Clay-colored stools
    Pruritus
    Increased PT
    Increased serum bilirubin and alkaline phosphatase
Rapid weight loss
Anorexia
Nausea, vomiting
Fatigue

Laboratory/diagnostic studies

Serum bilirubin, alkaline phosphatase, amylase, and lipase (elevated)
Electrolytes, FBS, liver function studies, PT
Percutaneous transhepatic cholangiography (PTC)
Endoscopic retrograde cholangiopancreatography (ERCP)
Arteriography, ultrasonography, CT scan
Percutaneous needle aspiration cytology, biopsy
Upper GI examination, abdominal radiologic study
Duodenal secretion, cytology

Potential complications

Hyperglycemia
Hyperinsulinism
Steatorrhea
Hepatomegaly
Bleeding tendencies (vitamin K deficiency)
Gastric ulcer–type symptoms
Ascites
Thrombophlebitis
Diabetes mellitus

Medical management

Analgesics, antiemetics, vitamin K, pancreatic enzymes, bile salts, insulin
Diet, parenteral nutrition with electrolytes, TPN
Nasogastric aspiration, urethral catheter
Activity, stool softeners
Chemotherapy, radiation therapy
Surgical interventions

Nursing diagnoses/goals/interventions*

ndx Potential fluid volume deficit related to abnormal loss of body fluids

GOAL: *Patient will remain hydrated; and electrolytes will be within normal limits*

Maintain NPO with discriminate use of ice chips
Administer parenteral fluids with electrolytes, vitamins, and insulin as ordered
Insert nasogastric tube as ordered; connect to low, intermittent suction apparatus; irrigate gently with measured amounts of normal saline
Measure intake and output q8h
Monitor vital signs q4h; take rectal temperature
Monitor electrolytes

ndx Potential for complications related to pancreatic dysfunction†

GOAL: *Patient will exhibit minimal or no complications*

Monitor glucose, bilirubin, PT, Hgb, Hct, and albumin
Monitor gastric aspirate and stools for bleeding; check each for occult blood with Hemastix
Test urine for sugar and acetone q4h
Monitor skin, sclera, and urine for jaundice
Observe for signs of vitamin K deficiency
Monitor ankles for peripheral edema and calves for tenderness or pain
Perform passive or assist with active ROM exercises q4h
Auscultate abdomen for bowel sounds and measure girth q8h
Monitor mental acuity and emotional state
Administer medications as ordered: antacids, vitamin K, salt-poor albumin, diuretics
Provide skin care, and oronasal hygiene q2h

ndx Alteration in comfort: pain related to disease process

GOAL: *Patient will verbalize minimal discomfort or absence of pain*

---

*Patient's condition dictates amount of care required; modify accordingly.
†Not a NANDA-approved nursing diagnosis.

Maintain bed rest in position of comfort and in quiet environment; no knee gatch
Assess location and type of pain
Administer analgesics as ordered; avoid opiates; methadone may be beneficial
Change position frequently; sitting up and leaning forward may alleviate pain
Avoid allowing pain to become too severe
Assist and teach patient to turn q2h and deep breathe q½h

ndx: Alteration in nutrition: less than body requirements related to anorexia, weight loss, and/or fatigue

GOAL: *Patient's nutritional status will be adequate within confines of disease process*

Administer TPN as ordered
Provide high-protein, high-carbohydrate, high-calorie diet as ordered when tolerated; amounts of nutrients may depend on liver involvement
Encourage small, frequent meals and assist as needed
Monitor intake and output q8h
Administer stool softeners
Weigh patient daily at same time with same clothing and scale
Administer medications as ordered: antiemetics, antacids, pancreatic enzymes, bile salts, and insulin

ndx: Ineffective family coping related to poor disease prognosis

GOAL: *Patient and/or significant other will express concerns and feelings and move toward adaptation of positive coping behaviors*

Reinforce physician's explanation of prognosis; clarify misconceptions
Encourage and allow time for verbalization of fears and concerns; listen attentively
Assess present coping behaviors and support past strengths that were successful
Encourage communication with significant other and assist in identifying problems
Promote feelings of self-worth and self-esteem

ndx: Grieving related to anticipated loss

GOAL: *Patient and/or significant other will express feelings and will be assisted in identifying grieving process in supportive manner*

Encourage expression of feelings about death with patient and significant other
Provide realistic hope by setting short-term goals
Assist in identifying grieving stages; promote them as normal and assist in working through them as they occur

ndx: Knowledge deficit regarding diabetes and home care management

GOAL: *Patient and/or significant other will demonstrate understanding or home care and follow-up instructions through interactive discussion and actual return demonstration*

Explain chemotherapy and/or radiation therapy schedule: where and when to report, length of procedure, and side effects
Provide written diet instructions, including amounts of rest and exercise
Demonstrate diabetes care: insulin administration (p. 444) and urine testing (p. 443)
Discuss medications: name, schedule, dosage, purpose, and side effects; explain importance of taking only medications prescribed by physician
Discuss signs and symptoms to report to physician
   Ascites, weight gain (abnormal)
   Jaundice, mucosal bleeding
   Increased pain
   Hematemesis, tarry stools
   Peripheral edema, dyspnea
Promote follow-up visits with physician

Evaluation

Nutrition and hydration are adequate within confines of disease process
Pain is manageable
Adaptive behaviors are demonstrated
Diabetes and home care management are understood

CHAPTER 7

Endocrine System

ENDOCRINE ASSESSMENT

Subjective Data

Change in stamina and ability to perform activities of daily living (ADLs)
Fatigue
Numbness
Tingling
Paresthesia
Bone pain
Change in height
Change in mental status
Headache
Syncope
Anorexia
Nausea
Abdominal pain
Change in weight
Change in body proportions
Palpitations
Shortness of breath
Hoarseness
Change in secondary sex characteristics
Change in menstrual cycle
Impotence
Decreased libido
Dysuria

Objective Data

General appearance: body development, proportion
Vital signs: BP, P, R, T
Skin
  Temperature
  Turgor
  Hydration
    Dry, scaly
    Excessive perspiration
    Excessive oiliness
  Texture
    Fine, smooth
    Coarse, leathery
  Color
    Increased pigmentation
      Gums
      Breast
      Abdomen
      Creases
    Yellow pigmentation
    Flushed
    Pale
    Cyanotic
    Purple striae over areas of fat
  Edema
    Face, eyelids
    Lower extremities
    Pitting, nonpitting
  Lipodystrophy
  Poor wound healing
Hair and nails
  Texture of nails
    Thick
    Brittle
    Thin
    Cracking
  Horizontal nail ridges
  Amount of hair
    Thin
    Increased
    Alopecia
  Distribution of hair
  Texture of hair
    Coarse, dry, brittle
    Fine, silky, soft
Musculoskeletal system
  Fat distribution
  Muscle mass distribution
  Buffalo hump
  Changes in height
  Changes in body proportions: enlarged hands and feet
  Height and weight age-related in children: segmental measurements
  Extremities
    Weakness

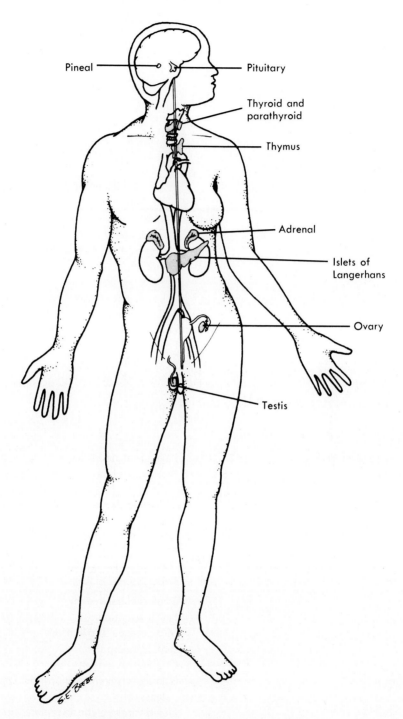

FIGURE 7-1. Endocrine system (male and female).

TABLE 7-1. The Endocrine Glands

Name	Hormones	Function	Endocrine disorders
Pituitary			

Anterior	Somatotropin (growth hormone)	Promotes growth and retention of nitrogen for protein metabolism; maintains established lactation	Hypofunction
			  Dwarfism
			Hyperfunction
			  Acromegaly

	Thyroid-stimulating hormone (TSH)	Promotes bone growth and function of thyroid; controls release of thyroxine	Increased or decreased function of thyroid gland
	Adrenocorticotropic hormone (ACTH)	Promotes growth and function of adrenal cortex; controls release of glucocorticoid	Increased or decreased function of adrenal cortex
	Follicle-stimulating hormone (FSH)	Promotes development of ovaries, secretion of estrogen, and sperm maturation	Increased or decreased function of gonads
	Luteinizing hormone (LH)	Promotes maturation of ovaries, ovulation, and secretion of progesterone	
	Interstitial cell-stimulating hormone (ICSH)	Promotes secretion of testosterone	
	Prolactin (luteotrophic hormone)	Maintains corpus luteum; initiates secretion of milk and progesterone	Hyperprolactinemia
Posterior	Antidiuretic hormone (ADH)	Promotes reabsorption of water	Hypofunction Diabetes insipidus
	Oxytocin	Contracts pregnant uterus	
Adrenal			

Cortex	Glucocorticoids (Cortisol)	Regulates metabolism of carbohydrates, fats, protein; acts as an antiinflammatory agent	Hypofunction
			  Addison's disease
			Hyperfunction
			  Cushing's syndrome

	Androgens	Masculinization of females (axillary and pubic hair); supplements the testes as major source of androgens in males	Hypofunction Delay of secondary sex characteristics
	Mineralocorticoids (Aldosterone)	Balances sodium, water, and potassium concentration; controls release of angiotension	Primary aldosteronism
Medulla	Epinephrine Norepinephrine	Increases blood sugar, stimulates ACTH production, controls vasoconstriction	Pheochromocytoma

Islet's of Langerhans	Insulin (beta cells)	Increases anabolism of carbohydrates; lowers blood glucose	Hypofunction
			  Diabetes mellitus
			Hyperfunction
			  Hyperinsulinism

	Glucagon (alpha cells)	Elevates blood glucose; increases fat metabolism (ketogenesis)	

Continued.

TABLE 7-1. The Endocrine Glands—cont'd

Name	Hormones	Function	Endocrine disorders
Thyroid	Thyroxine (T_4)	Regulates metabolic rate	Hypofunction
	Triiodothyronine (T_3)	Influences growth and development	Cretinism Hypothyroidism (myxedema)
	Calcitonin	Decreases serum calcium levels, bone remodeling	Hyperfunction Hyperthyroidism (Graves' disease)
Parathyroid	Parathyroid hormone (PTH)	Activates bone calcification; increases serum calcium levels	Hypofunction Tetany Hyperfunction Hyperparathyroidism—reabsorption of bone and formation of renal calculi
Gonads	Estrogen Testosterone	Influences secondary sex characteristics; sexual functioning	Hypofunction Lack of or regression of sexual development Hyperfunction Abnormal sexual development
	Progesterone	Prepares and maintains pregnancy; develops mammary secretory tissue	

    Twitching
    Tremors
    Spasms
    Tetany
    Ataxia
Central nervous system (CNS)
    Personality changes
        Complacent
        Dull
        Nervous
        Irritable
        Anxious
        Depressed
        Labile
            Euphoric to depressed
            Frank psychosis
    Alterations in consciousness
        Drowsy
        Slowing of cognitive ability
        Inappropriate response to questions
        Somnolence
        Stupor
        Seizures
        Confusion
        Coma
Small, reactive pupils
Position sense
Response to touch, vibration, and pain

    Speech
        Monotonous
        Slowed
        Weak
        Hoarse
    Reflexes
        Hyperreflexia
        Hyporeflexia
        Trousseau's sign
        Chvostek's sign
    Decreased Apgar score at birth
    Children: activity level related to age level
Head and neck
    Mouth
        Brown pigmentation
        Delayed eruption of permanent teeth
        Malocclusion of teeth
    Tongue
        Color
        Size: enlarged
        Tremors
    Face
        Coarse
        Protruding
        Moon face
        Edema
    Infants
        Short forehead

    Wide, puffy eyes
    Wrinkled eyelids
    Broad, short, upturned nose
    Enlarged lip and nose
    Related to age in children
Eyes
    Protruding eyeballs
    Drooping eyelids
    Cataracts
    Periorbital edema
    Ocular dysfunction
    Microaneurysms
    Hemorrhage
    Exudates
    Arteriolar narrowing
Thyroid
    Size
    Shape
    Symmetry
    Nodules
        Tenderness
        Systolic bruit
Gastrointestinal system
    Anorexia
    Polyphagia
    Polydipsia
    Vomiting
    Diarrhea
    Constipation
    Dehydration
    Weight change
    Increased abdominal girth
    Obesity
    Feeding problems in infants: jaundice
Cardiovascular system
    Tachycardia
    Bradycardia
    Hypotension
    Hypertension
    Arrhythmias
    Cardiomegaly
Respiratory system
    Tachypnea
    Kussmaul's respirations
    Acetone breath
    Stridorous respirations
    Supraclavicular retractions
Renal system
    Polyuria
    Oliguria
    Anuria
    Enuresis
Reproductive system
    Female masculinization
    Changes in secondary sex characteristics
        Genital atrophy
        Breast atrophy
        Precocious puberty
        Delayed puberty
        Enlargement of clitoris
        Infants
            Ambiguous genitalia
            Enlargement of genitalia
            Frequent erections
            Hypospadias

Pertinent Background Information
CONCURRENT DISEASES OR CONDITIONS

Cardiovascular disease
    Heart failure
    Pericardial effusion
    Myocardial infarction
Intestinal obstruction
Pulmonary edema
Mental retardation
Psychologic problems/stress
Pathologic fracture
Obesity

PREVIOUS SURGERY OR ILLNESS

Cancer
Pancreatic disease
Burns
Renal disease
Cardiovascular disease
Transplant
Sarcoidosis
Trauma
Oophorectomy
Neck surgery
Adrenalectomy
Hypophysectomy
Gestational diabetes
Irradiation
Meningitis
Encephalitis

FAMILY HISTORY

Diabetes mellitus
Thyroid disease
Hypertension
Pheochromocytoma
Delayed puberty

SOCIAL HISTORY

Physical environment
Psychologic environment

MEDICATION HISTORY

Corticosteroids
Diuretics
Medication for sleep, nerves, and/or anxiety
Alcohol

Diagnostic Aids

LABORATORY STUDIES

T_3 serum triiodothyronine
T_3 resin uptake
T_4 serum thyroxine
Thyroid-stimulating hormone (TSH)
I_{123} or I_{125} (radioactive iodine uptake)
Parathyroid hormone level (PTH)
Plasma adrenocorticotropic hormone (ACTH)
Growth hormone (somatotropin)
Plasma cortisol
Plasma ketones
Plasma testosterone or estrogen
Cholesterol
Prolactin levels
Triglyceride
Creatinine phosphokinase (CPK)
Catecholamine levels
Potassium
Sodium
Calcium
　Serum
　Urine
Phosphorus
Phosphate reabsorption test
pH
CO_2
Bicarbonate levels
Blood urea nitrogen (BUN)
Fasting blood sugar
Glucose tolerance test (GTT)
17-Hydroxycorticosteroids
17-Ketosteroids
Serum osmolality
Urine metanephrine
Urine specific gravity

PROCEDURES

X-ray examinations of bone
Water deprivation test
Thyroid scan/ultrasound
Thyroid stimulation test
Thyroid suppression test
Achilles tendon reflex recording
Twenty-four hour urine collections
Fractional urine testing
Chemstrip bG

Computed tomography (CT) scans
　Thyroid
　Adrenals
Adrenal angiography
Adrenal venography
Dexamethasone suppression test
ACTH stimulation test
Metyrapone test
Insulin tolerance test
Insulin stress test

HYPOTHYROIDISM: MYXEDEMA

hypothyroidism Lack of thyroid hormone in the adult due to removal or atrophy of the thyroid gland or hypofunction of the pituitary gland or the hypothalamus

myxedema A severe form of hypothyroidism; develops after a prolonged period of untreated or uncontrolled hypothyroidism and is due to deposition of mucopolysaccharides in the tissues

Assessment

Observations/findings

Neurologic
　Lethargy
　Slow, monotonous speech
　Hoarseness
　Memory impairment
　Slow cognition
　Personality changes: complacent, dull, apathetic
　Night blindness
　Perceptive hearing loss
　Paresthesia
　Slowed deep tendon reflexes
　Ataxia
　Somnolence
　Syncope
Musculoskeletal
　Muscle stiffness or aching
　Myalgia
　Arthralgia
　Fatigue
Cardiovascular
　Intolerance to cold
　Decreased sweating
　Low blood pressure, pulse, and temperature
　Narrow pulse pressure
　Diminished heart sounds
　Precordial pain
Respiratory
　Shortness of breath with mild exertion
　Pleural/pericardial effusions

Gastrointestinal/nutritional
  Weight gain
  Anorexia
  Constipation
  Intestinal obstruction
  Ascites
Sexuality/reproductive
  Menorrhagia, metrorrhagia, amenorrhea
  Decreased libido
  Decreased fertility: spontaneous abortion
  Impotence
Integumentary
  Skin: pale, cold, dry, coarse, scaling
  Nonpitting edema: hands, feet, periorbital, supraclavicular
  Enlarged tongue and lips
  Coarse, thinning hair
  Nails: brittle, slow growing

Laboratory/diagnostic studies

Electrocardiogram (ECG): low-voltage, nonspecific ST segment changes, prolonged PR interval, heart block, flat or inverted T wave
Decreased total and free T_4
Decreased ^{131}I resin uptake
Decreased serum sodium
Anemia
TSH levels: low if secondary hypothyroidism; elevated if primary hypothyroidism
Increased serum: cholesterol, triglycerides, CPK
Increased protein in cerebrospinal fluid (CSF)
Arterial blood gasses: hypoxia, elevated CO_2

Potential complications

Heart failure
Myocardial infarction
Stupor
Coma

Medical management

Thyroid hormone replacement with synthetic L-thyroxine
Glucocorticoids if myxedema develops

Nursing diagnoses/goals/interventions

ndx: Potential for physical injury related to changes in sensory perception and coordination

GOAL: *Patient will not incur preventable physical injury*

Assess for development or worsening of perception/coordination defects q8h
Assist patient with ambulation as necessary; provide aids to ambulation (walker, cane) as needed
Place articles patient may wish to use frequently within easy reach
Arrange environment simply; avoid unnecessary clutter
Reorient patient to environment as necessary
Serve foods at tepid temperature to avoid thermal injury
Assist with bathing, shaving, and toileting as necessary
Utilize safety measures (e.g., jacket restraint; avoid wrist restraints) as necessary
Remove potentially hazardous objects from patient's environment
Assess muscle strength and mobility daily
Instruct patient to call for assistance when getting out of bed
Keep call light within easy reach at all times

ndx: Fluid volume excess, extravascular, related to increased capillary permeability

GOAL: *Patient will exhibit a return to normal of the extravascular fluid volume*

Monitor intake and output q8h and prn
Weigh patient daily and report significant gain to physician (significant gain is greater than 0.5 g daily)
Monitor for signs and symptoms of excess extravascular volume: ascites
  Increasing abdominal girth
  Presence of abdominal fluid wave
  Pulmonary edema: dyspnea, orthopnea, and/or crackles in lungs; monitor chest x-ray results
Monitor serum albumin levels
Maintain high-protein diet to increase serum protein levels
Administer diuretics and IV albumin as ordered
Monitor vital signs q4h and observe for
  Increased pulse
  Labored respirations
  Development of S_3 gallop
Notify physician of development or worsening of any of the above signs or symptoms

ndx: Activity intolerance related to muscular stiffness and pain, and/or shortness of breath on exertion

GOAL: *Patient is able to complete required daily activities*

Plan care to allow sufficient time for patient to accomplish activities
  Do not hurry with activities
  Arrange materials and assist patient with hygiene
  Assist with active range-of-motion (ROM) exercises q8h

Encourage patient to walk and assist as necessary
Restrict activity to patient's level of tolerance
Discontinue activity at first signs of fatigue
Plan daily activity/rest pattern that will facilitate increasing tolerance for self-care

ndx: Altered bowel elimination: constipation related to decreased metabolic rate and/or decreased intestinal peristalsis

GOAL: *Patient will excrete stool that is soft and easily passed*

Maintain diet of preference that includes high-fiber foods
Administer fluids to tolerance; remind patient to drink fluids hourly
Administer laxatives, stool softeners, and/or enemas as ordered
Encourage exercise as tolerated
Teach patient to respond rapidly to urge to defecate
Assist patient with recognizing activities that stimulate urge to defecate (drinking warm liquids)
Encourage patient to attempt defecation at same time each day in order to establish a routine

ndx: Potential impairment of skin integrity: edema, dry, scaly skin

GOAL: *Patient will maintain smooth, supple skin free from breakdown*

Assess for redness or breakdown q24h; if patient is on bed rest, assess q8h
Administer skin care to pressure points four times daily and as necessary
Avoid use of harsh soaps
Use oil or lotion in bathwater
Use elbow and heel protectors
Place patient on decubitus-prevention mattress or bed
Elevate edematous extremities with pillows
Assist and encourage patient to change positions frequently
Maintain optimal nutritional status

ndx: Sexual dysfunction related to altered body functions

GOAL: *Patient, along with significant other (if appropriate), will develop a plan for satisfying sexual desires within limits of the disease process*

Explore with patient and significant other usual patterns of sexuality and how this disease may affect these patterns
Encourage patient and significant other to explore alternatives to usual patterns that consider disease limitations
Explore alternatives to becoming parents if appropriate
Initiate referral to appropriate personnel if patient and/or significant other wish therapy
Assist patient and/or significant other to redefine beliefs regarding sexual performance if necessary

ndx: Alteration in thought processes related to altered metabolic processes

GOAL: *Patient will maintain reality-based orientation, will take active interest in environment, and will participate in self-care*

Assess level of orientation q4h and reorient patient as necessary
Explain procedures clearly and slowly, and repeat as necessary
Provide a stable, calm, and nonstressful environment
  Be consistent in timing and performance of activities and procedures
  Restrict visitors as necessary
  Avoid frequent changing of personnel
  Prevent emotionally upsetting or confusing situations
Plan care with patient
Anticipate needs
Provide diversional activities and materials

ndx: Knowledge deficit regarding disease process, treatment, and self-care

GOAL: *Patient and/or significant other will demonstrate understanding of home care and follow-up instructions through interactive discussion and actual return demonstration, and will explain in own words basic concepts of the disease process*

Explain basic concepts of the disease
Give reasons for physical and emotional changes
Teach name of medication, dosage, time and method of administration, purpose, side effects, and toxic effects
Emphasize that medication must not be discontinued without consulting physician
Emphasize importance of telling all health care personnel about disease
Explain need to avoid taking over-the-counter medications without consulting physician
Explain that condition is potentially reversible if treatment regimen is followed
Emphasize importance of
  Ongoing outpatient follow-up

Understanding of slowness and dullness
Increasing self-care
Avoiding very cold environments and stressful situations
Adequate periods of rest alternating with increasing activity/exercise
Maintaining balanced diet and adequate fluid intake
Avoiding constipation
Discuss symptoms of infection to report to physician
    Temperature above patient's normal
    "Cold" or "flu" symptoms
    Redness or swelling around lesions
    Frequency of or burning on urination

Evaluation

Patient does not incur physical injury
Extravascular fluid volume remains within normal values
Effective activity and rest patterns are maintained
Bowel movements are regular without constipation
Skin remains intact
Alternatives to usual sexual patterns are developed
Patient remains oriented to environment and takes active role in care
Patient and/or significant other demonstrates understanding of disease process and principles of home and follow-up care

HYPERTHYROIDISM: THYROID CRISIS (STORM, THYROTOXIC CRISIS)

hyperthyroidism Characterized by excessive production of thyroid hormone; causes may be classified as autoimmune (Graves' disease), viral, hyperplastic, familial, or neoplastic, or it may be secondary to an acute systemic illness (Excess thyroid hormone results in enhanced sympathetic tone, which is responsible for many of the assessment findings listed below.)

Graves' disease Most prevalent form of hyperthyroidism; most commonly seen in women during the third and fourth decades of life

thyroid storm A medical emergency due to acute exacerbation of the symptoms of hyperthyroidism; usually precipitated by a stressful event such as surgery, infection, trauma, or acute cardiovascular disease

Assessment
Observations/findings

Neurologic
    Hyperthyroidism
        Irritability/nervousness
        Tremors
        Insomnia
        Emotional lability
        Diplopia
        Headache
        Large, protruding eyes
        Periorbital edema
        Tremor of eyelids
        Weakness or paralysis of extraocular muscles
        Brisk deep tendon reflexes
        Muscle weakness or atrophy
    Thyroid storm
        Extreme restlessness
        Confusion or disorientation
        Frank psychosis
        Apathy
        Stupor or delirium
        Coma
Cardiovascular
    Hyperthyroidism
        Palpitations
        Rapid, bounding pulses
        Wide pulse pressure
        Irregular pulse/dysrhythmias
        Systolic cardiac murmur
        Congestive heart failure
        Edema
    Thyroid storm
        Profuse diaphoresis
        Tachycardia disporportionate to change in BP
        Atrial fibrillation
        Weak pulses
        Hypotension
Respiratory
    Hyperthyroidism
        Dyspnea
        Increased depth of respiration
        Pulmonary edema
    Thyroid storm: pulmonary edema
Gastrointestinal
    Hyperthyroidism
        Weight loss
        Increased thirst and/or appetite
        Diarrhea
        Nausea, abdominal pain
        Hyperactive bowel sounds
    Thyroid storm
        Anorexia
        Protracted vomiting
        Severe abdominal pain
        Hepatomegaly
        Jaundice
Metabolic

Profuse sweating
  Sensitivity to heat
  Increased tolerance to cold
  Enlarged thyroid gland
  Bruit over neck
 Integumentary
  Skin: soft, warm, moist, shiny
  Reddened, hyperpigmented
  Hair: thinning, fine, straight
  Oily scalp
  Separation of nails from nail beds
 Sexuality/reproductive
  Changes in menstruation
  Changes in sexual activity or desires
  Gynecomastia in males

Laboratory/diagnostic studies

Elevated total and free T_3 and T_4
TSH response to thyrotropin-releasing hormone (TRH) is flat
Thyroid radioiodide uptake test (RAIU)
  Low uptake in thyroiditis or excess thyroid hormone medication
  High uptake in Graves' disease
TSH present in serum
Decreased T_3 resin uptake
Basal metabolism rate (BMR)
Decreased TSH

Potential complications

Fever
Marked elevation in P and BP
Dangerous dysrhythmias
Extreme restlessness
Widespread tremors
Circulatory collapse
Shock
Death

Medical management

Antithyroid medications
  Propylthiouracil
  Methimazole
Beta-blockers for control of symptoms of excessive sympathetic stimulation
Radioactive ^{131}I therapy
Subtotal thyroidectomy
Reserpine/guanethidine to deplete tissue catecholamines
Hyperthermia control (aspirin is contraindicated)
Cooling measures
Volume expanders and/or vasopressors for hypotension
Total parenteral nutrition
Glucocorticoids
Digoxin and/or diuretics for congestive heart failure

Nursing diagnoses/goals/interventions

ndx: Alteration in thought processes related to increased stimulation of the sympathetic nervous system by high levels of thyroid hormone

GOAL: *Patient will express emotions approriate to situation and will maintain a reality-based orientation*

Provide a stable, calm, nonstressful, and nonstimulating environment
  Be consistent in timing and performance of activities and procedures
  Restrict visitors as necessary
  Avoid frequent changing of personnel
  Prevent emotionally upsetting situations
Plan care with patient
Anticipate needs
Inform patient that activities may be restricted
Provide diversional activities and materials
Reorient patient to environment as needed
Administer medications as ordered; monitor for adverse reactions to medications (Table 7-2)

ndx: Activity intolerance related to ease of fatigability, increased resting metabolic rate, and intolerance to heat

GOAL: *Patient will maintain sufficient energy to complete required daily activities*

Restrict activity to patient's level of tolerance
Space procedures to allow adequate rest periods
Discontinue activity at onset of signs of intolerance: dyspnea, tachycardia, fatigue
Assist patient with those activities patient is unable to perform due to weakness or tremors
Plan daily activity and rest pattern that will facilitate increasing tolerance for self-care

ndx: Sleep pattern disturbance related to increased metabolic rate and/or activity intolerance

GOAL: *Patient will verbalize feelings of being well rested and ready for the day's activities*

Provide sleep aids requested by patient: warm drink, back rub, quiet music
Discourage frequent daytime sleeping
Avoid intake of stimulants in diet
Assist patient with establishing a regular pattern of physical activity

TABLE 7-2. Antithyroid Medications

Drug	Action	Adverse reactions	Comments
Sodium iodide (^{131}I)	Selectively destroys thyroid tissue, thereby decreasing secretion of thyroid hormone	Buccal edema Excess salivation Enlarged neck glands Coryza Skin eruptions Unusual irritability or tiredness	Begin after propylthiouracil (PTU) is begun Peak therapeutic effect in 2 to 4 months
Propylthiouracil (PTU) Methimazole	Inhibits synthesis of thyroid hormone	Transient: dermatitis, urticaria, pruritus Leukopenia Myalgia Arthralgia Elevated alkaline phosphatase Agranulocytosis Jaundice	Peak therapeutic effects in 6-10 weeks May enhance anticoagulant effects of heparin/coumadin Teach patient to report onset of sore throat or fever

Provide environment conducive to sleep: dim lighting; close door to room; maintain quiet; maintain privacy

Avoid disturbing patient during the night for unnecessary procedures

Schedule treatments and medications for daytime and evening hours when possible

ndx: Alteration in nutrition: less than body requirements related to diarrhea, nausea, abdominal pain, and/or elevated BMR

GOAL: *Patient will maintain caloric, nutritive, and fluid intake sufficient to meet metabolic needs*

Maintain high-calorie, high-protein, high-carbohydrate, high–vitamin B diet as ordered

Offer frequent small meals and between-meal supplements

Consult patient as to food preferences

Avoid stimulants: coffee, tea, colas or other beverages with caffeine or theobromine

Avoid highly bulky, highly seasoned foods

Encourage fluid intake to 3 to 4 L daily

Weigh patient daily

Medicate as necessary for nausea and abdominal pain as ordered

ndx: Potential for injury to the eyes related to compromised protective mechanisms

GOAL: *Patient's eyes will remain moist and free from abrasions*

Provide sunglasses during the day prn

Administer lubricants as ordered

Patch or tape eyes during sleep

Avoid getting foreign bodies in eyes (dirt, dust)

Assist and teach patient to perform eye motion exercises

ndx: Hyperthermia related to hypermetabolic state

GOAL: *Patient will attain or maintain a euthermic state*

Provide tepid sponge baths as necessary

Use light clothing and bed linens

Maintain cool environment

Use hypothermia blanket as ordered

Administer acetaminophen as ordered (aspirin is contraindicated)

Monitor temperature q2h and prn

ndx: Potential for injury: trauma related to altered mental status

GOAL: *Patient will not incur physical injury*

Utilize safety measures as necessary
  Pad side rails
    Avoid use of extremity restraints (may increase restlessness)

Remove potentially hazardous objects from patient's environment

Assess muscle strength and mobility

Assist patient when ambulating as needed

Instruct patient to call for assistance when getting out of bed

Keep call light within easy reach of patient

Keep personal articles patient may wish to use frequently within easy reach

ndx: Knowledge deficit regarding disease process, treatment, and self-care

GOAL: *Patient and/or significant other will demonstrate understanding of home care and follow-up instructions through interactive discussion and actual return demonstration, and will explain in own words basic concepts of the disease process*

Explain basic concepts of the disease process
Give reasons for physical and emotional changes
Teach name of medication, dosage, time and method of administration, purpose, side effects, and toxic effects
Explain need to avoid taking over-the-counter medications without checking with physician
Emphasize importance of ongoing outpatient care
Explain that symptoms of disease may be reversible if medical regimen is followed
Explain that nervous symptoms are part of the disease process and will decrease with treatment
Instruct patient to inform all health care givers of presence of disease (physician, dentist)
Emphasize importance of planned rest periods
Emphasize importance of avoiding stressful situations
Emphasize that high-calorie, high-protein, high-carbohydrate, and high–vitamin B diet with increased fluids must be maintained until discontinued by physician

Evaluation

Patient expresses appropriate emotions
Orientation to environment is maintained
Effective sleep and activity patterns are maintained
Nutritional needs are met
Eye injury is avoided
Euthermic state is maintained
Physical injury is prevented
Any compromised functioning of body systems is recognized early and referred to physician, and medical treatment is initiated without delay
Patient and/or significant other demonstrates understanding of disease process and principles of home and follow-up care

THYROIDECTOMY

Surgical removal of part (subtotal thyroidectomy) or all of the thyroid gland; usually reserved for patient who does not respond to medical treatment with antithyroid drugs; treatment of choice to remove very large goiters or those compressing surrounding structures; may also be performed for men and women of childbearing age for whom radiation exposure is unwanted, patients allergic to antithyroid medications, and pregnant women

Postoperative assessment
Observations/findings

Increasing hoarseness
Change in tone or pitch of voice
Weak voice, inability to speak
Hypoparathyroidism
   Numbness
   Tingling
   Twitching
   Spasm, tetany
Incision site
   Color (redness)
   Pain, guarding of site
   Swelling
   Drainage, bleeding
Airway
   Choking sensation
   Dysphagia
   Complaints of heaviness or fullness in throat
   Complaints of tight dressing
   Stridorous respirations
   Retraction of neck muscles
   Cyanosis

Laboratory/diagnostic studies

Serum: total and free T_3 and T_4; calcium levels

Potential complications

Airway obstruction
Hemorrhage
Paralysis of recurrent laryngeal nerves
Hypothyroidism
Hypoparathyroidism

Medical management

IV fluids progressing to po diet
Treatment of complications
Pain management

Nursing diagnoses/goals/interventions

ndx: Potential for ineffective airway clearance: bleeding; edema; presence of bulky dressing; painful, dysfunctional swallowing; vocal cord paralysis

GOAL: *Patient will maintain a patent upper airway*

Position patient on back with head elevated 30 degrees to 45 degrees
Have patient turn, cough, and deep breathe q2h and prn
Keep suction equipment at bedside; gently suction oropharynx only when necessary
Have tracheostomy tray immediately available

Monitor for signs of respiratory distress or obstructed airway qh: stridor, wheezing, coarse airway crackles, dyspnea, cyanosis, labored respirations
Check dressing for bleeding qh for first 24 hr
Notify physician if dressing requires reinforcement more than one time

ndx: Impaired skin integrity related to surgical incision

GOAL: *Patient will maintain surgical incision free from infection and well healed*

Prevent tension on suture line: use pillows to maintain head alignment; use sandbags if pillows are insufficient
Prevent flexion or extension of head and neck
Instruct patient to maintain head and neck in neutral position
Instruct patient to use hands to support neck during movement
Place articles within easy reach of patient
Change dressing daily and prn when wet; observe for signs and symptoms of infection or impaired healing: redness, swelling, foul drainage, fever
Promote incision healing: prevent stress on suture line, cleanse site daily as ordered, and apply dry, sterile dressing
Use only necessary dressing and tape; remove tape toward incision

ndx: Potential for impaired verbal communication related to damage and/or manipulation of laryngeal nerves

GOAL: *Patient will maintain effective communication*

Monitor voice quality q2h
Discourage talking for first 48 hr
Reassure patient that voice should return to normal after a few days
Provide alternate means of communication (e.g., pad and pencil)
Keep call bell within reach at all times
Report increasing hoarseness to physician
Anticipate patient's needs

ndx: Alteration in comfort: pain at surgical site

GOAL: *Patient will verbalize feeling of comfort*

Assess patient for verbal and nonverbal signs of pain
Discuss with patient factors that increase or relieve pain
Assist patient with finding physical position of comfort
Assist patient with using distraction as means of pain control: guided imagery, progressive relaxation, soft music, reading, visitors
Administer pain medications as necessary
Maintain support of surgical site
Administer analgesic throat spray or lozenges as ordered and as patient desires

ndx: Knowledge deficit regarding home and follow-up care

GOAL: *Patient and/or significant other will demonstrate understanding of home and follow-up care through interactive discussion and actual return demonstration*

Teach care of surgical incision
Emphasize importance of supporting incision until healed
Teach head and neck exercises: flexion, lateral movement, and hyperextension
Discuss symptoms of recurrent hyperthyroidism, hypothyroidism, or hypoparathyroidism to report to physician
Discuss symptoms of wound infection to report to physician
Emphasize importance of
  Rest and relaxation
    Avoiding stressful situations and emotional outbursts
  Proper nutrition and fluid intake
  Ongoing outpatient care
Teach name of medication, purpose, time and method of administration, dosage, side effects, and toxic effects
Explain need to avoid taking over-the-counter medications without consulting physician

Evaluation

Airway remains patent
Surgical incision begins to heal without complications of infection or disruption of suture line
Communication is maintained between patient and environment
Patient expresses feelings of comfort
Symptoms of hypothyroidism or hypoparathyroidism are recognized in a timely manner and referred to physician
Patient and/or significant other demonstrates understanding of home and follow-up care

HYPOPARATHYROIDISM

Rare condition characterized by a deficiency of parathyroid hormone; may be due to removal of or damage to parathyroid glands (e.g., during thyroid or other neck surgery), biologically ineffective parathyroid hormone, or impaired renal and/or skeletal response to parathyroid hormone

Assessment

Observations/findings

Neurologic
  Hyperreflexia
  Paresthesia
  Tingling
  Tremor
  Positive Chvostek's and/or Trousseau's signs
  Papilledema
  Emotional lability
  Irritability
  Anxiety
  Depression
  Delirium
  Delusions
  Changes in level of consciousness
  Tetany
  Seizures
  Cataracts
Musculoskeletal
  Stiffness
  Cramping
  Weakness
  Fatigue
Cardiovascular
  Cyanosis
  Palpitations
  Cardiac irregularities
  ECG changes: prolonged QT interval, peaked or inverted T waves, heart block
Respiratory
  Hoarseness
  Laryngeal stridor
Gastrointestinal
  Nausea, vomiting
  Abdominal pain
Renal: calculi formation
Integumentary
  Dystrophic, dry skin and nails
  Cutaneous pigmentation
  Alopecia
  Horizontal ridges on nails
In children
  Mental retardation
  Malformed teeth
  Poor physical growth and development

Laboratory/diagnostic studies

Decreased serum calcium
Increased serum phosphorus
Decreased serum bicarbonate
Decreased or absent serum parathyroid hormone
Hypocalciuria
Hypophosphaturia
Calcification of basal ganglia on CT scan

Potential complications

Acute tetany

Medical management

High-calcium, high–vitamin D diet and supplements
Phosphate binders (aluminum hydroxide)
Parenteral fluids
Medications
  Dihydrotachysterol
  Calcitrol
If acute tetany, IV calcium administration

Nursing diagnoses/goals/interventions

ndx: Potential for complication: hypocalcemia leading to acute tetany*

GOAL: *Patient will exhibit reduced risk factors for development of acute tetany*

Maintain high-calcium, high–vitamin D, low-phosphorous diet
Administer vitamin D and calcium supplements as ordered
Monitor serum levels of calcium and phosphorus q8h
Measure intake and output q4h
Monitor vital signs q2h to 4h
Monitor cardiac function continuously if ECG abnormalities are present
Force fluids to 3 to 4 L daily
Do not administer phosphate binders within 1 to 2 hr before or after calcium supplements or other medications
Monitor for signs and symptoms of acute tetany: tingling, paresthesia, numbness, seizures, laryngeal edema
Maintain seizure precautions
Monitor voice quality and respiratory effort q2h
Keep suction, padded tongue blade, and tracheostomy tray at bedside

---

*Not a NANDA-approved nursing diagnosis.

ndx: Potential for ineffective airway clearance related to laryngeal edema

GOAL: *Patient will exhibit decreased risk factors for development of ineffective airway clearance*

Keep suction at bedside at all times
Have tracheostomy tray readily available at all times
Assess respiratory efforts q2h and prn
Auscultate for subtle laryngeal stridor q4h
Have oral airway and manual resuscitation equipment readily available at all times
Instruct patient to inform nurse or physician at first sign of tightness in throat or shortness of breath
Position patient to optimize airway clearance: keep head in neutral position, midline
Hyperextend head and perform chin lift maneuver if necessary

ndx: Potential for injury: trauma related to musculoskeletal and neurologic changes associated with hypocalcemia

GOAL: *Patient will not incur preventable physical injury*

Assess for presence of or worsening of musculoskeltal symptoms q8h
Plan care to permit adequate rest periods
Assist patient with ambulation as needed
Provide aids to ambulation (walker, cane) as needed
Place articles required frequently within easy reach
Arrange environment simply; avoid unnecessary clutter
Provide night-light
Place call bell within easy reach at all times
Instruct patient to call for assistance prior to getting out of bed
Keep bed in low position and side rails up
Assist with personal hygiene (e.g., shaving) as needed
Utilize safety measures (e.g., soft restraints) as needed
Remove potentially hazardous objects from patient's immediate environment
Pad side rails to prevent injury during seizure
Do not attempt to insert airway or tongue blade after seizure has begun
Prevent patient from injuring self during seizure
Administer antiseizure medications as ordered

ndx: Alteration in nutrition: less than body requirements related to nausea, vomiting, and/or abdominal pain

GOAL: *Patient will maintain caloric, nutritive, and fluid intake sufficient to maintain a stable weight*

Offer frequent small meals and between-meal supplements
Consult patient as to food preferences
Ask patient's family to bring favorite foods from home
Weigh patient daily
Medicate for nausea or abdominal pain as needed 30 min prior to meals
Assist patient with arranging meal tray and feeding self if necessary

ndx: Alteration in thought processes related to neurologic changes (emotional lability, irritability, delirium, delusions)

GOAL: *Patient will maintain a reality-based orientation and will interact with environment in a logical, purposeful manner*

Provide a stable, calm, and nonstressful environment
  Be consistent in timing and performance of activities and procedures
  Avoid frequent changing of personnel
  Restrict visitors as necessary
  Prevent emotionally upsetting or confusing situations
Plan care with patient
Anticipate needs
Reorient patient to environment as necessary
Assess orientation and level of interaction q4h
Encourage patient to take an active role in care
Avoid administration of narcotics or sedatives if possible

ndx: Potential impairment of skin integrity: dry/dystrophic skin, decreased activity

GOAL: *Patient's skin will remain supple and free from breakdown*

Assess for redness, development of pressure areas, and breakdown q8h, (q4h if patient is on bed rest)
Administer skin care to pressure points q4h and as necessary
Avoid use of harsh soaps and rough towels
Use lotion or oil in bathwater
Use elbow and heel protectors
Place patient on decubitus-prevention mattress or bed
Encourage patient to change position frequently; assist as necessary
Maintain optimal nutritional status

ndx: Knowledge deficit regarding disease process, treatment, and self-care

GOAL: *Patient and/or significant other will demonstrate understanding of home care and follow-up instructions through interactive discussion and actual return demonstration, and will explain in own words basic concepts of the disease process*

Explain basic concepts of the disease process
Give reasons for physical and emotional changes
Teach name of medication, dosage, time and method of administration, purpose, side effects, and toxic effects
Explain need to avoid taking over-the-counter medications without consulting physician
Emphasize importance of ongoing follow-up care
Instruct patient to maintain high-calcium, high–vitamin D, low-phosphorous diet and increased fluid intake

Evaluation

Signs or symptoms of acute tetany are recognized early and reported to physician for appropriate orders
Airway patency is maintained
Preventable physical injury does not occur
Stable weight is maintained
Patient remains oriented and interactive with environment
Skin remains free from breakdown
Patient and/or significant other understands disease process and principles of home and follow up care

HYPERPARATHYROIDISM

Increased secretion of parathyroid hormone due to hypertrophy of parathyroid gland or as compensatory mechanism in presence of hypocalcemia

Assessment
Observations/findings

Neurologic
　Apathy
　Depression
　Malaise
　Easy fatigability
　Slow mentation
　Drowsiness
Musculoskeletal
　Bone pain with weight bearing
　Arthralgia
　Bone deformities, shortened stature
　Muscular weakness
　Myopathy
　Hyporeflexia
Cardiovascular
　Hypertension
　ECG changes: broad T wave, short or prolonged QT interval, bradycardia
Gastrointestinal/nutritional
　Anorexia
　Nausea
　Weight loss
　Gastric ulcers
　Constipation
Renal
　Polyuria
　Dysuria
　Dehydration
　Renal colic
　Uremia

Laboratory/diagnostic studies

Hypercalcemia
Hypophosphatemia
Hyperchloremia
Low serum HCO_3
Increased urine phosphate and urine calcium
Anemia
Elevated parathyroid hormone (PTH) radioimmunoassay
X-ray: subperiosteal bone resorption
Ultrasound: enlarged parathyroid gland

Potential complications

Renal failure
Pathologic bone fractures
Pancreatitis
Stupor
Coma

Medical management

Parenteral hydration: usually with normal saline
Avoidance of thiazide diuretics
Medications
　Sodium sulfate, sodium phosphate
　Glucocorticoids
　Calcitonin
　Mithramycin
Treatment of choice: surgical removal of the gland(s)

Nursing diagnoses/goals/interventions

ndx: Potential for complication: hypercalcemia leading to renal failure*

GOAL: *Patient will exhibit decreased risk factors for development of hypercalcemia (renal failure)*

---

*Not a NANDA-approved nursing diagnosis.

Monitor vital signs and central venous pressure (CVP) q4h

Monitor intake and output and electrolyte values q4h

Monitor cardiac rhythm for changes in T waves or QT intervals indicative of hypercalcemia

Assess muscle strength and mobility q4h

Assess reflexes q4h

Administer medications as ordered and observe for adverse reactions: hypotension with IV phosphates, extravasation with IV mithramycin

Strain urine if symptoms of renal calculi are present

Maintain low-calcium, high-phosphorous diet

Force fluids to 3 to 4 L daily

Provide diet to maintain acidic urine: cranberries, prunes, tomatoes, asparagus, grapes

Notify physician promptly of any changes in physical examination and carry out orders received

ndx: Potential for injury: trauma related to musculoskeletal weakness

GOAL: *Patient will remain free of preventable physical injury*

Plan care to permit adequate rest periods between activities

Assess for worsening of muscular weakness q8h

Assist patient with ambulation as needed

Provide aids to ambulation: walker, cane

Place articles patient may require frequently within easy reach

Arrange environment simply; avoid unnecessary clutter

Provide night-light

Place call bell within easy reach at all times

Instruct patient to call for assistance before getting out of bed

Keep bed in low position with side rails up

Assist with personal hygiene as needed

Utilize safety measures (e.g., jacket restraint) as necessary

Remove potentially hazardous objects from patient's environment

ndx: Alteration in nutrition: less than body requirements related to anorexia, nausea, and/or gastric ulcers

GOAL: *Patient will maintain caloric, nutritive, and fluid intake sufficient to maintain a stable weight*

Provide low-calcium, high-phosphorous, acidic ash diet

Encourage patient to eat several small meals daily when not nauseated

Consult patient as to food preferences and have them available if possible

Ask patient's family to bring favorite foods from home, within limitations of therapeutic diet

Encourage fluids to 3 to 4 L daily

Weigh patient daily

Medicate as necessary for nausea 30 min prior to meals

Assist patient with arranging meal tray and with feeding if necessary

ndx: Alteration in thought processes related to slow mentation, depression, and/or drowsiness

GOAL: *Patient will maintain a reality-based orientation and will interact with environment in a logical, purposeful manner*

Provide a stable, calm, and nonstressful environment
 Be consistent in timing and performance of activities and procedures
 Restrict patient's visitors as necessary
 Avoid frequent changing of personnel
 Prevent emotionally upsetting or confusing situations

Plan care with patient as appropriate

Anticipate needs

Reorient patient to environment as necessary

Assess level of consciousness and orientation q4h

Explain procedures slowly and clearly; repeat as necessary

Encourage patient to take active role in care

Avoid administration of narcotics or sedatives if possible

ndx: Knowledge deficit regarding disease process, treatment, and self-care

GOAL: *Patient and/or significant other will demonstrate understanding of home care and follow-up instructions through interactive discussion and actual return demonstration, and will explain in own words basic concepts of the disease process*

Explain basic concepts of the disease

Give reasons for physical and emotional changes

Teach name of medication, dosage, time and method of administration, purpose, side effects, and toxic effects

Explain need to avoid taking over-the-counter medications without consulting physician

Emphasize importance of ongoing outpatient follow-up

Instruct patient to maintain low-calcium/high-phosphorous diet

Instruct patient to maintain increased fluid intake
Discuss signs and symptoms of renal colic to report
Teach prevention of falls in home

Evaluation

Signs or symptoms of hypercalcemia or renal failure are recognized early and reported to physician so that treatment is begun in a timely manner
Preventable physical injury does not occur
Stable weight is maintained
Patient remains oriented to and interacts appropriately with environment
Patient and/or significant other demonstrates understanding of disease process and principles of home and follow-up care

PARATHYROIDECTOMY

Surgical removal of the parathyroid glands; if surgery is performed for adenoma, total removal of all involved glands is done; if the cause of hyperparathyroidism is hyperplasia, three total glands are removed and three fourths of the fourth gland is removed, leaving sufficient gland to prevent hypocalcemia in most patients

Postoperative assessment

Observations/findings

Signs and symptoms of hypocalcemia
   Paresthesia
   Tingling
   Stiffness
   Cramping
   Tremor
   Tetany
Respiratory
   Hoarseness
   Laryngeal stridor
   Cyanosis
Incision site
   Redness
   Pain
   Swelling
   Drainage
   Bleeding
   Choking sensation
   Complaints of heaviness or fullness in throat
   Dysphagia

Laboratory/diagnostic studies

Serum calcium levels
Serum phosphorus levels

Potential complications

Hemorrhage
Hypocalcemia: seizures, tetany
Respiratory arrest

Medical management

IV fluids, progressing to diet as tolerated
Treatment of complications
Pain management

Nursing diagnoses/goals/interventions

ndx: Potential for complication: hypocalcemia*

GOAL: *Patient will maintain serum calcium levels such that tetany or seizures do not occur*

In conjunction with physician
   Monitor serum calcium levels daily; expect return to normal or less than normal within first few days postoperatively
   Monitor vital signs, assessing for changes in cardiac rate and rhythm q4h for 48 hr
   Check deep tendon reflexes q2h for 24 hr and q8h thereafter until calcium levels are normal
   Monitor intake and output q8h
   Assess for signs and symptoms of hypoparathyroidism (p. 432)

ndx: Potential for ineffective airway clearance related to bleeding, edema, presence of bulky dressing, painful, dysfunctional swallowing, and/or vocal cord paralysis

GOAL: *Patient will maintain a patent upper airway and will exhibit decreased risk factors for development of airway obstruction*

Position patient on back with head elevated 30 to 45 degrees
Have patient turn, cough, and deep breathe q2h and prn
Keep suction equipment at bedside; gently suction oropharynx only when necessary
Have tracheostomy tray immediately available
Monitor for signs of respiratory distress or obstructed airway qh: stridor, wheezing, coarse airway crackles, dyspnea, cyanosis, labored respirations
Check dressing for bleeding qh for first 24 hr
Notify physician if dressing requires reinforcement more frequently than one time

ndx: Impaired skin integrity related to surgical incision

---

*Not a NANDA-approved nursing diagnosis.

GOAL: *Patient will maintain surgical incision free from infection and well healed*

Prevent tension on suture line: use pillows to maintain head alignment; use sandbags if pillows are insufficient

Prevent flexion or extension of head and neck

Instruct patient to maintain head and neck in neutral position

Instruct patient to use hands to support neck during movement

Place articles within easy reach of patient

Change dressing daily and prn when wet; observe for signs and symptoms of infection or impaired healing: redness, swelling, foul drainage, fever

Promote incision healing: prevent stress on suture line; cleanse site daily as ordered and apply dry, sterile dressing; use only necessary dressing and tape; remove tape toward incision

ndx: Potential for impaired verbal communication related to damage or manipulation of laryngeal nerves

GOAL: *Patient will maintain effective communication despite decreased verbal abilities*

Monitor voice quality q2h

Discourage talking for first 48 hr

Reassure patient that voice shows return to normal after a few days

Provide alternate means of communication (e.g., pad and pencil)

Keep call bell within reach at all times

Report increasing hoarseness to physician

Anticipate patient's needs

ndx: Alteration in comfort: acute pain related to surgical incision

GOAL: *Patient will verbalize feeling of comfort*

Assess patient for verbal and nonverbal signs of pain

Discuss with patient factors that increase or relieve pain

Assist patient with finding physical position of comfort

Assist patient with using distraction as means of pain control: guided imagery, progressive relaxation, soft music, reading, visitors

Administer pain medications as necessary

Maintain support of surgical site

Administer analgesic throat spray or lozenges as ordered and as patient desires

ndx: Knowledge deficit regarding home care and continued medical follow-up

GOAL: *Patient and/or significant other will demonstrate understanding of home and follow-up care through interactive discussion and actual return demonstration*

Discuss signs and symptoms of hypoparathyroidism/hypocalcemia to report to physician

Emphasize importance of maintaining special diet as ordered (high–vitamin D, low-phosphorous diet)

Teach care of surgical incision

Emphasize importance of supporting incision until healed

Teach head and neck exercises: flexion, lateral movement, and hyperextension

Discuss symptoms of wound infection to report to physician

Emphasize importance of
  Rest and relaxation
  Avoiding stressful situations and emotional outbursts
  Proper nutrition and fluid intake
  Ongoing outpatient care

Teach name of medication, purpose, time and method of administration, dosage, side effects, and toxic effects

Explain need to avoid taking over-the-counter medications without consulting physician

Evaluation

Airway remains patent

Surgical incision begins to heal without signs of infection or other complication

Patient is able to communicate needs effectively

Patient expresses feelings of comfort

Any symptoms of hypocalcemia are recognized in a timely manner and referred to physician

Patient and/or significant other understands home care and follow-up instructions

DIABETIC KETOACIDOSIS

Acute complication of diabetes mellitus, characterized by hyperglycemia, metabolic acidosis, increased plasma ketones, and severe dehydration; precipitating factors include stresses of all kinds (physical and emotional), omission of insulin dose, and infection; diabetic ketoacidosis occurs more frequently in type I insulin-dependent patients

Assessment
Observations/findings

Neurologic
  Listlessness

Lethargy
Drowsiness
Visual disturbances
Twitching, tremors
Paralysis
Paresthesia
Headache
Slowed reflexes
Confusion, disorientation
Musculoskeletal
  Decreased muscle tone
  Weakness
Cardiovascular
  Dehydration
  Hyperthermia
  Hypotension
  Tachycardia
  Weak pulses
Respiratory
  Complaints of air hunger
  Tachypnea, Kussmaul's respirations
  Sweet, acetone breath
Gastrointestinal/nutritional
  Anorexia
  Nausea, vomiting
  Abdominal bloating, pain
Renal
  Polydipsia
  Polyuria, osmotic diuresis
Metabolic: poor wound healing
Integumentary
  Hot, dry, flushed skin
  Dry mucous membranes
  Sunken eyes
  Pruritus

Laboratory/diagnostic studies

Elevated blood sugar (200 to 1000 mg/dl)
Elevated plasma ketones
Low pH (less than 7.2)
Low CO_2-combining power
Metabolic acidosis (serum bicarbonate less than 15)
Increased serum osmolality
Glucosuria
Ketonuria
Hyperkalemia initially, with treatment hypokalemia
Increased anion gap
ECG: increased P wave amplitude, flat T wave, prolonged QT interval

Potential complications

Shock
Anuria, renal failure
Cerebral edema
Coma
Heart failure

Medical management

Insulin IV or subcutaneously (5 to 10 units/hr)
Rapid IV hydration: 1 L/hr (approximately 6 L)
Normal saline initially, then as serum glucose decreases, glucose will be added to infusion
IV potassium replacement
$NaHCO_3$ replacement for pH less than 6.9

Nursing diagnoses/goals/interventions

ndx: Fluid volume deficit related to osmotic diuresis

GOAL: *Patient will attain or maintain normal intravascular fluid volume*

Infuse IV fluids as ordered; maintain large-bore IV for rapid infusion
Administer plasma expanders as ordered
Insert indwelling urinary catheter for exact assessment of urine output
Measure intake and output qh and report output less than 30 ml/hr
Monitor CVP if inserted q½h to 1h
Weigh patient daily, observing for weight loss
Assess for signs and symptoms of hypovolemia continuously: tachycardia; low blood pressure; weak, thready pulses; cool skin; increased body temperature; change in level of consciousness
Administer insulin therapy as ordered
Measure capillary blood glucose qh
Measure urine sugar and ketones every hour

ndx: Potential for complication: multisystem failure*

GOAL: *Patient will exhibit decreased risk factors for development of multisystem failure*

Perform cardiovascular, respiratory, and renal assessments q2h
Report changes or abnormal findings to physician
Assess vital signs q½h to 1h; report changes or abnormal findings to physician
Monitor intake and output qh
Monitor cardiac rhythm continuously; observe for signs of electrolyte abnormalities, conduction defects, and premature beats
Position patient to promote optimal cardiac and respiratory function

---

*Not a NANDA-approved nursing diagnosis.

Draw arterial blood gases as ordered; check results for worsening metabolic acidosis

Monitor serum blood sugar, ketones, and electrolytes q1h to 2h until within normal limits

Carry out medical orders received in a timely manner

ndx: Sensory-perceptual alterations: visual disturbances and/or paresthesia related to elevated serum osmolality

GOAL: *Patient will not incur preventable physical injury, will maintain a reality-based orientation, and will respond to or interact with environment in an appropriate manner*

Assess for presence of neurologic deficits q4h
Plan care to permit adequate rest periods
Place articles frequently required within easy reach
Instruct patient to call for assistance prior to getting out of bed
Keep call light within patient's reach at all times
Keep bed in low position with side rails up at all times
Utilize safety measures (soft restraints) as needed
Remove potentially hazardous materials from patient's immediate environment
Assist with ambulation and transfer patient from bed to chair as needed
Provide aids to ambulation and mobility (walker, cane, over-the-bed trapeze) as needed
Be aware that patient's vision may be affected; assist with feeding and personal hygiene as needed
Maintain orientation to environment: assess level of consciousness and orientation q4h and prn
Provide a stable, calm, and nonstressful environment
  Avoid frequent changing of personnel caring for patient
  Be consistent in timing and method of performance of procedures and activities
  Anticipate and avoid emotionally upsetting or confusing situations
Explain all procedures to patient clearly; repeat as necessary; solicit patient's assistance in the performance of procedures
Provide stimulation in the environment that will assist in maintaining orientation: pictures from home, calendar, clock, radio, television
Maintain eye contact while speaking with patient and while providing care
Allow frequent, brief visits from significant others of patient's choosing
Address patient by name, and review day, date, time, and current events with patient as necessary
Encourage and provide positive reinforcement to patient for participating in environment
Allow patient to participate in decisions regarding care

ndx: Potential for complication: electrolyte imbalance*

GOAL: *Patient will exhibit decreased risk factors for the development of electrolyte imbalance*

Administer fluid and electrolyte therapy as ordered
Monitor for hypokalemia: muscle weakness, flacidity, paralytic ileus, prolonged QT interval, cardiac arrest if severe
Monitor for signs of hyperkalemia: bradycardia, peaked T waves, loss of P waves, cardiac arrest if severe
Continuously monitor ECG rhythm
Monitor serum and urine electrolytes q4h; report abnormal values to physician
Maintain accurate intake and output record
Carry out medical orders received without delay

ndx: Potential impairment of skin integrity: dry skin and mucous membranes, dehydration, nutritional deficit, bed rest

GOAL: *Patient will maintain skin that is soft, supple, and free from breakdown*

Assess for redness, development of pressure areas, or breakdown q4h while patient is on bed rest
Administer skin care to pressure points q2h and prn
Avoid use of harsh soaps and rough towels
Use oil or lotion in bathwater
Place patient on decubitus-prevention mattress or bed
Encourage patient to change position frequently; assist as necessary
Maintain optimal nutritional status

ndx: Knowledge deficit regarding disease process, treatment, and self-care

GOAL: *Patient and/or significant other will demonstrate understanding of home and follow-up care through interactive discussion and actual return demonstration, and will explain in own words basic concepts of the disease process*

Ensure that patient and/or significant other understands the following in addition to diabetic teaching (p. 442)
  Basic concepts of the disease process
  Symptoms of early ketoacidosis: nausea; vomiting;

---

*Not a NANDA-approved nursing diagnosis.

abdominal pain; hot, dry, flushed skin; drowsiness; glycosuria; ketonuria

Symptoms of hypoglycemia

Need to report any of the above signs or symptoms to physician

Factors that predispose to ketoacidosis: increased food intake, omitted doses of insulin, failure to respond to increased need for insulin, decreased activity, exercise, stress, pregnancy, febrile illness, surgery

Symptoms of infection to report to physician: cuts, sores that do not heal, "cold" or "flu," coughing, burning on urination, fever

Importance of
  Balanced activity and rest cycle
  Regular urine and blood self-testing for glucose and ketones
  Accurate medication administration
  Weight control
  Avoiding contact with infectious persons
  General hygiene measures and foot care
  Wearing medical alert band or chain; carrying diabetic identification card
  Ongoing outpatient care

Evaluation

Patient will maintain intravascular fluid volume within normal limits

Any signs or symptoms of impending crisis are recognized in a timely manner, and medical orders are carried out without delay

Patient remains oriented to environment and takes an active role in care

Preventable physical injury is avoided

Electrolyte imbalances are recognized in a timely manner and reported to physician; are prevented if possible

Skin remains supple and intact

Patient and/or significant other understands basic concepts of disease process, and home and follow-up care

HYPEROSMOLAR HYPERGLYCEMIC NONKETOTIC COMA

Metabolic disorder in which the blood sugar level is extremely elevated, increasing the serum osmolality and resulting in hypertonic dehydration; serum ketosis is not significant; usually occurs in patients with type II diabetes mellitus but may occur with diabetes insipidus, GI hemorrhage, high-protein gastric tube feedings, or drugs such as diuretics, glucocorticoids, propranolol, diazoxide, or cimetidine

Assessment

Observations/findings

Neurologic
  Apprehension
  Lethargy
  Confusion
  Disorientation
  Small, equal, reactive pupils
Cardiovascular
  Hypertension to hypotension if untreated
  Tachycardia
Respiratory: normal to rapid respirations
Gastrointestinal
  Nausea, vomiting
  Abdominal pain
  Diarrhea
Renal: polyuria
Metabolic
  Polydipsia
  Elevated temperature
Integumentary
  Dry, flushed skin
  Decreased turgor
  Dry tongue and mucous membranes

Laboratory/diagnostic studies

Blood sugar 600 to 1200 mg/dl
Plasma ketones usually absent
Hyperosmolarity 350 to 475 mosm/L
Elevated BUN
Hypernatremia
Hyperkalemia
Slight metabolic alkalosis

Potential complications

Focal, grand mal seizures
Renal failure
Coma
Cardiovascular collapse
Thromboembolism

Medical management

IV insulin administration
IV fluid administration, plasma expanders as needed
Electrolyte replacement as needed
See Diabetic Ketoacidosis (p. 437)

Nursing diagnoses/goals/interventions

ndx: Fluid volume deficit related to osmotic diuresis

GOAL: *Patient will attain or maintain normal intravascular fluid volume*

Infuse IV fluids as ordered; maintain large-bore IV for rapid infusion

Administer plasma expanders as ordered

Insert indwelling urinary catheter for exact assessment of urine output when ordered

Measure intake and output qh and report output of less than 30 ml/hr

Monitor CVP q½h to 1h

Weigh patient daily, observing for weight loss

Assess for signs and symptoms of hypovolemia continuously: tachycardia; low blood pressure; weak, thready pulses; cool skin; increased body temperature; change in level of consciousness

Administer insulin therapy as ordered

Measure urine sugar and ketones qh

Measure capillary blood glucose qh

ndx: Potential for complication: multisystem failure*

GOAL: *Patient will exhibit decreased risk factors for development of multisystem failure*

Perform cardiovascular, respiratory, and renal assessments q2h

Report changes or abnormal findings to physician

Assess vital signs q½h to 1h; report changes or abnormal findings to physician

Monitor intake and output qh

Monitor cardiac rhythm continuously; observe for signs of electrolyte abnormalities, conduction defects, or premature beats

Position patient to promote optimal cardiac and respiratory function

Draw arterial blood gasses as ordered; check results for worsening metabolic acidosis

Monitor serum blood sugar, ketones, and electrolytes q1h to 2h until within normal limits

Carry out medical orders received in a timely manner

ndx: Potential for complication: electrolyte imbalance*

GOAL: *Patient will exhibit decreased risk factors for development of electrolyte imbalance*

Administer fluid and electrolyte therapy as ordered by physician

Monitor for hypokalemia: muscle weakness, flacidity, paralytic ileus, prolonged QT interval, cardiac arrest if severe

Monitor for signs of hyperkalemia: bradycardia, peaked T waves, loss of P waves, cardiac arrest if severe

Continuously monitor ECG rhythm

Monitor serum and urine electrolytes q4h; report abnormal values to physician

Maintain accurate intake and output record

Carry out medical orders received without delay

ndx: Alteration in thought processes related to increased serum osmolality

GOAL: *Patient will maintain a reality-based orientation and will take an active role in self-care, with consideration of physical limitations*

Provide a stable, calm, and nonstressful environment
  Be consistent in timing and performance of activities and procedures
  Restrict visitors as necessary
  Avoid frequent changing of health care personnel
  Anticipate and prevent emotionally stressful situations

Plan care with patient

Inform patient that activities may be restricted

Explain all procedures to patient and answer any questions

Explain planned activities for the day clearly; repeat as necessary

Assess patient's level of consciousness q4h and reorient patient to environment as needed

Encourage patient to keep personal articles at bedside: pictures of family, clock or watch, calendar

ndx: Knowledge deficit regarding disease process, and home and self-care

GOAL: *Patient and/or significant other will demonstrate understanding of home and follow-up care through interactive discussion and actual return demonstration, and will explain in own words basic concepts of the disease process*

Explain basic concepts of the disease process

Teach name of medication, purpose, time and method of administration, dosage, and side and toxic effects

Explain need to avoid taking over-the-counter medications without consulting physician

For specific patient teaching refer to standard for primary disease entity (e.g., Diabetic Ketoacidosis, p. 437)

Evaluation

Intravascular fluid volume is restored to within normal limits

Any signs or symptoms of severe dehydration are reported to physician, and medical orders are carried out without delay

Any signs or symptoms indicating pending multisystem

---

*Not a NANDA-approved nursing diagnosis.

failure are recognized in a timely manner, and medical orders are carried out without delay

Any electrolyte imbalances are recognized and treated in a timely manner, and are prevented when possible

Patient remains oriented to and interactive with environment

Patient and/or significant other demonstrates understanding of disease process, and home and follow-up care

TEACHING THE DIABETIC PATIENT

Assessment prior to teaching

Health
    Predisposing factors
    Length of present problem
    Past health care experience
    Laboratory data
Psychologic status
    Strengths and weaknesses
    Coping methods
    Self-concept
    Reaction to diagnosis
    Willingness to assume self-care
Social and economic status
    Life-style
        Factors consistent with recommended plan
        Areas of inconsistency
    Dietary habits
    Available support systems
    Home environment
        Physical setting
        Available resources
    Cultural influences leading to acceptance or rejection of care
    Occupation
        Type and hours
        Income level related to care
        Referral needs
    Learning
        Previous instruction, knowledge, and misconceptions
        Ability to learn at present time
        Present learning needs

Nursing diagnosis/goal/interventions

ndx: Knowledge deficit regarding home glucose monitoring, self-urine testing, self-administration of insulin, self-administration of oral hypoglycemic agents, alteration in diet and insulin requirements during illness or life-style changes, foot and leg (skin) care, personal hygiene, and precautions to take during travel

GOAL: *Patient and/or significant other will demonstrate understanding of home and follow-up care through interactive discussion and actual return demonstration*

Determine what to teach and when to start teaching program by
    Discussing "need to know" topics, procedures, and skills with patient
    Allowing patient to make choices of what to learn first to relieve anxiety, give control to patient, and maintain high interest level
    Formulating total plan of care with patient
Involve significant other in care and teaching very early, when appropriate, to give support to patient
Stress positive points
    Care program would benefit all: regular exercise, control of weight, and diet management conducive to health maintenance
    Discuss ways care program can be adapted to patient's life-style
    The more patient knows about disease process, daily activities, skills, procedures, and complications, the more control patient maintains over life
    Discuss importance of balance among diet, medication, and exercise/activity
        An alteration in one area requires changes in others to maintain control
        This balance and general health and hygiene measures can be achieved through joint effort of patient and staff
Stress that staff and others will be available to assist in learning and planning process as well as for later consultation as patient incorporates information, skills, and dietary plan into daily schedule
Include these topics and skills in teaching plan
    Disease process, predisposing factors, and presenting symptoms
    Physiology of pancreas, insulin, and metabolism
    Diet management
    Medications
        Insulin (p. 444)
        Oral hypoglycemics (p. 446)
        Urine testing (p. 443)
        Blood testing
            Laboratory preparation
            Home glucose monitoring (p. 443)
    Exercise
    Personal care (p. 449)
    Foot care (p. 448)
    Travel tips (p. 450)

Management of complications
   Sick day rules (p. 446)
   Ketoacidosis (p. 437)
   Nonketoic hyperosmolar ketoacidosis (p. 440)
   Hypoglycemia (p. 450)
   Cardiovascular system
   Neuropathy
   Renal system
Resources
   Community agencies and groups
   Literature
   Cookbooks
   Magazines
   Newspapers
Caution patient with regard to articles in newspapers and magazines written by nonauthoritative persons and to be sure to check with physician/nurse practitioner prior to adapting any new dietary or self-care practices

Home Glucose Monitoring Teaching Guide

Ensure that patient and/or significant other knows and understands
   Reasons for testing blood for glucose
   Frequency of testing blood: usually four times each day until stabilized, then twice each day (before first and last meal)
   Need to rotate sites of finger punctures: six sites on each finger (Figure 7-2)
   Importance of not using alcohol or povidone-iodine to clean finger prior to stick
   Care and storage of reagent strips
   Care and storage of finger puncture equipment
   Method for disposing of lancets
   Method of recording estimated blood glucose
   Importance of checking accuracy of test results by comparing with laboratory data
Ensure that the patient and/or significant other demonstrates
   Handwashing technique
   Method of obtaining blood sample by finger puncture
   Method of milking finger to obtain blood sample (Figure 7-3)
   Procedure for using and reading reagent strips or for using automated equipment
Ensure that patient and/or significant other demonstrates procedures using equipment that will be available at home

Diabetic Urine Testing Teaching Guide

Ensure that patient and/or significant other knows and understands
   Reason for testing second voided specimen and how to collect this urine specimen
      Void and discard first specimen
      Void again in 20 to 30 min (second voided specimen)
      Pass dipstick testing material through stream of urine or place urine specimen in clean, dry container if using Clinitest* and Acetest*
   Use this specimen to test for glucose and/or acetone

---

*Ames Co., Division of Miles Laboratories, Inc., Elkhart, Ind.

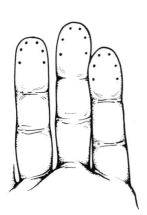

FIGURE 7-2. Finger puncture sites.

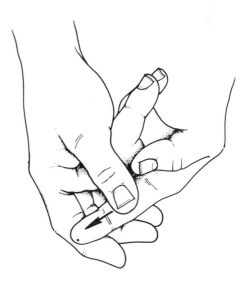

FIGURE 7-3. Milking finger to obtain blood sample.

Take no more than 240 ml of noncaloric fluids to obtain second specimen

Need for urine testing, renal threshold, and meaning of test results

Importance of testing urine at least twice daily, 30 min before first and last meal and more often as ordered or during periods of illness

Method of recording test results on home record and taking record to each appointment with physician

Instructions to follow when abnormal results are obtained
- Repeat test
- Change dietary intake, activity and exercise level, or insulin dosage as ordered
- Notify physician

Medication that may give false-positive or false-negative test results

Examples of medication that give false-positive results: ascorbic acid, cephalosporin, chloral hydrate, isoniazid, levodopa, salicylates, and tetracycline

Need to store testing materials in cool, dark area away from children and oral medication

Ensure that patient and/or significant other demonstrates urine testing procedure using equipment that will be available at home

GLUCOSE TESTS
Clinitest*

Follow directions with set
Use either two-drop or five-drop method as ordered
Avoid shaking test tube while boiling
Watch color change while boiling; more than 2% is indicated by change from orange to dark brown-green
Wait 15 sec after boiling stops and compare with color chart if this color change does not occur
Keep tablets in tightly sealed container
Avoid wetting or touching tablets with hands
Do not use if tablets turn blue

Tes-Tape†

Follow directions on tape container
Use end of tape not touched or exposed to light or air
    Compare strip with color chart
        Make another reading after 2 min if reading is 0.5% after 1 min

Avoid exposing tape to light, moisture, or heat
Observe expiration date

Diastix*

Follow directions on container
Compare strip to color chart after 30 sec

ACETONE TESTS
Acetest*

Follow directions on container
Pour tablet onto paper towel without touching
Compare tablet with color chart after 30 sec
Avoid exposing tablets to moisture or light

Ketostix*

Follow directions on container
Compare strip with color chart after 15 sec

COMBINED TEST
Keto-Diastic*

Follow directions on container
Compare ketone side of strip after 15 sec, glucose side after 30 sec

Insulin Therapy Teaching Guide
Observations

Hypoglycemia (p. 450)
Ketoacidosis (p. 437)
Insulin resistance: requires over 200 units
Ability to prepare injection with two types of insulin, when this is prescribed
    Equalize pressure in both vials of insulin by injecting air to equal amount of insulin to be withdrawn
    Withdraw regular insulin first, then longer-acting insulin
Use of special equipment if patient has difficulty seeing or has other handicaps
    Preset dosage syringe
    Needle guide for insulin vial
    Automatic injector

Site of injection

Ensure that patient and/or significant other knows and understands
    That most rapid absorption occurs in abdomen, arms, and thighs (in that order)
    Importance of rotating site of injection with each

---

*Ames Co., Division of Miles Laboratories, Inc., Elkhart, Ind.
†Eli Lilly & Co., Indianapolis, Ind.

*Ames Co., Division of Miles Laboratories, Inc., Elkhart, Ind.

dose of insulin to prevent atrophy, fibrosis, lipodystrophy, and decreased insulin absorption

Need to avoid injection into extremities just prior to exercise

Importance of using each site only once in 80 injections (Figure 7-4)

Importance of recording site used for each injection by location and number (Table 7-3)

Injection

Ensure that patient and/or significant other demonstrates injection technique

Select site for injection; may use abdomen or thigh for first injection

Prepare skin by cleaning with alcohol

Hold syringe filled with correct insulin dosage as one would a pencil or a dart

Pinch up skin

Insert needle at 45- or 90-degree angle (depends on amount of subcutaneous tissue) and quickly push into tissue up to hub of syringe; may need to guide patient's hand at this point

Release skin

Withdraw plunger to check for entry into blood vessel

Inject medication

Withdraw needle and hold alcohol swab on area for a few seconds

Record date and time given, type of insulin, dosage, and site of injection on record for home use

Types of insulin

Ensure that patient and/or significant other knows and understands

Action of the type(s) of insulin to be used (additional information may be confusing initially)

Time of day patient may expect to have reaction

Factors that precipitate reaction

Incorrect, increased dosage of insulin

Altered routine in diet or activity without pre-planning

Emotional stress

Other disease processes

"Cold"

"Flu"

Nausea, vomiting

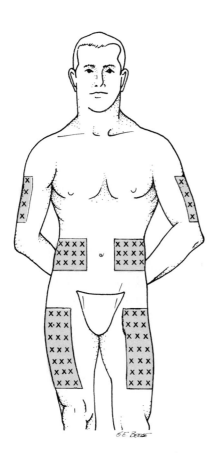
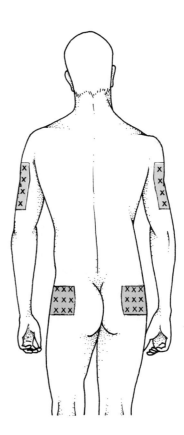

FIGURE 7-4. Rotation of insulin injection sites.

TABLE 7-3. Diabetic Flow Sheet

Date	Time	Urine test	Blood glucose test	Insulin type/dosage	Site	Comments
	Before first meal Before second meal Before third meal Bedtime					
	Before first meal Before second meal Before third meal Bedtime					

NOTE: Glucose test and urine test may not indicate same amount of glucose because of patient's renal threshold.

 That type and dosage of insulin will be adjusted as ordered by physician
 That dosage may be adjusted according to blood or urine test results only if ordered by physician

Care of equipment

Ensure that patient and/or significant other knows and understands
 Care of insulin
  Keep opened insulin vial currently in use at room temperature away from sunlight; keep no longer than 2 months
  Have at least one unopened vial stored in refrigerator—not in freezer
  Observe expiration date
 Types of syringes: care and disposal
  Be sure units marked on syringe match units of insulin being used
  Handle syringe and needles carefully to avoid self-puncture
  Disposable syringe and needle: demonstrate ability to maintain sterility of syringe and needle; dispose of syringe and needle in safe container after use
  Reusable syringe and needle: demonstrate ability to clean needle with alcohol swab after each use; store syringe and needle in refrigerator; follow procedure until needle becomes blunt (about four uses), then discard

Oral Hypoglycemic Therapy Teaching Guide
Sulfonylureas

Ensure that patient and/or significant other knows and understands
 Action and dosage of preparation of medication ordered
  Acetohexamide (Dymelor): usual daily dosage, 250 to 1500 mg
  Chlorpropamide (Diabinese): usual daily dosage, 100 to 500 mg
  Tolazamide (Tolinase): usual daily dosage, 100 to 1000 mg
  Tolbutamide (Orinase): usual daily dosage, 500 to 2000 mg
 Side and/or toxic effects to report to physician
  GI upset
  Weakness
  Paresthesia
  Headache
  Tinnitus
  Skin rash
  Jaundice
  Intolerance to alcohol
  Prolonged action of sedatives and hypnotics
  Hypoglycemia (p. 450)
 Importance of taking medication prior to meal
 Need to observe specific diet and control weight
 Importance of notifying physician immediately if pregnancy is suspected

Sick Day Rules

Ensure that patient and/or significant other knows and understands
 That any illness, injury, or change in body functioning causes an increased need for glucose, which the body will automatically produce
 That a change in medication and food usually is required

TABLE 7-4. Action of Insulin

Type	Company, product	Species source	Onset of action (hours)	Peak of action (hours)	Duration of action (hours)
CONVENTIONAL INSULINS					
Regular	Lilly (Iletin I)	B-P*	½	2-4	6-8
	Squibb	Pork	½	2½-5	6-8
Semilente	Lilly (Iletin I)	B-P	1-2	3-8	10-16
	Squibb	Beef	½-1	5-10	12-16
NPH (Isophane)	Lilly (Iletin I)	B-P	1-2	6-12	18-26
	Squibb	Beef	1-1½	4-12	24
Lente	Lilly (Iletin I)	B-P	1-3	6-12	18-26
	Squibb	Beef	1-1½	7-15	24
Protamine zinc	Lilly (Iletin I)	B-P	4-6	12-24	26-36
	Squibb	Beef	4-8	14-20	36
Ultralente	Lilly (Iletin I)	B-P	4-6	14-24	28-36
	Squibb	Beef	4-8	10-30	36
PURIFIED INSULINS†					
Regular	Lilly (Iletin II)	Beef or pork	½	2-4	6-8
	Nordisk (Velosulin)	Pork	½	1-3	8
	Novo (Actrapid)	Pork	½	2½-5	8
Semilente	Novo (Semitard)	Pork	½-1	5-10	16
NPH (Isophane)	Lilly (Iletin II)	Beef or pork	1-2	6-12	18-26
			1-3	6-12	24-28
	Nordisk (Insulatard)	Pork	1½	4-12	24
	Novo (Protaphane)	Pork	1½	4-12	24
Lente	Lilly (Iletin II)	Beef or pork	1-3	6-12	18-26
	Novo (Monotard)	Pork	2½	7-15	22
	Novo (Lentard)	B-P	2½	7-15	24
Protamine zinc	Lilly (Iletin II)	Beef or pork	4-6	14-24	26-36
Ultralente	Novo (Ultratard)	Beef	4	10-30	36
Biphasic (30% regular, 70% NPH)	Nordisk (Mixtard)	Pork	½	4-8	24
HUMAN INSULINS					
Regular	Lilly (Humulin-R)	Bacteria	½	2-4	6-8
	Squibb/Novo (Novolin-R)	Semisynthetic	½	2½-5	6-8
NPH (Isophane)	Lilly (Humulin-N)	Bacteria	1-2	6-12	18-24
	Squibb/Novo (Novolin-N)	Semisynthetic	1½	4-12	24
Lente	Squibb/Novo (Novolin-L)	Semisynthetic	2½	7-15	24

*B-P, mixed beef and pork insulin.
†The Food and Drug Administration recommends that purified insulins be considered in patients with local or systemic reactions to conventional insulins and in patients with lipodystrophy caused by conventional insulins.

Signs and symptoms of illness, injury, or functional change that may require changes in medication or food
Injuries
Infections
Nausea, vomiting
Diarrhea
Burns
Dental care
Surgery
Pregnancy
Emotional stress
Unaccustomed physical activities; periodic jogging, swimming, tennis
Importance of increasing testing of blood and/or urine to at least four times a day during this change

Need to notify physician when urine test results are 2% with or without ketones for two successive times
Unable to take oral feedings
Pregnant
Special diet to follow when ill

Skin, Foot, and Leg Care Teaching Guide

Skin care

Ensure that patient and/or significant other knows and understands
  Observations to make daily and report to physician if found
    Dry, scaly skin
    Itching
    Blueness, swelling around varicosities
    Hardened areas, corns, calluses
    Decreased sensitivity
    Pain
    Redness
    Swelling
    Cracking
    Blisters
    Abrasions
    Infection
    Thickened, discolored nails
  Daily care of feet
    Bathe feet daily in tepid water
    Check temperature of water with elbow or forearm before placing feet in water
    Use mild or superfatted soap
    Dry skin gently but thoroughly with soft towel; avoid vigorous rubbing
    Apply lanolin-based lotion starting at distal end of toes
      Remove extra lotion with dry towel
      Avoid use of alcohol preparations
    Keep feet dry at all times
      Wear clean, preferably cotton, socks daily
      Women wear hose with cotton feet
      Use clean lamb's wool or cotton between toes if perspiring; do not bunch—use only small amount; change daily or more frequently
      Avoid over-the-counter foot powders without checking with physician
  Inspect and feel areas of feet, especially around nails, and between and under toes for cracks, dry scaling, redness, swelling, itching, blisters, and ulcers daily
  Clean small areas of abrasion with soap and water; dry well
  Apply dry sterile dressing
  Notify physician if no improvement occurs in 24 to 36 hr

Nail care
  Soak feet in tepid water 3 to 5 min
  Cut long nails straight across; *do not cut* to level of tissue
    Never cut corners of nails
    File nails to just above soft tissue
  Have another person cut nails if patient has poor vision
  Have thickened, deformed nails cut by physician or podiatrist
  Care of hardened areas
    Soak feet in tepid water 3 to 5 min
    Use soft brush over area
    Rub with washcloth
    Do not attempt to remove with devices (e.g., razors, scissors, or medicated remedies)
    Never tear skin off
  Care of abrasions
    Notify physician of any
      Redness
      Blistering
      Break
      Swelling
      Pain
    Avoid use of strong antiseptics (tincture of iodine)
    Cover area with sterile gauze
    Elevate injured foot
    Avoid use of foot

Safety

Ensure that patient and/or significant other knows and understands
  To avoid trauma to feet and legs
    Do not walk barefoot
    Always use a light at night to prevent accidental bumps
    Do not scratch insect bites
    Do not use hot-water bottles or electric heating pads on extremities
    Avoid sunburn
    Dress warmly in cold weather
  To avoid use of constricting garments
    Avoid girdles, garters, hose or stockings with elastic tops, tight belts, and tight-fitting undergarments
    Tie shoes loosely but firmly

Shoes

Ensure that patient and/or significant other knows and understands
  To alternate wearing two pairs of shoes
  To air each pair between use; if wet, air-dry slowly on shoe trees

To wear leather-soled shoes; avoid rubber soles
To break in new shoes gradually
  Wear ½ hr first day
  Increase by 1 hr each day
  Check feet q2h
To have shoes well fitted
  One-half inch longer than largest toe
  Wide enough to prevent pressure and to avoid rubbing
    Snug fit at heel
    Check inside for cracks or bumps
To avoid sandals and slippers for working
That moderately high-heeled shoes may be worn if there are no pressure points

Rest and exercise

Ensure that patient and/or significant other knows and understands importance of
  Walking daily to tolerance
  Planning to exercise after meals
  Curling and stretching toes several times each day
  Rotating ankles
  Bending and straightening knees
  Following exercises prescribed by physician

Position

Ensure that patient and/or significant other knows and understands
  To avoid any one position for long periods of time: standing, sitting, or bed rest
  To alternate position with walking when able
  Sitting position
    Avoid more than right-angle bend when sitting
    Prevent pressure at back of knee from use of chair that is too high
    Rotate ankles occasionally
    Bend and straighten knees
    Never cross knees
  Standing position
    Walk in place
    Rotate ankles
    Shift weight from both legs to one leg occasionally
  Resting position: place pillow at foot of bed to prevent constricting toes with tight covers

Personal Care

Ensure that patient and/or significant other knows and understands
  Care of teeth
    Need to follow daily care regimen
      Brush after sleep and meals and before bedtime
      Floss at least daily
      Examine mouth for irritated gums, bleeding, and rough edges on teeth and report to dentist
    Importance of denture care
      Clean dentures after every meal and whenever removed
      Have ill-fitting or loose dentures correctly fitted
      Examine mouth daily for irritation, areas of pressure, or sores and report to dentist
    Need to schedule periodic dental examinations (usually every 6 months)
    Importance of telling dentist about condition and checking with primary physician before scheduling extensive dental care or surgery
  Care of eyes
    Knowledge that eye changes (vision) may be temporary if blood sugar is high
    Importance of scheduling yearly examinations with an ophthalmologist; more often if vision changes are noted
  Care of skin
    Importance of checking body daily for any skin changes, especially in neck, axilla, groin, or extremities
    Need to care for small skin breaks, irritation, or scratches immediately
      Wash with soap and water; dry well and cover with sterile dressing
      Check daily; if no improvement occurs within 24 hr, notify physician
      Avoid use of strong antiseptics with phenol, mercury, oil of mustard, cantharidin, or salicylic acid
    Importance of reporting other problems to physician immediately: large or deep cuts, boils, carbuncles, burns, abscesses, blisters, or ulcers
    Need to avoid use of harsh household cleaners; use only with protective gloves
    Need to avoid extremes in temperature without protective clothing for warmth or sunshielding
    Need to avoid sunburns; use sunscreen with level 15 protection
    Need to be knowledgeable and cautious when using machinery, tools, and equipment
    Importance of not using hot-water bottles or heating lamps if skin sensation is diminished
  Urinary and genital care
    Need to ensure adequate urinary output
      Drink six to eight glasses of water per day
      Importance of avoiding urinary tract or vaginal infections
      Avoid excessive amounts of fluids with caffeine or alcohol

Urinate as soon as urge is felt
Wash and dry genital area daily
Inspect for irritation and discharge
Uncircumcised males clean area under foreskin daily with soap and water; dry well
Females wipe from front to back after urination and bowel movements
Shower rather than use tub baths
Wear underwear and/or panty hose with cotton crotch
Avoid douching except as ordered by physician
Symptoms of infection to report to physician
  Urinary tract
    Difficulty in voiding
    Burning or pain on voiding
    Incontinence
  Vagina
    Heavy discharge
    Itching

Travel Tips

Ensure that patient and/or significant other knows and understands
  Need to prepare ahead
    Inform physician
    Obtain immunizations well in advance of trip when needed
    Have generic prescriptions in duplicate for
      Diabetic medications
      Syringes and needles
      Other medications needed
    Have letter describing condition and treatment (in language of country visiting if possible)
    Buy and "break-in" new shoes well in advance
    Obtain identification necklace or band if patient normally carries a card
    Arrange for special meals when flying
  Importance of carrying supply of insulin and syringes in hand luggage to prevent exposure to extreme temperature and to prevent loss
  Need to take supply of emergency medication to prevent or treat possible travel complications when ordered by physician
  Importance of carrying emergency carbohydrates and a meal
  Method to alter meal, medication, and activity needs when traveling to other time zones
  Where to obtain emergency assistance and how to express needs in language of country visited
  Importance of traveling with a companion when possible

HYPOGLYCEMIA

A low serum glucose level that can be caused by a multitude of factors, including insulinoma, extrapancreatic tumors, hepatic, renal, or endocrine disease, drugs, or gastric surgery; symptoms may be experienced at different levels by individual patients

Assessment
Observations/findings

Diagnostic "Whipple's" triad: low plasma glucose associated with symptoms of hypoglycemia, which resolve with administration of glucose (carbohydrate ingestion)
Fasting plasma glucose of less than 45 to 50 in men and less than 35 to 40 in women
The following signs and symptoms may be due to catecholamine release, central nervous system (CNS) dysfunction, or excessive administration of insulin
  Neurologic
    Lack of muscle coordination
    Lethargy, lassitude
    Headache (may occur in morning)
    Yawning
    Blurred or double vision
    Inability to concentrate
    Confusion
    Anxiety
    Irritability
    Vertigo
    Aphasia
    Numbness, tingling: lips, tongue
    Hyperreflexia, tremor
    Primitive movements: sucking, smacking lips, picking, grasping
    Inappropriate affect
    Abnormal behavior
    Change in personality, work performance, or study habits
    Psychotic behavior
    Nighttime: nightmares, crying out, sleepwalking, unusual sleep posture, restless sleep, difficulty in waking, night sweats, loud respirations during sleep
  Musculoskeletal: weakness
  Cardiovascular
    Pale, moist skin
    Bradycardia to tachycardia
    Hypotension to hypertension
    Diphoresis
    Palpitations
    Faintness

Gastrointestinal
  Hunger
  Nausea

Laboratory/diagnostic studies

Fasting blood sugar of less than 45 to 50 in men and less than 35 to 40 in women

Potential complications

Permanent brain damage if chronic and untreated
Seizures (may be presenting sign)
Coma
Shock

Medical management

50% glucose IV bolus
IV fluids $D_{10}W$
Diet: 300 g of carbohydrate daily

Nursing diagnoses/goals/interventions

ndx Potential for complication: insufficient glucose to meet metabolic needs*

GOAL: *Patient will exhibit decreased risk factors for development of severe hypoglycemia*

Perform neurologic, cardiovascular, and renal assessments q4h; observe for signs of hypoglycemia
Maintain patent IV line for administration of glucose as ordered
Monitor serum glucose levels q2h to 4h and prn
Assess vital signs q2h to 4h; ascultate heart and breath sounds q2h to 4h
Monitor cardiac rate and rhythm continuously if severe reaction occurs
Measure intake and output q2h
Test urine for sugar and acetone q2h
Be alert to factors affecting patient that may precipitate hypoglycemia: infection, fever, increased activity, stress, improper diet
Notify physician of signs and symptoms of hypoglycemia and carry out medical orders

ndx Potential for injury: trauma related to neurologic changes during hypoglycemic episode

GOAL: *Patient will not incur preventable physical injury*

Assess for presence or worsening of neurologic deficits q2h

Plan care to permit adequate rest periods
Assess insulin requirements during increased physical activity; adjust as ordered
Place articles frequently required within easy reach
Instruct patient to call for assistance before getting out of bed
Provide aids to ambulation or mobility (walker, cane, over-the-bed trapeze) as needed
Keep call light within easy reach at all times
Keep bed in low position with side rails up at all times
Maintain seizure precautions as needed
Remove potentially hazardous objects from patient's environment
Be aware that patient's vision may be affected; compensate as needed
Instruct patient to notify nurse of early signs or symptoms of hypoglycemia

ndx Sleep pattern disturbance related to occurrence of hypoglycemia during sleeping hours

GOAL: *Patient will verbalize feelings of being well rested and ready for daily activities*

Ensure adequate intake of carbohydrate during waking hours
Provide high-carbohydrate food source to have available at bedside if patient awakens during night
Check blood glucose prior to bedtime; provide supplemental glucose (carbohydrate) as needed
Encourage patient to establish regular hours of sleep and activity in order to regulate diet and insulin therapy
Provide sleep aids requested by patient
Avoid intake of stimulant in diet
Provide environment conducive to sleep: dim lighting; close door to room; maintain privacy; maintain quiet
Assure patient that you will check on him during the night and will provide needed assistance if sleepwalking or other abnormal sleep disturbances occur
Schedule treatments and medications during daytime and evening hours if possible

ndx Activity intolerance related to insufficient blood sugar levels to maintain energy level

GOAL: *Patient will maintain sufficient energy to complete required daily activities*

Restrict activity to patient's level of tolerance
Space procedures to allow for adequate rest
Discontinue activity at onset of signs or symptoms of hypoglycemia

---

*Not a NANDA-approved nursing diagnosis.

Assist with those activities patient is unable to perform independently

Plan daily activity/rest pattern that will facilitate increasing tolerance for self-care and that considers diet and insulin timing

ndx: Alteration in thought processes related to decreased available glucose for brain metabolism

GOAL: *Patient will maintain reality-based orientation and will interact appropriately with environment*

Provide a stable, calm, and nonstressful environment
    Be consistent in timing and method of treatments, and performance of activities
    Restrict visitors as necessary
    Avoid frequent changing of personnel assigned to care for patient
Explain all procedures to patient clearly and answer all questions; repeat information as necessary
Recognize that mental status changes are due to hypoglycemia; notify physician and initiate appropriate therapy to raise blood sugar
Reorient patient to environment as necessary
Provide clock, calendar, and other reminders of person, time, and place

ndx: Knowledge deficit regarding disease process, and home and self-care

GOAL: *Patient and/or significant other will demonstrate understanding of home and follow-up care through interactive discussion and actual return demonstration, and will explain in own words basic concepts of the disease process*

Discuss symptoms and observations of hypoglycemia, especially early symptoms *specifically* experienced by patient
Explain that hypoglycemic reactions may be different for each person
    Any unusual feeling or symptom must be considered
    Each patient must become familiar with initial reactions
Identify the time reactions will most likely occur; relate to type of insulin prescribed (see Table 7-4)
Emphasize importance of always carrying fast-acting sugar in same pocket, and keeping juice or other drink in same container in same place in refrigerator
Emphasize importance of avoiding reactions: potential complications to body systems
Emphasize importance of early treatment of symptoms
Advise patient to eat 10 g of quick-acting carbohydrate with appearance of initial symptoms

The following foods contain 10 g of quick-acting carbohydrate:

Orange juice	4 oz
Apple juice	4 oz
Grape juice	2 oz
Coca-Cola	3 oz
Ginger ale	4 oz
7-up	3 oz
Corn syrup	2 tsp
Honey	2 tsp
Granulated sugar	2½ tsp
Grape jam	2 tsp
Animal crackers	4
Space Food Stix	1
Gumdrops	10 small
Jelly beans	6
Hard candy such as Life Savers	5 or 6
Dextrose wafers or tablets as labeled	
Glucose paste, amount indicated on label	

Explain importance of eating slowly digested carbohydrate, such as milk, cottage cheese, bread, or peanut butter following response to fast-acting carbohydrate to offset a secondary reaction
Demonstrate method for glucagon administration; action and dosage if ordered
    Use if patient clamps mouth shut or is unable to swallow; patient should respond in 5 to 15 min
    Follow physician's orders if no response
        Phone physician if further orders are not indicated
        Give another injection of glucagon if ordered
        Phone for emergency help or take patient to emergency room of hospital
    Have patient eat slowly digested carbohydrate when he responds
Demonstrate alternate method of glucagon therapy: oral glucose in tube; squeeze directly between cheek and gum area
Explain need to observe closely for further reaction for 1 to 1½ hr; avoid strenuous activity during this time
Explain importance of assessing reason for reaction after reaction is controlled
    Length of time since last meal
    Correct amount of food eaten or meal omitted
    Correct dosage of insulin or oral hypoglycemic taken
    Kinds of activities, exercise, or situations that occurred prior to reaction, planned or unplanned
Discuss symptoms that predispose to reactions and must be reported to physician
"Cold"
"Flu"

Elevated temperature
Nausea, vomiting
Diarrhea
Emphasize importance of reporting reaction to physician as directed
   Give time of onset and length of time until response to care
   Discuss predisposing factor if known
Discuss prevention and early care
   Always carry some form of quick-acting carbohydrate (see list, p. 452); take when first symptoms appear
   Eat correct diet regularly; remember between-meal nourishment when included in diet
   Test urine or blood regularly for glucose and acetone (p. 443); anticipate probable reactions
   Be aware of more activity or emotional stress than normal; follow physician's directions to either notify physician, increase food intake, or decrease dosage of insulin
Discuss prevention of dosage errors
   Check dosage of insulin or oral hypoglycemic with another person when possible
   Record medication when it is taken to prevent duplication (see Table 7-3)
   Always wear medical alert band or chain and carry diabetic identification card

Evaluation

Any impending hypoglycemic reactions are recognized early, and measures to raise blood sugar are taken without delay

Physical injury that is preventable does not occur

Patient receives sufficient undisturbed sleep to promote feeling of being well rested

Patient maintains sufficient energy to complete daily activities

Patient remains oriented to and interactive with environment

Patient and/or significant other demonstrates understanding of home and follow-up care

HYPOPITUITARISM

Decreased or absent secretion of one or more of the anterior pituitary gland hormones; causes are varied and may include malignancies, infection, vascular changes, or physical injury such as head trauma; hypopituitarism may be a disorder of the pituitary gland itself or may be caused by insufficient pituitary stimulation by the hypothalamus

Assessment

*Observations/findings**

General
   Wrinkled, waxy skin
   Hypothermia
   Low blood pressure
   Low serum glucose
Gonadotropin deficiency
   Regression of secondary sex characteristics
   Decreased libido
   Impotence, infertility
   Loss of muscle tone
Thyrotropin deficiency: see Hypothyroidism (p. 427); symptoms will be less severe
ACTH deficiency
   See Adrenocortical Insufficiency (p. 457)
   No hyperpigmentation
   No sodium depletion
Growth hormone deficiency
   Mental retardation in children
   Dwarfism/short stature
   Lack of development of secondary sex characteristics
   High-pitched voice
Prolactin deficiency: absence of lactation in postpartum women

Laboratory/diagnostic studies

Deficiency of serum cortisol, thyroxine, testosterone, and/or estrogen

Lack of compensatory increased levels of serum ACTH, TSH, FSH, and LH

Potential complications

Deficiencies in adults are usually not severe (see specific disease entities)

Medical management

Hormone replacement
   Glucocorticoids
   Thyroxine
   Gonadal steroids
   Growth hormone in children
   GnRH therapy in women to restore fertility

Nursing diagnoses/goals/interventions†

ndx: Disturbance in self-concept: body image related to changes in physical characteristics and capabilities

---

*Findings depend on which hormonal deficiencies are present.
†For additional diagnoses see specific disease process.

GOAL: *Patient will verbalize feelings of self-worth and will take an active role in seeking positive outlook on the future*

Encourage verbalization by patient of feelings related to physical changes

Assist patient with developing coping mechanisms to deal with changes

Reinforce patient's qualities that have positive impact on self-image

Answer questions and clarify misunderstandings regarding diagnosis and permanence or regression of changes

Provide diversional activities of interest and enjoyment to patient

Encourage patient to participate in daily care activities

Assist patient with developing a plan to incorporate any permanent changes into life-style

Demonstrate acceptance of patient as he is and encourage others to do the same

Reinforce behaviors that demonstrate acceptance of changes

ndx: Altered patterns of sexuality related to hormonal deficiencies

GOAL: *Patient, along with significant other (if appropriate), will develop a plan for satisfying sexual desires within limits of the disease process*

Explore with patient and/or significant other usual patterns of sexuality and how current diagnosis may affect these patterns

Encourage patient and/or significant other to explore alternatives to usual patterns that consider limitations of the disease

Initiate referral to appropriate personnel if patient desires

Explore with patient and/or significant other alternatives to becoming parents if appropriate

ndx: Knowledge deficit regarding disease process, treatment, and self-care

GOAL: *Patient and/or significant other will demonstrate understanding of home and follow-up care through interactive discussion and actual return demonstration, and will explain in own words basic concepts of the disease process*

Ensure that patient and/or significant other responsible for patient understands the following*

---

*For further interventions refer to specific disease entity.

Basic concepts of the disease process
Name of medication, dosage, time and method of administration, purpose, side effects, and toxic effects
Importance of regular outpatient follow-up
Need to avoid taking over-the-counter medications without consulting physician
Importance of discussing feelings regarding body changes with significant other
Signs and symptoms of importance to report to physician

Evaluation

Beginning acceptance of physical characteristics and capabilities is demonstrated

Alternatives to usual sexual patterns are developed

Patient demonstrates understanding of disease process, and home and follow-up care

HYPOPHYSECTOMY

Surgical removal of pituitary gland to slow growth of endocrine-dependent tumors, to correct Cushing's disease, and as palliative therapy in certain types of breast and prostate cancer

Postoperative assessment

Observations/findings

Signs and symptoms of increased intracranial pressure (ICP)
  Increasing restlessness
  Decreasing level of consciousness
  Unequal pupils
  Visual changes
  Widened pulse pressure
  Bradycardia
  Respiratory arrest
Gum line incision
  Redness
  Swelling
  Edema
  Drainage or bleeding
Nasal packing
  Intact
  CSF drainage (may be postnasal drip): frequent swallowing, coughing
  Bleeding
  Patent airway

Laboratory/diagnostic studies

Hormone levels
Electrolyte levels
Blood sugar levels

Potential complications

Adrenal insufficiency (p. 457)
Addisonian crisis (p. 457)
Thyroid crisis (p. 427)
Severe hypoglycemia (p. 450)
Diabetes insipidus (p. 456)
Decreased levels of sex hormones

Medical management

IV fluids progressing to po diet
Treatment of complications
Pain management

Nursing diagnoses/goals/interventions

ndx Potential for complication: increased ICP*

GOAL: *Patient will maintain physiologic level of ICP*

In conjunction with physician
  Assess for signs and symptoms of increased ICP qh for first 24 hr, then q4h
  Notify physician at once if onset of restlessness, or pupillary or vital sign changes occur
  Perform neuro checks qh for first 24 hr, then q4h
  Monitor vital signs qh for first 24 hr, then q4h
  Maintain head of bed elevated 30 degrees
  Avoid turning, extending, and flexing head for first 24 hr
  Avoid having patient cough vigorously or strain for any reason
  Maintain calm, dimly lit environment
  Pace care to avoid excessive stimulation; allow adequate rest periods that are undisturbed

ndx Potential for ineffective airway clearance related to nasal packing, postnasal drip, and/or dry oropharynx

GOAL: *Patient will maintain a patent upper airway*

Assess for intactness of nasal packing q2h; determine if packing is slipping posteriorly
Patient must maintain mouth breathing; maintain oral mucous membranes in moist condition
Provide oral care with hydrogen peroxide and mouthwash q2h and prn
Supply humidity to room or via face mask if necessary
Keep suction at bedside; *gently* suction oropharynx only when absolutely necessary
Remind patient to deep breathe and turn q2h; to avoid forceful coughing

---

*Not a NANDA-approved nursing diagnosis.

Monitor for signs of respiratory distress: stridor, wheezing, labored respirations, cyanosis
Check dressing for bleeding and oropharynx for bleeding or CSF leakage q2h to 4h and prn

ndx Impaired skin integrity related to surgical incision

GOAL: *Patient will maintain surgical incision that is well healed and free from infection*

Monitor incision for signs and symptoms of infection q4h
Provide oral care q2h; do not use toothbrush until incision is healed
Avoid foods that would irritate incision

ndx Alteration in comfort: pain at surgical site, headache

GOAL: *Patient will express feelings of comfort*

Assess patient for verbal and nonverbal signs of pain
Be aware that severe headache may be a sign of increased ICP
Discuss with patient factors that relieve pain and facilitate use of these as possible
Assist patient with finding position of comfort, maintaining neutral head position and head elevated 30 degrees
Provide means of distraction from pain: guided imagery, relaxation, soft music, visitors as tolerated
Administer pain medications as ordered; be aware that they may mask signs of increased ICP

ndx Knowledge deficit regarding home and follow-up care

GOAL: *Patient and/or significant other will demonstrate understanding of home and follow-up care through interactive discussion and actual return demonstration*

Explain that decrease in taste and smell for several months is expected
Explain need to avoid persons with infections, especially upper urinary infections (URIs)
Discuss symptoms of incisional or systemic infection to report to physician
Emphasize importance of avoiding vigorous coughing, straining, and nose-blowing
Emphasize importance of ongoing patient care
Discuss signs and symptoms of hormonal imbalances to report to physician
Teach name of medication, dosage, time and method of administration, side effects, and toxic effects

Evaluation

Increased ICP is prevented if possible
Any signs or symptoms of increased ICP are detected and reported to physician without delay
Patient maintains patent upper airway
Surgical incision heals without infection
Patient expresses feeling of comfort
Patient and/or significant other understands home and follow-up care

CENTRAL DIABETES INSIPIDUS

Disorder of hypothalamus or posterior pituitary that results in insufficient synthesis or secretion of antidiuretic hormone; consequently, the renal mechanism for concentration of urine is impaired and large amounts of dilute urine are excreted; causes may include head injury, neurologic surgery, and hypothalamic tumors

Assessment
Observations/findings

Neurologic
    Headache
    Irritability
    Apathy
    General weakness
Gastrointestinal
    Thirst
    Weight loss
    Anorexia
    Constipation
Renal
    Polyuria to 10 L daily
    Frequency
    Nocturia
Integumentary
    Very dry skin
    Poor turgor

Laboratory/diagnostic studies

Increased serum osmolality
Urine specific gravity of less than 1.010
Urine osmolality of less than 300 mosm/L; increases with administration of pitressin
Electrolyte imbalances
Water deprivation studies
Hypertonic saline test

Potential complications

Severe dehydration
Hypotension

Medical management

ADH replacement therapy
    Pitressin tannate in oil
    Aqueous pitressin
    Lypressin nasal solution
Synthetic vasopressin: DDAVP

Nursing diagnoses/goals/interventions

ndx: Fluid volume deficit related to inability of renal tubules to concentrate urine in absence of ADH

GOAL: *Patient will exhibit decreased risk factors for developing severe hypovolemia*

Provide sufficient fluid of patient's preference to maintain equal intake and output per 24 hr
Supplement oral intake with IV fluids as ordered
Monitor intake and output q4h and notify physician if output is greater than 100 ml over intake
Weigh patient daily, observing for weight loss or gain
With each voiding check urine for specific gravity and send urine for osmolality daily
Assess for signs and symptoms of hypovolemia: tachycardia, poor skin turgor, weak pulses, low blood pressure, cool skin, increased body temperature, dry mucous membranes, changes in mental status
Report occurrence of any of the above signs or symptoms to physician and initiate medical orders without delay
Administer ADH replacement therapy as ordered

ndx: Alteration in bowel elimination: constipation related to excessive fluid loss

GOAL: *Patient will excrete stool that is soft and easily passed*

Maintain diet of preference that contains foods high in fiber
Maintain fluid intake equal to or slightly greater than output
Administer laxatives and stool softeners as ordered
Encourage regular exercise as tolerated
Instruct patient to respond immediately to urge to defecate
Assist patient with recognizing activities that stimulate urge to defecate (drinking warm liquids)
Encourage patient to attempt to defecate at same time daily in order to establish a routine

ndx: Knowledge deficit regarding disease process, treatment, and self-care

GOAL: *Patient and/or significant other will demonstrate understanding of home and follow-up care through interactive discussion and actual return demonstration, and will explain basic concepts of disease process in own words*

Explain basic concepts of disease process
Teach name of medication, purpose, time and method of administration, dosage, and toxic and side effects
Emphasize importance of maintaining fluid intake equal to output
Explain need to avoid liquids that may cause a diuretic effect: coffee, alcohol, tea
Emphasize importance of regular outpatient follow-up
Explain need to avoid taking over-the-counter medications without consulting physician

Evaluation

Intravascular fluid volume remains within normal limits (normal serum osmolality)
Bowel movements are regular, soft, and easily passed
Patient and/or significant other demonstrates understanding of disease process, and home and follow-up care

ADRENOCORTICAL INSUFFICIENCY

Hypofunction of the adrenal cortex; primary adrenocortical insufficiency results in a deficiency of mineralocorticoids and glucocorticoids; secondary insufficiency results in a deficiency of only glucocorticoids; primary insufficiency is usually due to idiopathic atrophy of the cortex, whereas secondary insufficiency may be due to pituitary tumor, postpartum pituitary necrosis, tumor of the third ventricle, head trauma, or optic gliomas

Assessment

Observations/findings

Neurologic
  Vertigo
  Syncope
  Mental fatigue
  Apathy
Musculoskeletal
  Weakness
  Fatigue
  Muscle wasting
  Muscle aching
Cardiovascular
  Hypotension
  Decreased contractility
  Decreased cardiac output
  Postural hypotension with reflex tachycardia
  Decreased tolerance to cold or stress
  Hypovolemia
Gastrointestinal
  Weight loss
  Anorexia
  Nausea, vomiting
  Salt craving
  Diarrhea
Integumentary
  Hyperpigmentation
  Decreased body hair
Sexuality/reproductive
  Loss of secondary sex characteristics (especially in females)
  Amenorrhea
  Decreased libido

Diagnostic/laboratory studies

Increased serum ADH
Markedly increased serum ACTH
Hyponatremia
Hyperkalemia
Increased BUN
Metabolic acidosis
Increased plasma renin levels
Decreased plasma cortisol, no response to administration of ACTH
Decreased plasma aldosterone
Subnormal excretion in urine of 17-hydroxycorticoids and aldosterone-18-glucuronide

Potential complications

Addisonian crisis: medical emergency involving intensification of symptoms of adrenal crisis; usually precipitated by acute infection, trauma, surgery, or excessive loss of body salts
  Observations/findings in adrenal crisis include
    Severe pain: back, abdomen, extremities
    Severe headache
    Lassitude
    Confusion
    Restlessness
    Profound asthenia
    Coma
    Hypopyrexia
    Severe hypotension
    Shock
    Cardiac arrest
    Renal failure
    Azotemia
    Death

Medical management

IV hydration and sodium replacement
Glucocorticoids: dexamethazone, hydrocortisone
Mineralocorticoids: fludrocortisone
In crisis: vasopressors, plasma expanders, supportive therapy
Antibiotics if infection is cause of episode

Nursing diagnoses/goals/interventions

ndx: Fluid volume deficit related to inability of renal tubules to retain sodium and water

GOAL: *Patient will exhibit decreased risk factors for development of fluid volume deficit*

Force fluid intake to 3000 ml/day or as ordered
Monitor serum sodium levels q8h as ordered
Measure intake and output q8h and prn; report intake less than output
Weigh patient daily; observe for weight loss
Administer IV fluids and sodium replacement as ordered
Assess for signs and symptoms of hypovolemia or dehydration: poor skin turgor, weak pulses, tachycardia, thirst, low blood pressure, cool skin, increased body temperature, dry mucous membranes, change in mental status
Report occurrence of any of the above signs or symptoms to physician without delay; carry out medical orders received
Administer antiemetics as ordered
Provide diet high in sodium

ndx: Potential for infection related to inability of adrenal cortex to produce steroids in times of stress

GOAL: *Patient will exhibit decreased risk factors for development of infection*

Maintain environment as stress free as possible
Monitor for signs and symptoms of infection; report if detected (especially URI or urinary tract infection [UTI])
Have patient turn, cough, and deep breathe q2h while on bed rest
Avoid unnecessary invasive procedures (urinary catheterization)
Use sterile technique when caring for any skin leisons, tubes, drains, or IV lines
Culture suspicious wounds or secretions
Maintain optimal nutritional status
Avoid placing patient in room with other potentially infectious patients
Avoid having nursing personnel with URI or other infection care for patient

ndx: Potential for injury related to inability to tolerate environmental stresses

GOAL: *Patient will exhibit improved ability to tolerate environmental stresses*

Select quiet, nonstimulating room with noninfectious roommate
Avoid exposure to cold: provide extra blankets; have patient wear bed socks and use warm robe when out of bed
Give consistent care
Explain all procedures
Provide emotional support: answer all questions, and discuss disease process and implications as patient desires
  Listen for expression of anxiety/fear
  Encourage communication with significant other
Administer steroid therapy as ordered
Medicate for pain or nausea as required
Encourage regular rest periods during activity
Anticipate stressful situations and diffuse as possible
Consider need for increased doses of steroids during periods of stress (consult physician)
Always administer steroid therapy on time; do not alter hours of administration of dose abruptly
Monitor for signs and symptoms of impending crisis
  Vital sign abnormalities (decreased blood pressure, high pulse rate, fever)
  Change in level of consciousness (confusion, restlessness, stupor)
  Abnormal fluid/electrolyte values

ndx: Activity intolerance related to decreased cardiac output

GOAL: *Patient will maintain sufficient energy to complete required daily activities and will perform required daily activities in such a manner as to conserve cardiac output*

Allow patient to move at own pace
Assist with active or perform passive ROM exercises while patient is on bed rest
Assist with ambulation and bed mobility as needed
Provide patient with assistive devices: walker, cane, over-the-bed trapeze, side rails
Anticipate need for help with daily activities (grooming, feeding, toileting)
Restrict patient's activities to level of tolerance

Discontinue activity at first signs of intolerance: tachycardia, fatigue, dyspnea, cardiac dysrhythmias, drop in blood pressure, complaints of vertigo

ndx: Alteration in comfort: pain (headache, back, extremity, abdominal) related to fluid and electrolyte imbalances

GOAL: *Patient will verbalize feeling of physical comfort*

Identify with patient location, severity of pain, and factors that worsen or improve pain

Explore with patient measures to reduce or relieve pain: positioning, use of pillows for support, warm or cold compresses, manipulation or massage of body part or area

Monitor effectiveness of above interventions at routine intervals

Assess need for and administer pain medication as ordered

Provide distraction from pain (conversation, visitors, reading materials, quiet music)

Assist patient with developing pain management techniques such as progressive relaxation or guided imagery

ndx: Alteration in thought processes related to deficient levels of adrenal steroids

GOAL: *Patient will maintain a reality-based orientation and will take an active role in self-care, with consideration of physical limitations*

Provide a stable, calm, and nonstressful environment
   Be consistent in timing and performance of activities and procedures
   Restrict visitors as necessary
   Avoid frequent changing of health care personnel
   Anticipate and prevent emotionally stressful situations

Plan care with patient

Inform patient that activities may be restricted

Explain all procedures to patient and answer any questions

Explain planned activities for the day clearly; repeat as necessary

Assess patient's level of consciousness q4h and reorient patient to environment as needed

Encourage patient to keep personal articles at bedside: pictures of family, clock or watch, calendar

ndx: Potential for complication: multisystem failure (adrenal crisis)*

GOAL: *Patient will exhibit decreased risk factors for development of adrenal crisis*

Perform cardiovascular, neurologic, respiratory, and renal assessments q4h; report changes or abnormal findings to physician

Assess vital signs q4h and prn; report abnormal findings to physician

Monitor cardiac rhythm continuously if dysrhythmias occur

Monitor intake and output q4h and prn; report output greater than intake

Position patient to promote cardiovascular and respiratory function

Carry out medical orders received if adrenal crisis develops

ndx: Knowledge deficit regarding disease process, treatment, and self-care

GOAL: *Patient and/or significant other will demonstrate understanding of home and follow-up care through interactive discussion and actual return demonstration, and will explain in own words basic concepts of the disease process*

Explain basic concepts of the disease process

Give reasons for physical and emotional changes

Teach name of medication, dosage, time and method of administration, and toxic and side effects

Explain need to avoid taking over-the-counter medications without consulting physician

Demonstrate method of administering IM injections in case of emergency

Emphasize importance of regular exercise alternating with rest periods and avoiding strenuous exercise

Teach patient to recognize and avoid stressful situations

Explain need to avoid persons with infectious diseases (especially URIs)

Instruct patient to wear medical alert band and inform all health care providers regarding disease

Explain need for high-sodium, low-potassium diet with plenty of fluids

Evaluation

Intravascular fluid volume remains within normal limits

Patient does not develop avoidable infection

Any signs or symptoms of impending crisis are recognized in a timely manner, and medical orders are carried out without delay

Patient is able to complete required daily activities

Patient verbalizes feeling of comfort

---

*Not a NANDA-approved nursing diagnosis.

Patient remains oriented to environment and takes an active role in own care

Patient and/or significant other demonstrates understanding of disease process and principles of home and follow-up care

CUSHING'S SYNDROME

Results from chronic exposure to excessive glucocorticoid hormones; affects carbohydrate, protein, and lipid metabolism; may be produced by various neoplasms or by exogenous glucocorticoid administration (When Cushing's syndrome is produced by bilateral adrenal hyperplasia due to excessive secretion of ACTH, it is called Cushing's disease.)

Assessment
Observations/findings

Neurologic
   Headache
   Lability of mood: depression to mania
Musculoskeletal
   Truncal obesity with thin extremities
   Supraclavicular fat pads
   Buffalo hump
   Moon face
   Backache
   Muscle weakness or wasting
   Osteoporosis
Cardiovascular
   Hypertension
   Pitting edema
Renal
   Renal calculi
   Polyuria
Metabolic
   Impaired wound healing
   Increased susceptibility to infection
   Carbohydrate intolerance
Integumentary
   Facial plethora
   Increased pigmentation
   Acne
   Red cheeks
   Striae
   Easily bruised
   Baldness/hairline recession
Sexuality/reproductive
   Female masculinization
   Menstrual disorders
   Male feminization
   Impotence
   Decreased libido

Laboratory/diagnostic studies

Hyperglycemia
Metabolic alkalosis
Hypokalemia
Elevated plasma ACTH
Elevated serum sodium and plasma cortisol
Plasma cortisol not suppressed with dexamethasone
White blood cell count (WBC) elevated
Hyperactive response to 8 hr ACTH stimulation test
Increased 24 hr urine cortisol and 17-hydroxycorticosteroids
Increased response to metyrapone

Potential complication

Congestive heart failure

Medical management

Removal or irradiation of pituitary adenoma if present (most common cause)
Medications
   Mitotane
   Aminogluthethimide
   Metyrapone
Adrenalectomy

Nursing diagnoses/goals/interventions

ndx: Disturbance in self-concept: body image related to musculoskeletal, integumentary, and sexuality/reproductive changes

GOAL: *Patient will verbalize beginning of acceptance of changes in body appearance*

Respect patient's wishes for privacy
Be sensitive to needs
Set aside time each shift for active listening and emotional support
Maintain environment conducive to discussing body image changes
Discuss with patient feelings related to body image changes
Assist patient with identifying and developing personal strengths and coping mechanisms for dealing with physical changes
Discuss palliative measures for hirsutism (hair removal)
Consult mental health nursing specialist

ndx: Potential for infection related to impaired immune responses

GOAL: *Patient will exhibit decreased risk factors for development of infection*

Monitor for and report any signs or symptoms of infection
Monitor temperature q4h
Have patient turn, cough, and deep breathe q2h while on bed rest
Avoid unnecessary invasive procedures (urinary catheterization)
Use sterile technique when caring for any skin lesions, tubes, drains, or IV sites
Culture suspicious wound sites or secretions
Maintain optimal nutritional status
Avoid placing patient in room with other potentially infectious patient
Avoid having personnel with URI or other infection care for patient

ndx: Alteration in thought processes related to excessive cortisol secretion

GOAL: *Patient will express emotions appropriate for situation and will maintain a reality-based orientation*

Provide a stable, calm, and nonstressful environment
  Be consistent in timing and performance of activities and procedures
  Restrict visitors as necessary
  Avoid frequent changing of personnel
  Prevent emotionally upsetting situations
Plan care with patient
Anticipate needs
Inform patient that activities may be restricted
Provide diversional activities and materials
Reorient patient to environment as needed
Explain procedures slowly and clearly; repeat as necessary

ndx: Activity intolerance related to musculoskeletal weakness (increased protein catabolism)

GOAL: *Patient will maintain sufficient energy to complete required daily activities*

Allow patient to move at own pace; use side rails and overhead trapeze
Assist with active or perform passive ROM exercises if patient is on bed rest
Assist with and provide aids to ambulation (walker, cane) as necessary
Anticipate need for help with daily activities: grooming, toileting
Restrict activities to patient's level of tolerance
Discontinue activity at first signs of intolerance: tachycardia, dyspnea, fatigue

ndx: Potential impairment of skin integrity related to less than optimal nutritional status and/or fragile capillaries

GOAL: *Patient will maintain skin free from breakdown*

Assess for redness or breakdown q8h; if patient is on bed rest, assess q4h
Administer skin care to pressure points q4h and as needed
Use oil or lotion in bathwater
Use elbow and heel protectors
Place patient on decubitus-prevention mattress or bed
Assist and encourage patient to change positions frequently
Maintain optimal nutritional status
Avoid use of harsh soaps or rough towels

ndx: Potential for electrolyte imbalance: hypernatremia, hypokalemia, hyperglycemia*

GOAL: *Patient will exhibit decreased risk factors for development of electrolyte imbalance*

Monitor electrolyte values q4h to 8h and report abnormal findings to physician
Monitor intake and output q4h
Check urine for sugar and acetone q24h
Check blood glucose q8h; administer insulin as ordered
Weigh patient daily
Avoid excessive fluid intake when patient is hypernatremic
Monitor ECG for abnormalities associated with electrolyte imbalances
Monitor blood pressure and pulse q4h and report significant changes from patient's baseline
Maintain high-protein, high-potassium, low-sodium diet

ndx: Potential for complication: hypertension*

GOAL: *Patient will exhibit decreased risk factors for development of hypertension*

Monitor blood pressure for orthostatic changes q8h
Observe for gradual elevations in blood pressure
Report elevations in blood pressure to physician
Administer diuretics as ordered; monitor for hypokalemia

---

*Not a NANDA-approved nursing diagnosis.

Administer supplemental potassium as ordered
Maintain a stress-free environment if possible

ndx: Knowledge deficit regarding disease process, treatment, and self-care

GOAL: *Patient and/or significant other will demonstrate understanding of home care and follow-up instructions through interactive discussion and actual return demonstration, and will explain in own words basic concepts of the disease process*

Explain basic concepts of the disease
Give reasons for physical and emotional changes
Teach name of medication, dosage, time and method of administration, purpose, side effects, and toxic effects
Explain that medication must not be discontinued without consulting physician
Explain need to avoid taking over-the-counter medications without consulting physician
Explain that condition is potentially controllable if treatment regimen is followed
Emphasize importance of ongoing outpatient care

Evaluation

Beginning acceptance of body image changes is manifested
Preventable infection does not occur
Patient remains oriented to environment and takes active role in care
Effective activity/rest patterns are maintained
Skin remains intact
Electrolytes remain within normal values
Any hypertension is recognized early, and interventions to resolve it are undertaken without delay
Patient and/or significant other demonstrate understanding of disease process and principles of home and follow-up care

PRIMARY ALDOSTERONISM

Overproduction of mineralocorticoids by the adrenal cortex caused by benign adenoma, or less commonly, by carcinoma or hyperplasia of the adrenal cortex

Assessment
Observations/findings

Neurologic
  Headache
  Retinopathy
  Muscle weakness
  Fatigue
  Paresthesia
  Paralysis of arms and legs
  Tetany
  Personality disturbances
  Autonomic dysfunction
Cardiovascular
  Hypertension
  Postural hypotension without reflex tachycardia
  Increased pulse when squatting
  Cardiomegaly
  Decreased conduction through myocardium
Renal
  Polyuria, especially nocturnal
  Polydipsia
  Azotemia

Laboratory/diagnostic studies

Elevated plasma aldosterone
Suppressed/nonstimulatable plasma renin activity
Failure to supress aldosterone with usual maneuvers
Hypernatremia
Hypokalemia
Hypervolemia
Metabolic alkalosis
Urine excretion (24 hr) of 18-glucuronide
ECG
  Depressed ST segments and T waves; appearance of U waves
  Premature ventricular contractions
Iodocholesterol scan
CT scan of adrenal glands to localize an adenoma or to differentiate hyperplasia from adenoma
Adrenal venous catheterization

Potential complications

Renal failure
Heart failure

Medical management

Adrenalectomy
  Unilateral for adenoma
  Bilateral for hyperplasia
Spironolactone
Low-sodium diet

Nursing diagnoses/goals/interventions

ndx: Alteration in fluid volume: excess intravascular volume related to hypernatremia

GOAL: *Patient will exhibit decreased risk factors for development of intravascular fluid volume overlaod*

Weigh patient daily; report to physician if gain of over 0.5 kg occurs

Measure intake and output q8h

Maintain low-sodium diet

Monitor serum sodium levels q8h

Monitor for signs and symptoms of fluid overload: pulmonary edema (dyspnea, orthopnea, crackles in lung fields)

Monitor chest x-ray results

Monitor vital signs q4h and prn; observe for increased pulse, development of S_3 gallop, and labored respirations

Notify physician of development or worsening of any of the above signs or symptoms

Administer diuretics as ordered

ndx: Potential for electrolyte imbalance related to hypokalemia*

GOAL: *Patient will exhibit decreased risk factors for development of injury related to hypokalemia*

Maintain high-potassium diet: avocado, apricots, bananas, meat, poultry, potatoes, milk

Administer potassium supplements as ordered

Monitor serum potassium levels q8h and prn

Monitor for signs and symptoms of hypokalemia
  ECG changes (ectopic beats, decreased T wave amplitude, increased U wave amplitude)
  Muscular weakness
  Neurologic impairments

Report development of any of the above signs or symptoms to physician and carry out medical orders received

ndx: Activity intolerance related to muscle weakness, fatigue, paresthesia, and/or autonomic dysfunction

GOAL: *Patient will maintain sufficient energy to complete required daily activities*

Allow patient to move at own pace; allow and encourage use of side rails and trapeze for assistance

Assist patient with active ROM exercises q8h if patient is on bed rest

Assist with and encourage ambulation if patient is able

Provide aids to ambulation such as a walker or cane

Anticipate postural hypotension when patient gets out of bed or chair; if it occurs, have patient sit or lie down with head lower than heart

Anticipate need for help with daily activities: grooming, feeding, toileting

Restrict activities to patient's level of tolerance

Discontinue activity at first signs of intolerance: tachycardia, dyspnea, fatigue, diaphoresis

ndx: Potential for physical injury related to neurologic and cardiovascular compromise

GOAL: *Patient will not incur preventable physical injury*

Assess for presence of or worsening of neurologic and/or cardiovascular symptoms q8h

Plan care to permit adequate rest periods

Place articles frequently required within easy reach at all times

Instruct patient to call for assistance before getting out of bed

Keep call light within patient's reach at all times

Keep bed in low position and side rails up at all times

Assist patient with personal hygiene (e.g., shaving)

Utilize safety measures (padded side rails for tetany, soft restraints) as needed

Remove potentially hazardous materials and objects from patient's environment

Assist with ambulation and transfer patient from bed to chair as needed

Be aware that patient's vision may be affected; assist as necessary

ndx: Knowledge deficit regarding disease process, treatment, and self-care

GOAL: *Patient and/or significant other will demonstrate understanding of home care and follow-up instructions through interactive discussion and actual return demonstration, and will explain in own words basic concepts of the disease process*

Explain basic concepts of the disease

Teach name of medication, dosage, time and method of administration, purpose, side effects, and toxic effects

Explain need to avoid taking over-the-counter medications without consulting physician

Emphasize importance of ongoing outpatient care

Emphasize importance of regular exercise alternating with rest periods

Instruct patient to maintain therapeutic low-sodium, high-potassium diet

Evaluation

Intravascular fluid volume excess is minimized

Any signs or symptoms of intravascular fluid volume excess are recognized and reported without delay; medical orders are carried out

---

*Not a NANDA-approved nursing diagnosis.

Risk factors for developing hypokalemia are minimized

Any signs or symptoms of hypokalemia are recognized and reported without delay; medical orders are carried out

Patient is able to complete daily physical activities that are required

Preventable physical injury does not occur

Patient and/or significant other demonstrates understanding of disease process and principles of home and follow-up care

PHEOCHROMOCYTOMA

A rare tumor that may occur in any sympathetic ganglion in the body; however, the vast majority (90%) arise from the adrenal medulla; tumors arising outside the adrenal medulla are called paragangliomas; these tumors usually secrete norepinephrine, which accounts for the most common clinical manifestations

Assessment
Observations/findings

Neurologic
   Headache
   Syncope
   Anxiety/nervousness
   Tremor
   Hyperreflexia
   Insomnia
   Paresthesia
   Tetany
   Blurred vision
Cardiovascular
   Hypertension
   Precordial pain
   Excess diaphoresis
   Tachycardia
   Palpitations
   Flushing
   Postural hypotension
   Arrhythmias
   Heat intolerance
Respiratory
   Tachypnea
   Dyspnea
Gastrointestinal/nutritional
   Abdominal pain
   Hyperglycemia
   Anorexia
   Nausea, vomiting
   Weight loss
   Constipation
Renal: decreased urine output

Laboratory/diagnostic studies

Elevated serum catecholamines
Elevated urine metanephrines and vanillylmandelic acid
Failure of serum catecholamines to respond by suppression after administration of clonidine
Glucosuria
Abdominal CT scan showing tumor location

Potential complications

Heart failure
Renal failure
Cerebrovascular accident (CVA)
Myocarditis
Arrhythmias
Surgical morbidity or mortality

Medical management

Surgical removal of the tumor(s)
Medications
   Alpha- and beta-adrenergic blockers
   Alpha-methylparatyrosine

Nursing diagnoses/goals/interventions

ndx: Alteration in tissue perfusion related to hypertensive episodes

GOAL: *Patient will maintain adequate tissue perfusion and diminish/control events that stimulate a hypertensive episode*

Remain with patient during episodes of hypertension
   Check blood pressure q10 to 15 min
   Be prepared to administer antihypertensive medications
   Position patient with head elevated 30 degrees to minimize effects on ICP
   Perform neuro checks; auscultate chest for heart sounds, rate, and rhythm
   Provide a calm, low-stimulus atmosphere
Review events prior to episode to determine etiology; discuss methods of avoiding precipitating events with patient
Provide quiet environment for adequate periods of rest
Avoid caffeine-containing foods and beverages
Administer antihypertensives as ordered

ndx: Sleep pattern disturbance: insomnia related to increased levels of circulating catecholamines

GOAL: *Patient will verbalize being well rested and ready for the day's activities*

Provide sleep aids requested by patient: quiet music, warm drink
Discourage frequent daytime sleeping
Avoid intake of stimulants in diet
Assist patient with establishing a regular pattern of activity
Provide environment conducive to sleep: dim lighting; close door to room; maintain quiet and privacy
Avoid disturbing patient at night for unnecessary procedures
Schedule treatments, procedures, and medications for daytime and evening hours when possible

ndx: Alteration in nutrition: less than body requirements related to abdominal pain, anorexia, nausea, and/or constipation

GOAL: *Patient will maintain caloric, nutritive, and fluid intake sufficient to maintain a stable weight*

Encourage patient to eat several small meals daily when not nauseated
Consult patient as to food preferences and have them available if possible
Ask patient's family to bring favorite foods from home, within limits of therapeutic diet
Weigh patient daily
Medicate as necessary for nausea 30 min prior to meals
Assist patient with arranging meal tray and with feeding self if necessary
Offer between-meal supplements
Assess for occurrence of bowel movement daily
Provide diet rich in fiber
Administer laxatives, stool softners, and enemas as ordered

ndx: Activity intolerance related to cardiovascular and neurologic changes

GOAL: *Patient will maintain sufficient energy to complete required daily activities*

Plan care to allow sufficient time for patient to accomplish activities
Do not hurry patient
Arrange articles and assist with personal hygiene
Assist with active or perform passive ROM exercises q8h
Encourage patient to ambulate and assist as necessary
Provide aids to ambulation (walker, cane) as needed
Restrict activity to patient's level of tolerance
Discontinue activity at first sign of fatigue
Plan daily activities and rest times that will facilitate increasing tolerance for self-care

ndx: Knowledge deficit regarding disease process, treatment, and self-care

GOAL: *Patient and/or significant other will demonstrate understanding of home care and follow-up instructions through interactive discussion and actual return demonstration, and will explain in own words basic concepts of the disease process*

Explain basic concepts of the disease process
Discuss methods for avoiding hypertensive episodes
Explain need to avoid tyramine-containing foods
Discuss pain management
Teach name of medication, dosage, time and method of administration, purpose, side effects, and toxic effects
Explain need to avoid taking over-the-counter medications without consulting physician
Emphasize importance of ongoing outpatient care
Refer to Adrenalectomy (below) for preoperative patient teaching

Evaluation

Hypertensive episodes are minimized
Hypertensive episodes are recognized in a timely manner, and medical interventions are carried out without delay
Effective activity/rest patterns are maintained
Stable weight is maintained
Patient and/or significant other demonstrates understanding of disease process and principles of home and follow-up care

ADRENALECTOMY

Surgical removal of the adrenal gland(s); unilateral removal may be performed for benign adenomas, whereas bilateral removal is done for malignant ACTH-producing tumors; other diseases of the adrenal glands, such as Cushing's disease, may also require removal

Postoperative assessment
Observations/findings

Signs of adrenal crisis (p. 457)
    Falling blood pressure
    Tachycardia; weak, thready pulses
    Elevated temperature
    Restlessness

Severe weakness
Lethargy
Headache
Hypoglycemia
Electrolyte imbalance
Seizures
Dehydration
Flatulence
Impaired wound healing
Site of incision
  Redness
  Pain
  Swelling
  Drainage, bleeding
Respiratory distress
  Atelectasis
  Decreased breath sounds
  Tachypnea, bradypnea

Laboratory/diagnostic studies

Decreased serum aldosterone levels
Decreased serum steroid levels
Hyperglycemia
Hyperkalemia

Potential complications

Adrenal crisis
Coma
Cardiac arrest

Medical management

IV fluids progressing to po diet when bowel sounds return
Treatment of complications
Pain management

Nursing diagnoses/goals/interventions

ndx: Potential for complication: adrenal crisis*

GOAL: *Patient will exhibit decreased risk factors for development of adrenal crisis*

Perform cardiovascular, neurologic, respiratory, and renal assessments q4h; report changes or abnormal findings to physician
Assess vital signs q4h and prn; report abnormal findings to physician
Monitor cardiac rhythm continuously if dysrhythmias occur
Monitor intake and output q4h and prn; report output that is greater than intake
Position patient to promote cardiovascular and respiratory function
Carry out medical orders received if adrenal crisis develops

ndx: Potential for fluid/electrolyte imbalance: unstable levels of circulating steroids*

GOAL: *Patient will exhibit decreased risk factors for development of fluid/electrolyte imbalances*

Force fluids; maintain IV fluids to 3000 ml/day
Monitor serum electrolytes q8h and prn as ordered
Measure intake and output as ordered; report intake less than output
Weigh patient daily; observe for weight loss
Administer sodium replacement as ordered in diet or IV fluids
Assess for signs and symptoms of fluid/electrolyte imbalance: poor skin turgor, weak pulses, tachycardia, thirst, low blood pressure, cool skin, cardiac arrhythmias, increased body temperature, change in mental status
Report any of the above signs or symptoms to physician without delay and carry out medical orders received
Check for urine sugar and acetone q8h or check blood sugar via fingerstick

ndx: Alteration in comfort: pain at surgical site

GOAL: *Patient will express feeling of comfort*

Assess for verbal and nonverbal signs of pain
Discuss with patient factors that increase or decrease pain
Assist patient with finding position of comfort
Assist patient with using distraction as means of pain control: guided imagery, progressive relaxation, soft music, visitors
Maintain support of surgical incision during movement or ambulation
Progress ambulation as tolerated
Administer pain medications as needed and ordered

ndx: Impaired skin integrity related to surgical incision

GOAL: *Patient will maintain surgical incision free from infection and well healed*

Prevent tension on suture line: maintain proper body alignment; use pillows for support during movement
Instruct patient in proper way to move from lying to sitting or standing position, using pillows for support

---

*Not a NANDA-approved nursing diagnosis.

Change dressing daily and when wet; observe for signs of infection or impaired healing: redness, foul drainage, fever

Promote incisional healing: prevent stress on suture line; remove sutures when ordered; use dry, sterile dressing when changing; use only necessary amount of tape and remove in direction of incision; cleanse site daily as ordered; instruct patient to avoid touching incision site

ndx: Knowledge deficit regarding home and follow-up care

GOAL: *Patient and/or significant other will demonstrate understanding of home and follow-up care through interactive discussion and actual return demonstration*

Discuss symptoms of adrenal crisis
Emphasize importance of reporting physical and emotional stress situations to physician immediately
    Gastroenteritis
    Elevated temperature
    "Flu"
    Infections, no matter how minor
    Emotionally upsetting situations (avoiding stressful situations when possible)
Teach care of incision
Discuss symptoms of infection to report to physician
    Incision
    General
Explain need to avoid persons with infections, especially URIs
Emphasize importance of
    Adequate rest
    Moderate exercise
    Good nutrition
    Ongoing outpatient care, being certain to inform all physicians and dentists of surgery and prescribed medications
Explain need to avoid strenuous, unaccustomed activity and fasting or fad diets
Emphasize importance of wearing medical alert band or chain and carrying identification card
Explain that if surgery was for Cushing's syndrome, these symptoms will slowly recede
Explain that if bilateral adrenalectomy was performed, steroid therapy will be needed for remainder of life

Evaluation

Any signs or symptoms of adrenal crisis are detected in a timely manner and referred to physician
Patient expresses feelings of comfort
Surgical incision heals without infection or other complication
Patient and/or significant other understands home and follow-up care

CORTICOSTEROID THERAPY

Observations

Sodium, water retention
    Weight gain
    Edema
    Hypertension
Potassium depletion
    Weakness
    Fatigue
    Alkalosis
Calcium, phosphorus depletion
    Pathologic fractures
    Bone pain
Iatrogenic Cushing's syndrome
    Moon face
    Truncal obesity
    Buffalo hump
Increased hydrochloric acid production
    Gastric ulcer
        Vomiting
        Tarry stools
        Abdominal pain
    Increased appetite
Eye: with local administration
    Corneal ulceration
    Herpetic infection
Skin
    Thin
    Purple-red striae
    Ecchymosis
    Acne
    Hirsutism
Increased ICP
    Mood alteration
        Euphoria
        Depression
        Weird dreams
        Withdrawal from social contact
        References to suicide
    Restlessness
    Insomnia
Symptoms of diabetes mellitus
Menstrual irregularities, usually amenorrhea
Increased susceptibility to infection
Adrenal crisis (p. 457)

Local reaction to injection
　Atrophy
　Abscess
　Hyperpigmentation, hypopigmentation
　Leukocytosis without a shift to the left

Interventions

Understand that if medication is given by parenteral route, correct dosage of solution and drops per minute must be maintained; *never alter rate or dosage* unless ordered

Understand that if medication is given by oral route, dose must be given as scheduled; *never alter time schedule or dosage* unless ordered

Understand that alternate-day therapy may be ordered to minimize side effects

Choose room placement carefully; place patient in noninfectious, nonstressful environment

Check BP and P q4h to 6h

Check T and R qid

Weigh patient daily at same time with same clothing and scale

Test urine for sugar daily or monitor glucose by fingerstick

Measure intake and output; note and report great discrepancies between intake and output

Maintain diet as permitted by primary disease process or low-sodium, high-protein, high-calcium, high-potassium diet

Check muscular strength qid

Encourage activity as permitted by primary disease process

Assist with active or perform passive ROM exercises q4h to 6h

Determine ability and tolerance for exercise; restrict activity to this level to prevent injury

Perform hygiene and mouth care gently
　Avoid skin abrasions or trauma
　Use sheepskin, foam pads, or heel and elbow guards for friable skin areas

Check for changes in skin color, tone, or edema bid

Check healing process daily if wound or incision is present

Use sterile technique for all invasive procedures and dressing changes

Promote sleep
　Soothing back rubs
　Warm drinks (avoid coffee, tea)
　Quiet environment
　Wrinkle-free bed
　Medication as ordered

Act as buffer between patient and environment to reduce stress

Plan care with patient
Avoid inconsistencies
Explain all procedures
Involve family or significant other in reducing stress
Provide atmosphere for discussion of feelings; explain reason for mood changes

Patient teaching/discharge outcome

Ensure that patient and/or significant other knows and understands
　Importance of medication
　　Do not alter dosage, time, or frequency of administration
　　Never stop taking medication abruptly
　　Take medication with food, milk, or antacid if ordered
　　Avoid excessive use of caffeine and nicotine products
　　Never take aspirin-containing medications
　　Avoid taking over-the-counter medications without checking with physician
　　Report toxic symptoms to physician
　Importance of intermittent therapy; report appearance of disease symptoms
　Need to maintain diet as ordered or high-protein, high-potassium, high-calcium, low-sodium diet
　Need to weigh routinely each week
　　Report 5 lb (11 kg) weight change associated with
　　　Dizziness
　　　Irregular heart rate
　　　Weakness
　　　Fatigue
　Method for IM injection of medication in emergencies if ordered
　Importance of
　　Quiet, nonstressful, safe environment
　　Avoiding persons with infections, especially URIs
　　Regular exercise and rest
　　Skin care
　　Avoiding trauma
　Need to tell all care givers about medication
　　Dentist
　　Podiatrist
　　Other physicians
　Importance of notifying physician about stressful events
　　Trauma
　　Immunizations
　　Pregnancy
　　Emotional upsets
　　Infection

- Fever
- Sore throat
- Pain or burning on urination
- Muscular aching
- Sputum production
- Delayed wound healing
- Unusual change in weight
- Gastric distress
  - Loss of appetite
  - Indigestion
  - Vomiting
  - Diarrhea
  - Bloody or black stools
- Pain, redness, or excessive bruising of legs
- Adrenal insufficiency
  - Weakness
  - Fatigue
  - Weight loss
  - Dizziness
  - Hypoglycemia
- Hyperglycemia
  - Increased thirst
  - Increased urination
  - Fatigue
  - Changes in emotional status
- Need to refill prescription 5 days before taking last pill
- Importance of taking medication in hand luggage and extra written prescription when traveling
- Importance of wearing medical alert band or chain and carrying identification card
- Importance of ongoing outpatient care

Chapter 8

Musculoskeletal System

MUSCULOSKELETAL ASSESSMENT

Subjective Data

Pain and/or edema in muscles, joints, or bones with or without movement
Weakness in extremities
Limited activity and movement
Sensory changes
Anorexia; loss of weight
Insomnia
Tires easily
Unsteady gait or stance
Frustration, anger at self

Objective Data

General appearance
Age
Vital signs: BP, T, P, and R
Joint(s) inflamed and/or warm to touch
Impaired neurovascular status of extremity(ies)
Difficulty in breathing
Deformities
Paralysis
Contractures
Posture
Abnormal body alignment
Limited ability or inability to move in bed
Abnormal gait; needs assistance
Decreased handgrip and range of motion (ROM)
Internal and external rotation of extremities
Ability to perform ROM exercises
Contusions, lacerations, scars
Wounds: amount and type of drainage
Foot-drop, wrist-drop
Facial and body gestures indicating pain
Loss of extremity
Decubitus ulcers
Skin rashes
Allergies
Tenseness
Presence of casts, braces, prostheses, crutches, traction, cane, or walker
Nutritional history
Ability to use trapeze in bed, to sit up, and to turn
Ability to perform activities of daily living (ADLs)
Constipation
Dependence, independence, and interdependence

Pertinent Background Information
CONCURRENT DISEASES AND/OR CONDITIONS

Spinal cord injury, nerve impairment
Cerebrovascular accident (CVA)
Rheumatoid arthritis
Arthritis
Bursitis
Polyneuritis
Multiple sclerosis
Muscular dystrophy
Myasthenia gravis
Fracture
Ruptured disc
Meniere's disease
Labyrinthitis
Osteoporosis
Congenital conditions
Low back pain
Lupus erythematosus
Gout
Blood dyscrasias

PREVIOUS SURGERY AND/OR ILLNESS

Poliomyelitis
Hemiplegia, paraplegia
Cerebral palsy
Orthopedic surgery
Spinal surgery
Parkinson's disease
Ataxia
Alcoholism
Syphilis
Impaired vision and/or hearing
CVA
Hyperparathyroidism
Osteoporosis
Rickets, osteomalacia
Tuberculosis

Musculoskeletal System

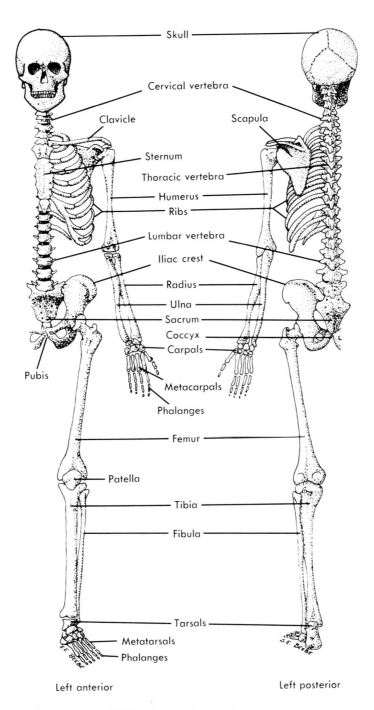

FIGURE 8-1. Musculosketetal system.

FAMILY HISTORY

Carcinoma
Diabetes
Tuberculosis

SOCIAL HISTORY

Hazardous job or recreation (e.g., construction work or contact sports)
Safety measures used
Accident prone
Alcohol, chemical substance, tobacco use

MEDICATION HISTORY

Antiinflammatory agents: steroid and nonsteroid
Sedatives
Tranquilizers
Analgesics
Acetylsalicylic acid
Antimalarials
Antiemetics
Anticoagulants
Psychotherapeutic agents
Antibiotics
Antihypertensive agents

Diagnostic Aids

LABORATORY STUDIES

Serum
   Calcium level
   Phosphorus level
   Alkaline phosphatase level
Urine
   Calcium level
   Phosphorus level

PROCEDURES

X-ray examinations of bones
Arthrogram
Arthroscopy
Myelograms
Fluoroscopy
Arteriograms
Venograms
Bone marrow aspiration
Bone or muscle biopsy
Incision and drainage of joint
Aspiration of joint
Electromyogram (EMG): muscle
Bone scan
Computed tomography (CT scan)
Thermography

RHEUMATOID ARTHRITIS

A chronic systemic disease of unknown cause characterized by an inflammatory reaction in the synovial membrane leading to destruction of joint cartilage and subsequent deformities

Assessment

Observations/findings

Fatigue
Malaise
Weight loss
Joint pain and stiffness, especially on rising
Joint inflammation and swelling
Impaired joint function
Shiny, taut skin over impaired joint
Elevated temperature (low grade)
Muscular weakness, spasms, atrophy, contractions
Subcutaneous nodules over bony prominences: hands, elbows, knees
Parasthesia of hands and feet

Laboratory/diagnostic studies

Complete blood cell count (CBC), white blood cell count (WBC), erythrocyte sedimentation rate (ESR)
ASO titer, rheumatoid factor
C-reactive protein (CRP)
Serum protein electrophoresis
Arthroscopy with synovial membrane biopsy
Joint radiologic study

Potential complications

Anemia
Gastrointestinal (GI) bleeding
Renal calculi
Pericarditis
Tenosynovitis

Medical management

Acetylsalicylic acid: buffered, enteric coated
Nonsteroid antiinflammatory agents: ibuprofen (Motrin) naproxen (Naprosyn)
Antirheumatic agents: gold, sodium thiomaleate, penicillamine
Corticosteroids
Tranquilizers, antidepressants
Physical therapy: paraffin glove, whirlpool, moist heat, cold or heat
Diet, activity
Surgical intervention: total arthroplasty, synovectomy, arthrodesis

Nursing diagnoses/goals/interventions

ndx: Alteration in comfort: pain related to joint inflammation

GOAL: *Patient will express minimal discomfort or absence of pain*

Maintain bed rest as ordered
Use firm mattress, bedboard, and footboard as indicated
Maintain proper body alignment; assist and teach patient to
    Extend joints as tolerated
    Avoid external rotation of extremities; utilize sandbags or trochanter rolls
    Avoid use of pillow under knees
    Place pillow between knees
    Avoid flexion of neck; use thin pillow beneath head
Keep bedclothes off feet
Use splints, braces, or traction as ordered
Immobilize and/or support joints
Avoid jarring or quick, jerky movements
Handle affected limbs gently, giving support above and below joint
Administer treatments as ordered
    Hot pack, tub baths
    Ice pack, paraffin, whirlpool
Administer skin care and gentle rubs
Use sheepskin, air mattress, egg-crate mattress, and/or elbow and heel guards
Administer acetylsalicylic acid as ordered
    Observe for overdose: tinnitus, GI upset, or bleeding
    Assess effectiveness of pain relief measures

ndx: Impaired physical mobility related to joint inflammation, swelling, and pain

GOAL: *Patient will demonstrate increasing mobility of joints*

Assist with and teach active and/or perform passive ROM exercises after heat treatments or apply passive ROM machine as ordered
Assist with and teach isometric and resistive exercises
Develop and teach planned daily exercise program as ordered
Observe patient's tolerance to exercise program and modify accordingly
Maintain planned rest periods
Maintain a safe environment
    Handrails, shower, tub, toilet
    Raised toilet seat
    Rubber-tipped walker, cane
    Raised chairs
    Wheelchair in locked position when stationary
Evaluate location and type of pain: chest, flank, tendons
Explain signs and symptoms of paresthesia of hands and feet

ndx: Potential for injury related to pharmacologic agents

GOAL: *Patient will remain free of complications, or they will be managed*

Monitor vital signs and observe for gastric bleeding: tarry stools, hematemesis
Monitor hemoglobin (Hgb) and hematocrit (Hct)
Monitor for aspirin toxicity: headache, nausea, tinnitis, bleeding gums

ndx: Alteration in self-concept related to body image change and self-esteem

GOAL: *Patient will verbalize understanding of changes in body image due to disease process and will exhibit increased confidence in dealing with self-esteem*

Encourage verbalization about fears and anxiety of disease process
Deal with behavioral changes: denial, powerlessness, anxiety, dependence
Be supportive, but firm, in setting goals
Encourage independence and give praise for tasks accomplished
Modify environment and allow time for patient to accomplish goals
Be aware of limitations and encourage discussion of feelings and concerns

ndx: Self-care deficit: feeding, bathing/hygiene, dressing/grooming, etc.

GOAL: *Patient's independence in self-care activities will increase within parameters of disability*

Teach self-care activities
Establish and teach routine plan for ADLs
Assist with feedings prn; have patient use large-grip handles for utensils as needed
Set goals with patient; encourage short-term, easily accomplished goals
Discuss use of snaps on clothing and slip-on shoes

ndx: Knowledge deficit regarding home care management

GOAL: *Patient and/or significant other will demonstrate understanding of home care and follow-up instructions through interactive discussion and actual return demonstration*

Stress importance of maintaining prescribed exercise, activity, and rest program
Reinforce physician's explanation of disease process, expectations, and limitations
Discuss diet management; stress importance of balanced diet and no undue weight gain
Provide medication schedule, including name, dosage, purpose, side effects, and signs of aspirin toxicity
Explain that constipation should be avoided; need to use stool softeners and natural laxatives
Promote follow-up visits with physician

Evaluation

Complications are managed
Pain is controlled within parameters of disability
Increased mobility is established
Confidence in ability to perform ADLs is demonstrated
Patient demonstrates adaptive behaviors related to self-concept
Home care management is understood

ORTHOPEDIC SEPSIS: ACUTE PYOGENIC ARTHRITIS, ACUTE OSTEOMYELITIS

acute pyogenic arthritis Acute bacterial infection affecting one or more joints caused by trauma or a penetrating wound; highest incidence is in children
acute osteomyelitis Infection of the long bones due to acute local infection or bone trauma, usually caused by Escherichia coli, Staphylococcus aureus, or Streptococcus pyogenes

Assessment

Observations/findings

Pain, redness, and swelling in affected joint; increases with motion
Chills
Rapid elevation of temperature
Diaphoresis
Muscular spasms around affected joint
Leukocytosis
Tachycardia
Headache
Restlessness
Irritability
Weakness

Laboratory/diagnostic studies

CBC, blood cultures
Joint radiologic study
Culture of joint aspirate

Potential complications

Limited motion, contractures
Ankylosing of joint
Degenerative joint changes
Chronic osteomyelitis

Medical management

Antibiotics, analgesics
Immobilization of joint
Excision, aspiration, drainage, irrigation of joint

Nursing diagnoses/goals/interventions

ndx: Impaired physical mobility related to pain, swelling, and fever

GOAL: *Patient's mobility will be maintained within limitations of impairment*

Maintain bedrest; handle affected extremity gently
Immobolize joint/extremity as ordered with use of cast, splint, and/or pillows; elevate as ordered
Assist with and teach active or perform passive ROM exercises to unaffected extremities q4h and deep breathe q½h
Administer skin care prn

ndx: Potential for complications related to disease and infection*

GOAL: *Patient will become afebrile, and complications will be minimal or nonexistent*

Order blood cultures immediately
Initiate parenteral fluids with antibiotics as ordered
Monitor vital signs q4h; institute cooling measures as ordered
Apply warm, moist compresses or alternate warm and cold compresses as ordered
Prepare patient for excision and drainage of area as ordered
  Take cultures of aspirate
  Irrigate area as ordered if irrigating catheter is in place; continuous irrigation with antibiotics may be ordered
    Monitor intake and output of irrigant
    Do not allow irrigating bottle to run dry

---

*Not a NANDA-approved nursing diagnosis.

Keep patient warm and dry
Observe for skin breakdown
Monitor incision for bleeding
Change dressing prn; maintain rigid aseptic technique
Measure intake and output q8h
Provide high-calorie, high-protein diet as tolerated; assist with meals as needed
Force fluids to upper limits for age and weight

ndx: Alteration in comfort: pain related to inflammation

GOAL: *Patient will verbalize minimal discomfort or absence of pain*

Assess location and type of pain
Provide analgesics as ordered; assess effectiveness of pain relief measures
Assist patient with changing position frequently; support affected extremity; administer back rubs
Provide diversional activities

ndx: Potential activity intolerance related to discomfort and physical impairment

GOAL: *Patient will demonstrate ability to obtain maximal activity levels*

Increase activity as ordered after fever and swelling subside or drainage decreases
Initiate ROM of affected joint/extremity as ordered
Monitor tolerance before increasing activity
Provide resistive exercises as ordered
Protect affected joint/extremity from trauma
Assist patient to chair; elevate affected extremity
Ambulate as ordered with crutches; advance to walker or cane as tolerated
Provide a safe environment
Instruct patient in weight bearing when ordered
Provide encouragement and support for each accomplishment

ndx: Knowledge deficit regarding home care management

GOAL: *Patient and/or significant other will demonstrate understanding of home care and follow-up instructions through interactive discussion and actual return demonstration*

Provide information on prescribed rehabilitation program: physical therapy and home instructions
Demonstrate incisional care and stress importance of aseptic technique and a daily shower
Discuss signs and symptoms to report to physician
Tenderness, pain, discomfort
Fever, malaise
Drainage from incision
Provide medication schedule, including name, dosage, purpose, and side effects; instruct patient to take all prescribed medications
Stress importance of nourishing diet and increased fluid intake
Promote regular visits with physician

Evaluation

Patient is afebrile
Mobility is increasing
Pain is manageable
Incision is clean and intact
Home care management is understood
There are no complications

OSTEOSARCOMA

A rapidly growing malignant bone tumor of unknown cause occurring most often in the long bones of young people; secondary malignant tumors of the bone often metastasize from other primary sites

Assessments

Observations/findings

Pain over affected area of extremity, especially at night
Limited use of extremity
Anorexia
Weight loss
Fatigue
Localized swelling with or without trauma
Increased skin temperature over affected area
Elevated temperature

Laboratory/diagnostic studies

Radiologic examinations of affected bones and chest
Bone scan, CT scan
Alkaline, acid phosphatase (elevated)
Serum calcium (decreased); urine calcium (increased)

Potential complications

Cough, hemoptysis (respiratory metastasis)
Pathologic fractures
Infection
Loss of limb

Medical management

Biopsy, amputation
Antineoplastic agents

Radiation therapy
Analgesics, tranquilizers
Diet, activity, immobilization of limb

Nursing diagnoses/goals/interventions

ndx: Impaired physical mobility related to pain, fatigue, and swelling

GOAL: *Patient's mobility will be maintained within limitations of immobilization*

Maintain bed rest in correct body alignment as ordered with splint, sandbags, and/or pillows
Assist with activity as tolerated and ordered
  Handle affected extremity gently and elevate as ordered
  Assist with and teach active or perform passive ROM exercises to unaffected extremity or use passive ROM machine as ordered
  Ambulate with assistance if tolerated; use crutches, cane, or walker as needed
Maintain planned rest periods

ndx: Alteration in nutrition: less than body requirements related to anorexia and fatigue

GOAL: *Patient's nutritional status will be maintained to meet body requirements*

Provide high-calorie, high-protein diet as ordered; encourage food selection
Provide small, frequent meals and snacks
Monitor intake and food tolerances
Weigh patient daily at same time with same clothing and scale
Force fluids to upper limits for age and weight

ndx: Potential for infection following biopsy

GOAL: *Patient will remain afebrile, and wound will be clean, dry, and intact*

Monitor vital signs q4h; provide cooling measures as needed
Monitor biopsy site q2h and observe for bleeding and drainage; change dressing prn

ndx: Potential for complication: metastasis to lung*

GOAL: *Patient's lungs will remain clear with no metastatic signs*

Assess respiratory status for cough and dyspnea
  Auscultate chest for breath sounds q8h

---

*Not a NANDA-approved nursing diagnosis.

Observe for productive cough and/or pink-tinged sputum
Elevate head of bed to facilitate breathing
Assist patient to turn and cough q4h and deep breathe q1h
Handle extremities with care and support well when moving or turning patient

ndx: Alteration in comfort: pain related to disease process

GOAL: *Patient will express minimal discomfort or absence of pain*

Assess type and location of pain; observe for increasing pain and/or dysfunction
Administer analgesics as ordered; assess effectiveness of pain relief measures
Assist patient with changing position frequently; administer back rubs
Provide diversional activities
Promote a safe environment

ndx: Knowledge deficit regarding amputation, chemotherapy, and/or radiotherapy

GOAL: *Patient and/or significant other will demonstrate understanding of surgical procedure, chemotherapy, and/or radiotherapy through interactive discussion and actual return demonstration*

Reinforce physician's explanation of surgical procedure, postoperative care, and rehabilitation; clarify any misconceptions
Provide information on chemotherapy and/or radiotherapy: possible side effects, support systems available
Encourage communication with significant other and allow time for expressions of fears and anxieties; provide supportive environment

Evaluation

Complications are managed
Nutrition is adequate
Pain is minimal or controlled
Biopsy site is clean, dry, and intact
Surgical procedure, postoperative care, rehabilitation program, as well as chemotherapy and/or radiotherapy plan are understood

SYSTEMIC LUPUS ERYTHEMATOSUS (SLE)

A chronic, autoimmune, inflammatory disease of the connective tissues that produces biochemical and

structural changes in skin, joints, and muscles, usually with multiple organ involvement; the number of organs involved makes the disease an imitator of many other diagnoses

Assessment

Observations/findings

Fever
Malaise
Weakness
Anorexia
Nausea
Vomiting
Diarrhea
Abdominal pain
Weight loss
Hepatosplenomegaly
Lymphadenopathy
Drug history of hydralazine, procainamide, and/or isoniazid
Allergies
Renal system
   Hematuria
   Cellular casts*
   Proteinuria*
   Hypertension
   Edema
   Azotemia
   Hypoproteinemia
   Renal failure
Central nervous system (CNS)
   Neuritis
   Headache
   Seizures*
   Personality changes
   CVA
   Psychosis*
Joints
   Nondeforming arthritis
   Joint warmth and swelling
Integumentary system
   Sensitivity to sun*
   Rash/erythema, "butterfly" over cheeks and bridge of nose*
   Partial alopecia*
   Oral or nasal ulcerations*
Respiratory system
   Pleuritis
   Parenchymal lung infiltrates
   Pneumonia
   Pulmonary hemorrhage
Cardiovascular system
   Pericarditis
   Murmurs
   Cardiomegaly
   Raynaud's phenomenon*
   Vasculitis: necrosis of small arteries
   Electrocardiogram (ECG) changes: arrhythmias
   Congestive heart failure (CHF)
   Myocardial infarction (MI)
Abdomen
   Peritonitis
Ocular system
   Retinal "cytoid" bodies
   Conjunctivitis
   Photophobia
   Diplopia
Behavioral changes
   Depression
   Psychosis
Hematologic system
   Positive antinuclear antibodies*
   Hemolytic anemia*
   Thrombocytopenia
   Leukopenia
   False positive serology*

Laboratory/diagnostic studies

LE prep (positive)
Antinuclear antibodies (ANA) (positive)
Anti-double-standard DNA antibody (positive)
Fluorescent treponemal antibody absorption (FTA-ABS) (negative)
Complement (C3 and C4)
CBC, C-reactive protein, ESR, coagulation profile, rheumatoid factor, urinalysis
Creatinine clearance test
Chest radiologic study
Skin and kidney biopsies

Potential complications

Infections from long-term steroid therapy
Complications from any one of the multisystems affected, such as renal failure, MI, pneumonia, CVA

Medical management

Nonsteroid antiinflammatory agents
Corticosteroid therapy

---

*Four or more support the diagnosis.

Antiinfective agents
Antineoplastic agents
Medications related to system(s) affected
Plasmapheresis, dialysis
Joint arthroplasty
Diet, activity, rest

Nursing diagnoses/goals/interventions*

ndx Alteration in tissue perfusion related to multisystem involvement: renal, cardiopulmonary, cerebral, musculoskeletal, integumentary

GOAL: *Patient's condition will stabilize, and complications will be managed or minimized*

Assess renal status; observe for signs of edema, nausea, hematuria, and hypertension
  Measure urine output as needed
  Provide antihypertensive medication and low-salt diet as ordered
  Monitor urinalysis and kidney function studies
Assess neurologic status; observe for alterations in orientation, judgment, mental acuity, speech, and muscle tone
  Provide a safe environment
  Assist as needed with activity, meals, and toileting
  Observe for personality changes; monitor for signs of suicide
  Encourage communication with significant other
Assess for muscle/joint involvement
  Monitor ability to move; observe for pain, swelling, and limited ROM
  Administer ROM exercises as ordered to unaffected joints or use passive ROM machine
  Apply warm or cold compresses to area as ordered
  Administer analgesics as ordered
Assess cardiopulmonary system; observe for dyspnea, cyanosis, decreased breath sounds, tachypnea, bradypnea, rales, and rhonchi
  Auscultate chest for breath sounds
  Elevate head of bed
  Encourage patient to turn, cough, and deep breathe
  Administer oxygen therapy, analgesics, and bronchodilators as ordered
  Monitor vital signs q4h prn; take apical pulse and observe for arrhythmias, tachycardia, and bradycardia
  Monitor arterial pulses for bruits
  Administer steroids and antiarrhythmic agents as ordered

---

*Patient's condition dictates amount and type of care required; modify accordingly.

Observe for peripheral edema
Assess integumentary status; observe skin and mucous membranes for color, temperature, turgor, edema, signs of infection, and rashes
  Administer topical steroid and antibiotic ointments as ordered
  Provide nonallergenic soaps and creams
  Promote sunscreen use if patient is photosensitive
  Administer skin care and oral hygiene prn
Assist patient with changing position frequently

ndx Alteration in nutrition: less than body requirements related to anorexia, fatigue, and/or electrolyte imbalance

GOAL: *Patient's nutritional status will improve and be maintained*

Assess nutritional status and monitor caloric intake as ordered
Provide well-balanced, small, frequent meals; encourage patient selection
Determine weight gain related to steroid therapy; sodium may be restricted
Weigh patient daily at same time with same clothing and scale
Provide vitamin supplement for pregnant or dieting patient
Monitor abdomen for distention, pain, and tenderness

ndx Potential activity intolerance related to fatigue and arthralgia

GOAL: *Patient will increase activities to tolerance within limitations of impairment*

Provide bed rest during exacerbation
Increase activity slowly; provide ROM exercises to unaffected joints q4h
Assist with chair sitting when allowed; support affected joint(s)
Increase ambulation as tolerated; use crutches, walker, or cane as needed

ndx Potential for infection related to steroid therapy

GOAL: *Patient will remain afebrile without signs of infection*

Monitor WBC and differential, ESR, C-reactive protein, urinalysis, and cultures for signs of sepsis
Culture drainage from skin rashes, breaks, injection sites, etc., and sputum, urine, etc.
Monitor temperature for febrile state
Maintain clean environment and good physical hygiene

Provide planned rest periods
Administer antipyretics, antibiotics, and analgesics as ordered

ndx: Disturbance in self-concept: body image change related to physical appearance

GOAL: *Patient will be allowed time for verbalization of concerns and assisted with forming adaptive behaviors in a supportive environment*

Encourage patient to express feelings and concerns; listen carefully
Reinforce physician's explanation of disease process: its chronicity, treatment, remissions, and exacerbations; clarify misconceptions
Provide a supportive environment, praising positive ideas and accomplishments
Identify present coping patterns and strengths that were successful in past experiences
Promote communication with significant other

ndx: Knowledge deficit regarding home care management

GOAL: *Patient and/or significant other will demonstrate understanding of home care and follow-up instructions through interactive discussion and actual return demonstration*

Provide written diet, activity, and rest instructions as prescribed
Stress importance of skin care; explain need to use only nonallergenic preparations on skin and hair, need to avoid exposure to sun or use sunscreen with protection factor of 15, and need to avoid hair spray and hair dyes
Provide instructions on medication schedule, including name, purpose, dosage, and side effects —especially for steroids; explain that they must be taken uninterrupted; explain need to avoid penicillin, sulfa, phenytoin, and oral contraceptives
Discuss signs and symptoms of exacerbation to report to physician: fever, rash, cough, joint pain
Promote and encourage patient to wear medical alert tag indicating dose of steroid and name and number of physician
Discuss advantages of assistance from Lupus Foundation*
Promote follow-up visits with physician

---

*Lupus Foundation of America, Inc., 1717 Massachusetts Ave., N.W., Suite 203, Washington, D.C., 20036.

Evaluation

Complications have been prevented or are controlled
Patient is afebrile
Nutritional status is adequate
Pain is manageable
Patient complies with treatment and understands home care management
Patient demonstrates adaptive behaviors toward body image change

PROGRESSIVE SYSTEMIC SCLEROSIS (SCLERODERMA)

A chronic inflammatory disease of the connective tissue (collagen) affecting many organs and other connective tissue in its later stages

Assessment
Observations/findings

Joints/skin
 Edema
 Weakness, muscle
 Tough, hard skin, progressing to taut and shiny
 Tenderness, pain in joints
 Skin rash (hands, feet)
Altered self-concept
History of pulmonary, cardiac, renal, and/or digestive disturbance

Laboratory/diagnostic studies

Skin biopsies, angiography
ESR, rheumatoid factor
Antinuclear antibody studies
Renal, GI, and pulmonary studies

Potential complications

Raynaud's phenomenon
Cardiac, renal, GI, and pulmonary dysfunction
Atrophic changes in skin

Medical management

Analgesics, antipyretics, anticholinergics, antibiotics
Corticosteroids, potassium (Potaba)
Diet, activity, rest
Physical therapy
Surgical intervention: joint arthroplasty

Nursing diagnoses/goals/interventions

ndx: Impaired physical mobility related to pain and edema of joints

GOAL: *Patient will progress to activities as tolerated within limitations of disease process*

Promote and perform prescribed exercise program
    Perform passive or assist with and teach active ROM exercises
    Provide and encourage planned rest periods
    Encourage use of affected joints to maintain function
    Keep joints warm
Ambulate with assistance as allowed

ndx: Alteration in tissue perfusion related to disease progression: renal, gastrointestinal, cardiopulmonary

GOAL: *Patient's vital signs, urine output, respirations, nutrition, and hydration will be maintained within confines of disease process*

Assess renal function
    Monitor and measure urinary output
    Monitor vital signs for hypertension
    Force fluids to upper limits for age and weight
Assess cardiopulmonary function
    Monitor vital signs q4h; take apical pulse and observe for arrhythmias
    Observe fingers and toes for signs of blanching, cyanosis, redness (Raynaud's phenomenon)
    Assess for paresthesia, numbness, or tingling
    Monitor and auscultate chest for breath sounds
    Observe for diminished breath sounds or dullness (pleurisy)
    Monitor respirations; observe for impaired gas exchange
    Monitor ECG and pulmonary function studies and arterial blood gases
    Administer corticosteroids as ordered
Assess GI function
    Monitor nutrition and fluid intake; observe for dysphasia, reflux, and esophageal stricture
    Administer Potaba and anticholinergics as ordered
Provide well-balanced, high-fiber diet and force fluids to upper limits for age and weight
    Encourage small, frequent meals
    Measure intake
    Assess ability to chew foods well
Auscultate abdomen for bowel sounds; observe stools for steatorrhea

ndx: Potential for infection of skin related to ulceration

GOAL: *Patient's skin integrity will be maintained, and infection will be absent or minimal*

Assess skin integrity and observe for rashes, excoriation, breaks, or ulcers
Provide skin care frequently, keeping skin well lubricated with lotions
Provide quiet, clean environment
Administer antipyretics and antibiotics as ordered

ndx: Disturbance in self-concept related to body image change

GOAL: *Patient will verbalize feelings and concerns and will progress toward adaptive behavior patterns*

Encourage and allow time for patient to discuss body image change; listen carefully
Assess present coping styles and provide support for strengths that assisted in the past
Encourage communication with significant other
Promote independence and provide positive feedback for tasks accomplished
Encourage social interaction with family and friends

ndx: Knowledge deficit regarding home care management and disease process

GOAL: *Patient and/or significant other will demonstrate understanding of disease process, home care, and follow-up instructions through interactive discussion*

Reinforce physician's explanation of progression of disease, treatment, and prognosis; clarify any misconceptions
Promote independence in ADLs to lessen complications
Explain signs and symptoms of specific organ involvement to report to physician
Discuss medications: name, purpose, schedule, dosage, and side effects; explain need to avoid medications not ordered by physician
Stress importance of nutritional diet, exercise schedule, and planned rest periods
Promote follow-up visits with physician

Evaluation

Complications are absent or minimal
Nutrition and hydration are adequate
Skin integrity is maintained
Mobility is adequate for self-care and ADLs
Home care management is understood

GOUTY ARTHRITIS

Acute and/or chronic arthritis of the joints due to impaired uric acid production

Assessment

Observations/findings

Affected joint (usually metatarsophalangeal joint of great toe)
   Excruciating pain
   Tenderness
   Redness
   Increased heat
   Swelling
   Shiny
   Vein distention
   Deformed
Anorexia
Headache
Elevated temperature
Chills
Constipation
Subcutaneous tophi: ears, joints, knuckles

Laboratory/diagnostic studies

Serum uric acid, WBC, ESR
Microscopic examination of joint aspirate

Potential complications

Decreased urine output
Hypertension
Renal calculi

Medical management

Antigout agents, probenecid (Benemid), colchicine (Colsalide)
Nonsteroid antiinflammatory agents, phenylbutazone (Butazolidin), indomethacin (Indocin)
Analgesics, antipyretics, allopurinol
Cold packs

Nursing diagnoses/goals/interventions

ndx: Alteration in comfort: pain related to disease process

GOAL: *Patient will express minimal discomfort or absence of pain*

Maintain patient in position of comfort with foot supported and in alignment; place cradle over foot; no weight bearing
Apply cold packs as ordered, keeping pressure off joint
Administer analgesics, and antigout and antiinflammatory agents as ordered; observe for side effects
   Colchicine: nausea, vomiting, bloody diarrhea, oliguria, hematuria
   Phenylbutazone: nausea, vomiting, diarrhea, rash, edema, hypertension, leukopenia
   Administer allopurinol as ordered to reduce serum uric acid levels

ndx: Impaired physical mobility related to joint pain and immobility

GOAL: *Patient will progress to activities as tolerated*

Increase activity as pain and swelling subside
Ambulate with assistance; use walker or cane
Perform gentle ROM exercises to affected joint
Promote return to normal activities

ndx: Knowledge deficit regarding medications and home care management

GOAL: *Patient and/or significant other will demonstrate understanding of medication therapy, home care, and follow-up instructions through interactive discussion*

Provide medication schedule, including name, dosage, purpose, and side effects, and explain necessity of taking colchicine hourly at onset of acute attacks
Discuss importance of diet, exercise, and rest program
Encourage follow-up visits with physician

Evaluation

There are no complications
Pain is managed
There are no side effects from maintenance medications
Medication schedule and home care management are understood

OSTEOPOROSIS

Overall reduction in bone mass and density, causing increased porosity and brittleness; suggested etiology—immobilization due to illness or aging process, decreased blood estrogen, increased ratio of blood calcium to phosphorus, excessive steroid therapy; disease predisposes patients to fractures and/or deformities

Assessment

Observations/findings

Backache, neck pain, decrease in height, kyphosis
Age and sex of patient (usually over 50 years and female)
History of inactivity or immobilization
Nutritional history
   Lack of vitamins D and C, and calcium
   Diets high in acids, alcohol, and caffeine
History of endocrine disease

Diabetes
Hyperthyroidism
Hyperparathroidism
Cushing's syndrome
Acromegaly
Hypogonadism

Anorexia nervosa
Hematologic malignancies
History of steroid therapy or smoking
Alteration in self-concept
Decreased mobility

Laboratory/diagnostic studies

Radiologic studies
Bone scan

Potential complications

Fractures: lower radius, femoral neck, vertebrae
Increased immobility

Medical management

Calcium, vitamin D supplements
Estrogen therapy if postmenopausal or hysterectomy
Increased activity
Back corset

Nursing diagnoses/goals/interventions*

ndx: Impaired physical mobility related to disease process

GOAL: *Patient will move toward increased mobility and activity*

Provide firm mattress with bedboard as necessary
Encourage ambulation with assistance; use walker or cane if indicated
Assist with and teach active ROM exercises q4h
Monitor and maintain body alignment; fractures can occur without patient's knowledge
Handle patient carefully and assist with and teach correct body mechanics
Assist with and teach patient application of braces or corset as applicable
Administer analgesics, estrogen, calcium, and vitamin D as ordered
Provide diet high in calcium and vitamins C and D
Monitor serum calcium levels

ndx: Disturbance in self-concept: body image change and impaired self-esteem related to disease process

---

*Nursing intervention is usually educational in hospital setting unless fractures occur.

GOAL: *Patient will express concerns and feelings and work toward positive coping behaviors in supportive environment*

Encourage and allow time for verbalization of feelings; listen attentively
Clarify any misconceptions about disease process and treatment
Assist patient in identifying strengths that were successful in past experience
Identify present coping behaviors and give praise for tasks accomplished
Encourage communication with significant other

ndx: Knowledge deficit regarding home care management

GOAL: *Patient and/or significant other will demonstrate understanding of home care and follow-up instructions through interactive discussion*

Stress importance of diet, activity, and rest; provide written aerobic exercise schedule; avoid jogging
Provide medication schedule, including name, dosage, purpose, and side effects
Discuss importance of safe environment
  Use ambulatory devices as needed; avoid slippery areas
  Maintain awareness of possible falls or fractures; avoid small rugs; use hand rails
  Avoid activity after taking analgesics or muscle relaxants
  Avoid quick movements that may cause fractures
Encourage reduction of caffeine, alcohol intake, and smoking
Promote follow-up visits with physician for medication adjustments, serum calcium levels, Pap smears, and mammography

Evaluation

There are no complications
Activity and mobility have been established to tolerance
Adaptive behaviors are demonstrated
Home care management is understood

LOW BACK PAIN

Pain in the lower back that may be caused by a variety of diseases that affect bone, but is generally due to stress on the vertebral process or a herniated disc

Assessment

Observations/findings

Back pain: low and intense
Radiating leg pain
Sciatica
Muscle spasms
Muscular weakness
Obesity
Faulty posture
Strenuous occupation
Decreased ROM of spine
    Flexion, extension
    Lateral bending, rotation

Laboratory/diagnostic studies

Myelogram, discogram
Radiologic examination of lower back
EMG
Biofeedback therapy
MRI

Potential complications

Ruptured vertebral disc
Neurologic dysfunction

Medical management

Diet, activity, rest
Analgesics, muscle relaxants, nonsteroid antiinflammatory agents, cortisones
Exercise program
Physical therapy intervention
TENS unit (transcutaneous electrical nerve stimulator)
Epidural injections of antiinflammatory agent
Facet joint injection of antiinflammatory agent with lidocaine

Nursing diagnoses/goals/interventions

ndx: Alteration in comfort: pain related to disease process

GOAL: *Patient will express minimal discomfort or absence of pain*

Maintain bed rest with firm mattress in position of comfort; usually with knees flexed and head elevated 30 degrees
Administer medications as ordered: analgesics, muscle relaxants, antiinflammatory agents
Apply hot or cold compresses as ordered
Provide and teach use of TENS unit as ordered
Involve physical therapy as ordered: hydrotherapy, deep heat, hot paraffin
Apply back brace or corset as ordered
Prepare patient for epidural or facet joint injections of antiinflammatory agent; assess sensation, mobility, pulses, color, and temperature postoperatively
Assist and teach ROM exercises q4h and abdominal and gluteal contractions 10 times qh
Increase activity as allowed; ambulate with assistance; observe gait and evidence of pain

ndx: Knowledge deficit regarding home care management

GOAL: *Patient and/or significant other will demonstrate understanding of home care and follow-up instructions through interactive discussion and actual return demonstration*

Stress importance of prescribed rehabilitation plan
    Maintain correct body alignment
        Flex knees and hips when bending
        Sleep on side or back with small pillow under head
        Keep knees flexed while in bed
        Use straight-backed chair or recliner when sitting
        Do not cross legs or sit with legs straight out on footstool
    Maintain planned rest periods and avoid fatigue
    Maintain normal weight
    Wear flat-heeled shoes
Demonstrate application and maintenance of body corset or brace
Demonstrate use of TENS unit
Provide diet instructions and fluid intake amount; avoid constipation with use of stool softeners and natural laxatives
Discuss medications: name, schedule, purpose, dosage, and side effects
Promote follow-up visits with physician

Evaluation

There are no complications
Mobility is restored to optimal level
Pain is controlled or decreased
Home care management is understood

FRACTURES

A break in bone continuity; there are many types of fractures—a few major ones are as follows
compound fracture *A break with bone protruding through the skin*
simple fracture *A break with the skin left intact*

complete fracture *A break through the entire bone; bone may be displaced*

incomplete fracture *A break through only part of the bone*

Assessment

Observations/findings

Fracture site
    Pain, tenderness, edema
    Skin open or intact
    Color and temperature of surrounding tissues
    Presence of pulse distal from break
    Numbness, tingling
    Bleeding, hematoma
    Restricted, limited mobility
Signs of shock: hypotension, tachycardia

Laboratory/diagnostic studies

Radiologic films of fracture
CBC, electrolytes
Arthroscopic aspirate studies

Potential complications

Malunion, delayed, or nonunion of fracture
Thrombophlebitis
Fat embolism
Compartmental syndrome (knee, elbow)
Infection
Nerve compression

Medical management

Open or closed reduction of fracture
Joint arthroplasty
Analgesics, narcotics, sedatives, antibiotics, muscle relaxants
Application of cast, traction, splint, and/or sling
Ice application
Bed rest in specific position
Diet, activity, rest, mobility restrictions
Physical therapy

Nursing diagnoses/goals/interventions

ndx: Impaired physical mobility related to fracture and injury to surrounding tissues

GOAL: *Patient's mobility will return to prefracture status*

Maintain bed rest in ordered position to facilitate healing
Elevate affected extremity and apply ice bags as ordered
Support affected extremity above and below fracture when moving, turning, and lifting
Monitor cast, traction, and sling q1h initially, then q4h; observe for cast integrity and position of traction and sling
Assist with and teach use of trapeze and other methods of moving and turning
Perform passive or assist with and teach active ROM exercises to unaffected joints
Explain restrictions and limitations in activity
Administer skin care q2h to 4h; observe for skin breaks around cast and traction
Assist with and teach patient use of urinal or bedpan for elimination; administer perineal care as needed

ndx: Alteration in tissue perfusion related to location of fracture and its effect on other organs or systems

GOAL: *Patient's condition will become and remain stable, and complications will be minimal or absent*

Assess neurologic status
    Monitor pulses distal from fracture q1h to 2h and observe color, temperature, and sensation
    Maintain body alignment and position as ordered
    Observe for signs of compartmental syndrome
Assess cardiopulmonary status
    Monitor vital signs q2h to 4h; take apical pulse as needed
    Auscultate chest for breath sounds q4h; observe for diminished sounds and dyspnea
    Assist and teach patient to turn and cough q2h and deep breathe q1h
    Apply antiembolic stockings as ordered
Assess GI and renal status
    Monitor stool and urine for blood
    Measure intake and output
    Provide high-protein diet with iron, calcium, and vitamin supplements; avoid weight gain
    Force fluids to upper limits for age and weight unless contraindicated

ndx: Potential for infection related to immobility and/or surgical reduction

GOAL: *Patient's skin/wound integrity will remain clean, dry, and intact*

Assess wound integrity and observe for signs of infection or drainage
    Administer antibiotics as ordered
    Monitor and change dressings prn
    Monitor temperature

ndx Alteration in comfort: pain related to fracture and/or other trauma

GOAL: *Patient will express minimal discomfort or absence of pain*

Assess location and type of pain

Administer narcotics, analgesics, and muscle relaxants as ordered; avoid allowing pain to become severe; assess effectiveness of pain relief measures

Provide quiet environment initially and encourage diversional activities

Change position frequently and administer back rubs and massages

Encourage chair sitting with legs elevated and ambulation with assistance when allowed

Involve physical therapy in instructions in use of crutches, walker, or cane

ndx Disturbance in self-concept related to body image change

GOAL: *Patient will verbalize feelings and concerns and strive for positive coping patterns in a supportive environment*

Reinforce physician's explanation of treatment and expected outcome; clarify misconceptions

Encourage and allow time for verbalization of feelings; listen attentively

Assess present coping behaviors and encourage use of behaviors that were successful in managing past experiences

Encourage interaction with significant other and with friends and relatives

Explain all procedures and treatments; involve patient in plan of care; provide options; encourage safe decision making

ndx Knowledge deficit regarding home care management

GOAL: *Patient and/or significant other will demonstrate understanding of home care and follow-up instructions through interactive discussion and actual return demonstration*

Stress importance of prescribed rehabilitation plan of activity, rest, and exercise

Provide diet instructions as to type and amount, and to avoid weight gain if applicable

Discuss medications: name, purpose, schedule, dosage, and side effects

Discuss signs and symptoms to report to physician: severe pain, changes in temperature, color or sensation in extremity, foul odor, drainage from wound

Encourage follow-up visits with physician

Evaluation

Complications are absent or controlled

Pain is manageable

Behavior indicates positive coping patterns

Mobility is at upper limits of restriction

Home care management is understood

MAXILLOMANDIBULAR FIXATION

Surgical procedure to reduce and repair jaw fractures

Preoperative assessment and care

Assess respiratory status; observe for signs of upper respiratory infection (URI)

Explain purpose of wires and rubber bands following surgery and provide method of communication: pad and pencil, Magic Slate

Assist with and teach patient method for pushing secretions and vomitus through clamped jaw (if possible) and demonstrate use of oral suction catheter

Discuss importance of oral hygiene and oral suctioning, and teach procedure

Demonstrate feeding procedure using straw or syringe

Explain possibility of nasopharyngeal airway and/or nasogastric tube and aspiration postoperatively

Perform facial scrub and oral hygiene preoperatively as ordered

Administer antibiotics as ordered

Answer all questions and allow time for verbalization of fears and anxieties

Postoperative assessment
Observations/findings

Edema of
  Face
  Base of tongue
  Front of neck
  Nose

Pain

Nausea, vomiting; aspiration of emesis

Dyspnea

Elevated temperature

Apprehension

Drainage from mouth

Location of wire cutters or scissors

Laboratory/diagnostic studies

CBC, electrolytes

Radiologic examinations for alignment of fracture

Potential complications

Respiratory distress
Aspiration pneumonia
Hemorrhage, shock

Medical management

Analgesics, sedatives, antibiotics
Parenteral fluids
Nasogastric aspiration
Oxygen therapy
Wire and band cutting procedure
Diet, activity, rest

Nursing diagnoses/goals/interventions

ndx Ineffective airway clearance related to inability to open mouth and expectorate

GOAL: *Patient's airway will be maintained*

Maintain bed rest with head elevated when reactive
Perform oral suctioning prn; assist and teach patient to clear airway and perform suctioning
Keep suction on at all times; observe for edema, drainage, and bleeding
Administer antiemetics as ordered
Connect nasogastric tube to low, intermittent suction apparatus if applicable; maintain patency with normal saline irrigations prn
Apply ice bags as ordered
Tape wire cutters or scissors to head of bed; if aspiration is imminent, cut wires and rubber bands as needed
Monitor vital signs q2h to 4h; observe for dyspnea, restlessness, and tachycardia; take axillary or rectal temperature
Auscultate chest for breath sounds as indicated
Administer nasal oxygen or vaporizer as ordered

ndx Alteration in comfort: pain related to surgical procedure

GOAL: *Patient will experience minimal discomfort or absence of pain*

Assess type and location of pain; administer analgesics as ordered; assess effectiveness
Assist patient with changing position frequently while in bed and maintain quiet environment
Administer frequent oral hygiene; use water jet if available or mouth swabs; keep lips well lubricated; apply dental wax to rubber bands as ordered
Ambulate with assistance when allowed
Establish means of communication: pad and pencil, Magic Slate

ndx Potential alteration in nutrition: less than body requirements due to surgical procedure

GOAL: *Patient's nutrition will be adequate for body needs*

Administer parenteral fluids as ordered; wean off as fluid intake increases
Provide clear liquid to full high-calorie diet as ordered and tolerated, and/or after nasogastric tube has been removed
　Assist and teach patient to use straw or feed with syringe
　Follow each feeding with water
　Provide small, frequent meals
　Consult dietitian (RD) regarding alternatives in food selections (i.e., commercially prepared formulas)
Measure intake and output and weigh patient q2d at same time with same clothing and scale
Monitor electrolytes

ndx Knowledge deficit regarding home care management

GOAL: *Patient and/or significant other will demonstrate understanding of home care and follow-up instructions through interactive discussion and actual return demonstration*

Provide diet instructions for full liquid diet and foods allowed: blended junior foods, eggnogs, and milk shakes; demonstrate use of straw or syringe
Discuss importance and purpose of small, frequent meals
Stress and teach oral hygiene; demonstrate use of water pic and dental wax and to keep lips moist
Demonstrate method for cutting wires or bands and under what circumstances to cut (wires and/or bands will remain for 6 to 8 weeks)
Explain signs and symptoms to report to physician: fever, increased pain, edema, foul odor from mouth
Discuss obtaining all medications in liquid form
Promote follow-up visits with physician

Evaluation

There are no complications
Jaw is in correct alignment
Pain is managed
Nutrition is adequate
Home care management is understood

SPINAL SURGERY

Surgery performed to relieve pressure on the spinal nerves and/or cord due to a herniated disc, trauma, displaced fracture, incomplete vertebral dislocation from rheumatoid arthritis, osteoporosis, or insertion of rods to correct scoliosis; incision may be anterior or posterior in cervical, thoracic, or lumbar areas

laminectomy *Removal of part of the disc lamina*

discectomy *Removal of part of the disc*

spinal fusion *Solidification of several vertebrae by grafting bone from the iliac crest of the tibia*

microsurgical doral root rhizotomy *Severing of the sensory nerve root to the painful area; provides symptomatic relief and causes loss of sensation and possible motor damage; performed when other treatments have been unsuccessful*

facet joint rhizotomy *Needle insertion into the facet joint with distruction of the nerve by microwave current; provides symptomatic relief*

Harrington rod instrumentation for scoliosis *Surgical correction of scoliosis by insertion and implantation of rods along either side of the spine to correct the existing concavity or convexity; a posterior spinal fusion is performed concurrently*

Preoperative assessment and care

Assess patient's neurovascular and respiratory status, and location, type, and duration of pain

Discuss with and teach patient postoperative care and rationale

    Definition and importance of prescribed postoperative position and good body alignment

    Methods for turning, coughing, and deep breathing

    Use of trapeze and method for getting in and out of bed

Necessary movement limitations and activities allowed ROM and isometric exercises

    Gluteal contractions, quadriceps setting

Provide firm mattress and bedboard if spinal fusion is to be performed

Cervical fusion or fracture patients may have head immobilized prior to surgery with head collar, brace, halo cast, or traction (Crutchfield tongs); these devices will accompany patient to operating room

Explain that body brace, cast, or mold will be in place after surgery for thoracic and lumbar fusion; these devices are made ready for patient prior to surgery

Explain that a Hemovac or a Jackson-Pratt drain will be in place, and drainage may be profuse

Explain that there will be a second incision from bone graft site for spinal fusion

Discuss possibility of nasogastric aspiration and urinary drainage catheter; for thoracoabdominal approach, chest tubes may be in place

Explain that pain may be less with laminectomy, discectomy, or rhizotomy, but more with spinal fusion; discuss pain management

Encourage patient to ask questions and provide emotional support

    Reinforce physician's explanation of surgical procedure

    Allow time for and discuss patient's fears and anxieties

Postoperative assessment

Observations/findings

Decreased sensation and motor activity of extremities

Circulatory status of extremities: change in color, temperature, or pulse

Respiratory status (especially in cervical surgery)

    Difficulty in breathing

    Cyanosis

    Tachypnea

    Diminished cough

Body alignment: presence of immobilization devices

Location and character of pain

Character and amount of

    Wound drainage

    Hemovac drainage if present

    Urinary output

Laboratory/diagnostic studies

CBC, electrolytes

Spinal radiologic examinations

Urine for culture/sensitivity

Potential complications

Neurologic damage

Hemorrhage

Shock

Urinary retention, infection

Abdominal distention

Paralytic ileus

Atelectasis, hypostatic pneumonia

Pulmonary embolus

Wound infection

Medical management

Analgesics, antibiotics, antiemetics, stool softeners

Parenteral fluids with electrolytes

Nasogastric aspiration, urinary drainage catheter

Hemovac drainage, dressing change

Oxygen therapy, incentive spirometer

Immobilization devices: brace, cast, corset
Diet, activity, rest
Antiembolic stockings

Nursing diagnoses/goals/interventions

ndx: Ineffective breathing pattern related to anesthesia, surgical incision, and pain

GOAL: *Patient's respirations will remain adequate to meet body requirements*

Assess respiratory status q2h
    Assist and teach patient to deep breathe q2h
    For cervical surgery
        Check respirations q½h for rate, quality, and distress signs
        Maintain endotracheal suction apparatus, tracheostomy set, and inspiratory positive pressure breathing (IPPB) respirator at bedside
        Observe for diminished cough reflex
        Assess face and neck for edema qh
Auscultate chest for breath sounds q2h
Monitor vital signs q2h for 8 hr, then q4h
Administer oxygen therapy; use incentive spirometer as ordered
Apply antiembolic stockings as ordered

ndx: Potential fluid volume deficit related to NPO status and/or abnormal fluid loss

GOAL: *Patient will remain hydrated with vital signs and adequate urine output being maintained*

Maintain NPO
Administer parenteral fluids with electrolytes as ordered
Connect nasogastric tube to low, intermittent suction apparatus; irrigate with measured amounts of normal saline to maintain patency
Connect indwelling urethral catheter to closed gravity drainage system as ordered
    Monitor output qh; if output is less than 20 to 30 ml/hr, notify physician
    Measure intake and output q8h
Monitor dressing(s) for drainage q2h for 24 hr, then q4h
    Patient may be in supine position for extended period; assessment must be made by feeling dressing
    Check Hemovac drainage and graft incision q1h to 2h
    Change dressing prn with initial change by physician
Monitor Hgb, Hct, and electrolytes
Administer naso-oral hygiene q2h; keep areas moist

Auscultate abdomen for bowel sounds q8h; report return to physician; observe for detention
Provide diet as tolerated when bowel sounds return or nasogastric tube is clamped or removed
    Initiate clear liquids and increase to soft or regular diet
    Measure intake and output until adequate
Remove indwelling urethral catheter as ordered
    Obtain specimen for culture
    Institute voiding measures as needed
Administer stool softeners as ordered

ndx: Impaired physical mobility related to postoperative restrictions and pain

GOAL: *Patient's mobility will be optimal within limitations of surgical outcome*

Maintain bed rest as ordered, usually in supine or prone position
Maintain immobilization of spine as ordered
    Placement of immobilization devices
    Good body alignment
    No knee flexion
    For cervical surgery, sandbags on both sides of head may be ordered if no immobilization device is present
    Do not flex head forward
    Elevate head of bed 40 to 60 degrees
Assess motor activity, sensation, color, pulse, and temperature of lower extremities q2h
    Report changes to physician
    For cervical surgery, assess upper extremities for color, pulse, and temperature q2h; report changes to physician
Turn patient only when ordered
    Administer pain medication 30 min prior to turning when possible
    Use logrolling method
    Keep head aligned with body at all times
    Turn q2h from back to side to side
    While turning, maintain alignment
        Support legs with pillow between knees
        Support head with small pillow
        Roll in one continuous motion
        Support back with pillows
    Administer skin care with each turn; assess for pressure points
    Observe dressing for drainage
    Encourage deep breathing while on side
Remove immobilization device as ordered and check for altered skin integrity
Maintain scheduled rest periods

Increase activity as ordered
  Initiate quadriceps setting and gluteal contractions
  Assist with and teach active or perform passive ROM exercises q4h as indicated according to surgical procedure
  Avoid sudden movements or twisting of extremities or neck
  Involve physical therapist if available
Ambulate with assistance when ordered
  Maintain patient in immbolization device or apply immobilization device as indicated; Harrington rod patients will have body cast or two-piece plastic shell (turtle shells)
  Assist with and reinforce teaching of method for sitting up and getting out of bed
  Maintain body alignment
  Have patient wear supportive shoes
  Assist patient in walking
    Observe for vertigo, nausea, and hypotension
    Observe gait
    Avoid shuffling feet
  Place patient in straight-backed chair with feet on floor
  Increase ambulation to tolerance; avoid standing, sudden movements, and twisting
Encourage self-care as tolerated; assit with and teach modified ADLs as needed

ndx: Alteration in comfort: pain related to surgical intervention

GOAL: *Patient will verbalize minimal discomfort or absence of pain*

Assess location, type, and duration of pain
Administer analgesics as ordered; avoid morphine for cervical surgery patients
Assist patient with changing position frequently, maintaining correct body alignment
Provide and teach use of TENS unit as ordered
Encourage diversional activities

ndx: Knowledge deficit regarding home care management

GOAL: *Patient and/or significant other will demonstrate understanding of home care and follow-up instructions through interactive discussion and actual return demonstration*

Stress importance of prescribed activity, exercises, and restrictions
  Degree of activity and self-care allowed; need to avoid overdependence
  Need to maintain good body alignment
  No heavy lifting or strenuous exercise, automobile driving or riding, stooping, or bending
  Methods of knee bending
  Need to avoid fatigue; to exercise to tolerance with frequent rest periods
  ROM exercises as allowed
  Straight-backed chair for sitting
  Convalescent period (may be an extended length of time: 2 to 9 months)
  Need to wear immobilization device as ordered; method of application, care, and removal of device; observance of device for areas that may cause skin irritation or breakdown
  Firm mattress with bedboard (essential)
Provide instructions on diet and fluid intake; explain need to avoid weight gain and constipation
Discuss and demonstrate incisional care
  Signs and symptoms of wound infection
  Need to shower daily with mild soap and to observe skin for signs of irritation (use lotion to heal)
  For tibial graft incision site: need to wear elastic bandage for edema and rewrap qid
Discuss signs and symptoms to report to physician
  Decreased motor activity and/or sensation in extremities
  Increased pain in surgical area
  Elevated temperature
Discuss medications: name, schedule, purpose, dosage, and side effects
Promote follow-up visits with physician

Evaluation

There are no complications
Mobility is restored to optimal level
Pain is managed
Nutrition and hydration are adequate
Home care management is understood

FRACTURE OR DISLOCATION OF CERVICAL SPINE

A condition of the cervical spine in which one or more vertebrae are fractured or dislocated; either may cause pressure on the spinal cord, manifesting neurologic dysfunction

Assessment
Observations/findings

Neck pain, headache
Signs of spinal cord compression
  Loss of mobility and sensation below compression

Urinary retention
Paroxysmal hypertension
Bradycardia
Dyspnea

Laboratory/diagnostic studies

Radiologic examination of cervical spine
Baseline CBC, urinalysis, electrolytes

Potential complications

Respiratory distress
Abdominal distention, paralytic ileus
Decreased bowel and urine function
Complete paralysis of all extremities and trunk

Medical management

Immobilization devices: sandbags, Crutchfield tongs, skeletal traction—amount of weight applied
Analgesics, muscle relaxants, antibiotics, stool softeners
Parenteral fluids with electrolytes
Nasogastric aspiration, urinary indwelling catheter
Oxygen therapy, incentive spirometer
Diet, activity, rest

Nursing diagnoses/goals/interventions

ndx: Impaired physical mobility related to location of fracture, dislocation, and/or bed rest

GOAL: *Patient's mobility will be restored within confines of residual effects of fracture or dislocation*

Maintain bed rest in correct body alignment; avoid lifting or twisting head; use sandbags until immobilization device is applied
Place patient in immobilization device as ordered: cervical head halter, skeletal traction, Stryker frame, or Circolectric bed; maintain cervical spine in extention
Assess neurovascular status q2h; monitor pulses, color, temperature, sensation, and mobility of all extremities
Perform passive or assist with and teach active ROM exercises for all extremities q2h
As fracture heals, traction is replaced with casts (halo, Minerva) or neck brace; it is worn continuously; monitor for comfort and correct fit
Ambulate with assistance when ordered; monitor for vertigo and weakness; progress slowly

ndx: Ineffective breathing pattern related to location of fracture and inactivity

GOAL: *Patient's respirations will be adequately maintained to meet body requirements*

Assess respiratory status q2h; observe for dyspnea, cyanosis, and decreased breath sounds
Auscultate chest for breath sounds q2h; assist with and teach patient to deep breathe q1h
Monitor vital signs q2h to 4h; observe for hypertension
Elevate head of bed as ordered; provide incentive spirometer as ordered

ndx: Potential impairment of skin integrity related to bed rest, pressure points, inactivity, and/or skeletal traction

GOAL: *Patient's skin will be maintained clean, dry, and intact without signs of inflammation*

Provide sheepskin or alternating pressure mattress to maintain skin integrity
Administer skin care q2h without turning if not permitted
Apply lanolin-based lotions and provide massage and back rubs
Maintain wrinkle-free bottom sheets
Monitor bilateral skull dressings and tong placement for skeletal traction; observe amount of drainage and cleanse areas q4h with half-strength hydrogen peroxide or normal saline; allow to dry and apply antibiotic ointment as ordered; redress
Monitor weights for correct amount and placement; never release traction, and keep them off floor

ndx: Potential fluid volume deficit related to decreased fluid intake and trauma

GOAL: *Patient will remain adequately hydrated to meet body needs*

Administer parenteral fluids with electrolytes as ordered
Monitor vital signs q2h to 4h
Measure intake and output q8h; observe for urine retention
Auscultate bowel sounds q4h; monitor for diminished sounds
Observe for signs of paralytic ileus: abdominal distention, decreased bowel sounds
Provide well-balanced diet when tolerated and ordered
 Initiate clear to full liquids and progress to soft or regular diet
 Provide foods easily chewed and swallowed
 Assist with feeding as needed
 Observe for signs of dysphagia
Avoid constipation with stool softeners as ordered

ndx: Alteration in comfort: pain related to condition

GOAL: *Patient will express minimal discomfort or absence of pain*

Assess location, type, and duration of pain
Administer analgesics and muscle relaxants as ordered; avoid morphine; assess effectiveness of pain relief measures
Encourage patient to change position slightly at frequent intervals; reinforce correct body alignment
Provide diversional activities

ndx: Knowledge deficit regarding home care management

GOAL: *Patient and/or significant other will demonstrate understanding of home care and follow-up instructions through interactive discussion and actual return demonstration*

Stress importance of prescribed activity and immobilization device
   Need to avoid fatigue with planned rest periods
   Signs and care of pressure points from device
   Length of time device is to be worn
Demonstrate application and care of immobilization device
Explain importance of well-balanced diet; need to avoid weight gain and constipation
Discuss maintaining a safe environment to prevent accidents and falls
Encourage diversional activities
Promote follow-up visits with physician

Evaluation

There are no complications
Pain is managed or controlled
Mobility is restored to optimal level
Home care management is understood

ANKYLOSING SPONDYLITIS

A progressive inflammatory disease of the vertebral column and surrounding tissues that begins in the low back and eventually causes ankylosing and deformity of the entire spinal column; etiology is unknown

Assessment

Observations/findings

Vertebral pain and stiffness on arising; may radiate to buttocks
Limited mobility
Fatigue, malaise, chest discomfort
Anorexia, weight loss
Conjunctivitis, urethritis, polyarthritis
Kyphosis

Laboratory/diagnostic studies

Radiologic examination of spine
Histocompatability antigen HLA: B27 (positive)
ESR (elevated)

Potential complications

Neurologic damage
Respiratory dysfunction depending on stage of progression
Thrombophlebitis
Fractured vertebrae

Medical management

Analgesics, antipyretics, nonsteroid antiinflammatory agents
Exercise program, physical therapy
Bedboard, firm mattress, small pillow
Back brace, corset
Surgical intervention: cervical spinal fusion, osteotomy

Nursing diagnoses/goals/interventions

ndx: Impaired physical mobility related to degree of vertebral involvement

GOAL: *Patient will attain optimal mobility within confines of disease process*

Assess present mobility and observe for increased or decreased impairment
Assist with and reinforce prescribed exercise program
   ROM exercises, ambulation, self-care, and ADLs as tolerated
   Discuss importance of infrequent rest periods, since they are not beneficial
   Provide diversional activities
Prepare bed with bedboard, firm mattress, and small pillow as ordered; administer frequent back rubs and massages
Monitor vital signs q4h
Assess neurologic status; monitor peripheral pulses and check extremities for color, warmth, sensation, edema, and weakness q4h
Monitor skin and mucous membranes for irritation, rashes, or breaks
Administer antiinflammatory agents as ordered

ndx: Alteration in comfort: pain related to inflammation/disease process

GOAL: *Patient will express minimal discomfort or absence of pain*

Assess location and type of pain; observe for progression of pain to new areas

Administer analgesics as ordered; assess effectiveness of pain relief measures

Apply back brace or corset as ordered

Assess respiratory status; auscultate chest for breath sounds; observe for chest pains and dyspnea; teach deep-breathing exercises qh

ndx Disturbance in self-concept related to body image change and lowered self-esteem

GOAL: *Patient will express feelings and concerns and move toward adaptive coping behaviors in a supportive environment*

Allow time for and encourage verbalization of feelings and concerns; listen attentively

Reinforce physician's explanation of disease process, treatment, and expected outcome; clarify misconceptions

Provide a supportive environment and assist patient with identifying positive coping styles

Provide realistic hope and set short-term goals to be attained; praise patient for each task accomplished

Encourage communication with significant other and socialization with family and friends

ndx Knowledge deficit regarding home care management

GOAL: *Patient and/or significant other will demonstrate understanding of home care and follow-up instructions through interactive discussion and actual return demonstration*

Stress importance and benefits of maintaining prescribed exercise program; add swimming as another exercise

Discuss medications: name, schedule, purpose, dosage, and side effects

Promote physical therapy visits if ordered

Demonstrate application and care of brace or corset

Encourage nutritious diet and fluid intake

Stress importance of safe environment to prevent fractures

Discuss signs and symptoms of disease progression: increased pain and immobility

Promote follow-up visits with physician

Evaluation

Mobility is at optimal level

Pain is managed

Adaptive behaviors are demonstrated as related to self-concept

There are no complications

Home care management is understood

CHEMONUCLEOLYSIS

Spinal injection of proteolytic enzyme chymopapain (Chymodiactin, Discase) into a vertebral disc to dissolve the gelatinous core material that is pressing on nerve roots

Preoperative assessment and care

Assess location, duration, and type of pain; relief measures used and activity tolerance

Assess allergies, especially to papaya juice, since injected enzyme is extracted from papaya; discuss also allergies to fast-food hamburgers, beer, and digestive acids

Reinforce physician's explanation of surgical procedure; explain that pain and muscle spasms may continue for months

Explain that patient will be awake during procedure, since local anesthetic is administered

Administer antihistamines and corticosteroids as ordered to prevent allergic reaction and as antiinflammatory agent respectively

Explain that procedure can only be performed once because of antibody formation to enzyme

Postoperative assessment
Observations/findings

Site of injection: edema, drainage

Location and character of pain

Circulatory and neurologic status of extremities: color, temperature, pulses, sensation, mobility

Position and body alignment

Allergic reaction to enzyme: hypotension, tachycardia, arrhythmia, skin rash, hives, perioral/ocular edema

Headache, nausea

Laboratory/diagnostic studies

Radiologic examination during procedure for placement of needle

Potential complications

Neurologic dysfunction

Anaphylactic shock

Thrombophlebitis

Medical management

Position and duration of position postoperatively
Analgesics, muscle relaxants, antiemetics
Diet, rest, activity

Nursing diagnoses/goals/interventions

ndx: Impaired physical mobility related to surgical procedure, pain, and restrictions postoperatively

GOAL: *Patient's mobility will be restored to optimal levels*

Maintain bed rest for 8 to 24 hr or as ordered; assist patient with assuming position of comfort: usually on side with pillow between flexed knees and at back
Provide a trapeze and assist with and teach its use
Change patient's position, using logrolling method q2h; monitor spinal injection site
Perform passive or assist with and teach active ROM exercises of ankles, feet, and calves: dorsiflexions and plantar flexions q1h to 2h
Assess neurovascular status of legs q2h: pedal pulses, color, temperature, sensation, mobility
Monitor vital signs q2h to 4h; observe urine for protein fragments (normal)
Ambulate with assistance when ordered; instruct patient to rise from side and use trapeze
Provide reclining chair, since it takes pressure off lower back, or have patient straddle straight-backed chair backward

ndx: Alteration in comfort: pain related to invasive procedure

GOAL: *Patient will express minimal discomfort or absence of pain*

Assess location and character of pain (muscle spasms are quite painful)
Administer analgesics and/or muscle relaxants as ordered; assess effectiveness of pain relief measures
Administer antiemetics as ordered for nausea; avoid prochlorperazine (Compazine), since it reacts with myelogram dye

ndx: Knowledge deficit regarding home care management

GOAL: *Patient and/or significant other will demonstrate understanding of home care and follow-up instructions through interactive discussion*

Stress importance of good body alignment to reduce pressure on back; review sitting positions and include
Place affected leg on stool while standing
Heavy lifting is contraindicated; bend knees and use leg muscles for moderate weights
Explain need to avoid pregnancy until healing is complete
Promote increasing activities to tolerance
Discuss signs and symptoms to report to physician: increasing pain, muscle spasm, muscle weakness
Explain that protein fragments in urine are normal
Promote follow-up visits with physician

Evaluation

There are no complications
Pain is minimal and controlled
Mobility has improved
Home care management is understood

HIP SURGERY

internal fixation *Surgical repair of hip fractures using an internal fixation device, such as a nail, pin, screw, or plate, or a combination thereof*

cup arthroplasty *Surgical repair of a diseased acetabulum; the head of the femur is covered with a metal cup or mold and is placed into the reconstructed acetabulum; the cup prevents the two surfaces from fusing and reestablishes joint function*

Preoperative assessment and care

Assess respiratory and neurovascular, nutritional, and integumentary status
Assess hearing, visual status, and presence of other diseases
Monitor traction (Buck's or Russell) as ordered
Discuss with and teach patient
  Method of coughing and deep breathing or use of incentive spirometer
  ROM exercises to unaffected extremities
  Postoperative position to be maintained
  Gluteal and abdominal contractions and quadriceps setting
  Dorsiflexion and plantar flexion of foot
  Importance of leg abduction postoperatively
  Use of trapeze
  Method of bladder and bowel elimination
  Method of pain management
Discuss and assist patient in dealing with fears and anxieties
  Reinforce physician's explanation of surgical procedure and follow-up care

Encourage communication with significant other
Elderly patients may need instructions repeated with each task or procedure
Provide praise or encouragement for tasks attempted and completed

Postoperative assessment
Observations/findings

Correct placement of affected leg
Location and character of pain
Neurovascular status of affected extremity
Urinary output, vital signs
Color and amount of wound drainage
Mental alertness
Respiratory status

Laboratory/diagnostic studies

CBC, electrolytes, CO_2
Radiologic examination of hip

Potential complications

Elevated temperature
Hemorrhage
Shock
Urinary retention, infection
Confusion, if elderly
Decubitus ulcers
Atelectasis
Thrombophlebitis
Pin or prosthesis slippage
    Extreme internal or external rotation
    Severe pain
    Localized edema of hip
Malunion of fracture
    Severe pain
    Elevated temperature
    Severe muscle spasms
Fat embolus
    Difficulty in breathing
    Cough
    Chest petechiae
    Tachycardia

Medical management

Position to be maintained
Analgesics, muscle relaxants, antibiotics
Parenteral therapy with electrolytes, urinary catheter
Oxygen therapy, incentive spirometer
Diet, activity, rest

Nursing diagnoses/goals/interventions

ndx Impaired physical mobility related to surgical incision and temporary absence of weight bearing

GOAL: *Patient's mobility will be restored to optimal level*

Maintain bed rest in prescribed position with firm mattress and trapeze
Monitor vital signs and urine output q4h
Perform neurovascular assessment q2h to 4h
Assist and teach patient to cough and deep breathe qh
    Auscultate chest for breath sounds q8h
    Provide incentive spirometer as ordered
    Observe for dyspnea and chest pain
Turn patient on unaffected side q2h as ordered; maintain body alignment with pillow between knees and at back; turn on affected side if ordered
Ambulate with assistance when ordered (cup arthroplasty patients are bedfast longer); assist patient with dangling at bedside, then with standing and pivoting on unaffected leg into chair (no weight bearing); involve physical therapy if available
Assist with and teach ROM exercises to unaffected extremities q4h, and with ROM exercises to knee, foot, and ankle of affected leg; passive continuous ROM machine may be ordered
Encourage and teach use of walker and increase ambulation as tolerated
Monitor incision for Hemovac placement and/or type of drainage; change dressings prn; observe for healing process and signs of infection
Maintain planned rest periods

ndx Alteration in comfort: pain related to surgical procedure

GOAL: *Patient will express minimal discomfort or absence of pain*

Assess location and character of pain
Administer analgesics as ordered; assess effectiveness of pain relief measures
Provide frequent skin care and back rubs; change position slightly to prevent skin breakdown
Monitor dosage of analgesics for the elderly patient, since confusion and disorientation may result with normal dosage
Encourage and increase self-care activities as tolerated
Provide diversional activities
Promote well-balanced diet and increase fluid intake to 2000 ml/day unless contraindicated after parenteral fluids and urinary catheter are discontinued; avoid weight gain and constipation

ndx Knowledge deficit regarding home care management

GOAL: *Patient and/or significant other will demonstrate understanding of home care and follow-up instructions through interactive discussion and actual return demonstration*

Stress importance of prescribed rehabilitation plan: amount of weight bearing and activities allowed; correct body alignment

Discuss need for nutritional diet and fluids to facilitate bone union and to maintain circulation and elimination

Discuss signs and symptoms to report to physician: increased incisional or leg pain, fever, decreased urinary output, signs of wound infection

Demonstrate incisional care

Promote increasing self-care and ADLs as tolerated

Encourage follow-up visits with physician

Evaluation

There are no complications
Pain is managed or controlled
Mobility is increasing to presurgical level
Home care management is understood

TOTAL JOINT ARTHROPLASTY: HIP, KNEE, ANKLE, SHOULDER, ELBOW, WRIST, FINGER

Replacement of a total joint with a prosthesis to provide stability and motion; performed on diseased or traumatized joints

Preoperative assessment and care

Assess respiratory, neurovascular, nutritional, and integumentary status

Assess hearing and visual status and presence of other diseases (diabetes, arthritis)

Discuss with and teach patient
- Method of coughing and deep breathing
- ROM exercises to unaffected extremities
- Postoperative restrictions or limitations; these may differ according to physician preference
- Total hip arthroplasty (Figure 8-2, A)
  - Gluteal and abdominal contractions and quadriceps setting
  - Dorsiflexion and plantar flexion of foot
  - Hip hiking, isometric exercises
  - Use of trapeze
  - Importance of leg abduction or adduction postoperatively, depending on surgical approach
- Total knee arthroplasty (Figure 8-2, B)
  - Quadriceps setting, gluteal contractions, and flexion-extension exercises
  - Straight leg lifts
- Total shoulder arthoplasty (Figure 8-2, C)
  - Presence of sling to support affected arm; no side elevation of arm
  - Prescribed exercises of fingers, wrist, and elbow
- Total elbow arthroplasty (Figure 8-2, D)
  - Presence of abduction humerus splint to prevent rotation
  - Elbow will be immobilized at 90 degrees of flexion
  - Prescribed wrist and finger exercises
- Total wrist arthroplasty (Figure 8-2, E)
  - Presence of volnar splint to prevent wrist flexion
  - Prescribed finger and arm exercises
- Total thumb replacement
  - Presence of immobilizing splint or brace to provide wrist and thumb support but allowing for movement of fingers
  - Prescribed finger and arm exercises
- Total finger arthroplasty (Figure 8-2, F)
  - Presence of immobilizing splint or brace that provides involved finger support but allows movement of other fingers
  - Prescribed exercises for arm and unaffected fingers
- Total ankle arthroplasty (Figure 8-2, G)
  - Presence of posterior plaster cast and Hemovac suction apparatus
  - Method of crutch walking
  - Prescribed exercises for toes and knee
- Involvement of physical therapy department in planning rehabilitation goals
- Methods of bladder and bowel elimination
- Methods of pain management

Administer antibiotics and anticoagulants as ordered
Measure for antiembolic stockings as ordered
Administer surgical scrub bid or as ordered
Discuss and assist patient in dealing with fears and anxieties
- Reinforce physician's explanation of surgical procedure and follow-up care
- Encourage communication with significant other
- Repeat instructions as needed with each procedure or task for elderly patients
- Provide praise and encouragement for tasks attempted and/or completed

Postoperative assessment
Observations/findings

Neurovascular status of involved extremity
- Peripheral pulse, pallor, cyanosis, edema
- Sensation, temperature, mobility

Site of incision
- Wound drains

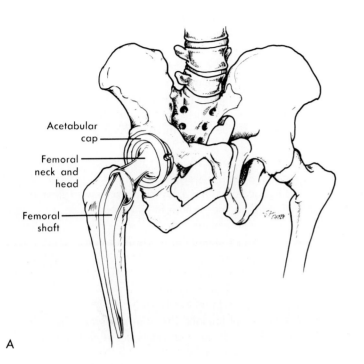
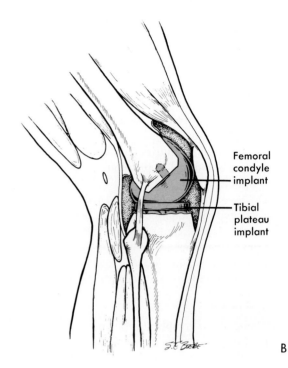
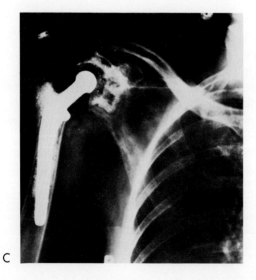
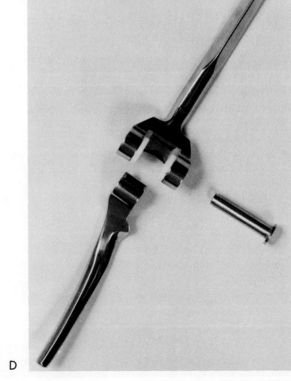

FIGURE 8-2. **A,** Oblique view of total hip arthroplasty. **B,** Total knee arthroplasty. **C,** Shoulder arthroplasty. **D,** Total elbow arthroplasty. **E,** Total wrist arthroplasty. **F,** Total finger arthroplasty. **G,** Total ankle arthroplasty.

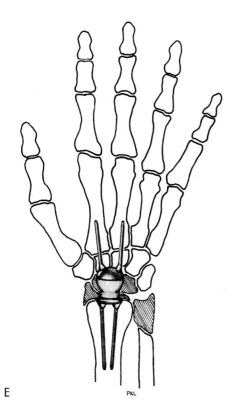
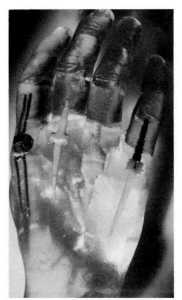
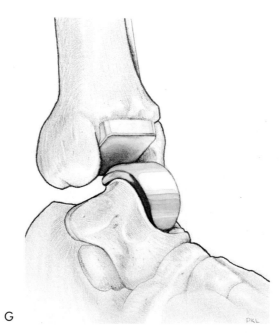

FIGURE 8–2, cont'd. For legend see opposite page.

Hemovac
Excessive bleeding or drainage
Location and character of pain
Respiratory status
Position of affected joint and extremity
Mental alertness

Laboratory/diagnostic studies

Electrolytes, CBC, prothrombin time (PT)
Joint radiologic study

Potential complications

Disorientation (elderly patient)
Elevated temperature
Tachycardia
Tachypnea
Chest pain
Atelectasis
Pneumonia
Thrombophlebitis
Pulmonary embolus
Hemorrhage
Shock
Fat embolus
Wound infection
Compartmental syndrome (knee, elbow)

Medical management

Postoperative position of involved extremity
Parenteral fluids with electrolytes until diet as tolerated
Incision and draining apparatus care
Analgesics, antibiotics, sedatives, antipyretics, anticoagulants, stool softeners, laxatives, antiinflammatory agents
Oxygen therapy: IPPB, incentive spirometer
Antiembolic stockings
Diet, rest
Physical therapy: exercise depends on joint replaced

Nursing diagnoses/goals/interventions

ndx: Impaired physical mobility related to surgical procedure of joint involved and pain

GOAL: *Patient will regain optimal mobility of involved joint*

Maintain bed rest with affected joint in prescribed position
 Provide firm mattress, trapeze, and overhead frame
 Support joint as ordered
Perform passive or assist with and teach active ROM exercises to unaffected joints
Turn patient as ordered; support joint to maintain body alignment
Ambulate with assistance as ordered (length of bed rest depends on joint replaced)
 Provide ambulatory aids as needed
 Observe weight-bearing restrictions as ordered
 Monitor for vertigo, weakness, and nausea
Continuous passive ROM machine may be ordered for affected extremity of hip arthroplasty patients

ndx: Alteration in tissue perfusion: peripheral related to surgical intervention and anesthesia

GOAL: *Patient's circulation will be maintained to fulfill body requirements*

Monitor vital signs q2h to 4h and prn
Assess neurovascular status of affected extremity q1h for 12 hr, then q4h; observe color, temperature, pulse, sensation, and mobility; observe for signs of thrombophlebitis (hip) and compartmental syndrome (elbow, knee)
Apply antiembolic stockings as ordered
Apply ice bags to affected joint as ordered
Monitor CBC, electrolytes, and PT
Administer parenteral fluids as ordered; monitor intake and output; observe for urinary retention
Administer anticoagulants as ordered
Provide high-protein, high-fiber diet when tolerated; force fluids to 2000 ml/day unless contraindicated; assist with feeding as indicated

ndx: Potential for infection (wound, pneumonia) related to surgical intervention and immobility

GOAL: *Patient will remain infection-free or will be successfully treated*

Monitor incision and dressings for drainage and presence of drain or Hemovac
 Attach drain or Hemovac to prescribed apparatus; monitor output for color and amount q4h
 Reinforce dressings prn and change when ordered; observe for signs of healing process or wound infection
 Administer wound irrigation with antibiotics as ordered
Assess respiratory status q4h; observe for pain, dyspnea, and tachyphea
 Auscultate chest for breath sounds q4h; observe for diminished breath sounds
 Provide oxygen therapy as ordered: incentive spirometer, IPPB

Assist patient with coughing and deep breathing qh
Administer antipyretics and/or antibiotics as ordered

ndx: Alteration in comfort: pain related to surgical intervention

GOAL: *Patient will verbalize minimal discomfort or absence of pain*

Assess location and character of pain
Administer analgesics, sedatives, and/or antiinflammatory agents as ordered; assess effectiveness of pain relief measures; monitor dosage for elderly patients, since prescribed dose may cause disorientation
Change position frequently to prevent fatigue and pressure on bony prominences; administer back rubs or massage as indicated
Provide diversional activities
Promote self-care activities as tolerated
Prevent constipation with stool softeners, laxatives, and/or enemas as ordered

ndx: Knowledge deficit regarding rehabilitation plan and home care management

GOAL: *Patient and/or significant other will demonstrate understanding of rehabilitation plan, home care, and follow-up instructions through interactive discussion and actual return demonstration*

Stress importance of and provide written instructions of prescribed rehabilitation program: daily exercises and/or ROM for affected joint, activity allowed, physical therapy involvement
Discuss and demonstrate incision care
Provide medication schedule, including name, purpose, dosage, and side effects; if patient is taking anticoagulants, explain need to have PT checked regularly and to observe for bleeding
Explain importance of diet and fluid intake to facilitate healing and prevent constipation
Discuss need for a safe environment
Discuss signs and symptoms of wound infection to report to physician: fever, inflammation, pain
Promote follow-up visits with physician

Evaluation

There are no complications
Pain is managed
Incision is clean, dry, and intact
Mobility is restored to optimal level
Rehabilitation program and home care management are understood

AMPUTATION OF LEG: ABOVE OR BELOW KNEE

Surgical removal of part of the leg due to trauma, disease, tumors, or congenital anomalies; a skin flap is generally constructed to facilitate healing and use of prosthetic equipment

Preoperative assessment and care

Monitor neurovascular status, both extremities
Observe affected extremity for open, draining sites
Obtain baseline vital signs
Administer skin preparation as ordered
Encourage and allow time for verbalization of fears and anxieties
  Reinforce physician's explanation of operative procedure and phantom limb sensation
  Begin to deal with body image change, loss, and grief; listen carefully and support positive coping behaviors; assist patient with expressing feelings to significant other
Explain process of and preparation for rehabilitation
  Strengthen muscles of upper extremities for crutch walking
    Push-ups from prone position
    Alteration of flexing and extending arms holding weights
    Sit-ups from seated position
  Practice crutch walking
  Practice quadriceps setting exercises, gluteal contraction exercises, and leg lift of affected extremity unless contraindicated
  Practice use of overhead trapeze attached to frame
  Explain types of prostheses available if appropriate
    Immediate postsurgical fitting (IPSF) and immediate postoperative prosthesis (IPOP); used for immediate or early ambulation and weight bearing; cast is applied to stump and prosthesis is attached to cast
    Delayed: dressing and elastic bandage are applied to stump; and prosthesis is not made for 2 to 3 months

Postoperative assessment
Observations/findings

Location and type of pain
Type of dressing or rigid plaster cast
Position of stump
Stump dressing, amount and color of drainage, presence of drains, Hemovac
Respiratory status, vital signs

Laboratory/diagnostic studies

CBC, fasting blood sugar (FBS; for diabetics)

Potential complications

Hemorrhage, dehiscence
Wound infection
Phantom pain
Contractures
Abduction deformity

Medical management

Position of stump postoperatively
Type of dressing and/or postsurgical fitting applied
Analgesics, antibiotics, antipyretics, sedatives
Exercises, physical therapy
Diet, activity, rest

Nursing diagnoses/goals/interventions

ndx: Impaired physical mobility related to amputation

GOAL: *Patient's mobility will improve to optimal level with use of crutches and/or prosthesis*

Maintain bed rest in prescribed position
    Elevate stump as ordered; usually for 24 hr; avoid pillow unless it is removed for 30 min q2h to prevent contractures; avoid outward rotation
    Elevate head no more than 30 degrees
Maintain heavy tourniquet at head of bed to apply if hemorrhage occurs
Turn from side to back to abdomen (after 24 hr) q2h as ordered
Assist with and teach active or perform passive ROM exercises q4h to unaffected extremities
Assist with and teach adduction and extension exercises to affected extremity q4h
Assist with ambulation when allowed
    No prosthesis
        Avoid long periods of chair-sitting
        Provide ambulation devices: crutches, walker
        Encourage use of good walking shoe and maintain stump in normal position—relaxed and in downward position—involve physical therapy
    Prosthesis
        Assist with measuring for prosthesis
        Provide ambulation device: crutches, walker
        Increase ambulation with prescribed amount of weight bearing; involve physical therapy
Assist with and reiterate postoperative conditioning exercises: trunk flexion, sit-ups, hopping in place, hopping with walker

ndx: Alteration in peripheral tissue perfusion related to surgical intervention and trauma

GOAL: *Patient's incision will remain clean, dry, and intact with no evidence of excessive bleeding*

Monitor vital signs q2h to 4h
Monitor dressings and incision for color and amount of drainage and for presence of drains or Hemovac; observe for bleeding; outline bleeding area on dressing with pen and write date and time
Monitor postsurgical cast for bleeding and mark area as above; observe for cast slippage and report to physician

ndx: Potential for infection related to bacterial invasion of incision

GOAL: *Patient's wound will be clean, dry, and intact*

Change stump dressing and elastic bandage, when allowed, to produce shrinkage and prepare for prosthesis
    Wash and dry area, and expose it to air before reapplying
    Perform at least bid
    Observe for signs of infection and increasing edema
    Begin stump strengthening and conditioning as ordered; push against pillow and increase to firmer surface as tolerated
Change postsurgical cast dressing; wash and dry area, and allow it to air dry bid
    Apply properly fitting stump sock daily and prn
    Observe incision and surrounding area for increasing edema and signs of wound infection
    Massage stump toward suture line as ordered: usually 1 week postoperatively
    Reapply postsurgical cast
Measure intake and output q8h
Monitor vital signs q4h
Provide high-protein diet and force fluids to upper limits for age and weight as ordered
Administer antibiotics and/or antipyretics as ordered

ndx: Alteration in comfort: pain related to surgical amputation

GOAL: *Patient will express minimal discomfort or absence of pain*

Assess character and location of pain; observe for compartmental syndrome in below-the-knee amputation
Administer analgesics and sedatives as ordered; assess effectiveness of pain relief measures
Assist patient with changing position slightly at frequent intervals to reduce fatigue and pressure; provide back rubs
Provide diversional activities

Discuss and explain phantom pain and that the pain is usually temporary

Coordinate care to provide rest periods

Prevent constipation with stool softeners, laxatives, and/or enemas as ordered

ndx: Alteration in self-concept related to body image change

GOAL: *Patient will express feelings and move toward adaptive coping patterns in a supportive environment*

Encourage and allow time for patient to express feelings of loss and grief

Assist in identifying positive coping behaviors and provide encouragement and praise for strengths observed

Provide praise for attempted and/or completed tasks

Encourage patient to perform self-care activities and involve patient in stump care as soon as tolerated; promote independence

Promote communication with significant other

Explain all procedures and treatments

ndx: Knowledge deficit regarding rehabilitation program and home care management

GOAL: *Patient and/or significant other will demonstrate understanding of rehabilitation program, home care, and follow-up instructions through interactive discussion and actual return demonstration*

Stress importance of rehabilitation program; involve physical therapy for daily exercises and stump strengthening and conditioning

Demonstrate dressing changes, incisional care, skin care, and massage technique of stump

Discuss and demonstrate care of IPSF/IPOP as indicated; consult physical therapy

Promote safe home environment; wear rubber-soled shoe(s) as indicated

Discuss signs and symptoms to report to physician: fever, inflammation of incision, prolonged phantom pain, increasing edema of stump

Discuss importance of well-balanced diet; avoid weight gain and constipation

Encourage follow-up visits with physician

Evaluation

There are no complications

Pain is controlled

Mobility is maintained to optimal level

Positive coping patterns are demonstrated

Rehabilitation program and home care management are understood

ARTHROSCOPIC SURGERY OF KNEE

Management of various knee disorders, using an arthroscope; small surgical instruments are introduced via a trocar and scope into the knee joint, and needed surgical procedures are performed; this technique allows for early rehabilitation and return to work, as well as decreased patient discomfort and confinement

Preoperative assessment and care

Determine presence or absence of both pedal pulses

Discuss with and teach patient
    ROM exercises to unaffected extremities
    Restrictions and limitations postoperatively
        These will vary with physicians and according to extent of surgery
            Usually patient is out of bed on evening of surgery, but with no weight bearing
    Method of crutch walking
    Methods of pain management

Administer antiseptic scrub to affected knee as ordered

Reinforce physician's explanation of procedure

Explain that local anesthetic is usually used

Postoperative assessment
Observations/findings

Position of knee and degree of elevation

Character and amount of drainage

Type of immobilization device (rarely used)

Neurovascular status of affected leg: pulse, color, temperature, sensation, mobility

Location and character of pain

Potential complications

Edema

Hemorrhage

Thrombophlebitis

Postoperative arthrosis

Compartmental syndrome

Medical management

Analgesics, antibiotics, sedatives

Position of knee postoperatively, exercises, ambulation

Ice bag to knee

Diet, activity, rest

Nursing diagnoses/goals/interventions

ndx: Alteration in peripheral tissue perfusion related to arthroscopy

GOAL: *Patient's circulation to affected extremity will be maintained*

Monitor neurovascular status of affected extremity q1h for 4hr, then q4h; check pulse, color, temperature, sensation, and mobility
Monitor vital signs q4h
Assess dressing, and color and amount of drainage (should be scant); change prn
Apply ice pack to knee as ordered

ndx: Impaired physical mobility related to procedure and discomfort

GOAL: *Patient will regain mobility to optimal level*

Maintain bed rest in position of comfort with involved knee elevated in slight flexion
Encourage ROM exercises of unaffected extremities q2h
Ambulate with assistance as ordered (usually on evening of surgery)
    Assist patient with getting out of bed, keeping affected leg elevated until standing; no weight bearing until ordered
    Assist patient with use of crutches
    Increase ambulation as ordered and tolerated
    Provide rest periods between ambulations
Initiate and assist with ordered exercises; these depend on physician preference and extent of surgery
    Involve physical therapy if available
    Teach dorsiflexion and plantar flexion of foot and increasing flexion of knee as ordered

ndx: Alteration in comfort: pain related to invasive procedure

GOAL: *Patient will express absence of pain or minimal discomfort*

Assess location and type of pain; severe unrelenting pain and edema may indicate compartmental syndrome
Administer analgesics and/or sedatives as ordered
Provide well-balanced diet and encourage fluid intake to upper levels for age and weight

ndx: Knowledge deficit regarding home care management and rehabilitation program

GOAL: *Patient and/or significant other will demonstrate understanding of rehabilitation program, home care, and follow-up instructions through interactive discussion*

Stress importance and goals of prescribed rehabilitation program
    Amount of weight bearing and knee flexion allowed
    Need to elevate leg while sitting
    Need to avoid twisting knee
    Dorsiflexion and plantar flexion exercises of feet
    Planned rest periods between exercises
    Ambulation with crutches
    Dates and times of physical therapy visits as ordered
    Swimming may be encouraged
Discuss signs of wound infection to report to physician
Promote follow-up care with physician

Evaluation

There are no complications
Mobility is at optimal level
Rehabilitation and home care management are understood

EXTERNAL FIXATION FOR COMPLICATED FRACTURES

A surgical procedure to immobilize and reduce complicated fractures; stabilizing pins or wires are inserted into and/or through the bone and attached to an external metal frame (Figure 8-3)

Preoperative assessment and care

Preoperative teaching may be limited, depending on urgency of needed treatment
Assess neurovascular and respiratory status
Discuss with and teach patient
    Methods of coughing and deep breathing and/or use of incentive spirometer
    Necessary ROM exercises, quadriceps setting, and gluteal contractions according to location of fracture
    Use of trapeze
    Necessary movement limitations and activities allowed
    Importance of external fixator
        Reinforce physician's explanation of procedure
        Fixator usually causes little pain or discomfort, and allows for early ambulation
        Device is unsightly, but long-range results are primary goal
Explain that extremity will be elevated postoperatively to reduce edema
Involve physical therapy department, if available, for crutch walking and exercises
Administer antibiotics and skin prep as ordered

Postoperative assessment
Observations/findings

Elevation and position of extremity
Edema of extremity at operative site and below
Presence of supportive dressings

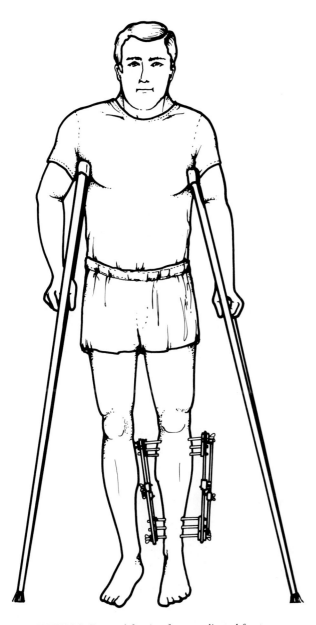

FIGURE 8-3. External fixation for complicated fractures.

Character and amount of drainage from wound and pin sites
Neurovascular status of affected extremity: color, sensation, mobility, peripheral pulse, temperature
Location and character of pain

Laboratory/diagnostic studies

CBC
Radiologic examination of affected bone

Potential complications

Hemorrhage
Shock
Wound or pin site infection
Nonunion, malunion
Neuromuscular dysfunction
Compartmental syndrome

Medical management

Position of affected extremity
Analgesics, antibiotics, antipyretics, sedatives
Ice bag to area
Diet, activity, ambulation, rest

Nursing diagnoses/goals/interventions

ndx: Impaired physical mobility related to surgical intervention and pain

GOAL: *Patient will regain mobility to optimal level*

Maintain bed rest in position of comfort with extremity elevated as ordered
Assist with and teach active ROM exercises to unaffected extremities q2h to 4h; initiate quadriceps setting, gluteal contractions, or palmar or dorsal flexion as needed
Assist and teach patient to cough and deep breathe qh
Monitor neurovascular status of affected extremity q1h for 24 hr, then q4h
Monitor vital signs q4h
Ambulate when ordered (usually when edema of soft tissues has decreased)
  Holding fixator with both hands, assist patient to sitting position on bed side; observe for vertigo and nausea
  Always support fixator, not extremity
  Assist patient with ambulation with crutches or sling as indicated
Do not change or adjust fixator bars (can cause misalignment)
  No weight bearing until ordered
  Physical therapy department will be involved where available
Elevate extremity while sitting up

ndx: Actual impairment of skin integrity related to pin and fixator insertion

GOAL: *Patient's pin sites and incisions will remain clean, dry, and intact*

Monitor pin sites, incision, and supportive dressing q1h to 2h for drainage and edema
Initiate pin site and incisional care bid
  Assess for pain, tenderness, redness, and tension around each pin site
  Cleanse around each pin site with hydrogen peroxide; rinse with normal saline

Apply nonocclusive antibacterial agent around each pin as ordered
Allow to air dry
Cover each pin head with cork or rubber tip to prevent injury
Cleanse fixator with sterile water
Assist with and teach patient wound, pin site, and fixator care as soon as patient is physically and emotionally able
Change incisional dressings bid prn; observe for wound healing
Apply ice bags to area as ordered
Administer antibiotics and antipyretics as ordered

ndx: Alteration in comfort: pain related to surgical intervention

GOAL: *Patient will verbalize minimal discomfort or absence of pain*

Assess location and character of pain; observe proximal joint for compartmental syndrome signs: unrelenting pain, edema
Administer analgesics and sedatives as ordered; assess effectiveness of pain relief measures
Assist patient with changing position frequently while in bed to prevent fatigue and pressure
Provide diversional activities
Prevent constipation with stool softeners as ordered

ndx: Disturbance in self-concept related to body image change (external fixator)

GOAL: *Patient will verbalize feelings and be assisted in learning adaptive behaviors in a supportive environment*

Promote and allow time for expression of feelings; encourage communication with significant other
Assist in identifying positive coping patterns; acknowledge strengths
Promote self-care activities and praise tasks attempted or completed
Stress that fixator is temporary and promote its positive aspects

ndx: Knowledge deficit regarding rehabilitation program, care of external device, and home management

GOAL: *Patient and/or significant other will demonstrate understanding of home care and follow-up instructions through interactive discussion and actual return demonstration*

Provide goals, restrictions, and activities of rehabilitation program as outlined by physician
Demonstrate care of pins, fixator, and incision
  Observe return demonstration
  Stress importance of not tampering with fixator, since it may alter alignment of fracture
  Explain that showering is permitted, but that patient needs to avoid swimming, since chlorine and salt corrode metal
Stress importance of diet and elimination
Discuss signs and symptoms of wound infection to report to physician
Encourage follow-up visits with physician

Evaluation

There are no complications
Mobility is regained to optimal level
Home care management of fixator and rehabilitation program are understood

DIGITAL REPLANTATION

Surgical reconnection of severed digit(s) following trauma by a sharp object, crushing blow, or avulsion; general criteria for replantation include thumb replacement, multiple digit replacement, or replacement if patient is a child or if patient's occupation requires manual skills; surgery must be performed within 24 hr

Preoperative assessment and care

Preservation of digit(s)
  Wrap digit(s) in gauze soaked with normal saline
  Place in plastic bag
  Place bag in ice
  Never place digit directly on ice
Care of amputated stump: apply sterile pressure dressing and elevate hand as ordered
Administer parenteral fluids with antibiotics as ordered
Administer anticoagulant and tetanus toxoid as ordered
Assess respiratory, cardiovascular, and neurologic status
Determine presence or absence of further trauma or injury
Assess medication and medical history; diseases such as diabetes, chronic obstructive pulmonary disease (COPD), vascular disease, rheumatoid arthritis, osteoarthritis, and bleeding tendencies inhibit replantation success

Determine dominant hand
Assess emotional status where possible
- Be alert for maladaptive behavior, since functional return depends on patient's motivation, emotional acceptance, and willingness to adapt to alterations in body image and life-style
- Reinforce physician's explanation of surgical procedure
- Discuss and deal with fears and anxieties
- Encourage communication with significant other

Discuss with and assist patient with understanding that because nicotine is a potent vasoconstrictor, smoking is prohibited for 3 weeks

Postoperative assessment

Observations/findings

Neurovascular status of digit
- Sensation, color, temperature
- Capillary refill, skin turgor
- Edema

Anatomic position of digit, wrist, and elbow, and elevation of each

Presence or absence of skin graft and graft site

Character and amount of drainage from incision

Location and character of pain

Laboratory/diagnostic studies

CBC, PT

Radiologic examination of replantation

Potential complications

Hemorrhage
Shock
Vascular thrombosis or occlusion
Wound infection
Inappropriate or maladaptive behavior
Nonunion or malunion of digit(s)

Medical management

Position and immobilization of wrist, hand, and digits
Analgesics, antibiotics, anticoagulants
Physical therapy involvement
Diet, activity, rest

Nursing diagnoses/goals/interventions

ndx Alteration in peripheral tissue perfusion related to surgical intervention/replantation

GOAL: *Patient's circulation to affected hand and digit(s) will become adequate to maintain perfusion*

Maintain bed rest in position of comfort within confines of prescribed position of affected arm

Elevate affected arm on pillow
- Wrist and hand elevation of 30 degrees
- Forearm in prone position
- Elbow flexion of no more than 10 to 15 degrees, since further flexion may impair venous return

Repositioning patient in bed may alter prescribed position of affected arm

Assess neurovascular status of digit(s) qh
- Check sensation, temperature, color, pulse, skin turgor, and capillary refill
- Digit is pinker and capillary refill is faster immediately after surgery; accurate assessment and recording are imperative
- Report alterations in color to physician immediately
  - Pink to white or mottled: arterial failure
  - Pink to dusky purple: venous failure
- Both nurses assess status at change of shift

Monitor vital signs q4h for 24 hr, then qid; monitor BP on unaffected arm

Check dressing qh for drainage; report excess bleeding to physician; change dressing as ordered

Monitor Hgb, Hct, and PT

Maintain NPO until fully reactive

Administer parenteral fluids with antibiotics and anticoagulants as ordered

Observe for occult bleeding: gums and injection sites

Measure intake and output

ndx Impaired physical mobility related to surgical procedure

GOAL: *Patient will regain digital mobility to an optimal level*

Assist and teach patient to cough and deep breathe qh while in bed

Perform passive or assist with and teach active ROM exercises q4h to unaffected extremities while in bed

Ambulate with assistance when ordered
- Maintain forearm and hand in sling
- Observe for vertigo and nausea

Involve patient, and physical and occupational therapy departments in establishing rehabilitation goals according to physician's order
- Goals are individualized according to
  - Healing process and progress
  - Patient's motivation to master manual skills
  - Patient's willingness to use replanted digit
  - Patient's acceptance of replanted digit into body image

Assist patient with and teach modified ADLs according to prescribed limitations dictated by surgery and if affected arm is dominant

Provide liquid to regular diet when tolerated
  Assist with eating if affected arm is dominant
  Force fluids to upper limits of normal for age unless contraindicated

ndx: Alteration in comfort: pain related to trauma and surgical procedure

GOAL: *Patient will verbalize minimal discomfort or absence of pain*

Assess location and character of pain
Administer analgesics as ordered; assess effectiveness of pain relief measures
Assist patient with changing position frequently to prevent pressure and fatigue; maintain elbow flexion at prescribed amount
Provide diversional activities

ndx: Disturbance in self-concept related to body image change

GOAL: *Patient will verbalize feelings and make strides in attaining adaptive coping patterns in a supportive environment*

Provide time for and assist patient in expressing feelings, encourage communication with significant other
Assess present coping behaviors and reinforce positive coping patterns that helped in the past
Stress positive aspects of replantation
Reinforce physician's explanation of expected outcome of surgical procedure
Involve patient in self-care as soon as patient is physically able

ndx: Knowledge deficit regarding home care management

GOAL: *Patient and/or significant other will demonstrate understanding of home care and follow-up instructions through interactive discussion and actual return demonstration*

Stress importance of prescribed rehabilitation program
  Degree of movement of digit allowed and duration and times of exercise
  Exercises for wrist, elbow, and arm
  Position of arm, elbow, and hand during rest and ambulation
Stress that using and wanting to use the digit are the most important factors in function return
Paresthesia may last 4 to 6 months, whereas return of function may take a year

Replanted digit(s) may be shorter than opposing digit(s)
Demonstrate incisional care and discuss signs of wound infection
Stress importance of well-balanced diet, rest, and daily exercise
Explain symptoms to report to physician
  Changes in color and temperature of digit
  Increased incisional pain and/or edema
  Wound infection
Promote importance of physical therapy and follow-up visits with physician

Evaluation

There are no complications
Circulation of digit is regained to optimal level
Pain is controlled
Home care management is understood

COMPARTMENTAL SYNDROME

Increased pressure in compartments of the forearm or lower leg following trauma; within compartments are muscles, blood vessels, and nerves, and any internal pressure (trauma, surgery, edema, bleeding) or external pressure (tight casts or dressings, IV infiltrations) can cause impaired circulation, nerve damage, and muscle weakness; if left unchecked, necrosis with loss of extremity and renal failure, acidosis, and shock (crush syndrome) can occur

Assessment
Observations/findings

Pain in compartment area: increasing, unrelenting, and unrelieved by narcotics
Swelling and localized redness
Pain with passive motion of fingers or toes
Paresthesia of hand or foot
Absent pulse below compartment
Progressive loss of motor function

Laboratory/diagnostic studies

Deep vein thrombosis (DVT) studies
Ankle or brachial index
Vascular occlusion studies
CBC, PT

Potential complications

Neurovascular dysfunction of extremity
Muscle weakness
Necrosis, amputation
Renal failure, acidosis
Shock

Medical management

Analgesics, antibiotics
Dressing and cast removal; cast window made
Neurovascular check q½h
Tissue pressure monitoring, fasciotomy

Nursing diagnoses/goals/interventions

ndx: Alteration in peripheral tissue perfusion related to syndrome

GOAL: *Patient's circulation to extremity will be maintained*

Monitor and assess pain q½h if syndrome is suspected
   Notify physician immediately if pain in extremity is
     Increasing
     Unrelenting
     Unrelieved by narcotics
     Occurring during passive motion of fingers or toes
   Be aware that this type of pain is primary indicator of compartmental syndrome; other symptoms may take longer to appear
Remove dressing or have windows cut in cast immediately as ordered
Assess neurovascular status of foot or hand bilaterally q15 to 30 min
Measure forearm or calf bilaterally for presence of or increase in edema q1h to 2h
If no improvement is noted, prepare for and assist with tissue pressure monitoring, a means to measure fascial pressure (normal fascial pressure is about 4 mm Hg, and when this pressure nears 30 mm Hg below diastolic pressure, capillaries and arteries will close, causing occlusion)
Prepare for fasciotomy as ordered (longitudinal incision into fascia surrounding compartment to release pressure)
Needle may be removed or left in place for continuous monitoring
Postoperatively, extremity will be immobilized in posterior cast or splint
Be aware that wound may be left open, with future grafting required, and that it may be a long, painful procedure
Change dressings as needed; observe for altered alignment of extremity
Continue neurovascular monitoring qh; observe for return of color, temperature, and capillary refill
Assess pain and observe for relief following analgesic administration

ndx: Anxiety/fear related to lack of knowledge of the syndrome and emergency procedure

GOAL: *Patient will express anxieties and fears and experience an increase in comfort following explanation of condition, procedure, and expected outcome*

Reinforce physician's explanation of syndrome, procedure, and outcome
Allow time for verbalization of fears and explain all treatments as much as possible
Following procedure assist patient in identifying coping strengths and discuss ways of dealing with wound and possible skin grafting
Encourage communication with significant other

Evaluation

There are no further complications
Wound heals with or without skin grafting
Circulation is restored to hand or foot

TISSUE PRESSURE MONITORING

A procedure for measuring fascial tissue pressure to diagnose compartmental syndrome

Preprocedure assessment and care

Explain procedure to patient (patient will have severe forearm or lower leg pain)
Check baseline BP
Equipment needed
   Local anesthetic, needle, and syringe
   Vial of bacteriostatic normal saline
   Three-way stopcock
   Mercury manometer
   20 ml sterile syringe
   Two 18-gauge needles
   Two IV extension tubes
Prepare muscle site for injection and equipment as shown below
Position patient as comfortably as possible

Interventions

Prepare site with antiseptic
Assist physician with anesthetizing exposed muscle site
Following diagram A (Figure 8-4)
   Withdraw enough saline with syringe to fill IV tube half full
   Close stopcock
Following diagram B (Figure 8-4)
   Assist physician with needle insertion into fascia
   Connect second IV tube to manometer and close stopcock

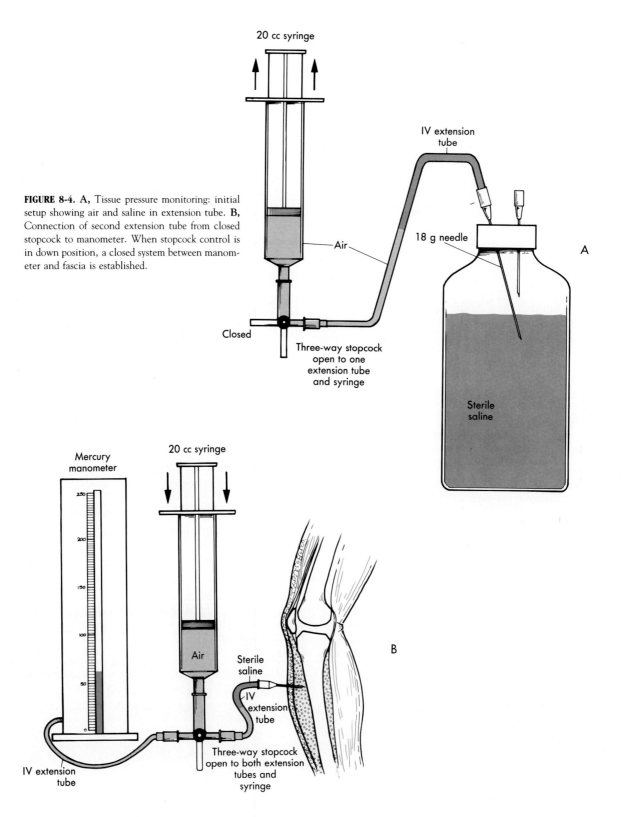

FIGURE 8-4. A, Tissue pressure monitoring: initial setup showing air and saline in extension tube. **B,** Connection of second extension tube from closed stopcock to manometer. When stopcock control is in down position, a closed system between manometer and fascia is established.

Move stopcock control to down position opposite syringe; this provides closed system

Gently depress syringe barrel to increase pressure in system; manometer will begin to register

When closed system pressure exceeds fascial pressure, some saline will enter fascia; amount of saline in IV tubing will decrease

Observe manometer at this point; this is tissue pressure reading

Assist with second fascial injection to verify initial reading

Normal fascial tissue pressure is about 4 mm Hg; readings of 30 mm Hg or more are usually diagnostic of compartmental syndrome, but this may vary according to physician

Monitor bilateral peripheral pulses and measure calf, forearm, thigh, or arm for edema

Needle may be removed or left in place for continuous monitoring

Assist patient with assuming position of comfort and prepare for fasciotomy as ordered

OPEN MENISECTOMY

Surgical removal of the meniscus of the knee joint following a traumatic injury; closed menisectomy may be performed using an arthroscope

Preoperative assessment and care

Determine presence or absence of bilateral pedal pulses
Discuss with and teach patient
- Quadriceps setting
- Straight leg lifts
- Crutch walking (p. 516)
- Use of trapeze
- ROM exercises

Postoperative assessment

Observations/findings

Neurovascular status of involved extremity: pulses, color, temperature, edema, sensation, and mobility
Location and character of pain
Site of incision: drainage, bleeding

Potential complications

Fever
Hemorrhage
Compartmental syndrome
Phlebitis
Wound infection
Peroneal nerve damage
Numbness in lower leg or foot
Inability to abduct foot
Inability to dorsiflex foot
Posterior tibial nerve damage
Sensory loss
Inability to abduct toes
Loss of ankle jerk

Medical management

Immobilization device (cast, splint, elastic bandage)
Ice bag to knee
Analgesics, antibiotics
Exercise, diet, ambulation

Nursing diagnoses/goals/interventions

ndx Alteration in peripheral tissue perfusion related to surgical intervention

GOAL: *Patient's circulation to affected extremity will remain adequate*

Monitor neurovascular status q1h to 2h; compare with other extremity as to color, pulses, temperature, edema, sensation, and mobility
Monitor vital signs q4h
Apply ice bag to affected knee as ordered
Elevate leg and knee as ordered
Monitor immobilization device: correct alignment, pressure areas, constriction of circulation
Encourage patient to deep breathe qh

ndx Impaired physical mobility related to pain and surgical intervention

GOAL: *Patient will regain mobility to optimal level*

Maintain bed rest until fully reactive with affected leg in extension
Assist patient with straight leg lifts and quadriceps setting exercises q1h to 2h as ordered, 5 to 20 times, holding quadriceps setting to count of 5
Assist patient up in chair with affected leg elevated as ordered; support leg when assisting patient to and from bed
Ambulate with assistance as ordered; assist with crutch walking (no weight bearing initially); increase as ordered
Inspect incision q4h; change dressing prn; report increasing edema and pain to physician (compartmental syndrome)
Demonstrate application and care of immobilization device; remove q8h, wash entire extremity, dry well, apply lotion lightly, and reapply device
Assist with ROM exercises to unaffected extremities q2h while patient is in bed

Promote self-care activities as tolerated and assist with ADLs as needed

ndx: Alteration in comfort: pain related to trauma and surgical procedure

GOAL: *Patient will verbalize minimal discomfort or absence of pain*

Assess location and character of pain
Administer analgesics as ordered; assess effectiveness of pain relief measures; observe for signs of thrombophlebitis or compartmental syndrome
Assist patient with changing position frequently to prevent pressure and fatigue; maintain correct alignment of extremity
Provide and encourage diversional activities

ndx: Knowledge deficit regarding rehabilitation program and home care management

GOAL: *Patient and/or significant other will demonstrate understanding of rehabilitation program and home care and follow-up instructions through interactive discussion and actual return demonstration*

Provide and discuss importance of rehabilitation goals: activities and exercises as ordered
Stress importance of avoiding strenuous exercises (running, climbing, squatting) that could retraumatize knee
Reiterate application and care of immobilization device
Demonstrate neurovascular check and explain signs to report to physician
Demonstrate incisional care and symptoms of wound infection to report to physician
Encourage follow-up visits with physician

Evaluation

There are no complications
Circulation to extremity is maintained
Pain is controlled
Mobility is restored to optimal level
Rehabilitation program and home care management are understood

BUNIONECTOMY

Surgical correction of hereditary or acquired hallux valgus: acute angulation of the first metatarsophalangeal joint; procedure is either Keller or Mayo arthroplasty

Preoperative assessment and care

Assess mobility, color, and sensation of toes
Discuss with and teach patient
    Crutch walking
    Use of walker
    Toe flexing
    Quadriceps setting
    ROM exercises

Postoperative assessment
Observations/findings

Neurovascular status of affected toes: color, temperature, sensation, edema
Location and character of pain
Site of incision for drainage and bleeding
Placement of plaster toe cap or splint

Potential complications

Fever
Wound infection
Recurrence of hallux valgus

Medical management

Analgesics, antipyretics
Type of immobilization device
Ambulation, weight bearing
Diet, activity, rest
Ice bags to affected site

Nursing diagnoses/goals/interventions

ndx: Altered physical mobility related to surgical intervention and pain

GOAL: *Patient will regain mobility of affected foot to optimal level*

Maintain bed rest until fully reactive
    Elevate foot as ordered
    Place bed cradle over feet
    Monitor immobilization device for pressure areas and circulatory constriction
Ambulate with assistance as ordered: usually 24 to 48 hr postoperatively
Monitor vital signs q4h and affected toe for color, temperature, sensation, and edema q2h for 24 hr, then qid
Assist patient with performing ROM exercises q4h while in bed
Monitor dressing and cast for drainage q2h
Assist and teach patient to turn and deep breathe q2h to 3h while in bed; hold affected foot during turn and place on pillow after turn has been completed

Apply plaster walking boot if ordered
Initiate flexing exercises of toes five times qh when edema subsides and as ordered

ndx Alteration in comfort: pain related to surgical intervention

GOAL: *Patient will express minimal discomfort or absence of pain*

Assess location and character of pain
Administer analgesics as ordered; assess effectiveness of pain relief measures
Apply ice bag to area as ordered
Assist patient with changing position frequently while on bed rest
Provide diet as tolerated

ndx Knowledge deficit regarding home care management

GOAL: *Patient and/or significant other will demonstrate understanding of home care and follow-up instructions through interactive discussion and actual return demonstration*

Stress importance of foot and incisional care, and prescribed exercises
  Demonstrate dressing change
  Explain need for foot soaks in warm, soapy water after sutures are removed; need to dry feet well
  Discuss care of plaster boot if applicable
  Demonstrate toe and foot ROM exercises
  Explain importance of proper footwear
Discuss activities allowed; encourage self-care and ADLs
Discuss signs of wound infection to report to physician: fever, pain, edema
Encourage follow-up care with physician

Evaluation

There are no complications
Pain is managed
Mobility is restored to optimal level
Home care management is understood

TRACTION

Method of providing a pulling effect to an extremity or body part while also maintaining a countertraction (pull in opposite direction)

balanced suspension with Thomas' splint and Pearson's attachment Skeletal or skin traction *applied to a lower extremity while weights and a splint simultaneously provide countertraction and suspension of that extremity*
skin traction *Light or temporary traction applied directly to the skin*
skeletal traction *Insertion of a pin or wire into a bone to provide continuous traction*
pelvic traction *Provides traction to the lower back as a means of reducing low back pain*
traction on the humerus (side arm traction) *Skin traction to the humerus to align the fracture after an open reduction procedure*
cervical traction *Application of a cervical halter with traction to reduce neck pain or when a fracture of the cervical spine is suspected*
Bryant's traction *Treatment for fractures of the femur shaft in young children*
halo traction *Metal brace attached to the skull and iliac crest or femur with pins; provides spinal support following fusion or as treatment for scoliosis*

Interventions
General

Maintain constant pull in line with deformity
Assess and maintain ropes and pulleys
  Taut
  Riding freely over pulleys
  Free of bedding
  Knots secure
  Adequate space between pulley and traction
Monitor and maintain weights
  Hanging free
  Off floor
  Away from bed
  NOTE: *Never remove weights; never lift weights*
Monitor and maintain countertraction
  Elevation of bed under part to which traction is applied
  Pull exerted against fixed point
  Pull exerted against traction in opposite direction

Balanced suspension with Thomas' splint and Pearson's attachment (Figure 8-5)

Maintain anatomic position of extremity
Maintain 20-degree angle between thigh and bed
Have heel clear of sling under calf
Maintain abduction of extremity
Monitor femoral and popliteal pulses

Skin traction

Observe carefully for slippage and bunching up of bandage

PATIENT CARE STANDARDS

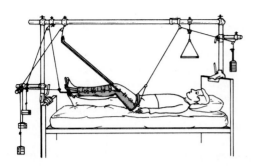

FIGURE 8-5. Balanced suspension with Thomas' splint and Pearson's attachment.

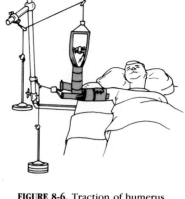

FIGURE 8-6. Traction of humerus.

Replace bandage prn
Observe for pressure areas at distal end of bandage (wrist or heel), especially if weight is greater than 7 pounds
Check neurovascular status q2h to 4h

Skeletal traction

Cover ends of pin with cork
Observe site of insertion
    Redness
    Swelling
    Discharge
    Odor
    Bleeding
Clean skin around puncture sites as ordered; do not remove crusts around pin sites
Monitor neurovascular status q2h to 4h

Pelvic traction

Ensure that pelvic girdle is proper size for patient and that pelvic girdle fits snugly over iliac crests and pelvis
Inspect skin areas over iliac crests for pressure points q4h
Pelvic straps must be equal in length and unrestricted

Traction on the humerus: side arm traction (Figure 8-6)

Maintain position as directed by physician
Check neurovascular status of affected arm q2h to 4h
Notify physician immediately if any change is noted
Apply chest restraint sheet for countertraction prn

Cervical traction (Figure 8-7)

Position without pillows
Take care that weight and pulley are free of wall

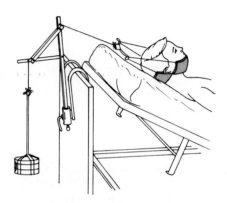

FIGURE 8-7. Cervical traction.

Observe for pressure areas
    Jaws and ears
    Site of head
    Back of head
Pad as necessary for comfort

Bryant's traction (Figure 8-8)

Raise buttocks slightly from mattress
Observe bandages carefully for slippage and bunching over heel cords
Observe for skin sloughing on both legs
Check feet for color, pulses, temperature, and sensation q2h to 4h
Use harness restraint to prevent turning over
Avoid thick, wide diapers between legs

Halo traction

Cover ends of pins with cork
Observe pin insertion sites
    Redness

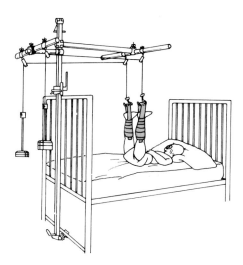

FIGURE 8-8. Bryant's traction.

Swelling
Drainage
Odor
Bleeding
Clean skin around pin sites as ordered; do not remove crusts
Monitor straps for areas of constriction
Pad pressure points as necessary for comfort
Do not alter amount of traction applied

CARE OF PATIENT IN TRACTION

Assessment

Observations/findings

Neurovascular status of affected extremity
Cardiopulmonary status
Integumentary status
Type of traction
Urinary retention
Fecal impaction
Location and type of pain

Laboratory/diagnostic studies

CBC, urinalysis
Radiologic study of affected bone and joint

Potential complications

Phlebitis
Compartmental syndrome (knee, elbow)
Infection if wounds are present
Fat embolism

Medical management

Analgesics, tranquilizers, muscle relaxants, stool softeners
Type of traction and weight
Ice bag, antiembolic stocking(s)
Physical therapy
Diet, activity, rest

Nursing diagnoses/goals/interventions

ndx: Alteration in comfort: pain related to physical immobility

GOAL: *Patient will express minimal discomfort or absence of pain*

Assess location and type of pain; observe for pain indicative of respiratory, circulatory, or integumentary problems
Administer analgesics as ordered; assess effectiveness of pain relief measures; report unrelenting pain in elbow or knee to physician immediately
Administer skin care q2h to 4h and prn
  Maintain skin integrity with applications of lanolin-based lotion
  Avoid vigorous rubbing of extremities
  Provide air mattress or convoluted foam (egg crate) mattress prn
  Assist patient with changing position frequently to prevent fatigue and pressure
  Change linen daily
Maintain proper body alignment at all times
Apply ice bag as ordered
Promote diversional activities
Monitor vital signs q4h and tissue pressure q1h if patient is being monitored (p. 507)

ndx: Alteration in physical mobility related to traction

GOAL: *Patient's mobility of unaffected extremities will be maintained, and mobility of affected extremity will return to optimal level*

Maintain bed rest in prescribed position
  Do not alter amount of traction applied
  Do not lift weights
  Keep weights off floor
  Maintain proper body alignment
Check neurovascular status of affected extremity q1h to 2h; report changes to physician immediately
Check cardiopulmonary status q2h to 4h; especially in halo and cervical traction patients
Apply antiembolic stockings as ordered
Assist with and teach patient allowed exercises and activities
  Provide trapeze bar if applicable
  ROM exercises of unaffected extremities

Muscular tone maintenance
  Isometric exercises
    Quadriceps setting
    Gluteal contractions
  Abdominal sets
  Dorsiflexion and plantar flexion of ankle
  Palmar flexion of wrist
  Provide footboard as needed
Provide high-protein diet as tolerated
  Avoid weight gain or loss
  Assist with feeding prn
Force fluids to upper limits of normal for age and weight if not contraindicated
Assist and teach voiding measures prn
  Provide fracture pan or female urinal
  Measure intake and output
  Observe for urine retention
Administer medications as ordered: antispasmodics, iron and vitamin therapy
Avoid constipation with use of stool softeners or natural food laxatives as ordered

ndx: Disturbance in self-concept related to body image change

GOAL: *Patient will express feelings and concerns and move toward positive coping patterns in a supportive environment*

Reinforce physician's explanation of traction: its purpose and expected outcome; clarify misconceptions
Explain all procedures and treatments
Allow time for and promote verbalization of concerns; encourage communication with significant other and visits from others
Assess present coping behaviors and assist patient with identifying patterns that were helpful in past
Promote self-care and assist with ADLs; praise tasks attempted and/or completed

ndx: Knowledge deficit regarding traction and patient care at home if applicable

GOAL: *Patient and/or significant other will demonstrate understanding of care of traction, patient care, home care, and follow-up instructions through interactive discussion and actual return demonstration*

Stress importance of diet, activity, and rest as prescribed
Demonstrate application of traction and provide instructions for care
Refer to social service or home health care agencies as needed

Explain medication schedule, including name, purpose, dosage, and side effects
Discuss neurovascular monitoring at home and symptoms to report to physician
Promote follow-up visits with physician

Evaluation

There are no complications
Mobility is restored to optimal level
Pain is managed
Home care and traction care are understood

CARE OF PATIENT IN CAST

Casts are applied to immobilize musculoskeletal tissues following trauma; they are made of plaster, fiberglass, plastic, or a new material—cast tape

Assessment
Observations/findings

Type of cast applied, moistness
Neurovascular status of affected extremity
Location and character of pain
Integumentary status at edges and under cast
GI, renal, and/or respiratory dysfunction (body or cervical cast)

Laboratory/diagnostic studies

Radiologic examination of healing fracture and muscle

Potential complications

Neurovascular impairment
Fever
Skin impairment
Infection
Compartmental syndrome

Medical management

Analgesics, antispasmodics, sedatives, stool softeners
Position of cast
Ice bags to area
Diet, activity, rest
Passive ROM exercise machine (for long-term patients)

Nursing diagnoses/goals/interventions

ndx: Altered physical mobility related to location and position of cast

GOAL: *Patient's mobility will be regained to optimal level*

Casts of extremities

Maintain bed rest as ordered, usually until cast dries; patients with plastic or fiberglass casts may ambulate as ordered

Expose cast to air until dry; warm, circulating air from cast dryer held 18 inches from cast is helpful

Elevate cast on firm pillow(s)

Explain that skin will feel warm under cast until cast dries

Elevate each joint higher than preceding joint (e.g., hand higher than elbow); avoid restriction of brachial artery

If blood or drainage appears on cast
   Mark spot with circle
   Note date and time
   NOTE: Use china or permanent marker on plastic or fiberglass cast
   Observe for further drainage q2h and report to physician

Assist with and teach active ROM exercises to unaffected extremities and flexion of hand or foot of affected extremity qid and prn

Avoid footdrop by use of footboard

Assist with and teach isometric exercises

Exercise forearm: clench and relax fist

Ambulate with assistance as ordered
   Provide support for arm cast as needed
   Allow no weight bearing on leg cast until ordered
   Assist with and teach crutch walking (p. 516)

Body, hip spica, cervical casts

Maintain bed rest in prescribed position until cast dries
   Use bedboard and firm mattress
   Provide trapeze on bed
   Support feet with footboard

Expose cast to air until dry unless quick-drying plaster is used
   Cover uncasted areas only; maintain warmth
   Protect privacy by covering perineal area with towel (hip spica)

Use palms of hands only when handling wet cast; handle cast as little as possible until dry (approximately 8 hr)

Assist and teach patient to turn, cough, and deep breathe q2h when cast dries sufficiently

When turning, encourage coughing and deep breathing
   Utilize enough personnel to maintain alignment
   Turn to unoperated side or as ordered
   Place side rails up
   Support chest and cast with pillows
   Turn entire body at one time
   Avoid twisting body beneath cast
   Do not use abduction crossbar (hip spica)
   Administer skin care to back, buttocks, and heels at each turning
   Observe for respiratory distress

Assist with and teach active ROM exercises q4h

For body or cervical cast, ambulate when ordered, usually when cast dries

Monitor neurovascular status of affected extremity q1h to 2h and vital signs q4h

Apply ice bags as ordered

Maintain correct alignment at all times

ndx: Potential impairment of skin integrity related to irritation and/or pressure from cast

GOAL: *Patient's skin will remain clean, dry, and intact*

Inspect skin under edges of cast for irritation q2h to 4h
   Apply lotion to reachable areas (no powder)
   Massage areas gently
   Keep cast dry
   Apply moleskin tape to cast edges to prevent irritation

Administer skin care to hands and/or feet of affected extremity
   Apply lotion to fingers and/or toes and heels prn
   Massage gently
   Check perineal opening for adequacy of elimination (hip spica)
      Protect edges of cast with thin plastic
      Replace as soiling occurs
      Use fracture pan or female urinal
      Provide perineal care
      Avoid constipation with stool softeners
      Observe for urine retention
      Measure intake and output

ndx: Alteration in comfort: pain related to fracture, dislocation, and/or physical immobility

GOAL: *Patient will verbalize minimal discomfort or absence of pain*

Assess location and character of pain; observe for signs of phlebitis and compartmental syndrome

Administer analgesics and antispasmodics as ordered; assess effectiveness of pain relief measures

Encourage diversional activities

Promote self-care when tolerated

Assist patient with changing position frequently to relieve pressure and fatigue

ndx: Knowledge deficit regarding home care and cast management

GOAL: *Patient and/or significant other will demonstrate understanding of cast care, home care, and follow-up instructions through interactive discussion and actual return demonstration*

Provide information on and stress importance of prescribed activities and exercises of rehabilitation
Demonstrate turning procedure for patient in spica cast and reiterate crutch walking procedure where appropriate
Provide information on well-balanced diet; need to avoid weight gain and constipation, need to force fluids to upper limits for age and weight
Promote self-care activities to optimal level
Demonstrate neurovascular monitoring of affected extremity(ies) as needed
Discuss signs and symptoms to report to physician
  Fever, foul odor from cast
  Increasing pain or decreased sensation
Demonstrate skin care around cast
Encourage follow-up visits with physician

Evaluation

There are no complications
Mobility is regained to optimal level
Pain is controlled
Home and cast care are understood

CRUTCH-WALKING PROCEDURE

Observations/findings

Correct body alignment and posture
Correct size and fit of crutches
Ability to use correct gait for condition
Brachial or radial nerve damage

Interventions

Measure accurately for proper fit
  Lying on back: measure from axilla to a point 6 to 8 inches out from bottom of foot or shoe to be used or subtract 16 inches from total height
  Standing: measure down 1½ inches from axilla; from that point measure to 4 inches in front of foot and 6 inches to side of toes
Prepare crutches to ensure safe use
  Use soft rubber suction tips
  Pad axilla bar with sponge rubber
  Adjust handgrip so elbow and wrist are in complete extension
  Allow for approximately 30% elbow flexion
Depending on patient's condition, certain exercises may be indicated prior to crutch walking
  Strengthening upper extremities
    Push-ups
    Pulling weights
    Extension of arms
    Rubber ball squeezing
    Sit-ups
  Standing exercises: use of tilt table
  Isometric exercises
    Quadriceps setting
    Gluteal contractions
  Use of parallel bars for balance
Teach crutch-walking gaits; determine gait by patient's disability and strength
Maintain body alignment and posture as disability allows
  Head erect
  Back straight
  Chest forward
  Hips and knees extended
  Pelvis over feet (depending on gait being used)
Monitor for safety factors

TABLE 8-1. Crutch-Walking Gaits

Gait	Condition for use	Procedure
Swing-to	When one leg can bear weight	Place crutches forward; swing body to crutches; repeat
Swing-through	When one leg can bear weight	Place crutches forward; swing body through crutches; repeat
Three-point	When one leg can bear weight	Place crutches and affected extremity forward; bear weight on good extremity; repeat
Four-point	When able to move each leg separately with some weight bearing	Place right crutch forward; bring left foot forward; swing weight to right side and repeat
Two-point	When able to move each leg separately with some weight bearing	As in four-point, only at faster pace
Tripod	When there is no ability to walk; legs are dragged	Place crutches forward at wide distance apart; drag legs to a point just behind crutches; maintain tripod position for balance; repeat

No weight bearing on axilla; carry weight with hands
Position crutches (where applicable)
  4 inches to side of feet
  4 inches in front of feet
Encourage short strides
Assist patient when first learning and remain with him
Check floors for hazards
  Extension cords
  Rugs
  Wet or oily spots
Keep area clear of furniture
Replace worn suction tips, axilla pads, and handgrips prn

EXERCISE TERMINOLOGY

ROM Exercises

Movement of a joint through its entire, normal range
  Passive ROM exercises: performed by nurse
  Active ROM exercises: performed by patient
  Resistive ROM exercises: performed by patient against a resistive force

POSITION OF ROM

Adduction: moving extremity toward body
Abduction: moving extremity away from body
Flexion: natural bending of a joint
Extension: natural straightening of an extremity
Hyperextension: extreme extension
Internal rotation: rotating an extremity from the joint toward the body
Extenal rotation: rotating an extremity from the joint away from the body
Continuous passive motion device

Isometric exercises

Tightening and relaxing of a muscle without moving the joint
  Quadriceps setting: isometric exercise of quadriceps muscle
  Gluteal contractions: isometric exercise of gluteus maximus muscle

CONTINUOUS PASSIVE MOTION DEVICE

A patient-guided machine that provides passive exercise to the hip and knee following surgery or trauma

Purpose

Facilitates early movement and increased flexion of joint
Prevents stiffness of joint and contractures of tissue
Enhances circulation
Reduces pain of or psychologic resistance to flexion

Assessment/procedure

Physician's order to include
  Initial degree of flexion; number of degrees to increase flexion per hour and number of hours per day to use
  Restrictions or special instructions for use
Assess patient's ability to operate and manage device
Explain purpose of machine and its advantages
Remove any splints before applying device
Following machine setup by physical therapist, or cast or traction technician
  Place extremity on device and check the following
    Lower buttock is against femur support
    Knee is directly over center of frame
    Foot is firmly against foot plate
  Apply Velcro safety straps to extremity; check that they do not interfere with gear assembly
  Set automatic flexion and/or extension motion as ordered by physician (usually at 10)
    Increase flexion 1 to 5 degrees qh as ordered
    Assess patient's tolerance prior to increasing flexion
  Adjust speed as prescribed (maximum speed to flex joint from 0 to 110 degrees is about 1 min, 40 sec; minimum speed is approximately 12 min; slow speeds are used initially and at night to facilitate sleep
  Set ROM limits as ordered by physician
  Instruct patient in use of controls
    Control has three settings: flexion, stop, and extension
    Once device is operating, patient can control movement, stop, or reverse at any point within preset range limits
Each time machine is applied, reduce flexion 5 degrees for about 15 min and then increase to original setting
Encourage patient to use machine as much as possible and as tolerated

Evaluation

Knee and hip flexion are at optimal levels

CHAPTER 9

Genitourinary System

GENITOURINARY ASSESSMENT

Subjective Data

Dysuria
Frequency
Urgency
Strangury
Burning on urination
Dribbling
Incontinence
    Functional
    Reflex
    Stress
    Total
    Urge
Hesitancy
Urinary stream decreased in size
Nocturia
Enuresis
Hematuria
Pneumaturia
Complaints of pain
    Back
    Flank
    Costovertebral angle
    Abdominal
    Bladder spasms
    Urethal
    Legs
    Genital
    Scrotal
    Testicular
    Perineal
    Rectal
Nausea, vomiting
Anorexia
Diarrhea
Constipation
Paralytic ileus
Painful intercourse

Objective Data

Physical examination
    Kidney (fullness, pain, bruits)
    Bladder (presence of distention, pain)
    Urethra (drainage, discharge)
    Vagina (drainage, discharge, redness, inflammation)
    External genitalia (redness, sores, ulcers/lesions, rash, inflammation, pain)
    Testes/scrotum (enlargement, tenderness)
    Prostate via rectum (enlargement)
Urine
    Color
    Odor
    Amount
        Polyuria
        Oliguria
        Anuria
    Voiding
    Presence of catheter
Pain (location, type, duration, precipitating and alleviating factors)
BP, T, P, and R
Weight
Fluid and electrolyte balance
Edema
Skin (dry, scaly, pale or yellow-tan)
Uremia
Anemia
Congestive heart failure (CHF)
Pericarditis

Pertinent Background Information

CONCURRENT DISEASES AND/OR CONDITIONS

Hypertension
Diabetes
Tuberculosis
Allergies
    Shellfish
    Iodine
    Isotope dyes
    Penicillin
    Nonsteroidal antiinflammatory agents
Hormonal imbalance
Systemic lupus erythematosus
Vascular disease: polyarteritis
Sickle cell disease
Amyloidosis

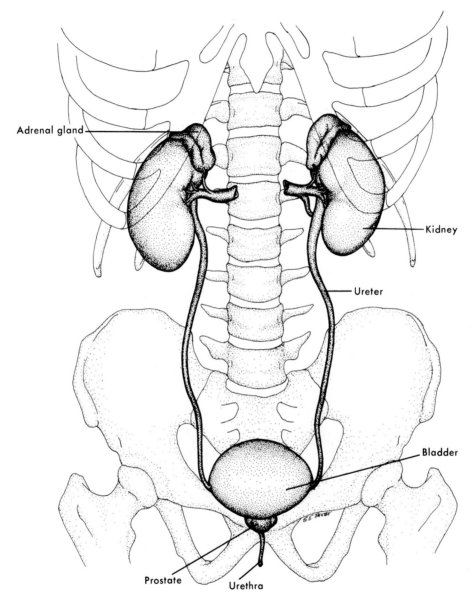

FIGURE 9-1. Genitourinary system.

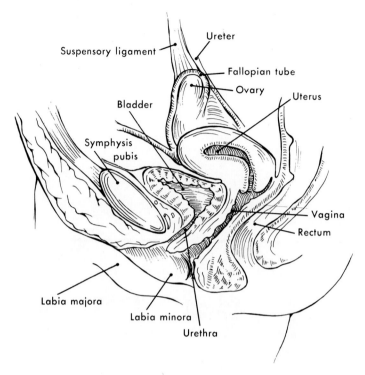

FIGURE 9-2. Female genitourinary and reproductive system. (From Gruendemann, B.J., and Meeker, M.H.: Alexander's care of the patient in surgery, ed. 8, St. Louis, 1987, The C.V. Mosby Co.; modified from Keuhnelian, J., and Sanders, V.: Urologic nursing, New York, 1970, Macmillan Publishing Co.)

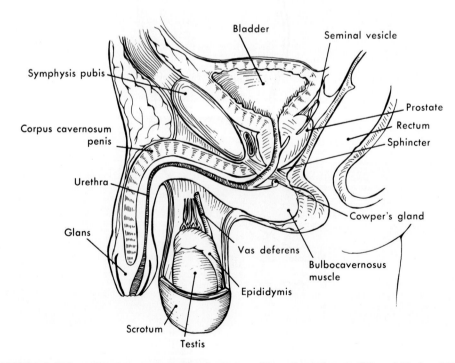

FIGURE 9-3. Male genitourinary and reproductive system. (From Gruendemann, B.J., and Meeker, M.H.: Alexander's care of the patient in surgery, ed. 8, St. Louis, 1987, The C.V. Mosby Co.; modified from Keuhnelian, J., and Sanders, V.: Urologic nursing, New York, 1970, Macmillan Publishing Co.)

Gout
Hyperparathyroidism
Chemotherapy
Trauma
Presence of continuous, indwelling catheter
Frequent intermittent catheterization
Renal radiologic procedures
Exposure to sexually transmitted diseases
Forceps delivery
Date of last menstrual period

PREVIOUS SURGERY OR ILLNESS

Genitourinary (GU) trauma/injury
Urologic and/or renal surgery
Congenital anomalies
Urinary tract infections
Hereditary and/or noninherited renal disease
Kidney transplant
Kidney and/or bladder stones
Tuberculosis
Recent blood transfusion
Sexually transmitted disease
Multiple births

FAMILY HISTORY

Hereditary and/or noninherited renal disease
Hypertension
Diabetes
Congenital anomalies
Cancer

SOCIAL HISTORY

Drinking of coffee, tea, cola, or alcoholic beverages
Smoking
Sexual activity
Occupation (e.g., contact with chemicals, plastic, pitch, tar, or rubber)
Use of feminine hygiene sprays
Use of perfumed soaps
Tub baths

MEDICATION HISTORY

Penicillin and/or other antibiotics
Hormones
Anticoagulants
Nonsteroidal antiinflammatory agents
Analgesics
Alpha-adrenergics
Beta-adrenergics
Diuretics

Laboratory Tests

Urinalysis
  Color
  Clarity
  Odor
  pH
  Specific gravity
  Osmolality
  Sediment
  Red blood cells
  Pus
  Bacteria
  White blood cells
  Casts
  Crystals/calculi
  Blood
  Protein
  Glucose
  Creatinine
  Urea
  Uric acid
  Electrolytes
    Sodium
    Potassium
    Chloride
    Calcium
    Phosphorus
    Magnesium
Urine culture and sensitivity
Urine collection (24 hr)
  Aldosterone
  17-Hydroxycorticosteroids
  17-Ketosteroids
  Catecholamines
    Norepinephrine
    Epinephrine
    Dopamine
  Calcium
  Phosphorus
  Uric acid
Urine clearance tests
  Inulin
  Creatinine
  Phenosulfonphthalein (PSP)
Serum analysis
  Osmolality
  Electrolytes
    Sodium
    Potassium
    Chloride
    Calcium

Phosphorus
Magnesium
Alkaline phosphatase
Blood urea nitrogen (BUN)
Creatinine
Uric acid
Total protein
Albumin
Complete blood cell count (CBC)
Coagulation factors
   Platelets
   Prothrombin time (PT)
   Partial thromboplastin time (PTT)

Diagnostic Tests

Radiographic studies
   Kidney, ureter, bladder (KUB) x-ray examination
   Excretory urogram
      Intravenous pyelogram (IVP)
      Intravenous urogram (IVU)
   Retrograde pyelogram
   Retrograde cystogram
   Retrograde urethrogram
   Voiding cystourethrogram (cystometrogram)
   Renal angiogram (renogram)
      Renal arteriogram
      Renal venogram
   Renal computed tomography (CT) scan
   Nephrotomogram
Renal ultrasonography
Radionuclide imaging
Endoscopic studies
   Cystoscopy
   Cystourethroscopy
   Percutaneous renal endoscopy (nephroscopy)
   Renal biopsy
Urodynamic studies
   Uroflowmetry
   Urethral pressure profile
   Electromyography

URINARY TRACT INFECTION (UTI)

An infection in any part of the urinary tract, caused by bacteria, primarily Escherichia coli; risk and severity are enhanced by conditions such as vesicourethral reflux, urinary tract obstruction, urinary stasis, catheterization, cystoscopy, and septicemia

lower urinary tract infections
   urethritis An infection of the urethra
   cystitis An infection localized in the bladder
   prostatitis An infection of the prostate gland due to an ascending urethral infection

upper urinary tract infection
   pyelonephritis *An infection causing inflammation of the renal parenchymal tissue, caused by an ascending infection of the lower urinary tract*

Assessment

Observations/findings

LOWER UTI

Suprapubic discomfort
Low back pain
Bladder spasms
Dysuria
Burning on urination
Urinary frequency
Urinary hesitancy
Urinary urgency
Nocturia
Hematuria
Pyuria
Malodorous urine
Elevated temperature

UPPER UTI*

Flank pain
Tender, enlarged kidney
Costovertebral tenderness
Abdominal rigidity
Fever
Chills
Malaise
Anorexia
Nausea, vomiting
Decreased urine output
Elevated leukocyte count
Positive urine culture

Laboratory/diagnostic studies

Urinalysis
   Cloudy
   Bacteria
   Pyuria
   White blood cell count (WBC)
   Red blood cell count (RBC)
Positive urine culture and sensitivity
Radiography
   KUB
   Excretory urography (IVP)
   Cystoscopy

Potential complications

Progression of UTI upward to kidney, resulting in
   Renal papillary necrosis

---

*Findings are in addition to those for lower UTI.

Renal abscess
Perinephric abscess
Recurrence (20% to 50% chance)
Fibrotic changes in bladder wall, resulting in decreased bladder capacity
Formation of urinary calculi
Sepsis

Medical management

Antibiotic therapy determined by urine culture and sensitivity
Fluids
Analgesics
Bed rest with gradual return to activities as tolerated
Surgical intervention if obstruction is present

Nursing diagnoses/goals/interventions

ndx: Infection related to presence of bacteria in the urinary tract

GOAL: *Patient will exhibit no signs of UTI, as evidenced by absence of flank pain, suprapubic tenderness, dysuria, fever, chills, and/or malaise; urine culture will be negative for bacteria*

Assess temperature q4h and report if greater than 101° F (38.5° C)
Note character of urine; report if cloudy and malodorous
Collect midstream and/or clean-voided urine for culture and sensitivity as ordered
Encourage high oral fluid intake, up to 3000 ml day, to flush out bacteria, unless contraindicated
Instruct patient to drink cranberry juice, prune juice, and/or plum juice to acidify urine
Administer antibiotics as ordered
Obtain repeat urine specimens for culture and sensitivity as ordered, to determine response to therapy
Teach patient to shower daily with antibacterial soap
Teach female patient to avoid tub baths
Provide good perineal hygiene; keep area clean and dry
Teach female patient to administer perianal care after each bowel movement, and to wipe from front to back

ndx: Alteration in pattern of urinary elimination (dysuria, urgency, frequency, and/or nocturia) related to UTI

GOAL: *Patient will void with pattern of urinary elimination as near normal as possible, as evidenced by absence of dysuria, urgency, frequency, nocturia, and balanced intake and output*

Measure and document urine output with each voiding
Encourage voiding every 2 to 3 hr
Palpate bladder q4h for distention
Provide easy access to bathroom, bedpan, or urinal
Help patient assume a comfortable position for urination
Provide well-lighted area for patients with nocturia
Instruct patient to avoid drinking fluid for 2 to 3 hr before bedtime and to void before bedtime to achieve maximal sleep
Encourage fluid intake up to 3000 ml/day unless contraindicated
Instruct patient to avoid coffee, tea, cola, and alcoholic beverages
Explain all diagnostic procedures used to further evaluate UTI
Prepare patient for cystoscopy and/or IVP as ordered

ndx: Alteration in comfort: pain related to UTI

GOAL: *Patient will report and experience a decrease in pain and a decrease in burning on urination, and will show a relaxed facial expression and body position*

Assess nature, intensity, location, duration, and precipitating and alleviating factors of pain
Provide bed rest; increase activities as ordered and tolerated
Provide nonpharmacologic comfort measures: assist patient with assuming comfortable position, provide sitz baths and warm perineal soaks, teach relaxation techniques and guided imagery, and/or provide diversional activity
Encourage high oral fluid intake to dilute urine
Administer urinary analgesic as ordered
Administer other pain medication as ordered
Assess vital signs prior to and after administering pain medications
Monitor and document pain relief and any undesirable side effects
Notify physician of unrelieved or increasing pain

ndx: Knowledge deficit regarding disease process, methods of prevention, and home care and follow-up instructions

GOAL: *Patient and/or significant other will verbalize understanding of disease process, methods of prevention, and home care and follow-up instructions, and will return-demonstrate Microstix urine test and midstream urine specimen techniques*

Instruct patient to drink 3000 ml of fluid per day unless contraindicated
Instruct patient to avoid coffee, tea, cola, and alcoholic beverages
Teach methods of preventing recurrence of UTI
  Empty bladder q4h; avoid prolonged bladder distention
  Women
    Keep perineal region clean and dry; wipe from front to back after each bowel movement
    Empty bladder before and after intercourse
    Shower with antibacterial soap; avoid perfumed soaps
    Avoid tub baths, especially bubble baths
    Report and treat vaginal discharge promptly
    Avoid use of feminine hygiene sprays and douches
    Wear cotton underpants; avoid nylon underpants
    Wear loose, nonrestrictive clothing
Teach symptoms of recurrence of UTI and instruct patient to report their presence to physician
Instruct patient to complete prescribed course of antibiotics
Teach method and importance of obtaining midstream urine specimen for culture and sensitivity after course of antibiotic therapy
Teach method of self-monitoring urine test for bacteria (Microstix)
Teach name of medication, dosage, schedule, purpose, and side effects
Instruct patient to avoid taking over-the-counter medications without checking with physician
Teach importance of ongoing outpatient care due to high incidence of recurrent infection

Evaluation

Patient is voiding clear, bacteria-free urine
No signs or symptoms of UTI are present
Patient's voiding pattern has returned to normal
Intake and output are balanced
Patient verbalizes a decrease in pain and absence of burning on urination, and has a relaxed facial expression and body position
Patient and/or significant other verbalizes understanding of disease process, methods of prevention, and home care and follow-up instructions; is able to state symptoms of recurrence of UTI to report to physician; and return-demonstrates self-monitoring urine test for bacteria (Microstix) and midstream urine collection technique

GONORRHEA

A sexually transmitted disease caused by a gram-negative diplococcus, Neisseria gonorrhoeae

Assessment

Observations/findings

FEMALE

Vaginal discharge
Nausea, vomiting
Abdominal pain

MALE

Hematuria
Pyuria
Enlarged lymph glands in groin
Prostatic abscess

BOTH SEXES

Urethral discharge
  Scant to thick
  White, creamy; may be yellow or green
Red, swollen urinary meatus
Pain on urination
Frequency of urination
Nocturia
Elevated temperature
Sore throat
Urethral stricture
Rectal discharge
  Mucopurulent
  Bleeding
Anal burning
Anal itching
Pain with defecation
Skin lesions
  Papules
  Hemorrhagic pustules

Laboratory/diagnostic studies

Gram's stain of urethra, urethral exudate, and endocervix
Culture of urethra, urethral exudate, and/or endocervix
Urine culture and sensitivity

Potential complications

FEMALE

Pelvic inflammatory disease
Abscess of Bartholin's gland

MALE

Periurethritis
Prostatitis
Epididymitis
Sterility due to vasoepididymal duct obstruction

BOTH SEXES

Gonococcal arthritis
Conjunctivitis
Meningitis
Endocarditis
Sterility

Medical management

Antibiotic therapy
   Penicillin G
   Tetracycline
   Ampicillin
   Amoxicillin
   Spectinomycin
Patient education

Nursing diagnoses/goals/interventions

ndx: Infection related to presence of *N. gonorrhoeae*

GOAL: *Patient will exhibit no signs of gonorrhea, as evidenced by absence of vaginal and/or urethral discharge, dysuria, and swelling of urinary meatus; Gram's stain and cultures will be negative for N. gonorrhoeae*

Be aware that many persons infected with gonorrhea are asymptomatic
Maintain sterile technique when coming in contact with open, draining lesions
Use good handwashing techniques before and after coming in contact with infected patient
Wear gloves if there is any broken skin on your (care giver's) hands
Place used dressings in waxed paper bags and dispose of as contaminated waste for 24 hr after treatment initiated with antibiotics
When emptying urine of a patient newly diagnosed with gonorrhea, take special precautions to avoid splashing urine in eyes
Monitor character of urine; report if cloudy and malodorous
Assess temperature q4h and report if greater than 101° F (38.5° C)
Keep perineal area clean and dry
Obtain cultures as ordered
Assist physician with obtaining cultures
Administer antibiotics as ordered

ndx: Anxiety related to diagnosis of venereal disease

GOAL: *Patient is able to discuss disease process, indentify contacts, and discuss feelings of embarrassment about having venereal disease with care giver or significant other*

Investigate your own feelings about veneral disease
Maintain a nonjudgmental attitude and an atmosphere of acceptance
Be aware that patient may be distressed about naming sexual contacts, and about family and friends finding out
Do not discuss patient's condition with other staff, family, or friends
Encourage patient to express feelings
Actively listen
Provide privacy during examinations
Educate patient about disease process and prevention

ndx: Knowledge deficit regarding disease process, and home care and follow-up instructions

GOAL: *Patient and/or significant other will verbalize understanding of disease process, prevention, and home care and follow-up instructions; patient's sexual contacts will present themselves for treatment*

Teach patient importance of completing full course of antibiotic therapy
Explain to patient that gonorrhea is a reportable disease
Encourage patient to identify sexual contacts
Instruct patient not to resume sexual activity until indicated by physician
Instruct patient to avoid sexual activity with untreated previous partners until they have been examined and treated
Urge patient to have sexual contacts present themselves for treatment
Instruct patient to use condom to help prevent infection in the future
Teach patient that there is no immunity to gonorrhea
Teach patient symptoms of gonorrhea and instruct patient to notify physician of presence of these symptoms
Teach name of medication, dosage, schedule, purpose, and side effects
Instruct patient not to take any over-the-counter medications without checking with physician
Teach patient importance of ongoing outpatient care

Evaluation

There are no signs or symptoms of gonorrhea present
Patient verbalizes feelings related to diagnosis of vene-

real disease and reports feeling less anxious about having venereal disease
Patient identifies sexual contacts
Sexual contacts present themselves for examination and treatment
Patient and/or significant other verbalizes understanding of disease process of gonorrhea and prevention; and is able to state symptoms to report to physician

URINARY INCONTINENCE

A symptom of urinary tract dysfunction; causes include urethral resistance, detrusor dysfunction, obstruction, neurologic abnormalities, degenerative changes, congenital malformations, and side effects of medications; may be categorized as stress, reflex, urgency, and/or overflow incontinence

Assessment
Observation/findings

Dribbling of urine
Urinary incontinence
    Frank
    Sneeze or cough
    Exercise
    Walking
Urinary urgency
Urinary frequency
Burning on urination
UTI
Bladder distention
Suprapubic tenderness
Cystocele
Prolapsed uterus
Urethral prolapse
Enlarged prostate
Mental status change
    Disorientation
    Comatose
Central nervous system (CNS) lesion
Disruption of nerves supplying bladder
Disturbance in self-concept: body image

Laboratory/diagnostic studies

Urinalysis
Urine for culture and sensitivity
Cystoscopy
Excretory urography
Urine flow rate measurement
Urethral pressure profile
Anal sphincter electromyogram
Bonney-Read-Marshall test (vesical neck elevation test)

Potential complications

Increasing incontinence
Frequent, recurrent, progressive UTIs

Medical management

No smoking, diuretics, ETOH, or caffeine
Reduction of intraabdominal pressure
    Weight loss/diet
    No heavy lifting
    Correct chair or bed if too low
Pelvic floor musculature training
    Kegel's exercises
    Electrotherapy
Bladder training
    Bladder drills
    Biofeedback
    Behavioral reinforcement
Catheterization: external condom catheter (male)
Mechanical/occlusive devices
    Pessaries
    Penile clamp
    Inflatable vaginal device
Drug therapy
    Estrogens (female)
    Cholinergics (neostigmine, bethanechol chloride [Urecholine]) for hypotonic bladder and overflow incontinence
    Anticholinergics (oxybutynin chloride [Ditropan]) for hypertonic bladder
    Alpha-adrenergics (Imipramine) for stress incontinence
    Alpha-adrenergic blocking agents (phenoxybenzamine hydrochloride [Dibenzyline]) for overflow incontinence
    Beta-adrenergic blocking agents (propranolol hydrochloride [Inderal]) for stress incontinence
Surgical interventions
    Vaginal repair of colporrhaphy
    Marshall-Marchetti-Kranz
    Modified Burch colposuspension and sling
    Pereya procedure
    Artificial urinary sphincter

Nursing diagnoses/goals/interventions

ndx: Alteration in pattern of urinary elimination: incontinence (type) related to urinary tract dysfunction

GOAL: *Patient will establish voiding pattern as near normal as possible*

Teach dietary restrictions; instruct patient to control weight as ordered
Instruct patient to avoid tea, coffee, ETOH, and smoking

Instruct patient to void at least q2h to 4h

Teach and encourage patient to perform Kegel's exercises

Suggest measures to decrease cough or control cough symptoms (lozenges) in order to decrease urine leakage

Teach proper body mechanics

Instruct patient to avoid heavy lifting or straining

Instruct patient to walk stairs slowly with good posture

Teach bladder training as ordered

Provide easy access to bathroom, bedpan, urinal, and call light

Provide positive reinforcement for continent behavior

Instruct patient to avoid drinking fluid for 2 to 3 hr before bedtime and to void before going to bed

Instruct patient to modify activities that precipitate stress

Instruct patient to avoid constipation

Administer medications as ordered

Monitor and document desired and side effects of medications

Explain and prepare patient for diagnostic procedures used to evaluate urinary incontinence

ndx: Potential impairment of skin integrity related to skin contact with urine

GOAL: *Patient will show no signs of skin redness, breakdown, and/or excoriation*

Inspect patient's skin for redness, breakdown, and/or excoriation

Report skin redness, breakdown, and/or excoriation to physician

Apply protective skin ointments and/or barriers as ordered

Provide good perineal hygiene; wash area with soap and water; rinse and dry thoroughly

Instruct female patient to wipe from front to back after bowel elimination

Keep perineal area dry

Maintain clean, unwrinkled linen and absorbent pads or briefs

ndx: Potential for infection (UTI) related to incontinence of urine

GOAL: *Patient will exhibit no signs of UTI, as evidenced by absence of flank pain, suprapubic tenderness, dysuria, fever, chills, and/or malaise; urine culture will be negative for bacteria*

Assess temperature q4h and report if greater than 101° F (38.5° C)

Note character of urine; report if cloudy and malodorous

Collect midstream and/or clean-voided urine for culture and sensitivity as ordered

Encourage high oral fluid intake, up to 3000 ml/day, to flush out bacteria unless contraindicated

Instruct patient to drink cranberry juice, prune juice, and/or plum juice to acidify urine

Administer antibiotics as ordered

Obtain repeat urine specimens for culture and sensitivity as ordered, to determine response to therapy

Teach patient to shower daily with antibacterial soap

Teach female patient to avoid tub baths

Provide good perineal hygiene; keep area clean and dry

Teach female to administer perianal care after each bowel movement and to wipe from front to back

ndx: Potential for disturbance in self-concept: altered body image related to incontinence of urine and odor

GOAL: *Patient will be able to discuss feelings of anxiety, embarrassment, and changes in life-style with care giver or significant other; will express feeling a decrease in anxiety related to body image and an increase in self-esteem; and will continue with activities of daily living (ADLs)*

Provide an accepting and supportive atmosphere

Determine how incontinence has affected patient's daily activities and sex life

Assess emotion regarding incontinence

Encourage expression of feelings of anxiety, fear, embarrassment, anger, frustration, and/or helplessness

Promote feelings of self-worth by stressing positive features in patient's life

Be nonjudgmental when cleaning patient after an episode of incontinence

Be realistic with patient regarding control of incontinence

Suggest methods to control odor
   Good perineal hygiene
   Change underclothing daily
   Avoid foods that cause a strong odor in urine

Provide suggestions to help patient maintain a satisfactory level of sexual expression
   Alternative positions
   Instruct patient to empty bladder before intercourse

Encourage communication with significant other

Provide assistance from other professionals to help patient to deal with emotional changes (psychiatry, sexual counselor)

ndx: Knowledge deficit regarding disease process, and home care and follow-up instructions

GOAL: *Patient and/or significant other will verbalize understanding of urinary incontinence and methods of prevention, symptoms to report to physician, and home care and follow-up instructions, and will return-demonstrate Kegel's exercise*

Explain to patient that urinary incontinence is a symptom of urinary tract dysfunction
Teach Kegel's exercises: instruct patient to tighten rectum and vagina, as if to stop urine stream, hold contraction for 5 sec, then relax; continue process for 5 min every 2 to 4 hr
Instruct patient to keep perineal area clean and dry
Instruct patient to change incontinent pads frequently
Instruct patient to monitor and report skin redness, breakdown, and excoriation to physician
Teach patient self-examination of perineal area with use of a mirror
Instruct patient to clean affected area with soap and water, then rinse and dry thoroughly
Teach patient ways to control odor
Teach methods of preventing incontinence
   Void q2h to 4h
   Use good body mechanics
   Avoid heavy lifting
   Control cough
   Avoid coffee, tea, ETOH, smoking, and diuretics
Teach symptoms of UTI and instruct patient to report their presence to physician (see Urinary Tract Infection [UTI], p. 522)
Teach name of medication, dosage, schedule, purpose, and side effects
Instruct patient to avoid over-the-counter medications without checking with physician
Teach importance of ongoing outpatient care

Evaluation

Patient has established as near normal voiding pattern as possible
There are no signs or symptoms of UTI
Patient verbalizes feelings related to urinary incontinence and changes in life-style to care giver or significant other
Patient verbalizes feeling less anxious about body image and an increase in feelings of self-esteem
Patient continues ADLs
Patient and/or significant other verbalizes understanding of urinary incontinence and methods of prevention, and home care and follow-up instructions; states symptoms to report to physician; and return-demonstrates Kegel's exercises

SURGERY FOR FEMALE URINARY INCONTINENCE

Marshall-Marchetti-Kranz A surgical procedure for correcting stress incontinence; the urethra and vesical neck of the bladder are suspended to restore the normal vesicourethral angle by suturing the paraurethral anterior vaginal wall to the periosteum of the symphysis pubis and to the lower rectal fascia via a suprapubic incision

Pereya procedure A surgical procedure performed vaginally to restore the normal vesicourethral angle, thus decreasing stress incontinence; the urethra and vesical neck are suspended by suturing the anterior vaginal wall to the rectal fascia

Assessment

Observations/findings

Urinary output
   Amount
   Color
   Character
UTI
Incision
   Redness
   Pain
   Swelling
   Drainage
Difficulty in voiding after removal of catheter

Laboratory/diagnostic studies

Urinalysis
Urine culture and sensitivity
Cystoscopy
Excretory urography
Urine flow rate measurement
Urethral pressure profile
Bonney-Read-Marshall test (vesical neck elevation test)

Potential complications

UTI
Postoperative complications
   Atelectasis
   Thrombophlebitis
   Pulmonary embolism
   Paralytic ileus
   Wound infection

Medical management

NPO until bowel sounds are audible
Parenteral fluids until liquids or diet is tolerated
Intake and output
BP, T, P, and R per postoperative procedure

Analgesics
Stool softeners
Indwelling urethral catheter or suprapubic tube for 4 to 6 days postoperatively (Marshall-Marchetti-Kranz)
Indwelling urethral catheter for 2 days postoperatively (Pereya procedure)

Nursing diagnoses/goals/interventions

ndx: Alteration in comfort: pain related to surgical incision and manipulation of organs, and to periostitis

GOAL: *Patient will verbalize feeling a decrease in pain and will have a relaxed facial expression and body position*

Assess nature, intensity, location, duration, and precipitating and alleviating factors of pain
Assess nonverbal signs of pain
Check urethral catheter and/or suprapubic tube for obstruction
Assess incisional site for redness, tenderness, swelling, and drainage
Provide nonpharmacologic comfort measures
  Assist patient with assuming a comfortable position
  Teach relaxation techniques
  Teach and assist with guided imagery techniques
  Provide diversional activity
  Provide a restful environment
Administer pain medication as ordered
Observe for desired effects and side effects of medications
Instruct patient to splint incision when turning, coughing, and deep breathing
Consult with physician if measures fail to provide adequate pain relief or if a dosage or interval change for pain medication is needed

ndx: Alteration in pattern of urinary elimination related to presence of urethral catheter and/or suprapubic tube

GOAL: *Patient will maintain patency of urethral catheter and/or suprapubic tube, as evidenced by no signs or symptoms of urinary retention and balanced intake and output; patient will not experience difficulty in voiding after catheter removal*

See nursing diagnosis of alteration in pattern of urinary elimination under Care of Patient with Indwelling Urethral Catheter (p. 540)
Keep tubings below level of patient's bladder
Keep urine draining freely, avoiding kinks in tubing
Anchor suprapubic tube to patient's abdomen
Irrigate suprapubic tube only under direct order
Measure and document urinary output q8h, or more frequently if necessary
Note character of urine; report abnormalities
Palpate bladder for distention if output is low
Explain to patient that presence of catheter may cause urge to urinate
Maintain patency of catheter
  Avoid clamping or occluding catheter
  Avoid irrigating catheter unless ordered
  Keep catheter below level of bladder
Maintain integrity of closed gravity drainage system at all times
Clean periurethral area bid
  Protect patient's privacy
  Remove all crusts and mucus from catheter
Reduce swelling of urinary meatus if present
  Apply anesthetic ointment to urethral meatus if ordered
  Avoid placing tension on catheter
Follow clamping routine as ordered
Remove indwelling catheter as soon as possible when ordered
Use voiding measures to facilitate voiding (see nursing diagnosis of alteration in pattern of urinary elimination under Acute Urinary Retention, p. 535)
Observe voiding pattern
Measure urinary output after each voiding
Note character of urine; report any abnormalities to physician
Report retention of urine with overflow to physician
If residual urine is greater than 100 ml postvoid, a postvoid catheter program may be ordered
Perform intermittent catheterization as ordered
Instruct patient to avoid staying in sitting position for prolonged periods of time
Administer stool softeners and laxatives as ordered
Instruct patient to avoid straining during bowel elimination

ndx: Potential for infection (UTI) related to presence of indwelling urethral catheter and/or suprapubic tube

GOAL: *Patient will show no signs of UTI*

See nursing diagnosis of potential for UTI under Care of Patient with Indwelling Urethral Catheter, p. 540
Monitor patient's temperature and report if greater than 101° F (38.5° C)
Maintain sterile technique when performing intermittent catheterization
Administer antibiotics as ordered
Note character of urine; report if cloudy and malodorous

Collect urine specimen for culture and sensitivity as ordered

Encourage high oral fluid intake, up to 3000 ml/day, to flush out bacteria unless contraindicated

Instruct patient to drink cranberry juice, prune juice, and/or plum juice to acidify urine

Administer antibiotics as ordered

Teach patient to shower daily with antibacterial soap

Teach female patient to avoid tub baths

Provide good perineal hygiene; keep area clean and dry

Teach female to administer perianal care after each bowel movement, and to wipe from front to back

ndx: Potential for complications: atelectasis, thrombophlebitis, pulmonary embolism, paralytic ileus, and wound infection*

GOAL: *Patient will exhibit no signs or symptoms of atelectasis, thrombophlebitis, pulmonary embolism, paralytic ileus, and/or wound infection*

Atelectasis

Assist patient with turning, coughing, and deep breathing q2h and prn

Assist patient with incentive spirometer to maximize lung expansion as ordered

Assess BP, heart rate, and heart rhythm q2h

Assess breath sounds q4h

Report diminished or absent breath sounds to physician

Assess skin for signs of cyanosis and diaphoresis

Monitor for and report symptoms of inpaired gas exchange (confusion, restlessness, irritability, decreased PO_2, and increased PCO_2)

Administer pain medication at proper intervals to manage pain and to help patient perform coughing and deep-breathing exercises more effectively

Administer O_2 as ordered

Thrombophlebitis

Monitor for and report signs of venous thrombosis (pain, tenderness, warmth or redness in extremity, positive Homan's sign)

Apply antiembolic stockings as ordered

Assist and teach patient to perform passive ROM exercises to extremities q2h to 4h; avoid straight leg exercises

Avoid placing patient in a sitting position for prolonged periods of time

Avoid pressure or putting pillows under knees

Instruct patient not to cross legs

Administer anticoagulants as ordered

Pulmonary embolism

Monitor for and report signs and symptoms of pulmonary embolism (sudden chest or shoulder pain, cough, hemoptysis, dyspnea, tachycardia, hypertension, cyanosis, restlessness, decreased PO_2)

If symptoms of pulmonary embolism occur
  Place patient in semi- or high-Fowler's position
  Administer O_2 as ordered
  Monitor vital signs qh
  Maintain strict bed rest
  Administer anticoagulants as ordered
  Prepare patient for diagnostic tests (lung scan, venography, pulmonary angiography)

Paralytic ileus

Monitor for and report signs of paralytic ileus (absent or diminished bowel sounds, persistent or worsening abdominal pain and cramping, distended, firm abdomen, failure to pass flatus)

Maintain NPO until active bowel sounds are audible or passage of flatus is noted

Auscultate for bowel sounds q4h

Insert and maintain nasogastric tube as ordered

Encourage early ambulation

Instruct patient to avoid smoking and/or chewing gum in order to reduce air swallowing

Administer stool softeners, laxatives, or enemas as ordered

Wound infection

Monitor for and report signs and symptoms of wound infection (fever, chills, redness, swelling, tenderness, purulent and/or malodorous wound drainage)

Check surgical incision q4h for redness, swelling, tenderness, and purulent drainage

Assess temperature q4h

Monitor WBC as ordered

Obtain wound culture as ordered

Use good handwashing technique and teach and encourage patient to do the same

Instruct patient to avoid touching incision, dressings, and drainage

Maintain sterile technique when changing dressings and performing wound care

Administer antibiotics as ordered

ndx: Knowledge deficit regarding postoperative routine, and home care and follow-up instructions

---

*Not a NANDA-approved nursing diagnosis.

GOAL: *Patient and/or significant other will verbalize understanding of postoperative care, symptoms to report to physician, and home care and follow-up instructions, and will return-demonstrate wound care and dressing change*

Teach postoperative routine; encourage patient to participate in care

Instruct patient to avoid persons with infections

Instruct patient to get plenty of rest; to exercise to tolerance and to plan frequent rest periods

Instruct patient to avoid heavy lifting and heavy housework for 6 weeks or as indicated by physician

Teach patient good body mechanics; instruct patient to bend knees to pick up items from the floor

Instruct patient to avoid standing or sitting for long periods of time

Instruct patient to avoid constipation and to avoid straining when having a bowel movement

Instruct patient to avoid sexual activity for 6 weeks or as indicated by physician

Instruct patient to avoid tub baths and to shower daily

Instruct patient to report signs and symptoms of UTI and methods to avoid UTI (see Urinary Tract Infection [UTI], p. 522)

Teach patient to perform wound care and dressing change as ordered

Instruct patient to monitor for and report signs and symptoms of wound infection (fever, chills, redness, swelling, tenderness, and purulent and/or malodorous drainage from incision)

Teach name of medication, dosage, schedule, purpose, and side effects

Instruct patient to avoid taking over-the-counter medications without checking with physician

Teach importance of ongoing outpatient care

Evaluation

Patient verbalizes a decrease in pain and has a relaxed facial expression and body position

Urethral catheter and suprapubic tube remain patent for their duration

Patient shows no signs or symptoms of urinary retention

Patient does not experience difficulty in voiding after urethral catheter removal

Intake and output are balanced

There are no signs or symptoms of UTI

There are no signs or symptoms of postoperative complications (atelectasis, thrombophlebitis, pulmonary embolism, paralytic ileus, wound infection)

Patient and/or significant other verbalizes an understanding of postoperative routine, and home care and follow-up instructions; states signs and symptoms to report to physician; and return-demonstrates wound care and dressing change

ARTIFICIAL URINARY SPHINCTER

A fluid-filled system with a silicone rubber cuff that surrounds the urethra and functions as a urinary sphincter; a pump is implanted in the labia of the female and in the scrotum of the male or may be external, and a balloon reservoir sits in the abdomen; when the pump is squeezed, the fluid leaves the cuff and flows into the balloon (reservoir), thus allowing the urethra to open and the patient to void (Figure 9-4)

Assessment
Observations/findings

Urine
  Amount
  Character
Incontinence
Leakage of urine
Scrotal swelling
Bladder spasms
Incision
  Redness
  Swelling
  Tenderness
  Purulent and/or malodorous drainage
Elevated temperature
UTI

Laboratory/diagnostic studies

Urinalysis
Urine for culture and sensitivity
See Urinary Incontinence, p. 526

Potential complications

UTI
Infection
Rejection of artificial urinary sphincter
Malfunctioning artificial urinary sphincter

Medical management

NPO until bowel sounds are audible
Parenteral fluids until liquids or diet is tolerated
Intake and output
BP, T, P, and R per postoperative routine
Analgesics
Stool softeners
Antibiotics

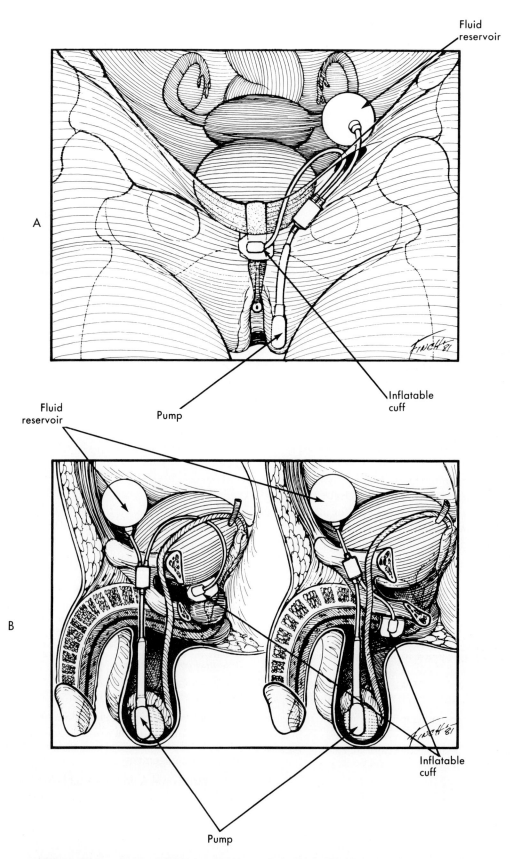

FIGURE 9-4. Artificial urinary sphincter. **A,** Location of artifical urinary sphincter in female. **B,** Location of artifical urinary sphincter in male; note that position of cuff may be around either bladder neck or bulbous urethra. (From Lerner, J., and Khan, Z.: Mosby's manual of Urologic nursing, St. Louis, 1982, The C.V. Mosby Co.; courtesy American Medical Systems, Inc., Minneapolis, Minn.)

Nursing diagnoses/goals/interventions

ndx: Alteration in comfort: pain related to low, transverse, deep, surgical incision and bladder spasms

GOAL: *Patient will verbalize a decrease in pain and will show a relaxed facial expression and body position*

Assess nature, intensity, location, duration, and precipitating and alleviating factors of pain
Assess nonverbal signs of pain
Monitor urine flow; check patency of urethral catheter
Report signs and symptoms of urinary retention to physician
Assess scrotum/labia for swelling
Assess incisional site for signs of wound infection
Provide nonpharmacologic comfort measures
    Assist patient with assuming a comfortable position
    Teach relaxation techniques
    Teach and assist with guided imagery
    Provide diversional activity
    Provide a restful environment
    Maintain Trendelenberg position, if ordered, to decrease scrotal swelling
    Apply ice bag to scrotum and/or perineal area for 12 to 48 hr or as indicated by physician
Administer pain medication as ordered
Take vital signs before and after administration of pain medication
Monitor and document pain relief and side effects of medication
Consult with physician if measures fail to provide pain relief, or if a dosage or interval change in pain medication is needed

ndx: Alteration in pattern of urinary elimination related to presence of artificial urinary sphincter and bladder spasms

GOAL: *Patient will establish a pattern of urinary elimination as near normal as possible*

Measure and document urinary output qh
Note character of urine; report any abnormalities to physician
Maintain patency of uninflated urethral catheter for 1 to 5 days or as ordered by physician
Monitor and report signs and symptoms of urinary retention
Locate pump qh postoperatively
Notify physician immediately if unable to palpate pump (it may have traveled into inguinal canal; this is an emergency)
Pull pump down into most dependent part of scrotum or labia and hold for 1 min
Remove urethral catheter as ordered when swelling goes down and patient can palpate and operate artificial urinary sphincter
Once urethral catheter is removed, use an external collecting device to prevent contact of urine with skin
Begin activating pump when ordered
    Pump bulb flat q2h during the day and once midway through the night
    Deflate device while patient is asleep and connect patient to an external urine collecting device
Teach patient to palpate and operate artificial urinary sphincter
Provide privacy while palpating, teaching, or activating pump
Explain to patient that he may experience some incontinence of urine at times
Report any leakage of urine to physician

ndx: Potential for infection (UTI, wound infection) and rejection of artificial urinary sphincter related to implantation of foreign body surrounding urinary tract

GOAL: *Patient will show no signs or symptoms of UTI, wound infection, or rejection*

Assess temperature q4h; report if greater than 101° F (38.5° C)
Assess site of incision for and report redness, swelling, tenderness, and purulent and/or malodorous drainage
Note character of urine; report abnormalities to physician
Monitor for and report signs and symptoms of UTI (see Urinary Tract Infection [UTI], p. 522)
Maintain a closed drainage system for duration of indwelling urethral catheter
Force fluids up to 3000 ml/day unless contraindicated
Maintain sterile technique when performing wound care and dressing changes
Monitor for and report signs and symptoms of rejection (erosion, increasing pain, abdominal tenderness, swelling, urinary retention)
Administer antibiotics as ordered

ndx: Knowledge deficit regarding activation of artificial urinary sphincter, and home care and follow-up instructions

GOAL: *Patient and/or significant other will verbalize understanding of artificial urinary sphincter, signs and symptoms to report to physician, and home care and follow-up instructions, and will return-demonstrate palpation of pump and activation of artificial urinary sphincter*

Instruct patient to force fluids up to 3000 ml/day unless contraindicated

Instruct patient to avoid smoking, tea, coffee, and alcohol

Teach patient to palpate pump and to activate artificial urinary sphincter
- Locate pump in labia or scrotum with thumb and forefinger of dominant hand
- Locate and gently support tubing above pump with nondominant hand to prevent pump from slipping away
- Using thumb and forefinger of dominant hand, squeeze pump until it reaches compressed state (usually three times); this opens cuff, allowing urine to flow

Explain to patient that within 3 to 5 min, cuff will automatically refill and compress urethra, thus maintaining continence

If urine does not flow
- Instruct patient to cough (this increases intraabdominal pressure and thus facilitates urine flow)
- Instruct patient to move from supine to sitting or standing position
- Instruct patient to use voiding measures (see nursing diagnosis of alteration in pattern of urinary elimination under Acute Urinary Retention, p. 535)
- Explain to patient that some patients may need to deflate pump twice to fully empty bladder

Instruct patient to pump bulb flat q2h during the day and once midway through the night for 3 weeks postoperatively or as ordered by physician; thereafter, patient may pump bulb to urinate only when sensation of bladder fullness occurs

Instruct patient not to leave device completely inflated while asleep; instruct patient to use smallest amount of fluid necessary for continence

Instruct patient to report leakage of urine to physician

Instruct patient to report if pump goes flat or if it requires more squeezes to inflate

Explain to patient that some incontinence may occur, especially with activities such as cycling or horseback riding

Teach and instruct patient to report signs and symptoms of UTI to physician

Teach and instruct patient to report signs and symptoms of rejection and wound infection to physician

Explain to patient that he may be catheterized with a deflated balloon only, but that it is not recommended

Instruct patient to wear a medical alert tag; therefore if patient ever unconscious, the pump may be activated and urine eliminated

Evaluation

Patient verbalizes a decrease in pain and has relaxed facial expression and body position

Patient establishes a near normal pattern of urinary elimination

There are no signs or symptoms of UTI, wound infection, or rejection of artificial urinary sphincter

Patient and/or significant other verbalizes function of artificial urinary sphincter, symptoms to report to physician, and home care and follow-up instructions; palpates pump; and operates artificial urinary sphincter

ACUTE URINARY RETENTION

A condition in which the bladder becomes distended with urine and the patient is unable to completely empty the bladder; major cause is obstruction; other causes include a neurogenic bladder, trauma, postoperative complications, anxiety, muscle tension, and side effects of medications

Assessment
Observations/findings

Suprapubic pain
Restlessness
Anxiety
Diaphoresis
Frequency of urination
Urgency of urination
Voiding of 20 to 50 ml at a time
Dribbling of urine
Straining to urinate
Inability to urinate
Bladder distention
Bladder tenderness
Cystitis
Administration of medications
- Anticholinergics
- Antihistamines

Fecal impaction

Laboratory/diagnostic studies

Urinalysis
Urine culture and sensitivity

Serum electrolytes
Serum creatinine
Serum BUN
Kidney, ureter, bladder (KUB) x-ray examination
IVP
Cystometrogram

Potential complications

UTI
Electrolyte imbalance
Hemorrhage
Shock

Medical management

Catheterization
Bladder decompression
Cholinergics to stimulate bladder contraction (neostigmine, urecholine)
Analgesics to control pain
Antibiotics in presence of infection
IV hydration
Surgery to remove or bypass obstruction

Nursing diagnoses/goals/interventions

ndx: Alteration in pattern of urinary elimination: inability to urinate related to obstruction or neuromuscular dysfunction

GOAL: *Patient will empty bladder using as near normal voiding method as possible; intake and output will be balanced*

Utilize voiding measures to facilitate bladder emptying
  Ensure privacy
  Place patient in comfortable position to urinate
  Run tap water near patient
  Flush toilet
  Place patient's hands in warm water
  Apply heat to suprapubic area as ordered
  Pour warm water over perineum
  Assist patient with using relaxation techniques
  Place a few drops of oil of peppermint in bedpan or on cotton ball and hold briefly in front of urinary meatus
  Pull pubic hairs slightly
  Stroke inner aspect of thigh gently
  Stroke inner aspect of thigh with ice
Administer cholinergic medications as ordered
Observe for and document desired effects and side effects
Catheterize patient as ordered
  Avoid use of wire catheter
  Notify physician if unable to pass catheter; do not force
  Slowly decompress bladder as ordered
  Notify physician if bright red urine occurs after decompression
  After decompression of bladder, monitor for signs and symptoms of shock (decreased BP, tachycardia, tachypnea, restlessness, diaphoresis, pallor)
Measure and record urinary output qh
Monitor for postobstructive diuresis; report urine output greater than 200 ml/hr
If postobstructive diuresis occurs
  Maintain IV hydration as ordered
  Monitor vital signs qh
  Monitor serum and urine electrolytes and osmolality as ordered
Monitor for signs and symptoms of electrolyte imbalance
Assist and teach patient technique of self-catheterization
  Teach purpose of procedure: to completely empty bladder on a regular time schedule, usually q3h to 4h
  Instruct patient to have necessary equipment available
    Magnifying mirror (female)
    Low stool (male)
    Two No. 14 French catheters
    Pan or toilet
    Water-soluble lubricant
    Soap and water
    Clean washcloth
    Clean towel
  Instruct patient to perform good handwashing technique before and after self-catheterization
  Teach self-catherization procedure
    Women
      Perform catheterization procedure in semi-Fowler's position initially; later can sit or stand over toilet
      Identify urinary meatus by looking in magnifying mirror initially; later can sit on or stand over toilet
    Men
      Perform catheterization procedure sitting on stool or toilet
    Both sexes
      Clean meatus, labia, or glans with soap and water
      Grasp catheter 3 to 4 inches from tip
      Lubricate tip of catheter
      Insert catheter in urethral meatus until urine flows out
      Women will insert catheter 3 to 5 cm

Men will insert catheter approximately 20 cm
Allow urine to flow into pan or toilet until bladder is empty
Remove catheter
Wash catheter in soap and water
Rinse well
Dry catheter; roll in clean towel
Place catheter in clean plastic or paper bag for storage

ndx: Alteration in comfort: pain related to bladder fullness and inability to void

GOAL: *Patient will report and experience a decrease in pain and a decrease in burning on urination, and will show a relaxed facial expression and body position*

Assess nature, intensity, location, duration, and precipitating and alleviating factors of pain
Provide bed rest; increase activities as ordered and tolerated.
Provide nonpharmacologic comfort measures: assist patient with assuming a comfortable position, provide sitz baths and warm perineal soaks, teach relaxation techniques and guided imagery, and/or provide diversional activity
Encourage high oral fluid intake
Administer other pain medication as ordered
Assess vital signs prior to and after administering pain medications
Monitor and document pain relief and any undesirable side effects
Notify physician of unrelieved or increasing pain

ndx: Potential for infection (UTI) related to urinary obstruction

GOAL: *Patient will exhibit no signs of UTI, as evidenced by absence of flank pain, suprapubic tenderness, dysuria, fever, chills, and/or malaise; urine culture will be negative for bacteria*

Assess temperature q4h and report if greater than 101° F (38.5° C)
Note character of urine; report if cloudy and malodorous
Collect midstream and/or clean-voided urine for culture and sensitivity as ordered
Encourage high oral fluid intake, up to 3000 ml/day, to flush out bacteria unless contraindicated
Instruct patient to drink cranberry juice, prune juice, and/or plum juice to acidify urine

Administer antibiotics as ordered
Obtain repeat urine specimens for culture and sensitivity as ordered, to determine response to therapy
Teach patient to shower daily with antibacterial soap
Teach female patient to avoid tub baths
Provide good perineal hygiene; keep area clean and dry
Teach female to administer perianal care after each bowel movement and to wipe from front to back

ndx: Knowledge deficit regarding disease process, and home care and follow-up instructions

GOAL: *Patient and/or significant other will verbalize understanding of disease process of acute urinary retention, symptoms to report to physician, and home care and follow-up instructions, and will return-demonstrate self-catheterization technique*

Instruct patient to force fluids up to 3000 ml/day unless contraindicated
Instruct patient to avoid alcohol, coffee, tea, and cola beverages
Instruct patient to avoid extreme cold
Instruct patient to measure urine after each void and to note character of urine
Teach voiding measures
Instruct patient to perform self-catheterization as ordered
Teach symptoms of recurrence and instruct patient to report these symptoms to physician
Teach symptoms of UTI and instruct patient to report these symptoms to physician (see Urinary Tract Infection [UTI], p. 522)
Teach name of medication, dosage, schedule, purpose, and side effects
Instruct patient to avoid over-the-counter medications without checking with physician
Teach importance of ongoing outpatient care

Evaluation

Patient empties bladder using as near normal voiding method as possible
Intake and output are balanced
Patient verbalizes a decrease in pain
There are no signs or symptoms of UTI
Patient and/or significant other verbalizes an understanding of acute urinary retention, and home care and follow-up instructions; states symptoms of recurrence and UTI to report to physician; and return-demonstrates self-catheterization technique

NEUROGENIC BLADDER

A dysfunction of the bladder due to lesion(s) of the CNS or nerves supplying the bladder; it usually results in some form of urinary incontinence and is associated with damage to the upper urinary tract, a high incidence of UTIs, and urolithiasis

upper motor neuron bladder, hyperreflexive bladder, hypertonic bladder, automatic bladder, reflex bladder, uninhibited neurogenic bladder *The lesion occurs high in the spinal cord; the reflex arc for voiding continues to function; however, its action is abnormal*

lower motor neuron bladder, hypotonic bladder, flaccid bladder, autonomous bladder, tabetic bladder, cord bladder, atonic bladder *Nerve damage in the sacral segments of the spinal cord or cauda equina interrupts afferent, efferent, and/or central components of the reflex arc; the bladder becomes overfilled and incapable of completely emptying; thus overflow voiding occurs*

Assessment

Observations/findings

UPPER MOTOR NEURON BLADDER, HYPERREFLEXIVE BLADDER, HYPERTONIC BLADDER, AUTOMATIC BLADDER, REFLEX BLADDER, UNINHIBITED NEUROGENIC BLADDER

Incontinence
Small bladder capacity
Uncontrolled frequent voiding
Hyperactive deep tendon reflexes
Dermatitis
Decubitus ulcers
UTI
Difficult initiation of bowel movement
Autonomic hyperreflexia
    Elevated BP
    Bradycardia
    Headache
    Flushed skin
    Diaphoresis
    Blurred vision
    Seizure
    Stroke

LOWER MOTOR NEURON BLADDER, HYPOTONIC BLADDER, FLACCID BLADDER, AUTONOMOUS BLADDER, TABETIC BLADDER, CORD BLADDER, ATONIC BLADDER

Large bladder capacity
Bladder distention
Overflow incontinence
Dribbling of urine
Stress incontinence
UTI
Absent deep tendon reflexes
Difficult initiation of bowel movement

SPINAL CORD INJURY ABOVE SACRAL REGION

Bladder distention
Chills
Tremors
Diaphoresis
Elevated BP
Headache
Spinal shock; there may be no reflex activity below level of lesion for days or weeks

Laboratory/diagnostic studies

Urinalysis
Urine culture and sensitivity
Urine creatinine clearance
Serum BUN
Serum creatinine
Cystoscopy
Cystogram
Urethrogram
Excretory urography

Potential complications

Progressive UTI
Hydronephrosis
Renal calculi
Renal failure
Autonomic dysreflexia

Medical management

Anticholinergics (propantheline bromide, oxybutynin chloride) for hyperreflexive bladder
Parasympathomimetics (bethanechol chloride) for hypotonic bladder
Alpha-adrenergics (phentolamine) for spastic bladder
Sympathomimetics (ephedrine) to improve bladder neck and urethral tone
Antibiotics in presence of infection
Fluid intake of 3000 ml/day, unless contraindicated
Low-calcium diet
Increased mobility
Bladder training
Penile clamp
Intermittent self-catheterization
Continuous indwelling catheter
Continent vesicostomy
Artificial urinary sphincter

Nursing diagnoses/goals/interventions

ndx: Alteration in urinary elimination related to lack of neuronal control of bladder

GOAL: *Patient will empty bladder using as near normal voiding method as possible*

Be aware that acute stage may last 3 to 6 months
Assess vaginal and rectal tone periodically for a period of 6 to 9 weeks
Catheterize patient as ordered
    Continuous, indwelling catheter
    Intermittent catheterization q2h to 4h
    See Care of Patient with Indwelling Urethral Catheter (p. 540)
Maintain a closed drainage system
Measure and document intake and output
Avoid use of penile clamp to control incontinence
Initiate bladder rehabilitation
    Clamp indwelling urethral catheter as ordered
    Assist and teach patient to establish voiding pattern
    Initiate voiding by manual stimulation q2h
        Be aware that bladder may become overdistended
        Monitor BP, P, and R q4h
        Perform Credés maneuver; exert manual pressure over suprapubic region
        Contract abdominal muscles while straining down
        Lean acutely forward
        Stretch anal sphincter
    Use voiding measures (see nursing diagnosis of alteration in pattern of urinary elimination under Acute Urinary Retention, p. 535)
    Record time and amount of fluid intake
    Record time and amount of urine voided
    Palpate and percuss bladder for evidence of urinary retention
    Catheterize for residual urine as necessary
Encourage patient to void twice during the night
Assist and teach patient to perform self-catheterization
Force fluids to 3000 ml/day unless contraindicated
Avoid coffee, tea, and alcoholic beverages
Provide majority of fluids during daytime hours
Space fluids to fill bladder for emptying at scheduled times
Maintain low-calcium diet as ordered
Maintain mobility
    Assist and teach patient to turn, cough, and deep breathe q2h
    Get patient up in wheelchair as soon as possible
    Perform active and passive ROM exercises to extremities
Administer acidifying agents as ordered to maintain urine pH below 6
Provide cranberry juice
Avoid citrus fruits and juices; vitamin C supplements may be necessary
Monitor urinary pH as ordered
Explain that bowel regularity must be maintained
Assist and teach digital stimulation of bowel as ordered
Administer stool softeners, suppositories, or enemas as ordered
Administer medications (anticholinergics, parasympathomimetics, alpha-adrenergics, and sympathomimetics) as ordered
Monitor and document desired effects and side effects of medications
Explain and prepare patient for cystoscopy, cystogram, urethrogram, or excretory urography as ordered

ndx: Potential for impairment of skin integrity related to incontinence

GOAL: *Patient will show no signs of skin redness, breakdown, and/or excoriation*

See nursing diagnosis of potential for impairment of skin integrity under Urinary Incontinence (p. 527)
Inspect patient's skin for redness, breakdown, and/or excoriation
Report skin redness, breakdown, and/or excoriation to physician
Apply protective skin ointments and/or barriers as ordered
Provide good perineal hygiene; wash area with soap and water; rinse and dry thoroughly
Instruct female patient to wipe from front to back after bowel elimination
Keep perineal area dry
Maintain clean, unwrinkled linen and absorbent pads or briefs

ndx: Potential for complications: UTI, autonomic dysreflexia*

GOAL: *Patient will show no signs or symptoms of UTI or of autonomic dysreflexia*

UTI

Monitor and report symptoms of UTI
Assess temperature q4h and report if greater than 101° F (38.5° C)
Note character of urine; report if cloudy and malodorous

---

*Not a NANDA-approved nursing diagnosis.

Collect midstream and/or clean-voided urine for culture and sensitivity as ordered

Encourage high oral fluid intake, up to 3000 ml/day, to flush out bacteria unless contraindicated

Instruct patient to drink cranberry juice, prune juice, and/or plum juice to acidify urine

Administer antibiotics as ordered

Obtain repeat urine specimens for culture and sensitivity as ordered, to determine response to therapy

Instruct patient to shower daily with antibacterial soap

Instruct female patient to avoid tub baths

Provide good perineal hygiene; keep area clean and dry

Instruct female patient to administer perianal care after each bowel movement and to wipe from front to back

Autonomic dysreflexia

Monitor for and report symptoms of autonomic dysreflexia (headache, hypertension, bradycardia, blurred vision, flushing of skin above level of injury, nausea, vomiting)

Have patient empty bladder and/or rectum

Notify physician if symptoms do not disappear after bladder and rectum are emptied

Check for patency of indwelling urethral catheter

Do not irrigate indwelling urethral catheter, because this increases pressure and may exacerbate condition

Administer medications as ordered (e.g., phenoxybenzamine hydrochloride—a long-acting vasodilator)

Monitor and document desired effects and side effects of medications

ndx: Potential for disturbance in self-concept: body image related to urinary incontinence

GOAL: *Patient will be able to discuss feelings of anxiety and embarrassment, and changes in life-style with care giver or significant other; will express feeling a decrease in anxiety related to body image and an increase in self-esteem; and will continue with ADLs*

Prepare patient with spastic bladder for life with a catheter

Answer questions honestly regarding return of urinary continence; support realistic hope

Provide an accepting and supportive atmosphere

Determine how incontinence has affected patient's daily activities and sex-life

Assess emotions regarding incontinence

Encourage expression of feelings of anxiety, fear, embarrassment, anger, frustration, and/or helplessness

Promote feelings of self-worth by stressing positive features of patient's life

Be nonjudgmental when cleaning patient after an episode of incontinence

Be realistic with patient regarding control of incontinence

Suggest methods to control odor
  Good perineal hygiene
  Change underclothing daily
  Avoid foods that cause a strong odor in urine

Provide suggestions to help patient maintain a satisfactory level of sexual expression
  Alternative positions
  Instruct patient to empty bladder before intercourse

Encourage communication with significant other

Provide assistance from other professionals to help patient to deal with emotional changes (psychiatry, sexual counselor)

ndx: Knowledge deficit regarding disease process, and home care and follow-up instructions

GOAL: *Patient and/or significant other will verbalize understanding of disease process of neurogenic bladder, symptoms to report to physician, and home care and follow-up instructions, and will return-demonstrate bladder exercises, palpation of bladder for distention, Credé's maneuver, stretching of anal sphincter, recording of time and amount of fluid intake and urine voided, testing of urine pH, application of condom catheter, and self-catheterization technique*

Instruct patient to avoid foods high in calcium

Instruct patient to drink at least 3000 ml of fluid per day unless contraindicated

Instruct patient to maintain an acidic urine by drinking cranberry juice and taking ascorbic acid if ordered

Instruct patient to avoid citrus juices, alcoholic beverages, coffee, and tea

Instruct patient to maintain as much mobility as possible

Teach signs of a full bladder

Instruct patient to avoid use of penile clamp to control incontinence if possible

Instruct patient to avoid persons with infections

Teach care of indwelling catheter (see Care of Patient with Indwelling Urethral Catheter, p. 540)

Instruct patient to monitor and report symptoms of UTI and calculi (see Urinary Tract Infection [UTI], p. 522; Renal Calculi/Urolithiasis, p. 553)

Explain to patient that rehabilitation may be a long process

Teach name of medication, dosage, schedule, purpose, and side effects

Instruct patient to avoid taking over-the-counter medications without checking with physician

Teach importance of ongoing outpatient care; explain that a referral to Visiting Nurses Association has been made

Teach and instruct patient to perform bladder exercises q2h to 4h

Teach and instruct patient to palpate bladder for distention q4h

Teach and instruct patient to perform Credé's maneuver to manually stimulate bladder and empty bladder q2h

Instruct patient to stretch anal sphincter
   Lean forward while sitting on commode
   Insert one or two gloved fingers into anus

Teach and instruct patient to record time and amount of fluid intake and urine voided

Teach and instruct patient to test urine for pH qd

Teach application of condom catheter if necessary

Teach self-catheterization technique (see nursing diagnosis of alteration in pattern of urinary elimination under Acute Urinary Retention, p. 535)

Evaluation

Patient empties bladder using a method that is as near normal as possible

There are no signs or symptoms of urinary tract infection

There are no signs or symptoms of autonomic dysreflexia

Patient discusses feelings with care giver or significant other

Patient verbalizes feeling less anxious about body image and changes in life-style and verbalizes an increase in feelings of self-esteem

Patient continues ADLs

Patient and/or significant other verbalizes understanding of neurogenic bladder disease, and home care and follow-up instructions; states symptoms to report to physician; and return-demonstrates bladder exercises, palpation of bladder for distention, Credé's maneuver, stretching of anal sphincter, recording of time and amount of fluid intake and urine voided, testing of urine pH, application of condom catheter, and self-catheterization technique

CARE OF PATIENT WITH INDWELLING URETHRAL CATHETER

A catheter inserted through the urethra into the bladder to drain urine

Assessment

Observations/findings

Distended bladder
Bladder spasms
UTI
  Cystitis
  Epididymitis
    Elevated temperature
    Chills
    Pyuria
Edema of urethral meatus: paraphimosis
Reflux of urine into bladder
After catheter removal
  Dysuria
  Frequency of urination
  Urinary retention with overflow
  Inability to urinate
  Urethral stricture
    Dribbling
    Difficulty in initiating urinary stream
    Small urinary stream
  Incontinence
  Hematuria

Laboratory/diagnostic studies

Urinalysis
Urine for culture and sensitivity

Potential complications

Progressive UTI
Septicemia
Urinary tract calculi
Difficulty in voiding after removal

Medical management

Fluid intake of 3000 ml/day unless contraindicated
Periodic catheter change
Antibiotics in presence of infection

Nursing diagnoses/goals/interventions

ndx: Alteration in pattern of urinary elimination related to presence of indwelling urethral catheter

GOAL: *Patient will maintain patency of indwelling urethral catheter, as evidenced by no signs or symptoms of urinary retention and by balanced intake and output; patient will not experience difficulty in voiding after catheter removal*

Force fluids to 3000 ml/day unless contraindicated
Measure and document urinary output q8h or more frequently if necessary

Note character of urine; report abnormalities
Palpate bladder for distention if output is low
Explain to patient that presence of catheter may cause urge to urinate
Maintain patency of catheter
　Avoid clamping or occluding catheter
　Avoid irrigating catheter unless ordered
　Keep catheter below level of bladder
Maintain integrity of closed gravity drainage system at all times
Maintain tension-free catheter
　Tape drainage tubing to inner aspect of lateral thigh (female)
　Tape catheter to abdomen or upper thigh (male)
Clean periurethral area bid
　Protect patient's privacy
　Remove all crusts and mucus from catheter
Reduce swelling of urinary meatus if present
　Apply anesthetic ointment to urethral meatus if ordered
　Avoid placing tension on catheter
Remove catheter as ordered
　Use voiding measures to facilitate voiding (see nursing diagnosis of alteration in pattern of urinary elimination under Acute Urinary Retention p. 535)
　Measure urinary output for 24 hr after catheter removal
　Note character of urine; report abnormalities to physician
　Observe voiding pattern; report retention of urine with overflow to physician

ndx: Potential for infection: UTI related to presence of indwelling urethral catheter

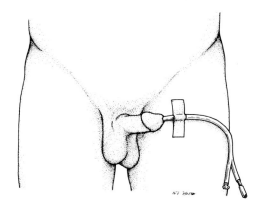

FIGURE 9-5. Indwelling urethral catheter.

GOAL: *Patient will show no signs of UTI*

Maintain closed gravity drainage system; avoid contamination when disconnecting and reconnecting catheter
Apply water-soluble bacteriostatic ointment to urethral meatus; avoid antibiotic ointments
Obtain urine specimen for culture as ordered
Collect urine specimens only by aspirating urine through catheter collection portal with sterile 10 ml syringe and 25-gauge needle
Note character of urine; report abnormalities to physician
Assess temperature q4h and report if greater than 101° F (38.5° C)
Note character of urine; report if cloudy and malodorous
Encourage high oral fluid intake, up to 3000 ml/day, to flush out bacteria unless contraindicated
Instruct patient to drink cranberry juice, prune juice, and/or plum juice to acidify urine
Administer antibiotics as ordered
Obtain repeat urine specimens for culture and sensitivity as ordered to determine response to therapy
Instruct patient to shower daily with antibacterial soap
Instruct female patient to avoid tub baths
Provide good perineal hygiene; keep area clean and dry
Instruct female patient to administer perianal care after each bowel movement and to wipe from front to back

ndx: Knowledge deficit regarding care of indwelling urethral catheter and follow-up instructions

GOAL: *Patient and/or significant other will verbalize understanding of care of indwelling catheter, follow-up instruction, and symptoms to report to physician; and will return-demonstrate attaching catheter to leg bag and to closed drainage system, and periurethral care*

Explain to patient that urge to urinate is caused by catheter
Instruct patient to drink up to 3000 ml of fluid per day unless contraindicated
Instruct patient to drink more fluid if heavy sweating occurs
Instruct patient to avoid diuretic beverages (i.e., alcohol, tea, coffee, and cola)
Instruct patient to avoid placing tension on catheter
Instruct patient to check for patency of catheter q4h

Instruct patient to avoid clamping or kinking tubing
Instruct patient to keep drainage system below level of bladder; may place drainage system in shopping bag when ambulating
Instruct patient to clean periurethral area bid
Teach patient care of collecting bags, bottles, leg bags, and tubing
Instruct patient to
  Wash daily with soap and water
  Soak for 15 min in a mild vinegar solution
  Rinse with lukewarm water
  Protect ends of catheter and tubing with clean gauze square when disconnecting or prior to reconnecting catheter to drainage system
Teach patient procedure for attaching catheter to leg bag
Teach patient procedure for attaching catheter to closed drainage system
Instruct patient to urinate as quickly as possible once catheter has been removed
  Explain to patient to expect some burning with urination
  Instruct patient to report inability to urinate to physician
  Instruct patient to report hematuria to physician
  Instruct patient to measure urine after each voiding
  Teach patient other symptoms to monitor for and report to physician
    Catheter accidentally comes out
    Absence of urine
    Persistent leakage of urine around catheter
    Back pain
    Elevated temperature
    Cloudy urine
Instruct patient to avoid exposure to cold temperatures
Teach name of medication, dosage, schedule, purpose, and side effects
Instruct patient to avoid taking over-the-counter medications without checking with physician
Teach importance of ongoing patient care

Evaluation

Indwelling catheter remains patent; intake and output are balanced
There are no signs or symptoms of UTI
Patient experiences no difficulty in voiding after removal of catheter
Patient and/or significant other states symptoms to report to physician and return-demonstrates attaching catheter to leg bag, attaching catheter to closed drainage system, and periurethral care

URINARY DIVERSION

Diversion of urinary flow from the bladder by transplanting the ureters into the skin, intestine, descending colon, or an isolated section of ileum, colon, or sigmoid colon

ileal conduit: Bricker procedure *A method of diverting urinary flow by anastomosing the ureters into a prepared segment of the ileum, which is sutured closed at one end, forming a blind pouch; the other end is connected to an opening in the abdominal wall; remaining bowel is reanastomosed to provide normal gastrointestinal (GI) function (Figure 9-6)*

continent ileal reservoir: Kock pouch *A method of diverting urine flow from the bladder by anastomosing the ureters into a prepared segment of the ileum, forming a pouch that contains two nipple valves: one nipple valve prevents reflux of urine, and the other nipple valve maintains continence; the pouch is then anchored to the abdominal wall; no external appliance is required (Figure 9-7)*

cutaneous ureterostomy *A surgical procedure in which one or both ureters are implanted into an opening in the abdominal wall (Figure 9-8)*

ureterosigmoidostomy *Surgical implantation of the ureters into the sigmoid flexure, thus allowing the urine to pass with feces through the rectum; no external appliance is required (Figure 9-9)*

Assessment
Observations/findings

Urine
  Color; hematuria

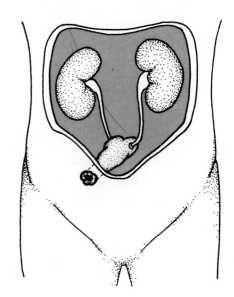

FIGURE 9-6. Ileal conduit.

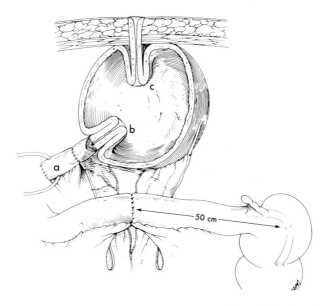

FIGURE 9-7. Kock continent ileal reservoir. *a,* Original ileal conduit with implanted ureters; *b,* reflux-preventing nipple valve; *c,* continence-maintaining nipple valve. (From Gerber, A.: J. Enterostom. Ther. **12**:15, 1985.)

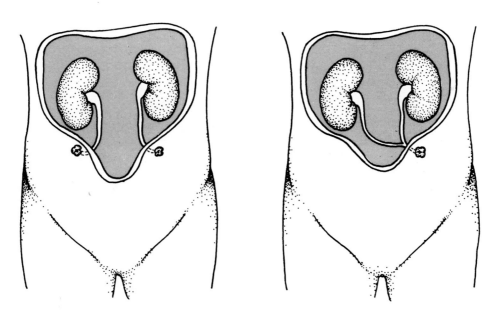

FIGURE 9-8. Cutaneous ureterostomies.

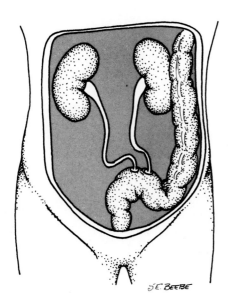

FIGURE 9-9. Ureterosigmoidostomy.

    Character
    Amount; oliguria
Intestinal obstruction
Diarrhea
Stoma/ureteral buds
    Placement
    Type
        Inverted
        Flush with skin
        Protruding
    Color
    Cyanosis
    Necrosis
    Prolapse
    Retraction
    Edema
    Stenosis
    Pouch in place
Skin excoriation
Pressure sores under faceplate
Infection at stomal site/ureteral buds
    Fungus
    Yeast
    Mold
Collection bag
    Kinks
    Compression
    Leakage around bag
    Offensive odor
Urinary fistula: urine from incision
Bowel fistula: feces from incision

Incision
    Redness
    Pain
    Swelling
    Drainage
    Dehiscence
    Evisceration
Elevated temperature
Back pain
UTI
Disturbance in self-concept: body image

Laboratory/diagnostic studies

Urinalysis
Urine culture and sensitivity
Serum BUN
Serum creatinine
Serum electrolytes

Potential complications

Hemorrhage
Shock
Atelectasis
Thrombophlebitis
Pulmonary embolism
Electrolyte imbalance
    Potassium loss
    Hyperchloremic acidosis
    Metabolic acidosis
    Paralytic ileus
    Peritonitis
    UTI: pyelonephritis
    Hydronephrosis
    Renal failure

Medical management

NPO until active bowel sounds are present
Connection of nasogastric tube to low, intermittent suction
BP and T, P, and R per postoperative routine
Serum electrolyte monitoring
Intake and output
Parenteral fluids with electrolytes as needed
Analgesics
Antibiotics

Nursing diagnoses/goals/interventions

ndx: Alteration in comfort: pain related to surgical incision and/or urinary obstruction

GOAL: *Patient will verbalize a decrease in pain and show a relaxed facial expression and body position*

Assess nature, intensity, location, duration, and precipitating and alleviating factors of pain
Assess nonverbal signs of pain
Monitor urine flow; check patency of urethral catheter
Report signs and symptoms of urinary retention to physician
Assess scrotum for swelling
Assess incisional site for signs of wound infection
Provide nonpharmacologic comfort measures
  Assist patient with assuming a comfortable position
  Teach relaxation techniques
  Teach and assist with guided imagery
  Provide diversional activity
  Provide a restful environment
Administer pain medication as ordered
Take vital signs before and after administration of pain medication
Monitor and document pain relief and side effects of medication
Consult with physician if measures fail to provide pain relief or if a dosage or interval change in pain medication is needed

ndx: Alteration in pattern of urinary elimination related to urinary diversion

GOAL: *Patient will establish a daily regimen as near normal as possible for urinary elimination and will show no signs or symptoms of urinary retention; intake and output will be balanced*

Measure and record urinary output qh
Report urine output of less than 30 ml/hr
Note character of urine; report presence of bright red or cloudy, foul-smelling urine (presence of mucous shreds is normal)
Monitor and report signs and symptoms of UTI (see Urinary Tract Infection [UTI], p. 522)
Encourage fluid intake of 3000 ml/day unless contraindicated
Maintain patency of urinary catheters
  Prevent kinking of drainage tubing
  Keep drainage bag below level of patient's bladder
  Position patient in bed so that flow of urine is not impeded
Assess size, shape, color, type, and placement of stoma/ureteral buds qh
Dilate stoma/ureteral buds as ordered
Notify physician if color of stoma/ureteral buds is not red or pink or if shape of stoma/ureteral buds appears to be changing
Check for presence and position of ureteral stents and catheters

Keep ureteral catheters securely taped to patient's thigh
Do not irrigate ureteral catheter unless directly ordered by physician
Label each collecting container and catheter as to "right" or "left," and type
Connect each catheter to a separate closed gravity drainage system
Keep separate, accurate output record for each source of drainage
Pay particular attention to urine output during first 24 hr after removal of ureteral catheter
Avoid having patient sitting in chair for long periods of time
Encourage early ambulation
For ureterosigmoidostomy
  Connect rectal tube to closed gravity drainage system
Measure output qh
  Be aware that rectal tube is usually in place for 7 to 8 days
  Anchor rectal tube to patient's buttocks with tape
  Irrigate rectal tube to free mucus with no more than 30 ml of normal saline solution prn; avoid overdistention
  Establish voiding schedule after rectal tube has been removed
  Have patient void q2h to 4h
  Understand that rectum will hold 200 ml of urine and that urine will combine with feces
  Explain that male patient will have to void in a sitting position
  Insert rectal tube gently into rectum approximately 4 inches and attach to closed gravity drainage system at night if ordered

ndx: Potential for impairment of skin integrity related to skin contact with urine

GOAL: *Patient will show no signs of skin redness, breakdown, and/or excoriation*

Inspect skin around stoma and report signs of redness, breakdown, and/or excoriation
Check for leakage of urine around ostomy bag, dressing, drains, or catheters
Notify physician if leaks occur around ureteral catheter
Keep skin clean and dry
Change dressings when wet
Change temporary appliance daily
  Clean skin around stoma/ureteral buds with soap and water; remove mucus present on and around stoma

Rinse thoroughly with water; pat dry

Place rolled 4 × 4 inch gauze over stomal/bud opening

Apply skin barrier; allow to dry completely

Measure stoma/bud size; bag opening should be 1/16 to 1/8 inch wider than stoma/bud

Make a pattern and leave at bedside

Check correctness of pattern q2d

Remove 4 × 4 inch gauze

Apply temporary bag directly to skin barrier around stoma/bud

Avoid wrinkles or creases in bag

Angle bag to patient's side when in bed and toward feet when ambulating

Attach ostomy bag to rubber or plastic bag attached to patient's leg if necessary during waking hours

Attach ostomy bag to bedside drainage system at night

Reapply ostomy bag prn if leakage or poor seal occurs

Assist and teach patient to empty appliance q2h

Fit patient with permanent appliance; be aware that 3 to 6 weeks after operation, stoma will shrink to normal size

Arrange a visit by hospital enterostomal therapist if available

ndx: Potential for disturbance in self-concept: body image related to loss of normal body function and presence of urinary stoma/bud on abdomen

GOAL: *Patient will be able to verbalize feelings related to change in body image to care giver or significant other; will be able to look at and care for urinary diversion; and will be able to resume ADLs*

Be aware that patients facing this type of surgery are under considerable emotional stress

Be sensitive to changes in patient's life-style

Encourage patient to express feelings

Actively listen

Explain to patient that feelings of grief are normal

Answer questions honestly

Be aware of coping mechanisms and expect that patient may exhibit irrational or inappropriate behaviors, irritability, and lack of motivation

Encourage adaptive coping behaviors

Set limits on maladaptive behaviors, especially if they are detrimental to patient's health

Instruct patient that there are no social limitations
  Patient may participate in any sport except boxing, and sports requiring body contact (football, wrestling) or heavy weight lifting should also be avoided

Explain to patient that there are no clothing limitations except bikinis or girdles

Explain to patient that there are no sexual limitations

Reassure patient that stoma will not smell bad; suggest methods to control odor

Encourage communication with significant other (one of the most common fears is that patient's family—especially patient's spouse—will not be able to accept stoma/bud)

Encourage patient to look at and touch stoma as soon as possible

Encourage patient to participate in emptying and changing appliance

Include spouse/significant other in teaching

Arrange for visit by an ostomate

Provide for psychiatric consultation if necessary

ndx: Potential for complications: infection, peritonitis, paralytic ileus, atelectasis/pneumonia, fluid and electrolyte imbalance (hyperchloremic acidosis, metabolic acidosis, hyponatremia, hypokalemia, reabsorption dehydration)*

GOAL: *Patient will show no signs or symptoms of complications*

Infection

Monitor temperature q4h and report if greater than 101° F (38.5° C)

Monitor and report signs and symptoms of UTI (see Urinary Tract Infection [UTI], p. 522)

Maintain closed drainage systems

Force fluids up to 3000 ml/day unless contraindicated

Administer oral hygiene q4h and prn

Check surgical incision q4h

Monitor for and report signs and symptoms of wound infection (fever, chills, redness, swelling tenderness, purulent and/or malodorous wound drainage)

Use good handwashing technique and teach and encourage patient to do the same

Instruct patient to avoid touching incision, dressings, or drainage

Maintain sterile technique when changing dressings and performing wound care

Obtain cultures as ordered

Monitor WBC as ordered

Administer antibiotics as ordered

Peritonitis

Monitor for and report signs and symptoms of peritonitis (abnormal drainage from wound or urethra,

---

*Not a NANDA-approved nursing diagnosis.

i.e., large quantities of cloudy, purulent fluid or stool in drainage; prolonged abdominal distention with rebound tenderness; prolonged absence of bowel sounds; sudden rise in temperature)

Administer antibiotics as ordered

Monitor results of methylene blue test as ordered

Prepare patient for surgery if necessary

Paralytic ileus

Monitor for and report signs and symptoms of paralytic ileus (absent or diminished bowel sounds; persistent or worsening abdominal pain and cramping; distended, firm abdomen; failure to pass flatus)

Maintain NPO until active bowel sounds are audible or passage of flatus is noted

Auscultate abdomen for bowel sounds q4h while patient is awake

Insert and maintain nasogastric tube to low, intermittent suction as ordered

Encourage early ambulation

Instruct patient to avoid smoking and/or chewing gum in order to reduce air swallowing

Administer stool softeners, laxatives, or enemas as ordered (except with ureterosigmoidostomy)

Atelectasis/pneumonia

Assist patient with turning, coughing, and deep breathing q1h to 2h

Assist patient with incentive spirometer to maximize lung expansion as ordered

Note character and amount of sputum; report any abnormalities to physician

Monitor for and report signs and symptoms of impaired gas exchange (confusion, restlessness, irritability, cyanosis, diaphoresis, decreased PO_2, increased PCO_2)

Administer pain medication at proper intervals to manage pain and to help patient perform coughing and deep-breathing exercises more effectively

Auscultate chest for and report diminished, absent, and adventitious breath sounds

Fluid and electrolyte imbalance

Monitor serum electrolytes as ordered

Measure and document intake and output

Inspect skin turgor

Administer parenteral fluids with electrolytes as ordered

Monitor for and report signs and symptoms of
  Hyperchloremic acidosis: nausea, vomiting, irregular pulse, muscle weakness, tachypnea, lethargy, diarrhea
  Metabolic acidosis: apathy, disorientation, weakness, Kussmaul's respirations
  Hyponatremia: apathy, twitching, seizures, nausea, vomiting, tachycardia, thready pulse
  Reabsorption dehydration: thirst, headache, diuresis

Encourage patient with ureterosigmoidostomy to evacuate rectum q4h to minimize absorption of urinary electrolytes through colonic mucosa

Monitor for signs and symptoms of hypokalemia and hyponatremia, especially in patient with ileal conduits

Encourage early ambulation to prevent urinary stasis and thus decrease risk of electrolyte imbalance

Utilize dietary sources for replacement of electrolytes

If patient is confused or has symptoms of increased neuromuscular activity, keep bed in low position and elevate side rails

ndx: Knowledge deficit regarding postoperative routine, symptoms to report to physician, and home care and follow-up instructions

GOAL: *Patient and/or significant other will verbalize understanding of postoperative routine, symptoms to report to physician, and home care and follow-up instructions; and will return-demonstrate wound and skin care, as well as emptying and changing of appliance*

Teach postoperative routine

Instruct patient to maintain diet as ordered

Instruct patient to force fluids

Teach patient effects of diuretic substances such as alcoholic beverages, tea, and coffee

Instruct patient to exercise to tolerance, to avoid heavy lifting, and to plan frequent rest periods

Instruct patient to shower daily

Teach methods of controlling urinary odor
  Avoid foods that give a strong odor to urine
  Drink cranberry juice several times a day
  Use a deodorizing tablet or drops in ostomy bag

Instruct patient to empty appliance q2h to 3h; instruct patient not to allow more than 100 ml of urine to accumulate at one time

Instruct patient to attach appliance to bedside closed gravity drainage system at night

Teach patient how to change appliance
  Instruct patient to change appliance early in morning or after fluids have been restricted for 2 to 3 hr or prn if leakage occurs
  Have patient sit in front of mirror
  Have patient bend over to allow conduit to empty
  Moisten edge of faceplate with adhesive solvent and gently remove it

Clean cement from skin with adhesive solvent
Wash skin with soap and water and rinse well (patient may shower); pat dry
Inspect skin for signs of irritation
Be aware that urine melts karaya
Keep skin free from direct contact with urine; place rolled 4 × 4 inch gauze over stoma/bud
Apply cement to faceplate and skin
Place appliance over stoma/bud
Center stoma over faceplate and skin
Have appliance extend down, toward thigh
Attach belt to appliance if necessary

Teach patient to dilate ureteral buds with sterile catheter as ordered

Teach patient to dilate stoma by using finger cot and water-soluble jelly; instruct patient to gently insert tip of finger close to size of stoma into stoma

Teach methods of managing appliance
Explain that when patient is lying down, drainage apparatus must be at a level lower than tube
Wash appliance with soap and lukewarm water
Soak in distilled vinegar
Rinse well with lukewarm water
Air dry overnight

Instruct patient to have two well-fitted appliances and two disposable appliances on hand
Instruct patient where to purchase supplies
Teach importance of meticulous skin care
Instruct patient to clip hairs; to never shave around stoma/buds
Instruct patient to avoid constipation
Explain importance of not irrigating ileal stoma or ureteral buds
Instruct patient not to put gauze or tampon in stoma/buds
Teach importance of resuming normal sexual activity
Instruct patient to report the following symptoms to physician
Absence of urine
UTI
Hematuria
Pain in back or abdomen
Elevated temperature
Incisional redness, pain, swelling, or drainage
Severe skin excoriation
Retraction of stoma
Malaise
Nausea, vomiting
Abdominal distention; pain

Instruct patient not to smoke or be near an open flame when removing appliance (adhesive solvent is flammable)

Teach care of ureterosigmoidostomy
Instruct patient to maintain voiding schedule once established
Instruct patient to avoid laxatives, suppositories, and rectal x-ray examinations
Instruct patient *never* to take an enema
Instruct patient to avoid gas-forming foods
Instruct patient to expel flatus only in a toilet
Instruct patient to shower daily and avoid taking tub baths

Evaluation

Patient verbalizes a decrease in pain and has a relaxed facial expression and body position
Patient has established a daily regimen as near normal as possible for urinary elimination
Patient shows no signs or symptoms of urinary retention
Intake and output are balanced
Patient shows no signs or symptoms of skin redness, breakdown, or excoriation
Patient verbalizes feelings related to body image and is able to look at and care for stoma/buds
Patient resumes ADLs
Patient shows no signs or symptoms of complications
Patient and/or significant other verbalizes understanding of postoperative routine, symptoms to report to physician, and home care and follow-up instructions; and return-demonstrates wound and skin care, as well as emptying and changing of appliance

POLYCYSTIC KIDNEY DISEASE

A hereditary, incurable renal disease in which multiple outpouchings (cysts) of the nephrons occur in both kidneys; the cysts may be filled with urine, serous fluid, blood, or a combination; as the cysts enlarge, they distort and compress surrounding renal tissue and blood vessels, causing ischemia and necrosis; eventually, too few normal nephrons remain to support patient, and end-stage renal disease slowly develops

Assessment
Observations/findings

Family history of polycystic kidney disease
Abdominal fullness
Palpable abdominal mass
Pain
Flank
Abdominal
Hypertension

Intracranial aneurysm in circle of Willis
Variable urine output
Proteinuria
Hematuria
Recurrent UTI
Progressive renal failure (see Renal Failure, p. 557)
Susceptibility to other infections
Anemia
Other cystic organs
    Pancreas
    Lung
    Spleen
    Liver
Psychosocial problems
    Hopelessness
    Depression
    Anxiety
    Fear of death

Laboratory/diagnostic studies

Urinalysis
Urine culture and sensitivity
Serum electrolytes
Urine electrolytes
BUN
Serum creatinine
Urine creatinine clearance
CBC
KUB
Renal ultrasound
Renal biopsy
Infusion nephrotomogram

Potential complications

Ruptured cysts causing infection and hemorrhage
Intracranial bleeding
Renal calculi
End-stage renal disease

Medical management*

Control of hypertension: antihypertensive medications
Analgesics
Dietary restriction of protein and sodium
Antibiotics for infection
Dialysis and renal transplant if renal failure occurs (see Renal Failure, p. 557)
Genetic counseling

Nursing diagnoses/goals/interventions

ndx: Alteration in comfort: pain related to renal cysts

---

*Medical management is preventive, supportive, and symptomatic in nature.

GOAL: *Patient will verbalize a decrease in pain and will exhibit a relaxed facial expression and body position*

Assess nature, intensity, location, duration, and precipitating and alleviating factors of pain
Assess nonverbal signs of pain
Provide nonpharmacologic comfort measures
    Assist patient with assuming a comfortable position
    Teach relaxation techniques
    Teach and assist with guided imagery technique
    Provide diversional activity
    Provide a restful environment
Administer pain medication as ordered
Observe for desired effects and side effects of medication
Take and document vital signs before and after administering pain medication
Consult with physician if measures fail to provide adequate pain relief or if a dosage or interval change for pain medication is needed

ndx: Potential for fluid excess or deficit and for electrolyte imbalance related to incompetence of kidney

GOAL: *Patient will show no signs of fluid or electrolyte imbalance; intake and output will be balanced*

Monitor for and report signs of fluid deficit (hypotension, poor skin turgor, decreased urinary output, thirst, dry mucous membranes, weight loss)
Monitor for and report signs of fluid excess (CHF, hypertension, weight gain, edema, decreased urine output, S_3, S_4, distended neck veins)
Monitor serum and urine electrolytes and osmolality; report abnormal laboratory values to physician
Monitor for and report signs and symtoms of electrolyte imbalance
Measure and document intake and output qh
Note character of urine
Measure urine specific gravity q8h
Weigh patient daily at same time with same clothing and scale
Avoid fluid dehydration; administer parenteral and oral fluids as ordered
Avoid fluid excess
    Restrict fluids as ordered
    Administer diuretics as ordered
Maintain dietary restrictions as ordered (low sodium, low protein)
Administer electrolytes parenterally and orally as ordered

ndx: Potential for infection (UTI, local, systemic) related to disease process, depressed immune system, and/or presence and rupture of fluid-filled cysts

GOAL: *Patient will show no signs of UTI, or local or systemic infection*

Monitor for and report signs and symptoms of infection (elevated temperature; chills; flushed skin; sore throat; adventitious breath sounds; cough; thick, colored, sputum; cloudy, malodorous urine; redness, swelling, tenderness, or drainage from wound)

Check temperature q4h and report if above 101° F (38.5° C)

Note character of urine; report if cloudy and malodorous

Avoid instrumentation and/or catheterization of urinary tract

If urethral catheter is present, maintain closed gravity drainage system

Monitor for and report signs and symptoms of UTI, and take measures to prevent UTI (see Urinary Tract Infection [UTI], p. 522)

Auscultate chest for breath sounds q4h; report adventitious breath sounds to physician

Encourage coughing and deep breathing

Use good handwashing technique; teach and encourage patient to do the same

Instruct patient to avoid persons with infections

Instruct patient to avoid chilling

Take measures to prevent skin breakdown

Encourage early ambulation

ndx: Grieving related to loss of function of major organ system, changes in life-style, decision of having no children, and life-threatening prognosis

GOAL: *Patient will begin progression through grieving process as evidenced by expression of feelings to care giver or significant other, utilization of support system and adaptive coping mechanisms, and by compliance with treatment plan and participation in self-care activities*

See nursing diagnosis of grieving under Renal Failure (p. 561)

Encourage and provide genetic counseling

ndx: Potential for complications: hypertensive crisis, hemorrhage, and renal failure*

GOAL: *Patient will show no signs or symptoms of complications*

---

*Not a NANDA-approved nursing diagnosis.

Hypertensive crisis

Monitor for and report signs and symptoms of hypertensive crisis (hypertension, tachycardia or bradycardia, confusion, decreased level of consciousness, headache, tinnitus, nausea, vomiting, seizures, arrythmias, cerebrovascular accident [CVA])

Monitor BP and heart rate q4h; report systolic BP greater than 160 and diastolic BP greater than 90 to physician

Administer antihypertensive medication as ordered

Maintain bed in a low position with side rails elevated

Hemorrhage

Monitor for and report signs and symptoms of hemorrhage (hypotension; tachycardia; dyspnea; cool, clammy skin; syncope; hematuria)

Report hematuria immediately (a cyst may have ruptured)

Monitor hematocrit (Hct) and hemoglobin (Hgb) as ordered

If hemorrhage occurs
  Place patient flat in bed
  Administer fluid replacement as ordered
  Transfuse with blood products as ordered
  Prepare patient for surgery if necessary

Renal failure

See Renal Failure (p. 557)

ndx: Knowledge deficit regarding disease process, and home care and follow-up instructions

GOAL: *Patient and/or significant other will verbalize signs of disease progression, symptoms to report, and home care and follow-up instructions*

Instruct patient to maintain dietary and fluid restrictions

Instruct patient to observe character of urine after each voiding

Instruct patient to report hematuria to physician

Teach methods of preventing UTI (see Urinary Tract Infection [UTI], p. 522)

Instruct patient to exercise to tolerance, plan frequent rest periods, and sleep 6 to 8 hr per night

Instruct patient to keep warm and dry and to avoid chilling

Teach importance of genetic counseling prior to having children

Teach and instruct patient to report symptoms of disease progression

Teach name of medication, dosage, schedule, purpose, and side effects

Instruct patient to avoid taking over-the-counter medications without checking with physician

Teach importance of ongoing outpatient care

Evaluation

Patient verbalizes a decrease in pain and has a relaxed facial expression and body position

Patient shows no signs or symptoms of fluid or electrolyte imbalance

Intake and output are balanced

Patient shows no signs or symptoms of UTI, or local or systemic infection

Patient has begun progression through grieving process and expresses feelings of grief to others

Patient utilizes adaptive coping mechanisms and support system

Patient complies with treatment plan and participates in self-care activities

Patient and/or significant other verbalizes symptoms to report to physician, and home care and follow-up instructions

GLOMERULONEPHRITIS

A group of diseases that result in an inflammatory reaction and/or necrotizing lesions within the glomeruli; usually caused by an immunologic response

Assessment

Observations/findings

History of beta-hemolytic streptococcal infection
History of systemic lupus erythematosus or other autoimmune disease
Dull flank pain
Headache
Low-grade fever
Fatigue
Anorexia
Nausea
Elevated BP
Urine
   RBC
   Casts
   Nocturia
   Proteinuria
Azotemia
Edema
   Facial in morning
   Sacrum with bed rest
   Ankles in evening
Circulatory overload
Sodium retention
Water retention
Dyspnea
   On exertion
   Supine position
Crackles, rales, pulmonary edema

Laboratory/diagnostic studies

Urinalysis
Urine protein excretion (24-hr)
BUN
Serum creatinine
Serum protein
Serum complement (decreased)
Antistreptolysin O titer (increased)
Renal biopsy
Throat and blood cultures
Hepatitis B antigen
Immunoelectrophoresis of serum and urine
Fibrin split products

Potential complications

Infection
Renal failure
Hypertensive encephalopathy
Cardiac failure, CHF

Medical management

Bed rest
BP, T, P, and R q4h
BUN, creatinine, and urine protein monitoring
Intake and output
Fluid replacement according to fluid loss
Dietary sodium and fluid restriction: high-carbohydrate, low-protein diet in presence of renal failure and/or low potassium
Antibiotics in presence of infection
Corticosteroids and cytotoxic agent to decrease immune system response and antibody formation
Anticoagulants
Antihypertensives to control BP
Diuretics to remove fluid
Plasmapheresis to remove antibodies

Nursing diagnoses/goals/interventions

ndx: Activity intolerance related to protein depletion and/or renal dysfunction

GOAL: *Patient will demonstrate ability to resume normal activity level*

Monitor for excessive body depletion of protein (proteinuria, hypoalbuminemia)

Utilize dietary protein to replace protein loss
Provide high-calorie, high-carbohydrate diet
Enforce bed rest as ordered
Provide exercise within prescribed activity restriction
Plan activities with frequent rest periods
Plan a progressive regimen (as tolerated) to return to normal level of activity

ndx: Potential for fluid volume excess related to sodium and water retention, and renal dysfunction

GOAL: *Patient will not exhibit signs or symptoms of fluid excess, as evidenced by stable weight, usual mental status, normal breath sounds, absence of hypertension, and edema; intake and output will be balanced*

Monitor for and report signs and symptoms of fluid excess (hypertension, CHF, weight gain, edema, S_3, S_4, and neck vein distention)
Measure and document intake and output qh
Note amount and character of urine; report decreased urine output to physician
Measure urine specific gravity q8h; report if elevated
Weigh patient daily at same time with same clothing and scale
Restrict sodium as ordered
Replace fluids according to fluid loss as ordered
Provide ice chips to control thirst
Administer diuretics as ordered
Monitor electrolytes and report abnormal laboratory values, and signs and symptoms of electrolyte imbalance
  Hypokalemia: abdominal cramps, lethargy, arrythmias
  Hyperkalemia: muscle cramps and weakness
  Hypocalcemia: neuromuscular irritability
  Hyperphosphatemia: hyperreflexia, paresthesias, muscle cramps, itching, seizures
  Uremia: confusion, lethargy, restlessness
Administer electrolytes parenterally and orally as ordered
See nursing diagnosis of potential for fluid volume excess under Renal Failure (p. 559)

ndx: Potential for infection (UTI, local, systemic) related to depressed immune system

GOAL: *Patient will show no signs of UTI, or local or systemic infection*

Administer immunosuppressive medications and cytotoxic agents as ordered
Monitor serum WBC, antibodies, and T cell values; report abnormal lab values to physician
Check temperature q4h and report if above 101° F (38.5° C)
Note character of urine; report if cloudy and malodorous
Avoid instrumentation and/or catheterization of urinary tract
If urethral catheter is present, maintain closed gravity drainage system
Monitor for and report signs and symptoms of UTI and take measures to prevent UTI (see Urinary Tract Infection [UTI], p. 522)
Auscultate chest for breath sounds q4h; report adventitious breath sounds to physician
Encourage coughing and deep breathing
Use good handwashing technique; teach and encourage patient to do the same
Instruct patient to avoid persons with infections
Instruct patient to avoid chilling
Take measures to prevent skin breakdown
Encourage early ambulation

ndx: Potential for complications: hypertensive crisis, hemorrhage, renal failure*

GOAL: *Patient will show no signs or symptoms of complications*

Hypertensive crisis

Monitor for and report signs and symptoms of hypertensive crisis (hypertension, tachycardia or bradycardia, confusion, decreased level of consciousness, headache, tinnitus, nausea, vomiting, seizures, arrythmias, CVA)
Monitor BP and heart rate q4h; report systolic BP greater than 160 and diastolic BP greater than 90 to physician
Administer antihypertensive medication as ordered
Maintain bed in a low position with side rails elevated

Hemorrhage

Monitor for and report signs and symptoms of hemorrhage (hypotension; tachycardia; dyspnea; cool, clammy skin; syncope; hematuria)
Report hematuria immediately (a cyst may have ruptured)
Monitor Hct and Hgb as ordered
If hemorrhage occurs

---

*Not a NANDA-approved nursing diagnosis.

Place patient flat in bed
Administer fluid replacement as ordered
Transfuse with blood products as ordered
Prepare patient for surgery if necessary

Renal failure

See Renal Failure (p. 557)

ndx: Knowledge deficit regarding disease process, and home care and follow-up instructions

GOAL: *Patient and/or significant other will verbalize understanding of disease process and progression, symptoms to report to physician, and home care and follow-up instructions; and will return-demonstrate measuring and recording of intake and output, taking and recording of BP, taking and recording of weight, and handwashing technique*

Instruct patient to maintain high-carbohydrate, low-protein, low-sodium diet as ordered
Instruct patient to maintain fluid restriction as ordered
Instruct patient to weigh self daily at same time with same clothing and scale
Instruct patient to report weight gain to physician
Instruct patient to take and record temperature daily
Teach and instruct patient to measure and record intake and output
Teach and instruct patient to use good handwashing technique
Teach and instruct patient to take BP daily at same time in same position and in same arm, and to rest 5 min before taking BP
Teach and instruct patient to report symptoms of recurrence and progression of disease to physician
  Rapid weight gain
  Progressive edema: puffy eyes, swollen extremities
  Elevated BP
  Lethargy
  Decreased urine output: less than 600 ml in 24 hr
Instruct patient to avoid fatigue: to exercise only to tolerance, to plan frequent rest periods, and to sleep 6 to 8 hr per night
Instruct patient to avoid persons with infections, especially upper respiratory, strep throat, and UTI; crowds; and chilling
Instruct patient to report symptoms of infection to physician
  Elevated temperature
  Sore throat
  Flu
  Cough

Teach methods for preventing UTI (see Urinary Tract Infection [UTI], p. 522)
Instruct patient to shower daily with antibacterial soap; women should avoid tub baths
Instruct patient to avoid pregnancy
Instruct patient to avoid overeating (appetite may be increased because of medications)
Instruct patient to avoid constipation
Teach medication name, dosage, schedule, purpose, and side effects
Instruct patient to avoid taking over-the-counter medications without checking with physician
Teach importance of ongoing outpatient care; teach need for long-term medical care, even though patient may feel well

Evaluation

Patient resumes normal activity level
Patient shows no signs or symptoms of fluid excess
Intake and output are balanced
Patient shows no signs or symptoms of infection (UTI, local, or systemic)
Patient shows no signs of complications
Patient and/or significant other verbalizes understanding of disease process and progression, and home care and follow-up instructions; and return-demonstrates measuring and recording of intake and output, taking and recording of BP, taking and recording of weight, and good handwashing technique

RENAL CALCULI/UROLITHIASIS

Formation of stones in the kidney (pelvis or calyx) and their passage in the path of urine flow; renal calculi are classified according to their composition—they are usually composed of calcium, uric acid, cystine, or struvite; the stones may vary in size from a few centimeters up to a size that occupies the entire renal pelvis

Assessment
Observations/findings
Pain
  Back
  Flank
  Abdominal
  Groin
  Renal colic
  Ureteral colic
Distress
Anxiety

Nausea, vomiting
Urine
    Hematuria
    Oliguria
    Incomplete bladder emptying
    Decreasing urine with each void
UTI
    Elevated temperature
    Chills
    Dysuria
    Pyuria
    Frequency of urination
    Urgency of urination

Laboratory/diagnostic studies

Serum
    BUN
    Creatinine
    Calcium
    Phosphorus
    Uric acid
Urine
    Urinalysis
    Urine culture and sensitivity
    Urine collection (24-hr)
        Creatinine clearance
        Calcium excretion
        Phosphorus excretion
        Magnesium excretion
        Uric acid excretion
        Cystine excretion
        Oxalate excretion
Chemical analysis of stones passed or extracted
Radiologic studies
    KUB
    Excretory urography
    Renal ultrasound
    Renal CT scan
    Nephrotomogram

Potential complications

UTI: pyelonephritis
Complete urinary obstruction
Hydronephrosis
Renal failure
Loss of a kidney: nephrectomy

Medical management

Treatment according to chemical composition of stone
    Calcium stone
        Thiazide diuretics
        Low-calcium diet
        Drugs to acidify urine (ammonium chloride, methenamine mandelate (Mandelamine) and vitamin C)
    Uric acid stone
        Allopurinol
        Sodium bicarbonate to alkalinize urine
        Sodium citrate
        Potassium phosphate
        Low-purine diet
    Cystine stone
        D-Penicillamine
        Sodium bicarbonate to alkalinize urine
        Low–animal protein diet
    Struvite stone
        Penicillin
        Drugs to acidify urine
Analgesics and antispasmodics for pain management
Antiemetics for nausea and vomiting
Antibiotics in presence of infection
Intake and output
Fluid intake up to 3000 ml/day unless contraindicated
Catheterization
Urine culture
Straining of all urine for stones and analysis
Evaluation of parathyroid function
Evaluation for absorptive hypercalcuric state

Surgical interventions

Percutaneous nephrostomy/nephrolithotripsy

Insertion of a tube into the renal calyx and through the parenchyma to the other side of the kidney

endoscopic removal of stone   Twenty-four hours after percutaneous nephrostomy, an endoscope is passed and the stone is extracted

percutaneous stone dissolution   Lithotriptic agents that dissolve the stone are injected into a nephrostomy tube

Surgical stone extraction

pyelolithotomy   Removal of stone through an incision into the renal pelvis

nephrolithotomy   Removal of stone through a longitudinal incison across the middle two thirds of the kidney, requiring a parenchymal incision

ureterolithotomy   Removal of stone by incision into the ureter

cystolithotomy   Removal of stone by incision into the bladder

nephrectomy   Removal of a kidney

Stone destruction

extracorporeal shock wave lithotripsy (ESWL)   A noninvasive procedure in which patient is anesthetized and is immersed into a tub of water; an electric spark generator is positioned over the affected area and creates high-energy shock waves, which shatter the stone; patient then passes the stone through the urine

percutaneous ultrasonic lithotripsy (PUL) A procedure in which, using local anesthesia, an ultrasonic probe is inserted into the renal pelvis via a nephrostomy and is positioned against the stone; pulses of ultrasound are administered and disintegrate the stone, which is then suctioned or irrigated out through the nephrostomy

Nursing diagnoses/goals/interventions

ndx: Alteration in comfort: pain related to passage of renal stone and/or surgical incision

GOAL: *Patient will verbalize a decrease in pain and will show a relaxed facial expression and body position*

Assess nature, intensity, location, duration, and precipitating and alleviating factors of pain
Monitor for syncopal episodes associated with renal colic (intense pain)
Assess for nonverbal signs of pain (restlessness, wrinkled brow, clenched fists, elevated BP and heart rate)
Monitor urine flow; check patency of catheters
Report signs and symptoms of urinary retention to physician
Assess incisional site for redness, swelling, tenderness, and drainage
Provide nonpharmacologic comfort measures
   Assist patient with assuming a comfortable position
   Teach relaxation techniques
   Teach and assist with guided imagery
   Provide diversional activity
   Provide a restful environment
   Encourage forcing fluids to dilute urine and flush stone
   Assist patient with ambulation, if tolerated, to promote movement of stone
Administer corticosteroids as ordered to decrease tissue swelling around stone
Administer antispasmodics and analgesics as ordered
Assess vital signs prior to and after administering pain medications
Monitor and document pain relief and side effects of medications
Consult with physician if measures fail to provide adequate pain relief or if a dosage or interval change for pain medication is needed

ndx: Alteration in comfort: nausea and vomiting related to pain and/or anatomic relation of kidney to stomach

GOAL: *Patient will verbalize a decrease in nausea and absence of vomiting*

Assess factors that contribute to nausea
Remove noxious sights and smells from room
Perform measures to relieve pain and anxiety
Provide a quiet, restful environment
Administer antiemetics as ordered
Monitor and document effects of medication
Instruct patient to change positions slowly
If emesis occurs, assess and document character and amount
Provide oral hygiene with each emesis
Provide small, frequent meals
Encourage patient to eat dry foods (toast, crackers)
Encourage patient to eat slowly

ndx: Alteration in pattern of urinary elimination due to presence of stone in path of urine flow

GOAL: *Patient will void normally; intake and output will be balanced; patient will pass stone*

Assess patient's "normal" voiding pattern
Monitor and document complaints of dysuria, frequency of urination, urgency of urination, and hematuria
Measure urine output qh or with each voiding
Measure and record output from all catheters, drains, and tubes separately, if present
Monitor and report signs of urinary retention
Assess bladder for distention q4h
Insert Foley catheter if ordered
Maintain patency of all catheters; avoid kinks or loops in catheters or tubing
Instruct patient to avoid Fowler's position and to move about carefully in order to avoid dislodging catheters
Ensure that all catheters, tubes, and drains are patent and draining tension-free q2h
Ensure that all collecting systems are below level of patient's bladder
Care of tubes and catheters
   Tape securely
   Label type, and "right" or "left" to avoid errors
   Secure connection sites
   Use sterile technique when disconnecting and reconnecting
Maintain nephrostomy tube
   Tape to patient's thigh

Never clamp
Irrigate only with a direct physician's order; be aware that irrigating may cause bleeding, infection, or mechanical damage to kidney
Irrigate q1h to 2h very gently with 5 to 10 ml of sterile normal saline using sterile syringe as ordered
Have a similar tube available at bedside
Notify physician immediately if nephrostomy tube becomes dislodged

Maintain ureteral catheter
Tape to urethral catheter or patient's thigh
Never clamp
Irrigate only with a direct physician's order
Irrigate gently with no more than 5 ml of sterile normal saline, using sterile syringe as ordered

Note character of urine; report abnormalities
Strain all urine and send for crystallographic analysis
Describe and report passage of stone
Force fluids up to 3000 ml/day unless contraindicated
Teach and instruct patient to collect urine for stones, urinalysis, culture and sensitivity, and 24-hr urine collection
Explain and prepare patient for diagnostic tests
Administer drugs to acidify or alkalinize urine as ordered

ndx: Potential for alteration in skin integrity related to wound drainage

GOAL: *Patient shows no signs or symptoms of skin redness, breakdown, or excoriation*

Monitor surgical dressings for drainage; change dressings when wet
Note and document wound drainage, odor, color, and consistency
Inspect skin around catheters and tubes and report redness, breakdown, and excoriation
Apply an ostomy appliance and skin barrier around wounds where there is prolonged or copious drainage
Maintain patency of catheters; avoid kinks in drainage appliances

ndx: Potential for complications: infection (UTI, local, systemic), hemorrhage*

GOAL: *Patient will show no signs or symptoms of complications*

---

*Not a NANDA-approved nursing diagnosis.

Infection

Monitor for, prevent, treat, and report signs and symptoms of infection (see nursing diagnosis of potential for infection under Polycystic Kidney Disease, p. 550)
Be alert for signs and symptoms of septic shock if patient had an infection around stone
Maintain sterile technique when emptying, disconnecting, and connecting drainage bags
Avoid backflow of urine

Hemorrhage

Monitor for, prevent, report, and treat signs and symptoms of hemorrhage (see nursing diagnosis of potential for complications: hemorrhage, under Polycystic Kidney Disease, p. 550)
Monitor color and amount of drainage from nephrostomy tube and ureteral catheter qh for first 24 hr and q shift thereafter (light bleeding is normal; report hemorrhage)
Monitor for and notify physician immediately of hematuria
Monitor for and report bruising at surgical/procedural site

ndx: Knowledge deficit regarding disease process, postoperative routine, symptoms to report to physician, and home care and follow-up instructions

GOAL: *Patient and/or significant other will verbalize understanding of disease process, postoperative routine, and home care and follow-up instructions; and will return-demonstrate wound care, dressing change, measuring and recording of urine output, and straining of all urine*

Instruct patient to force fluids to 3000 ml/day
Instruct patient to maintain diet as ordered
Teach and instruct patient to measure and strain urine
Instruct patient to save stone
Instruct patient to report passage of stone to physician
Instruct patient to observe character of urine and to report abnormalities to physician
Teach patient methods to avoid UTI (see Urinary Tract Infection [UTI], p. 522)
Instruct patient to avoid persons with infections
Teach and instruct patient to use good handwashing technique
Instruct patient to exercise to tolerance, to take frequent rest periods, and to sleep 6 to 8 hr per day
Instruct patient to monitor and report
Elevated temperature

UTI
  Incisional redness, swelling, tenderness, or drainage
  Hematuria
  Symptoms of recurrence
Teach care of incision and dressing change
Teach medication name, dosage, schedule, purpose, and side effects
Instruct patient to avoid taking over-the-counter medications without checking with physician
Teach importance of ongoing outpatient care

Evaluation

Patient verbalizes a decrease in pain and shows a relaxed facial expression and body position
Patient verbalizes a decrease in nausea and no vomiting
Patient is voiding normally and passes stone
Intake and output are balanced
Patient shows no signs of skin breakdown
Patient shows no signs or symptoms of complications
Patient and/or significant other verbalizes understanding of disease process, postoperative routine, and home care and follow-up instructions; and return-demonstrates wound care, dressing change, measuring and recording of urine output, and straining of all urine

RENAL FAILURE

acute renal failure A sudden decrease in renal function; causes are classified into three major categories: (1) prerenal hypoperfusion (decreased cardiac output, shock, vascular disorders), (2) intrarenal syndrome (acute tubular necrosis [ATN], acute allergic interstitial nephritis, glomerulonephritis), and (3) postrenal syndrome (obstruction of urine flow); acute renal failure can be divided into three phases (1) oliguric, (2) diuretic, and (3) recovery; with proper management acute renal failure is reversible, but it has a high mortality rate (40% to 60%)

chronic renal failure An irreversible disease of the kidney, characterized by a progressive loss of renal function, leading to end-stage renal disease and death; most common causes of chronic renal failure include glomerulonephritis, pyelonephritis, congenital hypoplasia, polycystic kidney disease, diabetes, hypertension, systemic lupus, Alport's syndrome, and amyloidosis

Assessment
Observations/findings

Neurologic
  Headache
  Blurred vision
  Nystagmus
  Personality changes
  Irritability
  Malaise
  Peripheral neuropathy
    Paresthesias
    Motor weakness
  Decreased level of consciousness
    Drowsiness
    Confusion
    Stupor
    Coma
  Seizure activity
Respiratory
  Pulmonary edema
  Pneumonia
  Cheyne-Stokes respirations
  Ammonia breath
  Uremic lung
Cardiovascular
  Hypertension
  Tachycardia
  CHF
  Arrythmias
  Myocardiopathy
  Pericarditis
  Cardiac tamponade
Fluid and electrolytes
  Oliguria
  Anuria
  Edema: weight gain
  Dehydration: weight loss
  Hyperkalemia
  Hyperphosphatemia
  Hypermagnesemia
  Hypocalcemia
  Hypoproteinemia
  Hyperlipidemia
  Metabolic acidosis
Gastrointestinal
  Bitter, metallic taste in mouth
  Oral ulcerations
  Anorexia
  Malnutrition
  Nausea, vomiting
  Diarrhea
  Constipation
  Pancreatitis
  Hemorrhage
Integumentary
  Dry, scaly skin

Pale, sallow, yellow, or bronze color
Brittle, pale nail beds
Petechiae
Bruising
Uremic frost
Pruritis
Hematologic
  Anemia
  Coagulopathy
Musculoskeletal
  Osteomalacia
  Osteitis fibrosis
  Osteosclerosis
  Loss of muscle mass
Endocrine
  Amenorrhea
  Sexual dysfunction
  Infertility
  Hyperparathyroidism
  Glucose intolerance
Immunologic
  Elevated temperature
  Elevated WBC
  Infection
  Septicemia
Drug toxicity
Psychosocial
  Anxiety
  Fear
  Powerlessness
  Grieving
  Denial
  Noncompliance
  Depression
  Alteration in relationship with significant others

Laboratory/diagnostic studies

Serum BUN
Serum creatinine
Serum electrolytes
Urinalysis
Urine osmolality
Urine electrolytes
Creatinine clearance
Uric acid serum and urine
KUB
Renal ultrasound
Renal CT scan
IVP
Renal biopsy

Potential complications

Progressive loss of renal function
Fluid and electrolyte imbalance
Infection/sepsis
Hemorrhage
Cardiovascular failure
Respiratory failure

Medical management

Maintenance of fluid and electrolyte balance
  Fluid restriction
  Daily weights
Medications*
  Diuretics
  Antihypertensives
  Aluminum hydroxide antacids
  Kayexalate
  Vitamin D
  Multivitamins
  Ferrous sulfate
  Calcium
  Sodium bicarbonate
  Diphrenhydramine
Dietary management
  High carbohydrate
  Low protein
  Low potassium
  Low sodium
  Total parenteral nutrition (TPN)
Blood transfusion
Peritoneal dialysis
Hemodialysis
Renal transplant
Treatment of complications

Nursing diagnoses/goals/interventions

ndx: Alteration in urinary elimination (oliguria, anuria, diuresis) related to decreasing renal function

GOAL: *Patient will maintain present level of urinary elimination or better (as near normal as possible), as evidenced by absence of further renal deterioration*

Measure urine output qh
Note character of urine and report abnormalities
Monitor urine specific gravity
Measure intake and output accurately
Weigh patient daily at same time with same clothing and scale

---

*Dosages of medications may need to be altered depending on whether they are excreted primarily by the kidney, are nephrotoxic, or are dialyzed out.

Avoid dehydration; replace fluids orally or parenterally as ordered
Avoid fluid excess; restrict fluids as ordered
Administer diuretics as ordered
Use extreme caution when administering nephrotoxic drugs
Monitor serum BUN and creatinine as ordered
Dialyze patient as ordered

ndx: Potential for electrolyte imbalance (hyperkalemia, hyperphosphatemia, hypermagnesemia, hypocalcemia) related to decreasing renal ability to regulate and excrete electrolytes*

GOAL: *Patient will maintain a safe serum level of electrolytes as evidenced by absence of signs and symptoms of electrolyte imbalance*

Monitor serum electrolytes as ordered
Report abnormal serum electrolyte values to physician
Dialyze as ordered

Hyperkalemia

Monitor for signs and symptoms of irritability, nausea, diarrhea, intestinal colic, arrythmias, and peaked T wave on electrocardiogram (ECG)
Restrict dietary potassium as ordered
Administer polystyrene sulfonate (Kayexalate) as ordered
Avoid administration of whole blood; use washed packed cells
Administer blood during dialysis to remove excess potassium

Hyperphosphatemia

Monitor for signs and symptoms of hyperreflexia, paresthesias, muscle cramps, and seizures
Administer aluminum hydroxide antacids as ordered
Restrict dietary phosphorus (peanuts, poultry, milk, cheese, corn, peas)

Hypermagnesemia

Monitor for signs and symptoms of hypoactive deep tendon reflexes, decreasing level of consciousness, hypotension, decreased respirations, bradycardia, flushed skin, nausea, and vomiting
Restrict dietary magnesium (nuts, whole-grain breads and cereals, meat, milk, and legumes)
Avoid use of laxatives and antacids containing magnesium

---
*Not a NANDA-approved nursing diagnosis.

Hypocalcemia

Monitor for signs and symptoms of abdominal cramps; muscle cramps; carpopedal spasm; tingling of fingertips, toes, and circumoral area; positive Chvostek's and Trousseau's signs; tetany; change in mental status; seizures; and arrythmias
Provide sources of dietary calcium (e.g., dairy products)
Administer vitamin D and calcium supplements
Prevent hyperphosphatemia

ndx: Potential for fluid volume excess related to decreased ability of kidney to extract water and to retain sodium

GOAL: *Patient will not exhibit signs of fluid excess as evidenced by balanced intake and output, stable weight, usual mental status, normal breath sounds, and absence of hypertension and edema*

Monitor and document intake and output accurately qh
Weigh patient daily at the same time with same clothing and scale
Monitor for elevated BP
Monitor serum electrolytes; report abnormal laboratory values or signs and symptoms of electrolyte imbalance
Assess level of consciousness; note changes in mental status
Assess heart sounds for presence of S_3 and/or S_4
Assess breath sounds for rales
Obtain chest x-ray film as ordered
Assess for peripheral edema
Assess for distended neck veins
Restrict fluids as ordered
Administer diuretics as ordered
Provide ice chips to control thirst

ndx: Alteration in skin integrity related to immobility, uremia, capillary fragility, and edema

GOAL: *Patient will maintain skin integrity as evidenced by absence of skin breakdown or bruising*

Assess patient's skin for redness, bruising or breakdown, turgor, and temperature
Keep skin clean and dry
Assist patient with cleansing and drying perineal area after bowel elimination
Administer skin care with lotion to avoid dryness
Avoid use of harsh soaps on patient's skin
Instruct patient not to scratch pruritic areas

Apply emollient lotion or cream to pruritic areas
Administer antihistamines or minor tranquilizers to relieve pruritis
Encourage ambulation as tolerated
Assist patient with turning and changing position q2h if on bed rest
Keep bed linen wrinkle-free
Use an egg-crate mattress or sheepskin to decrease skin irritation
Apply protectors to heels and elbows
Remove any clothes, jewelry, etc., that may compromise skin circulation
Handle edematous areas carefully
Instruct and assist patient with ROM exercises
Administer IM injections with caution to minimize bruising
Provide direct pressure to venipuncture sites for 5 min or longer to prevent bleeding or bruising
Maintain adequate nutrition; administer TPN if necessary
Notify physician if skin breakdown or signs of infection occur at sight
Administer decubitus care as ordered

ndx: Alteration in nutrition: less than body requirements related to anorexia, nausea and vomiting, dietary restrictions, and oral ulcerations

GOAL: *Patient will maintain adequate nutritional status as evidenced by weight within normal range for height, age, and body type, and by normal serum albumin, total protein, iron, Hgb, and Hct levels*

Assess nutritional status
Monitor patient's weight daily
Consult with dietitian to plan menus incorporating dietary restrictions, calorie requirements, and patient's preferences
Encourage patient to control menu planning as much as possible
Encourage patient to express feelings about dietary restrictions
Encourage meals from home as long as they follow dietary restrictions
Be empathetic and reexplain purpose of dietary restrictions
Provide good oral hygiene before and after meals and prn
Provide smaller, more frequent meals if patient is nauseated or experiences early satiety
Administer antiemetics on a timely basis before meals as ordered
Provide a pleasant environment during meals
Monitor percentage of meals eaten
Administer vitamin supplements and iron as ordered
Administer TPN as ordered

ndx: Activity intolerance: fatigue related to inadequate tissue oxygenation, anemia, inadequate nutrition, and difficulty in resting and sleeping

GOAL: *Patient will demonstrate an increase in activity tolerance as evidenced by verbalization of feeling less fatigued and getting adequate rest, and by as near-normal resumption of ADLs as possible*

Identify factors that reduce patient's activity tolerance
Assess patient's present daily schedule
Adjust patient's schedule to provide rest periods between activities and adequate nocturnal sleep
Limit visitors or length of stay as necessary
Maintain activity restrictions as ordered
Allow patient to set daily activity goals
Encourage gradual progression of activities as tolerated
Encourage self-care activities; assist as needed
Provide praise for all attempts to increase activity
Assess patient's response to increases in activity
Maintain adequate nutrition

ndx: Potential for infection related to depressed immune system, inadequate nutrition, and hospitalization

GOAL: *Patient will remain free of local or systemic infection as evidenced by absence of fever or leukocytosis; negative urine, sputum, and blood cultures; and absence of inflammation or drainage where there is a break in skin integrity or in oral mucosa*

Monitor for and report signs and symptoms of infection (fever, chills, elevated WBC, increased heart rate, adventitious breath sounds, colored or increased sputum, cloudy and foul-smelling urine, redness, swelling or drainage where there is skin breakdown, vaginal or urethral drainage, or ulceration of oral mucosa)
Monitor T, P, R, and BP every shift or more often if necessary
Obtain culture specimens as ordered
Use excellent handwashing technique and teach patient the same
Maintain sterile technique with all invasive procedures and when caring for catheters, tubes, lines, dressings, and dialysis accesses
Maintain skin and mucosal integrity by providing good skin care and oral hygiene

Avoid invasive procedures and indwelling catheters if possible
Maintain adequate nutrition
Discourage contact with persons having an infection
Maintain a clean environment
Encourage activity (ambulation if possible)
Encourage patient to take deep breaths and cough
Instruct patient to perform good perineal care

ndx: Potential for complications: hemorrhage, CHF, pericarditis, hypertension, arrythmias, uremia*

GOAL: *Patient will show no signs of complications of renal failure, as evidenced by absence of hemorrhage, CHF, pericarditis, hypertension, arrythmias, atelectasis/pneumonia, and uremia*

Hemorrhage

Assess patient for and report signs of unusual bleeding (petechiae, prolonged bleeding with venipuncture, bleeding gums, increased abdominal girth, significant drop in BP)
Guiac all GI tract fluids; report positive results
Monitor coagulation times (PT, PTT, platelets) and Hgb and Hct
Use smallest-gauge needle possible for all venipunctures and injections
Apply pressure to site after injections, and venous and arterial punctures, until bleeding stops
Caution patient to avoid activities that increase potential for trauma and bleeding

CHF

Monitor for and report signs and symptoms of CHF (tachycardia, muffled heart tones, S_3 and/or S_4, rales, shortness of breath [SOB], distended neck veins, peripheral edema, decreased urine output)
Obtain chest x-ray examination as ordered
Measure and record intake and output accurately
Maintain balanced intake and output
Administer oxygen as ordered
Administer diuretics as ordered

Pericarditis

Monitor for and report signs of pericarditis (sharp chest pain increased with deep inspiration; pericardial friction rub; elevated temperature, WBC, and sedimentation rate)
Administer medications to decrease pain and inflammation as ordered
Assist with pericardiocentesis if performed

Hypertension

Monitor BP and report systolic BP above 140 and diastolic BP above 90
Administer antihypertensives as ordered
Monitor for signs of myocardial infarction (MI) and CVA

Arrythmias

Monitor for and report irregular apical pulse, pulse rate below 60 or above 100, palpitations, dizziness, or syncope
Maintain fluid and electrolyte balance
Initiate cardiac monitoring as ordered
Administer oxygen as ordered
Administer antiarrythmics as ordered

Uremia

Monitor for and report signs and symptoms of uremia (arrhythmias, decreasing level of consciousness, confusion, paranoid delusions, hallucinations, seizures, nausea, vomiting, itching, muscle cramps, tingling of extremities, bleeding, stomatitis)
Monitor serum creatinine and BUN as ordered
Reorient patient to person, place, time, and situation
Initiate seizure precautions
Dialyze as ordered

ndx: Grieving related to loss of function of major organ systems, changes in life-style, and life-threatening prognosis

GOAL: *Patient will begin progression through the grieving process as evidenced by expression of feelings to care giver or significant other, utilization of support system, and effective coping mechanisms, and by compliance with treatment plan and participation in self-care activities*

Be sensitive to changes and restrictions in patient's life-style
Encourage patient to express feelings of frustration, anger, fear, and uncertainty
Actively listen
Observe for behavioral and emotional signs of grieving (denial, anger, crying, withdrawal, noncompliance, dependency, etc.)
Be patient and empathetic as patient experiences emotional changes and develops coping mechanisms
Set limits on maladaptive coping mechanisms if they interfere with patient's well-being
Support adaptive behaviors that suggest a progression and resolution of grieving process
Support realistic hope; answer questions honestly, providing requested information

---

*Not a NANDA-approved nursing diagnosis.

Provide assistance from other professionals to help patient with emotional changes (social worker, clergy, psychiatry)

Teach and reteach about disease process and management

Involve family and significant others in teaching process

ndx: Knowledge deficit regarding disease process of renal failure, home care, and follow-up instructions

GOAL: *Patient and/or significant other will verbalize understanding of renal failure, home care, follow-up instructions, and signs and symptoms to report to physician; and will return-demonstrate ability to weigh self, measure intake and output, and take BP accurately*

Instruct patient to eat high-carbohydrate, low-protein, low-sodium diet as ordered

Instruct patient to avoid salt substitutes

Teach amount of daily fluid allowed in diet, and that thirst is not a reliable indicator of fluid needs

Teach importance of and instruct patient to measure all output (urine, stools, and emesis)

Instruct patient to note character of urine, stool, and emesis

Instruct patient to report inability to urinate to physician

Instruct patient to weigh self daily at same time with same clothing and scale and to accurately record weight

Instruct patient to take BP daily at same time in same arm and in same position, and to rest briefly before taking it

Teach signs and symptoms of infection and instruct patient to notify physician of their occurrence

Instruct patient to avoid persons with infections, to avoid crowds, and to use good handwashing technique

Instruct patient to maintain good skin care
  Shower daily
  Avoid detergent soaps
  Apply lanolin-based lotion or cream to skin
  Avoid scratching skin

Teach and instruct patient to report symptoms of disease progression (rapid weight gain, lethargy, decreased urine output, absence of urine output for 24 hr, elevated BP, presence of edema)

Instruct patient to avoid fatigue: to exercise to tolerance, to plan frequent rest periods, and to sleep 6 to 8 hr per night

Teach name of medication, dosage, schedule, purpose, and side effects

Instruct need to avoid taking over-the-counter medications without checking with physician

Teach importance of ongoing outpatient care

Evaluation

There is no indication of further renal damage

There are no signs or symptoms of fluid or electrolyte imbalance

Skin remains intact with no evidence of breakdown

Adequate nutrition is maintained

Activity increase is well tolerated

There are no signs of local or systemic infection

There are no signs of complications: hemorrhage, CHF, pericarditis, hypertension, arrythmias, or uremia

There is progession of the grieving process with signs suggesting resolution

Patient and/or significant other is able to verbalize understanding of renal failure, fluid and dietary restrictions, and plan of follow-up care; identify ways to decrease the risk of further kidney damage, infection, and bleeding; state signs and symptoms to report to physician; and demonstrate ability to weigh self, measure intake and output, and take BP accurately

PERITONEAL DIALYSIS

A treatment indicated in renal failure, using the peritoneum as the dialyzing membrane to correct electrolyte and fluid imbalances and to remove toxic waste or drugs normally excreted by the kidneys; a catheter is inserted into the peritoneal cavity, and a hypertonic, warmed solution (dialysate) is infused by gravity into the peritoneal cavity and allowed to dwell; during the dwell time, osmosis occurs, moving water from the blood into the dialysate, and diffusion occurs, moving toxins and waste across the peritoneal membrane into the dialysate; after the appropriate dwell time, the dialysate and excess fluid are drained from the peritoneal cavity (Figure 9-10)

intermittent peritoneal dialysis (IPD) *Can be performed manually or with a cycler; patient is dialyzed for 6 to 10 hr periods, four to five times per week, using a predetermined amount of dialysate with a set dwell time*

continuous ambulatory peritoneal dialysis (CAPD) *Used to treat chronic renal failure and performed by the patient; dialysis changes are done continuously (24 hr a day, 7 days a week); dialysate*

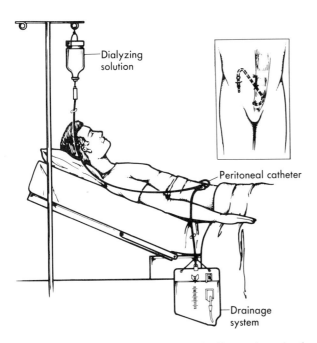

FIGURE 9-10. Peritoneal dialysis. *Insert,* Indwelling peritoneal catheter.

dwells in peritoneal cavity for 4 hr during the day and 8 hr during the night

continuous cycling peritoneal dialysis (CCPD) A combination of IPD and CAPD; a cycler performs three dialysate exchanges at night; during the day, dialysate is instilled and allowed to dwell in the peritoneal cavity the entire day and is drained at the end of the day

Assessment
Observations/findings

Fluid imbalance
  Overhydration
    Rapid weight gain
    Edema
  Dehydration
    Rapid weight loss
    Hypovolemia
Respiratory system
  Tachypnea
  Rales
  Pulmonary edema
  Pneumonia
Cardiovascular system
  Tachycardia
  Bradycardia
  Cardiac arrythmias
  Shock
  Pericardial friction rub
  Congestive heart failure (CHF)
GI system
  Abdominal pain
  Nausea, vomiting
  Diarrhea
Neurologic system
  Confusion
  Decreased level of consciousness
  Seizure activity
Metabolism: hyperglycemia
Hypothermia
Catheter insertion site
  Redness
  Pain
  Swelling
  Drainage
  Drainage of dialysate around catheter
  Bleeding
Retention of dialysate
Dialysate
  Cloudy
  Bright red
  Fecal colored
  Foul smelling
Psychologic
  Anxiety
  Disturbance in self-concept
  Fear of death

Laboratory/diagnostic studies

Serum electrolytes
Serum creatinine
Serum BUN
Serum protein
Urine glucose
See Renal Failure (p. 557)

Potential complications

See Renal Failure (p. 557)
Perforated bladder
Perforated bowel
Infection
Peritonitis
Hemorrhage

Medical management

Maintenance of fluid and electrolyte balance
  Restriction of fluids
  Daily weights

Medications*
  Diuretics
  Antihypertensives
  Aluminum hydroxide antacids
  Polystyrene sulfonate (Kayexalate)
  Vitamin D
  Multivitamins
  Ferrous sulfate
  Calcium
  Sodium bicarbonate
  Diphenhydramine
Dietary management
  High carbohydrate
  Low protein
  Low potassium
  Low sodium
  TPN

Nursing diagnoses/goals/interventions

ndx: Alteration in fluid balance (fluid excess or fluid deficit) related to fluid retention, abnormal loss due to hypertonicity of dialysate, or inadequate fluid replacement

GOAL: *Patient will not exhibit signs of fluid excess or deficit as evidenced by balanced intake and output, stable weight, usual mental status, and normal serum electrolytes*

Monitor baseline vital signs at beginning of each dialysis treatment, q15 min during first exchange, and q1h thereafter
Report elevated BP, decreased BP, bounding pulse, tachycardia, or dyspnea to physician
Maintain dialysis record
  Amount of solution instilled
  Amount of solution returned; notify physician if patient retains 500 ml or more
  Time of beginning and end of dialysis cycle
  Fluid balance
  Number of exchanges
  Medication used in dialyzing solution
  Patient's weight
Completely drain peritoneal cavity when weighing patient
Replace or restrict IV or oral fluid according to previous day's output + 400 ml to replace insensible loss as ordered
Monitor serum electrolytes; report abnormal laboratory values or signs and symptoms of electrolyte imbalance
Assess skin turgor
Assess mucous membranes
Assess level of consciousness; note changes in mental status
Assess heart sounds for presence of S_3 and/or S_4
Assess breath sounds for rales
Obtain chest x-ray film as ordered
Assess for peripheral edema
Assess for distended neck veins
Restrict fluids as ordered
Administer diuretics as ordered
Provide ice chips to control thirst

ndx: Ineffective breathing pattern related to fluid overload, pain, or rapid infusion of peritoneal dialysate

GOAL: *Patient will breathe comfortably*

Assess rate, rhythm, and depth of respirations qh
Auscultate chest for adventitious breath sounds q4h
Report tachypnea, dyspnea, or rales to physician
Raise head of bed 45 degrees so patient can maximally expand his chest
Assist with and teach frequent turning; turn onto side nearest closed drainage unit
Encourage patient to cough and deep breathe q2h and prn
Medicate as necessary to alleviate incisional pain at peritoneal catheter site, thus promoting comfortable deep breathing
Instruct patient to splint incision for effective coughing
Dialyze as ordered to remove excess fluid
Prevent air from entering peritoneum by keeping drip chamber three-fourths full
Check outflow tubing for kinks or poor connections to ensure proper drainage
If patient becomes dyspneic, notify physician; slow infusion rate; make sure tubing is patent and not kinked and assist patient with turning, coughing, and deep breathing
If patient has difficulty in breathing with instillation of peritoneal dialysate, consult with physician regarding instillation of smaller volumes, more frequently

ndx: Potential for infection (UTI, local, systemic) related to presence of peritoneal catheter

GOAL: *Patient will show no signs or symptoms of UTI, or local or systemic infection*

---

*Dosages of medications may need to be altered depending on whether they are excreted primarily by the kidney, are nephrotoxic, or are dialyzed out.

Use sterile technique when connecting and disconnecting peritoneal catheter from dialysis system and when adding medication to dialysate

Maintain closed drainage system; use distal emptying valve to empty collecting unit

Wear clean masks and sterile gowns when catheter is manipulated

Use povidone-iodine to clean connection site between catheter and dialysis tubing

Disconnect dialysis tubing from catheter and insert a sterile male Luer-Lok cap into open end of dialysis catheter

Apply antibacterial ointment to catheter insertion site

Apply sterile dressing to insertion site

Change dressing q24h or whenever wet or soiled

Monitor and report cloudy outflow

Avoid use of indwelling urethral catheter; use intermittent catheterization instead as ordered

Monitor and report catheter site redness, swelling, or drainage

Monitor and report leakage of dialysate around catheter site

Check temperature q4h and report if above 101° F (38.5° C)

Auscultate chest for breath sounds q4h; report adventitious breath sounds to physician

Encourage coughing and deep breathing

Use good handwashing technique; teach and encourage patient to do the same

Instruct patient to avoid persons with infections

Instruct patient to avoid chilling

Take measures to prevent skin breakdown

Encourage early ambulation

Prevent UTI (see Urinary Tract Infection [UTI], p. 522)

ndx: Activity intolerance: fatigue related to inadequate tissue oxygenation, anemia, inadequate nutrition, and/or difficulty in resting and sleeping

GOAL: *Patient will demonstrate an increase in activity tolerance as evidenced by verbalization of feeling less fatigued and of getting adequate rest, and by as near-normal resumption of ADLs as possible*

Identify factors that reduce patient's activity tolerance

Assess patient's present daily schedule

Adjust patient's schedule to provide rest periods between activities and adequate nocturnal sleep

Limit visitors or length of stay as necessary

Maintain activity restrictions as ordered

Allow patient to set daily activity goals

Encourage gradual progression of activities as tolerated

Encourage self-care activities; assist as needed

Provide praise for all attempts to increase activity

Assess patient's response to increases in activity

Maintain adequate nutrition

ndx: Alteration in comfort: pain related to cold or acidic dialysate, rapid infusion, or peritoneal infection

GOAL: *Patient will verbalize a decrease in pain and will show a relaxed facial expression and body position*

See nursing diagnosis of alteration in comfort: pain, under Polycystic Kidney Disease (p. 549)

Assist patient with assuming a comfortable position during dialysis

Warm dialysate solution prior to infusion

Prevent air from entering peritoneal cavity during infusion of dialyzing solution; keep drip chamber three-fourths full

Monitor for pain radiating to shoulder, which may result from air accumulation under diaphragm

Monitor for signs of peritonitis and report (see nursing diagnosis of potential for complications: peritonitis, under Urinary Diversion, p. 546)

Monitor for rectal pain (may indicate improper catheter placement)

Be aware that dialysis cycle usually takes 1 hr to complete
  Fluid time 10 min
  Equilibration time 30 min
  Drainage time 20 min

Instill no more than 2000 ml of dialyzing solution at one time

If pain occurs during infusion, slow infusion rate

Maintain tension-free patent drainage system

Add lidocaine to dialyzing solution as ordered

When administering CAPD, leave some dialyzing solution in peritoneal cavity (this prevents dialysis catheter from becoming plugged, thus facilitating infusion and drainage)

ndx: Potential for complications: electrolyte imbalance, hemorrhage, perforated bladder, perforated bowel*

GOAL: *Patient will show no signs of complications associated with peritoneal dialysis*

Electrolyte imbalance

Add electrolytes to dialysate as ordered

Monitor serum electrolytes as ordered

Report abnormal serum electrolyte values to physician

---

*Not a NANDA-approved nursing diagnosis.

HYPERKALEMIA

Monitor for signs and symptoms of irritability, nausea, diarrhea, intestinal colic, arrythmias, and peaked T wave on ECG

Restrict dietary potassium as ordered

Administer polystyrene sulfunate (Kayexalate) as ordered

Avoid administration of whole blood; use washed packed cells

HYPERPHOSPHATEMIA

Monitor for signs and symptoms of hyperreflexia, paresthesias, muscle cramps, and seizures

Administer aluminum hydroxide antacids as ordered

Restrict dietary phosphorus (peanuts, poultry, milk, cheese, corn, peas)

HYPERMAGNESEMIA

Monitor for signs and symptoms of hypoactive deep tendon reflexes, decreasing level of consciousness, hypotension, decreased respirations, bradycardia, flushed skin, nausea, and vomiting

Restrict dietary magnesium (nuts, whole-grain breads and cereals, meat, milk, and legumes)

Avoid use of laxatives and antacids containing magnesium

HYPOCALCEMIA

Monitor for signs and symptoms of abdominal cramps; muscle cramps; carpopedal spasm; tingling of fingertips, toes, and circumoral area; positive Chvostek's and Trousseau's signs; tetany; change in mental status; seizures; and arrythmias

Provide sources of dietary calcium (e.g., dairy products)

Administer vitamin D and calcium supplements

Prevent hyperphosphatemia

Hemorrhage

Examine outflow fluid q1h for color and clarity (normally it is clear and pale yellow and may be pink-tinged during first three to four cycles)

If gross blood is noted in outflow fluid, discontinue dialysis; notify physician immediately

Monitor Hct and Hgb as ordered

If hemorrhage occurs
  Place patient flat in bed
  Administer fluid replacement as ordered
  Transfuse with blood products as ordered
  Prepare patient for surgery if necessary

Perforated bowel

Monitor for and report signs and symptoms of perforated bowel to physician immediately (abdominal pain, flatus in outflow, foul-smelling dialysate drainage, fecal-colored dialysate drainage, diarrhea, poor outflow drainage)

Perforated bladder

Monitor for and report signs and symptoms of perforated bladder to physician immediately (bladder distention, abdominal pain, urination of dialysate, abrupt onset of polyuria, incomplete dialysate drainage)

ndx: Potential for fear related to life-threatening complications of disease process and peritoneal dialysis

GOAL: *Patient will be able to verbalize feelings of fear and uncertainty to care giver or significant other, will identify adaptive coping mechanisms, and will verbalize feeling increased psychologic comfort*

Teach patient about renal failure

Orient patient to environment

Announce any changes in routine; explain delays

Explain all procedures of peritoneal dialysis (i.e., implantation of catheter, exchanges, etc.)

Stress simplicity of peritoneal dialysis

Reinforce physician's explanation of procedure

Stress advantages to patient: more liberal diet and fluid intake

Encourage patient to verbalize feelings

Actively listen

Support adaptive coping mechanisms

Remain with patient until fear subsides

Encourage communication with significant other

Encourage sharing common problems with others (group of renal failure patients)

ndx: Potential alteration in self-concept: body image related to presence of peritoneal catheter

GOAL: *Patient will verbalize feelings related to change in body image to care giver or significant other, will be able to look at and care for peritoneal catheter, and will resume ADLs*

Be aware that patient is under considerable emotional stress

Be sensitive to changes in patient's life-style

Encourage patient to express feelings

Actively listen

Answer questions honestly

Be aware of coping mechanisms and expect that patient may exhibit irrational or inappropriate behaviors, irritability, and lack of motivation
Encourage adaptive coping behaviors
Set limits on maladaptive behaviors, especially if they are detrimental to patient's health
Instruct patient that there are no social limitations; patient may participate in any sport except boxing or sports requiring body contact (football, wrestling), and heavy weight lifting should also be avoided
Explain to patient that there are no clothing limitations except bikinis or girdles
Explain to patient that there are no sexual limitations
Encourage communication with significant other
Encourage patient to look at and touch catheter as soon as possible
Encourage patient to participate in caring for catheter
Include spouse/significant other in teaching
Provide for a psychiatric consultation if necessary

ndx: Knowledge deficit regarding renal failure, peritoneal dialysis procedure, and home care and follow-up instructions

GOAL: *Patient and/or significant other will verbalize understanding of renal failure, peritoneal dialysis procedure, symptoms to report to physician, and home care and follow-up instructions, and will return-demonstrate care of peritoneal catheter*

Teach about disease process and progression of renal failure (see Renal Failure, p. 557)
Teach need and procedure for peritoneal dialysis
Instruct patient to maintain fluid intake and diet as ordered
Instruct patient to measure and record urine output
Instruct patient to weigh self daily at same time with same clothing and scale, and with empty peritoneal cavity
Instruct patient to take BP, T, and P daily
Instruct patient to take measures to prevent UTI (see Urinary Tract Infection [UTI], p. 522)
Teach and instruct patient to report the following symptoms to physician
　Elevated temperature
　Elevated or decreased BP
　Abdominal pain
　Abdominal distention
　Nausea, vomiting
　Vertigo
　Rapid weight gain
　Edema
　Catheter insertion site
　　Redness
　　Pain
　　Swelling
　　Drainage
　Symptoms of progression of renal failure
Teach and instruct peritoneal catheter care
　Instruct patient to protect catheter from injury
　Instruct patient to keep sterile cap and dressing in place
　Teach patient to perform peritoneal dialysis exchanges at home
　Instruct patient to wash catheter insertion site gently with soap and water, rinse well, and pat dry
　Instruct patient to apply antibacterial ointment to catheter site daily
　Instruct patient to cover site with sterile dressing
Teach name of medication, dosage, purpose, schedule, and side effects
Instruct patient to avoid taking over-the-counter medications without checking with physician
Instruct patient to have blood drawn for laboratory analysis as ordered by physician
Teach importance of ongoing outpatient care

Evaluation

Patient shows no signs or symptoms of fluid excess of deficit
Patient breathes comfortably
Patient shows no signs of infection
Patient verbalizes a decrease in pain and has a relaxed facial expression and body position
Patient shows no signs of complications associated with peritoneal dialysis
Patient verbalizes feelings of fear and uncertainty to others, identifies adaptive coping mechanisms, and verbalizes increased psychologic comfort
Patient verbalizes feelings related to change in body image to others, looks at and cares for peritoneal catheter, and resumes ADLs
Patient and/or significant other verbalizes understanding of renal failure, peritoneal dialysis procedure, symptoms to report to physician, home care, and follow-up instructions; and return-demonstrates care of peritoneal catheter

HEMODIALYSIS

A treatment used in renal failure to remove toxic wastes and excess water and fluid, and to correct

electrolyte balance, by the principles of filtration, osmosis, and diffusion, using an external dialyzing system

Assessment

Observations/findings

See Renal Failure (p. 557)
See Peritoneal Dialysis (p. 562)
Low back pain
Muscle cramping
Patency of vascular access
    Bruits
    Thrills
    Color of blood in shunt
    Unrelieved pain, numbness, or tingling of extremity
    Poor capillary refill in extremity
Disequilibrium syndrome
    Headache
    Fatigue
    Confusion
    Muscle irritability
    Twitching
    Seizure

Laboratory/diagnostic studies

See Renal Failure (p. 557)
Coagulation studies
    PT
    PTT
    Platelets

Potential complications

See Renal Failure (p. 557)
Disequilibrium syndrome
Hemorrhage
Air embolism
    Cyanosis
    Hypotension
    Weak, rapid pulse
Severe hypotension
Hepatitis

Medical management

Maintenance of fluid and electrolyte balance
    Restriction of fluids
    Daily weights
    Medications*
        Diuretics
        Antihypertensives
        Aluminum hydroxide antacids
        Polystyrene sulfonate (Kayexalate)
        Vitamin D
        Multivitamins
        Ferrous sulfate
        Calcium
        Sodium bicarbonate
        Diphenhydramine
    Dietary management
        High carbohydrate
        Low protein
        Low potassium
        Low sodium
        TPN
Blood transfusion
Treatment of complications
Prescription of dialysis treatment

Nursing diagnoses/goals/interventions

ndx: Alteration in comfort: low back pain and muscle cramping related to rapid blood flow and to shift of fluid and sodium levels

GOAL: *Patient will verbalize a decrease in pain and muscle cramping and will show a relaxed facial expression and body position*

If low back pain occurs, reduce blood flow rate and provide comfort measures
If muscle cramping occurs
    Check BP and report if decreased
    Administer 100 ml of normal saline with 25% mannitol, 10 ml of 23% sodium chloride, or 50 ml of 50% dextrose as ordered to elevated BP
    Adjust sodium concentration in dialysate as ordered
Assess nature, intensity, location, duration, and precipitating and alleviating factors of pain
Assess nonverbal signs of pain
Provide nonpharmacologic comfort measures
    Assist patient with assuming a comfortable position
    Teach relaxation techniques
    Teach and assist with guided imagery technique
    Provide diversional activity
    Provide a restful environment
Administer pain medication as ordered
Observe for desired effects and side effects of medication
Take and document vital signs before and after administering pain medication
Consult with physician if measures fail to provide adequate pain relief or if dosage or interval change for pain medication is needed

---

*Dosages of medications may need to be altered depending on whether they are excreted primarily by the kidney, are nephrotoxic, or are dialyzed out.

ndx: Alteration in fluid volume: fluid excess or deficit related to kidney's inability to regulate fluid balance, inadequate fluid replacement, and/or excessive fluid removal during dialysis

GOAL: *Patient will not exhibit signs of fluid excess or deficit as evidenced by balanced intake and output, stable weight, usual mental status, and normal serum electrolytes*

Monitor and document intake and output accurately qh
Weigh patient daily at the same time with same clothing and scale
Monitor for elevated BP
Monitor serum electrolytes; report abnormal laboratory values or signs and symptoms of electrolyte imbalance
Assess level of consciousness; note changes in mental status
Assess skin turgor
Assess oral mucous membranes for moisture
Assess heart sounds for presence of S_3 and/or S_4
Assess breath sounds for rales
Obtain chest x-ray film as ordered
Assess for peripheral edema
Assess for distended neck veins
Restrict fluids as ordered
Administer diuretics as ordered
Provide ice chips to control thirst

ndx: Potential for infection related to vascular access, depressed immune system, inadequate nutrition, and hospitalization

GOAL: *Patient will show no signs of infection (UTI, local, or systemic)*

Monitor and report signs and symptoms of infection (fever; chills; elevated WBC; increased heart rate; adventitious breath sounds; colored or increased sputum; cloudy and foul-smelling urine; redness, swelling, or drainage where there is skin breakdown; vaginal or urethral drainage; ulceration of oral mucosa)
Monitor T, P, R, and BP q shift or more often if necessary
Obtain culture specimens as ordered
Use excellent handwashing technique and teach patient to do the same
Maintain sterile technique with all invasive procedures and when caring for catheters, tubes, lines, dressings, and dialysis accesses
Maintain skin and mucosal integrity by providing good skin care and oral hygiene
Avoid invasive procedures and indwelling catheters if possible
Maintain adequate nutrition
Discourage contact with persons having an infection
Maintain a clean environment
Encourage activity (ambulation if possible)
Encourage patient to take deep breaths and cough
Instruct patient to perform good perineal care

ndx: Grieving related to loss of kidney function, changes and restrictions in life-style, and life-threatening prognosis

GOAL: *Patient will show signs of progression through the grieving process as evidenced by expression of feelings to care giver or significant other, utilization of support system and coping mechanisms, and compliance with treatment plan*

Be sensitive to changes and restrictions in patient's life-style
Encourage patient to express feelings of frustration, anger, fear, and uncertainty
Actively listen
Observe for behavioral and emotional signs of grieving (denial, anger, crying, withdrawal, noncompliance, dependency, etc.)
Be patient and empathetic as patient experiences emotional changes and develops coping mechanisms
Set limits on maladaptive coping mechanisms if they interfere with patient's well-being
Support adaptive behaviors that suggest a progression and resolution of the grieving process
Support realistic hope; answer questions honestly, providing requested information
Provide assistance from other professionals to help patient with emotional changes (social worker, clergy, psychiatry)
Teach and reteach about disease process and management
Involve family and significant others in teaching process

ndx: Potential for complications: clotting of vascular access, disequilibrium syndrome, hemorrhage (internal, external), severe hypotension, air embolism*

GOAL: *Patient will show no signs or symptoms of complications of hemodialysis*

---

*Not a NANDA-approved nursing diagnosis.

Clotting of vascular access

Assess for and document patency of venous access by auscultating for bruits and palpating for thrills q shift

Monitor for and report signs and symptoms of clotting of venous access (dark or separated blood within shunt, site cool to touch, absence of bruits and/or thrills)

Monitor for and report signs and symptoms of inadequate peripheral perfusion (sudden, unrelieved pain; numbness; tingling of extremity distal to access site)

Prime line with heparin as ordered

Heparinize patient as ordered

Never kink tubing

Do not take BP, start IV lines, or draw blood from shunt arm

Avoid tight clothing, jewelry, and name bands on extremity of access site

Disequilibrium syndrome

Monitor for and report signs and symptoms of disequilibrium syndrome (headache, fatigue, confusion, muscle agitation, twitching, seizure)

Perform neuro checks q½h during dialysis

Monitor and report cardiac arrythmias

If disequilibrium syndrome occurs
  Reduce blood flow and inform physician immediately
  Administer diazepam and phenytoin as ordered
  Observe and document desired effects and side effects of medication administered
  Stay with patient

Maintain seizure precautions during hemodialysis: bed in low position, side rails elevated, tongue blade at bedside

Monitor serum electrolytes as ordered and report abnormal laboratory values to physician

Hemorrhage

See nursing diagnosis of potential for complications: hemorrhage, under Renal Failure (p. 561)

Maintain tight connection sites; tape shunt connection

Monitor blood line for leakage

Keep smooth clamps and tourniquet at bedside in case of line disconnection

Keep shunt securely wrapped with gauze, exposing only a portion of loop to evaluate patency

Never cut off dressings at access site

If disconnection occurs, clamp tubing and apply tourniquet proximal to site; notify physician immediately

Transfuse patient with blood products as ordered

Severe hypotension

Monitor BP q15 min during first hour of dialysis, then q30 min and prn

Report decreased BP to physician

If severe hypotension occurs
  Place patient supine or in Trendelenburg position
  Infuse normal saline to restore blood volume
  Administer plasma or albumin as ordered
  Monitor for angina due to decreased cardiac output

Assess patient for and report signs of unusual bleeding (petechiae, prolonged bleeding with venipuncture, bleeding gums, increased abdominal girth, significant drop in BP)

Guiac all GI tract fluids; report positive results

Monitor coagulation times (PT, PTT, platelets) and Hgb and Hct

Use smallest-gauge needle possible for all venipunctures and injections

Apply pressure to site after injections and venous and arterial punctures until bleeding stops

Caution patient to avoid activities that increase potential for trauma and bleeding

Air embolism

Monitor for and report signs and symptoms of air embolism (cyanosis; hypotension; weak, rapid pulse)

Monitor blood flow rate continuously for air

Always clamp IV bag before bag empties

Maintain tight connections

If air embolism occurs
  Notify physician immediately
  Turn patient onto left side; lower head of bed to Trendelenburg position (this keeps air on right side of heart, allowing pulmonary artery to absorb bubbles)

ndx: Knowledge deficit regarding hemodialysis procedure, home care follow-up instructions, and care of access site

GOAL: *Patient and/or significant other will verbalize understanding of hemodialysis procedure, symptoms to report to physician, and home care and follow-up instructions; and will return-demonstrate care of access site*

See nursing diagnosis of knowledge deficit under Renal Failure (p. 562) and under Peritoneal Dialysis (p. 567)

Teach about disease process and progression of renal failure

Teach need and procedure for hemodialysis
Instruct patient to measure and record urine output
Instruct patient to avoid wearing tight clothes or jewelry on access site extremity
Instruct patient to never have BP taken or blood drawn in extremity of access site
Teach and instruct patient to palpate for thrills over access site qd
Teach and instruct patient on symptoms to report to physician
  Decreased urine output
  Rapid weight gain
  Clotting of access site
    Absence of thrills
    Cool site
    Dark or separated blood
    Pain, numbness, tingling, and/or swelling of extremity distal to access site
  Elevated temperature
  Catheter insertion site
    Redness
    Pain
    Swelling
    Drainage
  Symptoms of progression of renal failure (see Renal Failure, p. 557)
Instruct patient to protect site from injury
Instruct patient to keep sterile dressing over site
Teach name of medication, dosage, purpose, schedule, and side effects
Instruct patient to have blood drawn for laboratory analysis as ordered by physician
Teach importance of ongoing outpatient care

Evaluation

Patient verbalizes a decrease in pain and has a relaxed facial expression and body position
Patient shows no signs or symptoms of infection
Patient shows no signs or symptoms of fluid excess or fluid deficit
Patient shows progression through the grieving process, expresses feelings of grief to others, utilizes adaptive coping mechanisms and support system, and is compliant with treatment plan
Patient shows no signs or symptoms of complications of hemodialysis
Patient and/or significant other verbalizes understanding of hemodialysis procedure, symptoms to report to physician, and home care and follow-up instructions; and return-demonstrates care of access site

NEPHRECTOMY

Surgical removal of a kidney, via a flank, transabdominal, or thoracoabdominal incision; indicated in the treatment of renal malignancy, chronic pyelonephritis, trauma, polycystic kidney disease, renal vascular disease, congenital deformity, or renal calculi, or for the purpose of donation

Assessment

Observations/findings

Urine output
  Character
  Amount
  Color
    Hematuria
    Pyuria
    Oliguria
    Sediment
Status of other kidney
  Present
    Ability to urinate
Tension-free catheters
Patent drainage system, below level of kidney
  Urethral catheter
  Ureteral catheter
  Nephrostomy tube
  Drains
Hemorrhage
Shock
Site of incision
  Redness
  Pain
  Swelling
  Drainage
Elevated temperature
Grieving

Laboratory/diagnostic studies

BUN
Serum creatinine
Serum electrolytes
CBC
Coagulation studies
Blood typing and cross matching
Tissue compatability testing
  Human leukocyte antigen (HLA)
  Mixed lymphocyte culture (MLC)
Urinalysis
Urine culture and sensitivity

KUB
Urine creatinine clearance (24-hr)
IVP
Renal perfusion scan
Renal ultrasound
Renal arteriography
Chest x-ray examination

Potential complications

Pneumonia
Pneumothorax
   Tachypnea
   Absent breath sounds
   Adventitious breath sounds
Atelectasis
Hemorrhage/shock
Paralytic ileus
Infection

Medical management

T, P, and R per postoperative routine
NPO until bowel sounds are audible
Nasogastric tube to low, intermittent suction
Chest x-ray examination
Incentive spirometry
Parenteral fluids until liquids and/or diet is tolerated
Monitoring of fluid and electrolyte balance
Intake and output
Wound management
Urethral and ureteral catheters
Nephrostomy tube
Antibiotics
Analgesics
Stool softeners, laxatives

Nursing diagnoses/goals/interventions

ndx: Potential alteration in tissue perfusion related to hemorrhage, hypovolemia, and/or shock

GOAL: *Patient will maintain circulation and perfusion to vital organs, as evidenced by normotensive BP, heart rate of 60 to 100, unlabored respirations, usual mental status, and urine output greater than 30 ml/hr*

See nursing diagnosis of potential for complications: hemorrhage, under Renal Failure (p. 561) and Polycystic Kidney Disease (p. 550)
Assess surgical dressing, tubes, and catheters for bleeding qh and report to physician
Instruct patient to take caution not to dislodge tubes or catheters when turning and repositioning

ndx: Potential for ineffective breathing pattern related to depressant effects of anesthetics and pain medications, or to reluctance of patient to breathe deeply due to incisional pain

GOAL: *Patient will maintain an effective breathing pattern as evidenced by unlabored respirations, full chest expansion, absence of diminished or adventitious breath sounds, ability to clear secretions, and normal arterial blood gas values (ABGs)*

Avoid positioning patient on unoperative side for 48 hr
Assist patient with turning, coughing, and deep breathing q2h and prn
Assist patient with incentive spirometer to maximize lung expansion as ordered
Assess BP, heart rate, and heart rhythm q2h
Assess breath sounds q4h
Report diminished or absent breath sounds to physician
Assess skin for signs of cyanosis and diaphoresis
Monitor for and report symptoms of impaired gas exchange (confusion, restlessness, irritability, decreased PO_2, increased PCO_2)
Administer pain medication at proper intervals to manage pain and to help patient perform coughing and deep-breathing exercises more effectively
Administer O_2 as ordered
If pneumothorax or atelectasis is suspected, obtain a STAT chest x-ray film as ordered
Assist in insertion of chest tubes if necessary
Maintain patency and integrity of chest tubes if present

ndx: Alteration in comfort: pain related to surgical incision

GOAL: *Patient will verbalize a decrease in pain and will show a relaxed facial expression and body position*

Assess nature, intensity, location, duration, and precipitating and alleviating factors of pain
Assess nonverbal signs of pain
Check catheters and/or drainage tubes for obstruction
Assess incisional site for redness, tenderness, swelling, and drainage
Provide nonpharmacologic comfort measures
   Assist patient with assuming a comfortable position
   Teach relaxation techniques
   Teach and assist with guided imagery techniques

Provide diversional activity
Provide a restful environment
Administer pain medication as ordered
Observe for desired effects and side effects of medications
Instruct patient to splint incision when turning, coughing, and deep breathing
Consult with physician if measures fail to provide adequate pain relief or if dosage or interval change for pain medication is needed

ndx: Alteration in urinary elimination: temporary urinary diversion or urinary retention related to nephrostomy tube, ureteral catheter, and surgical intervention

GOAL: *Patency of catheters will be maintained, patient will show no signs of urinary retention, and intake and output will be balanced*

Assess patient's "normal" voiding pattern
Monitor for and document complaints of dysuria, frequency of urination, urgency of urination, and hematuria
Measure urine output qh or with each voiding
Measure and record output from all catheters, drains, and tubes separately, if present
Monitor for and report signs of urinary retention
  Assess bladder for distention q4h
  Insert Foley catheter if ordered
  Maintain patency of all catheters; avoid kinks or loops in catheters or tubing
  Instruct patient to avoid Fowler's position and to move about carefully in order to avoid dislodging catheters
  Ensure that all catheters, tubes, and drains are patent and draining tension-free q2h
  Ensure that all collecting systems are below level of patient's bladder
  Care of tubes and catheters
    Tape securely
    Label type and "right" or "left" to avoid errors
    Secure connection sites
    Use sterile technique when disconnecting or reconnecting
  Maintain nephrostomy tube
    Tape to patient's thigh
    Never clamp
    Irrigate only with a direct physician's order; be aware that irrigating may cause bleeding, infection, or mechanical damage to kidney
    Irrigate q1h to 2h very gently with 5 to 10 ml of sterile normal saline and sterile syringe
    Have a similar tube available at bedside
    Notify physician immediately if nephrostomy tube becomes dislodged
  Maintain ureteral catheter
    Tape to urethral catheter or patient's thigh
    Never clamp
    Irrigate only with a direct physician's order
    Irrigate gently with no more than 5 ml of sterile normal saline, using a sterile syringe as ordered
  Note character of urine; report abnormalities
  Force fluids up to 3000 ml/day unless contraindicated
  Administer drugs to acidify or alkalinize urine as ordered
  Maintain nephrostomy and ureteral drainage system below level of patient's kidney

ndx: Potential for complications related to thrombophlebitis, pulmonary embolism, paralytic ileus, and wound infection*

GOAL: *Patient will show no signs or symptoms of postoperative complications*

Thrombophlebitis

Monitor for and report signs of venous thrombosis (pain, tenderness, warmth or redness in extremity; positive Homans' sign)
Apply antiembolic stockings as ordered
Assist and teach patient to perform passive ROM exercises to extremities q2h to 4h; avoid straight leg exercises
Avoid placing patient in a sitting position for prolonged periods of time
Avoid pressure or putting pillows under knees
Instruct patient not to cross legs
Administer anticoagulants as ordered

Pulmonary embolism

Monitor for and report signs and symptoms of pulmonary embolism (sudden chest or shoulder pain, cough, hemoptysis, dyspnea, tachycardia, hypertension, cyanosis, restlessness, decreased PO_2)
If symptoms of pulmonary embolism occur
  Place patient in semi- or high-Fowler's position
  Administer O_2 as ordered
  Monitor vital signs qh
  Maintain strict bed rest
  Administer anticoagulants as ordered
  Prepare patient for diagnostic tests (lung scan, venography, pulmonary angiography)

---

*Not a NANDA-approved nursing diagnosis.

Paralytic ileus

Monitor for and report signs of paralytic ileus (absent or diminished bowel sounds; persistent or worsening abdominal pain and cramping; distended, firm abdomen; failure to pass flatus)

Maintain NPO until active bowel sounds are audible or passage of flatus is noted

Auscultate for bowel sounds q4h

Insert and/or maintain nasogastric tube as ordered

Encourage early ambulation

Instruct patient to avoid smoking and/or chewing gum in order to reduce air swallowing

Administer stool softeners, laxatives, or enemas as ordered

Wound infection

Monitor for and report signs and symptoms of wound infection (fever, chills, redness, swelling, tenderness, purulent and/or malodorous wound drainage)

Check surgical incision q4h for redness, swelling, tenderness, and purulent drainage

Assess temperature q4h

Monitor WBC as ordered

Obtain wound culture as ordered

Use good handwashing technique and teach and encourage patient to do the same

Instruct patient to avoid touching incision, dressings, and drainage

Maintain sterile technique when changing dressings and performing wound care

Administer antibiotics as ordered

ndx: Grieving related to loss of major body organ; fear that recipient may reject kidney

GOAL: *Patient will show signs of progression through the grieving process, will express feelings to care giver or significant other, will participate in care, and will identify and utilize adaptive coping mechanisms and support system*

See nursing diagnosis of grieving under Renal Failure (p. 561)

Assess patient's perception of impact of loss of a kidney

Explain that remaining kidney will take over

If kidney is being used for transplantation

    Explore concerns with donor and donor's family that kidney may be rejected

    Provide emotional support to donor and donor's family

    Prepare donor and donor's family with possibility that donated kidney may be rejected and explain that this does not mean that donated kidney was inadequate

    Refer donor and donor's family for counseling if necessary

ndx: Knowledge deficit regarding postoperative routine, symptoms to report to physician, and home care and follow-up instructions

GOAL: *Patient and/or significant other will verbalize understanding of postoperative routine, symptoms to report to physician, and home care and follow-up instructions; and will return-demonstrate care of incision and nephrostomy/ureteral catheter*

Instruct patient to take measures to prevent UTI (see Urinary Tract Infection [UTI], p. 522)

Instruct patient to force fluids up to 3000 ml/day unless contraindicated

Instruct patient to maintain acid-ash diet

Instruct patient to avoid activities that may endanger remaining kidney

Instruct patient to exercise to tolerance, to plan frequent rest periods, and to avoid heavy lifting for at least 1 year

Teach care of incision

Teach patient to change surgical dressing

Teach care of nephrostomy tube or ureteral catheter if present

Teach symptoms and instruct patient to report UTI

    Elevated temperature

    Incisional and nephrostomy/ureteral catheter site redness, swelling, pain, or drainage

Teach medication name, dosage, schedule, purpose, and side effects

Instruct patient to avoid taking over-the-counter medications without checking with physician

Teach importance of ongoing outpatient care

Instruct patient to inform health care providers of presence of nephrostomy or ureteral catheter and history of nephrectomy

Evaluation

Patient maintains adequate circulation and perfusion to vital organs

Patient maintains an effective breathing pattern

Patient verbalizes a decrease in pain and has a relaxed facial expression and body position

Catheters and tubes remain patent, and patient shows no signs or symptoms of urinary retention

Intake and output are balanced

Patient shows progression through the stages of grieving

Patient expresses feelings of grief to others, participates in care, and identifies and utilizes adaptive coping mechanisms and support system

Patient and/or significant other verbalizes understanding of postoperative routine, symptoms to report to physician, and home care and follow-up instructions; and return-demonstrates care of incision, nephrostomy, and ureteral catheter

RENAL TRANSPLANT: CARE OF RECIPIENT*

A functioning kidney is removed from a living donor or a human cadaver and is transplanted into the right or left iliac fossa of the recipient; the renal blood vessels of the donor organ are anastomosed to the recipient's iliac artery and vein, and the ureter is transplanted into the bladder or anastomosed to the recipient's ureter, to establish urinary tract continuity

Assessment
Observations/findings

See Renal Failure (p. 557)
Rejection of kidney (Table 9-1)
    Transplant site: redness, swelling, tenderness
    Elevated temperature
    Elevated WBC
    Decreased urinary output
    Hematuria
    Increased proteinuria
    Sudden weight gain of over 2 lb (0.9 kg) in 24 hr
    Acute onset of hypertension

---

*See Nephrectomy (p. 571) for care of donor.

    Restlessness
    Irritability
    Lethargy
    Increased serum BUN
    Increased serum creatinine
Atelectasis: diminished or absent breath sounds
Tachycardia
Tachypnea
Pulmonary edema
Cardiac arrythmias
Thrombophlebitis
Pulmonary embolism
Hemorrhage
Infection (UTI, local, systemic)
    Incision
        Redness
        Pain
        Swelling
        Drainage
        Dehiscence
Character and amount of urine output
    Oliguria to anuria
    Large quantities of dilute urine
Location and patency of arteriovenous (AV) shunt
    Bruits
    Thrills
Cataracts
Psychosocial problems
    Grieving
    Disturbance in self-concept
    Anxiety
    Depression
Sensory deprivation
Sensory overload

TABLE 9-1. Classification of Rejection

Hyperacute	Acute	Chronic
Rejection occurs as soon as new kidney is implanted	Rejection occurs 1 week to 3 months after kidney has been implanted	Rejection occurs at any time after surgery
Rejection is caused by presence of antibodies in recipient that cause polymorphonuclear leukocytes to clot, thus blocking glomerular and peritubular capillaries	Immune response leukocytes and red blood cells invade vascular endothelium and intertubular vasculature; renal blood flow is decreased; therefore necrosis of renal tubules occurs	There is gradual decline in kidney function; glomerular filtration is decreased, and serum creatinine and serum urea nitrogen are elevated; proteinuria occurs, and sodium is decreased in urine
Rejection is usually irreversible	Rejection may be reversible	Early detection and treatment may decrease decline in kidney function
Transplanted kidney is removed immediately	Attempt is made to save new kidney	Attempt is made to save kidney
Patient resumes hemodialysis	Patient may need to resume dialysis treatments	Patient may need to resume dialysis treatments

Laboratory/diagnostic studies

See Renal Failure, p. 557
Blood typing and cross matching
Tissue compatibility testing
CXR
ECG

Potential complications

Rejection
Renal artery stenosis, thrombosis, aneurysm
Shock
Paralytic ileus
Side effects of immunosuppressive drugs
Diabetes
Cushing's syndrome
GI bleeding
Glaucoma

Medical management

BP, T, P, and R per postoperative routine
Intake and output
Monitoring of BUN, creatinine, and electrolytes
Parenteral fluids with electrolytes
NPO until bowel sounds are audible
Chest x-ray examination
Incentive spirometry
Reverse isolation
Hemodialysis
Immunosuppressive medications
Analgesics
Stool softeners, laxatives

Nursing diagnoses/goals/interventions

ndx: Alteration in comfort: pain related to surgical incision

GOAL: *Patient will verbalize a decrease in pain and will show a relaxed facial expression and body position*

See nursing diagnosis of alteration in comfort: pain, under Surgery for Female Urinary Incontinence (p. 529) and Artificial Urinary Sphincter (p. 533)

ndx: Potential for alteration in fluid volume: fluid excess or fluid deficit related to kidney's inability to regulate fluid balance and inadequate fluid replacement

GOAL: *Patient will not exhibit signs or symptoms of fluid excess or fluid deficit as evidenced by balanced intake and output, stable weight, usual mental status, and normal serum electrolytes*

Maintain patency of drainage catheters
Monitor for and report excessive drainage at surgical site
Monitor urine output and report no urine output after 24 h or large quantities of dilute urine
Monitor and document intake and output accurately qh
Weigh patient daily at the same time with same clothing and scale
Monitor for elevated BP
Monitor serum electrolytes; report abnormal laboratory values or signs and symptoms of electrolyte imbalance
Assess level of consciousness; note changes in mental status
Assess skin turgor
Assess oral mucous membrane for moisture
Assess heart sounds for presence of S_3 and/or S_4
Assess breath sounds for rales
Obtain chest x-ray film as ordered
Assess for peripheral edema
Assess for distended neck veins
Restrict fluids as ordered
Administer diuretics as ordered
Provide ice chips to control thirst

ndx: Potential for infection related to immunosuppression

GOAL: *Patient will show no signs of infection (UTI, local, or systemic)*

Administer immunosuppressive medications as ordered
Monitor for bone marrow suppression (leukopenia, anemia, thrombocytopenia)
Maintain reverse isolation as ordered
Remove all invasive lines and catheters as soon as possible
Assess temperature q4h and report if greater than 101° F (38.5° C)
Note character of urine; report if cloudy and malodorous
Avoid instrumentation/catheterization of urinary tract
If urethral catheter is present, maintain closed gravity drainage system
Monitor for and report signs and symptoms of UTI, and take measures to prevent UTI (see Urinary Tract Infection [UTI], p. 522)
Encourage high oral fluid intake, up to 3000 ml/day, to flush out bacteria unless contraindicated
Auscultate chest for breath sounds q4h; report adventitious breath sounds to physician
Encourage coughing and deep breathing
Use good handwashing technique; teach and encourage patient to do the same

Instruct patient to avoid persons with infections
Instruct patient to avoid chilling
Take measures to prevent skin breakdown
Encourage early ambulation
Administer antibiotics as ordered
Obtain specimens for culture and sensitivity as ordered

ndx: Potential for diversional activity deficit related to reverse isolation

GOAL: *Patient will verbalize decreased feelings of isolation and boredom, and will identify and participate in diversional activities*

Monitor for signs of diversional activity deficit (boredom, apathy, frequent napping during the day, etc.)
Explain rationale for reverse isolation
Familiarize patient with environment
Suggest and provide appropriate diversional activities (puzzles, books, model kits, handicrafts, cards, etc.)
Encourage patient to become involved in self-care activities to provide a sense of accomplishment (i.e., leg exercises, coughing and deep breathing, measuring and recording intake and output)
Encourage patient to verbalize feelings
Spend extra time with patient
Allow patient some control over scheduling of activities, treatments, and visitation
Encourage significant others to stagger visits throughout the day
Suggest that significant other bring radio, tape player, or other favorite items from home
Request consultation from psychiatry or pastoral care if necessary

ndx: Potential for complications: rejection, renal artery occlusion (stenosis, thrombosis, aneurysm), atelectasis, paralytic ileus, and/or side effects of immunosuppressive medications*

GOAL: *Patient will show no signs or symptoms of complications related to renal transplant*

Rejection

Monitor for and immediately report signs and symptoms of rejection (redness, swelling, and tenderness over transplant site; elevated temperature; elevated WBC; decreased urine output; increased proteinuria; sudden weight gain; simultaneously increased BUN and serum creatinine; acute onset of hypertension; symptoms of sodium retention; edema)

---
*Not a NANDA-approved nursing diagnosis.

Measure and document intake and output qh
Measure BP qh
Measure temperature q2h and report if greater than 101° F (38.5° C)
Monitor results of serum blood tests (BUN, creatinine, WBC) and report abnormal laboratory values to physician
Administer immunosuppressive medications as ordered
Dialyze patient as ordered
Prepare patient for surgery to remove rejected kidney if hyperacute reaction occurs
Support patient and family

Renal artery occlusion

Assess patency of catheters qh; note and report presence of blood clots
Measure urine output qh
Note character of urine (color, consistency, pH, and specific gravity)
Notify physician immediately if patient becomes anuric
Irrigate catheters with normal saline only with direct physician's order

Atelectasis

See nursing diagnosis of potential for complications: atelectasis, under Surgery for Female Urinary Incontinence (p. 530) and Urinary Diversion (p. 546)

Paralytic ileus

See nursing diagnosis of potential for complications: paralytic ileus, under Surgery for Female Urinary Incontinence (p. 530) and Urinary Diversion (p. 546)

Side effects of immunosuppressive medications

Monitor for and report signs and symptoms of infection
Monitor for and report symptoms of bone marrow suppression, leukopenia, anemia, and thrombocytopenia azathioprine [Imuran], cyclophosphamide [Cytoxan]
Monitor for and report nausea and vomiting (azathioprine, cyclophosphamide); if nausea and vomiting occur, administer antiemetics as ordered
Monitor for and report symptoms of hepatotoxicity (azathioprine, cyclosporine); monitor bilirubin and CBC; report abnormal laboratory values
Monitor for and report symptoms of nephrotoxicity, gingival hyperplasia, tremors, and hirsutism (cyclosporine)
Monitor for and report signs of adrenal insufficiency, depressive and/or psychotic episodes, and GI bleeding (steroids)

ndx: Potential for ineffective coping related to prolonged hospitalization, stages of transplant organ acceptance, and possibility of rejection

GOAL: *Patient will show signs of progression through the stages of transplant organ acceptance and will identify and utilize adaptive coping mechanisms and support system*

Assess patient's present coping mechanisms and what has worked in patient's past
Support adaptive coping mechanisms
Set limits on maladaptive coping mechanisms if they interfere with patient's health and well-being
Monitor for progression through stages of acceptance of transplant organ
   Foreign body stage: kidney feels strange; patient feels that kidney is sticking out of body
   Partial internalization stage: patient moves about cautiously; overemphasizes kidney's fragility
   Complete internalization: patient accepts kidney and focuses on it only during direct conversation related to kidney
Recognize that patient may regress to previous stage(s)
Encourage patient to express feelings
Encourage family support and involvement
Consult with clergy, social service, and psychiatry if necessary

ndx: Knowledge deficit regarding postoperative routine, symptoms to report to physician, home care, and follow-up instructions

GOAL: *Patient and/or significant other will verbalize understanding of postoperative routine, symptoms to report to physician, and home care and follow-up instructions; and will return-demonstrate handwashing technique, care of incision, taking and recording of temperature, weight, and BP, and measuring and recording of intake and output*

Instruct patient to prevent infections
   Instruct patient to limit visitors and to avoid large groups of people
   Instruct patient to avoid persons with infections
   Teach methods to prevent UTI (see Urinary Tract Infection [UTI], p. 522)
   Teach and instruct patient to use good handwashing technique
   Teach wound care and dressing change
   Instruct patient to take temperature at same time twice a day
Teach and instruct patient to report to physician
   Hematuria
   Temperature over 101° F (38.5° C)
   Increased pulse rate
   Weight gain of over 2 lb (0.9 kg) in 1 day or 4 lb (1.8 kg) in 1 week
   Lethargy
   Decreased urine output: <600 ml in 24 hr
   Tenderness over new kidney
   Respiratory distress
   Restlessness or irritability
   Sudden change in BP
   Edema
   Symptoms of rejection
Instruct patient to weigh self daily at same time with same clothing and scale
Instruct patient to take BP daily at same time in same position and in same arm, and to rest 5 min before taking it
Instruct patient to maintain dietary and fluid restrictions
Instruct patient to avoid overeating (appetite may increase because of medications)
Teach and instruct patient to measure and record intake and output
Instruct patient to exercise to tolerance, to avoid strenuous exercise, to plan frequent rest periods, and to avoid heavy lifting and excessive bending
Instruct patient to wait 2 weeks before driving a car and to avoid use of seat belts that may press on new kidney
Instruct patient to avoid drinking alcoholic beverages until allowed to do so by physician
Instruct patient to avoid sexual activity for 6 weeks or as indicated by physician
Teach importance of avoiding pregnancy until indicated by physician
Explain that symptoms of original disease may develop in new kidney
Explain that there is an increased risk of developing a malignancy—especially lymphomas, skin, and lip cancers
Teach name of medication, dosage, schedule, purpose, and side effects
Instruct patient to never stop taking immunosuppressive drugs without a physician's order
Instruct patient to avoid taking over-the-counter medications without checking with physician
Teach importance of ongoing outpatient care
   Instruct patient to have blood drawn for laboratory tests at regular intervals as ordered by physician
   Instruct patient to have eye examinations q6 months for glaucoma and cataracts

Instruct patient to notify physician before going to dentist

Instruct patient to wear a medical alert bracelet

Evaluation

Patient verbalizes a decrease in pain and shows a relaxed facial expression and body position

Patient shows no signs or symptoms of fluid excess or fluid deficit

Patient shows no signs or symptoms of infection

Patient verbalizes decreasing feelings of isolation and boredom, and participates in diversional activities

Patient shows no signs or symptoms of complications related to renal transplant

Patient shows signs of progression through the stages of acceptance of a transplant organ, and identifies and utilizes adaptive coping mechanisms and support system

Patient and/or significant other verbalizes an understanding of postoperative routine, symptoms to report to physician, and home care and follow-up instructions; and return-demonstrates handwashing technique, care of incision, taking and recording of BP, T, and weight, and measuring and recording of intake and output

PROSTATIC HYPERTROPHY

Enlargement of glandular and cellular tissue of the prostate gland related to endocrine changes associated with aging; the prostate gland surrounds the neck of the bladder and urethra; therefore, prostatic hypertrophy frequently prevents the bladder from emptying

Assessment

Observations/findings

Hesitancy in starting flow of urine
Stream of urine reduced
  Force
  Size
Incomplete emptying of bladder: residual urine
Urgency of urination
Frequency of urination
Nocturia: three times or more
Dysuria
Hematuria
Sciatica
  Low back pain
  Hip pain
  Leg pain
Bladder neck obstruction: acute retention of urine
UTI: cystitis
Enlargement and tenderness of prostate

Laboratory/diagnostic studies

Urinalysis
Urine culture and sensitivity
Serum creatinine
Serum BUN
Cystoscopy
Excretory urography
Retrograde studies

Potential complications

Pyelonephritis
Hydronephrosis
Azotemia
Uremia

Medical management

Fluid intake up to 3000 ml/day unless contraindicated
Antibiotics
Intake and output
See Acute Urinary Retention (p. 534)
Surgery
  Transurethral resesction of prostate
  Suprapubic prostatectomy
  Retropubic prostatectomy
  Radical retropubic prostatectomy
  Cystostomy drainage of bladder

Nursing diagnoses/goals/interventions

ndx: Alteration in urinary elimination: urinary retention related to enlarged prostate

GOAL: *Patient will empty bladder completely*

See nursing diagnosis of alteration in pattern of urinary elimination under Acute Urinary Retention (p. 535)

Encourage patient to void q2h to 4h and to obey impulse to void

Take caution when administering medications that may cause urinary retention

Restrict dietary alcohol, coffee, tea, and cola

Catheterize patient after each voiding as ordered to determine amount of residual urine; report if greater than 100 ml

Use voiding measures

Monitor serum BUN and creatinine

ndx: Potential for infection related to presence of indwelling catheter and/or urinary retention

GOAL: *Patient will show no signs or symptoms of UTI, or local or systemic infection*

Check temperature q4h and report if above 101° F (38.5° C)
Note character or urine; report if cloudy and malodorous
Avoid instrumentation/catheterization of urinary tract
If urethral catheter is present, maintain closed gravity drainage system
Monitor for and report signs and symptoms of UTI; take measures to prevent UTI (see Urinary Tract Infection [UTI], p. 522)
Auscultate chest for breath sounds q4h; report adventitious breath sounds to physician
Encourage coughing and deep breathing
Use good handwashing technique; teach and encourage patient to do the same
Instruct patient to avoid persons with infections
Instruct patient to avoid chilling
Take measures to prevent skin breakdown
Encourage early ambulation

ndx: Alteration in comfort: pain related to acute urinary retention

GOAL: *Patient will verbalize a decrease in pain and will show a relaxed facial expression and body position*

Assess nature, intensity, location, duration, and precipitating and alleviating factors of pain
Provide bed rest; increase activities as ordered and/or tolerated
Provide nonpharmacologic comfort measures: assist patient to comfortable position, provide sitz baths and warm perineal soaks, teach relaxation techniques and guided imagery, and/or provide diversional activity
Encourage high oral fluid intake
Administer other pain medication as ordered
Assess vital signs prior to and after administering pain medications
Monitor and document pain relief and any undesirable side effects
Notify physician of unrelieved or increasing pain

ndx: Knowledge deficit regarding disease process, symptoms to report to physician, and home care and follow-up instructions

GOAL: *Patient and/or significant other will verbalize understanding of disease process, symptoms to report to physician, and home care and follow-up instructions; and will return-demonstrate measuring urine output*

Instruct patient to force fluids up to 3000 ml unless contraindicated
Teach and instruct patient to measure urine output after each voiding
Instruct patient to not allow bladder to become too full
Instruct patient to urinate q2h to 4h and to obey impulse to void as quickly as possible
Teach and instruct patient symptoms to report to physician
  Inability to void
  UTI
  Urinary retention
Instruct patient to remain as active and mobile as possible
Instruct patient to sit in hard chair whenever possible
Instruct patient to avoid cold temperatures
Instruct patient to avoid long automobile, bus, or train rides unless voiding is possible at any time
Teach medication name, dosage, schedule, purpose, and side effects
Instruct patient to avoid taking over-the-counter medications without checking with physician
Teach importance of ongoing outpatient care

Evaluation

Patient empties bladder completely
Patient shows no signs or symptoms of UTI or of local or systemic infection
Patient verbalizes a decrease in pain and has a relaxed facial expression and body position
Patient and/or significant other verbalizes understanding of disease process, symptoms to report to physician, and home care and follow-up instructions; and return-demonstrates measuring urine output

PROSTATECTOMY

Removal of part or all of the prostate gland
transurethral resection of prostate (TURP) *Removal of part or all of the prostate gland via a cystoscope or resectoscope inserted through the urethra*
suprapubic prostatectomy *Removal of the prostate gland through an incision made in the bladder. (Figure 9-11)*
retropubic prostatectomy *Removal of the prostate gland via an incision in the lower abdomen through the anterior prostatic fossa (Figure 9-12)*

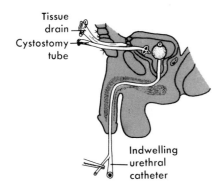

FIGURE 9-11. Suprapubic prostatectomy.

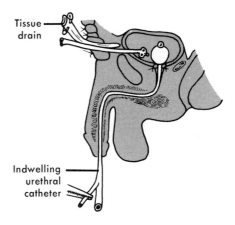

FIGURE 9-13. Radical retropubic prostatectomy.

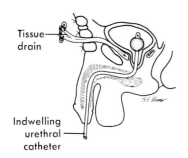

FIGURE 9-12. Retropubic prostatectomy.

radical retropubic prostatectomy *Removal of the prostate gland, including the capsule, seminal vesicles, and adjacent tissue through an incision in the lower abdomen; the urethra is anastomosed to the bladder neck (Figure 9-13)*

Assessment

Observations/findings

Urinary output
    Character
    Amount
Hemorrhage: bright red drainage and clots from catheter
Shock
Bladder spasms
Distended bladder
    Suprapubic pain
    Elevated BP
    Tachycardia
    Diaphoresis
    Restlessness
Absorption of irrigating solution during operation
    Elevated BP
    Headache
    Disorientation
    Pulmonary edema
    Hyponatremia
    Muscular weakness
    Apprehension
Extravasation of urine into abdominal cavity
    Tense, rigid abdomen
    Elevated temperature
    Renal failure
Patent, tension-free catheters
    Kinking
        Mucous plugs
        Blood clots
    Closed gravity drainage system
    Continuous bladder irrigation
    Leakage of urine around suprapubic catheter
Removal of indwelling catheter
    Incontinence
    Dysuria
    Hematuria
    Urethral stricture
        Dribbling
        Frequency of urination
        Difficulty in initiating urinary stream
        Small urinary stream
    Urinary retention with overflow
    Urinary fistula
    Inability to urinate
    Incisional redness, swelling, pain, drainage

Laboratory/diagnostic studies

See Prostatic Hypertrophy (p. 579)
Hgb, Hct
Serum electrolytes

Potential complications

Dilutional hyponatremia
Infection
Circulatory complication involving testicle
Hydrocele
Shock
Acute urinary retention
Paralytic ileus
Pelvic abscess
- Elevated temperature
- Pain on walking

Medical management

BP, T, P, and R per postoperative routine
Analgesics
Antispasmodics
Continuous bladder irrigation
Intermittent bladder irrigation
Parenteral IV therapy
Intake and output
NPO until bowel sounds are audible

Nursing diagnoses/goals/interventions

ndx: Alteration in comfort: pain related to surgical incision, bladder spasms, and urinary retention

GOAL: *Patient will verbalize a decrease in pain and will show a relaxed facial expression and body position*

See nursing diagnosis of alteration in comfort: pain under Urinary Tract Infection (UTI) (p. 523), Renal Calculi/Urolithiasis (p. 555) and Surgery for Female Urinary Incontinence (p. 529).
Administer antispasmodics as ordered
Administer anticholinergics as ordered
Observe and document desired and side effects of medications
Intermittently irrigate urethral/suprapubic catheters as ordered; use sterile normal saline and sterile syringe
   Instill solution gently; never force
   Aspirate gently
   Continue irrigation until urine is clear

ndx: Alteration in pattern of urinary elimination: hematuria, acute urinary retention, urinary diversion

GOAL: *Patient will show no signs or symptoms of urinary retention; urine will flow freely through catheters; intake and output will be balanced; and patient will void normally after catheter removal*

See nursing diagnosis of alteration in pattern of urinary elimination under Acute Urinary Tract Infection (UTI) (p. 523), Acute Urinary Retention (p. 535), Care of Patient with Indwelling Urethral Catheter (p. 540), and Renal Calculi/Urolithiasis (p. 555)
Maintain patent urethral and/or suprapubic catheters
Apply external traction to urethral catheter as ordered
Avoid inadvertent removal of catheters
Observe character and flow of urine through catheters q2h
Monitor for and report gross hematuria to physician
Notify physician should complete occlusion of catheter occur
Irrigate catheters as ordered
Maintain continuous bladder irrigation (CBI) as ordered
   Use sterile normal saline as ordered for irrigation
   Maintain sterile technique
   Maintain sterile irrigating equipment
   Instill irrigating solution through smallest lumen of catheter
   Regulate flow of solution at 40 to 60 drops/min or to maintain clear urine
Measure urinary output q1h
Measure and record intake and output q shift
   Measure urine output
   Record amount of irrigating solution instilled
   Subtract this amount from total urinary output
   If a significant difference in totals occurs, notify physician
Monitor for and report signs of urinary retention to physician
After catheter removal
   Measure urine after each voiding
   Use voiding measures
   Perform intermittent catheterization to check for residual urine as ordered; report if greater than 100 ml

ndx: Potential for infection related to presence of catheters in bladder and presence of wound

GOAL: *Patient will show no signs of UTI, or local or systemic infection*

Check temperature q4h and report if above 101° F (38.5° C)
Note character of urine; report if cloudy and malodorous
Maintain closed gravity drainage system
Monitor for and report signs and symptoms of UTI; take measures to prevent UTI (see Urinary Tract Infection [UTI], p. 522)
Auscultate chest for breath sounds q4h; report adventitious breath sounds to physician

Encourage coughing and deep breathing
Use good handwashing technique; teach and encourage patient to do the same
Instruct patient to avoid persons with infections
Instruct patient to avoid chilling
Take measures to prevent skin breakdown
Encourage early ambulation
Remove catheters as soon as possible
Monitor for and report redness, swelling, pain, or leakage around suprapubic catheter

ndx: Potential for complications: dilutional hyponatremia, hemorrhage/shock, and/or atelectasis/pneumonia*

GOAL: *Patient will show no signs or symptoms of complications related to prostatectomy*

Dilutional hyponatremia

Monitor for and report signs and symptoms of dilutional hyponatremia (low serum sodium, change in mental status, confusion, restlessness, muscles twitching, convulsions, nausea, vomiting, SOB, elevated BP)
Administer parenteral fluids as ordered
Administer hypertonic saline as ordered
Administer diuretics as ordered
Administer sodium bicarbonate as ordered

Hemorrhage/shock

Monitor for and report signs and symptoms of hemorrhage (hypotension; tachycardia; dyspnea; cool, clammy skin; syncope; hematuria)
Monitor abdominal/suprapubic dressing q2h for bleeding
Monitor urethral and suprapubic catheters q2h for bleeding
Report excessive bleeding and/or gross hematuria to physician
Monitor Hct and Hgb as ordered
If hemorrhage occurs
  Place patient flat in bed
  Administer fluid replacement as ordered
  Transfuse with blood products as ordered
  Prepare patient for surgery if necessary

Atelectasis/pneumonia

Assist patient with turning, coughing, and deep breathing q2h and prn

---

*Not a NANDA-approved nursing diagnosis.

Assist patient with incentive spirometer to maximize lung expansion as ordered
Assess BP, heart rate, and heart rhythm q2h
Assess breath sounds q4h
Report diminished or absent breath sounds to physician
Assess skin for signs of cyanosis and diaphoresis
Monitor for and report symptoms of inpaired gas exchange (confusion, restlessness, irritability, decreased PO_2, increased PCO_2
Administer pain medication at proper intervals to manage pain and to help patient perform coughing and deep breathing exercises more effectively
Administer O_2 as ordered

ndx: Potential for disturbance in self-concept related to fear of impotence, loss of male identity, and urinary incontinence

GOAL: *Patient will verbalize feelings related to change in body image to care giver or significant other and will be able to resume ADLs*

Be aware that patients facing this type of surgery are under considerable emotional stress
Be sensitive to changes in patient's life-style
Encourage patient to express feelings
Actively listen
Explain to patient that feelings of grief are normal
Answer questions honestly
Be aware of coping mechanisms and expect that patient may exhibit irrational or inappropriate behaviors, irritability, and lack of motivation
Encourage adaptive coping behaviors
Set limits on maladaptive behaviors, especially if they are detrimental to patient's health
Explain that some urinary incontinence is normal at first
Provide reassurance that as surgical site heals, good urinary control will return
Teach and encourage patient to practice perineal exercises
Include spouse/significant other in teaching
Reassure that potency should be unaltered
Explain that a dry ejaculation will occur for the first few months
Reassure that normal ejaculation will be restored
Explain that ability of conception is gone, with exception of simple TURP
Encourage communication with significant other

ndx: Knowledge deficit regarding postoperative routine, symptoms to report to physician, and home care and follow-up instructions

GOAL: *Patient and/or significant other will verbalize understanding of postoperative routine, symptoms to report to physician, and home care and follow-up instructions, and will return-demonstrate perineal exercises and care of incision*

Instruct patient to avoid sitting for long periods of time
Teach and instruct patient to perform perineal exercises 10 to 20 times qh once urethral catheter has been removed
   Tense perineal muscles by contracting rectal sphincter
   Hold position, then relax
Instruct patient to maintain diet as ordered and to avoid coffee, tea, and cola; instruct patient to avoid alcohol for 1 month or as indicated by physician
Instruct patient to exercise to tolerance, to avoid strenuous exercise, and to plan frequent rest periods
Instruct patient to shower daily
Instruct patient to avoid sexual activity for 1 month or as indicated by physician; reinforce physician's explanation of retrograde ejaculation
Instruct patient to avoid long automobile trips
Teach and instruct patient to report symptoms to physician
   Heavy bleeding (intermittent hematuria is expected for 2 to 4 weeks)
   Difficulty in voiding
   Incisional redness, swelling, pain, drainage
   Elevated temperature
   Pain on walking
Instruct patient to avoid constipation
Teach care of incision and dressing change
Teach name of medication, dosage, schedule, purpose, and side effects
Instruct patient to avoid taking over-the-counter medications without checking with physician
Teach importance of ongoing outpatient care

Evaluation

Patient verbalizes a decrease in pain and has a relaxed facial expression and body position
Patient shows no signs or symptoms of urinary retention
Urine flows freely through catheters
Intake and output are balanced
Patient voids normally once catheter is removed
Patient shows no signs or symptoms of UTI, or local or systemic infection
Patient shows no signs or symptoms of postoperative complications related to prostatectomy
Patient verbalizes feelings about change in body image to others and resumes normal daily activities
Patient and/or significant other verbalizes understanding of postoperative routine, symptoms to report to physician, and home care and follow-up instructions; and return-demonstrates perineal exercises and care of incision

PENILE IMPLANT

Surgical implantation of a prosthesis in the penis for the treatment of impotence; two types of prostheses are used: a silicone rubber prosthesis, which leaves the penis in a constant state of semierection, and an inflatable penile prosthesis that contains two cylinders in the corpora cavernosa (penile shaft), a balloon reservoir in the extraperitoneal space beside the bladder, and a pump in a subcutaneous pouch in the lower scrotum

Assessment
Observations/findings

Scrotal edema
Scrotal discoloration
Incisional
   Pain
   Redness
   Swelling
   Drainage
Elevated temperature
Mechanical failure of prosthesis
Urinary retention
Hematuria
Incontinence
Psychosocial problems
   Anxiety
   Fear that prosthesis will fail

Laboratory/diagnostic studies

Snap guage test
Nocturnal penile tumescence test
Doppler ultrasound flow meter for penile blood flow
Penile arteriogram
Sacral evoked response
Bulbocavernous reflex/artery time
Urodynamic studies
Cystometrogram
Electromyogram
Cystoscopy
Carpocavernosogram

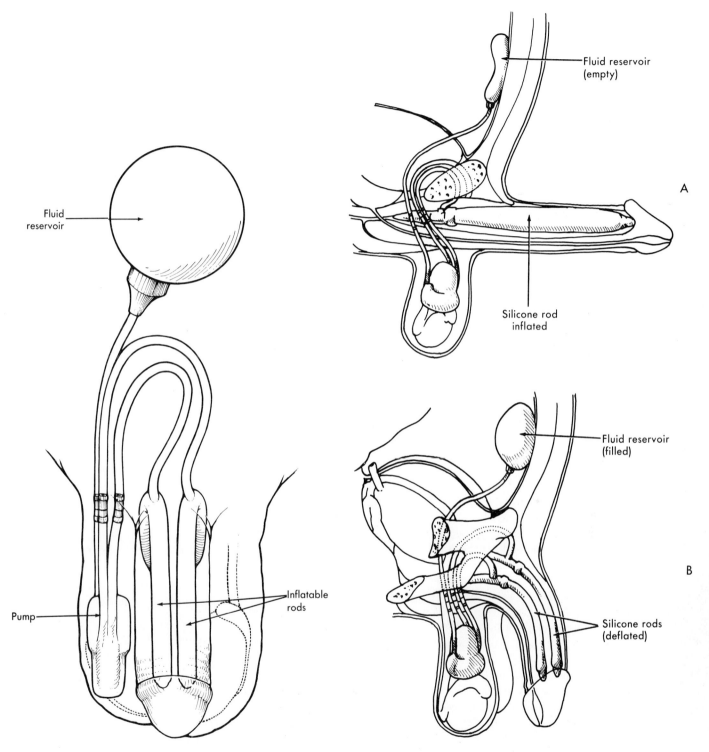

FIGURE 9-14. Implantation of penile prosthesis. Inflatable penile prosthesis, frontal view. (From Lerner, J., and Khan, Z.: Mosby's manual of urologic nursing, St. Louis, 1982, The C.V. Mosby Co.; courtesy American Medical Systems, Inc., Minneapolis, Minn.)

FIGURE 9-15. Inflatable prosthesis, sagittal view. **A,** Penis in erect position. **B,** Penis in flaccid position. (From Lerner, J., and Khan, Z.: Mosby's manual of urologic nursing, St. Louis, 1982, The C.V. Mosby Co.; courtesy American Medical Systems, Inc., Minneapolis, Minn.)

Potential complications

Rejection of prosthesis
Mechanical failure of prosthesis
Extravasation of fluid of prosthesis reservoir into surrounding tissue
Testicular necrosis

Medical management

Counseling therapy
Hormonal therapy
Revascularization
Penile prosthesis implantation
    Semirigid penile prosthesis
    Inflatable penile prosthesis
Postoperative care
    NPO until bowel sounds are audible
    Parenteral IV until liquids and/or diet is tolerated
    Monitoring of BP, T, P, and R per postoperative routine
    Analgesics
    Ice to scrotum
    Antibiotics
    Stool softeners, laxatives

Nursing diagnoses/goals/interventions

ndx Alteration in comfort: pain related to surgical incision

GOAL: *Patient will verbalize a decrease in pain and will show a relaxed facial expression and body position*

Elevate scrotum as ordered
Pack scrotum in ice as ordered
Explain to patient that some scrotal swelling and discoloration is normal and may last for 7 to 10 days
For inflatable implants, keep patient in Trendelenburg position for 24 hr to prevent scrotal edema
Assess nature, intensity, location, duration, and precipitating and alleviating factors of pain
Assess nonverbal signs of pain
Check urethral catheter for obstruction
Provide nonpharmacologic comfort measures
    Assist patient with assuming a comfortable position
    Teach relaxation techniques
    Teach and assist with guided imagery techniques
    Provide diversional activity
    Provide a restful environment
Administer pain medication as ordered
Observe for desired effects and side effects of medications
Consult with physician if measures fail to provide adequate pain relief or if dosage or interval change for pain medication is needed

ndx Potential for infection and/or rejection related to surgical incision and implantation of a foreign object

GOAL: *Patient will show no signs of UTI, or local or systemic infection and will show no signs of rejection*

Monitor for and report signs and symptoms of rejection (elevated temperature; elevated WBC; pain, redness, and swelling over implant site; urinary retention)
Check temperature q4h and report if above 101° F (38.5° C)
Note character of urine; report if cloudy and malodorous
Avoid instrumentation/catheterization of urinary tract
If urethral catheter is present, maintain closed gravity drainage system
Monitor and report signs and symptoms of UTI; take measures to prevent UTI (see Urinary Tract Infection [UTI], p. 522)
Encourage high oral fluid intake, up to 3000 ml/day, to flush out bacteria unless contraindicated
Instruct patient to drink cranberry juice, prune juice, and/or plum juice to acidify urine
Auscultate chest for breath sounds q4h; report adventitious breath sounds to physician
Encourage coughing and deep breathing
Use good handwashing technique; teach and encourage patient to do the same
Instruct patient to avoid persons with infections
Instruct patient to avoid chilling
Take measures to prevent skin breakdown
Encourage early ambulation
Administer antibiotics as ordered
Obtain specimens for culture and sensitivity as ordered

ndx Anxiety related to embarrassment, fear that implant will fail, and/or previous experiences with impotence

GOAL: *Patient will verbalize feelings of anxiety to care giver or significant other and will verbalize feeling less anxious*

Maintain a matter-of-fact attitude when discussing impotence or implant
Encourage patient to verbalize feeling of embarrassment or anxiety, and fears and concerns
Provide privacy when teaching or activating prosthesis
Include significant other in teaching
Encourage communication with significant other
Be aware that patient and/or significant other may need sexual counseling

ndx: Potential for complications: urinary retention, migration of pump into inguinal canal, mechanical failure, testicular necrosis*

GOAL: *Patient will show no signs or symptoms of complications*

Urinary retention

See nursing diagnosis of alteration in pattern of urinary elimination under Acute Urinary Retention (p. 535)
Monitor and report signs and symptoms of urinary retention

Migration of pump into inguinal canal

Beginning with the second day postoperatively, pull pump down into most dependent part of scrotum
Notify physician if unable to locate pump

Mechanical failure

Leave prosthesis deflated for 5 to 7 days postoperatively, or until scrotal discomfort is minimal
After sixth day postoperatively inflate and deflate prosthesis once per day for first week
Notify physician if unable to inflate or deflate pump
Mechanical failure of pump may require correction using local anesthetic or further surgery

Testicular necrosis

Monitor for and report penile and scrotal discoloration, hematoma, sudden absence of pain, or coolness
Instruct patient not to wear underclothing until swelling has subsided

ndx: Knowledge deficit regarding inflation of prosthesis, symptoms to report to physician, and home care and follow-up instructions

GOAL: *Patient and/or significant other will verbalize understanding of penile prosthesis, symptoms to report to physician, and home care and follow-up instructions; and will return-demonstrate inflation of penile prosthesis*

Teach patient to inflate penile prosthesis
  Use model or picture
  Instruct patient to locate pump in scrotum between thumb and forefinger
  Instruct patient to inflate prosthesis by squeezing bulb 10 to 15 times between thumb and index finger
  To deflate pump, press release valve on side of pump between thumb and forefinger
Explain to patient that prosthesis need not be deflated all the way; do not squeeze penis to completely empty cylinders
Inflation schedule
  First week: qd
  Second week: bid
    Third week: qd plus firmly inflate and leave inflated for 30 min qd
    Fourth week: qd plus firmly inflate and leave inflated for 30 min bid
Explain to patient that prosthesis will not interfere with physiologic mechanism of intercourse, orgasm, or ejaculation
Explain to patient that previous ability to have a partial erection may diminish
Explain to patient that implant erection will probably not be exactly the same as that achieved naturally before onset of impotence
Explain to patient that if sperm production is normal, he may father a child
Instruct patient to avoid intercourse for 6 weeks, or until incision heals, or as indicated by physician
Instruct patient to avoid tight, restrictive underclothing for 2 to 3 weeks postoperatively
Instruct patient that he may shower or bathe
Instruct patient to avoid strenuous activity, heavy lifting, jogging, or sports for about 3 weeks
Teach and instruct patient to report symptoms to physician
  Incisional redness, pain, swelling, drainage
  Elevated temperature
  Inability to urinate
Teach medication name, dosage, schedule, purpose, and side effects
Instruct patient to avoid taking over-the-counter medications without checking with physician
Teach importance of ongoing outpatient care

Evaluation

Patient verbalizes a decrease in pain and has a relaxed facial expression and body position
Patient shows no signs or symptoms of UTI, or local or systemic infection, and no signs or symptoms of rejection
Patient verbalizes feelings of anxiety to others and verbalizes feeling less anxious
Patient shows no signs or symptoms of complications related to penile implant
Patient and/or significant other verbalizes an understanding of penile prosthesis, symptoms to report to physician, and home care and follow-up instruc-

---

*Not a NANDA-approved nursing diagnosis.

tions; and return-demonstrates inflation and deflation of penile prosthesis

TORSION OF SPERMATIC CORD

Twisting of the spermatic cord, which causes blockage of blood to the testes (Each spermatic cord consists of the vas deferens, spermatic blood vessels, and nerves of the testis and is surrounded by the cremaster muscle.)

Assessment
Observations/findings

Severe localized testicular pain
Nausea, vomiting
Scrotal edema
Scrotal redness
Elevated temperature
Body image disturbance
    Fear of castration
    Fear of loss of male identity
    Fears of sterility and/or impotence

Laboratory/diagnostic studies

Transillumination of cord with use of external flashlight for black dot

Potential complications

Testicular necrosis

Medical management

NPO
Analgesics
Surgical exploration of scrotum

Nursing diagnoses/goals/interventions

ndx: Alteration in comfort: pain related to torsion of spermatic cord

GOAL: *Patient will verbalize a decrease in pain and will show a relaxed facial expression and body position*

Provide scrotal support as ordered
Elevate scrotum
Apply ice bags to scrotum as ordered
Observe for testicular necrosis qh (a sudden absence of pain)
Prepare patient for exploration of scrotum and surgical fixation of testes
Explain that surgery is usually performed within 10 hr
Assess nature, intensity, location, duration, and precipitating and alleviating factors of pain

Assess nonverbal signs of pain
Provide nonpharmacologic comfort measures
    Assist patient with assuming comfortable position
    Teach relaxation techniques
    Teach and assist with guided imagery techniques
    Provide diversional activity
    Provide a restful environment
Administer pain medication as ordered
Observe for desired effects and side effects of medications
Consult with physician if measures fail to provide adequate pain relief or if a dosage or interval change for pain medication is needed

ndx: Anxiety related to fear of impotence, fear of castration, and fear of loosing male identity

GOAL: *Patient will verbalize fears to care giver or significant other and will report feeling less anxious*

Encourage patient to verbalize fears
Encourage communication with significant other
Provide privacy when assessing scrotal area
Ensure patient that everything possible will be done to prevent testicular necrosis
Manage pain

ndx: Knowledge deficit regarding disease process, symptoms to report to physician, and home care and follow-up instructions

GOAL: *Patient and/or significant other will verbalize understanding of disease process, symptoms to report to physician and home care and follow-up instructions*

Teach and instruct patient to report the following to physician
    Progression of edema or discoloration of scrotum
    Incisional redness, pain, swelling, drainage
    Elevated temperature
Instruct patient not to touch incisional area postoperatively
Instruct patient to avoid tight, restrictive underclothing
Teach name of medication, dosage, schedule, purpose, and side effects

Evaluation

Patient verbalizes a decrease in pain and has a relaxed facial expression and body position
Patient expresses fears to others and reports feeling less anxious
Patient and/or significant other verbalizes understand-

ing of torsion of spermatic cord, symptoms to report to physician, and home care and follow-up instructions

ORCHIOPEXY

Surgical fixation of testes to scrotal sac

Assessment
Observations/findings

Scrotal edema
Scrotal discoloration
Site of incision
    Redness
    Pain
    Swelling
    Drainage
Elevated temperature
Disturbance in self-concept
    Fear of castration
    Fear of loss of male identity
    Fear of sterility and/or impotence

Laboratory/diagnostic studies

Physical examination
Radiography

Potential complications

Testicular necrosis
Atelectasis and/or pneumonia
Hemorrhage
Wound infection

Medical management

NPO until bowel sounds are audible
Parenteral IV fluids until liquids and/or diet is tolerated
BP, T, P, and R per postoperative routine
Analgesics
Antibiotics
Scrotal support
Ice packs to scrotum

Nursing diagnoses/goals/interventions

ndx: Alteration in comfort: pain related to surgical incision and scrotal swelling

GOAL: *Patient will verbalize a decrease in pain and will show a relaxed facial expression and body position*

Provide scrotal support as ordered
Apply ice bags to scrotum as ordered
Assess nature, intensity, location, duration, and precipitating and alleviating factors of pain
Assess nonverbal signs of pain
Check urethral catheter and/or suprapubic tube for obstruction
Assess incisional site for redness, tenderness, swelling, and drainage
Provide nonpharmacologic comfort measures
    Assist patient with assuming a comfortable position
    Teach relaxation techiques
    Teach and assist with guided imagery techniques
    Provide diversional activity
    Provide a restful environment
Administer pain medication as ordered
Observe for desired effects and side effects of medications
Consult with physician if measures fail to provide adequate pain relief or if dosage or interval change for pain medication is needed
Observe for testicular necrosis qh for 4 hr, then q8h

ndx: Potential alteration in pattern of urinary elimination: urinary retention related to postoperative scrotal edema

GOAL: *Patient will show no signs or symptoms of urinary retention and will empty bladder using a method as close to usual voiding method as possible; intake and output will be balanced*

Utilize voiding measures to facilitate bladder emptying
    Ensure privacy
    Place patient in comfortable position to urinate
    Run tap water near patient
    Flush toilet
    Place hands in warm water
    Apply heat to suprapubic area as ordered
    Pour warm water over perineum
    Assist patient with using relaxation techniques
    Place a few drops of oil of peppermint in bedpan, on cottonball, and hold briefly in front of urinary meatus
    Pull pubic hairs slightly
    Stroke inner aspect of thigh gently
    Stroke inner aspect of thigh with ice
    Catheterize patient as ordered

ndx: Potential disturbance in self-concept: body image related to fear of castration, impotence, and loss of masculinity

GOAL: *Patient will verbalize feelings to care giver or significant other, will report feelings of increased self-esteem, and will resume ADLs*

Provide an accepting and supportive atmosphere
Encourage expression of feelings of anxiety, fear, embarrassment, anger, frustration, and/or helplessness
Promote feelings of self-worth by stressing positive features in patient's life
Provide suggestions to help patient maintain a satisfactory level of sexual expression
Encourage communication with significant other
Provide assistance from other professionals to help patient to deal with emotional changes (psychiatry, sexual counselor)

ndx Potential for postoperative complications: hemorrhage, wound infection, paralytic ileus, atelectasis/pneumonia*

GOAL: *Patient will show no signs or symptoms of hemorrhage, wound infection, paralytic ileus, or atelectasis/pneumonia*

Hemorrhage

Monitor and report signs and symptoms of hemorrhage (hypotension, tachycardia, dyspnea, cool, clammy skin, syncope)
Check incision for bleeding q4h
Monitor Hct and Hgb as ordered
If hemorrhage occurs
   Place patient flat in bed
   Administer fluid replacement as ordered
   Transfuse with blood products as ordered
   Prepare patient for surgery if necessary

Wound infection

Monitor for and report signs and symptoms of wound infection (fever, chills, redness, swelling, tenderness, purulent and/or malodorous wound drainage)
Check surgical incision q4h for redness, swelling, tenderness, and purulent drainage
Assess temperature q4h
Monitor WBC as ordered
Obtain wound culture as ordered
Use good handwashing technique and teach and encourage patient to do the same
Instruct patient to avoid touching incision, dressings, and drainage
Maintain sterile technique when changing dressings and performing wound care
Administer antibiotics as ordered

Paralytic ileus

Monitor for and report signs of paralytic ileus (absent or diminished bowel sounds; persistent or worsening abdominal pain and cramping; distended, firm abdomen; failure to pass flatus)
Maintain NPO until active bowel sounds are audible or passage of flatus is noted
Auscultate for bowel sounds q4h
Insert and/or maintain nasogastric tube as ordered
Encourage early ambulation
Instruct patient to avoid smoking and/or chewing gum in order to reduce air swallowing
Administer stool softeners, laxatives, or enemas as ordered

Atelectasis/pneumonia

Assist patient with turning, coughing, and deep breathing q2h and prn
Assist patient with incentive spirometer to maximize lung expansion as ordered
Assess BP, heart rate, and heart rhythm q2h
Assess breath sounds q4h
Report diminished or absent breath sounds to physician
Assess skin for signs of cyanosis and diaphoresis
Monitor for and report symptoms of inpaired gas exchange (confusion, restlessness, irritability, decreased PO_2, increased PCO_2)
Administer pain medication at proper intervals to manage pain and to help patient perform coughing and deep-breathing exercises more effectively
Administer O_2 as ordered

ndx Knowledge deficit regarding postoperative routine, symptoms to report to physician, and home care and follow-up instructions

GOAL: *Patient and/or signigicant other will verbalize understanding of disease process, symptoms to report to physician, and home care and follow-up instructions, and will return-demonstrate care of incision*

Instruct patient to exercise to tolerance, to avoid heavy lifting and strenuous activity for 6 months, and to plan frequent rest periods
Instruct patient to avoid constipation
Teach and instruct patient to care for incision
Teach and instruct symptoms to report to physician
   Elevated temperature
   Scrotal pain
   Inability to void
   Incisional redness, swelling, pain, drainage
   Testicular necrosis

---

*Not a NANDA-approved nursing diagnosis.

Reinforce physician's explanation regarding sterility or impotence

Instruct patient to resume normal sexual activity as indicated by physician

Instruct patient to avoid wearing tight undergarments until scrotal swelling subsides

Teach name of medication, dosage, schedule, purpose, and side effects

Instruct patient to avoid taking over-the-counter medications without checking with physician

Teach importance of ongoing outpatient care

Evaluation

Patient verbalizes a decrease in pain and has a relaxed facial expression and body position

Patient voids normally and shows no signs or symptoms of urinary retention

Patient verbalizes feelings to others

Patient reports feeling an increase in self-esteem and resumes ADLs

Patient shows no signs or symptoms of postoperative complications

Patient and/or significant other verbalizes understanding of disease process, symptoms to report to physician, and home care and follow-up instructions; and return-demonstrates care of incision

ORCHIECTOMY FOR TESTICULAR TUMOR

Surgical removal of the testis; most commonly performed in the presence of advanced prostatic cancer and in testicular cancer

Assessment

Observations/findings

Scrotal mass
Testicular swelling
Groin pain
Backache
Weight loss
Malaise
Gynecomastia
Urine: positive reaction to any standard pregnancy test
Elevated temperature
Scrotum
    Edema
    Discoloration
Incision
    Redness
    Pain
    Swelling
    Drainage
Disturbance in self-concept

Laboratory/diagnostic studies

IVU
CT scan of abdomen
Urine pregnancy test
Lymphangiogram

Potential complications

Hemorrhage
Shock
Wound infection
Atelectasis and/or pneumonia

Medical management

NPO until bowel sounds are audible
Parental IV fluids until liquids and/or diet is tolerated
BP, T, P, and R per postoperative routine
Analgesics
Antibiotics
Scrotal support
Chemotherapy
Radiation therapy
Radical lymph node dissection

Nursing diagnoses/goals/interventions

ndx: Alteration in comfort: pain related to surgical incision and scrotal swelling

GOAL: *Patient will verbalize a decrease in pain and will show a relaxed facial expression and body position*

Provide scrotal support as ordered
Assess nature, intensity, location, duration, and precipitating and alleviating factors of pain
Assess nonverbal signs of pain
Assess incisional site for redness, tenderness, swelling, and drainage
Provide nonpharmacologic comfort measures
    Assist patient with assuming a comfortable position
    Teach relaxation techniques
    Teach and assist with guided imagery techniques
    Provide diversional activity
    Provide a restful environment
Administer pain medication as ordered
Observe for desired effects and side effects of medications
Consult with physician if measures fail to provide adequate pain relief or if dosage or interval change for pain medication is needed

ndx: Potential alteration in urinary elimination: urinary retention related to postoperative scrotal swelling

GOAL: *Patient will void normally postoperatively and will show no signs or symptoms of urinary retention*

Utilize voiding measures to facilitate bladder emptying
  Ensure privacy
  Place patient in comfortable position to urinate
  Run tap water near patient
  Flush toilet
  Place hands in warm water
  Apply heat to suprapubic area as ordered
  Pour warm water over perineum
  Assist patient with using relaxation techniques
  Place a few drops of oil or peppermint in bedpan, on cottonball, and hold briefly in front of urinary meatus
  Pull pubic hairs slightly
  Stroke inner aspect of thigh gently
  Stroke inner aspect of thigh with ice
Catheterize patient as ordered
Measure and record urinary output qh

ndx: Potential disturbance in self-concept: body image related to gynecomastia, fear of loss of masculinity, and potency

GOAL: *Patient will express feelings to care giver or significant other, will report feelings of increased self-esteem, and will resume ADLs*

Provide an accepting and supportive atmosphere
Encourage expression of feelings of anxiety, fear, embarrassment, anger, frustration, and/or helplessness
Promote feelings of self-worth by stressing positive features in patient's life
Provide suggestions to help patient maintain satisfactory sexual expression
Encourage communication with significant other
Provide assistance from other professionals to help patient to deal with emotional changes (psychiatry, sexual counselor)
Emphasize positive results of surgery

ndx: Potential for complications: hemorrhage, wound infection, paralytic ileus, atelectasis/pneumonia*

GOAL: *Patient will show no signs of postoperative complications*

Wound infection

Monitor for and report signs and symptoms of wound infection (fever, chills, redness, swelling, tenderness, purulent and/or malodorous wound drainage)
Check surgical incision q4h for redness, swelling, tenderness, and purulent drainage

---

*Not a NANDA-approved nursing diagnosis.

Assess temperature q4h
Monitor WBC as ordered
Obtain wound culture as ordered
Use good handwashing technique and teach and encourage patient to do the same
Instruct patient to avoid touching incision, dressings, and drainage
Maintain sterile technique when changing dressings and performing wound care
Administer antibiotics as ordered

Paralytic ileus

Monitor for and report signs of paralytic ileus (absent or diminished bowel sounds; persistent or worsening abdominal pain and cramping; distended, firm abdomen; failure to pass flatus)
Maintain NPO until active bowel sounds are audible or passage of flatus is noted
Auscultate for bowel sounds q4h
Insert and/or maintain nasogastric tube as ordered
Encourage early ambulation
Instruct patient to avoid smoking and/or chewing gum in order to reduce air swallowing
Administer stool softeners, laxatives, or enemas as ordered

Atelectasis/pneumonia

Assist patient with turning, coughing, and deep breathing q2h and prn
Assist patient with incentive spirometer to maximize lung expansion as ordered
Assess BP, heart rate, and heart rhythm q2h
Assess breath sounds q4h
Report diminished or absent breath sounds to physician
Assess skin for signs of cyanosis and diaphoresis
Monitor for and report symptoms of inpaired gas exchange (confusion, restlessness, irritability, decreased PO_2, and increased PCO_2)
Administer pain medication at proper intervals to manage pain and to help patient perform coughing and deep breathing exercises more effectively
Administer O_2 as ordered

ndx: Knowledge deficit regarding postoperative routine, symptoms to report to physician, and home care and follow-up instructions

GOAL: *Patient and/or significant other will verbalize understanding of disease process, symptoms to report to physician, and home care and follow-up instructions; and will return-demonstrate care of incision and testicular self-examination*

Instruct patient to maintain diet as ordered

Instruct patient to avoid constipation

Instruct patient to exercise to tolerance, avoid fatigue, avoid heavy lifting, and plan frequent rest periods

Teach and prepare patient for chemotherapy, radiation therapy, or radical lymph node dissection

Teach and instruct patient to report the following symptoms to physician

    Incisional redness, pain, swelling, drainage

    Pain on walking

    Thickening or any abnormality in remaining testicle

Teach and instruct patient to perform testicular self-examination once a month

Teach and instruct patient to care for incision

Teach medication name, dosage, schedule, purpose, and side effects

Instruct patient to avoid taking over-the-counter medication without checking with physician

Teach importance of ongoing outpatient care

Evaluation

Patient verbalizes a decrease in pain and has a relaxed facial expression and body position

Patient voids normally and shows no signs or symptoms of urinary retention

Patient verbalizes feelings to others and reports feeling an increase in self-esteem

Patient resumes ADLs

Patient shows no signs or symptoms of postoperative complications

Patient and/or significant other verbalizes understanding of the disease process, symptoms to report to physician, and home care, and follow-up instructions; and return-demonstrates care of incision and testicular self-examination

CHAPTER 10

Female Reproductive System

FEMALE REPRODUCTIVE SYSTEM ASSESSMENT

Subjective Data

Lower abdominal pain
Cramps
Vaginal bleeding
Vaginal discharge
   Mucoid
   Thick white
   Frothy, watery, yellow-green
   Thick, yellow-green or brown, and bloody
   Yellow
   Odoriferous
   Duration
Itching
Swelling
Redness
Painful intercourse
Painful urination
Stress incontinence
Burning on urination
Breasts
   Tenderness
   Pain
   Stinging sensation
   Burning

Objective Data

General appearance
Vital signs, weight
Breasts
   Size
   Symmetry
   Contour
   Lumps, bumps
   "Orange peel" texture
   Venous pattern
   Moles, nevi
   Dimpling
   Erythema
Nipples
   Color
   Discharge (serous, bloody, purulent)
Abdomen
   Contour
   Lesions
   Scars
   Stretch marks
   Symmetry
   Visible pulsations
   Visible peristaltic waves
   Presence of bowel sounds in each quadrant
External genitalia
   Labia majora
      Edema
      Redness
      Lumps
      Lesions
   Clitoris
      Edema
      Redness
   Urethral orifice
      Size
      Redness
   Discharge
      Bloody
      Purulent
      Odoriferous
   Introitus
      Presence or absence of hymenal ring
      Hymenal tags
      Edema
      Redness
      Drainage
      Mucoid (normal)
      Thick, white, cheesy (typical of moniliasis)
      Purulent
      Frothy, water, yellow-green (typical of trichomoniasis)
      Thick, yellow-green or brown, and bloody (typical of upper genital tract infection)
      Bloody
      Yellow
   Perineum
      Scars
      Redness
      Edema
      Excoriation

Female Reproductive System

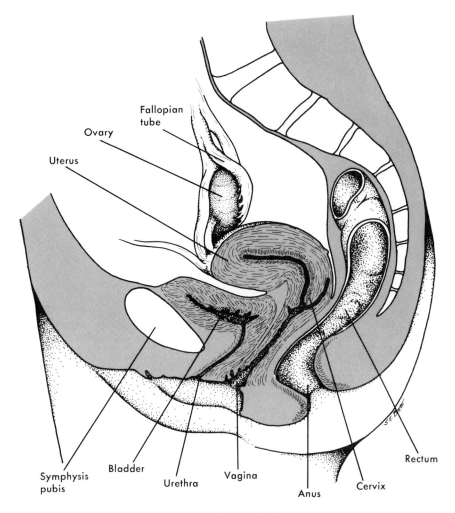

FIGURE 10-1. Female reproductive system.

Pertinent Background Information
CONCURRENT DISEASES OR CONDITIONS

Menstrual cycle
  Age at onset
  Length of cycles (duration)
  Interval between cycles
  Regularity of cycles
  Amount and type of flow
    Number of tampons or napkins used
    Date of most recent douching
    Type of contraceptive used
  Date of last menstrual period (LMP)
  Associated symptoms (pain, menorrhagia, metrorrhagia, etc.)
Pregnancy
  Number of pregnancies and outcome of each
  Complications of pregnancy and delivery and/or abortion

Menopause
  When occurred
  Related symptoms
    Hot flashes
    Dry vaginal mucosa
Gastrointestinal (GI) system
  Constipation
  Hemorrhoids
Endocrine system
  Hypothyroidism
  Hyperthyroidism
  Stein-Leventhal syndrome
Blood dyscrasias
Hypertension

PREVIOUS SURGERY OR ILLNESS

Gynecologic surgery
Other major surgery of illness (of abdomen or endocrine system, etc.)

595

FAMILY HISTORY

Cancer
Sickle cell disease
Thyroid disorder
Diabetes
Other diseases
Death due to gynecologic-related conditions
Maternal diethylstilbestrol (DES) usage

SOCIAL HISTORY

Smoking
Sexual activity; abnormal lesions or discharge in sexual partner
Contraception

MEDICATION HISTORY

Oral contraceptives
Estrogen therapy
Intrauterine contraceptive device (IUD)
Phenothiazines
Digitalis
Diuretics

Diagnostic Aids

Bimanual examination
Basal body temperature
Papanicolaou (Pap) test
Wet mount
Culture
Punch biopsy
Endobiopsy
Dilation and curettage (D & C)
Cold-knife conization
Colposcopy
Hysteroscopy
Culdoscopy
Culpotomy
Laparoscopy
Ultrasound
Insufflation
Mammography
Thermography
Radionuclide imaging
Galactography
Hysterosalpingography

LABORATORY STUDIES

Human chorionic gonadotropin (HCG) level
Serum luteinizing hormone (LH) and follicle-stimulating hormone level (FSH)
Thyroid function studies
Basal metabolic rate (BMR)
Protein-bound iodine (PBI) level
Adrenal function
   17-Ketosteroids
   Corticosteroids
Venereal disease research laboratory (VDRL) test

PELVIC INFLAMMATORY DISEASE (PID)

An infectious process of the pelvic cavity that may include the fallopian tubes, ovaries, pelvic peritoneum, veins, and pelvic connective tissue

Assessment

Observations/findings

Abdominal and pelvic pain
Low back pain
Dyspareunia
Fever
Maladorous, purulent vaginal discharge
Malaise, general aching
Nausea, vomiting
Pruritis or maceration of vulva
Diarrhea

Laboratory/diagnostic studies

Elevated white blood cell count (WBC)
Elevated erythrocyte sedimentation rate
Culture of purulent secretions positive for organisms
Laparoscopic visualization of pelvic inflammation
Ultrasound of tubo-ovarian abscess, if present
Needle culdocentesis of WBCs or nonclotting blood

Potential complications

Urinary tract infection
Peritonitis
Tubo-ovarian abscess
Infertility
Paralytic ileus

Medical management

Antibiotics as determined by sensitivity
Bed rest in semi-Fowler's position or position of comfort
Local heat application to abdomen
Warm douches
Parenteral fluids
Nasogastric suctioning if ileus is present
Removal of intrauterine device if present
Analgesics

Nursing diagnoses/goals/interventions

ndx: Alteration in comfort: pain related to disease process

GOAL: *Patient will state that pain is relieved*

Maintain complete bed rest in semi-Fowler's position or position of comfort
Administer analgesics as needed
Apply local heat to abdomen as ordered
Increase activity as tolerated

ndx: Impairment of skin integrity secondary to drainage

GOAL: *Patient's skin integrity will be maintained*

Assist and teach patient to perform gentle perineal care q3h to 4h and prn; blot skin dry (avoid rubbing)
Teach patient to wipe from front to back after elimination
Prevent excessive warmth of perineal area with bed covers

ndx: Impaired home maintenance management related to lack of knowledge

GOAL: *The patient will manage self–health care needs*

Explain importance of handwashing both before and after contact with perineum
Explain need to use perineal pads, to change them as needed, and to wrap and properly dispose of them; avoid use of tampons
Explain that a shower is preferred to a tub bath
Promote good nutrition with diet as tolerated

ndx: Knowledge deficit regarding disease process

GOAL: *Patient and/or significant other will demonstrate understanding of home care and follow-up instructions through interactive discussion and actual return demonstration*

Teach measures to prevent venereal disease if condition is caused by gonococcus or chlamydia
Emphasize need for sexual partner to be examined or treated
Discuss alternative methods of conception control if condition is related to an intrauterine device
Explain importance of avoiding douching, intercourse, or use of tampons for 1 week following antibiotic therapy or as directed by physician
Discuss symptoms of recurrence that should be reported to physician

Evaluation

Comfort is achieved
Skin integrity is maintained
Body temperature is normal
Infection is resolved
Knowledge about self-care and prevention of recurrence is verbalized

TOXIC SHOCK SYNDROME (TSS)

An acute bacterial infection caused by penicillinase-resistant Staphylococcus aureus; most often associated with continuous use of super-absorbent tampons during menses

Assessment

Observations/findings

Sudden onset of high fever
Myalgia
Vomiting
Watery diarrhea
Sore throat
Profound tiredness
Macular erythematous rash (sunburn-like) on palms and soles
Eventual desquamation within 1 to 2 weeks
Impaired joint mobility
Decreased circulation of fingers and toes
Alterations in level of consciousness: disorientation
Vaginal, oropharyngeal, or conjunctival hyperemia
Severe peripheral edema

Laboratory/diagnostic studies

Elevated
  WBC
  Blood urea nitrogen (BUN)
  Creatinine
  Bilirubin
  Serum glutamic-oxaloacetic transaminase (SGOT)
  Creatinine phosphokinase (CPK)
Decreased
  Platelets

Potential complications

Pulmonary edema
Adult respiratory distress syndrome (ARDS)
Sudden hypotension progressing to shock
Disseminated intravascular coagulation (DIC)

Medical management

Antibiotics
Parenteral fluids to 3000 ml daily unless containdicated
Septic shock management as indicated

Nursing diagnoses/goals/interventions

ndx: Alteration in tissue perfusion related to septic shock and/or ARDS

For specific goals and interventions, see Shock Syndrome (p. 104) and Adult Respiratory Distress Syndrome (ARDS) (p. 263)

ndx: Knowledge deficit regarding home care needs

GOAL: *Patient will demonstrate understanding of home care and follow-up instructions through interactive discussion and actual return demonstration*

Explain need to avoid use of tampons until vaginal cultures are negative
Instruct patient to thoroughly wash hands prior to tampon insertion
Instruct patient to use tampons made of cotton, avoiding the super-absorbent, noncotton type
Explain need to change tampons frequently and need to rotate using tampons and sanitary napkins (consider wearing napkins at night)
Emphasize importance of avoiding tampons altogether if there is a concurrent skin infection such as a boil due to *Staphylococcus aureus*
If the following symptoms occur, instruct patient to discontinue use of tampons immediately and report symptoms to physician
  Nausea
  Vomiting
  Diarrhea
  Fever

GENITAL HERPES

An infection caused by type 2 herpes simplex virus usually transmitted by sexual contact, sometimes occurring in immunocompromised patients, that causes painful vesicular eruptions on the skin and mucous membranes of the genitalia of males and females (this contrasts with herpes virus type 1, which produces small, fluid-filled blisters most commonly around the mouth and nose)

Assessment

Observations/findings

Localized infection
  Fluid-filled vesicle surrounded by erythematous tissue
  Edema: local and of lymph glands
  Tissue tenderness
  Pain, with or without burning sensation
  Thin, white vaginal discharge (females)
  Urine retention secondary to edema
  Dyspareunia
  Dysuria

Laboratory/diagnostic studies

Positive tissue culture of fluid smear

Potential complications

Disseminated infection
Signs of local infection as well as
  Elevated temperature
  Malaise
  Headache
  Anorexia
  Myalgia

Medical management

Antiinfective agents as ordered, including Acyclovir
Topical steroids, anesthetics, or antibiotics
Cesarean delivery before rupture of membranes when condition occurs in late pregnancy, especially if active lesions are present

Nursing diagnoses/goals/interventions

ndx: Alteration in comfort related to tender and painful lesions

GOAL: *Patient will not experience pain*

Keep perineal area clean and dry
Apply topical anesthetics as ordered
Maintain patient in position of comfort

ndx: Potential for (superimposed) infection related to impaired skin integrity

GOAL: *Patient will not develop a superimposed infection and will not transmit herpes to others*

Administer perineal care as indicated
Implement drainage and secretion precautions
Wear gloves when in contact with lesions or secretions

ndx: Knowledge deficit regarding home care management

GOAL: *Patient will demonstrate understanding of home care and follow-up instructions through interactive discussion and actual return demonstration*

Relate importance of abstaining from sexual activities while lesions are present during initial and recurrent infections
Discuss use of condoms during latent periods
Instruct patient to notify physician of genital herpes should conception occur
Relate importance of handwashing after elimination
Explain importance of follow-up outpatient care, including routine gynecologic examination with Pap smear
Emphasize importance of avoiding situations that contribute to recurrence, including fever, ultraviolet light, trauma, and physical and emotional stress
Explain nature of illness/condition and mode of transmission
Explain that recurrence with menses is common
Emphasize importance of utilizing stress reduction techniques
Explain that the disease becomes communicable when lesions reappear and that recurrence may be preceded by local symptoms, including tingling, itching, or burning
Explain importance of follow-up outpatient care

Evaluation

Patient denies discomfort
Patient does not develop a superimposed infection
Infection is not spread to others
Patient demonstrates understanding of self-care instructions

PREMENSTRUAL SYNDROME (PMS)

A condition characterized by nervousness, irritability, weight gain, edema, headache, mastalgia, dysphoria, and lack of coordination before the onset of menstruation

Assessment

Observations/findings

Edema: weight gain, breast tenderness, mastalgia, backache
Abdominal bloating; diarrhea or constipation; nausea, vomiting; food craving, compulsive eating
Irritability, anxiety, fatigue, depression, lethargy, agitation, insomnia
Headache, vertigo, fainting, migraine, paresthesia of head and feet
Increase in colds, asthma, or allergic rhinitis
Cystitis, enuresis, urethritis
Conjunctivitis, styes
Recurrence of herpes; acne, urticaria, boils; easy bruising

Laboratory/diagnostic studies

There are none specific for PMS

Medical management

Diuretics
Vitamins, particularly B_6 and E
Limitation of salt, refined sugars, or animal fat intake

Nursing diagnosis/goal/interventions

ndx: Knowledge deficit regarding self-help measures

GOAL: *Patient will demonstrate understanding of home care and follow-up instructions through interactive discussion and change of behavior*

Explain importance of adequate rest and sleep to avoid fatigue, which exaggerates symptoms
Encourage avoidance of stressful activities or situations during the premenstrual period
Explain importance of avoiding glucose fluctuations by consuming small, frequent amounts of high-protein, complex carbohydrate diet
Explain importance of decreasing salt intake and need to avoid foods with "hidden salt" (e.g., luncheon meats, dried meats, hotdogs, tomato juice, cheeses, crackers)
Explain other dietary modifications to reduce symptoms, including
  Avoidance of dairy products
  Restriction of caffeine sources of coffee, tea, cola, and chocolate
  Restriction of alcohol intake
  Increased intake of leafy green vegetables and whole-grain cereals
Instruct patient to take medications as prescribed and rationale for same (e.g., vitamin B_6 to increase blood progesterone and promote diuresis and vitamin E to reduce breast tenderness)

Evaluation

Patient verbalizes understanding of self-care instructions
Patient describes a feeling of well-being and absence of symptoms of PMS

MENOPAUSE AND CLIMACTERIC

menopause *Physiologic cessation of menses*
climateric *Transitional period during which reproductive function diminishes and eventually ceases*

Assessment

Observations/findings

Irregular menses or amenorrhea
Hot flashes, night sweats

Diaphoresis
Insomnia
Headache
Chilly sensations
Abdominal fat deposition
Tachycardia
Palpitations
Vertigo, syncope
Vague abdominal pain
Constipation or diarrhea
Nausea, vomiting
Flatulence
Fatigability
Lack of appetite or weight gain
Numbness, tingling, or pain in joints
Irritability
Nervousness
Depression or crying spells
Forgetfulness
Difficulty in concentrating
Temporary distortions in close personal relationships
Changes in sexual desire
Dyspareunia

Laboratory/diagnostic studies

Papanicolaou smear
Blood chemistries: estradiol, estrogen, estrone, luteinizing hormone, follicle-stimulating hormone
Urine chemistries: estrogens, pregnanediol, luteinizing hormone, follicle-stimulating hormone

Medical management

Estrogen, oral therapy
Estrogen-based vaginal cream
Progestin or progestogens

Nursing diagnoses/goals/interventions

ndx: Disturbance in self-concept related to concerns about femininity, sexuality, and aging

GOAL: *Patient will verbalize acceptance of altered body image and self concept*

Encourage patient and/or significant other to verbalize concerns
Confirm accurate information and correct information related to self-concept issues

ndx: Knowledge deficit regarding physiologic and psychologic changes

GOAL: *Patient will verbalize an understanding of physiologic and psychologic changes related to climacteric and menopause*

Explain physiologic process of climacteric and menopause
Explain importance of keeping fit and eating a well-balanced diet, getting adequate rest and sleep, avoiding stress and fatigue, and continuing contraception until not indicated by health care provider
Inform patient about side effects of estrogen replacement therapy if ordered
Instruct patient to report any vaginal bleeding occurring 6 months or more after last menstrual period
Relate availability of water-soluble lubricants if needed before coitus

Evaluation

Patient verbalizes understanding of physiology and desired health behaviors
Patient verbalizes understanding of importance of taking medications as prescribed and knows dosage, route of administration, frequency, and potential side effects
Conversations indicate adaptive responses in self-concept and movement toward acceptance of physiologic and psychologic phenomena

HYDATIDIFORM MOLE

Tumor mass of chorionic cells in the uterus that mimics pregnancy; about 10% become malignant

Assessment

Observations/findings

Vaginal bleeding
Uterine cramping
Enlarged uterus (larger than pregnant uterus for same date)
Absence of fetal heart tones
Absence of fetal movement
Vaginal expulsion of vesicular tissue
Hypertension
Hyperthyroidism
Nausea, vomiting
Excessive weight loss

Laboratory/diagnostic studies

Elevated HCG titer
Ultrasonography

Medical management

Evacuation of mole by suction curettage
Routine preprocedural and postprocedural care

Nursing diagnoses/goals/interventions

ndx: Anxiety related to situational crisis

GOAL: *Patient will demonstrate a reduction in anxiety and appropriate coping behaviors*

Encourage verbalization about outcome of diagnosis and treatment

Use active listening skills and assist patient and family with use of adaptive coping strategies to reduce anxiety about pseudocyesis

ndx: Knowledge deficit regarding preprocedural and postprocedural care and risk of choriocarcinoma

GOAL: *Patient and/or significant other will demonstrate understanding of home care and follow-up instructions through interactive discussion*

Explain preoperative and postoperative vital sign and care routines

Reinforce physician's explanation of current condition, risk factors, avoidance of pregnancy (usually for 1 year), need for periodic HCG titers and chest x-ray examinations, and follow-up outpatient care

Evaluation

Anxiety is recognized, and adaptive coping strategies are used for its reduction

Patient verbalizes understanding of home care and follow-up instructions

CHORIOCARCINOMA

Highly malignant neoplasm derived from chorionic epithelium; may develop after a hydatidiform mole, a miscarriage, or a full-term delivery

Assessment

Observations/findings

Profuse and/or intermittent vaginal bleeding
Malodorous vaginal discharge between menses
Cough
Hemoptysis
Headache
Irritability
Nausea, vomiting
Hypertension
Tachypnea
Orthopnea
Vaginal or vulvar lesion
Anemia
Sepsis
Cachexia
Weight loss

Laboratory/diagnostic studies

Rising HCG titer
Ultrasonography
Curettage

Potential complications

Metastasis (lung, vagina, oral cavity, GI tract, central nervous system, liver)

Medical management

Total abdominal hysterectomy and bilateral salpingo-oophorectomy (TAH-BSO)
Antineoplastic chemotherapy (methotrexate, actinomycin D, chlorambucil)

Nursing diagnoses/goals/interventions

See Total Abdominal Hysterectomy and Bilateral Salpingo-oophorectomy (TAH-BSO) (p. 606)
See Antineoplastic Chemotherapy (p. 666)

Evaluation

See Total Abdominal Hysterectomy and Bilateral Salpingo-oophorectomy (TAH-BSO) (p. 606)
See Antineoplastic Chemotherapy (p. 666)

DILATION AND CURETTAGE (D & C)

Expansion of the cervix and scraping of the endometrial lining of the uterus for diagnostic and/or therapeutic purposes

Assessment

Observations/findings

Vaginal hemorrhage
Pelvic and low back pain
Hematuria
Foul odor of vaginal drainage
Elevated temperature

Potential complications

Endometritis
Sepsis
Uterine rupture

Medical management

T, P, R, and BP monitoring
Intake and output for 2 to 4 hr; notation of amount and color of first-voided urine following procedure
Analgesics as indicated

Nursing diagnoses/goals/interventions

ndx: Alteration in comfort: pain related to uterine cramping

GOAL: *Patient will experience minimal discomfort*

Administer analgesics as ordered
Maintain bed rest immediately following procedure, progressing to activity as tolerated

ndx: Potential for infection related to intrauterine curettage

GOAL: *Patient will not develop endometritis or vaginitis*

Administer perineal care after elimination as necessary
Explain importance of wiping from front to back after elimination
Explain that shower is preferred to tub bath for 3 to 4 days
Note amount, color, and odor of vaginal drainage and change perineal pads as necessary q2h and prn
Understand that vaginal packing, if used, is usually removed by physician

ndx: Knowledge deficit regarding home/self-care management

GOAL: *Patient will demonstrate understanding of home care and follow-up instructions through interactive discussion and actual return demonstration*

Explain that vaginal bleeding or spotting may continue for a week and that mild cramps may continue for 2 to 3 days
Explain that minimal activity is preferred for 2 to 3 days
Explain that coitus and/or douching should be delayed for 2 to 3 weeks or as indicated by physician
Discuss symptoms that should be reported to the physician
  Excessive bleeding, heavier than a menstrual period
  Foul odor of vaginal drainage
  Temperature over 100° F (37.8° C)
  Severe lower abdominal cramps or pain

Evaluation

Patient has experienced minimal to no discomfort
There is no infection
There is no excessive bleeding

COLD-KNIFE CONIZATION OF CERVIX

Surgical removal of cervical tissue in the shape of a cone for biopsy or treatment of cervical infection and/or carcinoma in situ

Assessment

Observations/findings

Vaginal hemorrhage
Foul odor of vaginal drainage
Elevated temperature
Pelvic pain and/or low back pain
Expulsion of vaginal packing

Laboratory/diagnostic studies

Tissue examination
Papanicolaou test
Cytologic examination

Potential complications

Hemorrhage
Infection

Medical management

BP and TPR monitoring
Intake and output

Nursing diagnosis/goal/interventions*

ndx: Knowledge deficit regarding home/self-care management

GOAL: *Patient will demonstrate understanding of home care and follow-up instructions through interactive discussion and actual return demonstration*

Explain that no coitus, douching, or tampons are allowed for 6 weeks or as indicated by physician
Teach perineal hygiene; instruct patient to wipe from front to back after each elimination
Discuss symptoms of infection to report to physician (e.g., purulent and/or foul-smelling drainage)
To avoid constipation, instruct patient to use stool softeners or mild laxatives as needed
Explain need to report to physician any bleeding (of a greater amount than a normal period) that occurs 7 to 10 days postoperatively
Emphasize importance of follow-up outpatient care

Evaluation

Patient has experienced minimal to no discomfort
There is no infection
There is no excessive bleeding

---

*See Dilation and Curettage (D & C) for routine care; in addition, note that any vaginal packing should be removed only by physician.

ABORTION: SALINE OR PROSTAGLANDIN INFUSION

Termination of pregnancy after the sixteenth week of gestation by intraamniotic injection of hypertonic saline solution or by administration of prostaglandin suppositories or infusion

Preprocedure nursing diagnoses/goals/interventions

ndx: Disturbance in self-esteem (self-concept) related to termination of pregnancy

GOAL: *Patient will demonstrate problem-solving skills that promote a positive level of self-esteem*

Encourage patient to verbalize and identify strengths, assets, and adaptive coping measures
Be aware of own feelings that may affect nonverbal communication
Avoid evaluative statements when providing information
Provide factual information related to procedure and care
Give empathetic responses to expression of feelings to encourage acceptance of these feelings
Assist patient in working through denial or other defense mechanisms

ndx: Knowledge deficit regarding procedure

GOAL: *Patient will demonstrate understanding of information through interactive discussion*

Reinforce physician's explanation as to how procedure is done
Explain that patient will experience "mini" labor for which analgesia will be available
Explain that fetus is usually aborted within 18 to 36 hr following saline infusion, with fetus delivered first, followed by placenta
Explain that fetus is usually aborted within 8 to 12 hr following prostaglandin administration, with fetus delivered first, followed by placenta
Explain that a D & C may be done if any products of conception are retained longer than 2 hr after expulsion of fetus

Assessment
Observations/findings
GENERAL

Emotional stress
  Extremely talkative
  Crying
  Uncommunicative
Hypertonicity or flaccidity of uterine fundus

SALINE INTRAAMNIOTIC INFUSION

Intravascular injection of saline solution
  Sensation of heat
  Dry mouth
  Tinnitus
  Tachycardia
  Severe headache
Gradual or sudden onset of elevated BP
Signs of water intoxication
  Urine output <200 ml q8h
  Edema
  Shortness of breath
  Difficulty in breathing
  Thirst
  Restlessness

PROSTAGLANDIN VAGINAL SUPPOSITORIES OR INFUSION

Nausea, vomiting
Diarrhea

Potential complications

Hemorrhage
Shock
Uterine rupture

Medical management

Parenteral oxytocin following procedure
Vital signs
Clear liquid intake progressing to regular diet following placenta expulsion
Intake and output
Monitoring of contraction pattern, time, frequency, and duration

Nursing diagnoses/goals/interventions

ndx: Alteration in comfort: pain due to uterine contractions

GOAL: *Patient will experience minimal discomfort*

Assist patient with assuming position of comfort
Teach and demonstrate breathing patterns and relaxation techniques
Administer analgesics as ordered

Concurrent care

Check BP, P, and R q15 min for four times, then q4h and prn

Check T, P, and R q4h
Encourage activity as ordered
Empty bladder q4h to 6h if patient does not have an indwelling catheter connected to closed gravity drainage
Give clear liquids as ordered
Administer parenteral fluids with oxytocic as ordered

Postfetal expulsion care

Maintain complete bed rest
Clamp and cut cord and remove fetus from bedside
    Tell patient sex of fetus if it is discernible and she desires to know
    Show fetus to patient at her request
Check BP, P, and R q15 min for four times, then qh until placenta is expelled
Change pad under buttocks q30 to 60 min and prn
Measure intake and output
Control pain as ordered
Notify physician if placenta is not expelled or if excessive vaginal bleeding occurs within 2 hr

Postplacental expulsion care

Check BP and P q15 min for four times, then qh for 2h, then q8h
Check T, P, and R q4h
Palpate and massage fundus if necessary q15 min for four times, then q4h for three times and prn
Change perineal pads q2h and prn
Administer perineal care with antiseptic solution q4h for two times and prn
Increase activity as tolerated
Administer medication as ordered
    Anti-Rh globulin
    Lactation suppressant
Retain products of conception until checked by physician to determine whether or not fragments have been retained; prepare for D & C as indicated
Maintain diet as tolerated

ndx: Knowledge deficit regarding home and follow-up care

GOAL: *Patient will demonstrate understanding of information through interactive discussion*

Emphasize importance of reporting bleeding that lasts longer than 7 to 10 days or excessive bright red bleeding with clots
Discuss symptoms of infection to report
    Nausea, vomiting
    Severe uterine cramping
    Temperature above 100° F (37.8° C)
    Foul odor of vaginal discharge
Instruct patient on careful cleaning of perineal area; wipe from front to back after each elimination
Instruct patient to avoid douching, tampons, and coitus for 4 to 6 weeks or as indicated by physician
Explain that normal menstrual period should begin in 4 to 6 weeks
Emphasize importance of follow-up outpatient care
Discuss contraceptive method of choice, since pregnancy is possible within 2 to 3 weeks

Evaluation

Patient demonstrates adaptive coping behaviors and positive self-esteem
There is no evidence of hemorrhage, and blood loss is normal
Patient is knowledgeable about home care and signs and symptoms that should be reported to physician
Patient verbalizes a plan for conception control

TUBAL LIGATION (ABDOMINAL)

Tying of the fallopian tubes, usually with excision of a portion of the tube, to interrupt tubal continuity, thereby providing sterilization; this procedure contrasts with laparoscopic tubal ligation, which is usually done on an outpatient basis

Assessment

Observations/findings

Abdominal pain
Site of incision
    Redness
    Pain
    Swelling
    Drainage
Elevated temperature
Abdominal distention
Absence of bowel sounds
Changes in body image
Feelings of loss of sexuality

Potential complication

Infection

Medical management

Parenteral fluids until diet is resumed as tolerated
Analgesics
Intake and output until patient is voiding clear urine in sufficient quantity
Vital signs

Nursing diagnoses/goals/interventions

ndx: Alteration in comfort due to incision and abdominal distention

GOAL: *Patient will verbalize that discomfort is absent or minimal*

Assist patient with assuming position of comfort
Administer analgesics as indicated
Insert rectal tube or give Harris flush if ordered
Progressively increase activity

ndx: Disturbance in self-concept: body image related to loss of reproductive potential and gender identity

GOAL: *Patient will accept body change in a positive and realistic manner*

Encourage patient to verbalize feelings regarding body image
Inform patient that sexual desire will not be decreased; it is often increased, with the knowledge that pregnancy is not possible
Correct any misconceptions; explain that hormonal therapy is not necessary, because ovaries are not removed and continue to function

Evaluation

Comfort is achieved
Patient expresses positive acceptance of body image
There is no infection

TUBAL PREGNANCY AND SALPINGECTOMY

Implantation of the fertilized ovum in the fallopian tube is the most common type of ectopic pregnancy; incidence has increased because of the greater incidence of pelvic inflammatory disease resulting in tubal stricture following salpingitis

Assessment

Preoperative observations/findings
UNRUPTURED TUBE

Low abdominal pain and tenderness: unilateral or generalized
Vaginal bleeding: usually scanty and dark brown; intermittent or continuous
Signs of pregnancy
   Amenorrhea
   Nausea, vomiting
   Urinary frequency
   Breast changes

RUPTURED TUBE

Severe lower abdominal pain: may be sudden and stabbing
Vaginal bleeding may or may not be present
Dizziness
Fainting
Pallor
Progressive supine hypotension
Referred supraclavicular pain

Laboratory/diagnostic studies

Culdocentesis (positive for free blood)
Laparoscopy
Ultrasonography
Complete blood cell count (CBC), electrolytes, type and screen/cross
Urinalysis

Postoperative observations/findings

Site of incision
   Redness
   Pain
   Swelling
   Drainage
Elevated temperature
Feelings of loss and grief

Potential complications

Paralytic ileus
Pneumonia
Hemorrhage, anemia
Shock

Medical management

Parenteral fluids
Analgesics
Indwelling catheter to closed gravity drainage
Vital signs
Intake and output
Anti-Rh globulin

Nursing diagnoses/goals/interventions

ndx: Alteration in comfort: pain related to incision and abdominal distention

GOAL: *Patient will verbalize that discomfort is minimal*

Assist patient with assuming position of comfort
Administer analgesics as ordered
Auscultate abdomen for bowel sounds; insert rectal tube and/or give Harris flush as ordered for abdominal distention

ndx: Anticipatory grief related to loss of pregnancy

GOAL: *Patient will demonstrate successful progress through grieving process with absence of characteristics of dysfunctional grieving*

Encourage verbalization of feelings
Assist patient with working through grieving process by using supportive statements
Involve spouse or significant other with loss and grief

ndx: Self-care deficit related to discomfort

GOAL: *Patient will perform self-care activities, including feeding, hygiene measures, and toileting prior to discharge*

Observe site of incision and reinforce and change dressing as necessary
Demonstrate same and assist patient with performing care
Progress from clear liquid to regular diet as tolerated
Encourage and assist patient as needed with early ambulation; increase activity to tolerance
Involve social service worker regarding placement of other children at home if necessary, since emergency surgery of mother prohibits preoperative planning for their care

ndx: Knowledge deficit regarding ectopic pregnancy

GOAL: *Patient and/or significant other will demonstrate understanding of home care and follow-up instructions through interactive discussion*

Discuss symptoms of wound infection to report to physician
Explain need for activity to tolerance
Explain importance of planned rest periods
Emphasize importance of prevention of pregnancy for 2 to 4 months or as indicated by physician
Explain that childbearing ability is usually diminished, especially if tubal pregnancy was a result of PID or anomaly of the tube resulting in bilateral obstruction

Evaluation

Comfort is achieved
Patient demonstrates progress in grieving process
Patient performs self-care activities
Patient verbalizes understanding of home care instructions

TOTAL ABDOMINAL HYSTERECTOMY AND BILATERAL SALPINGO-OOPHORECTOMY (TAH-BSO)

Surgical removal of the uterus, cervix, both fallopian tubes, and ovaries through an abdominal incision to treat malignant neoplastic disease, leiomyomas, and chronic endometriosis

Assessment

Observations/findings

Vaginal discharge other than serosanguineous and/or with foul odor
Redness, pain, swelling, or drainage at incision site
Fever
Difficulty in voiding
Diminished or absent bowel sounds
Maladaptive comments related to self-concept

Laboratory/diagnostic studies

Urine culture and sensitivity following catheter removal
Hemoglobin and hematocrit postsurgically

Potential complications

Infection: intraabdominal or incisional
Urinary tract infection
Paralytic ileus
Pneumonia
Hemorrhage
Thrombophlebitis
Pulmonary embolus

Medical management

NPO until bowel sounds are audible
Parenteral fluids until liquids or diet is tolerated
Indwelling catheter to low-gravity drainage system
Intake and output
BP, T, P, and R per postoperative procedure
Analgesics and stool softeners
Hormone replacement as indicated

Nursing diagnoses/goals/interventions

ndx: Alteration in tissue perfusion secondary to surgical intervention

GOAL: *Patient's vital signs will remain within normal presurgical limits; circulation will remain normal without evidence of pelvic stasis or peripheral thrombophlebitis; bowel sounds will remain active*

Monitor vital signs as ordered

Avoid placing patient in high-Fowler's position and placing pressure under knees
Avoid sitting with knees bent and/or crossing legs
Apply antiembolic stockings as ordered
Auscultate bowel sounds q6h to 8h; maintain NPO status until bowel sounds are active
Assist with initial ambulation as needed

ndx: Alteration in comfort related to pain in operative site

GOAL: *Patient will verbalize that she is comfortable, and pain will be reduced*

Assist patient in assuming a position of comfort
Place pillow on abdomen for support when patient is coughing
Assist with bed bath until patient is able to bathe or shower

ndx: Ineffective breathing pattern related to discomfort and postsurgical status

GOAL: *Patient will have clear breath sounds on auscultation*

Assist with turning, coughing, and deep breathing q2h and prn, decreasing frequency as patient becomes more active
Assist and teach patient to use incentive spirometer as indicated
Auscultate chest for breath sounds qid for 2 days, then prn

ndx: Actual impairment of skin integrity related to surgical incision

GOAL: *Patient's incision will remain clean, dry, and intact without signs of inflammation*

Observe incision for condition q4h or as indicated
Cleanse incisional area as indicated; keep it clean and dry
Change or reinforce dressing as necessary
Explain to patient importance of avoiding lifting or placing strain on abdominal muscles; avoid straining at stool

ndx: Alteration in bowel elimination related to NPO status and manipulation of pelvic and abdominal structures during surgery

GOAL: *Patient will expel flatus and defecate prior to discharge*

Progress to high-protein or high-residue diet as ordered
Encourage adequate fluid intake
Give Harris flush or insert rectal tube for gas as indicated
Assist patient with assuming lateral Sim's position if this promotes expulsion of flatus
Encourage ambulation
Give stool softeners or mild laxatives as ordered

ndx: Alteration in urinary elimination related to postsurgical sensory motor impairment

GOAL: *Patient will void qs without difficulty*

Connect indwelling catheter to closed gravity drainage bag
Give catheter care as indicated
Promote micturation at regular intervals when catheter is removed

ndx: Potential disturbance in self-concept related to body image change and value of reproductive organs

GOAL: *Patient will demonstrate adaptive responses related to self-concept: she will ask appropriate questions, give correct information related to procedures and prognosis, and will indicate that she has discussed concerns with partner*

Encourage patient's comments and questions about surgery, progress, and prognosis
Reinforce correct information and provide factual information to correct any misconceptions: common misconceptions are that after a hysterectomy a woman grows fat and flabby, develops facial hair, becomes wrinkled, old, and masculine, loses her mind, or becomes depressed and nervous; normal concerns usually in need of discussion are fear of death, disfigurement, cancer, loss of femininity, pain, loss of childbearing ability, and changes in sexuality
Encourage verbalization with significant others
Discuss hormone replacement therapy

ndx: Knowledge deficit regarding home care needs

GOAL: *Patient and/or significant other will demonstrate understanding of home care and follow-up instructions through interactive discussion and actual return demonstration*

Explain need to avoid coitus or douching, tampons, or anything in vagina for 6 weeks or as indicated by physician

Instruct patient to ambulate at regular intervals and to avoid sitting for prolonged periods at home or when traveling

Instruct patient to care for incision with general cleanliness and daily bathing; to report signs of infection to physician, including redness, swelling, pain, discharge or increase in vaginal drainage, and foul odor

Explain need to avoid heavy lifting and vigorous activities for 6 weeks after surgery

Explain need to avoid constipation and straining at stool

Emphasize importance of maintaining regular outpatient gynecologic examinations

Explain need to take estrogen-progesterone hormones as ordered (if surgical menopause is caused by removal of all ovarian tissue)

Evaluation

There are no complications

Presurgical dietary and elimination patterns have resumed

Patient performs hygienic self-care activities

Pain is controlled with comfort measures and oral medication as needed

Patient verbalizes understanding of surgically induced menopause (if all ovarian tissue has been removed)

Patient verbalizes understanding that childbearing is no longer possible

Patient demonstrates adaptive response related to self-concept and sexuality

Patient and/or significant other demonstrates understanding of principles of home and follow-up care

RADICAL HYSTERECTOMY

Surgical removal of the ovaries, tubes, uterus with the cervix, and parametrial tissue, and lymph node dissection; ovarian tissue is often preserved in premenopausal patients

Preoperative teaching and care

For 2 days before surgery maintain clear liquid diet as ordered

Administer cleansing enema the evening before surgery

Teach postoperative breathing exercises

Have practice sessions with intermittent positive pressure breathing (IPPB) or incentive spirometer

Explain that patient will have an indwelling catheter for 24 hr and/or suprapubic catheter for 1 to 8 weeks because of denervation of bladder, causing large amounts of residual urine; reinforce that bladder function probably will resume

Explain that patient may have Jackson-Pratt or other drains present

Postoperative assessment
Observations/findings

Hemorrhage
Vaginal drainage
   Other than serosanguineous fluid
   Foul odor of discharge
Site of incision
   Redness
   Pain
   Swelling
   Drainage
Elevated temperature
Tachycardia
Jackson-Pratt or Hemovac drains
   Leakage of urine
   Hemorrhage
Hematuria
Urinary retention
Vaginal leakage of urine
Suprapubic leakage of urine
Abdominal distention

Potential complications

Hemorrhage
Urinary tract infection
Paralytic ileus
Pneumonia
Thrombophlebitis
Constipation
Pulmonary embolus
Infection
Ureteral fistula
Ureter ligation (iatrogenic)
   Low back pain
   Decreased urine output
Lymphocyst

Immediate postoperative care

Check BP, T, P, and R q4h for 48 hr, then qid
Maintain NPO status until patient is passing flatus
Progress from NPO to clear liquid diet as ordered; administer mouth care q2h while patient is NPO
Provide parenteral fluids as ordered
Connect indwelling catheter(s) to closed gravity drainage system
Measure intake and output
Assist and teach patient to turn, cough, and deep breathe q2h

Administer incentive spirometer
Auscultate chest for breath sounds q4h and prn
Empty Jackson-Pratt q1h to 2h and prn (decrease frequency as amount of drainage decreases)
Observe site of incision q2h to 4h
Change dressing as ordered; reinforce dressing prn
Assist patient with getting out of bed on first postoperative day as ordered
Decrease pelvic congestion
  Avoid high-Fowler's position
  Place head of bed flat q2h for 5 to 10 min during first 24 hr
  Avoid pressure under knees
  Apply antiembolic stockings as ordered; reapply q6h to 8h and prn
  Perform passive leg exercises
Manage pain; provide medication as ordered
Administer perineal care with antiseptic solution q4h and prn
Auscultate abdomen for bowel sounds each shift
Give complete bed bath until activity is increased

Convalescent management

Continue with immediate postoperative care and decrease frequency of nursing functions as patient's condition improves
Progress from clear liquid diet to high-protein or high-residue diet
Encourage fluid intake
Use voiding measures; check for residual urine
Provide abdominal support or binder as indicated
Ambulate as ordered; avoid sitting for long periods
Insert rectal tube and/or give Harris flush prn
Administer stool softeners, mild laxatives, suppositories, or small enema prn
Administer hormone therapy as ordered
Give partial bed bath progressing to self-bath or shower as indicated

Nursing diagnosis/goal/interventions*

ndx: Knowledge deficit regarding home care management

GOAL: *Patient and/or significant other will demonstrate understanding of home care and follow-up instructions through interactive discussion and actual return demonstration*

Ensure that patient and/or significant other demonstrates care of suprapubic catheter if patient is discharged with one in place

---

*See Total Abdominal Hysterectomy and Bilateral Salpingo-oophorectomy (TAH-BSO) (p. 606).

Give reasons for estrogen therapy if ordered: necessitated by surgically induced menopause
Explain that no intercourse, tampons, douching, or tub baths are allowed for 6 weeks or as indicated by physician
Caution patient to avoid sitting for long periods of time
Relate that supportive hosiery may be indicated
Caution patient to avoid constipation
Explain importance of exercise and activity to tolerance
Caution patient to avoid jarring activities, driving, and heavy lifting for 6 weeks or as indicated by physician
Explain importance of planned rest periods
Relate that abdominal support or binder may be indicated
Discuss symptoms to report to physician
  Elevated temperature over 100° F (37.8° C)
  Vaginal bleeding (more than slight bloody discharge)
  Abdominal cramps or change in bowel habits
Explain that menstruation will no longer occur
Emphasize importance of involving family or significant other in dealing with body image changes
Caution patient to avoid activities that increase pelvic congestion (e.g., dancing, horseback riding) until allowed to do so by physician
Relate that counseling for sexually active woman and her partner is available
  Coitus is usually possible if a wide cuff of vagina has been removed; remaining vagina stretches with use
  Alternate methods of achieving sexual satisfaction can be explored if indicated
Teach name of medication, dosage, time of administration, purpose, and side effects
Emphasize importance of follow-up outpatient care

Evaluation

See Total Abdominal Hysterectomy and Bilateral Salpingo-oophorectomy (TAH-BSO) (p. 606)

VULVECTOMY

vulvectomy with lymphadenectomy Excision of the vulva (labia majora, labia minora, clitoris, the surrounding tissues) and the pelvic lymph nodes as a treatment for cancer
skinning vulvectomy with skin graft Excision of the upper skin layers of the vulva and placement of a skin graft from the buttock or thigh as a treatment for cancer in situ

Preoperative teaching and care

Be aware that patient is usually admitted 1 day prior to surgery

Maintain clear liquid diet as ordered for 48 hr prior to surgery

Administer antibiotic therapy as ordered for 24 to 48 hr prior to surgery

Provide emotional support; encourage communication with spouse or significant other

Explain the following to patient

    Bed rest will be maintained for 24 to 48 hr postoperatively

    Indwelling catheter will be present

    Bulky dressing may be present on surgical site; dressing may be removed 24 to 48 hr postoperatively to irrigate perineal/groin area

    Alternating pressure air mattress, convoluted foam (egg-crate) mattress, or water mattress will be used

    Antiembolic stockings may be on legs

    Hemovac or other drains may be present

Teach postoperative breathing exercises

Have practice sessions with IPPB or incentive spirometer

Teach leg exercises

Teach use of overhead trapeze

Explain that pain will be managed

Postoperative assessment

Observations/findings

Perineal hemorrhage

Purulent drainage and/or foul odor from surgical site; sloughing of skin flap or graft

Elevated temperature

Body image disturbances

Psychologic changes

    Anger

    Depression

    Anxiety

    Withdrawal

    Hostility

Edema of lower extremities

Absence of popliteal or pedal pulses (especially with lymphadenectomy)

Skin

    Excoriation

    Decubiti

Constipation or impaction

Anemia

Potential complications

Hemorrhage

Paralytic ileus

Thrombophlebitis

Infection (sepsis)

Pulmonary embolus

Pneumonia

Urinary tract infection

Immediate postoperative care

Provide overhead trapeze; convoluted foam (egg-crate) mattress, alternating-pressure air mattress, or water mattress; and bed cradle

Maintain complete bed rest in flat position unless otherwise ordered

Check BP, T, P, and R q2h for 6 hr, then q4h for 4 days, then q8h; do not take temperature rectally

Assist and teach patient to turn, cough, and deep breathe q2h; use pillow between legs when turning

Administer IPPB or incentive spirometer

Auscultate chest for breath sounds q2h to 4h and prn

Manage pain with analgesics

Maintain NPO status; provide mouth care q2h

Administer parenteral fluids with antibiotics as ordered

Administer low-dose heparin therapy as ordered

Connect indwelling catheter to closed gravity drainage system

Administer catheter care q6h to 8h and prn

Measure intake and output

Administer skin care to back and sides q2h to 4h and prn

Auscultate abdomen for bowel sounds each shift

Check popliteal and pedal pulses q2h to 4h and prn

Perform passive range-of-motion (ROM) exercises to all extremities

Apply antiembolic stockings as ordered; reapply q6h to 8h and prn

Check circulation in extremities; report edema

Skinning volvectomy with skin graft

Irrigate vulvar sponge dressing with solution ordered (frequently this is chloramphenicol 1 g in 150 ml of normal saline used qd)

Report excessive drainage

Observe dressing of graft donor site (usually buttock or thigh); report any untoward signs to physician when dressing is removed; place bed cradle over area to prevent linens from touching area

Maintain bulky dressing in place with patient on bed rest for 7 days

Vulvectomy with lymphadenectomy

Observe Jackson-Pratt drains and empty as indicated q2h to 4h, then each shift and prn

Observe dressing

Reinforce if necessary q1h to 2h
Report excessive drainage
Do not change dressing

Convalescent management

Maintain clear liquid diet progressing to low-residue and/or high-protein, high carbohydrate diet
Avoid defecation with dressings in place; give diphenoxylate or paregoric as indicated
When dressings have been removed
   Irrigate surgical site (usually with half-saline solution and half-peroxide solution or plain saline solution) for vulvectomy with lymphadenectomy
   Irrigate skinning vulvectomy site with antibiotic solution
   Dry with hand-held dryer on low or use heat lamp
   Apply clean fluff or cotton-free gauze and change prn when wet
   Use sitz baths or whirlpool as ordered bid and prn
   Check for bowel movement within 24 hr
     Avoid straining
     Administer stool softeners, laxatives, suppositories, or enemas as indicated
Elevate head of bed from 30 to 60 degrees or position patient on side with pillow between legs (upper leg bent and slightly forward)
Avoid pressure under knees; no knee gatch
Assist with active ROM exercises to all extremities tid and prn
Ambulate
   Avoid chair sitting
   Avoid crossing legs
Use voiding measures after removal of indwelling catheter (between the fifth and tenth postoperative days)
Encourage fluid intake to 2500 ml daily
Provide high-protein between-meal snacks and a variety of liquids as ordered, such as milk shakes, custards, and eggnog

Nursing diagnoses/goals/interventions

ndx: Potential disturbance in self-concept related to body image change and value of reproductive organs

GOAL: *Patient will verbalize acceptance of altered body image and will confirm that she has shared her feelings with partner*

Encourage patient's comments and questions about surgery, progress, and prognosis
Reinforce correct information and provide factual information to correct any misconceptions
Relate importance of communicating anything that causes anxiety
Encourage patient to verbalize and explore feelings regarding what impact the missing body part might have on assuming activities of daily living (ADLs)
Encourage patient to look at and touch the changed body part
Encourage use of rehabilitative services (e.g., ostomy club, wellness community, etc.)

ndx: Knowledge deficit regarding home care management

GOAL: *Patient and/or significant other will demonstrate understanding of home care and follow-up instructions through interactive discussion and actual return demonstration*

Involve family or significant other in all aspects of care and instruction
Emphasize importance of communicating anything that causes anxiety
Explain need for exercise and activity to tolerance
Explain need for planned rest periods
Instruct patient to take sitz baths bid and prn
Demonstrate wound irrigation and dressing change; give written instructions to patient
Discuss symptoms of wound infection to report to physician
   Unusual odor
   Fresh bleeding
   Perineal pain
   Elevated temperature above 100° F (37.8° C)
   Increased swelling of groin
   Urinary tract infection
     Frequency and urgency of urination
     Burning and pain on urination
Relate that low-dose prophylactic antibiotics may be ordered (possibly for as long as a year)
Relate that antiembolic stockings or supportive hosiery may be indicated
Instruct patient to elevate legs periodically at home (elevate lower end of mattress or consider using 1- to 2-inch blocks at foot of bed)
Caution patient to avoid sitting or standing for long periods of time or crossing legs
Caution patient to avoid constipation
Caution patient to avoid heavy lifting
Relate that counseling for sexually active woman and her partner is available
   No coitus until indicated by physician
   Alternate methods of achieving sexual satisfaction can be explored if clitoris has been removed; vaginal orgasm may be achieved
   Water-soluble lubricant may be necessary
   Fertility is not affected in woman of childbearing age

Explain need for high-protein, high-carbohydrate diet
Teach name of medication, dosage, time of administration, purpose, and side effects
Relate that referrals may be indicated for Visiting Nurses Association, social service worker, or clergy
Emphasize importance of follow-up outpatient care

Evaluation

There are no complications
Pain is controlled and minimized
Intake and output are balanced
Patient verbalizes understanding of home care management instructions
Patient demonstrates adaptive response related to self-concept and sexuality

PELVIC EXENTERATION

total exenteration *Removal of all reproductive organs and adjacent tissues: radical hysterectomy, pelvic node dissection, cystectomy with formation of ileal conduit, vaginectomy, and rectal resection with colostomy*
anterior exenteration *Excludes rectal resection with colostomy*
posterior exenteration *Excludes cystectomy with formation of ileal conduit*

Preoperative teaching and care

Be aware that patient is usually admitted 1 day prior to surgery
Maintain clear liquid diet until patient is NPO
Administer cathartics as ordered 48 hr before surgery
Prepare bowel
　Give cleansing enemas hs for 2 days (24 to 48 hr) before surgery
　Give antibiotics as ordered 48 to 72 hr before surgery
Inform enterostomal therapist of patient's admission
Administer vitamin K as ordered 24 hr before surgery
Explain that bed rest will be maintained for 3 to 7 days postoperatively
Teach postoperative breathing exercises
Have practice sessions with IPPB
Teach use of overhead trapeze
Explain the following to patient
　Bulky dressings may be present on surgical site; pelvic pack may be used
　Urethral catheters, colostomy, ileostomy, or urinary conduit may be present
　Patient may have Jackson-Pratt or Hemovac and other drains
　Antiembolic stockings may be on legs
　Pain will be managed
Encourage communication with enterostomal therapist, psychiatric nurse, or patient recovered from same surgery
Encourage communication with spouse or significant other
Explore sexual needs; vaginal reconstruction may be performed during exenteration or at a later time

Postoperative assessment
Observations/findings

Site of incision
　Redness
　Pain
　Swelling
　Drainage
Colostomy, ileostomy, urinary diversion
　Necrosis
　Edema
　Stenosis
　Excoriation of skin around stoma
Oliguria progressing to anuria
Body image disturbances
Psychologic changes
　Anger
　Depression
　Withdrawal
　Anxiety
　Hostility
Elevated temperature
Tachycardia
Edema of lower extremities
Absence of popliteal or pedal pulses

Potential complications

Major complications
　First 48 hr: hemorrhage
　Days 2 to 4: infection
　Days 5 to 21: urinary or GI fistula
Shock
Electrolyte imbalance
Dehydration
Paralytic ileus
Thrombophlebitis
Pulmonary embolus
Pneumonia
Sepsis

Immediate postoperative care

Use overhead trapeze; convoluted foam (egg-crate) mattress, alternating-pressure air mattress, or water mattress; and bed cradle as necessary

Check BP, P, and R qh for 48 hr, then q4h for 7 days, and as indicated by patient's condition

Check axillary or oral temperature q4h and prn; do not take temperature rectally

Measure intake and output

Maintain bed rest

Assist and teach patient to turn, cough, and deep breathe q2h

Administer incentive spirometer q4h and prn

Auscultate chest for breath sounds q4h and prn

Manage pain; administer medications as ordered

Maintain NPO status; provide mouth care q2h

Connect intestinal decompression tube to intermittent, low-suction apparatus; measure carefully to calculate fluid replacement

Administer parenteral fluids with electrolytes to 3000 to 4000 ml daily; provide total parenteral nutrition (TPN) as indicated

Give blood or blood component transfusions q2d to 3d for a week

Check popliteal and pedal pulses q2h to 4h and prn

Apply antiembolic stockings as ordered; reapply q6h to 8h

Perform passive ROM exercises to all extremities q4h and prn

Observe surgical site, dressings, and drainage apparatus qh for 48 hr
  Reinforce dressings as necessary
  Change dressings as ordered
  Measure and empty drainage receptacles prn
  Weigh dressings before applying and after changing if indicated; report excessive drainage to physician

Administer skin care to pressure areas q2h to 4h

Auscultate abdomen for bowel sounds each shift

See appropriate standard of care
  Ostomy care
  Urinary diversion

Do not remove pelvic packing; assist physician in its removal
  Administer analgesic prior to removal of packing; observe closely for signs of hemorrhage

Maintain therapeutic environment
  Adequate ventilation
  Privacy during all nursing care activities
  Room deodorants
  Immediate removal of soiled dressings

Maintain planned rest periods

Convalescent management

Continue with immediate postoperative care and decrease frequency of nursing functions as patient's condition improves

Check BP, T, P, and R q4h, decreasing to qid

Clamp intestinal decompression tube 24 hr prior to clear liquid diet as ordered; physician will remove tube

Assess nutritional status; TPN may be indicated

Slowly increase to high-protein, high-carbohydrate diet as ordered

Administer oral medication after removal of tube; include oral vitamins
  Iron
  Urinary antiseptics
  Antibiotics

Encourage oral fluids to 3000 ml daily unless contraindicated

Provide high-protein between-meal snacks and a variety of liquids as ordered, such as milk shakes, custards, and eggnog

When dressings and packings have been removed
  Irrigate perineal area with half-saline and half-peroxide solution
  Pat dry with sterile towel
  Dry with hand-held hair dryer on low or use heat lamp
  Give sitz baths as ordered tid and prn
  Ambulate after removal of pelvic packing and progress according to patient's tolerance (at least bid); avoid chair sitting

Assist with active ROM exercises to all extremities qid and prn

Administer ostomy care; see Ostomy Management and Care (p. 391)
  Measure and empty ileostomy appliance q2h to 4h; never irrigate
  Measure and empty ileal conduit appliance q2h to 4h
  Irrigate colostomy daily or every other day after 8 to 10 days postoperatively

Nursing diagnoses/goals/interventions*

ndx: Potential disturbance in self-concept related to body image change and value of reproductive organs

GOAL: *Patient will verbalize acceptance of altered body image and will confirm that she has shared her feelings with partner*

Encourage patient's comments and questions about surgery, progress, and prognosis; reinforce correct information and provide factual information to correct any misconceptions

---

*See Ostomy Management and Care (p. 391) and Urinary Diversion (p. 542).

Relate importance of communicating anything that causes anxiety

Encourage patient to verbalize and explore feelings regarding what impact the missing body part might have on assuming ADLs
- Encourage patient to look at and touch the changed body part
- Encourage use of rehabilitation services (e.g., ostomy club, wellness community, etc.)

ndx: Knowledge deficit regarding home care management

GOAL: *Patient and/or significant other will demonstrate understanding of home care and follow-up instructions through interactive discussion and actual return demonstration*

Demonstrate ostomy care
Demonstrate uirinary diversion care
Demonstrate wound irrigation procedure: give written instructions
Explain importance of sitz baths bid and prn
Discuss symptoms of wound infection to report to physician
- Unusual odor and/or discharge
- Fresh bleeding
- Unusual pain
- Elevated temperature above 100° F (37.8° C)
- Upper respiratory infection (URI)
- Increased swelling at groin or elsewhere

Relate that antiembolic stockings or supportive hosiery may be indicated
Explain importance of exercise and activity to tolerance; caution patient to avoid prolonged sitting
Explain need to plan rest periods
Explain need for high-protein, high-carbohydrate diet
Relate that estrogen therapy may be indicated
Relate that referrals may be indicated for Visiting Nurses Association, social service worker, clergy, or ostomy association
Relate that counseling for sexually active woman and her partner is available
- Functional vagina may be possible; check with physician
- Alternate methods of achieving sexual satisfaction can be explored

Teach name of medication, dosage, time of administration, purpose, and side effects
Emphasize importance of follow-up outpatient care

Evaluation

There are no complications
Pain is controlled
Intake and output are balanced
Patient verbalizes understanding of home care management instructions
Patient demonstrates adaptive response related to self-concept and sexuality

CARE OF PATIENT RECEIVING RADIUM (CESIUM) THERAPY SEALED IN A MOULD, AFTERLOADER, COLPOSTAT, OR ERNST APPLICATOR

Sealed source of radiation is inserted through the vagina and left in place for a specific length of time to treat cancer of the cervix

Preinsertion teaching and care

Give low-residue diet as ordered
Administer bowel sedatives as ordered
Assess for potential problems with skin care and positioning
Give povidone-iodine douche as ordered
Administer enemas until clear as ordered
Insert indwelling bladder catheter as ordered
Explain need for bed rest; that head of bed may be elevated slightly
Explain importance of
- Low-residue diet
- Bowel sedation
- Reporting pain
- Private room and limited visitors
- Minimal exposure to nursing staff

Explain that pain will be managed
Place patient in private room
Place needed items within patient's reach

Postinsertion assessment
Observations/findings

Anorexia
Nausea, vomiting
Diarrhea
Elevated temperature: over 100° F (37.8° C)
Abdominal distention
Dehydration
Tachycardia
Decreased BP
Rectal bleeding
Vaginal bleeding
Uterine contractions
Skin over pelvic area
- Red
- Blistered

Position of radium
Sensory deprivation

Potential complications

Profuse bleeding
Atelectasis
Oliguria
Hematuria

Postinsertion care

Place lead shield next to patient's pelvic area
Keep lead-lined container in room in case cesium is accidentally dislodged
Elevate head of bed 35 degrees
Maintain clear liquid diet; force fluids to 3000 ml daily unless contraindicated
Administer parenteral fluids
Measure intake and output
Manage pain; give analgesics
Administer bowel and other sedation
Check BP, P, and R, and oral temperature q4h
Give partial bath daily
    Wash hands, face, and upper chest
    Do not bathe below waist
    Do not give routine perineal or catheter care
    Do not rub back; may massage shoulders and neck
    Avoid routine linen change
Check position of radium q4h
    Notify physician and radiation officer if dislodged
    Wear rubber gloves
    Use long-handled (12-inch) forceps to retrieve
Check for vaginal and rectal bleeding q2h to 4h and prn; copious discharge is common
    Report bleeding to physician
    Change perineal pads only when necessary
If irrigating catheter has been placed in vagina, irrigate with bacteriostatic solution
Connect indwelling urethral catheter to closed gravity drainage system
    Note character of urine
    Report hematuria to physician
Use room deodorizer as needed
Keep all used linen and trash in room
Removal of radium
    Remove catheter as ordered; voiding measures may be necessary
    Maintain adequate fluid intake to 3000 ml daily unless contraindicated
    Douche as indicated
    Enema as indicated
    Shower
    Apply analgesic ointment to anal area as ordered
    Increase activity and ambulate without assistance prior to discharge

Nursing diagnoses/goals/interventions

ndx: Impaired physical mobility secondary to placement of afterloader

GOAL: *Patient will maintain skin integrity and musculoskeletal, cardiorespiratory, and psychosocial function*

Assist and teach patient to deep breathe q2h during the day and evening
Auscultate chest for breath sounds q2h to 4h
Assist with active ROM exercises to upper extremities q4h
Flex knees slightly and prop with pillow
Do *not* turn patient from side to side; tilt shoulders and prop with pillow q1h to 2h
Cautiously change perineal pad *only* when necessary
Provide emotional support
    Visit often for short periods of time
    Encourage verbalization of fears
    Provide diversional activities
        Reading
        Watching television
    Encourage family visits for short periods (exclude pregnant visitors and children); encourage communication with significant other
Place needed items within patient's reach

ndx: Knowledge deficit regarding home care management

GOAL: *Patient and/or significant other will demonstrate understanding of home care and follow-up instructions through interactive discussion and actual return demonstration*

Explain need to maintain diet as ordered
Explain importance of drinking fluids to 3000 ml daily unless contraindicated
Relate that isolation will end as soon as radium is removed and that patient is not radioactive once radium is removed
Explain need to exercise to tolerance; to plan rest periods
Instruct patient to douche daily if vaginal discharge is present
Discuss symptoms to report to physician
    Vaginal bleeding
    Rectal bleeding
    Stool or urine from vagina
    Foul-smelling vaginal discharge
    Abdominal distention
    Abdominal pain
    Nausea, vomiting, or diarrhea
    Elevated temperature

Hematuria
Signs of menopause

Instruct patient to shower daily (avoid extremes in water temperature)

Caution patient to avoid exposure of pelvic area to direct sunlight; instruct patient to apply lanolin-based cream or baby oil to dry areas

Relate that sterilization and cessation of menses usually occur

Relate that sexual intercourse may be resumed 6 weeks after course of treatment has ended or as indicated by physician

Demonstrate method of using vaginal dilator if ordered

Instruct patient on how to prevent urinary tract infection (UTI)

Caution patient to avoid constipation

Emphasize importance of follow-up outpatient care

Evaluation

There are no complications
Body hydration is normal
Perineal skin integrity has been maintained
Patient demonstrates adaptive psychosocial behavior

MODIFIED RADICAL MASTECTOMY

Surgical removal of the entire breast, axillary lymph nodes, and all fat, fascia, and adjacent tissues as treatment for carcinoma

Preoperative observations

Emotional aberrations related to feelings of
    Loss of femininity
    Fear of mutilation and death

Preoperative care

See General Preoperative Care/Teaching (p. 29)
Provide emotional support
    Encourage verbalization of fears
    Encourage communication with significant other
    Avoid false reassurances
    Help anticipate future
    Arrange for visit from Reach for Recovery, Inc.
Explain that arm will feel tight after surgery

Postoperative assessment
Observations/findings

Hemorrhage
Edema of affected arm: lymphedema
Atelectasis
Emotional/behavioral changes related to
    Anxiety
    Depression
    Anger
    Withdrawal
    Feeling of hopelessness
    Body image change
Incision: skin donor site; nipple-grafted site
    Redness
    Pain
    Swelling
    Drainage
Wound drains
    Sump drain
    Hemovac or Jackson-Pratt

Potential complications

Hemorrhagic shock
Infection
Brachial plexus damage
    Contractures
    Shortening of muscles
Pneumonia

Immediate postoperative care

Place patient in position of comfort
Administer parenteral fluids as ordered; *avoid drawing blood from or administering parenteral fluids in affected arm*
Administer oral fluids as ordered
Measure intake and output; empty wound drains and measure drainage q8h and prn
Assist and teach patient to turn, cough, and deep breathe q2h
    Alternate back and unaffected side
    Support chest when coughing
Auscultate chest for breath sounds q4h
Check BP, T, P, and R q4h for 48 hr, then qid; *take BP in unaffected arm only*
Reinforce dressing prn; report excessive drainage or blood to physician
Apply pressure dressing as necessary
    Check color, sensation, and motion in fingers and hand q1h to 8h as indicated; notify physician of impaired color, sensation, or motion
    Do not release pressure dressing
If skin graft is done
    Check donor site q4h
    Reinforce dressing prn
    Notify physician if drainage is excessive
If nipple has been relocated pending future cosmetic surgery, check site q1h to 2h as ordered and perform care as explicitly as ordered by plastic surgeon
Control pain with analgesics

Perform wrist and elbow ROM exercises; gradually abduct arm and gradually raise arm over head
Ambulate prn
Monitor edema present in affected arm; measure upper arm and forearm bid

Convalescent management

Maintain progressive diet
Encourage oral fluids to 2500 ml daily unless contraindicated
Ambulate on first postoperative day
Assist and teach arm exercises qid
    Gradually increase extent of exercises daily
    Perform hand exercises: alternately clench and extend fingers
Involve patient in care; encourage use of affected arm to wash face, brush teeth, and eat
Provide physical therapy as indicated
Notify Reach to Recovery, Inc.

Nursing diagnoses/goals/interventions

ndx: Potential disturbance in self-concept related to body image change and value of reproductive organs

GOAL: *Patient will verbalize acceptance of altered body image and will confirm that she has shared her feelings with partner*

Encourage patient's comments and questions about surgery, progress, and prognosis
Reinforce correct information and provide factual information to correct any misconceptions
Relate importance of communicating anything that causes anxiety
Encourage patient to verbalize and explore feelings regarding what impact missing body part might have on assuming ADLs
Encourage patient to look at and touch the changed body part
Encourage use of rehabilitation services (e.g., Reach for Recovery, wellness community, etc.)

ndx: Knowledge deficit regarding home care management

GOAL: *Patient and/or significant other will demonstrate understanding of home care and follow-up instructions through interactive discussion and actual return demonstration*

Explain importance of exercise to tolerance; instruct patient to stop at point of pain
Discuss types of prostheses available
Discuss types of reconstruction available
Teach care of incision
Discuss symptoms to report to physician
    Redness
    Pain
    Swelling
    Drainage
    Elevated temperature
Emphasize need to gradually resume housekeeping duties
Explain that incision and/or chest wall may feel numb
Instruct patient to shower daily
Have patient check with physician regarding use of deodorant under affected arm
Instruct patient to examine remaining breast once a month
Caution patient to avoid allowing *blood to be drawn from or IV to be started in affected arm*
Caution patient to avoid injections, vaccinations, and taking of BP in affected arm
Instruct patient to carry handbag with unaffected arm
Relate that sexual activity may be resumed when desired; position of partner should avoid any pressure on chest wall
Refer patient to Visiting Nurses Association as needed
Emphasize importance of follow-up outpatient care

Evaluation

There are no complications
Pain is controlled and minimized
Intake and output are balanced
Patient verbalizes understanding of home care management instructions
Patient demonstrates adaptive response related to self-concept and sexuality

CHAPTER 11

Integumentary System

INTEGUMENTARY SYSTEM ASSESSMENT

Subjective Data

Skin
  Itching
  Pain
  Rash
  Oily
  Dry
  Rough
  Bumpy
  Thin
  Peeling
  Puffy
  Blisters
  Hot
  Cold
  Changes in skin color
  Liver spots: aging spots
  Boils

Objective Data

Skin
  Color
    Cyanosis
      Lips
      Circumoral area
      Mucous membranes
      Earlobes
      Nail beds
    Jaundice: sclera
    Plethora
    Pallor: conjunctiva, nail beds
    Pigmentation distribution
  Turgor
  Elasticity
  Intactness
  Rashes
  Moisture
  Temperature
  Cleanliness
  Odor
  Edema
  Needle marks
  Insect bites
  Scabies
  Acne, calluses, corns
  Exudate
  Uremic frost: beard, eyebrows
  Sclerema
  Striae
  Pressure areas over bony prominences
  Decubitus ulcers
Nails
  Cleanliness
  Brittleness
  Condition of surrounding tissue
  Clubbing of fingers and toes
  Lines
  Ram's horn shape: turning under fingertip
  Spoon shape: concave
Hair
  Distribution and configuration
  Texture
  Color
  Quantity
  Parasites
  Alopecia
Lesions
  Macula
    Flat
    Discolored
  Papule
    Elevated
    Discolored
  Exanthema
    Macular
    Papular
  Vesicle
    Blister
    Serous exudate
  Pustule
    Blister
    Purulent exudate
  Bulla
    Large blister

Serous or purulent exudate
Crusts: dried exudate
Scales: flakes of dead epidermis
Hive
  Swollen
  Hot
  Raised
  Itchy
Wart
  Elevated
  Brown
Mole
  Flat or raised
  Excessive pigment
Comedo: blackhead
Chancre
  Small
  Hard or ulcerated
Excoriation: break
Ulcer: necrosis
Cicatrix: scar
Keloid: excessive tissue formation around lesion or scar
Petechia
  Small
  Bright red
  Flat
Lipoma: subcutaneous fatty lump
Nodule
Fissure
Telangiectasia
Erosion

Pertinent Background Information
FAMILY HISTORY AND CONCURRENT DISEASES

Allergies
Exposures to external allergens
  Cosmetics
  Soaps
  Medication
  Plants
Exposures to internal allergens
  Drugs
  Food
Travel history
Exposure to parasites
Response to sun

MEDICATION PRESENTLY BEING TAKEN

Injectable medication
Prescription medication
Over-the-counter medication
Creams, lotions, ointments
Hygienic practices
Sexual practices

Diagnostic Aids

Diagnosis of causative disease
Skin and lesion cultures
Electron microscopy
Diascopy
Immunofluorescence (I.F.)
Lupus erythematosus prep
Punch biopsies, cytology
Allergy skin testing
Blood culture
Skin scraping

DECUBITUS (PRESSURE) ULCER

An area of cellular necrosis, usually over a bony prominence, that results from tissue hypoxia due to pressure

Assessment
Observations/findings

Location of pressure area
  Ear rims
  Shoulder blades
  Elbows, heels
  Sacrum
  Hips
  Inner knee
  Outer ankle
Stage of Necrosis
  I: Transient circulatory disturbance; redness or blanching with pressure that disappears when pressure is removed
  II: Reddened or blanched area with no break in skin integrity
  III: Erythema and edema with blister and/or break in integrity
  IV: Full-thickness lesion extending to subcutaneous fat with or without serosanguinous drainage
  V: Full-thickness lesion extending to deep fascia muscle and bone
Immobility
Elevated temperature
Medical history (diabetes, carcinoma, anemia)
Pain, numbness
Nutritional status
Age, weight, mental acuity

Laboratory/diagnostic studies

Lesion culture
Complete blood cell count (CBC), electrolytes
Serum albumin

Potential complications

Infection
Further necrosis

Medical management

Diet, topical antibiotics, ointments, powders
Surgical debridement

Nursing diagnoses/goals/interventions

ndx: Potential impairment of skin integrity related to immobility

GOAL: *Patient's skin integrity will be maintained*

Preventive measures
   Maintain skin integrity by keeping skin clean and dry
   Perform skin care daily and prn
   Bathe with mild soap and warm water; remove powder and ointments
   Rinse skin thoroughly and pat dry
   Apply lotion to feet, elbows, and back, and massage gently
   Administer perineal care following elimination
   Turn patient q2h: side, back, to side
   Assess and monitor pressure points qid and prn
   Assist and teach patient to change position slightly every 30 to 60 min to avoid pressure and fatigue
   Maintain clean, comfortable bed with wrinkle-free sheets
   Lift patient with turn sheet; avoid sliding
   Administer back rubs and massage bony prominences with lanolin-based lotion; avoid alcohol
   Prevent and eliminate pressure and friction by placing pillows between pressure areas (knees, ankles)
   Prevent pressure with the following devices
     Alternating pressure mattress
     Convoluted (egg-crate) mattress
     Flotation mattress
     Sheepskin
     Silicone pads
     Heel and elbow guards
   Assist with and teach active or perform passive range-of-motion (ROM) exercises to all extremities q4h
   Increase activity as allowed: assist patient out of bed and into chair; avoid sitting for more than 30 min; alternate chairs

ndx: Actual impairment of skin integrity related to pressure ulcer (Stages I, II, III)

GOAL: *Patient's skin will return to optimal integrity, and further necrosis and infection will be prevented*

Assess skin and identify stage of ulcer development
Involve enterostomal therapist if available
Eliminate causative factors and initiate appropriate ulcer care
   Cleanse area at least q8h with mild soap and water and pat dry
   Massage area gently to increase circulation; avoid vigorous rubbing
   Expose area to sunlight and air q2h to 4h or to heat lamp qd for 15 min; observe area frequently to prevent burning
   Position patient on unaffected areas
Protect skin surface and affected area with one of, or combination of, the following
   Apply Karaya powder lightly; dust off excess
   Apply skin prep/skin gel
   Cover area with moisture-permeable adhesive or wafer barrier
   Apply Granulex spray q8h or commercial fat pad according to manufacturer's directions
   Continue one type of application, or combination, for 48 to 72 hr; if improvement is apparent, continue applications; if no improvement is noted, begin another type of treatment

ndx: Actual impairment of skin integrity related to pressure ulcer (Stages IV and V)

GOAL: *Patient's skin integrity will return to optimal level following cleansing routine and/or debridement of ulcer*

Assess ulcer for size, color, odor, and amount and type of drainage
Monitor temperature for elevation
Culture ulcer as needed
Continue applications to promote healing
If healing is not evident, prepare for debridement as ordered
Following debridement, change dressings as ordered
Administer antibiotics as ordered
Involve enterostomal therapist

ndx: Alteration in nutrition: more than body requirements related to promotion of ulcer healing

GOAL: *Patient's nutritional intake will be increased to promote wound healing and prevent further loss of skin integrity*

Assess patient's ability to chew and swallow food, determine dietary preferences, and provide appropriate type of diet
Explain diet rationale to patient and the need for high-protein, high-carbohydrate foods to promote healing
Offer frequent small feedings on attractive trays
Administer vitamins and daily mineral supplements as ordered
Increase fluid intake to 2500 ml/day if not contraindicated
Weigh patient daily at same time with same clothing and scale
Monitor CBC, electrolytes, and serum albumin
Measure intake and output q8h

ndx: Knowledge deficit regarding home management and care

GOAL: *Patient and/or significant other will demonstrate understanding of home care and follow-up instructions through interactive discussion and actual return demonstration*

Provide written instructions for ulcer care
Demonstrate cleansing procedure and application of medication and dressings as ordered; observe return demonstrations
Explain dietary regimen and provide written instructions
Stress importance of daily weights
Discuss signs and symptoms to report to physician
 Weight loss
 Increased drainage from ulcer
 Foul odor from dressing
 Further necrosis around ulcer
 Reddened areas at other pressure points
Explain importance of increasing activity as tolerated, of changing positions frequently while in bed, and of avoiding pressure on affected area
Promote follow-up visits with physician

Evaluation

There are no complications
Skin integrity is improving
Nutritional intake is adequate for age, weight, and healing process
Home care management is understood

CELLULITIS

An acute streptococcal, staphylococcal infection of the skin and subcutaneous tissue, usually due to bacterial invasion through a broken area in the skin; however, it may occur with no site of entry evident, and it usually occurs on the lower extremities

Assessment

Observations/findings

Localized pain, redness, swelling, tenderness of skin
Lymphangitic streaks
Skin resembling skin of orange (peau d'orange)
Presence of open wound
Amount, color, odor of drainage
Fever, chills, malaise
Headache, tachycardia
Hypotension
Leukocytosis

Laboratory/diagnostic studies

CBC: increased white blood cell count (WBC), eosinophils, lymphocytes
Erythrocyte sedimentation rate (ESR) increased
Cultures: lesion and blood

Potential complications

Systemic infection
Ulceration

Medical management

Antibiotics, analgesics, antipyretics
Position and immobilization of extremity
Alternate cool/warm compresses

Nursing diagnoses/goals/interventions

ndx: Actual impairment of skin integrity related to altered turgor, circulation, and edema

GOAL: *Patient's skin integrity will return to optimal level, and further infection/involvement will be prevented*

Maintain bed rest with extremity elevated and immobilized as ordered
Assess area for ulceration or skin breaks
 Apply sterile dressings as ordered
 Administer compresses as ordered
 Maintain aseptic techniques and wound isolation
Administer antibiotics as ordered
Monitor temperature q4h; administer antipyretic as ordered

ndx: Alteration in comfort: pain related to tissue inflammation

GOAL: *Patient will express minimal discomfort or absence of pain*

Maintain affected extremity in ordered position
Explain need for immobilization for 48 to 72 hr
Administer analgesic as ordered
Change position frequently, maintaining alignment, to prevent pressure and fatigue
Promote diversional activities
Encourage active ROM exercises to unaffected extremities

ndx: Knowledge deficit regarding home care management

GOAL: *Patient and/or significant other will demonstrate understanding of home care and follow-up instructions through interactive discussion and actual return demonstration*

Demonstrate wound care and dressing-change procedure; stress importance of aseptic technique
Discuss maintaining elevation and immobilization of extremity as ordered
Encourage activity to tolerance utilizing supportive devices: sling, crutches
Explain signs and symptoms to report to physician
  Wound pain or increased drainage
  Fever, chills, headache
  Odor from dressings and wound
Discuss medication schedule, including name, purpose, dosage, and side effects
Stress importance of nutritional diet to promote wound healing
Promote follow-up visits with physician

Evaluation

There are no complications
Skin integrity is improving
Mobility is regained to optimal level
Home care is understood

HERPES TYPE 1 VIRAL INFECTION

An infection caused by the herpes simplex virus; the virus usually infects the skin, especially the facial area around the nose and mouth, and the nervous system; less frequently, the eye is infected; herpes viruses are extremely contagious, may remain latent, and can be reactivated by a variety of stimuli

Assessment
Observations/findings

Early sensations at edges of lips or nose or other site of contact
  Pruritus
  Paresthesia
  Anesthetic sensation
  Feeling of pressure
  Pulselike throb
  Tingling sensation
  Ache
Later observations
  Red macules
  Fluid-filled vesicles (fever blisters)
  Bullae
  Yellow-crusted lesions
  Necrotic areas
Generalized symptoms
  Chills
  Elevated temperature
  Headache
  Lymphadenopathy
Herpes keratitis
  Feeling of having something in the eye
  Irritation
  Photophobia
  Pain
  Conjunctivitis
  Lesions on eyeball
Herpes encephalitis
  Flulike symptoms
  Personality change
  Speech difficulties
  Motor difficulties
  Seizures
  Coma

Laboratory/diagnostic studies

Pap smear or Tzanck test positive
Tissue culture positive

Potential complications

Recurrent infection

Medical management

Zoster immune globulin or plasma
Acyclovir: ointment or parenteral
Vidarabine
Idoxuridine

Nursing diagnoses/goals/interventions

ndx: Impairment of skin integrity related to contagious lesions

GOAL: *Patient will exhibit healing of lesions, which will remain localized*

Initiate procedure for wound and skin precautions

Wear gloves when contact is made at site of lesions or with secretions, especially if performing any suctioning techniques or applying medication

Instruct patient not to touch lesions or secretions and to wear gloves when washing face or performing oral care

Use disposable dishes and utensils

Teach and assist with oral care q2h to 4h

Gently wash lesions

Apply acyclovir ointment as ordered (½-inch ribbon per 4 square inches of surface is usually ordered)

Apply ice to lesions for local management of pain

Assess condition of skin, mucous membranes, or eyes for extension of infection q8h

Check T q4h; report elevation

Keep patient dry; avoid chills

Administer antipyretics and antibiotics as ordered

Administer acyclovir IV as ordered

Provide soft, bland diet for oral lesions
- Avoid hot, spicy, or acidic foods
- Provide cool or iced liquids and flavored ice pops
- Straws are usually helpful to avoid contact with lesions

Wash crusts (if present) from eyes with clear water; dry gently

Administer vidarabine or idoxuridine as ordered for herpes keratitis

ndx: Knowledge deficit regarding disease process, precautions, and home care

GOAL: *Patient will verbalize understanding of home care instructions and demonstrate skin or eye care procedures, and temperature taking and reading*

Disease process

Explain about infective virus transmission, reactivation, symptoms to report to physician, and importance of avoiding persons with herpes viral infections, "flu," or chickenpox

Precautions

Instruct patient to wash hands prior to care

Have patient wear gloves or finger cots when cleaning or applying medication to affected area to avoid autoinfection or infection of others

Explain need to keep materials for cleaning lesions separate: towels, cloths, soap; launder after each use or use disposables

Explain need to keep dishes and utensils separate; to wash immediately after use; to consider use of disposables

Advise patient to keep toothbrush away from others and use own dentrifrice

Caution patient to avoid direct contact with others (i.e., kissing) from time of early symptoms until lesions have completely healed

Care

Instruct patient to wash skin area with soap and water or eye with clear water; dry gently

Explain need to perform oral care q2h to 4h while awake; to rinse mouth and lips well; to dry gently

Demonstrate how to apply medication as ordered

Instruct patient to always use gloves when touching infected area

Demonstrate how to take temperature; instruct patient to report elevations

Evaluation

Lesions remain localized, are healed, or are in process of healing; no symptoms are noted in other areas

Patient demonstrates cleaning of and medication application to affected areas, and follows procedure for taking temperature and reading thermometer

HERPES ZOSTER (SHINGLES)

Acute viral infection characterized by crops of vesicles, usually confined to a specific nerve tract, and by neuralgic pain in the affected nerve area; may be the response of a partially immune host to the varicella virus; severity of symptoms is in direct relationship to age

Assessment
Observations/findings

Preeruptive phase (last days of 7- to 21-day incubation period)
- Pain along involved nerve tract
- Malaise
- Fever
- Anorexia
- History of recent trauma to area or exposure to chickenpox

Posteruptive phase
- Raised, papular, reddened vesicles along affected nerve tract unilaterally
- Pain, itching along tract
- Regional lymph node enlargement
- Ruptured vesicles, necrosis

Areas of involvement
- Sacral nerve
  - Neuralgia

Transient paralysis of affected limb
Permanent weakness of affected limb
Trigemenal nerve
    Keratitis
    Uveitis
    Corneal scarring
Facial nerve: paralysis of facial muscles
Thoracic nerve: neuralgia

Laboratory/diagnostic studies

Culture of vesicles
CBC, electrolytes, ESR
Pregnancy test
Chest x-ray examination
Spinal fluid analysis

Potential complications

Malnutrition
Dehydration
Bacterial infection of vesicles
Central nervous system (CNS) inflammation
Pneumonia

Medical management

Analgesics, topical anesthetics, corticosteroids, gamma globulin, barbiturates, antihistamines, antibiotics
Ganglia nerve block
Warm saline compresses
Specific vesicle care
Transcutaneous electrical nerve stimulation (TENS) unit

Nursing diagnoses/goals/interventions

ndx Alteration in comfort: pain related to disease process

GOAL: *Patient will express minimal discomfort or absence of pain*

Assess location, type, and severity of pain
Administer analgesics and sedatives as ordered; assess effectiveness of pain relief measures
Administer corticosteroids, antihistamines, and topical anesthetics as ordered
Apply cool compresses/sprays as ordered
Change position frequently to prevent pressure and fatigue; avoid pressure on affected areas
Promote diversional activities

ndx Impairment of skin integrity related to pruritus and skin lesions

GOAL: *Patient's skin will return to normal integrity, and areas of involvement will decrease*

Assess areas of involvement for color, drainage, odor, and size
Administer warm tub baths with baking soda or Burow's solution
Avoid rubbing skin and extremes in temperature
Pat skin dry with soft towel
Apply medications as ordered
Promote wearing loose garments and provide bed cradle as indicated
Cleanse lesions as ordered; keep affected areas dry and dressing-free except when compresses are in place

ndx Potential for infection related to inadequate primary defense; skin lesions

GOAL: *Patient's skin lesions will heal, and further infection will be prevented*

Provide protective isolation as indicated
Dispose of dressings, linen, etc., according to hospital policy
Explain and teach handwashing technique
Advise patient not to scratch lesions
Monitor vital signs q4h
Observe for signs of complications
    Neuromuscular disturbance
    Eye involvement
    Pneumonia
    Bacterial infection
Obtain lesion and blood cultures as applicable
Administer antibiotics as ordered

ndx Alteration in nutrition: less than body requirements related to anorexia/malaise

GOAL: *Patient's nutritional intake will be adequate to meet body requirements*

Provide diet high in protein and carbohydrates to promote healing
Serve food attractively in six small meals
Assist patient with menu selection and explain which foods will promote healing
Weigh patient biweekly at same time with same clothing and scale
Force fluids to 2000 ml/day unless contraindicated
Measure intake and output

ndx Ineffective individual coping related to longevity of neuralgia and/or sequelae

GOAL: *Patient will express understanding of disease process and required treatment, and move toward positive coping behavior*

Reinforce physician's explanation of disease and rationale of treatment; clarify misconceptions
Explain that one attack generally confers immunity
Explain and discuss methods of pain management: position, medications, TENS unit, loose-fitting garments
Assess present coping patterns and assist patient with identifying positive patterns from past experience
Encourage and allow time for verbalization of concerns and feelings; include significant other

ndx: Knowledge deficit regarding home care management

GOAL: *Patient and/or significant other will demonstrate understanding of home care management through interactive discussion and actual return demonstration*

Provide nutritional information and need for increased fluid intake
Explain and demonstrate care of pruritis/lesions
Discuss importance of exercise/activity to maintain strength, and rest to promote healing
Explain medication schedule, including name, dosage, purpose, and side effects, and caution patient to avoid over-the-counter medications without physician's permission
Discuss signs and symptoms to report to physician
　Increased pain
　Fever
　Exacerbation of pruritis

Evaluation

There are no complications
Lesions are healed or are healing
Nutrition and fluid intake are adequate
Positive coping behavior is demonstrated
Home care management is understood

CARE OF PATIENT WITH BURNS

Classification of Burns
PARTIAL THICKNESS

First degree: epidermis is red, with no blister formation
Second degree: epidermal and dermal layers are blistered, with subcutaneous edema and pain

FULL THICKNESS

Third degree: all layers of skin are involved, and fat, muscle, nerves, and blood supply may be affected
Fourth degree: all layers of skin, fat, muscle, nerves, blood supply, and bone are involved

Assessment: full-thickness burns
Observations/findings

Percentage of body surface involved (Figure 11-1)
Classification and anatomic location
Age of patient
Cause of burn
　Hot liquid: usually partial thickness
　Flame: some areas may be full thickness
　Explosion: may be full or partial thickness
　Chemical: difficult to evaluate
　Electrical: usually full thickness
History of preexisting illness
Other body trauma
　Fractures
　Deep tissue destruction
　Respiratory tract trauma
　Respiratory distress due to toxic inhalation
　Hypotension, tachycardia, shock
　Presence of pain

Laboratory/diagnostic studies

CBC, electrolytes, serum albumin, oxyhemoglobin
Arterial blood gases, glucose
Urinalysis for hemoglobin, albumin, glucose, acetone, specific gravity
Chest and body radiology, bronchoscopy, lung scan
Electrocardiogram (ECG)

Potential complications

Hyponatremia (first 48 hr)
Hypernatremia (after 48 hr)
Hyperkalemia (first 48 hr)
Hypokalemia (after 48 hr)
Hypoproteinemia
Dehydration
Hypoxia
Circulatory collapse
Hematuria, oliguria
Anemia
Adult respiratory distress syndrome (ARDS)
Gastric atony
Septic shock
Curling's ulcer (as early as first week; as late as ninth week)
Fecal impaction
Emotional shock
Disseminated intravascular coagulation (DIC)

	Age in years					
	0	1	5	10	15	Adult
A, One half of head	9½	8½	6½	5½	4½	3½
B, One half of one thigh	2¾	3¼	4	4¼	4½	4¾
C, One half of one leg	2½	2½	2¾	3	3¼	3½

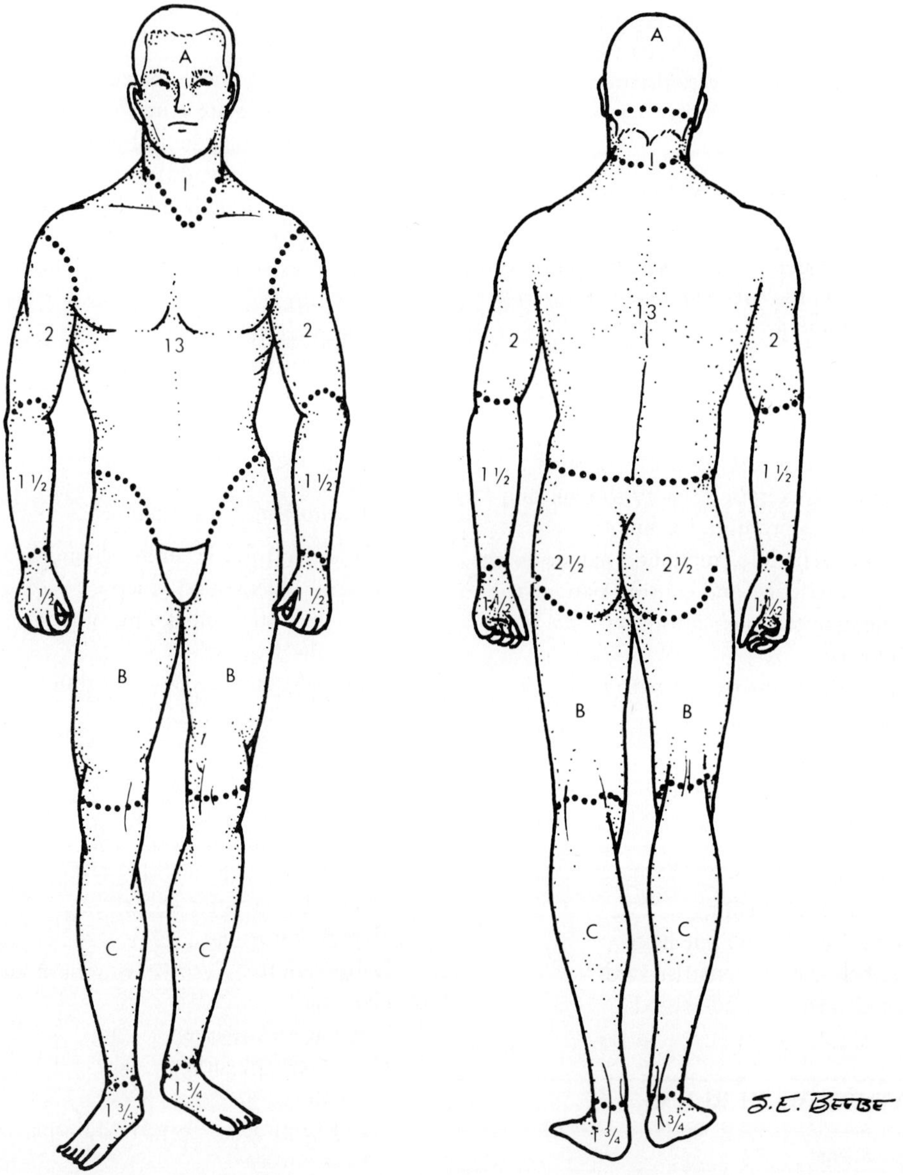

FIGURE 11-1. Calculation of percentage of burn surface.

Medical management

Narcotics, sedatives, analgesics, insulin, tetanus
Broncholytic agents, steroids, diuretics, antacids
Antibiotics, vasodilators
Oxygen therapy, postural drainage, tracheal aspiration
Mechanical ventilation, endotracheal tube
Parenteral fluids with electrolytes and vitamins
Hemodynamic monitoring
Transfusion/plasma
Nasogastric aspiration/indwelling urinary catheter
Diet, total parenteral nutrition (TPN), fluid-replacement formula
Burn care, hydrotherapy, physiotherapy
Escharotomy, fasciotomy
Skin graft

Nursing diagnoses/goals/interventions

ndx: Ineffective airway clearance related to inhalation of smoke/heat

GOAL: *Patient's airway will be maintained, and arterial blood gas levels will remain adequate*

Assess respiratory status qh; observe for decreased breath sounds, tachypnea, dyspnea, cough, pallor, and cyanosis
Monitor arterial blood gases (ABGs) as needed
Maintain patent airway; perform orotracheal suction as needed; place patient on mechanical ventilation as ordered
Assist patient with turning and coughing q2h and deep breathing qh
Administer oxygen therapy as ordered
Administer broncholytic agents as ordered

ndx: Actual fluid volume deficit related to abnormal fluid loss (first 48 hr)

GOAL: *Patient's fluid volume and intake will be adequate to meet body requirements*

Maintain NPO
Administer parenteral fluids with electrolytes as ordered
Administer blood transfusions as ordered
Monitor intake and output carefully
Connect indwelling catheter to closed gravity drainage system as ordered
Measure output qh; report less than 30 to 50 ml/hr in adults; 1 to 1.5 ml/kg/hr in children
  Observe for hematuria; monitor with Hemastix
  Monitor specific gravity
Monitor central venous pressure (CVP) line q1h to 2h
Administer diuretics as ordered
Connect nasogastric tube to low, intermittent suction apparatus as ordered; irrigate gently with measured amounts of normal saline as ordered; observe drainage for amount, consistency, and color
Weigh patient daily at same time with same clothing and scale

ndx: Alteration in tissue perfusion related to decreased circulating blood volume

GOAL: *Patient's cardiac output/tissue perfusion will be maintained*

Monitor vital signs q1h to 2h (first 48 hr); observe for signs of reduced cardiac output, changes in sensorium, neurologic deficits, and renal disturbance
Place patient on cardiac monitor if applicable
Administer vasodilators as ordered
Monitor CBC

ndx: Actual impairment of skin integrity related to full-thickness burn

GOAL: *Patient's destroyed skin will return to optimal integrity*

Implement isolation precautions as ordered
Initiate local burn therapy using the following principles; these are general considerations
  Culture burn areas
  Cleanse burn and remove all pieces of detached epithelium; cleanse with saline or mild soap and tap water (hexachlorophene is not recommended)
  Debride, using sterile equipment
    Remove dirt and blood
    Break blisters
    Shave surrounding area
  Prevent destruction of viable epithelium
  Produce environment unfavorable to bacterial growth
  Aid separation of burn slough
  Apply skin coverage as soon as possible
Initiate one of the following burn care methods as ordered
  Open air–exposure method
    Maintain isolation with sterile linen, gloves, and masks
    Monitor humidity and temperature of room to maintain comfort
    Provide bed cradle with warm covering
    Bathe only unaffected areas
    Observe burns for exudate
    Culture burns q5 to 7 days
  Silver nitrate method

Remove dressings daily; observe for infection
Administer tap water tub bath with electrolytes and mild detergent
Debride loose epithelium
Apply dressings moistened with silver nitrate 0.5% solution; keep saturated with solution q3h to 4h or as ordered
Culture burn q5 to 7 days
   Monitor serum electrolytes and calcium
Silver sulfadiazine 1% (Silvadene) method
   Administer tub bath biweekly
   Debride loose epithelium
   Allow burn area to air dry
   Apply thick layer of silver sulfadiazine with sterile tongue blade and gloves
   Place mesh dressing as needed to keep ointment in place
   Monitor serum chloride and pH
Skin graft method
   Homograft: from deceased person
   Autograft: from unburned area
   Heterograft: pigskin or synthetic
   Autologous: epithelium cells cultured into sheets
   Maintain graft site per physician's order
   Change dressings as ordered
   Culture burn area weekly

ndx: Potential for infection related to inadequate primary defenses; lack of skin integrity

GOAL: *Patient will remain infection free or infection will be managed*

Maintain isolation precautions and initiate aseptic technique
Monitor vital signs and electrolytes
Observe for signs of infection: monitor burn for amount, color, and odor of drainage
Monitor invasive hemodynamic monitoring lines for infection
Culture exudate as ordered
Administer antibiotics as ordered
Limit visitors to patient's significant others, especially exclude people with upper respiratory infections (URIs)
Monitor and observe for abdominal distention and decreased bowel sounds
Monitor urine for sugar, acetone, and hematuria
Observe mental acuity

ndx: Impaired physical mobility related to burn hypertrophy and possible contractures

GOAL: *Patient's mobility will be maintained to optimal level, and contractures will be prevented*

Maintain bed rest with affected extremity elevated and immobilized as ordered
Monitor neuromuscular status q2h to 4h
Maintain body alignment within parameters of treatment
Prevent contractures and/or hypertrophy
   Head and neck: do not use pillows (Figure 11-2)
   Hand (Figure 11-3)
   Upper chest, axilla, and arms (Figure 11-4): maintain arm at 90-degree angle, away from body and slightly above shoulder
   Ankles and feet (Figure 11-5): use footboard with patient in supine position
   Legs: traction/splints may be used
Explain necessity of positions, since they can be uncomfortable; position of comfort can be position of contracture
Assist with and teach active or perform passive ROM exercises on unaffected extremities
Coordinate care to allow for rest periods
Encourage patient to perform self-care activities
Change position frequently to prevent fatigue and pressure; CircOlectric bed may be required
Refer patient for physiotherapy and/or hydrotherapy as ordered
Ambulate as soon as possible

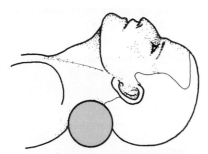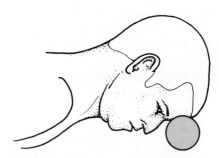

FIGURE 11-2. Head and neck burns.

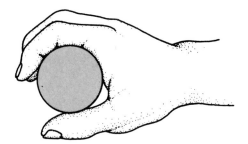

FIGURE 11-3. Hand burns.

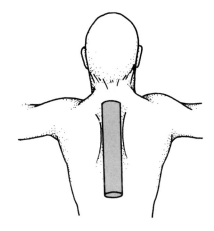

FIGURE 11-4. Upper chest, axilla, and arm burns.

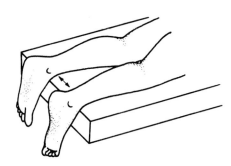

FIGURE 11-5. Ankle and foot burns.

ndx Alteration in nutrition related to increased body requirements

GOAL: *Patient's nutritional intake will be increased to promote healing and meet body requirements*

Calculate and initiate fluid replacement formula as ordered (p. 630)
Provide high-protein, high-calorie diet as ordered and tolerated
  Protein: 3g/kg/day
  Fat: 20% of calories
  Carbohydrate: remainder of calories

Administer supplemental vitamin therapy as ordered
Provide attractive trays in frequent small meals
Encourage oral fluids as ordered: milk, juice, carbonated beverages; no water if burns are covered with cream or dressings
Administer TPN as ordered
Assist patient in menu selection; explain need for certain foods

ndx Alteration in comfort: pain related to burn therapy and required position

GOAL: *Patient will verbalize minimal discomfort or absence of pain*

Assess location, type, and severity of pain
Administer analgesics as ordered; assess effectiveness of pain relief measures; decrease narcotics as soon as possible
Perform dressing changes after patient is medicated and/or in hydrotherapy
Provide diversional activities

ndx Disturbance in self-concept related to body image change and lowered self-esteem

GOAL: *Patient will move toward body image acceptance and demonstrate positive coping behaviors and increased self-esteem*

Discuss and explain all care, treatments, and procedures
Maintain continuity of all care
Set realistic short-term goals and acknowledge tasks attempted and/or completed
Allow patient to progress through stages of grief at own pace
Encourage and allow time for verbalization of concerns/feelings; include significant others
Maintain nonjudgmental attitude and avoid nonverbal rejection
Assess present coping attitudes and assist patient with identifying successful past behaviors
Promote self-care activities as soon as possible
Involve patient with unit routine and other burn patients
Refer to social service agencies for financial, family, and educational assistance

ndx Knowledge deficit regarding home care management

GOAL: *Patient and/or significant other will demonstrate understanding of home care management through interactive discussion and actual return demonstration*

Provide written dietary instructions; discuss importance of maintaining normal weight
Explain rehabilitation plan and use of splints or other immobilizing devices
Discuss maintaining normal activity with planned rest periods
Demonstrate burn care as necessary; avoid sunlight, detergents, and fabric softeners
Explain symptoms to report to physician
  Fever, malaise
  Bleeding, odor, and drainage from burn area
Discuss medication schedule, including name, purpose, dosage, and side effects; caution patient to avoid over-the-counter medication unless approved by physician

Evaluation

There are no complications
Burns are healing or are healed
Nutrition is adequate
Patient demonstrates positive coping behaviors, and self-esteem is increasing
Home care is understood

Calculation of Fluid Replacement for Burns: Brooke Formula

NOTE: Many formulas are in use; Brooke formula is moderate and most frequently used

Calculation for adults

First 24 hr (calculated from time of burn, not admission)
  Colloids (blood, dextran, or plasma): 0.5 ml/kg/percentage body surface burned
  Lactated Ringer's solution: 1.5 ml/kg/percentage body surface burned
  Five percent dextrose in water: 2000 ml
  Half of each solution is to be given in the first 8 hr, a fourth in the second 8 hr, and a fourth in the third 8 hr
Second 24 hr
  Colloids (blood, dextran, or plasma): half the amount is given in the first 24 hr
  Lactated Ringer's solution: half the amount is given in the first 24 hr
  Five percent dextrose in water: 2000 ml

Calculation for children

First 24 hr (calculated from time of burn, not admission)
  Colloids (dextran or plasma; use blood cautiously): 0.5 ml/kg/percentage body surface burned
  Electrolyte solution (1:3 with 5% dextrose in water): 1.5 ml/kg/percentage body surface burned
Five percent dextrose in water
  Up to 2 years of age: 150 ml/kg
  2 to 5 years of age: 100 ml/kg
  5 to 8 years of age: 75 ml/kg
  8 to 12 years of age: 50 ml/kg

CHAPTER 12

Optic and Auditory Systems

Optic System

EYE ASSESSMENT

Subjective Data

Blurred or double vision
Light, flashes, rainbows, or halos seen
Decreased or absent vision
Decreased night or peripheral vision
Objects held too near or far
Collides with unfamiliar objects
Eye fatigue and strain
Tenderness or pain: sudden or gradual onset
Eyes water and itch
Trauma to head, face, or eyes
Inability to see in bright light
Headache
Squinting
Frequent falls
Head tilt
Clumsiness

Objective Data

General appearance
Age of patient
Vital signs: elevated BP, T, P, or R
Wears glasses, contact lenses, or eye patch
Position of reading material
Conjunctivitis
Drainage
  Amount
  Type
Hemorrhage
Rubbing eyes
Edema of eyelids
Amount of dependence or independence
Visual acuity
Exophthalmos
Ability to close eyelid(s)
Ability to blink
Abnormal eye movement
Opaqueness of eyeball
Amount of tearing

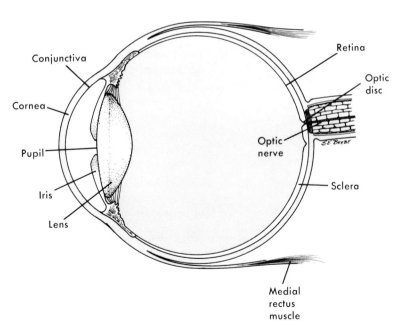

FIGURE 12-1. The eye.

631

Ptosis of eyelid(s)
Medication, eye drops used
Allergies
Strabismus
Nystagmus
Scleral edema, infection, jaundice
Chalazion
Foreign body
Laceration, contusion
Enucleation

Pertinent Background Information
CONCURRENT DISEASES OR CONDITIONS

Multiple sclerosis
Diabetes mellitus
Hypothyroidism
Hyperthyroidism
Sinus problems
Hypertension
Cerebral associated diseases, trauma, or tumors
Venereal disease
Myasthenia gravis
Glaucoma
Cataract
Retinal detachment

PREVIOUS SURGERY OR ILLNESS

Eye surgery or treatments
Head or face trauma
Oxygen therapy as newborn
Coma
Hypertension
Substance abuse
Retinal degeneration

FAMILY HISTORY

Glaucoma
Diabetes mellitus
Cataracts
Retinitis pigmentosa

SOCIAL HISTORY

Hazardous job or recreation
Safety precautions taken
Alcohol or drug abuse
Venereal disease

MEDICATION HISTORY

Antibiotics
Antiemetics
Miotics
Acetazolamide
Mydriatics

Diagnostic Aids
PROCEDURES

Visual fields and acuity
Incision and drainage
X-ray studies of orbit and skull
Ophthalmoscopic evaluation
Tonometry
FLuorescein angiography
Ultrasonography
Gonioscopy
Brain scan
Ultrasound
Electroretinogram (ERG)
Color vision test
Refraction
Microscopic procedures
Conjunctival scrapings

GLAUCOMA: ADULT ONSET

acute (narrow-angle) glaucoma Disease characterized by sudden impaired vision due to intraocular tension caused by imbalance in production and excretion of aqueous humor

chronic (wide-angle) glaucoma Disease characterized by impaired vision due to intraocular tension caused by an actual obstruction in the excretion of aqueous humor

Assessment
Observations/findings

Acute glaucoma
  Rapid onset of severe pain in eye(s)
  Blurred vision
  Headache
  Rainbows in artificial light
  Halos around lights
  Nausea, vomiting
  Dilated pupil(s)
Chronic glaucoma
  Insidious onset: generally no discomfort
  Gradual loss of peripheral vision
  Patient rarely admitted to hospital; seen only when admitted for some other reason

Laboratory/diagnostic studies

Tonometry
Gonioscopy
Visual fields

Potential complications

Infection
Increased intraocular pressure

Increased visual impairment
Blindness if untreated

Medical management

Myotic eye drops
Carbonic anhydrase inhibitors
Hyperosmotic agents
Antiemetics
Sympathomimetics
Beta-blockers
Analgesics

Nursing diagnoses/goals/interventions

ndx: Alteration in comfort: pain related to disease process

GOAL: *Patient will indicate that pain is reduced or alleviated*

Maintain bed rest in quiet, darkened room with head elevated 30 degrees or in position of comfort
Administer analgesics and other medications as ordered
Avoid nausea and vomiting; administer antiemetics as ordered
Assess visual acuity
Administer back rubs, position changes, and oral hygiene as indicated
Assess type and location of pain; be alert for signs of increased intraocular pressure

ndx: Anxiety related to hospitalization and loss of visual acuity

GOAL: *Patient will verbalize anxieties and demonstrate understanding of disease and disease process*

Provide emotional support
   Answer questions honestly
   Explain all procedures
   Reinforce physician's explanation of disease process and surgery if indicated
   Visit frequently, especially at night
   Explain nursing care plan
   Discuss visual limitations as needed
Place all needed articles within reach and strive to keep them in same place at all times
Assist with self-care as indicated and teach altered activities of daily living (ADLs)
Provide nutritious diet and adequate fluid intake as tolerated; assist with feeding as needed

ndx: Knowledge deficit regarding self-care and disease process

GOAL: *Patient and/or significant other will demonstrate understanding of disease process, and home and follow-up care through interactive discussion and actual return demonstration*

Teach eye drop instillation procedure to patient and significant other
   Always count drops and do not miss a dose
   Keep extra bottle of drops in case of loss or breakage
   Wear and carry medical alert band and card
   Never take medication containing atropine or over-the-counter medications
Discuss symptoms to report to physician
   Severe pain in eye(s)
   Blurred vision
   Headache
   Halos or rainbows
   Nausea, vomiting
Explain importance of follow-up care with physician

Evaluation

There are no complications
Intraocular pressure is stabilized
Patient demonstrates understanding of disease and disease process, and anxiety is reduced
Patient demonstrates ability to instill eye drops and performs self-care activities

EYE SURGERY

cataract removal with or without intraocular lens transplant Surgical removal of a lens that has become opaque due to senile degenerative changes, trauma, or systemic disease (diabetes) or a congenitally opaque lens; an intraocular lens may be implanted simultaneously as an alternative to wearing cataract glasses or contact lenses postoperatively

corneal transplant Surgical procedure to replace a damaged cornea with a healthy, clear donor cornea of equal size

scleral buckling, retinal cryopexy, photocoagulation Surgical repair of a detached retina

enucleation Surgical removal of a blind, painful eye globe while maintaining orbital integrity for insertion of a prosthesis

iridectomy, iridencleisis, trabeculectomy, sclerotomy Surgical incision to release accumulated pressure due to glaucoma by creating a channel for the drainage of the aqueous humor

radial keratotomy Surgical procedure to correct myopia

keratophakia Surgical procedure to correct hyperopia

global decompression *Surgical procedure to correct exophthalmos*

NOTE: Be aware that patients with retinal detachment may need special positioning in bed, patching of the eye, and restrictions on activity to prevent further or complete detachment

Preoperative assessment and care

Reinforce physician's explanation of surgical procedure
Encourage and allow time for verbalization of fears and anxieties
Answer all questions with honesty, empathy, and understanding
Explain postoperative nursing care plan and that staff is always available
Assess present degree of sight and assist as needed
Provide a safe environment; orient patient to room floor plan, placement of call bell, personal articles, etc.
Explain surgical preparation of eye according to hospital policy and physician's order
Explain that all eye makeup is removed and hair braided if long

Postoperative assessment
Observations/findings

Nausea, vomiting
Placement of eye bandage(s)
Sudden, severe eye pain
Restlessness
Position to be maintained while in bed

Potential complications

Hemorrhage
Shock
Infection
Decreased visual acuity
Blindness

Medical management

Analgesics
Antiemetics
Antibiotics
Stool softeners
Eye drops, eye shield or patch
NPO until fully reactive, increase to presurgery diet
Ambulation and activities
Dressing changes/warm or cold sterile compresses
Prescription glasses

Nursing diagnoses/goals/interventions

ndx: Potential for infection related to invasive surgical procedure

GOAL: *Patient will exhibit no signs of wound dehiscence or symptoms of intraocular pressure or infection*

Check dressing q2h for 12 hr, then q4h
Observe for drainage, bleeding, and/or pain; report immediately
Apply eye shield or patch as ordered
Caution patient not to touch, squeeze, or rub eye
Monitor vital signs q4h, then qid
Enucleation patients have clean plastic conformer in eye socket to retain eye shape

ndx: Potential for injury related to altered visual acuity

GOAL: *Patient will not have evidence of any injury*

Keep side rails up at all times
Plan all care with patient; explain routines of what will happen and when
Visit frequently and announce yourself on entering room
Assist with and teach deep-breathing exercises
  Avoid coughing
  Check with physician for any special positioning and/or precautions
Elevate head of bed 30 degrees or as ordered
Assist with and teach active or perform passive range-of-motion (ROM) exercises q4h
Avoid vomiting; administer antiemetics as ordered
Increase activities and ambulation as ordered
Assist with ambulation as needed
Teach self-care activities and assist as needed

ndx: Alteration in comfort: pain related to surgical procedure

GOAL: *Patient will verbalize reduction in pain and/or discomfort*

Administer back care and position changes to relieve discomfort
Administer analgesics as ordered; assess pain to ensure that it is not due to angled intraocular pressure or bleeding

ndx: Alteration in sensory perception related to impaired vision

GOAL: *Patient will express positive feelings and show no untoward reactions due to limited visual acuity*

Visit frequently to determine needs and allay anxiety—especially at night
Keep things needed in same place at bedside
Place call bell within reach

Encourage self-care with assistance
Provide diversional activities
Assist with feeding of diet as ordered

ndx: Knowledge deficit regarding home care and complications

GOAL: *Patient and/or significant other will demonstrate understanding of home care, follow-up care, and possible complications through interactive discussion and actual return demonstration*

Instruct patient and/or significant other in care of the eyes
  Dressing changes using aseptic techniques
  Use of eye patch or shield at night
  Method of eye drop instillation
  Need to avoid rubbing, squeezing, or touching eye
  Use of eyeglasses as ordered; sunglasses to reduce glare
  Need to keep an extra bottle of eye drops in case of loss or breakage, and while traveling
  Need to use eye only according to physician's orders
Caution patient to avoid constipation, bending, straining, and lifting heavy objects
Provide list of organizations that can assist with sight problems
Discuss home care with patient and family/significant other
  Arrange furniture for safety and convenience
  Encourage self-care
  Avoid being overprotective
  Provide nutritional diet for age and weight
  Avoid emotional upsets and stress
  Provide diversional activities: records, tapes, talking books; television and reading if able
  Know name of medication, dosage, time of administration, purpose, and side effects
  Avoid using over-the-counter medications, eye drops, or ointments without checking with physician
  Make and keep follow-up appointments with physician
Discuss symptoms to report to physician
  Increased pain in eye
  Redness
  Drainage
  Decreased visual acuity
  Floaters
  Halos, sparks
If patient has had cataract removal surgery
  Without lens transplant, using glasses: explain that glasses
    Usually magnify objects 25% to 30%
    Can cause visual disturbance if fit is incorrect
    Allow patient to focus; patient will be unable to focus without them
    Are temporary glasses and new ones will be prescribed in about 3 months
    Sometimes alter distance judgment
  Without lens transplant, using contact lenses: explain that contact lenses
    Will be fitted and worn after 3 months
    Allow patient to focus, but patient will need glasses for close vision
  With intraocular lens implant: explain that lens implant
    Aids in focusing and accommodation, but glasses will be needed for close vision
    Does not cause depth perception loss
If patient has had enucleation
  Conformer may become dislodged; explain that this is of little consequence and it need not be reinserted
  Discuss use of antibiotic drops and to wear eye shield until prosthesis is fitted (in about 1 month)

Evaluation

No complications are evident
Nutrition is adequate for age and weight
Patient demonstrates ability to perform self-care activities with assistance as needed
Patient demonstrates understanding of needed alterations in life-style
Patient understands signs of complications and/or disease progression
Patient understands need for follow-up care with physician

VISUALLY IMPAIRED PATIENT

Assessment
Observations/findings

Status of impairment
  Temporary (eye patch, shield)
  Permanent
Length of impairment
Degree of visual loss
Degree of acceptance of impairment
Cause of visual impairment: diabetes, stroke, aneurysms, brain tumor, trauma, glaucoma, etc.
Condition of eyes: drainage, redness, pain, edema, squinting, abnormal eye movements, rubbing, opacities
Ability to perform ADLs

Nursing diagnoses/goals/interventions

ndx: Alteration in sensory perception related to visual impairment

GOAL: *Patient will demonstrate ability to function adequately within confines of visual impairment*

Familiarize patient to surroundings
    Place all utensils and personal articles within easy reach and maintain consistency
    Utilize patient's sense of touch and smell during orientation
    Explain location of doors, windows, furniture, bathroom, and other patients
Establish effective lines of communication
    Always identify self when approaching or touching patient
    Call patient by name
    Explain purpose of visit and visit often, especially at night
    Utilize visual aids: magnifying glasses, large print
Encourage and assist with independence
    Provide nutritious meals according to diet ordered and tolerance
    Feed as indicated
    Explain position of food on tray and prepare food as necessary; use clock sequence (e.g., plate at 6 o'clock, fruit at 10 o'clock, milk at 1 o'clock)
Initiate grooming procedures as tolerated
    Explain position of articles and place in same position each time
    Withdraw assistance gradually

ndx: Potential for injury: trauma related to visual impairment

GOAL: *Patient will avoid activities that could precipitate injury*

Maintain safe environment
    Place side rails up while patient is in bed
    Keep bed in locked, low position
    Place call bell and needed articles within easy reach
    Maintain environment as described (e.g., furniture, footstools, IV poles, wastebaskets)
    Keep doors fully open or closed
Flag chart with sticker indicating degree and type of visual impairment
Encourage patient to call nurse prior to ambulating; assist as needed
Avoid sharp items such as razors, scissors, and glass
Remain with patient if smoking is allowed

ndx: Anxiety related to visual impairment

GOAL: *Patient will verbalize anxieties and strive toward adaptive coping mechanisms to decrease level of anxiety*

Assess level of anxiety and normal coping mechanisms
Encourage and allow time for verbalization of feelings
Explain daily plan of care
Involve patient in care, allowing as much independence as safety permits
Explain all procedures
Provide reassurance by being available and answering all questions
Provide planned rest periods
Encourage visitors and communication with significant others
Avoid being oversympathetic or overprotective
Present a calm, caring attitude
Provide diversional activities

ndx: Disturbance in self-concept related to visual impairment

GOAL: *Patient will express positive feelings of self-esteem and self-worth*

Discuss with patient and significant others alternatives in managing ADLs
Assess present coping mechanisms
Encourage independence as tolerated
Involve outside organizations: Braille Institute, Seeing Eye Dog
Encourage use of other senses: touch, smell, hearing

ndx: Knowledge deficit regarding self-care and home management

GOAL: *Patient and/or significant other will demonstrate understanding of home care and follow-up instructions through interactive discussion and actual return demonstration*

Reinforce safety precautions as to furniture placement, sharp objects and corners, scatter rugs, objects on floor, etc.
Reinforce physician's explanation of disease and disease process and need to notify physician of any changes in condition
Assist patient and/or significant other in managing ADLs
Promote self-care within limits of visual impairment
Demonstrate instillation of eye drops procedure
Refer to home health care agency and/or organizations for the visually impaired
Maintain regular outpatient care visits with physician

Evaluation

Patient

Performs self-care within limits of visual impairment

Demonstrates understanding of home and follow-up care

Demonstrates adaptive responses as related to self-concept and self-esteem

Demonstrates understanding of what constitutes a safe environment

CONTACT LENS REMOVAL

Occasionally unconscious, paralyzed, disoriented, or elderly patients and patients with limited or restricted use of their arms may be wearing contact lenses; lenses must be removed to avoid eye damage

Assessment

Level of consciousness/ability to cooperate

Presence of contact lenses in unconscious patient: shine flashlight into eye from outer canthus; lenses will appear around iris or slightly beyond

Type of lenses

   Hard: covers iris, may be tinted

   Soft: covers iris, may be tinted

   Scleral: covers iris and sclera

Small suction cup apparatus for removing contact lenses is often kept in emergency room

Removal procedure

Wash hands thoroughly prior to procedure

Removal of hard lenses

   Place forefinger at outer canthus of eye

   Gently push finger up and then down

   Lens will appear from under lid

   Store in distilled water, keeping right and left lenses separate and containers marked

Removal of soft lenses

   Place thumb and forefinger on lower and upper lid, respectively

   Gently open eye

   With other hand gently lift lens off iris, using thumb and forefinger

   Store in normal saline solution, keeping right and left lenses separate and containers marked

Removal of scleral lenses

   Place forefinger at edge of and parallel to lower lid

   Gently press lid downward until lower edge of lens is visible

   Continue gentle pressure, pulling lid toward ear

   Lens will slide out from under lid

   Store in distilled water, keeping right and left lenses separate and containers marked

Removal of lenses using suction cup apparatus

   Depress bulb between thumb and forefinger

   Position cup over lens

   Slowly release pressure on bulb

   Lens will adhere to cup

   Remove lens and store in marked containers with appropriate solution

If lenses are not visible (eye rolled back) or difficulty is experienced in removal procedure, notify ophthalmologist to remove lenses

INSTILLATION OF EYE DROPS/OINTMENTS

Preinstillation assessment

Assess patient's ability to hold eyes open and cooperate

Explain purpose of medication, procedure, and side effects

Perform medication assessment

   Correct medication, patient, dosage, time, and eye

   Check dropper for defects

   Understand abbreviations

      OD: right eye

      OS: left eye

      OU: both eyes

Instillation procedure (Figure 12-2)

Eye drops are sterile, and any contamination of the dropper or squeeze bottle can cause infection

   Always discard when contamination occurs

Position patient in chair with head tilted back or in dorsal recumbent position in bed

Wash hands prior to procedure

Draw medication into dropper (keep medication from going into bulb end) or open squeeze bottle of drops or tube of ointment

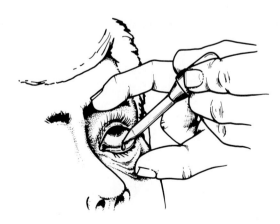

FIGURE 12-2. Instillation of eye drops.

Gently pull down skin beneath lower lid with forefinger and tissue
Instruct patient to look upward
Instill drops or dab ointment into pocket formation in lower lid; do not touch conjunctiva with dropper or tube
Instruct patient to close eye gently and not to squeeze eye closed or to rub it
Wipe off excess medication with tissue
Instruct patient to open and close eye slowly for a few minutes to distribute medication evenly

Auditory System

EAR ASSESSMENT

Subjective Data

Earache
Decreased, absent hearing acuity in one or both ears
Tinnitus
Feeling of fullness in ear
Own voice echoes
Popping noise when yawning or swallowing
Vertigo, dizziness
Itching in ear
Heart pulsating in ear
Ear drainage
  Dark
  Red
  Clear
  Yellow
Use of oils, cotton swabs, hairpins to clean ears

Objective Data

General appearance
Vital signs: elevated BP, T, P, and R
Ability to hear; use of hearing aid
Ability to lip-read or use sign language
Startle reflex
Tolerance of loud sounds
Type, color, and amount of ear drainage
Medication used (streptomycin, salicylates, quinine, gentamycin)
Allergies

Pertinent Background Information
CONCURRENT DISEASES OR CONDITIONS

Otitis media
Otosclerosis
Acoustic nerve tumor
Labyrinthitis
Meniere's disease
Cerebral tumors, contusion, diseases, fractures

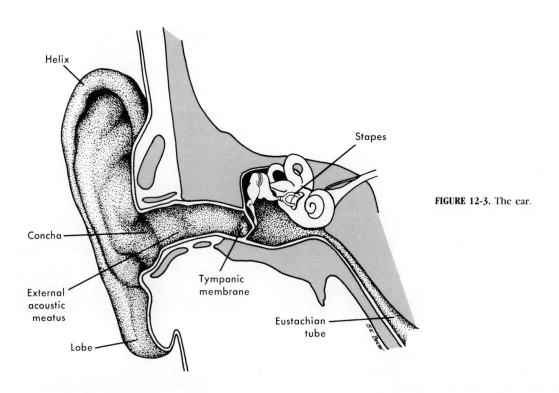

FIGURE 12-3. The ear.

Diabetes mellitus
Arteriosclerosis
Hypertension
Hypotension
Mastoiditis

PREVIOUS SURGERY OR ILLNESS

Stapes mobilization
Syphilis
Otitis media
Head trauma
Mastoidectomy

SOCIAL HISTORY

Venereal diseases
Recreational hazards: swimming
Exposure to loud noises
Safety precautions taken
Use of tobacco or coffee

MEDICATION HISTORY

Ear drops
Antibiotics
Salicylates
Quinine

Diagnostic aids
PROCEDURES

Audiogram, audiometry
Mastoid x-ray examination
Tuning fork test (Rinne)
Otologic examination
"Lateralization" tuning fork test (Weber)
Pneumatic otoscopy
Tympanometry
Caloric examination
Electronystagmography (ENG)
Electrocochleography
Tomogram
Cerebral arteriography
Computed tomography (CT) scan
Magnetic resonance imaging (MRI) scan

MICROBIOLOGIC PROCEDURES

Culture for pathogens

MENIERE'S SYNDROME (ENDOLYMPHATIC HYDROPS)

Disease of the inner ear thought to be caused by an overproduction of endolymph or malabsorption of endolymph, producing labyrinthine dysfunction

Assessment
Observations/findings
ACUTE ATTACK

Rapid onset: recurrent deafness
Tinnitus: usually roaring sensation
Vertigo and incoordination
Nausea, vomiting
Unsteady on feet: falls toward affected ear
Blurred vision
Photophobia
Nystagmus
History of
    Otitis media
    Arteriosclerosis
    Allergies
    Leukemia
    Smoking
Medication use
    Quinine
    Salicylates
    Streptomycin
Maladaptive behavior during attack

Laboratory/diagnostic studies

Audiologic testing
Audiogram
Caloric tests
X-ray examination of petrous bone

Potential complications

Increased hearing impairment
Deafness
Fractures caused by falling

Medical management

Anticholinergic agents: atropine, scopolamine
Antihistamines: dyphenhydramine, meclizine, cyclizine
Antianxiety agents: diazepam
Antiemetics: prochlorperazine
Diuretics: hydrochlorothiazide, furosemide
Adrenergic agents: epinephrine
Surgical interventions: labyrinthectomy, vestibular neurectomy, sacculotomy, endolymphatic-subarachnoid shunt

Nursing diagnoses/goals/interventions

ndx: Alteration in sensory perception related to auditory impairment

GOAL: *Patient will identify and understand factors that cause impairment*

Assess patient's auditory acuity
Flag chart to indicate impairment
Stand so that patient can see you
Speak slowly and enunciate well
Explain all procedures and nursing care plan
Maintain quiet environment
    Minimize activities in room
    Avoid bumping bed
Assist with personal care and activities as needed
Assist and teach patient to deep breathe q2h to 4h and to turn on affected side when symptoms subside
Administer antianxiety agents as ordered

ndx: Potential for injury related to trauma

GOAL: *Patient will express understanding of safety precautions needed during attacks of vertigo*

Maintain bed rest in position of comfort
Keep side rails of bed up and bed in low position
Discourage smoking
Instruct patient to call nurse before getting up
Ambulate as ordered
    Observe for vertigo, nausea, and nystagmus
    Assist with ambulation
    Increase distance as tolerated
Instruct patient to turn head slowly to prevent vertigo

ndx: Potential fluid volume deficit related to vomiting

GOAL: *Patient's fluid intake will be adequate to maintain hydration*

Monitor intake and output for severe vomiting
Administer antiemetics as ordered
Monitor vital signs qid
Provide low-sodium diet as ordered
    Assist with eating
    Restrict fluid intake as ordered

ndx: Knowledge deficit regarding disease process and home care management

GOAL: *Patient and/or significant other will demonstrate understanding of disease, home care, and follow-up instructions through interactive discussion*

Reinforce physician's explanation of disease process and procedures to follow when attacks occur
    Explain that vertigo is usually first symptom
    Patient should
        Take medication as ordered
        Lie or sit down when vertigo appears
        Not walk unassisted
        Notify physician of recurrence

Stress to patient that progressive hearing loss may occur if treatment is not initiated or successful
Explain that tinnitus may always be present; advise patient to utilize background music, radio, or TV to overcome tinnitus
Discuss importance of following low-sodium diet or neutral ash diet as ordered
Warn patient to avoid ototoxic medications: salicylates, quinine, some diuretics, and aminoglycoside antibiotics
Avoid smoking
Have periodic audiologic examinations

Evaluation

There are no complications or injuries
Auditory acuity is stablized
Nutritious low-sodium or neutral ash diet is understood, and diet instructions have been given
Patient demonstrates understanding of disease process, home care and follow-up care

STAPEDECTOMY

Surgical removal of all or part of the stapes footplate and creation of a patent oval window and pathway for sound transmission utilizing natural or artificial materials

Postoperative assessment
Observations/findings

Nausea
Vertigo
Character and amount of ear drainage
Headache
Fever
Location and character of pain
Excessive pain
Acoustic acuity

Potential complications

Facial paresis
Granuloma at surgical site
Infection

Medical management

Analgesics
Antiemetics
Antibiotics
Dressing change schedule

Nursing diagnoses/goals/interventions

ndx: Alteration in comfort: pain related to surgical procedure and discomfort related to position restriction

GOAL: *Patient will express understanding of position rationale and verbalize a reduction in pain*

Maintain bed rest in quiet environment
    Supine position with operative side up
    Keep side rails up
    Do not turn unless ordered
    Provide back rubs prn
    Perform passive exercises q4h
Administer analgesics as ordered
Avoid vomiting with use of antiemetics
Assist with ambulation after 24 hr
    Observe for vertigo and/or nausea
    Avoid rapid turning

ndx: Potential for infection related to invasive surgical procedure

GOAL: *Patient will verbalize and demonstrate understanding of ear care procedure*

Keep outer ear plug clean and dry
Change ear plugs prn
Report excessive bleeding to physician
Monitor vital signs q4h
Report fever, headache, or increased ear pain to physician

ndx: Alteration in sensory perception related to auditory impairment

GOAL: *Patient will identify and understand factors causing impairment*

Assess auditory impairment
Explain that hearing may not improve immediately and that this is not abnormal
    Ear plugs and bleeding decrease hearing acuity
    Hearing usually improves after plugs are removed

ndx: Knowledge deficit regarding home and follow-up care

GOAL: *Patient and/or significant other will demonstrate understanding of home care and follow-up instructions through interactive discussion and actual return demonstration*

Instruct patient on ear care
    Change only outer ear plug prn
    Keep plug clean and dry
    Avoid nose-blowing for 1 week
    Keep ear covered while outside
    Avoid sneezing; if unavoidable, open mouth wide and sneeze gently
    Wash hair only after 2 weeks
    No air travel or diving for 6 months
    Plugs and packing are removed after 1 week
Caution patient that smoking is contraindicated
Caution patient to avoid persons with infections, especially upper respiratory infections (URIs)
Advise patient to report symptoms of ear infection to physician immediately
Encourage patient to make and keep follow-up appointments with physician

Evaluation

There are no complications
Acoustic ability has improved
Activity level is normal for patient
Patient demonstrates understanding of principles of home and follow-up care

MYRINGOTOMY WITH TUBE INSERTION

Surgical incision into the tympanic membrane to aspirate collected fluid and insertion of a ventilating tube to keep the pressure equal between the middle and outer ear; performed to correct serous otitis media

Preoperative assessment and care

Assess hearing acuity in both ears
Reinforce physician's explanation of procedure—performed mostly on children
Establish means of communication, since hearing may be impaired
Use pictures of tubes to help with explanation
Explain that patient will not be aware that tube is in place
Discuss with patient that discomfort will not disappear immediately
Explain that impaired hearing may not improve for 1 to 2 weeks

Postoperative assessment
Observations/findings

Character and amount of ear drainage
Restlessness due to hearing loss
Nausea, vomiting
Location and character of pain
Hearing acuity

Potential complications

Decreased hearing acuity
Hemorrhage
Further infection

Medical management

Analgesics
Antibiotics
Antibiotic ear drops
Antiemetics
Dressing change schedule
Position following surgery

Nursing diagnoses/goals/interventions

ndx: Alteration in comfort: pain related to surgical intervention, nausea, and discomfort related to position restriction

GOAL: *Patient will express that comfort is maximal*

Maintain bed rest in quiet environment in position as ordered until fully reactive
Administer analgesics and antiemetics as ordered
Assist and teach patient to deep breathe qh

ndx: Potential for infection at surgical site related to surgical intervention

GOAL: *Patient will remain free of infection*

Keep external ear clean and dry
Change dressings as ordered and prn
Maintain aseptic technique, since drainage is usually purulent
Observe amount and type of drainage
Administer antibiotics as ordered
Monitor vital signs q4h
Observe for signs of infection
  Increased drainage/ear pain
  Fever
  Headache
  Nausea

ndx: Knowledge deficit regarding home and follow-up care

GOAL: *Patient and/or parent(s) will demonstrate understanding of home care and follow-up instructions through interactive discussion and actual return demonstration*

Discuss special precautions and restrictions
  Keep water out of ear
  Place petroleum jelly–covered cotton or lamb's wool pledget in ear before showering or shampooing
  Wear well-fitting ear plugs when swimming is allowed or wear a cap
  Do not dive
Explain that tube will come out naturally in 2 to 8 months and there may be bloody drainage; if tube is dislodged earlier, instruct patient or parent(s) to notify physician
Demonstrate ear drop instillation and instruct patient or parent(s) to complete prescribed course of oral or ear drop antibiotic therapy
Explain need to avoid contact with persons with URIs
Discuss symptoms to report to physician
  Fever and/or increased pain
  Increased drainage or bleeding
  Decreased hearing acuity
  Encourage patient to make and keep follow-up appointments with physician

Evaluation

There are no complications
Pain or discomfort is controlled
Patient and/or parent(s) demonstrate(s) knowledge of home and follow-up care

TYMPANOPLASTY: TYPES I THROUGH V

Surgical repair of perforated or largely destroyed tympanic membrane due to infection, trauma, otosclerosis, stenosis, or necrosis of the middle ear; type performed depends on degree of perforation and destruction as well as ossicular involvement and damage (Table 12-1)

Preoperative assessment and care

Assess hearing acuity in both ears; establish means of communication as necessary
Administer antibiotics as ordered
Discuss with and teach patient
  That large, bulky dressing may be in place and hearing acuity will be decreased temporarily
  Methods of deep breathing
  Not to blow nose, since graft may be dislodged
  To cough and sneeze with mouth open
  That vertigo and/or nausea may be present postoperatively
  That hearing acuity may not return immediately

Postoperative assessment
Observations/findings

Placement of ear dressing
Character and amount of ear drainage
Location and character of pain
Nausea, vomiting
Restlessness
Vertigo
Nystagmus

TABLE 12-1. Types of Tympanoplasty

Type	Damage to middle ear	Methods of repair
I	Perforation of tympanic membrane with normal ossicular chain	Closure of perforation; type I same as myringoplasty
II	Perforation of tympanic membrane with erosion of malleus	Closure with graft against incus or remains of malleus
III	Destruction of tympanic membrane and ossicular chain but with intact and mobile stapes	Graft contacts normal stapes; also gives sound protection for round window
IV	Similar to type III but with head, neck, and crura of stapes missing; footplate mobile	Mobile footplate left exposed; air pocket between round window and graft provides sound protection for round window
V	Similar to type IV but with fixed footplate	Fenestra in horizontal semicircular canal; graft seals off middle ear to give sound protection for round window

From Saunders, W., et al.: Nursing care in eye, ear, nose and throat disorders, ed. 4, St. Louis, 1979, The C.V. Mosby Co.

Potential complications

Infection
Hemorrhage, shock
Decreased hearing acuity
Deafness

Medical management

Analgesics
Antiemetics
Antibiotics
Dressing change schedule

Nursing diagnoses/goals/interventions

ndx: Alteration in comfort: pain related to surgical intervention and discomfort related to limited activity

GOAL: *Patient will express minimal discomfort or absence of pain*

Maintain bed rest until fully reactive, then elevate head to position of comfort
Administer analgesics as ordered; assess effectiveness of pain relief measures
Assist and teach deep-breathing exercises qh
Assist with ambulation; observe for vertigo, nausea, and nystagmus
Administer antiemetics as ordered

ndx: Potential for infection related to inadequate primary defense; traumatized tissue at surgical site

GOAL: *Patient's wound and dressings will be clean, dry, and intact*

Assess auditory acuity
Check ear dressing frequently and change outer dressing prn; report excessive drainage to physician
Monitor vital signs as needed
Administer antibiotics as ordered

ndx: Knowledge deficit regarding home care needs

GOAL: *Patient and/or significant other will demonstrate understanding of home care needs and follow-up instructions through interactive discussion and actual return demonstration*

Discuss precautions and restrictions in ear care
  Wear shower cap when bathing or place lamb's wool pledget in ear to protect ear from water
  Avoid blowing nose and sneeze through mouth
  Remove inner ear dressing only if prescribed by physician
  May swim or fly once healing has taken place
Explain importance of nutritional diet, fluid intake, rest, and activity
Discuss signs and symptoms to report to physician
  Elevated temperature
  Increased pain and/or ear drainage
  Decrease in hearing acuity
Discuss medications: name, dosage, time of administration, purpose, and side effects
Encourage follow-up visits with physician

Evaluation

There are no complications
Pain is controlled
Hearing acuity has improved
Home care instructions are understood

AUDITORY-IMPAIRED PATIENT

Assessment

Observations/findings

Assess hearing acuity and communication skills
  Lipreading or sign language
  Hearing aid
  Pad and pencil

Determine status and length of impairment
Assess acceptance of impairment
  Well-adjusted
  Fear/anxiety
  Frustration, depression
  Anger, hostility
Examine ears for drainage, crusts, cerumen accumulation, and deformities

Nursing diagnoses/goals/interventions

ndx: Alteration in sensory perception related to hearing impairment

GOAL: *Patient will express understanding of cause(s) of auditory impairment and will function optimally within limits of impairment*

Reinforce physician's explanation of hearing impairment
Assess and establish means of communication
  Lipreading (speech reading)
    Speak slowly and enunciate well
    Do not exaggerate sounds
    Have only one person speak at a time
    Stand so patient can see your mouth clearly
    Speak in simple phrases first to determine expertise in the skill
    Point to objects of conversation where appropriate
    Avoid chewing gum and shouting
    Rephrase statements if not first understood
  Sign language
    Determine if patient can communicate with pad and pencil, since most hospital personnel are not skilled in this technique
    Enlist cooperation of family/significant other in communication
  Hearing aid
    Assess patient's ability to use and care for appliance
    Make certain aid is in place and turned on before speaking
    Establish a pitch that is comfortable for patient
    Avoid shouting
  Pad and pencil
    Write messages clearly, in short, simple phrases
    Develop a checklist of phrases most often used and instruct patient to check appropriate one(s)
    Allow time for patient to understand and answer

ndx: Potential for injury related to hearing impairment

GOAL: *Patient will identify and understand risk factors of hearing impairment*

Maintain safe environment
  Locate bed so door is visible, when possible
  Orient patient to surroundings; have call bell within reach
  Answer call light promptly
  Keep side rails up if appropriate
  Approach patient carefully if eyes are closed; a gentle touch on patient's arm will arouse but not startle
Explain all procedures
Flag chart indicating type of impairment

ndx: Anxiety/fear related to hearing impairment

GOAL: *Patient will verbalize feelings and demonstrate adaptive responses to those feelings*

Maintain quiet, nonstressful environment
Assess level of anxiety/fear
Encourage and allow time for verbalization
Explain nursing plan of care and involve patient in planning care
Display confidence and a caring, patient manner
Visit frequently
Utilize pictures when explaining procedures or treatment
Encourage communication with significant other
Avoid using nurse-patient intercommunication system if patient has partial hearing, since it can cause frustration
Evaluate patient's ability to use other senses (sight and touch especially) as an aid in daily living
Provide diversional activities: puzzles, cards, hobbies

ndx: Knowledge deficit regarding home and follow-up care

GOAL: *Patient and/or significant other will demonstrate understanding of home care and follow-up instructions through interactive discussion and actual return demonstration*

Reinforce physician's explanation of cause of impairment and prescribed treatment
Explain safety factors important in home environment
Discuss availability of hearing devices: amplifiers, flashing lights on telephones, and door bells
Refer to local telephone company and/or hearing institute for assistance
Refer to local schools for classes on lipreading and/or sign language

Instruct patient in care of hearing aid
Demonstrate care of ear dressings and ear drop instillation
Encourage patient to make and keep appointments with physician

Evaluation

There are no complications
Patient demonstrates knowledge of risk factors involved from a safety standpoint
Patient demonstrates adaptive responses to feelings of anxiety/fear
Patient demonstrates understanding of home and follow-up care

Chapter 13

Oncology

ONCOLOGY ASSESSMENT

Current Condition

General appearance
  Posture
  Body movements
  Hygiene
General survey of mental status
  Orientation
  Attention span
  Speech
Behavior/mannerisms
Chief complaint
Vital signs
Weight and height
Patient's concerns
Patient's problems or needs
Patient's knowledge of
  Disease process
  Treatment
  Outcome

Physical Assessment

Hematologic system
  Monitor complete blood cell count (CBC), hemoglobin, platelet count
  Bleeding/hemorrhage
    Petechiae
    Unexplained bruises or ecchymoses
  Hematomas
  Bleeding from any body orifice
  Prolonged oozing of blood from IM or IV sites
  Change in vital signs
  Change in neurologic status (headache, disorientation)
  Pad count high for menstruating females
  Anemia
    Palpitations, chest pain on exertion
    Dyspnea
    Dizziness, syncope
    Fatigue, weakness
    Glossitis, anorexia, indigestion
    Insomnia, hypersensitivity to cold

Infection(s), present and past
  Temperature
  White blood cell count (WBC), including differential
  Skin integrity/mucous membranes
    Skin folds (axillae, buttocks, perineum)
    Body cavities (mouth, vagina, rectum)
    Venous access sites
    Surgical wounds
  Respiratory tract
  Genitourinary system
  Eyes
    Conjunctivitis, iritis
    Infection of eyelid or lacrimal gland
Pain (p. 8)
  Type
    Acute
    Chronic
    Emotional
  Location, circumstances of onset
  Intensity, quality
  Activities that increase pain: eating, separation from significant other
  Effects on patient and family
  Relief measures
    Medication
    Distraction, meditation, relaxation, exercises
    Imagery; psychosocial and/or spiritual counseling
    Variables affecting response
      Anxiety/fear
      Ethnic/cultural background
      Past experiences with pain management
      Meaning of pain (recurrence of disease, death)
      Perceptions of pain therapy (fear of addictions)
Skin
  Color: pallor, duskiness, jaundice
  Integrity
    Breaks, lesions, ulcers
    Petechiae, bruises, erythema, ecchymosis
  Temperature
    Local and systemic
    Feeling of warmth and/or cold
  Hydration: tugor, edema, perspiration

Hair: distribution, alopecia
Nails: color, texture, clubbing
Eyes
    Pupil size and response
    Color
    Sclera
    Cataract formation
Nose: bleeding, drainage, crusting
Mouth, tongue, lips
    Color, moisture; presence of lesions on palate, tongue, buccal mucosa, inner surface of lips, and/or oral pharynx
    Color, amount, and consistency of saliva
    Condition of teeth
        Dental caries, rough edges
        Plaque, dental fit
    Mobility of tongue
    Ability to chew and taste
    Breath odor
Parotid gland: size, tenderness, pain
Lymph nodes
    Neck, axilla, groin
    Size, tenderness, pain
    Thyroid size
Gastrointestinal system
    Appetite
    Food and fluid intake
        Type, consistency, amount
        Frequency, preferences
    See Alteration in Nutrition: Less Than Body Requirements (p. 59)
    Nausea, vomiting
        Frequency, character
        Color, amount
        Factors affecting occurrence
            Anticipation
            Activities, treatments, time of day
            Other associated factors
    Relief measures used; variables affecting response
    Abdomen
        Distention
        Bowel sounds
            Present: type, frequency, character
            Absent
        Rigid, flaccid, tender
    Spleen and liver: size, tenderness, pain
    Stool
        Normal pattern; frequency (time of last stool), amount, color, consistency
        Aids to normal elimination
            Dietary (food and fluid)
            Medications (laxatives)
            Enemas
        Method of elimination: toilet, commode, bedpan
        Artificial orifices
            Colostomy, ileostomy
            Ileal conduit
        Method of care for excretions from artificial orifices
        Pain related to defecation
        Presence of blood (on surface or mixed throughout)
        Mucus, pus
        Level of mobility-immobility
        Stress
    Diarrhea/constipation
        Frequency, amount
        Consistency, color
        Bleeding, occult bleeding
        Associated factors
        Flatulence
        Relief measures, methods of coping
Genitourinary system
    Urine, urination
        Usual pattern
        Frequency, amount
        Color, odor, specific gravity
        Presence of usual constituents
        Character, bleeding
        Any urgency felt
        Effort in starting and stopping
        Pain, burning, itching
        Nocturia
        Incontinence
        Retention
        Method of urine elimination (void, in-and-out catheter, Foley, urinary diversion)
        Care measures, methods of coping
    Fluid intake
    Medications (diuretics)
    History of urinary tract infection
Respiratory system
    Respiratory rate; depth and character of breathing
    Type of airway
    Patency of airway
    Breath sounds (normal, adventitious, increased, decreased)
    Color of skin and mucous membrane
    Chest size and shape
    Chest excursion and symmetry
    Position of trachea
    Shortness of breath on exertion

Use of accessory muscles
Nasal flaring, pursed lip breathing, clubbing of extremities
Cough: ability, frequency, depth, force, productivity
Sputum: color, amount, odor, consistency, time of day produced
Audible grunting, snoring, stridor
Frequency of suctioning
Present level and tolerance of activity
History of
    Smoking, pulmonary infection, exposure to air pollutants
    Chemotherapy (bleomycin), radiation therapy to thorax
Laboratory tests: blood gas, sputum, blood cultures, WBC
Diagnostic studies: chest x-ray examination, pulmonary function test

Cardiovascular system
    Heart rate, blood pressure, temperature
    Heart sounds
    Peripheral pulses: rate, rhythm, volume
    Skin color, dryness, moistness
    Decreased cardiac output
        Tachycardia
        Electrocardiogram (ECG) changes
        Dyspnea on exertion, exercise tolerance
        Rales, wheezing, cough
        Edema: location, type

Neurologic system
    Sensorium (awake, alert, lethargic, stuporous, comatose)
    Orientation to time, person, place, and situation
    Ability to follow commands
    Memory (recent, remote)
    Attentiveness, distractibility
    Language spoken, clarity, appropriateness
    Ability to read and write
    Motor response
        Voluntary, involuntary
        Gait, balance, paralysis, weakness
    Reflex response: pupil, gag, cough, Babinski's sign, deep tendon reflex
    Tics, trembling, seizures
    Pain
        Location, onset, duration, type
        Precipitating factors, relief measures
    Sensations: tingling, numbness, leg cramps
    Foot-drop, wrist-drop, handgrip
    Sensory
        Visual
        Auditory
        Olfactory
        Taste
        Tactile
    Safety measures used

Pertinent Background Information

Sleep/rest
    Usual pattern; hours of sleep at night
    Difficulties
    Number and duration of daily naps
    Use of sleep aids: name, dosage of drug, frequency of use, length of time used
    Symptoms that may affect sleep: pain, anxiety, night sweats
    Signs and symptoms of sleep disturbance: irritability, anxiety, loss of train of thought
    Care measures
Sexuality
    Sexual history
    Current practices, reproductive history
    Impact of therapies on sexuality/sexual function; reaction of partner to illness
    Expressions of affection
    Methods of coping
Social
    Support system; most significant other
    Role function
    Housing/living arrangement
    Presence of dependent behaviors; presence of independent behaviors
Spirituality (p. 6): beliefs, faith, concerns
Activities of daily living (ADLs)
    Life-style (active, sedentary); exercise tolerance
    Degree of immobility
    Household assistance
    Employment, leisure/hobbies
    Other activities and concerns
Home environment
    Care giver, facilities, and equipment available for meeting care needs
    Pets
    Concerns
Teaching needs
    During hospitalization
    Self-care
Previous conditions
Acute or chronic diseases or conditions
Surgery
Radiation therapy
Chemotherapy
Trauma
    Physical
    Emotional

Psychosocial Assessment*

PREDIAGNOSTIC PERIOD (DETERMINATION OF FEELINGS AND PRIOR KNOWLEDGE)

Awareness of signs and symptoms; length of time known
Delay in seeking treatment
    Threats to
        Independence
        Group belongingness
        Influence on others
        Adaptive functioning
        Preexisting stability
        Decision-making ability
        Cherished values
        Desired roles
        Limitless future
        Control over destiny
    Information about treatment
        Knowledge deficits
        Level of understanding
        Misconceptions and myths
        Ethnic/cultural beliefs
    Knowledge of resources

DIAGNOSTIC PERIOD

Fears of outcome
Perceptions of threat
Significance of studies
Information about cancer and body functions
    Factual
    Deficits
    Misconceptions
        Myths
        Fantasies
Knowledge and level of understanding
    Diagnostic tests and examinations
    Schedule of tests and examinations
    Reasons for studies and preparation
    Role of patient in studies
    Physical effect of studies; expected symptoms and responses
Continuously validate patient's understanding and perceptions
Coping methods of patient, significant other, or family
    Daily activities
    Utilization of work and leisure activities
    Relationships
    Methods of communication
    Ability to disclose: open with family, peers, counselors, and/or medical and nursing staff
    Inability to communicate; awareness of significance
Behavioral responses
    Anxiety
        Apprehensive expectation
        Fear and worry about negative outcome
    Vigilance and scanning
        Hyperattentiveness
        Distractibility
        Concentration problems
        Impatience
        Feeling "on edge"
    Motor tension
        Jumpiness
        Restlessness
        Inability to relax
        Insomnia
        Strained facies
        Easily startled
Autonomic hyperactivity
    Tachycardia
    Tachypnea
    Dry mouth
    Sweating
    Cold, clammy hands
    Upset stomach
    Nightmares

CONFIRMATION OF DIAGNOSIS

Knowledge of results and meaning of diagnostic studies
    X-ray examinations
    Computed tomography (CT) scans
    Isotope studies
    Ultrasound examinations
    Endoscopy
    Cytology
    Laboratory data
    Biopsy
Meaning of illness
    Threat to
        Independence
        Job and economic security
        Career goals
        Relationships
        Integrity of body
        Body functions
        Recreational activities
        Sexual attractiveness and functioning
        Intimacy
    Fears of disfigurement and pain

---

*Adapted from Marino, L.B.: Cancer nursing, St. Louis, 1981, The C.V. Mosby Co.

Secondary gains: alteration in behavior
    Acting out
    Demands for attention
    Controlling behaviors
  Methods for handling past crises
Availability of knowledgeable and supportive resources
  Family
  Significant others
  Co-workers
  Social contacts
  Religious counsel
  Community
Behavioral responses
  Shock/denial
    Rejection of reality
    Increased perspiration
    Pallor
    Faintness
    Nausea
    Anorexia
    Insomnia
    Confusion
    Difficulty in concentrating
    Difficulty in working
  Anger
    Impatience
    Bitterness
    Jealousy
    Helplessness
    Increased awareness
    Limited attention span
    Uncooperative behavior
    Attention-seeking behavior
    Loud talking
    Vulgar language
    Multiple complaints
  Guilt/punishment
    Underlying reasons
    Misconceptions about cancer: seen as unclean, contagious
    Diagnosis attributed to something they did or did not do
  Hopelessness (p. 16)
    Quiet
    Withdrawn
    Melancholy
    Older appearance
    Poor posture
    Gait: slow, dragging
    Decreased respiration
    Feeling of fullness
    Belching
    Constipation
  Bargaining
    Depression
    Exhaustion
    Attempts to avoid reality
    Self-questioning
    Shortness of breath
    Feelings of weakness
  Panic attack
    Dyspnea
    Palpitations
    Chest pain
    Feelings of choking or smothering
    Dizziness
    Feelings of unreality
    Tingling of hands and/or feet
    Hot and cold flashes
    Sweating
    Faintness
    Trembling or shaking
    Fear of dying, "going crazy," or doing something uncontrollable during an attack
  Be aware of importance of need to rapidly initiate appropriate interventions when the following are observed
    Agitation
    Uncharacteristic, unexplained extreme behavior
    Unrealistic perceptions and expectations
    Feelings of
      Worthlessness
      Extreme guilt
      Suicide (p. 20)
    Inappropriate resistance to treatment
    Use of controversial treatments (e.g., laetrile, megavitamins, mechanical devices, miracle drugs, psychic surgeons, Hoxsey and Krebiozen potions)
  Acceptance
    Contemplativeness
    Serenity
    Talks about condition

TREATMENT PHASE

Adequate information for informed decision making
  Types of surgery
  Radiotherapy
  Chemotherapy
  Immunotherapy
  Benefits and complications of each type of treatment
  Risks of each therapy

Results of research: outcome not predictable
Prognosis associated with each type
Level of understanding of chosen therapy
  Preparation
  Physical changes
  Complications
  Local and systemic effects
Reactions to treatment
  Follows directions
  Alterations in ADLs
Expresses needs for
  Hope associated with cure
    Future pleasurable experiences
    Ability to reach some goals
    Others being available for support
    Idea that life had meaning
  Honesty
    In answers to questions
    No protection from the truth
    In not withholding information
  Information about
    Treatment; side or toxic effects
    Expectations of patient during procedures or treatment
    Changes in expected outcomes
    Availability and support of resources
    Whether patient can share what he has learned about care
Expresses feelings or conveys
  Anger
  Fear
  Sadness
  Helplessness
  Dependency (p. 28)
  Powerlessness

PREPARATION FOR DISCHARGE

Knowledge of continuing care
Methods for dealing with pain (p. 8)
  Increase or decrease in functioning
  Complications of treatment as disease progresses
  Special procedures
  Psychologic needs
Daily activity allowances
Signs and symptoms of recurrence or progression
Need for follow-up care
Support groups and counselors: specific information, especially regarding contact person
Emergency care

Recurrence

Expresses fears of
  Increased dependency
  Increased weakness
  Increased immobility
  Isolation
  Disintegration of relationships
Communicates need for
  Being told death is close
  Information about practical things to do before death
  Discussing pain, pain relief measures, and fear of loss of control
  Discussion of beliefs
Ability to continue treatment

Advanced or terminal condition

Knowledge of present diagnosis and prognosis
Symptom control methods; patient and family participation
Responsibilities
  Relationships
  Completion of unfinished business
Ability to discuss fears of
  Inability to continue with life's activities and relationships
  Being abandoned
Hospice: alternative methods of care
Meaning of death
  Shameful
  Peaceful
Disengagement
  Life's business finished
  Goodbyes said
  Psychologic withdrawal
  Few interactions

CANCER DETECTION AND PREVENTION

General

Obtain health history through interview
Establish rapport
Identify risk factors and symptoms of specific cancers
Determine emotional needs
Provide information on self-examination
Warning signs of cancer
  Change in bowel or bladder habits
  A sore that does not heal
  Unusual bleeding or discharge
  Thickening or lump in breast or elsewhere
  Indigestion or difficulty in swallowing
  Obvious change in wart or mole
  Nagging cough or hoarseness

Skin Cancer
Determination of risk factors

Excessive exposure to sunlight (amount of absorption is dependent on time of day, season of year, and atmospheric conditions)
Occupational exposure to chemical irritants, such as tar, creosote, arsenic, or paraffin
Familial incidence
Fair-skinned, light-colored eyes and hair
Scars from previous burns and trauma
Precancerous dermatoses and conditions
    Actinic keratoses
    Xeroderma pigmentosum
    Lupus erythematosus
    Erythroplasia
    Leukoplasia
Ionizing radiation exposure: x-rays, radium, atom bomb exposure

Signs and symptoms

Skin lesion or rash
Firm, red or red-gray pearly lesion on face
Scaly, keratotic, slightly elevated lesion
Persistent skin growth with definite progression and/or elevation or ulceration
Any sore that does not heal
Change in a wart
Change in a mole

Nursing diagnosis/goal/interventions

ndx: Knowledge deficit regarding prevention and early detection of skin cancers

GOAL: *Patient and/or significant other will demonstrate knowledge of definition and risk factors of skin cancer, measures for prevention of skin cancer, and measures for early detection of skin cancer*

Prevention

Assess knowledge level
Assess readiness and ability to learn
Ensure that patient and/or significant other is knowledgeable about
    Factors that place an individual at risk
    Skin cancers and their types
    Importance of reducing exposure to sunlight, especially around noon
    Need to protect skin when exposed to sunlight
        Wear sunscreen at all times
        Cover exposed body parts
        Wear broad-brimmed hat
    Need to reduce exposure to chemical carcinogens: wear protective equipment
    Importance of reporting any skin changes to physician
    Importance of follow-up care q3 to 6 months if history of previous skin cancer

Detection

Obtain history of any recent change in skin, mole, or lesion
Assess skin for suspicious lesions
    Head and neck area are common sites of occurrence of skin cancers
    Basal cell cancers commonly have pearly, shiny translucent appearance
    Squamous cell cancers occur predominantly on sun-exposed skin; most appear as a solitary nodule with inflamed base and indistinct margin
Discuss procedure for and importance of monthly skin self-examination
Stress importance of medical follow-up

Evaluation

Patient demonstrates knowledge of definition and risk factors of skin cancer, and measures for prevention and early detection of skin cancer

Cancer of Head and Neck
Determination of risk factors

Heavy tobacco use: cigarettes, cigars, snuff, chewing tobacco, pipe
Chronic use of alcohol
Sun exposure
Chronic intake of extremely hot or cold liquids
History of exposure: nickel, wood dust, hydrocarbon gas, asbestos, mustard gas, radiation, uranium, syphilis, herpes simplex, Epstein-Barr virus
History of chronic inflammatory disease, chronic irritation to oral mucosa from ill-fitting dentures or defective teeth, or poor oral hygiene
Premalignant lesions
    Erythroplasia
    Leukoplasia

Signs and symptoms

Leukoplakia
Erythroplakia
Chronic, nonhealing, often painless sores
Positive submaxillary and digastric nodes
Nasal discharge
Earache
Enlarged cervical lymph nodes
Alteration in voice tone
    Hoarseness, cough

Glossitis
Dysphagia
Sore throat lasting longer than 2 weeks

Nursing diagnosis/goal/interventions

ndx: Knowledge deficit regarding prevention and early detection of head and neck cancer

GOAL: *Patient and/or significant other will demonstrate knowledge of risk factors associated with head and neck cancer, measures to reduce the risk of head and neck cancer, and modalities for early detection of head and neck cancer*

Prevention

Ensure that patient and/or significant other is knowledgeable about risk factors
Evaluate patient's potential for developing head and neck cancer by obtaining health history to include
  Exposure to risk factors
  Work history
  Alcohol and tobacco use
  Dental hygiene measures
Stress importance of avoiding
  Tobacco, heavy alcohol use
  Ill-fitting dentures or defective teeth
  Chemical carcinogens
  Excessive sun exposure
Stress importance of oral care with routine dental follow-up
Emphasize nutritional and fluid intake
Suggest programs to eliminate smoking and alcohol abuse
Refer patient to support groups for counseling and for help in coping

Detection

Obtain history of subjective symptoms: pain, visual changes (diplopia), hearing loss, taste or smell changes, changes in swallowing ability
Assess skin, eyelids, external ear and canal, and scalp and lips for lesions and visible swellings or adenopathy
Inspect external nose for loss of structure and support: test potency of nostrils by compressing one nostril at a time while patient inhales with mouth closed
Inspect oral cavity for areas of leukoplakia (white patches), erythema, or lesions that may appear infiltrating, ulcerative, or exophytic
Assess parotid, submaxillary, and sublingual glands for swelling and adenopathy; normally, thyroid gland is barely palpable
To examine thyroid, patient's neck should be slightly extended; assess for swelling; assess regional lymph nodes—observations of palpable lymph nodes include size, consistency, mobility, attachment, discoloration of overlying skin, and deep fixation to surrounding structures

Evaluation

Patient demonstrates knowledge of risk factors associated with head and neck cancer, and measures for prevention and early detection of head and neck cancer

Lung Cancer

Determination of risk factors

History of tobacco use
  Number of cigarettes or cigars per day
  Number of years patient has smoked, depth of inhalation, amount of tar in cigarettes smoked
Exposure to tobacco smoke
  Hours per day
  Number of years
Exposure to radiation
Exposure to carcinogens
  Asbestos
  Aromatic hydrocarbons
  Radioactive ores
  Bis ether
  Inorganic arsenic
  Nickel, silver, chromium, cadmium, beryllium, cobalt, selenium, steel
Exposure to atmospheric pollution
History of chronic lung disease
Low intake of vitamin A

Signs and symptoms

Change in pulmonary habits
Respiratory infections
Productive cough, usually at night
Rust-streaked sputum
Hemoptysis
Chest pain, tightness in chest
Unilateral wheeze
Dyspnea
Pneumonitis lasting longer than 2 weeks with treatment
Shoulder or arm pain
Weight loss
Extrapulmonary
  Hypercalcemia
  Cushing's syndrome
  Dermatomyositis
  Clubbed fingers

Migratory thrombophlebitis
Nonbacterial endocarditis
Anemia
Disseminated intravascular coagulation (DIC)

Nursing diagnosis/goal/interventions

ndx: Knowledge deficit regarding prevention and detection of lung cancer

GOAL: *Patient and/or significant other will demonstrate knowledge of factors associated with lung cancer, measures to reduce the risk of lung cancer, and measures for detection of lung cancer*

Prevention

Assess knowledge level
Assess readiness and ability to learn
Ensure that patient and/or significant other is knowledgeable about risk factors
Obtain patient's smoking history
Obtain patient's history of exposure to environmental carcinogens
Assess patient's history of lung disease
Ensure that patient and/or family is knowledgeable about
    Need to avoid exposure to tobacco smoke
    Correlation of smoking to lung cancer
    High-risk occupations
    Resources to help stop smoking

Detection

Obtain history of subjective symptoms: change in cough, chest pain, dyspnea, tightness in chest
Assess objective symptoms: increased sputum, hemoptysis, unilateral wheeze
Ascertain results of laboratory values: arterial blood gases, pulmonary function studies
Explain extrapulmonary signs and symptoms of lung cancer that may occur prior to pulmonary signs
    Superior vena cava syndrome
    Symptoms of metastatic lung tumor
        Lymph node adenopathy
        Enlarged liver, anorexia, pain in right upper quadrant
        Bone pain
        Change in mental status, seizures, headaches
    Conditions that result from ectopic hormone productions
        Inappropriate antidiuretic hormone (ADH) syndrome
        Hypercalcemia
        Cushing's syndrome

Ensure that patient and/or significant other is knowledgeable about methods of detection of lung cancer
    History and physical examination
    Sputum cytology
    Bronchoscopy and bronchial biopsy
    Brushings and washings
    Mediastinoscopy, lymph node biopsy
    Lung, brain, and bone scan when indicated

Evaluation

Patient demonstrates knowledge of risk factors associated with lung cancer, measures to reduce the risk of lung cancer, and measures for detection of lung cancer

Cancer of Esophagus and Stomach

Determination of risk factors

Chronic irritation from
    Heavy smoking
    Excessive use of alcohol
    Drinking and eating very hot foods
    Excessive use of hot, spicy foods
Exposure to foods containing nitrites and nitrates
Nutritional deficiency
Type A blood type
History of head and neck tumors, strictures, or peptic ulcer
Family history of
    Pernicious anemia
    Gastric polyps
    Gastritis
    Achlorhydria
    Gastric cancer

Signs and symptoms

Esophagus
    Dysphagia
        Early with swallowing hard, solid food
        Constantly with swallowing saliva
    Hoarseness
    Coughing
    Glossopharyngeal neuralgia
    Foul breath
    Hiccups
    Esophageal obstruction
        Sialism
        Nocturnal aspiration
        Regurgitation of saliva and food
Stomach
    Vague epigastric discomfort
    Vague feelings of fullness after meals
    Severe steady pain

Anorexia
Weight loss

Nursing diagnosis/goal/interventions

ndx: Knowledge deficit regarding prevention and detection of cancer of esophagus and stomach

GOAL: *Patient and/or significant other will demonstrate knowledge of risk factors associated with esophageal and stomach cancer, measures to reduce the risk of esophageal and stomach cancer, and measures for detection of esophageal and stomach cancer*

Prevention/detection

Ensure that patient and/or significant other is knowledgeable about risk factors
Obtain patient history of
  Smoking
  Alcohol
  Nutrition
Ensure that patient and/or significant other is knowledgeable about
  Signs and symptoms to report to physician
  Importance of periodic, regular physical examinations
  Need to avoid foods containing nitrite and nitrate preservatives
  Need to avoid chronic irritation by tobacco, alcohol, hot and spicy foods, and tea
  Importance of increasing dietary intake of vitamin C

Evaluation

Patient demonstrates knowledge of definition and risk factors of esophageal and stomach cancer, measures to reduce the risk of esophageal and stomach cancer, and measures for detection of esophageal and stomach cancer

Colorectal Cancer

Determination of risk factors

Age: over 40 years
High-fat, low-fiber diet
History of familial polyposis, Gardner's syndrome, adenomatous polyps, or villous adenomas
History of ulcerative colitis or Crohn's disease

Signs and symptoms

Recent changes in bowel habits
  Alternating diarrhea and constipation
  Note frequency, time of day, size
Symptoms depend on location of tumor
  Right colon
    Anemia and gastrointestinal (GI) tract bleeding
    Abdominal pain
    Weight loss, weakness, nausea
  Sigmoid colon
    Obstruction
    Blood per rectum
  Left colon
    Mucus in stool
    Constipation
    Decreased-caliber stools
    Blood or blood mixed with stools
    Intermittent abdominal pain
    Nausea, vomiting
  Rectum
    Rectal bleeding
    Mucous diarrhea
    Feeling of incomplete evacuation
    Tenesmus
    Abdominal and low back pain

Nursing diagnosis/goal/interventions

ndx: Knowledge deficit regarding prevention and early detection of colorectal cancer

GOAL: *Patient and/or significant other will demonstrate knowledge of risk factors associated with colorectal cancer, measures to reduce the risk of colorectal cancer, signs and symptoms that require health care evaluation, and detection methods to determine colorectal cancer*

Prevention

Assess knowledge level
Assess readiness and ability to learn
Ensure that patient and/or significant other knows and understands
  Risk factors
  Need to schedule regular, periodic examinations that include rectal examination and Hemoccult slide test if patient is 40 years of age or older
  Measures to promote bowel health
    Inspect stools regularly
    Include fresh vegetables and fruit in diet; avoid excessive fat in diet
    Drink at least 8 glasses of water per day
    Exercise regularly

Detection

Ensure that patient and/or significant other is knowledgeable about
  Signs and symptoms to report to physician
  Self-detection methods
    Observation of stools (describe abnormal stools)
    Stool guaiac testing

Ensure that patient and/or significant other demonstrates
  Hemoccult slide test
    Eat meat-free, high-residue diet for 24 hr before test
    Discontinue vitamin C use 72 hr prior to test
    Obtain stool in specimen container
    Place sample on one side of guaiac paper with tongue blade
    Place 2 drops of Hemoccult developer on other side of guaiac paper
    Bluish color indicates presence of occult blood
    Report positive results to physician
  Hematest tablets
    Obtain stool in specimen container
    Place stool sample on developer paper using tongue blade
    Place tablet on top of stool specimen
    Drop 2 to 3 drops of tap water on tablet
    Bluish discoloration indicates presence of occult blood
    Report positive results to physician
Provide written information on American Cancer Society (ACS) screening guidelines
  Annual digital rectal examination after age 40
  Guaiac stool testing annually after age 50
  Sigmoidoscopy every 2 to 5 years after two negative tests a year apart
Provide teaching and written guidelines on detection measures
  Sigmoidoscopy
  Colonoscopy
  Rectal examination
  Barium examination
  Carcinoembryonic antigen (CEA)

Evaluation

Patient demonstrates knowledge of risk factors associated with colorectal cancer, measures to reduce the risk of colorectal cancer, signs and symptoms that require health care follow-up, and methods to detect colorectal cancer

Renal, Pelvis, and Bladder Cancer and Cancer of Ureter and Urethra

Determination of risk factors

Age group: 50 to 70 years of age
Exposure to carcinogens through skin or vapor
  Aniline dye: rubber and cable industry
  Beta-naphthylamine
  4-Amino diphenyl
  Tobacco tar
  Benzedine
Exposure to pelvic irradiation
Chronic bacterial cystitis with
  Calculi
  Urethral strictures
  Diverticuli
  Paralytic stasis
Linked with but not proved
  Coffee drinking
  High use of sodium saccharin
  Urine stasis
  Incidence high in tobacco smokers

Signs and symptoms

Gross, painless hematuria: often intermittent
Microhematuria
Urinary
  Frequency
  Burning
  Urgency
  Pain
Dysuria
Weight loss and anemia
Back pain
Paraneoplastic syndrome associated with renal cancer
  Hypercalcemia
  Hypertension
  Polycythemia

Nursing diagnosis/goal/interventions

ndx: Knowledge deficit regarding prevention and detection of renal, pelvis, and bladder cancer and cancer of ureter and urethra

GOAL: *Patient and/or significant other will demonstrate knowledge of risk factors associated with renal, pelvis, and bladder cancer and cancer of ureter and urethra; measures to prevent renal, pelvis, and bladder cancer and cancer of ureter and urethra; signs and symptoms that require health care evaluation; and detection methods to determine renal, pelvis, and bladder cancer and cancer of ureter and urethra*

Prevention

Ensure that patient and/or significant other knows and understands
  Risk factors
  Importance of giving detailed occupation history
    Length of time of exposure
    Dates
    Hours per week
    Protective equipment
  Need to use safety equipment when exposed to carcinogens

Importance of reporting signs and symptoms to physician

Need to schedule periodic physical examinations, including rectal examination and bimanual pelvic examination for females; examinations at least q4 months for high-risk patients, including cystoscopy and cytology

Detection

Ensure that patient and/or significant other
- Recognizes signs and symptoms that require health care evaluation
- Describes detection methods to determine renal, pelvis, and bladder cancer and cancer of ureter and urethra
  - Urinalysis (for hematuria)
  - Intravenous pyelography (IVP), cystoscopy
  - Retrograde pyelography
  - Nephrotomogram
  - Ultrasound
  - CT scan
  - Renal arteriogram

Evaluation

Patient demonstrates understanding of risk factors associated with renal, pelvis, and bladder cancer and cancer of ureter and urethra; measures for prevention; signs and symptoms requiring health care evaluation; and detection measures for renal, pelvis, and bladder cancer and cancer of ureter and urethra

Testicular Cancer
Determination of risk factors

Between ages of 20 and 40 years
Cryptorchism (undescended testis)
Previously atrophic testes
Childhood hernia and other genitourinary anomalies
Contributing factors
- Trauma
- Orchitis, especially mumps

Family history of testicular cancer: father, brother
Klinefelter's syndrome
In utero exposure to diethystilbestrol (DES)

Signs and symptoms

Feelings of discomfort in testes
Swelling
- Painless
- Intermittent
- Scrotal heaviness

Testicular mass
Gynecomastia
Nipple pigmentation
Scrotal mass with or without pain
"Dragging" pain in lower back and abdomen
Endocrine disturbances: virilization to feminization
Metastatic
- Ureteral obstruction
- Abdominal mass
- Pulmonary lesion

Nursing diagnosis/goal/interventions

ndx: Knowledge deficit regarding early detection of testicular cancer

GOAL: *Patient and/or significant other will demonstrate knowledge of measures for early detection of testicular cancer*

Detection

Ensure that patient and/or significant other knows and understands
- Need to schedule regular, periodic physical examinations, including testicular and abdominal palpation
- High-risk factors
- Signs and symptoms to report to physician immediately
- Importance of performing testicular self-examination every month after age 15 or earlier if history of genitourinary anomalies (Figure 13-1)
- Facts about sexuality after surgery and availability of sperm banks

Ensure that patient and/or significant other demonstrates testicular self-examination
- Perform after warm shower or bath with relaxed scrotal skin

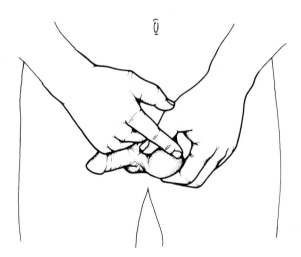

FIGURE 13-1. Testicular self-examination.

Perform in standing position
   Place middle and index fingers below one testis with thumb on top
   Gently roll testis between thumb and fingers
   Palpate for
      Normal findings
         Rubbery, spongy consistency
         Smooth, without lumps
         Abnormal finding: hard, painless tumor, usually on lateral or anterior surface
   Hold one testicle in palm of each hand; report weight differences to physician

Evaluation

Patient demonstrates testicular self-examination and knowledge of signs and symptoms requiring health care evaluation

Prostate Cancer

Determination of risk factors

Advancing age: usually over 50 years
Black population
Urban environment
Family history of prostatic cancer
Linked with but not proved
   First coitus at early age
   Multiple sex partners
   History of venereal disease

Signs and symptoms

Early signs
   Urinary hesitancy
   Dysuria
   Urgency
   Straining to start stream
Later signs
   Hematuria
   Chronic urinary retention with dribbling
   Bone and neuritic pain
   Weight loss, lethargy
   Low back pain

Nursing diagnosis/goal/interventions

ndx: Knowledge deficit regarding detection of prostate cancer

GOAL: *Patient and/or significant other will demonstrate knowledge of signs and symptoms that require health care evaluation and detection methods to determine prostate cancer*

Detection

Ensure that patient and/or significant other knows and understands
   Risk factors
   Need to schedule annual physical examinations that include digital rectal examination
      Yearly for men under 50 years of age
      Every 6 months for men 50 years of age and older
   Importance of reporting signs and symptoms to physician
   Detection measures
      Rectal examination
      Biopsy (needle or open)
      Laboratory studies
         Acid phosphatase
         Alkaline phosphatase

Evaluation

Patient demonstrates knowledge of signs and symptoms requiring health care evaluation, and measures for detection of prostate cancer

Breast Cancer

Determination of risk factors

Increased after 40 years of age
Upper socioeconomic status
Nulliparous or first parity after 30 to 35 years of age
Family history of breast cancer: sister, mother
Personal history of breast disease
Adverse hormone milieu
   Early menarche
   Late menopause
   Thyroid disorders
   Diabetes
   Postmenopausal hormone therapy
Lowered immunologic competence
   Thymic atrophy
   Decreased thymus-dependent (T) lymphocytes
   Exposure to excessive radiation
   Use of chemotherapy
   Use of immunosuppressants
Obesity
High dietary fat intake
Chronic psychologic stress

Signs and symptoms

Palpable lump
   Usually painless
   Most commonly found in upper outer quadrant
Nipple discharge
Nipple retraction
Dimpling of skin
Edema (peau d'orange) erythema
Change in contour of breast
Axillary adenopathy

Symptoms associated with metastasis
  Bone pain
  Pleural effusions

Nursing diagnosis/goal/interventions

ndx: Knowledge deficit regarding prevention and early detection of breast cancer

GOAL: *Patient will verbalize fears related to breast cancer and will demonstrate knowledge of risk factors for developing breast cancer and measures for early detection of breast cancer (i.e., breast self-examination)*

Prevention

Assess level of anxiety
  Observe verbal and nonverbal behaviors
  Explore concerns regarding breast disease
Assess readiness and ability to learn
Ensure that patient and/or significant other knows and understands
  Risk factors
  Personal risks
  Importance of breast self-examination (most women discover own breast lesions)
  That most breast lumps prove to be benign on biopsy
  That prognosis for breast cancer is more favorable when discovered early
  Importance of low-fat, high-fiber diet
  Importance of weight control or reduction

Detection

Ensure that patient and/or significant other knows and understands
  Methods of early detection of breast cancer
  Breast self-examination (monthly for all women over 20)
  ACS recommendations for clinical examination by health care professional
    Every 3 years for women 20 to 40 years of age
    Every year for women over 40
  ACS recommendations for mammography
    Baseline for women 35 to 40 years of age
    Every 1-2 years for women aged 40 to 49
    Annual for women over age 50
  Need for more frequent examinations and earlier mammograms for women with personal or family histories of breast cancer or who are at high risk
Ensure that patient and/or significant other demonstrates breast self-examination (Figure 13-2)
  Stand in front of mirror
    Inspect breasts in four positions
      Standing straight with arms at side
      Placing hands on waist and pressing in
      Arms elevated
      Leaning forward

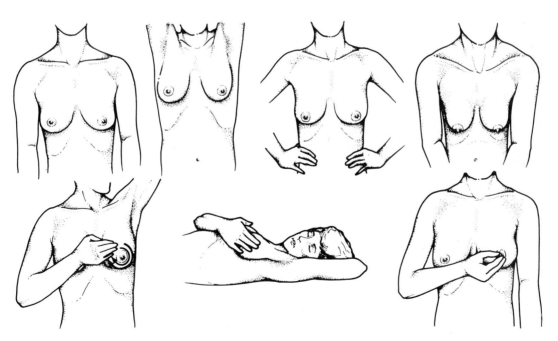

FIGURE 13-2. Breast self-examination.

Observe for size, differences in veins and skin, nipple irregularities, and contour
Palpate breasts
  Place one arm over head and palpate that breast with other hand
  Use flat part of fingers, beginning in upper, outer portion and continuing in circular movement to nipple
  Gently milk nipple for discharge
  Reverse position and palpate other breast
  Lie in supine position and repeat palpation steps
Premenopausal: perform breast self-examination 1 week after menses begin
Postmenopausal: perform breast self-examination once a month; usually easiest to remember either first or last day of month

Evaluation

Patient verbalizes fears and risk factors associated with breast cancer, demonstrates breast self-examination, and verbalizes signs and symptoms requiring follow-up health care

Vaginal Cancer
Determination of risk factors

Exposure to diethylstilbestrol (DES) in utero

Signs and symptoms

Abnormal bleeding
Vivid red areas in vagina
Firm, indurated, cystic areas in vagina or on cervix

Nursing diagnosis/goal/interventions

ndx: Knowledge deficit regarding prevention and early detection of vaginal cancer

GOAL: *Patient and/or significant other will demonstrate knowledge of risk factors associated with vaginal cancer, signs and symptoms that require health care evaluation, and detection measures for determining vaginal cancer*

Prevention/detection

Ensure that patient and/or significant other knows and understands
  Importance of maintaining accurate menstrual cycle history
    Frequency
    Length of menses
    Amount
    Color
  Need to maintain good gynecologic hygiene
  Need to avoid frequent douching, especially during adolescent and pregnant periods
  Importance of delaying sexual function in early teen years
  Need for regular, periodic gynecologic examinations
  Importance of cytologic Papanicolaou (Pap) examinations
    First smear at onset of sexual activity or age 18
    Second 1 year later, then q3 years to age 35, then q5 years to age 60
    Annual smears if at high risk
  Signs and symptoms to report to physician
  Method to inspect vulva for
    Skin excoriation
    Ulcers
    Lumps
    Leukoplakia
    Narrowing of introitus
    Atrophy

Evaluation

Patient demonstrates knowledge of risk factors associated with vaginal cancer, signs and symptoms requiring health care follow-up, and detection measures for determining vaginal cancer

Ovarian Cancer
Determination of risk factors

Upper socioeconomic status
Nulliparous
Older at first parity
Reduced fertility
Infertility
Exposure to carcinogens
  Radiation
  Asbestos
History of breast cancer
Family history of breast, colon, or ovarian cancer
History of
  Pentz-Jeghers syndrome
  Mucocutaneous pigmentation
  Intestinal polyps

Signs and symptoms

Dyspepsia
Vague abdominal discomfort
Change in abdominal girth
Bilateral, irregular, immobile ovarian mass
GI symptoms: weight loss is frequent in advanced disease
Palpable ovaries postmenopause
Adnexal thickening: postmenopausal or nulliparous women

Nursing diagnosis/goal/interventions

ndx: Knowledge deficit regarding detection of ovarian cancer

GOAL: *Patient and/or significant other will demonstrate knowledge of risk factors associated with ovarian cancer, signs and symptoms that require health care evaluation, and detection measures for determining ovarian cancer*

Prevention/detection

Ensure that patient and/or significant other knows and understands
   Risk factors
   Importance of maintaining accurate menstrual cycle
      history
      Frequency
      Length of menses
      Amount
      Color
   Need to maintain good gynecologic hygiene
   Need to avoid frequent douching, especially during adolescent and pregnant periods
   Importance of delaying sexual function in early teen years
   Need for regular, periodic gynecologic examinations
   Importance of cytologic Pap examinations
      First smear at onset of sexual activity or age 18
      Second 1 year later, then q3 years to age 35, then q5 years to age 60
      Annual smears if at high risk
   Signs and symptoms to report to physician
   Method to inspect vulva for
      Skin excoriation
      Ulcers
      Lumps
      Leukoplakia
      Narrowing of introitus
      Atrophy
   That early detection is rare (no early symptoms)

Evaluation

Patient demonstrates knowledge of risk factors associated with ovarian cancer, signs and symptoms requiring health care follow-up, and detection measures for determining ovarian cancer

Cervical Cancer
Determination of risk factors

Low socioeconomic status
First coitus at early age
Multiple sex partners
Frequent genital infections
Mismanaged parturition
Nonbarrier-type contraceptive
Chronic vaginal douching
Exposure to herpes simplex II virus

Signs and symptoms

Early
   Unexplained vaginal bleeding or spotting
   Postcoital, postdouche bleeding
   Vaginal discharge: watery, purulent, or mucoid
Late
   Pelvic pain
   Irritation, vulvitis
   Yellow, frequently foul-smelling vaginal discharge
   Urinary symptoms, leakage of urine or feces from vagina
   Anorexia, weight loss

Nursing diagnosis/goal/interventions

ndx: Knowledge deficit regarding prevention and early detection of cervical cancer

GOAL: *Patient and/or significant other will demonstrate knowledge of measures to reduce the risk of cervical cancer and detection measures for determining cervical cancer*

Prevention/detection

Ensure that patient and/or significant other knows and understands
   Importance of maintaining accurate menstrual cycle
      history
      Frequency
      Length of menses
      Amount
      Color
   Risk factors and importance of realistic modifications
   Need to maintain good personal hygiene
   Need to maintain good gynecologic hygiene
   Need to avoid frequent douching, especially during adolescent and pregnant periods
   Importance of delaying sexual function in early teen years
   Need for regular, periodic gynecologic examinations
   Importance of cytologic Pap examinations
      First smear at onset of sexual activity or age 18
      ACS states that women who have had normal Pap smear for 2 consecutive years can then have one every third year
      American College of Obstetrics and Gynecology recommends that sexually active women have a Pap smear annually

That Pap screening is the most effective measure of early detection and proper follow-up care to prevent cervical cancer

Signs and symptoms to report to physician

Methods to inspect vulva for
- Skin excoriation
- Ulcers
- Lumps
- Leukoplakia
- Narrowing of introitus
- Atrophy

Evaluation

Patient demonstrates knowledge of risk factors associated with cervical cancer, signs and symptoms requiring health care evaluation, and detection measures for determining cervical cancer

Uterine Cancer (Endometrial)
Determination of risk factors

Menstrual irregularities
Infertility, anovulatory
Nulliparous
Late menopause
Long-term use of estrogen drugs after menopause
History of
- Obesity
- Diabetes
- Hypertension
- Adenomatous hyperplasia

Signs and symptoms

Any abnormal vaginal bleeding
Purulent discharge
Endometrial polyps
Enlarged, boggy uterus on examination
Lower abdominal and low back pain in late-stage disease

Nursing diagnosis/goal/interventions

ndx: Knowledge deficit regarding prevention and early detection of uterine (endometrial) cancer

GOAL: *Patient and/or significant other will demonstrate knowledge of risk factors associated with uterine cancer, signs and symptoms that require health care evaluation, and detection measures for determining uterine cancer*

Prevention/detection

Ensure that patient and/or significant other knows and understands

Importance of maintaining accurate menstrual cycle history
- Frequency
- Length of menses
- Amount
- Color

Need to maintain good gynecologic hygiene
Need to avoid frequent douching
That detection by Pap smear is of low reliability
High-risk profile
- Over 50 years of age
- No pregnancies, obesity, diabetes, hypertension with increased estrogen exposure

Early detection helped by routine pelvic examinations

Signs and symptoms to report to physician

Method to inspect vulva for
- Skin excoriation
- Ulcers
- Lumps
- Leukoplakia
- Narrowing of introitus
- Atrophy

Evaluation

Patient demonstrates knowledge of risk factors associated with uterine cancer, signs and symptoms requiring health care follow-up, and detection measures for determining uterine cancer

Leukemia
Determination of risk factors

Exposure to ionizing radiation
- Work environment
- Prenatal
- Medical diagnosis or therapy

Genetic factors
- Bloom's syndrome
- Trisomy 21 (Down's syndrome: 15 to 20 times the risk)
- Trisomy G (Klinefelter's syndrome)
- Fanconi's syndrome
- Philadelphia chromosome: positive
- Ataxia telangiectasis

Chemical exposure
- Benzene
- Phenylbutazone
- Arsenic
- Chloramphenicol
- Alkylating chemotherapeutic agents and radiotherapy

Immunodeficiency
Viral

Signs and symptoms

Anemia: pallor, fatigue, dyspnea, palpitations, headache, syncope, anorexia
Thrombocytopenia: petechiae, epistaxis, blood in excreta, bleeding gums, ecchymosis, hematoma formation, purpura
Leukopenia
    Skin infections: may appear red or dark without pus
    Fever, stomatitis, upper respiratory infection (URI) symptoms, urinary infection
Bone and joint pain
Cervical lymphadenopathy
Oropharyngeal lesions
Peridontal infections
Ocular lesions and hemorrhage
Gingival hypertrophy
GI manifestation
    Dysphagia
    Esophagitis
    Perirectal abscess
Genitourinary: uric acid nephropathy
Cardiopulmonary manifestation
    Impaired respiration
    Pneumonia
Nervous system manifestation
Lymphadenopathy
Hepatomegaly
Splenomegaly

Nursing diagnosis/goal/interventions

ndx: Knowledge deficit regarding prevention and detection of leukemia

GOAL: *Patient and/or significant other will demonstrate knowledge of risk factors associated with leukemia, signs and symptoms that require health care evaluation, and detection methods for determining leukemia*

Prevention

Ensure that patient and/or significant other knows and understands
    Importance of decreasing exposure time to x-rays, especially in young children
        Be certain diagnostic studies are essential
        Careful preparation and positioning to prevent retakes
        Shielding of gonads and other body parts during x-ray examination
        Proper shielding of health care workers when assisting with x-ray examination

Detection

Ensure that patient and/or significant other knows and understands
    Importance of regular, periodic physical examinations, including
        Palpation of lymph nodes, liver, and spleen
        Inspection of skin and mucous membranes
        Palpation of sternum, bones, and joints
    Importance of reporting signs and symptoms to physician
Ensure that patient/significant other is knowledgeable about detection methods
    Bone marrow aspiration
    Laboratory tests
    Radiologic tests

Evaluation

Patient demonstrates knowledge of risk factors associated with leukemia, signs and symptoms requiring health care follow-up, and methods for detection of leukemia

Hodgkin's Disease

Determination of risk factors

Male
White
Young adult or over 70 years of age
High socioeconomic status
No or few siblings
History of
    Infectious mononucleosis
    Immunodeficiency syndrome
Use of amphetamines is questionable; not proven

Signs and symptoms

Painless lymphadenopathy (usually supraclavicular or cervical area)
    Mediastinal, axillary, and inguinal less commonly
    Fever, night sweats, weight loss, lethargy, malaise, anorexia
Lymphadenopathy can cause obstruction, resulting in edema and pain
Cervical node enlargement: venous occlusion, neck edema, airway obstruction
Mediastinal adenopathy: dyspnea, cough
Inguinal involvement: dysuria, frequency, painful urination, and lumbar discomfort

Nursing diagnosis/goal/interventions

ndx: Knowledge deficit regarding detection of Hodgkin's disease

GOAL: *Patient will demonstrate knowledge of risk factors associated with Hodgkin's disease, signs and symptoms requiring health care evaluation, and detection methods for determining Hodgkin's disease*

Detection

Ensure that patient and/or significant other knows and understands
  Importance of reporting symptoms to physician
  Importance of scheduling periodic physical examinations
  Detection methods
    Laboratory tests
    Staging laparotomy

Evaluation

Patient demonstrates knowledge of risk factors associated with Hodgkin's disease, signs and symptoms requiring health care follow-up, and methods for detection of Hodgkin's disease

---

TNM CLASSIFICATIONS

T: Primary tumor
  T_X: Minimum requirements to assess the primary tumor cannot be met
  T_0: No evidence of primary tumor
  T_{IS}: Carcinoma in situ
  T_1, T_2, T_3, T_4: Progressive increase in tumor size or involvement
N: Regional lymph nodes
  N_0: No evidence of regional nodal involvement
  N_1, N_2, N_3, N_4: Increasing degree of demonstrable abnormality of regional lymph nodes
M: Distant metastasis
  M_0: Indicates absence
  M_+: Indicates presence

HISTOPATHOLOGY

G_1: Well-differentiated grade
G_2: Moderately well-differentiated grade
G_3 and G_4: Poorly- to very poorly-differentiated grade

RESIDUAL TUMOR

R_0: No residual tumor
R_1: Microscopic residual tumor
R_2: Macroscopic residual tumor

STAGING METHOD

cTNM: Staging determined by clinical noninvasive physical examination, laboratory, and radiographic studies
sTNM: Staging information based on surgical procedures, biopsies, and histopathologic analysis
pTNM: Staging determined by correlation of clinical, pathologic, and residual tumor findings

HOST PERFORMANCE STATUS*

The host performance status is determined at the time of classification; the condition of the patient does not enter into determination of stage but may be a factor in deciding type and time of treatment

	ECOG/Zubrod	Karnofsky %
H_0: Normal activity	0	90-100
H_1: Symptomatic and ambulatory; cares for self	1	70-80
H_2: Ambulatory more than 50% of time; occasionally needs assistance	2	50-60
H_3: Ambulatory less than 50% of time; requires special nursing and/or medical assistance	3	30-40
H_4: Bedridden; may need hospitalization	4	10-20

*American Joint Committee for Cancer Staging.

TABLE 13-1. Classification of Tumors

Tissue of origin	Benign	Malignant
Epithelium: surface skin and mucous membranes	Papilloma Polyp	Squamous cell or epidermoid carcinoma Basal cell carcinoma
Glands	Adenoma Cystadenoma	Adenocarcinoma
Connective tissue		
Embryonic fibrous tissue	Myxoma	Myxosarcoma
Fibrous tissue	Fibroma	Fibrosarcoma
Cartilage	Chondroma	Chondrosarcoma
Bone	Osteoma	Osteosarcoma
Fat	Lipoma	Liposarcoma
Synovial membrane	Synovioma	Synovial sarcoma
Blood vessels	Hemangioma	Hemangiosarcoma
Lymph vessels	Lymphangioma	Lymphangiosarcoma
Muscle tissue		
Smooth muscle	Leiomyoma	Leiomyosarcoma
Striated muscle	Rhabdomyoma	Rhabdomyosarcoma
Hematopoietic tissue		
Lymphoid tissue		Malignant lymphoma Non-Hodgkin's lymphoma Lymphocytic leukemia
Granulocytic tissue		Myelocytic leukemia
Erythrocytic tissue		Erythroleukemia
Plasma cells		Multiple myeloma
Nerve tissue		
Glial cells	Glioma	Glioblastoma (astrocytoma) Spongioblastoma
Meninges	Meningioma	Meningeal sarcoma
Nerve cells	Neuroma; ganglioneuroma	Neurogenic sarcoma
Neuroectoderm	Nevus	Neuroblastoma
Fibers	Neurofibroma	Neurofibrosarcoma
Retina		Retinoblastoma
Adrenal medulla	Pheochromocytoma	Pheochromocytoma
Nerve sheaths	Neurilemmoma	Neurilemmal sarcoma
Tumors of more than one tissue		
Breast	Fibroadenoma	Cystosarcoma phyllodes
Embryonic kidney		Nephroblastoma (Wilms')
Multipotent cells	Teratoma	
Uterus		Mixed mesodermal
Miscellaneous		
Melanoblasts	Pigmented nevus	Malignant melanoma Melanocarcinoma
Placenta	Hydatidiform mole	Choriocarcinoma (chorionepithelioma)
Ovary	Granulosa-theca cell tumor	Carcinoma
Testes	Interstitial cell tumor	Seminoma (spermatocytic) Carcinoma (embryonal)
Thymus	Thymoma	Thymoma

TABLE 13-2. Cancer Staging Utilizing TNM* Classifications

Stage	T	N	M	Survival	Comments
I	1	0	0	70%-90%	Mass limited to organ of origin; nodes not involved; operable and resectable
II	2	1	0	50%±	Local spread to surrounding tissue; nodal involvement suspected or proven; operable but without certainty of total resection
III	3	2	0	20%±	Extensive primary tumor with fixation to deeper structures; nodes involved; operable but not resectable
IV	4	3	+	<5%	Distant metastases; inoperable

*T, Primary tumor; N, regional lymph nodes; M, metastasis by vascular dissemination.

ANTINEOPLASTIC CHEMOTHERAPY

chemotherapy Systemic cancer treatment using drugs to treat cancer; useful when there is disseminated disease or when there is a high risk of recurrence in the body; can be curative, can prolong life, or can be palliative; is often used as an adjuvant to surgery and/or radiation therapy

Assessment
Observations/findings

Physical response to specific condition
    Ability and desire to learn
    Barriers to learning: fatigue, denial
    Knowledge level related to cancer and cancer treatment
    Attitude and expected outcome related to chemotherapy
Psychosocial response based on patient's coping mechanisms, support system, previous experience with chemotherapy, and amount of information received about disease process
Obtain baseline assessment prior to beginning chemotherapy and continue throughout treatment period (see Oncology Assessment, p. 646)

Laboratory/diagnostic studies

Specific to each medication and expected responses (see Table 13-4)

Potential complications

Side effects or toxicities specific to each medication (see Table 13-4)
Consider the following
    Bone marrow suppression
    Cutaneous manifestations
    GI dysfunction
    Respiratory dysfunction
    Renal dysfunction
    Cardiac dysfunction
    Sexual and reproductive dysfunction
    Electrolyte/chemical imbalance
    Musculoskeletal dysfunction

Medical management

Antineoplastic medications ordered according to protocol
Laboratory diagnostic/monitoring studies
Vital signs
Antiemetics, antacids, oral anesthetics
Parenteral fluids

Nursing diagnoses/goals/interventions

ndx: Fear related to disease process and/or treatment

GOAL: *Patient will verbalize fears and begin to deal with them effectively*

Assess previous experience with chemotherapy
Assist patient and/or significant other with recognizing and clarifying fears and with developing coping strategies for those fears
May be helpful to role play and/or coach patient by using examples of coping skills used by others

ndx: Alteration in comfort: pain related to disease process

GOAL: *Patient's pain will be minimized, and comfort level will be maintained*

Monitor and document pain characteristics, as well as associated factors such as anxiety
Establish a trusting relationship with patient
Administer prescribed analgesic q3h to 4h at regular intervals to control pain
Provide environment conducive to rest
Evaluate patient's fears and perceptions regarding pain and pain therapy
Evaluate the meaning of the pain to patient (metastasis, punishment, recurrence, death)
Evaluate level of consciousness and note changes in sensorium
Involve significant other in care planning as much as possible

ndx: Alteration in nutrition: less than body requirements related to nausea and vomiting, anorexia, stomatitis, disease process and/or treatment

GOAL: *Patient will maintain adequate nutritional intake and control of nausea and vomiting; weight loss and other side effects of stomatitis and chemotherapy will be minimized*

Evaluate nutritional status
    Measure height and weight and compare with ideal body weight
    Assess laboratory values (CBC, serum albumin)
Obtain history of food preferences
Perform baseline oral assessment and daily oral assessment throughout treatment period
Evaluate for presence of fatigue, depression, anxiety, and/or pain
Describe signs and symptoms that could alter nutritional intake, such as nausea and vomiting, sore mouth, and pain

Describe measures to alter above signs and symptoms
Explain measures to maintain adequate nutritional intake (maintain ideal weight)
  Frequent oral hygiene
  Avoidance of extreme temperatures of foods, and spicy foods
  Encouraging significant other to make patient's favorite foods
  Include basic food group in diet
  Maintain fluid intake to 3000 ml daily unless contraindicated
  Provide suggestions for increasing calories and protein in diet
  Weigh patient weekly
Describe ways to overcome alteration in taste
  Experiment with different seasonings
  Cold foods may be more appealing
  Avoid preparation of foods with strong odors
Explain measures to prevent abdominal feeling of fullness or bloating
  Limit fluid intake at meals
  Avoid gas-producing foods (beans, cabbage)
  Encourage small, frequent meals
  Avoid greasy or spicy foods
Explain measures to control diarrhea
  Reduce amount of fiber in diet
  Assist patient in identifying foods, beverages, and medications that cause loose stools
  Explain use of antidiarrheal medication
Evaluate hydration status and skin turgor
Monitor intake and output
Describe measures to prevent constipation
  Increase liquids in diet
  Eat foods with high-fiber content
Assess history of nausea and vomiting: cause, time of occurrence, frequency
  Administer antiemetics before, during, and after chemotherapy as needed
  Medicate according to pattern of nausea and vomiting
  Administer chemotherapy in late afternoon or at night when possible
Encourage prophylactic oral hygiene measures before and after meals and at bedtime
Check for oral burning, pain, and changes in tolerance to foods
Teach signs and symptoms that may need health care follow-up, such as uncontrolled nausea and vomiting, diarrhea, weakness, and malaise

ndx: Actual impairment of skin integrity related to chemotherapy

GOAL: *Patient will verbalize measures to improve or heal impaired skin integrity*

Assess skin: color, temperature, rash, tenderness, itching, turgor, peeling of palms, drainage
Inspect skin folds, especially axillary, groin, and perineum
Determine fluid and nutritional status
Teach skin care
  Use mild soap and water, rinse, pat dry
  Keep skin and nails meticulously clean (prevent infection)
Avoid sun exposure: wear sunscreen, long sleeves, and hats
Teach patient signs and symptoms of skin changes, indicating those to report to physician
If skin tenderness or dryness is present, use water-based topical ointments
Dust on cornstarch
Wear soft cotton clothing

ndx: Alteration in fluid volume: deficit related to disease process and chemotherapy

GOAL: *Patient will exhibit stabilization of fluid volume*

Assess fluid intake and output
Inspect skin turgor and integrity
Inspect mucous membranes for moistness and integrity
Assess weight and vital signs
Evaluate laboratory values
Encourage oral fluids to 2 to 3 L/day unless contraindicated
Obtain order for parenteral fluids as needed
Identify and manage side effects that may interfere with fluid intake
Assess for factors that may contribute to fluid loss (fever, diarrhea)
Teach signs and symptoms to report to health care team

ndx: Alteration in fluid volume: potential excess related to disease process and/or chemotherapy

GOAL: *Patient will not have signs of fluid overload*

Regulate flow of IV at least hourly
Maintain accurate intake and output
Carefully observe for signs of fluid overload
  Increased respirations
  Moist rales
Auscultate chest q2h to 4h during hydration
Monitor blood pressure and pulse
Weigh patient daily

Observe for signs of edema, especially in ankles and fingers
Monitor laboratory data (usually no change in hematocrit but may be significant drop in serum sodium)
Teach patient signs and symptoms of fluid overload to report to health care team (increased respirations, increase in weight, finger and ankle edema, puffy eyelids)

ndx: Disturbance in self-concept related to disease process and/or treatment

GOAL: *Patient will verbalize concerns and develop coping mechanisms to deal effectively with problems*

Assess patient's level of knowledge related to the disease process and treatment
Evaluate how diagnosis and treatment are affecting patient's life-style
Evaluate support system/significant other
Determine patient and/or significant other's coping strategies
Provide opportunity for discussion of concerns regarding physical self (feelings: physically, feelings about one's body), role function (wife, mother, wage earner), and dependence/independence
Assess need for professional counseling if patient's support system is deteriorating; give information regarding necessary counseling in adaptation process
Refer patient and/or significant other to supportive group programs such as I Can Cope and Reach for Recovery

ndx: Self-care deficit (specify feeding, bathing/hygiene, dressing/grooming, toileting) related to weakness

GOAL: *Patient will function at maximal level of ability*

Determine nature, extent, and duration of self-care deficits
Determine patient's coping techniques
Assess family/significant other's availability, willingness, and readiness to assist patient if needed
Maintain a patient, supportive attitude
Allow patient to do things that he is capable of doing
Provide self-help devices as needed
Praise patient for progress and emphasize achievements
Recognize dependency needs and plan care accordingly with patient/significant other input
Assist patient/significant other in planning for long-term care if needed
Arrange for nursing services as needed at home
Teach patient/significant other skills needed for home care

ndx: Knowledge deficit regarding chemotherapy

GOAL: *Patient and/or significant other will demonstrate knowledge of disease process, treatment, and potential side effects of chemotherapy*

Assess ability and desire to learn
Assess knowledge and level of understanding related to the disease process (factual, misconceptions)
Assess knowledge and level of understanding related to treatment (misconceptions, myths, cultural beliefs, previous experience)
Ascertain expectations of outcome of treatment
With help of audiovisual aids, explain how drugs work and expected therapeutic effects of chemotherapy treatment
Provide patient and/or significant other with written material regarding name of drug, action of drug, and potential side effects
Explain method, frequency, and duration of administration of each drug
Provide verbal and written material regarding management of side effects/toxicity
Instruct patient regarding early side effects, such as nausea and vomiting, and side effects that will be delayed, such as myelosuppression
Discuss side effects that are reversible
Instruct patient regarding side effects to report to physician
Give written information on how and where to reach health care personnel if necessary
Involve significant other in care planning as much as possible

Evaluation

Patient expresses and discusses feelings about disease and treatment, and seeks out resources and assistance from others when needed
Patient verbalizes that pain is adequately controlled
Patient maintains adequate nutrition, has control of nausea and vomiting, and manages side effects
Patient verbalizes measures to improve or heal impaired skin integrity and demonstrates healing of impaired skin integrity
Patient verbalizes methods to correct fluid volume deficit and exhibits stabilization
Accurate intake and output are maintained; weight is stable
Patient verbalizes concerns and demonstrates successful positive coping and problem-solving techniques
Patient performs self-care tasks according to physical capacity and uses support system/resources effectively

Patient demonstrates knowledge of disease process, treatment and side effects, and measures to manage adverse effects

Administration of Chemotherapeutic Drugs

Verify patient's identification
Review patient's allergy history
Assess learning needs and concerns, and answer questions appropriately
Review educational materials with patient and family (films, pamphlets)
Check physician's order for drug dose, route, rate, and time of administration
Verify that informed consent has been given
Review laboratory data with knowledge of acceptable parameters
Review immediate and long-term side effects of drugs
Calculate dosage, double-check calculation, and ascertain if dosage is within normal administration range
Know amount and type of diluent to use for reconstitution (mix in biologic safety hood and observe safety precautions [p. 670])
Verify drug dosage with another nurse, a pharmacist, or physician
Correctly label drug with patient's name, dose, and route of administration
Select site for venipuncture with regard to previous trauma to arm (blood drawing or lymphatic resection) and drug to be given (vesicant vs. nonvesicant); begin at distal portion of extremity
Avoid use of preexisting IV for vesicant drugs
Avoid use of lower extremities
Wash hands
Start IV, following guidelines of facility's policy and procedures; needle gauge usually No. 23 or No. 25 scalp vein
Avoid multiple sticks; test patency of IV—blood backflows easily
Stabilize arm or hand; use pillow or board if necessary
Ensure patient's comfort
Instruct patient to notify nurse immediately of adverse effects
Administer antiemetic 30 min prior to administration of chemotherapy if indicated
Have emergency medications and antidote readily available for adverse reaction
Nonvesicants
  Can be given by IV bolus through side arm of free-flowing IV containing no additives, by continuous IV drip through a peripheral vein, or by two-syringe technique, with one syringe containing 10 ml of normal saline to test vein prior to drug administration and to flush vein following injection of drug
  When administering through side arm of IV by bolus, check for blood backflow by pinching IV tubing and quickly releasing, prior to administration of drug, at half-way mark, and at end of administration; before removing needle from injection port, place 4 × 4 with alcohol swab beneath injection port to catch drop
  When giving drug by continuous infusion, ensure vein patency throughout infusion period; before removing needle from injection port, place 4 × 4 and alcohol swab beneath infection port to catch drop (prevent spill)
Irritants
  Can be given by infusion over 30 to 60 min depending on dosage
  Check for blood backflow prior to administration and assure vein patency throughout infusion period; apply ice pack prophylactically at infusion site to prevent discomfort
Vesicants
  See Extravasation (p. 704)
  Can be safely administered through side arm of newly inserted, free-flowing peripheral IV containing no additives
  Check for blood backflow prior to instillation of each milliliter (as described above for nonvesicants)
  These drugs are not given as continuous infusions except through a well-established central venous access device
  When administering by central venous device, obtain blood backflow prior to instillation of chemotherapeutic drug (see Care of Patient with Central Venous Catheter, p. 55)
  Use mechanical or electrical controller for continuous chemotherapy infusion
  Keep IV site and as much of limb as possible visible
    Avoid obstructing view of site and vein with tape
    Keep clothing well above site; remove arm from clothing when possible
  Monitor for allergic reaction: anaphylaxis and extravasation (p. 704) on initiation, continuously during infusion, and then q4h to 8h for 24 hr
  Manage pain as indicated and ordered; adjust flow rate of "painful" medication to patient tolerance if possible
  Know and observe for side or toxic effects and complications during administration, then for 24 to 48 hr; be aware of nadir of drugs ordered

Differentiate between effect of drug and reaction to disease when possible

Infuse parenteral fluids after drug administration to flush tubing, needle, and vein

Apply pressure over site for 3 to 4 min following removal of needle

Document medication, site, and responses or untoward effects of interventions

Intrathecal or intraventricular administration

    Assist with lumbar puncture or ventricular puncture

    Be aware that intraventricular injection may be done through subcutaneously implanted reservoir

    Observe strict aseptic technique

    Be aware that a sterile isotonic diluent without preservatives is essential in minimizing neurotoxicity

Intraarterial administration

    May be given in one of several arteries (e.g., hepatic artery)

    See Electronic Infusion Devices (p. 60)

    Teach patient to call staff immediately if warning symptoms are noticed

Arterial perfusion

    Intraarterial administration of chemotherapeutic agent to an isolated extremity or body area

    See above

Intraperitoneal administration: administration of chemotherapeutic agent directly into peritoneal cavity by dialysis (p. 562)

Intracavitary administration

    Administration of chemotherapeutic agent into a body space to control malignant effusions

    Usually excess fluid is removed from cavity prior to instillation of drug

    Ensure free flow of medication during administration

    Aspirate frequently throughout instillation for fluid return to ensure that drug is being instilled into cavity

    Turn patient from side to side q15 min for four times then q2h to 4h to ensure maximal distribution throughout cavity

    Drain fluids from cavity q12h to 24h after instillation and then daily or as ordered

Implantable drug delivery systems

    Implantable drug infusion pumps are delivery systems intended to administer long-term chemotherapy in ambulatory patients

    Device delivers a precise, continuous drug flow to selected organs or sites via a pliable, radiopaque, silicone rubber catheter

    Pump is refilled by percutaneous injection and powered by a self-contained inexhaustible energy supply

Safety in Handling Cancer Chemotherapy Agents

Only pharmacists, physicians, and nurses with special training should prepare chemotherapeutic agents for administration

Text continued on p. 684.

TABLE 13-3. Hazards Associated with Chemotherapeutic Drugs

Medication	Route	Hazard	Precaution and action
ALKYLATING AGENTS			
Cyclophosphamide (Cytoxan)	IV, po	Teratogenic and carcinogenic; skin irritation is rare	Wear protective gloves; flush spills with large amounts of water
Mechlorethamine hydrochloride (Mustargen, nitrogen mustard)	IV, intracavitary, topical, intralesional	Strong vesicant, nasal irritant, highly toxic	Wear protective gloves; protect eyes; wash skin with large amounts of water, sodium carbonate (3%), or isotonic solution of sodium thiosulfate (2.5%); wash eyes out with large amounts of water; irrigate with sodium thiosulfate in isotonic solution (contact physician)
ANTIMETABOLITES			
Cytarabine (Ara-C, cytosar)	IV, SC, IM, intrathecal	Teratogenic; not absorbed through intact skin	Wear protective gloves; wash spills with water
5-Fluorouracil (Fluoroplex, Fluorouracil, Adrucil)	IV, po, topical	Minor inflammatory reaction if skin is broken	Flush spills with large amounts of water

TABLE 13-3. Hazards Associated with Chemotherapeutic Drugs—cont'd

Medication	Route	Hazard	Precaution and action
Methotrexate (Mexate, Amethopterin MTX)	IV, IM, intrathecal	Teratogenic, carcinogenic skin irritant	Wear protective gloves; wash spills with water; apply nonmedicated cream for stinging; for systemic absorption of significant quantity notify physician; give folinic acid (leucovorin calcium)
ANTIBIOTICS			
Dactinomycin (Cosmegen, actinomycin D)	IV	Teratogenic; corrosive to soft tissues	Wear protective gloves; protect eyes; rinse spillage off in running water for 10 min; rinse with buffered phosphate solution
Bleomycin (Blenoxane)	IV, IM, subcutaneous, intraarterial, intratumoral, intracavitary	Cytostatic: local, toxic, or allergic reaction	Wear protective gloves; wash spills thoroughly with water
Daunomycin (Cerubidin, Daunorubicin, DNR)	IV	Skin and mucous membrane irritant	Wear protective gloves; wash spills immediately with water or isotonic saline
Doxorubicin (Adriamycin)	IV	Potential teratogenic; suspected carcinogenic skin irritant—but not absorbed into bloodstream	Wear protective gloves; wash spills immediately with large amounts of water
Mithramycin (Mithracin)	IV	Rare skin irritation	Wash spills with water
Mitomycin (Mitomycin C, Mutamycin)		Teratogenic; suspected carcinogenic skin irritant	Wear protective gloves; wash spills thoroughly and immediately with large quantities of water; irrigate contaminated eyes with large amounts of water; notify physician
PODOPHYLLOTOXINS			
Etoposide (VP-16) Teniposide (VM-26)	IV	Suspected teratogenic and carcinogenic irritants	Wear protective gloves; wash spills with large amounts of water
VINCA ALKALOIDS			
Vinblastine (Velban)	IV	Suspected teratogenic skin irritant	Wear protective gloves; wash spills thoroughly and immediately with large amounts of water
Vincristine (Oncovin)	IV	Suspected teratogenic skin irritant	Wear protective gloves; wash skin with large amounts of water
Vindesine	IV	Suspected teratogenic skin irritant; may produce corneal ulcers	Wear protective gloves; protect eyes; wash areas with large amounts of water
MISCELLANEOUS			
Asparaginase (L-Asparaginase)	IV, IM	Potentially teratogenic	
Azathioprine (Imuran)	IV (Investigational)	Potentially teratogenic, suspected carcinogenic skin irritant	Wear protective gloves; protect eyes; wash spills off with water immediately
Cisplatin (Platinol)	IV	Suspected teratogen and carcinogen; skin reaction in sensitive patients	Wear protective gloves; rinse spills thoroughly with water
Dacarbazine (DTIC)	IV	Teratogenic, carcinogenic irritant to skin and mucous membranes	Wear protective gloves; wash spills with soap and water immediately; irrigate eyes with water

TABLE 13-4. Chemotherapeutic Drugs

Medication	Dosage	Routes of administration	Side effects and toxicities
ALKYLATING AGENTS			

Busulfan (Myleran)	4-6 mg/day (initially); 1-3 mg/day (maintenance); given according to protocol	po	Myelosuppression
			Low doses
			    Granulocytopenia
			    Platelets, lymphoid elements spared
			Hyperpigmentation
			High doses
			    Leukopenia (p. 684)
			Delayed-refractory
			    Pancytopenia
			Long-term therapy
			    Pulmonary fibrosis (rare)

Chlorambucil (Leukeran)	0.1-0.2 mg/kg; given according to protocol
	2 mg/day maintenance
		po	Myelosuppression
			    Leukopenia
			Nausea and vomiting, mild
			Amenorrhea
			Depressed spermatogenesis
			Long-term therapy
			    Alveolar dysplasia
			    Pulmonary fibrosis
			    Nausea and vomiting
			    Metallic taste
			    Sinus burning

Cyclophosphamide (Cytoxan, Endoxana, CTX)	40-50 mg/kg; given according to protocol
	1-5 mg/kg/day Oral
		po; IV	Myelosuppression
			    Leukopenia (p. 684)
			    Thrombocytopenia may occur
			Common with high doses
			    Stomatitis (p. 692)
			    Alopecia (p. 702)
			    Hemorrhagic cystitis (p. 698)
			        Dose-limiting
			Amenorrhea
			Testicular atrophy

Mechlorethamine (nitrogen mustard, HN_2)	0.4 mg/kg; given according to protocol	IV; intracavitary; topical; intralesional	Myelosuppression; dose-limiting
			    Lymphocytopenia; dose-limiting
			    Thrombocytopenia (p. 688)
			    Granulocytopenia (leukocytopenia, p. 684)
			Nausea and vomiting, severe (p. 690) onset 1-2 hr—lasting 8 hr
			Diarrhea (p. 694)
			Skin rash
			Amenorrhea
			Impaired spermatogenesis
			Vesicant; pain and tissue necrosis if extravasated

Nadir	Recovery after nadir (days)	Indications	Administration and nursing implications
10-12 days	42-50	Chronic myelogenous leukemia	Oral tablets may be taken any time of the day
11-30 days	24-54		
1-10 yr			
14-28 days	28-42	Chronic lymphocytic leukemia, ovarian cancer, Hodgkin's and non-Hodgkin's lymphoma	Give oral medication as ordered; no specific directions
8-14 days	18-25	Non-Hodgkin's lymphoma, sarcoma, breast, lung, and ovarian cancer: acute and chronic lymphocytic leukemia	Give IV push over 3-5 min through side port of patent IV
Give oral doses with or immediately after meals
Administer antiemetic prior to therapy and as indicated
Force fluids to 3000 ml/day prior to administration and 48 hr after
24 hr to several weeks			Check output; if falling, notify physician for parenteral therapy orders
IV hydration and bladder irrigation usually ordered when high doses given
Give within 15 to 30 min after reconstitution
7-15 days
Within 24 hr	28	Hodgkin's disease, non-Hodgkin's lymphomas, lung cancer, malignant pleural effusions	Give IV push through side port of patent IV; check blood backflow prior to instilling each ml; flush line with 30 ml IV fluid prior to each blood check; flush line after administration; monitor for extravasation (p. 704); give antidote as ordered
6-8 days	10-20		
	Several days		Administer antiemetic prior to therapy and then as indicated
Tell patient a metallic taste may be experienced just after drug injection
Inform patient that veins may become discolored
Reposition patient q15 min for four times after intracavitary instillation

Continued.

TABLE 13-4. Chemotherapeutic Drugs—cont'd

Medication	Dosage	Routes of administration	Side effects and toxicities

Melphalan (Alkeran)	0.25 mg/kg/day for daily dosage; 0.1-0.15 mg/kg for interval dosage; given according to protocol	po	Myelosuppression
			  Leukopenia (p. 684)
			  Thrombocytopenia (p. 688)
			High-dose therapy
			  Nausea and vomiting (p. 690)
			Long-term therapy
			  Acute leukemia (p. 177)
			  Alopecia (p. 702)
			  Dermatitis (p. 703)
			  Stomatitis (p. 692)

Thio-tepa (triethylene-thio-phosphoramide)	0.2 mg/kg/day
	60 mg instillations/60 ml
	Given according to protocol; dosage reduced with hepatic or renal dysfunction
		IV intracavitary, bladder instillation	Myelosuppression
			  Leukopenia (p. 684)
			  Thrombocytopenia (p. 688)
			  Anemia (p. 689)
			Mild
			  Local pain
			  Nausea, vomiting
			  Dizziness
			  Headache

NITROSOUREAS			

Carmustine (BCNU)	75-100 mg/m^2 or up to 200 mg/m^2; given according to protocol	IV
		Topical (investigational)
			Myelosuppression, dose-limiting
			  Leukopenia (p. 684)
			  Thrombocytopenia (p. 688)
			Immediate
			  Burning pain at IV site
			  Facial flushing
			  Severe nausea and vomiting onset 2 hr lasting 4-6 hr
			Long-term therapy
			  Pulmonary fibrosis

Lomustine (CCNU)	100-130 mg/m^2; given according to protocol	po	Myelosuppression, dose-limiting
			  Thrombocytopenia (p. 688)
			  Leukopenia (p. 684)
			Nausea, vomiting; onset 2-4 hr
			Anorexia
			Diarrhea

Semustin (investigational) (methyl CCNU)	125-200 mg/m^2; given according to protocol; dosage reduced with liver dysfunction and impaired marrow function	po	Myelosuppression, dose-limiting
			  May be cumulative
			  Thrombocytopenia (p. 688)
			  Leukopenia (p. 684)
			  Erythrocytopenia
			Nausea and vomiting; onset 4-6 hr

ANTIMETABOLITES			

Cytarabine (Ara-C, Cytosar)	1-3 mg/kg/day given according to protocol; dosage reduced with severe hepatic dysfunction	IV, intrathecal	Myelosuppression, dose-limiting
			  Leukopenia (p. 684)
			  Thrombocytopenia (p. 688)
			Nausea and vomiting especially with rapid infusion
			Stomatitis (p. 692)
			High dose
			  Flulike syndrome

Nadir	Recovery after nadir (days)	Indications	Administration and nursing implications
10-12 days	42-50	Breast, ovarian, and testicular cancer, myeloma, melanoma	Give oral doses 2 hr after meals
5-30 days	21-28	Papillary bladder tumors, malignant serous effusions Formerly breast and ovarian cancer and Hodgkin's lymphoma	Give IV push over 2-3 min through side port of patent IV Reposition patient q15 min for four times after intracavitary administration Bladder instillation is retained for 2 hr; reposition patient q15 min during this period

4-6 weeks
3-5 weeks
	7-14	Multiple myeloma, Hodgkin's disease, non-Hodgkin's lymphoma; brain tumor, colorectal adenocarcinoma; gastric adenocarcinoma, melanoma, hepatoma.	Give IV small volume for 15-45 min
			  Apply ice pack at IV site
			  Teach patient to report pain to staff immediately
			Flush vein before and after administration
			Administer antiemetics prior to administration and as ordered after

40-50 days 26-34 days 28-42 days	60 6-10 9-14 24 hr	Palliative: brain tumors, Hodgkin's disease, lung cancer, coorectal adenocarcinoma	Protect oral drug from heat and moisture Teach patient to take on an empty stomach; avoid alcohol after dose
28-63 days 21-35 days 28-42 days	82-89 6-8 hr	GI cancer, brain cancer, Hodgkin's disease, non-Hodgkin's lymphoma	Teach patient to take on an empty stomach (may lessen nausea and vomiting), observe patient preference Absorbed in 30-60 min if stomach is empty
12-14 days	22-24	Acute lymphocytic leukemia; acute granulocytic leukemia	Give IV push over 3-5 min through side port of patent IV; may be given as a continuous infusion Keep patient flat 4-6 hr after intrathecal administration

Continued.

TABLE 13-4. Chemotherapeutic Drugs—cont'd

Medication	Dosage	Routes of administration	Side effects and toxicities
5-Fluorouracil (5-FU, fluorouracil)	12 mg/kg/day, not to exceed 800 mg/day; given according to protocol Maintenance dosage; 6-15 mg/kg; given according to protocol; dosage adjusted with liver or kidney dysfunction	IV, topical, po	Myelosuppression, dose-limiting Leukopenia (p. 684) (granulocytes) Thrombocytopenia (p. 688) Nausea and vomiting Alopecia (p. 702) Neurotoxicity (p. 700) Diarrhea Stomatitis
Mercaptopurine (Purinethol, 6-mercaptopurine)	2.5-5 mg/kg/day; given po according to protocol; dosage reduced one third to one fourth with allopurinol	po	Myelosuppression Thrombocytopenia; mild Leukopenia; mild Mild nausea and vomiting Cumulative hyperbilirubinemia
Methotrexate (MTX, amethopterin)	2.5-5 mg po daily 50-70 mg/m² IV (low dose) 100-150 mg/m² IV (high dose) Given according to protocol	po Intrathecal Intraarterial IV	Myelosuppression Leukopenia (p. 684) Thrombocytopenia (p. 688) Anemia (p. 689) Hgb effect Reticulocytes Nausea and vomiting (p. 690) Anorexia Mucositis (p. 692) Hepatoxicity (p. 701) Dermatitis (p. 703) Alopecia (p. 702) Increased intracranial pressure Nephrotoxicity (p. 698)
Azacytidine (t-Azacytidine) (investigational)	100-150 mg/m²/day times 5; given according to protocol	IV	Myelosuppression Leukopenia (p. 684) Stomatitis (p. 692) Nausea and vomiting; onset 1-3 hr and lasting 3-4 hr Rash (p. 703) Diarrhea Neurotoxicity (p. 700) Hepatoxicity Hypotension
Thioguanine (6-thioguanine)	2-3 mg/kg/day; given according to protocol; dosage reduced with liver or kidney dysfunction	po	Leukopenia (p. 684) Thrombocytopenia (p. 688) Anemia (p. 689)
VINCA ALKALOIDS			
Vinblastine sulfate (Velban)	0.1-0.4 mg/kg/wk; given according to protocol; dosage decreased with liver disease and neurologic problems	IV	Leukopenia (p. 684), dose-limiting Thrombocytopenia, mild Mild nausea and vomiting Alopecia, mild Mucositis (p. 692)

Nadir	Recovery after nadir (days)	Indications	Administration and nursing implications
7-14 days	16-24	Breast cancer, oral lesions, gastric tumors, and colorectal cancer; topically—basal cell carcinomas	Give IV push over 3-5 min through side port of patent IV using two-syringe technique; flush line after therapy Tell patient to expect vein discoloration
7-14 days 12-21 days 11-23 days	14-21	Acute lymphocytic leukemia, chronic granulocytic leukemia	Give oral dose daily

7-14 days
4-7 days
5 days
6-13 days
2-7 days
	14-21	Acute lymphoblastic and myeloblastic leukemia, trophoblastic tumors, osteogenic sarcoma, epidermoid cancer of head and neck, multiple myeloma, lung, breast, and ovarian cancer	Ensure that patient knows not to take *any* medication before checking with physician when taking methotrexate po
			Check patency of IV prior to administration; flush IV after administration
			High-dose (investigational)
			  Force fluids to 3000-4000 ml/day to ensure high-volume output
			  Check creatinine results with increased dosage, sodium bicarbonate may be ordered to maintain urine pH 7.0
			  Administer citrovorum (leucovorin) rescue factor on time as ordered
			  After intrathecal administration keep patient flat 4-6 hr
			  Never give with salicylates, sulfonamide, phenytoin, *p*-aminobenzoic acid (PABA), alcohol, warfarin, amphotericin B

12-14 days	—	Acute granulocytic leukemia	Give within 8 hr of preparation; usually dilute in Ringer's lactate solution; administer IV push through side port of patent IV; may be ordered as continuous infusion
14-28 days	—	Acute granulocytic and lymphocytic leukemia.	Give total oral dose at one time between meals
4-10 days	7-14	Breast and testicular cancer, choriocarcinoma, Hodgkin's disease and lymphoma	Give IV push over through side port of freely running IV; Check blood backflow prior to instilling each ml; flush line with 30 ml IV fluid prior to each blood check; flush line after administration

Continued.

TABLE 13-4. Chemotherapeutic Drugs—cont'd

Medication	Dosage	Routes of administration	Side effects and toxicities
Vinblastine sulfate (Velban)—cont'd			Constipation Ileus Abdominal pain Long-term therapy Neurotoxicity (p. 700)
Vincristine sulfate (Oncovin)	1-2 mg/m^2—adult; given according to protocol; dosage decreased with liver disease	IV	Myelosuppression, unusual Neurotoxicity, dose-limiting Peripheral neuropathy, dose-limiting Constipation Ileus Alopecia
Vindesine (Eldesine) (investigational)	2-4 mg/m^2; given according to protocol; dosage decreased with impaired liver function	IV	Neutropenia, dose-limiting Thrombocytopenia Leukopenia Neurotoxicity, dose-limiting at low doses Alopecia Constipation Paralytic ileus
PODOPHYLLOTOXINS			

VM-26 (Teniposide) (investigational)	100 mg/m^2/wk, 45-50 mg/m^2/day; given according to protocol; dosage reduced with prior irradiation/chemotherapy	IV
		
		Bladder instillation investigational
			Myelosuppression, dose-limiting
			  Leukopenia (p. 684)
			  Thrombocytopenia (p. 688)
			Hypotension especially with rapid infusion
			Rare anaphylaxis

Etoposide	75-200 mg/m^2/day×3; given according to protocol	IV	Myelosuppression; dose-limiting
			  Leukopenia
			  Thrombocytopenia
			Mild nausea and vomiting
			Alopecia
			Severe hypotension with rapid infusion

ANTIBIOTICS			
Bleomycin sulfate (Blenoxane, "Bleo")	10-30 units/m^2 given according to protocol; dosage decreased with renal failure; test dose may be ordered Total cumulative lifetime dose not to exceed 400 units	IV Intracavitary Intraarterial—investigational	Anaphylaxis Elevated temperature with or without chills Hypotension Pulmonary toxicity (p. 697) Mild nausea and vomiting, dose-limiting Cutaneous reactions Alopecia (p. 702)

Nadir	Recovery after nadir (days)	Indications	Administration and nursing implications
			Monitor closely for extravasation (p. 704) Give antidote as ordered Avoid eye contact Experimentally given by IV infusion over 24 hr period; monitor site closely Administer stool softeners and laxatives as ordered
4-5 days	7	Acute lymphocytic leukemia, breast cancer, sarcomas, Hodgkin's disease, neuroblastoma, non-Hodgkin's lymphoma, small cell lung carcinoma	Assure patent IV; give IV push over 3-5 min through side port; check blood backflow prior to instilling each ml; flush line with 30 ml IV fluid prior to each blood check; Monitor for extravasation (p. 704) Give antidote if extravasation occurs Administer stool softeners and laxatives as ordered
5-10 days 5-10 days	—	Acute leukemia, lung cancer, esophageal cancer, melanoma	Give IV push over 3-5 min through side port of newly inserted patent IV; flush tubing with 50-100 ml after administration Monitor for extravasation (p. 704) Administer stool softeners and laxatives as ordered
3-14 days	28	Hodgkin's disease, non-Hodgkin's lymphoma, malignant pleural effusions, bladder cancer, cancer of central nervous system (CNS)	Give IV infusion in volume five times medication volume; over at least 45 min period through patent IV Take baseline BP prior to therapy then 15 min into administration and at conclusion Flush line after administration
16 days	20-22	Leukemia, lung cancer, lymphoma, testicular cancer	Give through side port of patent IV over at least 30 min to avoid severe hypotension Take baseline BP prior to therapy then 15 min into administration and at conclusion
—	—	Squamous cell carcinoma, Hodgkin's disease, non-Hodgkin's lymphoma, mycosis fungoides, lung cancer, testicular cancer, malignant effusions	Give IV push or IV infusion as ordered after obtaining baseline Be prepared to treat anaphylaxis; have life support equipment and medications available Take T and BP q4h during infusion Assess breath sounds and respiratory function Teach patient to report signs of respiratory difficulty immediately to staff Reposition patient q15 min for four times when administering intracavitary doses

Continued.

TABLE 13-4. Chemotherapeutic Drugs—cont'd

Medication	Dosage	Routes of administration	Side effects and toxicities

Dactinomycin (actinomycin D, Cosmegen)	0.5 mg/day for adult; 0.015-0.5 mg/kg for children; both given according to protocol	IV	Myelosuppression
			  Thrombocytopenia (p. 688)
			  Leukocytopenia (p. 684)
			  Anemia
			Nausea and vomiting (p. 690), onset 1-2 hr, lasting several days
			Mucositis (p. 692)
			Alopecia (p. 702)
			Skin changes, especially irradiated areas (p. 703)

Daunorubicin (Daunomycin, rubidomycin)	30-60 mg/m^2; given according to protocol; dosage reduced with impaired renal or liver function	IV	Myelosuppression; dose-limiting Nausea and vomiting (p. 690) Alopecia
Doxotrubicin (Adriamycin)	60-70 mg/m^2 single dose; given according to protocol; dosage decreased with hepatic dysfunction Total cumulative lifetime dose not to exceed 450-550 mg/m^2	IV Intraarterial—investigational	Myelosuppression Leukopenia (p. 684), dose-limiting Nausea and vomiting (p. 690), onset 3-4 hr Stomatitis (p. 692) Marked alopecia (p. 702) Reactivation of irradiated skin areas Cardiotoxicity (p. 696), dose-limiting

Mithramycin (Mithracin)	0.025-0.050 mg/kg; given according to protocol	IV	Myelosuppression
			  Thrombocytopenia (p. 688)
			  Decreased clotting factors
			  Mild leukopenia (p. 684)
			Nausea and vomiting (p. 690)
			Diarrhea (p. 694)
			Stomatitis (p. 692)
			Neurotoxicity (p. 700)
			Dermatologic reactions
			Nephrotoxicity (p. 698)
			Hepatoxicity (p. 701)

Mitomycin (Mutamycin, Mitomycin C)	10-20 mg/m^2—dose; given according to protocol	IV	Myelosuppression cumulative
			  Leukopenia (p. 684)
			  Thrombocytopenia
			  Erythrocytopenia
			Nausea and vomiting (p. 690), onset 1-2 hr, lasting 6-8 hr
			Stomatitis (p. 692)
			Alopecia (p. 702)
			Purple bands on nails
			Mild nephrotoxicity (p. 698)

Nadir	Recovery after nadir (days)	Indications	Administration and nursing implications
14-21 days	22-25	Choriocarcinoma, Wilms' tumor, sarcoma, testicular cancer	Give IV push through side port of patent IV; check blood backflow prior to instilling each ml, flush line with 30 ml IV fluid prior to each blood check; flush line after administration Monitor for extravasation (p. 704); give antidote if extravasation occurs Establish oral and skin hygiene care prior to therapy Administer antiemetic prior to administration and as indicated and ordered
7-14 days	—	Acute lymphocytic leukemia; acute granulocytic leukemia; neuroblastoma	Administer IV push through side port of patent IV Monitor closely for extravasation (p. 704); give antidote as ordered Tell patient that urine will be colored red
10-14 days	21-24	Acute leukemia, Hodgkin's disease, non-Hodgkin's lymphoma, sarcomas, Wilms' tumor, ovarian, breast, lung, thyroid, and bladder cancer	Give IV push through side port of patent IV; check blood backflow prior to instilling each ml; flush line with 30 ml IV fluid prior to each blood check; monitor carefully to prevent extravasation (p. 704) that may cause severe ulceration; flush line after administration with 50-100 ml solution Teach patient to report *any sensation* during administration to staff Give antiemetics prior to administration and as indicated after Assess cardiac status prior to administration Institute oral hygiene care prior to administration
14 days	21-28	Testicular cancer, hypercalcemia in malignancy	Give in small volume IV over 30-45 min through side port of patent IV; may be ordered as IV infusion given over 4-6 hr for hypercalcemia Observe for extravasation (p. 704); give antidote as ordered
28-42 days	42-56	Cancer of stomach and pancreas	Give IV push over 3-5 min through side port of patent IV; check blood backflow prior to instilling each ml; flush line with 30 ml IV fluid prior to each blood check; flush line after administration Monitor closely for extravasation (p. 704); give antidote if extravasation occurs Administer antiemetics prior to administration and then as indicated Institute oral hygiene care prior to therapy Observe for skin changes at IV site or distal to site for 6 weeks

Continued.

TABLE 13-4. Chemotherapeutic Drugs—cont'd

Medication	Dosage	Routes of administration	Side effects and toxicities
Streptozocin (Zanosar)	1.0-1.5 g/m^2/wk; 500 mg-1.0 g/m^2/day; given according to protocol	IV	Severe nausea and vomiting (p. 690) Nephrotoxicity (p. 698), dose-limiting Mild hepatotoxicity (p. 701) Immediate burning pain at IV site; decreases after 15-20 min of infusion
MISCELLANEOUS			
Asparaginase (Elspar, L-Asparaginase)	10,000-40,000 IU/m^2/day, q2-3 weeks; given according to protocol Skin test may be ordered prior to administration	IV, IM	Anaphylaxis Mild nausea and vomiting Neurotoxicity (p. 700) Hepatotoxicity (p. 701) Pancreatitis Hyperosmolar, nonketotic hyperglycemia (p. 440)
Cisplatin	80-120 mg/m^2; given according to protocol Higher doses may be mixed in hypertonic saline solution to prevent nephrotoxicity	IV	Anaphylaxis Nephrotoxicity (p. 698) Ototoxicity Severe nausea and vomiting (p. 690) Hypomagnesium
Dacarbazine (DTIC)	250 mg/m^2; given according to protocol	IV	Myelosuppression, dose-limiting Leukopenia (p. 684) Thrombocytopenia (p. 688) Severe nausea and vomiting, onset 1 hr, lasting to 12 hr Immediate burning pain at IV site, decreased with further dilution
Procarbazine (Matulane)	50-200 mg/day; given according to protocol	po	Myelosuppression, dose-limiting Thrombocytopenia (p. 688) Leukopenia (p. 684) Anemia

Nadir	Recovery after nadir (days)	Indications	Administration and nursing implications
—	—	Pancreatic islet cell tumors, non beta cell pancreatic tumors, stomach, carcinoid, colon	Give IV push through side port of patent IV; check blood backflow prior to instilling each ml; flush line with 30 ml IV fluid prior to each blood check; flush line after administration; monitor for extravasation (p. 704), give antidote if extravasation occurs Administer antiemetics prior to therapy and then as indicated Tell patient burning sensation may be experienced; slow infusion to decrease burning Force fluids to 3000 ml/day, unless contraindicated, to ensure adequate urine output Observe for hypoglycemia reactions immediately after administration Have glucose 50% available
—	—	Acute lymphocytic leukemia	Give IV push over 3-5 min through side port of patent IV Take baseline, T, P, R, and BP prior to administration Be prepared to treat anaphylaxis; have life support equipment readily available
—	—	Testicular and ovarian cancer, squamous cell carcinoma, lung, head and neck cancer	Assess baseline T, P, R, and BP Give by continuous IV infusion Force fluids to 3000 ml/day and give parenteral therapy as ordered 12-24 hr prior to drug administration Monitor intake and output Mannitol may be ordered with or after administration Ensure output of 100-150 ml/hr before giving medication Give antiemetics as ordered and indicated Be prepared to treat anaphylaxis Have life support equipment and medications available *High-dose*—investigational Parenteral hydration and bladder irrigation may be ordered
21-28 days	36-50	Malignant melanoma, Sarcoma, Hodgkin's Disease	Administer small volume IV over 30-60 min through side port of patent IV Flush line after therapy Apply ice pack at IV site Give antiemetics prior to therapy, then as indicated
25-36 days	36-50	Hodgkin's disease and non-Hodgkin's lymphomas, malignant melanoma, lung and brain cancer	Avoid use of alcohol, sympathomimetic drugs, trycyclic antidepressants, CNS depressants, and heavy intake of dark beer, cheese, bananas

Continued.

TABLE 13-4. Chemotherapeutic Drugs—cont'd

Medication	Dosage	Routes of administration	Side effects and toxicities

Amsacrine (AMSA)	75 mg/m²/day; 120 mg/m²/wk; given according to protocol; dosage reduced with hepatic dysfunctions	IV	Myelosuppression
			  Leukopenia (p. 684), dose-limiting
			Neurotoxicity (p. 700) (cerebellar dysfunction, grand mal seizures)
			Conjunctivitis
			  Nausea and vomiting, mild mucositis (p. 690)
			Dermatologic toxicity (p. 703)
			Cardiac arrhythmias
			Phlebitis

Interferon (Intron A, Roferon)	2 million units/m² three times weekly	SC, IM, IV	Flulike syndrome—fever, malaise, fatigue, myalgia Skin disorders—dry skin GI disorders—diarrhea, constipation, nausea, vomiting

All equipment and unused drug(s) should be treated as hazardous waste and disposed of according to facility's policy and procedure: place linen in double bag marked "Caution, Chemotherapy"; instruct personnel to observe precautions in handling; wash twice

Personnel who are planning to become or who may be pregnant should not handle these medications

Be aware that all parenteral agents should be prepared in biologic safety cabinet

Transport parenteral drugs in plastic cover to prevent spillage and contamination

Avoid eating, drinking, smoking, and using cosmetics while preparing and/or administering drug

Wear disposable cover gowns with closed front and cuffed, long sleeves and latex gloves throughout preparation, administration, and disposal period when handling medication or equipment

Wear protective garment and gloves when handling patient excreta during administration and for 48 hr following administration

Syringes and IV sets with Leur-Lok fitting should be used whenever possible to prevent spillage

When priming IV line and removing needle from injection port, place alcohol swab and 4 × 4 beneath site to collect small spills; discard in hazardous waste container

Occupational Safety and Health Administration (OSHA) recommends
  Prime IV tubing with compatible solution (normal saline or dextrose in water) prior to attaching prepared chemotherapy for infusion

Wipe up spills immediately; contain spills by gently covering them with disposable absorbent material; be careful to prevent aerosolization (wear gown, mask, double gloves); place absorbent material in double plastic bag marked "Hazardous Waste"

COMPLICATIONS IN CHEMOTHERAPY

Myelosuppression

Inhibition of bone marrow activity resulting in decreased production of blood cells and platelets due to the effects of chemotherapy, the disease state, or radiation therapy; the majority of chemotherapeutic agents produce some degree of myelosuppression; since the blood count nadirs produced by most chemotherapeutic agents can be predicted, the schedule of drug delivery is designed to coincide with the recovery of the bone marrow; the nurse must be aware of the nadir (the point of lowest drop in blood count) for each chemotherapeutic drug

LEUKOPENIA

Temporary reduction in the total number of circulating white blood cells; since the life span of the leukocyte is very brief (12 hr), leukopenias occur frequently in patients receiving chemotherapy, placing them at risk for infections; a good indication of a patient's ability

Nadir	Recovery after nadir (days)	Indications	Administration and nursing implications
	—	Acute myeloblastic leukemia, lymphoma, sarcoma, lung and breast cancer	Give within 30-60 min of preparation Dilute only in D$_5$W, never use saline Administer through side port of patent IV Administer corticosteroid eye medication as ordered Tell patient skin may have yellow-orange tinge

	—	Approved
		  Hairy cell leukemia
		Unapproved
		  Kaposi's sarcoma
		  Melanoma
		  Lymphoma
		  Myeloma
		  Chronic myelogenous leukemia
			Side effects may be minimized with evening administration and acetaminophen
			Tolerance to side effects usually occurs in 2 weeks

to fight infection is the absolute granulocyte count (AGC), which is calculated by multiplying the total WBC count by the percent of granulocytes in the differential:

$$AGC = WBC \times \%\ granulocytes$$

When AGC is below 1000 cells/mm^3, patient is at risk of infection; opportunistic endogenous organisms can cause systemic and severe infections

Assessment
Observations/findings

Elevated temperature if not masked by corticosteroids or antiinflammatory drugs
Any sudden rise or fall of temperature of even 1° F
Elevated temperature of 100.4° F (38.3° C) lasting 24 hr or longer, not associated with blood products or drugs
Elevated temperature may be caused by other factors, such as atelectasis or response of disease process
Sudden rise and fall in neutrophils; may be indicative of infection
Respiratory
  Dyspnea, especially on exertion
  Cough, sore throat, sputum production
  Changes in breath sounds (wheezes, rales, rhonchi)
  "Colds" and "flu"
Skin and mucous membrane
  Skin breaks, puncture sites
  Redness
  Swelling
  Drainage
  Ulceration
Oral cavity
  Fissures
  Redness
  Swelling
  Ulceration
Perineum
  Discomfort
  Pain
  Excoriation
Rectum
  Tenderness
  Fissures
  Abscess
Vaginal discharge
In neutropenic patients inflammatory response (redness, heat, edema, pus formation, and pain) may be diminished or absent
Genitourinary
  Frequency, dysuria, urgency
  Neurologic deficit: monitor residual urine; check urine for clarity and odor
  Assess vaginal hygiene and contraceptive techniques
  Prostate enlargement
Eye or ear drainage

Laboratory/diagnostic studies

WBC
Differential values
  Granulocytes
    Comprise 60% of total WBC
    Responsible for fighting bacterial and fungal infection
    Half-life of 6 to 7 hr
    Type: neutrophils, eosinophils, basophils
  Lymphocytes
    Comprise 2% to 4% of total WBC
    Responsible for immune defenses
  Monocytes
    Comprise 40% of total WBC
    Defense against bacteria and fungi
Chest x-ray examination
Pulmonary function test
Urinalysis
Cultures, blood, sputum

Potential complications

Septicemia

Medical management

Antibiotics
Antifungal medications
Granulocyte infusion
Intake and output
Cultures of blood, sputum, urine, skin, drainage, etc.

Nursing diagnoses/goals/interventions

ndx: Potential for infection related to cytotoxic effects of chemotherapy

GOAL: *Patient will remain free of infection*

Check results of WBC and differential to ensure that they are within acceptable limits
Check vital signs and assess skin and mucous membranes for signs and symptoms of infection; give special attention to skin folds and body cavities
Assess respiratory and genitourinary tract for evidence of infection
Document findings and interventions
Instruct patient and/or significant other that it is not uncommon for WBC count to decrease following most chemotherapy; WBC count usually recovers before next dose; however, recovery may be delayed and an occasional dose of chemotherapy may be delayed
Teach patient to guard against infection by
  Maintaining meticulous total body hygiene, including perineal care
  Avoiding crowds and persons with infections
  Maintaining good nutrition and fluid intake
  Practicing good oral hygiene after meals
  Getting adequate rest and exercise
  Reporting signs and symptoms of infection to health care personnel immediately
Place patient in noninfectious environment if AGC is <1000/mm or as ordered; use of reverse isolation or laminar flow room are controversial based on research findings
Use physical means to reduce exposure to microbes
  Instruct and ensure that personnel and visitors follow handwashing procedure with povidone-iodine before entering room
  No one with infectious condition ("cold," "flu," skin rash, etc.) may enter room
  Staff assigned to care for patient must not be assigned to care for patients who have infections, if possible
  Care for neutropenic patient first and take other precautions to avoid transferring any infectious agents to neutropenic patient
  Keep room clean
    Avoid any trash in room and bathroom
    Remove food and examination trays immediately after use
    Maintain furniture, fixtures, floor, and equipment dust-free and spill-free
  Ensure that allied health personnel (i.e., laboratory technicians) do not bring into patient's room equipment that has been in other areas of hospital
  If patient requires transportation, avoid using elevator with potentially infectious passengers present; mask for patient may be required
Maintain skin integrity
  Avoid IM injections
  Observe IV or central line site q4h
  Change dressing daily if nonporous type is used, using aseptic technique
  Change IV tubing and bottles daily
  Avoid infiltrations that necessitate restarting IV; position IV site to prevent stress and movement at site of insertion
  Consolidate laboratory work; clean skin with povidone-iodine scrub prior to puncture
  Assess previous puncture sites each shift
  Assess and record condition of oral cavity each shift
    Teach or assist with oral hygiene measures in morning, after food ingestion, at bedtime, and q2h to 4h when patient is awake at night
    Administer antifungal medication as ordered

Assess and record condition of perineum daily
Initiate and teach perineal care to be performed after each bowel movement; use povidone-iodine wash, ABDs, or very soft cloths; rinse and dry well
Prevent constipation (p. 695) and diarrhea
  Administer medications as ordered
  Avoid use of enemas and suppositories
Monitor and record vital signs q4h; take temperature more frequently if trend is beginning; report any change in temperature immediately
Institute comfort and cooling measures as indicated by condition
  Change linen and clothing to keep patient dry
  Avoid chilling
  Administer antipyretics as ordered
  Mechanical cooling blanket may be ordered
Monitor intake and output; report urinary frequency, burning, or changes in character of urine
Use voiding measures when indicated to avoid catheterization
If catheterization is necessary
  Use strict aseptic technique for insertion
  Perform catheter care each shift
Obtain cultures as ordered: blood, urine, sputum, skin, drainage, etc.
Assess and record respiratory status q4h; report changes in breath sounds, cough, and sputum, or increases in respiratory rate, or presence of sore throat immediately
Assist and teach patient to turn, cough, and deep breathe q2h
Administer oxygen if ordered
Encourage mobility q2h
Turn and position immobile patient q2h to prevent pressure sores
Provide mild antibacterial soaps and soft cloths and towels for skin hygiene, daily and prn
Administer IV antibiotics as ordered
Monitor laboratory data daily; report changes
Administer granulocyte transfusions as ordered (p. 218); monitor migration of transfused granulocytes to site of infection (e.g., complaints of pain at site of infection, such as anal lesion; respiratory complications requiring ventilatory assistance, etc.)
Instruct patient about low-bacterial diet
Instruct about need to remove flowers and plants from environment during neutropenic phase

ndx: Knowledge deficit regarding infection, activities, prevention of injury, and daily care

GOAL: *Patient and/or significant other will demonstrate understanding of activities, daily care, and measures to prevent infection*

Discuss signs and symptoms of infection to report to physician or nurse
Emphasize importance of avoiding persons who may be infectious or who may have potentially contagious conditions
Explain need to avoid persons who have been recently vaccinated
Explain need to avoid multiple sexual partners
Explain need to wash hands after using bathroom, before eating, and before performing any procedures
Emphasize importance of preventing injury to skin
  Use electric razors
  Handle knives and sharp objects carefully
  Wear protective gloves when gardening and when using strong household cleaning solutions
  Wear broad-brimmed hat and sunscreen when in sun
  Avoid going barefoot
  Wear warm clothing and boots in cold weather
  Avoid cutting cuticles, corns, or calluses
  Wear padded gloves when using oven
Explain need to perform oral hygiene periodically throughout the day
Emphasize importance of daily hygiene, including perineal and rectal care
Emphasize importance of drinking up to 3000 ml of fluid each day unless contraindicated; explain need to avoid using common drinking fountain
Explain need to maintain clean home environment and handle food properly
Caution patient to avoid contact with pets or other animals
Teach name of medication, dosage, time of administration, purpose, and side effects
Explain need to tell all health care personnel, especially dentists, about need to avoid infections
Emphasize importance of follow-up outpatient care
Ensure that patient and/or significant other demonstrates
  Method for taking and recording temperature
  Procedure for caring for very small cuts or breaks in skin

Evaluation

Patient demonstrates knowledge regarding prevention of infection and remains infection free

THROMBOCYTOPENIA

Reduction in the number of circulating platelets caused by destruction of bone marrow during chemotherapy; platelets circulate for about 10 days before removal from circulation

Assessment

Observations/findings

Petechiae, easy bruising, bleeding gums or nose, purpura (especially lower extremities), hypermenorrhea, tarry stools, blood in urine and/or emesis, abdominal pain, distention, prolonged bleeding from invasive procedures, vaginal or rectal bleeding, blurred vision, headache, disorientation, decreased platelet count

Certain drugs such as mitomycin and the nitrosoureas are associated with delayed, cumulative thrombocytopenia

Laboratory/diagnostic studies

CBC and platelet count
ABO, Rh and HLA compatability

Potential complications

Spontaneous bleeding
   <10,000 platelets: fatal central nervous system (CNS) hemorrhage or massive GI hemorrhage
   <20,000 platelets: hemorrhage in any system

Medical management

Platelet infusion (can be random or type specific)
Intake and output
Neurologic assessment
Stool softeners

Nursing diagnoses/goals/interventions

ndx: Potential alteration in tissue perfusion related to thrombocytopenia

GOAL: *Patient will demonstrate absence of bleeding*

Monitor CBC and platelet count
Anticipate nadir of platelet count
Identify drugs and/or other factors that may lower platelet count and predispose patient to bleeding
Assess and report any signs and symptoms of bleeding
Inspect gums and oral cavity for bleeding q2h to 4h
Inspect skin each shift for increased bruising, petechiae, ecchymosis, and swelling
Inspect and palpate joints each shift for increased size and decreased mobility
Assess sensorium and neurologic status each shift
Inspect nasal cavity at least once each shift

If epistaxis occurs
   Have patient sit at 90-degree angle
   Apply pressure to nose
   Place ice pack at back of neck
   If nasal bleeding is not controlled in 10 to 15 min
     Notify physician
     Have nasal packing tray available
Institute safety measures as platelet count decreases below 50,000/mm^3
   Avoid needle sticks when possible
   Consolidate laboratory work; apply pressure to site for 5 min and observe site q15 min for at least 1 hr
   Avoid IM injections, aspirin, and aspirin-containing products
   Do not take rectal temperatures or administer medications rectally; avoid enemas
   Avoid bladder catheterization when possible
   Take BP only when necessary and pump cuff only as high as necessary
   Avoid use of
     Rough towels and washcloths
     Razors
     Restraints
     Tight clothing
   Maintain clutter-free environment
   Provide nightlight to prevent bumping into objects or falling
Administer careful oral hygiene
   Use toothettes or gauze pads
   Avoid use of dental floss or toothpicks
   Encourage use of mouth rinse q2h to 4h
     Half saline and half water
     Half saline and half hydrogen peroxide followed by saline rinse
Administer platelets as ordered
   Inspect IV or central line site q20 to 30 min for hematoma or oozing
   Maintain pressure at site for 5 min when IV is discontinued
   Inspect q15 min for four times
Administer antacids as ordered
Test stool for blood after each movement
Test urine for blood each time patient voids
Administer stool softeners as ordered to prevent bleeding from constipation
Avoid vaginal douches

ndx: Knowledge deficit regarding prevention and bleeding measures

GOAL: *Patient and/or significant other will demonstrate knowledge of prevention and bleeding measures*

Discuss signs and symptoms of bleeding to be reported to physician in any of the following areas
  Skin
  Oral
  Nasal
  Rectal
  Stomach
  Cerebral
  Urinary tract
Discuss emergency plan to follow if spontaneous hemorrhage occurs
  Have emergency numbers on hand
  Call paramedics
  Go to nearest emergency area
Emphasize importance of telling dentist and other medical personnel about chemotherapy and low platelet count
Emphasize importance of maintaining safe, clutter-free environment
Explain need to apply pressure at blood withdrawal site after laboratory work is completed
Emphasize importance of avoiding over-the-counter medications, especially those containing acetylsalicylic acid (i.e., aspirin), without checking with physician
Caution patient to avoid use of sharp objects when possible
  Use electric razor
  Use caution when handling knives or other equipment
Explain need to avoid harsh coughing and blowing of nose
  If cough persists, notify physician
  Take cough medication as ordered
Emphasize importance of follow-up outpatient care
  Routine laboratory appointments
  Return physician and nurse appointments
Ensure that patient and/or significant other demonstrates
  Method for applying pressure to bleeding site
    Apply dressing or clean material directly over site
    Apply pressure for 5 min
    Apply ice in covered plastic bag over site once bleeding stops
    Check site for further bleeding q15 min for 1 hr
  Method for testing stool and urine for occult blood

Evaluation

Patient recognizes significance of being at risk for bleeding, demonstrates knowledge of measures necessary to prevent bleeding, and has no signs of bleeding

ANEMIA

Temporary reduction in the number of circulating red blood cells and the level of hemoglobin caused by destruction of cells during chemotherapy, leading to tissue hypoxia due to impaired oxygen-carrying capacity

Assessment
Observations/findings

Headache, dizziness, fainting, fatigue, irritability, difficulty in concentrating, dyspnea, palpitations, syncope, complaints of feeling cold, loss of color in nails and palms of hands

Laboratory/diagnostic studies

Decreased hemoglobin (Hgb) and hematocrit (Hct) (dehydration may raise Hgb/Hct); if precipitious drop in Hgb, may be due to hemorrhaging
CBC and platelet count
Reticulocyte count
ABO, Rh compatability
Mean cell volume (MCV)
Mean cell hemoglobin (MCH)
Mean cell hemoglobin concentration (MCHC)
Bone marrow aspirate
Total iron-binding capacity (TIBC)

Potential complications

Severe anemia can result in hypotension and myocardial infarction

Medical management

Packed cells
IV fluids
Intake and output
Electrocardiogram

Nursing diagnoses/goals/interventions

ndx: Potential activity intolerance related to anemia

GOAL: *Patient will return to preepisode activity level*

Monitor laboratory data
  Hgb and Hct
  MCV, MCH, MCHC, reticulocyte count
Anticipate nadir of red blood cell count (RBC)
Provide adequate periods of rest and sleep
  Plan nursing activities to avoid interrupting sleep
  Provide activity-free periods throughout the day for rest
  Schedule examinations and tests carefully
Conserve patient's energy for desired activities
  Assist with meal preparation

Keep needed items within reach
Assist with hygiene measures
Plan activities after rest periods

Keep patient warm
Encourage use of warm robes, socks, and clothing
Provide extra blankets; cotton sheets are often more comfortable

Assess neurologic status each shift
Skin: pallor, petechiae, purpura, jaundice
Nail beds: pallor, blanching
Mucous membranes: pallor, petechiae
Bones: tenderness over ribs and sternum

Take and record vital signs each shift

Assess respiratory and cardiac status each shift; report tachycardia, irregular cardiac sounds, and presence of wheezes or rales

Place patient at 60-degree angle to facilitate breathing; position with pillows if indicated

Administer oxygen therapy as ordered

Assess extremities, abdomen, and sacrum for presence of edema; report positive findings

Observe safety precautions: instruct patient to sit at side of bed before getting up; change position slowly

Provide nutritious diet high in iron

Plan rest periods after meals

Administer blood products when ordered (p. 218); one unit of blood will usually raise Hgb 1 g/dl

Monitor for
Hives
Chills
Elevated temperature

ndx: Knowledge deficit regarding anemia and home care management

GOAL: *Patient and/or significant other will demonstrate understanding of home care and follow-up instructions through interactive discussion*

Discuss signs and symptoms of anemia to report to physician

Discuss importance of maintaining normal Hgb level as it relates to overall health and cardiorespiratory status

Emphasize importance of eating foods high in protein, vitamins, and minerals, which are necessary for RBC production

Explain need to include foods high in iron, vitamin B_{12}, and folic acid

Arrange for dietitian to teach patient and significant other foods to include in diet

Discuss methods to conserve energy
Planned rest periods
Adequate rest
Activities planned after rest periods
Assisting with ADLs
Keeping needed items within reach

Explain need to change position slowly; use appliances (walker, bars, etc.) for movement if indicated

Emphasize importance of continuing to perform ADLs and other desired activities to tolerance

Emphasize importance of follow-up care

Evaluation

Patient demonstrates knowledge of factors that contribute to anemia and measures to prevent anemia, and demonstrates adequate oxygen saturation of tissue

Nausea and Vomiting

Caused by physiologic changes due to cancer, the toxicities of radiation therapy or chemotherapy, and/or psychologic expectation

Assessment

Observations/findings

Time of onset of nausea and vomiting before or after chemotherapy administration
Duration
Severity
Possible cause
Anticipation
Foods
Bowel obstruction
Other medications
Brain metastasis

Vomitus: amount, frequency, character, color

Nutritional status (p. 59): weight loss, decreased food/fluid intake

Dehydration
Dry mucous membranes and skin
Poor skin turgor
Sunken, soft eyeballs
Concentrated urine; decreased output

Antiemetics: type, frequency, and method of administration

Laboratory/diagnostic studies

Electrolytes
CBC

Potential complications

Severe dehydration
Electrolyte imbalance
Malnutrition

Medical management

Antiemetics
Barbiturates
IV fluids/parenteral nutrition

Nursing diagnoses/goals/interventions

ndx: Alteration in nutrition: less than body requirements related to nausea and vomiting

GOAL: *Patient will demonstrate measures to maintain improved nutritional status*

Instruct patient and/or significant other about drugs that are known to cause severe emetic action, such as cisplatin and nitrogen mustard
Instruct patient and/or significant other about measures used to minimize side effects
Assess history of nausea and vomiting
Assess for known or probable preexisting disease states such as diabetes or hypercalcemia
Administer antiemetics before administration of agents and every 4 to 6 hr for 24 hr rather than as needed
Administer antihistamines or barbiturates combined with an antiemetic as ordered to decrease stimulation of the vomiting center in the brain
    If metoclopramide (Reglan) is given, assess for extrapyramidal side effects; keep diphenhydramine (Benadryl) available to counteract side effects
    If dexamethasone (Decadron) is given, administer slowly to prevent sensations of hot flushes and burning in perineal area
    Lorazepam (Ativan) may be given as an amnesic during chemotherapy administration to help control nausea and vomiting
Provide safety measures when administering these medications
Give chemotherapy in late afternoon or at night when possible
Continually evaluate effectiveness of antiemetics to help patient find the most effective combinations of drugs
Teach patient and/or significant other methods to prevent nausea and vomiting
    Small, frequent meals
    Small dietary intake before treatment
    Avoidance of greasy or spicy foods
    Rest periods before and after meals
    Quiet, restful environment
Monitor laboratory values, CBC, electrolytes
Monitor vital signs
Maintain chart of onset of symptoms, reaction to varying dosage of medication, and frequency of administration
Marijuana may be prescribed
Monitor intake and output
Administer IV replacement fluids as ordered
Weigh patient daily at same time with same clothing and scale
Experiment with several methods to reduce or alleviate nausea and/or vomiting prior to or after chemotherapy
    Withhold food and fluids for 4 to 6 hr
    Eat a light, bland meal
    Eat a normal meal
    Take only fluids for 4 to 6 hr
    Eat dry foods only
Plan appetizing meals based on patient's preference
    Serve food attractively arranged and at proper temperature
    Avoid liquids with meals
    Provide foods high in carbohydrates to promote earlier emptying of stomach
    Cool foods that are bland, soft, and odorless may be tolerated
    Sweet foods are often preferred
    Add calories and nutrients by adding supplements to food (i.e., high-protein supplements, dry milk products, etc.)
    Encourage patient to chew food well to ensure easier digestion
    Serve main meal when patient can best tolerate food
Assist patient with belching air swallowed during feeding
Avoid motions conducive to nausea (rapid or frequent change of position)
After chemotherapy
    Take liquids only
    Eat dry foods only
    Use methods of diversion to distract patient
        Animated conversation
        Absorbing projects or activities
    Use other methods to prevent onset or reduce severity of symptoms
        Relaxation methods
        Rhythmic breathing exercises
        Imagery experiences
        Self-hypnosis
        Behavior modification techniques
Place patient in well-ventilated room and control odors
    Room should be away from food preparation area, and soiled linen and waste product storage
    Remove trash frequently
    Empty and remove emesis basin, bedpans, and urinals after use

Remove food trays as soon as patient has eaten
Be aware that flowers and scents may be noxious
Instruct personnel and visitors to avoid wearing colognes and perfumes or using tobacco products if these are noxious to patient
Provide oral hygiene materials
Keep dentifrice and mouth rinse pleasing to patient within reach
Encourage and assist with dental and oral care before and after meals and especially after vomiting

ndx: Knowledge deficit regarding control of nausea and vomiting and measures to improve nutrition

GOAL: *Patient and/or significant other will demonstrate knowledge of measures to control nausea and vomiting and to improve nutrition*

Teach method and rationale of all aspects of ongoing care to be implemented at home
Emphasize importance of maintaining adequate food and fluid intake
Emphasize importance of reporting the following to physician or nurse
Continuous vomiting for 24 hr without food or fluid intake
Signs and symptoms of dehydration (p. 46)
Feeling of extreme stomach fullness and/or abdominal pain relieved by vomiting
Teach name of medication, dosage, frequency of administration, purpose, and toxic or side effects; if medication causes drowsiness, caution patient to avoid driving and participating in activities that require mental alertness for safety
Emphasize importance of follow-up outpatient care

Evaluation

Patient demonstrates knowledge of measures to control nausea and vomiting and measures to improve nutritional status, and exhibits clinical improvement in nutritional/hydration status

Stomatitis/Mucositis

stomatitis *Temporary inflammatory response of the oral mucosa to the cytotoxic effects of chemotherapy and/or radiation; may progress to ulcerative bleeding and secondary infection*
mucositis *Temporary inflammatory response of mucous membrane*

Assessment
Observations/findings

Buccal mucosa
General erythema
Swelling
Pain
Bleeding
Ulceration
Infected lesions
Candida albicans: soft whitish patches; may be localized or extensive
Herpes simplex: painful clusters of vesicles or ulceration
Gram-positive: dry, brownish-yellow, circular, raised eruptions
Gram-negative: creamy white, raised, moist, nonpurulent painful ulcer
Lips
Red fissures at corners of mouth
Edema
Surface abnormalities on palpation
Changes in taste
Ability to chew and swallow
Hydration status

Laboratory/diagnostic studies

CBC, platelet count
Cultures of oral cavity

Potential complications

Infections caused by bacteria, fungi, and/or viruses
Pain associated with mucositis
Malnutrition
Dehydration
Electrolyte imbalance

Medical management

Antibacterial agents
Antifungal agents
Antiviral agents
Diet: may require parenteral nutrition
Analgesics

Nursing diagnoses/goals/interventions

ndx: Potential for impaired tissue integrity related to chemotherapy*

GOAL: *Patient will demonstrate knowledge regarding oral hygiene regimen and exhibit oral mucosa free of irritation and ulceration.*

Establish oral hygiene regimen at initiation of chemotherapy, especially if patient is receiving 5-fluouracil (5-FU), methotrexate, or bleomycin
Assess oral cavity daily with tongue blade and light, noting color, moisture, and presence of lesions

---

*Nursing management will depend on severity of condition.

Note color, amount, and consistency of saliva
Encourage prophylactic oral hygiene regimen before, within 30 min after each meal, and q2h to 4h during waking hours
- Brush with soft-bristled toothbrush and nonabrasive toothpaste
- Floss daily with unwaxed dental floss if there is no danger of bleeding
- Avoid mouthwashes with high alcohol content
- Remove dentures and bridges, and cleanse following oral hygiene regimen

Assess history of alcohol use, tobacco use, radiation therapy, and previous and current treatment with chemotherapy
Teach patient about oral complications of chemotherapy, how to examine mouth, and care

ndx: Impaired tissue integrity related to stomatitis, pharyngitis/esophagitis, and/or rectal or vaginal mucositis secondary to chemotherapy

GOAL: *Patient will exhibit healing of mucus membrane and other tissues within 5 to 10 days, will remain free from infection, and will experience relief from pain*

Stomatitis

NOTE: Stomatitis generally occurs 5 to 7 days after chemotherapy and persists for up to 10 days

If mild stomatitis occurs
- Request physician order for culture of oral cavity
- Assess oral cavity q8h

Encourage oral hygiene regimen q2h during waking hours and q6h during the night
- Brush with soft-bristled toothbrush and nonabrasive toothpaste q4h
- Use dilute nonalcohol mouthwash
  - Hydrogen peroxide and normal saline: swish, gargle, and expectorate
  - Baking soda (1 tsp in 8 oz of water): swish, gargle, and expectorate
- Use toothette or cotton-tipped applicator to remove mucus and debris
- Apply lip lubricant q2h during waking hours

Assess need for use of antifungal or antibacterial agents
Topical anesthetics such as viscous lidocaine (Xylocaine) or Orabase may be used before meals for discomfort
Use mild analgesic q3h to 4h
Encourage bland diet high in protein
Encourage fluid to 2 L/day; avoid citrus juices

If severe stomatitis occurs:
- Request order for culture for oral cavity
- Assess oral cavity q8h
- Practice oral hygiene q1h to 2h, including
  - Cleaning of teeth with soft-bristled toothbrush, toothette, or gauze soaked in mouthwash—hydrogen peroxide—normal saline mixture
  - Use of antifungal and/or antibacterial agents
  - Use of topical anesthetics such as equal parts diphenhydramine (Benadryl) elixir (25 mg), Maalox, and viscous lidocaine (Xylocaine)
  - Use of moderate to strong analgesic q3h to 4h

Encourage diet (pureed) and liquids high in protein
If patient has difficulty in eating and maintaining fluid intake, parenteral nutrition may be necessary
If oral hygiene is difficult because of pain in oral cavity, encourage patient to rinse with 1 tsp viscous lidocaine 15 min before oral hygiene
If patient is unable to brush or rinse, irrigate mouth with syringe or soft rubber catheter using hydrogen peroxide and water q3h to 4h
- Gently clean lips with hydrogen peroxide solution followed by a saline rinse

If oral candidiasis is present, instruct patient to swish and swallow an oral suspension of nystatin (Mycostatin)
Teach patient how to examine mouth and do oral care

Pharyngitis/esophagitis

Assess for difficulty in swallowing and for infection
Antacids may be helpful

Rectal or vaginal mucositis

Instruct female patients to report any pain, ulceration, or bleeding of mucous membrane lining perineum or vagina
Instruct patient to include frequent perineal washing after voiding; pat dry
Instruct patient to use sitz baths
Caution patient to avoid douches
Instruct male patient to report signs and symptoms involving perineum
Follow above regimen

Evaluation

Patient
- Demonstrates oral care regimen and intact oral mucosa, states relief of oral and esophageal pain, and exhibits healing of stomatitis and esophagus
- Demonstrates rectal and vaginal mucosa care and exhibits healing of mucositis

Diarrhea

Passage of frequent stools of a soft or liquid consistency with or without discomfort due to effects of chemotherapy on epithelium

Assessment

Observations/findings

Frequent stools
  Watery
  Bloody
  Containing mucus
  Tarry
Dehydration
  Dry mucous membranes
  Poor skin turgor
  Decreased urine output

Laboratory/diagnostic studies

CBC, electrolytes
Stool cultures

Potential complications

Electolyte imbalance
Dehydration
Malnutrition
GI bleeding

Medical management

Antidiarrheals
Antispasmodics
IV fluids/parenteral nutrition

Nursing diagnoses/goals/interventions

ndx: Alteration in bowel elimination: diarrhea related to chemotherapy

GOAL: *Patient will achieve normal bowel consistency and pattern*

Assess usual pattern of elimination, including use of laxatives
Determine other probable causes of diarrhea such as inappropriate diet, treatment side effects, infection, and stress
Evaluate hydration and electrolyte status
Monitor intake and output, weight, and electrolytes
Assess frequency, character, and volume of stool
Do abdominal assessment including bowel sounds; note distention, cramping, or flatus
Assess perineal/perianal region for skin status
Adjust diet as appropriate; include bananas and cheese; avoid hot liquids, coffee, fresh fruits, and prune juice
Include foods high in potassium if weakness is present and laboratory values indicate a low potassium level
Encourage increased fluid intake of 3 L/day if not contraindicated; suggest liquids that contain electrolytes, such as Gatorade, grape juice, and fruit drinks
Administer medications that control diarrhea, such as Kaopectate or Lomotil as ordered
Observe and report early signs of constipation
Establish protocol for care of perineal area
  Gently clean area with water and mild soap after each stool; dry thoroughly and inspect for breakdown
  Apply ointments as indicated
  Use sitz baths as indicated
  Use skin barrier as needed
Check and record all stools for
  Frequency
  Amount
  Consistency
  Presence of blood, overt or occult
Teach patient to perform perineal care after each defecation
  Use povidone-iodine wash or mild soap and water
  Wash with soft cloths, front to back for women
  Dry by gentle patting with soft toweling
  Wash and dry hands well
Perform perineal care if patient is unable to do
Apply medication to perineum as ordered
Teach patient to test stool for blood after each bowel movement
Assess and record status of perineal area at least each shift; q4h if frequency of stools increases
Weigh patient daily at same time with same clothing and scale
Consult with physician to determine possibility of interrupting treatment until diarrhea is controlled
Assess for edema; third spacing of fluids may occur due to protein deficiency and electrolyte imbalances

ndx: Knowledge deficit regarding methods for control of diarrhea

GOAL: *Patient and/or significant other will demonstrate knowledge of methods for control of diarrhea and testing stools for occult blood*

Discuss signs and symptoms of diarrhea that must be reported to physician
Emphasize importance of maintaining oral fluid intake of 3000 ml/day unless contraindicated
Explain need to avoid diet high in fiber and roughage
Explain need to take prescribed medication during episodes of diarrhea

Discuss signs and symptoms of constipation to report
Explain need to avoid over-the-counter medications without checking with physician or nurse
Ensure that patient and/or significant other demonstrates
  Method of performing perineal care after each bowel movement; soft cloths or tissues may be used
  Handwashing technique
  Method of testing stools for occult blood

Evaluation

Patient demonstrates knowledge of methods to correct and control diarrhea; achieves normal elimination pattern and consistency of stool

Constipation

Passage of irregular, infrequent hard feces; may be due to disease process, chemotherapy, or other factors

Assessment

Observations/findings

Absence of stool for more than 3 days
Difficult, painful stool evacuation
Stool
  Hard, dry
  Red-streaked
Absence of bowel sounds

Laboratory/diagnostic studies

Depends on cause

Potential complications

Ileus

Medical management

Stool softeners
Hydration: oral or parenteral
Laxatives or enemas if not contraindicated

Nursing diagnoses/goals/interventions

ndx: Alteration in bowel elimination: constipation related to chemotherapy

GOAL: *Patient will achieve normal pattern of elimination*

Assess usual pattern of elimination, including use of laxatives
Identify factors that could alter usual pattern of elimination such as immobility, chemotherapeutic drugs (vincristine, vinblastine), opiate/narcotic analgesics, low-bulk diet, or inadequate fluid intake
Assess for presence of associated signs and symptoms such as flatus, distention, or discomfort
Assess for fecal impaction
Evaluate and record time and character of bowel elimination daily
Auscultate abdomen for bowel sounds each shift
Administer enema type, amount, and solution as ordered; digital removal of feces may be necessary—follow hospital policy and procedure
If no spontaneous stool occurs within 24 hr after enema, administer stool softeners, laxative, or suppository as ordered
Monitor intake and output
Force fluids to 3000 ml/24 hr unless contraindicated
Maintain diet high in fiber and bulk
Encourage ambulation and exercise to tolerance
Perform range-of-motion (ROM) exercises q4h to 8h if patient is immobile
Provide privacy when needed
  Assist with ambulation to bathroom
  Screen patient in bed
  Do not schedule appointments or examinations at time of patient's usual evacuation
Perform perineal care after bowel movement
Assess condition of perineum daily
Apply medication to rectal area as ordered

ndx: Knowledge deficit regarding methods to prevent constipation

GOAL: *Patient and/or significant other will demonstrate knowledge of methods to prevent constipation*

Emphasize importance of noting daily bowel function and consistency of stool
Discuss/demonstrate methods to enhance daily bowel movements, especially when taking vinca alkaloid medication
  Take stool softener and laxative as ordered
  Maintain fluid level at 3000 ml/24 hr unless contraindicated
  Eat diet high in fiber and bulk
  Administer enema if no bowel movement occurs in 3 days
Explain need to report to physician if these methods fail
Explain need to avoid over-the-counter medications without checking with physician

Evaluation

Patient demonstrates knowledge of methods to promote adequate bowel elimination; achieves regular elimination pattern and consistency of stools

Gonadal Dysfunction

Testicular or ovarian dysfunction due to adverse effects of chemotherapeutic drugs (e.g., nitrogen mustard, cyclophosphamide, chlorambucil)

Assessment

Observations/findings

Reduction of spermatocytes
Irregular menses
Amenorrhea
Menopausal symptoms: hot flushes, insomnia, irritability, dyspareunia, vaginal dryness

Laboratory/diagnostic studies

Serum follicle-stimulating hormone (FSH)
Sperm count

Potential complications

Permanent sterility

Medical management

Estrogen (menopausal symptoms)

Nursing diagnosis/goal/interventions

ndx: Sexual dysfunction: infertility related to chemotherapy

GOAL: *Patient will verbalize feelings regarding potential or actual infertility and affirm appropriate sexual identity to achieve perceived sex role*

Obtain brief sexual history, including sexual practices, sex education and attitude, and effects of disease and treatment on sexual function
Advise male patients regarding sperm banking before chemotherapy administration
Provide contraceptive information to patients before they initiate chemotherapy if appropriate
Initiate discussion related to infertility
Encourage ventilation of feelings
Evaluate patient's and/or partner's coping skills and response to infertility
Instruct patient that infertility may be temporary or permanent (dose related)
Inform patient that sexual drive and capability usually are not physically impaired as a result of chemotherapy
Advise that antifertility effects may be reversible in some cases after therapy is terminated
Refer patient for counseling if appropriate

Evaluation

Patient achieves improving or satisfying sexual role function

Cardiotoxicity

Cardiac damage due to toxicity of antineoplastic medications

Assessment

Observations/findings

Tachycardia
Extrasystoles
ST-T wave changes
Transient ECG changes
Thirty percent decrease in limb-lead QRS voltage
Predisposing medications
    Doxorubicin (Adriamycin)
    Daunorubicin (Daunomycin)
    Concurrent use of cyclophosphamide
Predisposing factors
    Previous radiation therapy near heart
    Aortic stenosis
    Uncontrolled hypertension
    Distended neck veins
    Gallop heart rhythm
    Ankle edema

Laboratory/diagnostic studies

Electrocardiogram (ECG)
Cardiac enzymes
Chest x-ray examination
Echocardiogram
Radionuclide angiography
Percutaneous endomyocardial biopsy

Potential complications

CHF
Cardiomyopathy

Medical management

Serial electrocardiogram
Oxygen therapy
Cardiac glycosides

Nursing diagnosis/goal/interventions

ndx: Alteration in tissue perfusion: cardiopulmonary related to chemotherapy

GOAL: *Patient will have minimized or controlled arrhythmias or cardiac decompensation*

Monitor pulse rate and rhythm
Note significant variation in vital signs, skin color, temperature, sensorium, decreased urine output, and dyspnea
Be aware that by the time cardiac toxicity is clinically detectable, it is often irreversible and debilitating

Be aware of agents that place patient at risk for cardiotoxicity, such as doxorubicin (adult total cumulative dose not to exceed 450 to 550 mg/m^2) and daunorubicin (total cumulative dose is 550 mg/m^2); see Heart Failure (p. 101)

Be aware that weekly low-dose injection of doxorubicin and continuous infusions may be associated with less cardiotoxicity

Evaluation

Patient demonstrates minimized cardiac arrhythmias or decompensation

Pulmonary Toxicity

Respiratory difficulties, temporary or chronic, related to chemotherapeutic toxicities; chemotherapeutic drugs commonly associated with pulmonary toxicity include bleomycin, busulfan, and carmustine

Assessment

Observations/findings

Toxicities associated with bleomycin include pneumonitis and interstitial fibrosis

Persons over 70 years of age who receive total cumulative dose of greater than 400 to 500 units are at greatest risk

Fine, crackling basilar rales

Dyspnea at rest, hypoxemia

Tachypnea, fever

Headache

Malaise

Pneumonia (noninfectious)

Pulmonary edema

Pulmonary fibrosis

Predisposing factors
  Preexisting pulmonary disease
  Radiation therapy
  Pulmonary conditions: infection, edema, emboli
  Dry, hacking cough
  Adverse pulmonary changes are also associated with cyclophosphamide (Cytoxan) in combination with bleomycin, mitomycin, melphalan, and procarbazine
  History of smoking

Laboratory/diagnostic studies

Pulmonary function tests

Arterial blood gases

Chest x-ray examination

Potential complications

Pneumonitis

Interstitial fibrosis

Medical management

Steroids

Antimicrobials

Bronchodilators

Nursing diagnoses/goals/interventions

ndx: Impaired gas exchange related to adverse effects of chemotherapy

GOAL: *Patient will have improved ventilation and adequate oxygenation of tissues*

Be aware that once pulmonary changes are clinically detected, the disease course is often progressive

Observe for shortness of breath

Auscultate chest for breath sounds q4h during course of chemotherapy; report abnormal breath sounds immediately

Check T, P, R, and BP q4h; report temperature of 100.4° F (38° C) or above

Monitor pulmonary function tests as ordered

Teach and assist patient to turn, cough, and deep breathe q4h

Administer oxygen cautiously when ordered; high-dose oxygen may increase reaction, especially that due to bleomycin

Force fluids to 3000 ml/day unless contraindicated

Administer IV fluid therapy as ordered

Measure intake and output q8h

Administer medications as ordered: corticosteroids, bronchodilators, antimicrobials

See Adult Respiratory Distress Syndrome (ARDS) (p. 263)

ndx: Ineffective airway clearance related to adverse effects of chemotherapy

GOAL: *Patient will have adequate expectoration of secretions from airway*

Encourage fluids to 2 to 3 L/day if not contraindicated

Assist with turning, coughing, and deep-breathing exercises q2h to 4h

Assess chest sounds and respiratory movement q8h

Teach necessity of raising secretions and expectorating versus swallowing

Assist with nebulizer treatments and respiratory physiotherapy

Evaluation

Patient demonstrates improved ventilations and oxygenation of tissue

Secretions are removed, and airway patency is maintained

Urologic Toxicity
NEPHROTOXICITY

Dysfunction in any part of the renal system in the presence of chemotherapeutic agents that are excreted through the kidneys or act on the lining of the renal system; antineoplastic agents associated with renal dysfunction include cisplatin, methotrexate, mitomycin, 5-azatadine, nitrosoureas, and high-dose cyclophosphamide

Assessment
Observations/findings

Dysuria, frequency, urgency
Hematuria (mild to severe), proteinuria
Oliguria, anuria
Neuromuscular irritability
Muscle weakness
Tremors, personality change
Elevated uric acid
Hyperkalemia, hyperphosphatemia
Hypocalcemia, hypomagnesemia
Hyponatremia
Elevated blood urea nitrogen (BUN), serum creatinine, and creatinine clearance
Hypertension, headache, nausea, vomiting

Laboratory/diagnostic studies

Electrolytes, serum BUN and creatinine
Creatinine clearance
Uric acid, calcium, magnesium
Cystoscopy

Potential complications

Renal damage

Medical management

IV fluid (titrate according to output)
Intake and output
Medications
    Bicarbonate
    Allopurinol
    Antihypertensives
    Osmotic diuretics
    Antiemetics

Nursing diagnoses/goals/interventions

ndx: Alteration in tissue perfusion: renal related to chemotherapy

GOAL: *Patient will achieve and maintain adequate renal function*

Ensure adequate hydration and diuresis 24 hr prior to, during, and 24 to 48 hr after medication administration
Force fluids to 3000 to 4000 ml/day unless contraindicated
Enlist patient's assistance
    Provide fluids of choice and temperature
    Dietary restrictions of protein, potassium, and sodium may be necessary
    Offering small amounts frequently makes taking fluids less of a chore
    Serve attractively
If gastric distress is present, antacids may alleviate it
Use antiemetics for control of nausea
Administer IV fluids as ordered: usually dextrose in saline with electrolytes; often ordered at 200 mg/hr for 5 to 6 hr prior to, during, and after chemotherapy infusion
Measure intake and output; report discrepancies and output of 120 ml/hr
Test urine for occult bleeding q2h to 4h during chemotherapy infusion; then q4h to 8h if there is no bleeding; slow infusion and report overt hemorrhaging to physician
Monitor vital signs
Administer antihypertensive drugs as ordered
Test urine pH as ordered
Administer sodium bicarbonate as ordered to maintain urine ph of 7

ndx: Knowledge deficit regarding measures to enhance renal function

GOAL: *Patient and/or significant other will demonstrate knowledge of measures to enhance renal function*

Explain need to measure intake and output
Emphasize importance of maintaining fluid intake to 3000 to 4000 ml/day
Discuss signs and symptoms of nephrotoxicity to report to physician
Teach name of medication, dosage, frequency, and toxic or side effects to report to physician
Emphasize importance of follow-up outpatient care
Emphasize importance of taking antihypertensive drugs when ordered

Evaluation

Adequate renal function is maintained
Laboratory tests are within normal limits

HEMORRHAGIC CYSTITIS

Dose-related chemical cystitis due to toxic effects of cyclophosphamide's metabolite on bladder mucosa

Assessment

Observations/findings

Urinary frequency
Loss of bladder tone
Occult or gross hematuria

Laboratory/diagnostic studies

Urinalysis
CBC

Potential complications

Permanent bladder damage

Medical management

IV fluid
Bladder irrigation
Intake and output
Antiemetics
Sedatives

Nursing diagnosis/goal/interventions

ndx: Alteration in pattern of urinary elimination: bladder irritation related to chemotherapy

GOAL: *Patient will maintain urinary elimination within normal limits*

Encourage high fluid intake to 3 L/day (if not contraindicated) prior to and 48 hr following drug administration
Encourage frequent voiding q3h to 4h; bladder should be emptied before bedtime and when patient is awake at night
Observe and report signs and symptoms of cystitis
    Test urine for hematuria (dipstick)
        Monitor output closely; report decrease in urine (may be indicative of syndrome of inappropriate antidiuretic hormone secondary to drug)
Administer cyclophosphamide early in the day to prevent urine from pooling in bladder overnight
Indwelling catheter may be ordered
Through-and-through bladder irrigation may be ordered
Administer antiemetics and sedatives as needed
Teach exercises to regain bladder tone

Evaluation

Urinary elimination is within normal limits

Hyperuricemia

Increased uric acid levels as a result of rapid lysis of tumor cells induced by antineoplastic medications or radiation therapy; it often occurs in leukemia and/or diffuse histiocytic lymphoma

Assessment

Observations/findings

Lethargy, nausea, vomiting
Hematuria, renal colic
Oliguria, anuria

Laboratory/diagnostic studies

Uric acid >15 mg/ml

Potential complications

Renal damage

Medical management

IV fluids
Medication
    Allopurinol
    Bicarbonate
Intake and output

Nursing diagnosis/goal/intervention

ndx: Alteration in tissue perfusion: renal related to cytotoxic effects of chemotherapy

GOAL: *Patient will have adequate renal function with balanced intake and output*

Encourage high fluid intake to 4 L/day unless contraindicated (reduces the concentration of uric acid in the urine)
Initiate administration of allopurinol 12 to 24 hr prior to antineoplastic administration as ordered
    Assess patient for side and/or toxic effects
        Maculopapular rash
        Urticaria
        Purpura
        Exfoliative, erythema multiforme lesions
        Nausea, vomiting
        Abdominal pain
        Vasculitis
        Toxic epidermal necrolysis
        Cardiac standstill
NOTE: Mercaptopurine effects are enhanced when given with allopurinol; dosage of mercaptopurine is usually decreased by one third to one half to avoid toxic reactions
Ensure hydration of patient beginning 48 hr prior to antineoplastic medication administration (output >100 ml/m^2/hr)
Measure intake and output

Urine alkalinization may be ordered if patient is unable to take allopurinol
    Administer sodium bicarbonate IV as ordered to maintain urine pH of 7 to 7.5
    Check urine pH q2h to 4h
Monitor uric acid, creatinine, and creatinine levels

Emergent/crisis situation (serum urate levels >25 to 30 mg/100 ml)

Initiate IV fluid administration as ordered
Initiate urinary catheter when ordered; connect to closed gravity drainage system
Administer osmotic diuretics IV and/or acetazolamide as ordered
Prepare patient for peritoneal dialysis (p. 562) or hemodialysis (p. 567)
Provide emotional support for patient and/or significant other

Evaluation

Urine output is appropriate to intake
Laboratory tests are within normal limits

Neurotoxicity

Damage to myelin sheath, paralysis of autonomic nerves, or central nervous system (CNS) damage due to effects of chemotherapeutic medications; antineoplastic agents commonly associated with neurotoxicity are the Vinca (plant) alkaloids: vincristine, vinblastine, and vindesine

Assessment
Observations/findings

Tingling
Paresthesia
Tremors
Muscle aches/pain
Muscle weakness
    Difficulty in heel walking
    Inability to get out of chair
Foot-drop
Ptosis
Hyporeflexia to loss of deep tendon reflexes
Ataxia
Hemiplegia
Slurred speech
Jaw pain
Hoarseness
Irritability
Seizures
Somnolence
Personality change
Coma
Arachnoiditis (in relation to intrathecal administration)
    Fever
    Back pain
    Dizziness
    Headache
    Stiff neck
    Vomiting
Ototoxicity
Constipation and colicky pain
Ileus
Urinary retention

Laboratory/diagnostic studies

Neurologic examination
Neuroradiologic studies

Potential complications

Paralytic ileus
Obstipation
Adynamic ileus
Raynaud's phenomenon (with combination vinblastine and bleomycin)

Medical management

Medications
Stool softeners
Laxatives

Nursing diagnoses/goals/interventions

ndx: Impaired physical mobility related to toxic effects of chemotherapy

GOAL: *Patient will achieve and maintain mobility within normal limits*

Perform neurologic assessment prior to administration of medication, then q4h to 8h after infusion is completed; report changes to physician immediately
Assess ability to perform ADLs
Evaluate for discomfort or pain associated with movement
Assess pain, cardiac, respiratory, and elimination status
Provide safe, uncluttered environment to prevent falls
Instruct patient to sit on side of bed, stand, and then begin to walk; provide walkers, etc., as indicated
Instruct patient to report numbness and tingling or other signs of toxicity immediately
Assure patient and significant other that changes are usually reversible when medication is stopped; discuss specifics with physician—motor weakness may take many months to resolve

Provide environment and time conducive to discussing concerns and fears

Assess color and temperature of extremities, especially hands

Assess for CNS toxicity if methotrexate or cytarabine is given intrathecally; have patient lie flat for at least 1 hr following instillation of drug

ndx: Alteration in bowel elimination: constipation related to chemotherapy

GOAL: *Patient will achieve and maintain normal pattern of elimination*

Auscultate abdomen for bowel sounds q4h to 8h

Check and record daily bowel elimination (constipation and colicky pain that develop within 2 days of drug administration are early manifestations of toxicity)

Administer stool softeners and laxatives prophylactically

Encourage fluid to 3 L/day unless contraindicated

Encourage diet high in fiber and bulk

Measure intake and output

Administer enemas as ordered

Encourage mobility as tolerated

Evaluation

Patient
  Maintains mobility within normal limits
  Maintains normal bowel elimination

Hepatotoxicity

Dysfunction of the liver induced by chemotherapeutic medications, other hepatotoxic drugs, or preexisting hepatic conditions; because the hepatocytes are not rapidly dividing cells, they are less affected by many drugs; antineoplastic agents associated with hepatic toxicity include nitrosoureas, methotrexate, 6-mercaptopurine (6-MP), cytosine arabinoside, mithramycin, asparaginase, and interferon

Assessment

Observations/findings

Lethargy
Weakness
Pruritus (itching)
Jaundice
Dark urine
Sweet or sour odor of urine and breath
Clay-colored stools
Bleeding tendency
  Purpura
  Epistaxis
  Melena
Abdominal tenderness
Right upper quadrant pain
Anorexia
Digestive discomfort
Ascites
Generalized edema
Palmar erythema
Spider angiomas
Irritability
Apathy
Memory defects
Asterixis
Coma
Associated factors, preexisting or concurrent
  Viral hepatitis
  Abdominal radiotherapy
  Hepatic metastasis
  Hepatotoxic drugs
  Transfusion of blood products
  Graft vs. host disease (GVHD) (p. 189)

Laboratory/diagnostic studies

Elevated
  Serum transaminase
  Bilirubin
  Alkaline phosphatase
  Cholesterol
  Fibrinogen
Decreased
  Hepatic clotting factors
  Albumin
Liver function tests
Blood clotting test, CBC
Liver biopsy
Radiologic examination

Potential complications

Cirrhosis
Ascites
Hepatomegaly

Medical management

IV fluids
Blood products
Nasogastric tube

Nursing diagnosis/goal/interventions

ndx: Potential for complications: hemorrhage, pruritus*

---

*Not a NANDA-approved nursing diagnosis.

GOAL: *Patient will have minimized or controlled bleeding and/or pruritus*

Assess sensorium q2h to 4h
Report changes of increased lethargy
Avoid use of drugs such as narcotics and barbiturates that cause CNS depression
Observe for signs of bleeding: hematemesis, melena, petechiae
Assess for abdominal distention; measure abdominal girth
Assess bowel sounds
Monitor vital signs and laboratory studies; if nasogastric tube is being used, maintain patency
Provide oral care; keep nostrils clean and lubricated
Maintain proper position of tube
Place in semi-Fowler's position unless contraindicated
Report changes in color, bleeding, and edema to physician
Bathe patient daily; use soothing baths (i.e., use starch or oil) to relieve itching
Administer skin care as needed to decrease itching; antihistamine drugs may be ordered
Keep nails short to prevent scratching skin
Encourage fluids to 3000 to 4000 ml/24 hr unless contraindicated; fluids may be limited in presence of edema
Measure intake and output
Report changes in color of urine and stool
Manage pain as indicated or ordered
Assess response to relief measure(s)
If bleeding tendency
  Avoid IM injections
  Consolidate laboratory work
  Use fingersticks when possible
  Apply pressure at puncture or IV site for 5 min after procedure has been completed; check site q15 min for four times
  Place furniture, equipment, and personal items so as to prevent injuries from falls or bumping into objects
  Administer gentle oral hygiene using toothettes or swabs
  Avoid use of harsh soaps and rough towels and cloths
  Test urine and stool for occult bleeding
Provide diet with amount of calories, carbohydrate, and protein as ordered; avoid high-fat foods
Serve meals attractively and at correct temperature; small feedings may be more tempting
Weigh patient daily at same time with same clothing and scale
Encourage activity to tolerance; assist with and teach active ROM exercises q4h
Administer medications as ordered for itching
Continue nursing measures as indicated for primary condition

Evaluation

Bleeding and pruritus are controlled

Alopecia

Temporary loss of body hair as a result of chemotherapeutic agents that interact with cells that are in the anagen phase of cell cycle (85% to 90% of total scalp hair cells at any one time); permanent hair loss in area of radiotherapy; antineoplastics associated with alopecia include cyclophosphamide, doxorubicin, and vinblastine; antineoplastics associated with thinning rather than total hair loss include bleomycin, vincristine, 5-FU, and etoposide

Assessment
Observations/findings

Hair loss
  Scalp especially affected early
  Long-term therapy
    Axilla
    Extremities
    Pubis
Alterations in body image

Medical management

Ice cap (patient with solid tumors)

Nursing diagnoses/goals/interventions

ndx Disturbance in self-concept: body image, self-esteem

GOAL: *Patient will verbalize realistic view and acceptance of body as it is, and will focus on remaining strength and view of self as a capable, valuable person*

Establish therapeutic nurse-patient relationship
Inform patient in advance about impending hair loss
Have patient obtain wigs, scarves, hats, or caps before hair loss begins
Understand that hair loss cannot be controlled or minimized when it is a result of radiotherapy
Understand that hair loss usually begins 1 to 2 weeks after single dose of chemotherapy; maximum loss will occur 1 to 2 months after beginning therapy
Stress temporary nature of hair loss
  Complete regrowth is usual after chemotherapy is completed

Regrowth can begin during treatment
Tell patient to expect alterations in texture and color (physiology of hair follicle is changed by drugs)
Assess patient's perception of effect of hair loss
Short hairstyles may be preferred
  Beginning hair loss may not be readily noticeable
  Patient comfort may be increased by a short hair style when maximum amount of hair is falling out
  Stress importance of periodic rather than continuous use of wigs to allow scalp to "breathe"
Assist with gentle scalp care during susceptible period
  Wash hair with pH-balanced shampoo
  Expose hair and scalp to air as much as possible
Application of ice bags and tourniquets around hairline may assist in minimizing hair loss
  Be aware that efficacy of these procedures has not been proved
  Understand that these procedures are never used when patient has a widely metastatic tumor such as leukemia, lymphoma, myeloma, etc., or scalp tumor implants
  Be aware that these procedures, if used, could possibly create a tumor cell sanctuary in the scalp
  Use procedure only when administering IV push drugs that have a transiently elevated blood concentration
  Never use these procedures when administering drugs by IV infusion or oral route
  Apply ice cap or ice bag (i.e., chipped ice in plastic bag) to scalp when ordered; usually applied 20 to 30 min prior to administration of IV push medication and for 20 min after completion of administration
  Apply tourniquet or inflatable scalp pressure cuff when ordered
    Usually applied during drug administration and for 5 to 10 min after completion
    Ensure that extra pressure is applied at pinna of head
Manage pain as indicated and/or ordered
  Headache is usually experienced
  Assess effectiveness of pain relief measure(s)
Ensure that patient and/or significant other knows and understands
  Need to discuss feelings related to perceptions of hair loss
  Importance of gentle hair and scalp care
  To expose scalp to air as much as possible
  That hair loss will be temporary throughout course of treatment
  To avoid use of dyes, color rinses, permanents, and bleaches until such time as indicated by condition of scalp, hair, and physician's direction

ndx: Potential alteration in skin integrity related to total loss of hair

GOAL: *Patient will verbalize knowledge of scalp care*

Wash scalp with mild soap and water
Use soft-bristled hairbrush to reduce pull on hair
Use mild oil (mineral) to lubricate scalp and reduce itching
Reduce exposure to sun by using a sunscreen and/or wearing hat or cap

Evaluation

Patient
  Verbalizes acceptance of temporary body change
  Demonstrates care of scalp area

Dermatologic Toxicity

hypersensitivity reactions *Reactions to antineoplastic agents; can be very serious and/or life threatening, particularly if an anaphylactic reaction occurs; drugs most commonly associated with an anaphylactoid reaction include asparaginase, cisplatin (infrequent), and bleomycin*
hyperpyrexia *Associated with bleomycin, especially in patients with lymphoma*
erythema (Adria flaré) *Associated with doxorubicin; the flare usually results when the drug is too concentrated or if the patient has very sensitive skin*

Assessment
Observations/findings
GENERAL

Urticaria
Angioedema
Bronchospasm
Abdominal cramping
Hypotension
Hyperpigmentation
Maculopapular rash
Vesicle formation
Acne
Thinning of skin and striae
Petechiae
Ecchymosis
Hives
Pruritus
Desquamation
Jaundice
Photosensitivity
Nail changes
  Horizontal or longitudinal banding
  Thickening of nail bed
Radiation "recall" phenomena
Blue discoloration of vein

HYPERPYREXIA

High fever

ERYTHEMA (ADRIA FLARÉ)

Itching
Redness (diffuse or streak above the vein)
Urticaria

Medical management

GENERAL

Diphenhydramine (Benadryl)
Epinephrine
Parenteral corticosteroids

HYPERPYREXIA

Acetaminophen
Fluid intake

ERYTHEMA (ADRIA FLARÉ)

Ice pack to affected area

Nursing diagnosis/goal/interventions

ndx: Impairment of skin integrity related to adverse effects of antineoplastic agents

GOAL: *Patient will achieve and maintain skin integrity*

Review patient's allergy history
Monitor vital signs and mental status
Observe patient throughout administration of drug
Ensure that appropriate drugs and equipment are immediately available for possible emergency use; in the event of an anaphylactoid reaction, have the following available
    Diphenhydramine (Benadryl)
    Epinephrine
    Oxygen
    Airway
    Suction equipment
Be fully aware of facility procedure to follow in the event of such a reaction
For Adria flaré
    At first signs of itching or redness, reduce the amount of drug being given (i.e., if giving 1 ml, reduce to ½ ml); flush vein well and continue administering drug; if erythema and urticaria occur, stop IV and apply ice pack; start fresh IV and administer additional drug
For hyperpyrexia
    Give acetaminophen q4h as ordered
    Push oral fluids
Advise patient to report adverse reactions immediately

Assess skin condition q8h, especially axillary and breast folds, groin, perirectal area, and dependent extremities
Assist with daily bath prn
    Use antibacterial soaps and soft cloths
    Rinse and dry well
    If using lotions, do not leave skin moist
Keep linens dry and wrinkle-free
Teach and assist with perianal care after each elimination
    Use soft towels or cloths
    Wash with povidone-iodine wash
    Ensure that area is kept dry
    Advise patient to wear cotton clothing and underwear
Teach handwashing technique to be used after elimination and prn
Caution patient to avoid bumps, bruising, cuts, and scratches
    Explain importance of skin care to patient
    Caution patient to avoid use of sharp objects: razors, cuticle scissors, etc.
    Explain need to always wear slippers or shoes when out of bed
    Caution patient to avoid tight or constricting clothing
    Caution patient to avoid use of jewelry when possible; moisture and bacteria collect underneath, and sharp edges can cause scratches or cuts
Avoid IM injections when possible
Central line may be ordered and inserted to avoid multiple IV injections—perform daily central line care if inserted
Consolidate laboratory work; use fingersticks when possible; cleanse skin with povidone-iodine prior to venipuncture
Avoid excessive sunlight for photosensitivity; use of sunscreens is helpful

Evaluation

Patient achieves and maintains skin integrity

Extravasation

Escape of agents from a vein into the tissue; escape of certain antineoplastic agents can cause necrosis of local tissue; care must be taken when giving these agents (see Administration of Chemotherapeutic Drugs, p. 669); vesicant drugs, which can cause tissue necrosis if they infiltrate, include vincristine, vinblastine, doxorubicin (Adriamycin), dactinomycin, daunorubicin, dacarbazine, mitomycin, nitrogen mustard, mithramycin, and streptozocin

Assessment

Observations/findings

Venipuncture site
  During infusion
    Burning
    Pain
    Swelling
    Induration
    No blood return or questionable blood return (blood return is obtained, but patient questions or complains of pain—drug escape could be above injection site)
  Postinfusion
    Ulceration
    Desquamation
    Necrosis
  Phlebitis
    Pain
    Increased temperature
    Redness
    Swelling
  Predisposing factors
    Sclerotic vascular disease
    Multiple venipunctures

Medical management

Orders to institute extravasation procedure
Sodium thiosulfate
Hydrocortisone
Hyaluronidase
Ice or warm packs

Nursing diagnosis/goal/interventions

ndx: Impairment of skin integrity related to adverse effects of antineoplastic agents

GOAL: *Patient will have intact skin free from redness, swelling, and necrosis*

Prevention of extravasation

Administer vesicant medication through a freshly inserted IV site with a good blood return
Select large veins in region with large amount of soft tissue to avoid possible involvement of tendons should IV infiltrate
Check medication dosage and dilution carefully
Administer at rate ordered; monitor closely
Monitor IV site continuously during infusion
Instruct patient to notify staff immediately if burning sensation is felt at site or IV slows or stops
After infusing medication, infuse neutral solution through IV line as ordered
Observe for possible clinical signs of extravasation: pain, burning, swelling, no blood return or questionable blood return
Observe for possible clinical signs of tissue necrosis: erythema, induration, tenderness, pain, eventual ulceration with tissue breakdown
Steps in management of extravasation once confirmed
  Discontinue IV immediately
  Apply appropriate pack (hot or cold)
  Infiltrate area with antidote using interdermal technique
  Instruct patient on follow-up

Recommended protocol

Vesicants, when extravasated, produce local necrosis; recommended treatment is
  Mechlorethamine (mustargen, nitrogen mustard)
    Discontinue IV
    Infiltrate local area with 1/6 molar (isotonic) sodium thiosulfate using intradermal technique
    Apply ice for 20 min qh for 24 hr
    Notify physician
  Dactinomycin (actinomycin D, Cosmegen); mithramycin (Mithracin, Plycamycin); mitomycin C (Mutamycin); daunorubicin (Daunomycin); doxorubicin (Adriamycin); streptozocin (Zanosar); amsacrine *(investigational)*
    Discontinue IV
    Infiltrate area with hydrocortisone sodium succinate 50 mg or other water-soluble corticosteroid (using intradermal technique)
    Apply ice for 20 min qh for 24 hr
    Notify physician
  Vinblastine (Velban); vincristine (Oncovin)
    Discontinue IV
    Infiltrate area with hyaluronidase 150 units using intradermal technique
    Apply warm, moist packs for 24 hr
    Notify physician

Ongoing care

Instruct patient on follow-up
Continue to observe site
Notify physician of skin changes

Evaluation

Skin is intact; there is no redness, swelling, or necrosis

RADIOTHERAPY

Treatment of neoplastic disease by use of gamma rays to disturb proliferation of cells by decreasing the rate

of mitosis or impairing DNA synthesis, thereby reducing tumor mass; radiotherapy is administered externally (source outside of the body) or internally (source of radiation inside the body)

Assessment

Observations/findings

NOTE: Symptoms will vary depending on area(s) being irradiated; intensity of symptoms will also be affected

Skin, site of radiation
- Erythema
- Pruritus
- Edema
- Desquamation (dry or moist)
- Hyperpigmentation
- Atrophy
- Pain

Mucositis, dental caries
Altered taste
Nausea, vomiting
Anorexia, dysphagia, esophagitis
Diarrhea
Weight loss
Alteration in nutrition: less than body requirements (p. 59)
Headache
Malaise
Fatigue
Loss of hair, itching, scaling and tanning of scalp
Tachycardia
Pericarditis
Muocarditis
Pneumonitis
Decreased fertility
Increased susceptibility to infection

Laboratory/diagnostic studies

CBC
Decreased Hgb
Leukopenia
Thrombocytopenia
Pancytopenia
Electrolytes

Potential complications

Infection
Anemia

Medical management

Antiemetics
Antifungals
Viscous lidocaine
Antacids
IV fluids
Antidiarrheals
Urinary anesthesia
Antibiotics
Foley catheter
Blood products

Nursing diagnoses/goals/interventions

ndx: Anxiety/fear related to treatment

GOAL: *Patient will verbalize fears and concerns regarding treatment*

Pretreatment care

Patient will be seen by radiologist to determine if radiotherapy will be a useful treatment
Understand that patient is usually very anxious and fearful until treatment decision is made
Reinforce physician's explanation of procedure and benefits
Encourage discussion of fears, fantasies, and misconceptions surrounding treatment
Patient will be seen by radiologist once decision is made to administer radiotherapy
Understand that during this visit, area(s) to be irradiated will be marked with indelible dye
Explain procedure and what is expected of patient
- Equipment is similar to but larger than that used for x-ray examinations
- Radiologist or radiotherapist will be close by for communication during treatment
- Patient will be positioned on a table in a room by himself
- After positioning, patient must remain absolutely still
- Positioning may take 10 min or more
- Understand that treatment of one field usually lasts 1 to 3 min
- No pain results from treatment, but patient may experience discomfort from maintaining position

ndx: Potential for impaired skin integrity related to radiation

GOAL: *Patient will demonstrate understanding of methods to prevent or minimize skin problems*

Assess skin carefully
Teach importance of skin care
- Avoid tub bath or shower until ordered
- Do not wash skin in area being irradiated
- Do not remove skin markings between treatments

Avoid use of any product, including soap, on skin area being irradiated without checking with physician

Wear loose clothing to prevent rubbing

Avoid extremes in temperature and exposure to sunlight; do not use hot-water bottle or heating pad

Dry desquamation
   Avoid suntan lotion or powder
   Use cornstarch

Moist desquamation
   May use water/saline 1½ strength peroxide to clean
   Keep clean and dry (slow healing)

Precautions to prevent infection
   Expose skin to air when possible
   Cover broken skin areas with a dressing when ordered; use a stretch-type tubular dressing to hold in place
   Avoid use of tape; use nonallergic or paper tape applied to nontreated skin areas when required
   Avoid use of cosmetics and use wigs, hairpieces, or scarves as needed
   Avoid use of deodorants if treatment is to axilla

ndx: Alteration in nutrition: less than body requirements related to radiation

GOAL: *Patient will not lose more than 5% to 10% of body weight*

Assess nutritional status

Weigh patient daily at same time with same clothing and scale

Teach patient to maintain nutritious, high-protein diet
   Provide high-protein supplements
   Provide food when patient desires it; six small bland feedings may be more easily tolerated
   Experiment with foods
   Serve food attractively arranged and at proper temperature
   Provide cold foods, such as ice cream and gelatins, which are more soothing to patient with stomatitis; see Stomatitis/Mucositis (p. 692)
   Avoid smoking
   Avoid spicy or hot foods

Administer tube feedings or total parenteral nutrition (TPN) as ordered with severe decrease in intake

Administer vitamins as ordered

Maintain quiet periods before and after meals

Keep room odor free and fresh

Maintain high fluid intake, to 2000 to 3000 ml/day, unless contraindicated

Administer antiemetics as ordered

Administer antacid

Do calorie count when appropriate

Assess abdomen, including bowel sounds

Assess elimination status (diarrhea or constipation)

Administer antidiarrheal/laxative as needed

ndx: Impaired tissue integrity: oral mucous membrane related to radiation

GOAL: *Patient will prevent or minimize infection*

Assess oral cavity q8h

Administer oral hygiene before and after meals, morning and night, and after vomiting
   Increase to q2h with stomatitis (p. 692)
   Use soft-bristled toothbrush
   Use foam or sponge swabs as needed
   Use dilute mouthwash
   Use saline rinse as needed

Administer Nystatin (Mycostatin) as ordered

May need saliva substitutes

Assess for painful or difficulty in swallowing; administer viscous lidocaine as needed

ndx: Alteration in pattern of urinary elimination related to radiation

GOAL: *Patient will maintain balanced intake and output*

Assess genitourinary status

Monitor intake and output and for painful urination

Force fluids to 3 L/day unless contraindicated

Assist with and teach care of perianal area, especially if diarrhea is present

Protect from infection if WBC decreases (p. 684)

ndx: Potential complication: myelosuppression*

GOAL: *Patient will verbalize understanding of and demonstrate methods to control complications*

Monitor CBC (see Myelosuppression, p. 684)

Pace activities with frequent rest periods

May need to put radiation therapy on hold

If blood counts are very low
   Observe for signs and symptoms of bleeding and infection
   Administer antibiotics and blood products as ordered

---

*Not a NANDA-approved nursing diagnosis.

Interventions for specific types of implants

Brain implants

Assess for adverse reaction, fatigue, anorexia, possible tissue damage, neurologic side effects; perform neurologic assessment

Inform patient of hair loss

Gynecologic cesium implants

Assess and manage adverse effects: diarrhea, cystitis, dysuria, vaginal fibrosis, and dryness

Instruct patient of immobility
- Bed rest for 48 hr
- Elevate head 30 degrees only
- No baths or pericare until unloaded; patient to have minimal care
- Encourage fluid and low residue diet
- May need Lomotil to stop bowel movement
- Administer pain medication as needed

Breast implants

Assess for skin erythema

Provide insertion site care

Head and neck implants

Assess for side effects and manage dryness of mucous membrane of the oral cavity
- Stomatitis
- Dry desquamation
- Hair loss
- Possible infection
- Xerostomia

Assess and maintain patent airway

Assess for and manage bleeding

Manage pain

Provide means of communicating, such as writing pad or Magic Slate

Assess for alteration in body image
- Skin markers, especially on face
- Weight loss, loss of muscle mass
- Alopecia

Assess psychologic aspects and intervene
- Isolation: be attentive to patient's needs
- Allow verbalization and provide time for discussion of pains and anxieties

If implant, inform patient of need for personnel to observe time, distance, and shielding precautions

Personnel should wear film badges

No pregnant visitors

ndx: Knowledge deficit regarding potential complications and effects of radiation

GOAL: *Patient will demonstrate understanding of potential complications and effects of radiation through interactive discussion*

Explain need to avoid persons with infections, especially URIs

Discuss symptoms of infection to report to physician
"Cold," "flu," elevated temperature
- Diarrhea and frequency of or burning on urination
- Reddened, painful skin areas
- Mouth redness, swelling, ulceration, bleeding, increased salivation

Emphasize importance of maintaining nutritious diet and fluid intake to 3000 ml daily unless contraindicated
- Take six to eight small feedings
- Avoid eating immediately before or after treatment

Explain that radiation effects continue for 10 to 14 days after last treatment; tell patient signs of healing will not be seen until 18 to 21 days after last treatment

Explain need for daily oral hygiene—in the morning, after meals, and at bedtime—to keep mouth fresh and clean

Discuss the following symptoms to report to physician
- Mucositis (p. 692)
- Nausea and vomiting (p. 690)
- Inability to eat
- Increasing headache or tiredness
- Severe diarrhea (p. 694)
- Increasing redness, swelling, pain, or pruritus at site of therapy

Emphasize importance of follow-up outpatient care

Teach name of medication, dosage, time of administration, purpose, and side effects

Explain need to avoid taking over-the-counter medications without checking with physician

Evaluation

Patient freely discusses fears and concerns

Patient uses measures to decrease skin problems; skin is intact or is healing

Weight is stable at pretreatment level

There are no signs of oral infection; mucous membranes are moist and pink

Patient achieves normal elimination pattern; intake and output are balanced

Patient verbalizes symptoms to report and discusses home and follow-up care

UNSEALED RADIOACTIVE CHEMOTHERAPY

Preparation of room

Furniture convenient and functioning
Bed on external wall of building
   Bed freshly made
   Extra covers available
Lighting adequate
Phone and television functioning
Reading and/or hobby materials available
Flowers arranged and watered
Oral hygiene and bath equipment available
Trash baskets and linen hamper in room
Lead-lined urine containers in room
Saturated solution of potassium iodide in bathroom
Radioactive tags posted
   On door
   On chart cover and available for patient's use
Radioactive badges at room entrance

RADIOACTIVE IODINE

NOTE: *Pregnant staff members must not be assigned to care for patient*

Prior to administration of medication

Check room for needed equipment
Place items conveniently for patient's use
Order disposable dishes, utensils, and tray for diet

Ongoing care

Wear correct badge when entering room
Limit time spent in room; plan before entering room
   Observations to be made
   Equipment needed
   Care to be done
Handle urine or stool with rubber or plastic gloves when necessary
Dispose of excreta in toilet; place one dropperful of saturated solution of potassium iodide in toilet and flush
If excreta (urine, feces, sputum, vomitus) is spilled on skin
   Run water over area for 2 min
   Wash with soap and water for 3 min
   Have area monitored by radiation therapy department
If excreta is spilled on bed or other surface in room
   Notify radiation therapy department
   Clean in usual manner after area is cleared by monitoring
Handle dressings with rubber or plastic gloves when present; discard in plastic bag and keep in room
Handle bed linens with rubber or plastic gloves if they contain excreta or perspiration; place in linen hamper in room
Do not remove linen or trash from room
Do not perform routine nursing functions for ambulatory patients
Plan care to limit exposure if patient is debilitated
   Be efficient
   Have all needed equipment on hand
   Use turn sheets; bathe soiled areas only
   Prepare and cut foods prior to entering room
Collect and place specimens for laboratory in lead-lined containers
After discharge or discontinuation of isolation
   Have room equipment, linen, and trash monitored by radiation therapy department
   Remove equipment, linen, and trash when permission is given by radiation therapy department; handle in usual manner

RADIOACTIVE PHOSPHORUS

Follow care as for radioactive iodine except
   No special precautions are needed for disposal of urine, feces, or sputum
   No precautions are needed for disposal of vomitus unless ^{32}P is given orally
   If chromic phosphate is given into pleural or peritoneal cavity and leakage develops, notify radiation therapy department for monitoring and instructions

Care of Patient Receiving Unsealed Radioactive Chemotherapy
RADIOACTIVE IODINE

Administration of metabolized or absorbed radiation to treat such conditions as hyperthyroidism or thyroid cancer; usually ^{131}I or ^{32}P is administered

Assessment
Observations/findings

Response to isolation
   Depressed
   Euphoric
   Accepting
   Complaints of tender area in neck
   Progression of ophthalmopathy
   Transient productive cough
   Hypothyroidism (p. 424)
   Hyperthyroidism (p. 427)
   Hypoparathyroidism (p. 432)

Care prior to administration of medication

NOTE: *Pregnant staff members are not to care for patient*

Acute care

Bathe or have patient shower
Clean and arrange linen and furniture
- Have personal hygiene items, reading materials, television, hobby materials, and phone accessible to patient
- Remove unwanted items from room

Note food and fluid preferences and order from dietary department
Assist patient in notifying family and friends concerning visiting limitations
- Allow no visiting for 24 hr after administration of medication
- Allow 2 hr visiting per person thereafter, if visitor remains 6 feet away from patient

Patient teaching

Reinforce physician's explanation of procedure and need for isolation
Involve family or significant other in care and instructions
Orient patient to plan of care
- Relate that personnel will be in room for very short periods of time only
- Assure patient that necessary care will be done
- Reinforce that patient is to call for needed items or care

Daily hygienic measures are to be performed by patient if able
Hospital garments must be worn; medication is excreted via perspiration and saliva
Describe method to be used to collect 24-hr urine specimens; laboratory value of radioactivity level determines length of stay in isolation
Disposable dishes, utensils, and trays will be used for meals
Linen and waste material will remain in room
Communication with staff will be via call bell and intercommunications system
Visiting privileges will be limited
- No visitors will be allowed during first 24 hr
- Visitors will be allowed 2 hr/day thereafter, if visitor remains 6 feet away from patient

Routine housekeeping functions will not be performed

Care after administration of medication

Ongoing care

If patient vomits ^{32}P or ^{131}I immediately or within 4 hr of administration
- Notify radiation safety officer and physician
- All contaminated persons, materials, and surfaces must be decontaminated

Intracavity instillation

Place patient on side opposite incision after instillation
Turn patient q15 min for 2 to 3 hr
Check incision for leakage of solution q15 min for eight times, q30 min for two times, then q4h
If leakage occurs, notify radiation safety officer and physician
Visit patient briefly at least qh from doorway
Assess, anticipate, and fulfill needs and requests promptly
Deliver mail, paper, and flowers as they arrive
Provide additional diversionary activities as needed
See that additional materials and equipment are available when needed by patient for disposal of trash, excreta, and linen
Do not remove any items from room except laboratory specimens in lead-lined containers
Provide emotional support
- Assess patient's reaction to therapy and isolation
- Assure patient that isolation will last no longer than 8 days
- Discuss concerns about radioactivity remaining after therapy is completed

Patient teaching/discharge outcome

Ensure that patient and/or significant other knows and understands
- That patient is not continuing source of danger from radioactivity to family or others; majority of medication is excreted in 8 days
- Symptoms of recurrence of hyperthyroidism to report to physician
- Symptoms of hypothyroidism to report to physician
- Importance of
  - Balanced activity and rest periods
  - Ongoing outpatient care

Evaluation

Patient identifies and manages adverse effects of radiation

CHAPTER 14

Perinatal/Neonatal Standards

Mother

ANTEPARTUM ASSESSMENT

Observations/findings

Age
Height
Prepregnancy weight
History of infertility
Menstrual history
   Last menstrual period (LMP)
   Interval between periods
   Expected date of confinement (EDC)
Pregnancy history
   Gravida
   Term deliveries
   Premature deliveries
   Abortions
   Stillbirths
   Date of each delivery (month and year)
      Weeks of gestation
      Length of labor in hours
      Spontaneous or induced labor
      Type of delivery
      Children living (ages, any developmental problems)
      Multiple births
      Maternal, fetal, or neonatal complications
BP, T, P, and R
Fetal heart rate (FHR)
Blood type and Rh factor
Rubella titer
Urine protein and glucose
Date and results of last Papanicolaou (Pap) test
Previous major illnesses and surgeries
Current health problems
Breast changes
   Fullness
   Tingling
   Heaviness
   Darkening of areola
   Presence of colostrum
   Turgid nipples and engorged areolas with sexual stimulation
Cardiovascular changes
   Increase in heart rate of 10 beats/min from baseline from 14 to 30 weeks of pregnancy
   Slight decrease in BP during second trimester with increase in third trimester <15 mm Hg in either systolic or diastolic
   Tendency toward dependent edema
Hematologic changes during pregnancy
   Blood volume increases and peaks by 30 to 34 weeks
   Red blood cell (RBC) production accelerates
   Hgb declines due to hemodilution
   Reticulocyte count increases due to hematopoiesis
   White blood cell count (WBC) increases up to 25,000 mm^3
   Total plasma proteins decrease to 3 to 3.5 g/dl (normal = 4 to 4.5 g/dl) due to fall in albumin level
   Sedimentation rate increases due to decrease in total plasma proteins
Respiratory changes
   Nasal stuffiness due to estrogen-initiated hyperemia
   Increased oxygen consumption
   Decreased functional residual capacity and residual volume of air
   Increased tidal volume, minute ventilatory volume, and minute oxygen uptake
   Increased respiratory rate
Urinary changes
   Frequency of urination
   Increased bladder capacity
   Increased glomerular filtration rate
   Mild proteinuria
   Mild glycosuria
Gastrointestinal (GI) changes
   Tender gums
   Transitory nausea and vomiting in first trimester
   Heartburn and acid indigestion (esophageal regurgitation and decreased emptying time)
   Unusual food preferences
   Constipation
   Hypercholesterolemia
   Decreased gallbladder emptying time
Neurologic changes

Lightheadedness or faintness in early pregnancy
Headache associated with pregnancy-induced hypertension
Sensory changes in legs with compression of pelvic nerves
Musculoskeletal changes
  Decreased abdominal muscle tone
  Increase in lumbosacral curve
  Hypermobility of pelvic joints
  Waddling gait near term
Integumentary changes
  Thickened skin
  Increased subdermal fat
  Hyperpigmentation
  Increased hair and nail growth
  Accelerated sebacous and sweat gland activity
  Increased fragility of cutaneous elastic tissues (stretch marks)
  Chloasma
  Acne vulgaris (preexisting)
    Aggravated in first trimester
    Improved in third trimester
Patterns of tobacco, alcohol, and prescription/nonprescription drug use
Patterns of nutrient intake
Planned method of feeding infant
Self-concept and perceived ability to cope with life situations
Body image due to physiologic changes of pregnancy
Desire for participation in prepared childbirth classes
Plans for postdischarge infant care at home
Concurrent conditions
  Diabetes
  Cardiovascular conditions
  Severe anemia
  Epilepsy
  Asthma or other pulmonary conditions
  Drug sensitivities
  Renal disorders
  Sexually transmitted disease
Patterns of work or employment

Laboratory/diagnostic studies

Pregnancy test confirmation
Blood typing and Rh factor identification
Hemoglobin (Hgb) and hematocrit (Hct)
VDRL (Veneral disease research laboratories) test
Pap test (cervical cytology test)
Urinalysis
Irregular antibody screen
Rubella antibody titer
TORCH screen as indicated
Fasting blood sugar (FBS) screening (at 26 weeks gestation if no high-risk factors are present for diabetes)
Glucose tolerance tests for diabetes as indicated and per facility protocol

Medical management

Uncomplicated pregnancy visit schedule
  Every 4 weeks during first 28 weeks
  Every 2 to 3 weeks until 36 weeks
  Weekly until delivery
Diabetic screening as indicated
Other diagnostic tests as indicated
Laboratory tests as indicated
Nonstress testing (NST) (p. 737)
Contraction stress testing (CST) (p. 738)
Antibiotics for treatment as indicated
Prenatal vitamins and iron supplements
Counseling and other referrals as indicated for high-risk pregnancy
Genetic counseling as indicated

Nursing diagnosis/goal/interventions

ndx: Knowledge deficit regarding changes of pregnancy

GOAL: *Mother and significant other will demonstrate ability to adapt and adjust to changes of pregnancy; family will prepare appropriately for role transitions to parenthood*

Discuss danger signals to report to physician immediately
  Any vaginal bleeding
  Swelling of face or fingers
  Severe or continuous headache
  Dimness or blurring of vision
  Abdominal pain
  Persistent vomiting
  Chills or fever
  Dysuria
  Escape of fluid from vagina
  Abrupt decrease in fetal movements during last trimester
Emphasize importance of avoiding smoking, alcohol, and "hard" drugs, including opium derivatives, barbiturates, and amphetamines
Emphasize importance of avoiding any nonprescription drugs, including aspirin and nose drops, without checking with physician
Explain need to check with physician before traveling
Discuss methods to alleviate nausea, hemorrhoids, and/or varicose veins
Emphasize importance of ongoing outpatient care
Explain need to avoid excessive fatigue when exercising

Explain need to maintain good body mechanics when bending, lifting, or walking

Explain need to rest periodically with legs elevated

Emphasize importance of being sedentary if pregnant with two or more fetuses or if pregnancy-induced hypertension is present

Explain need to avoid use of constricting garments, especially on lower extremities

Explain need to drink adequate amounts of fluid to 3000 ml daily unless contraindicated

Emphasize importance of well-balanced diet

Explain need to wear well-fitting, supportive brassiere

Explain need to wear only low-heeled shoes if backache or unstable balance occurs with higher-heeled shoes

Emphasize importance of maintaining normal bowel habits with adequate fluid intake, reasonable exercise, and diet high in fiber
- Mild laxatives such as prune juice, milk of magnesia, bulk-producing substances, or stool softeners may be taken when necessary
- Avoid use of nonabsorable oil preparations and any other nonprescription medications without checking with physician

Emphasize importance of avoiding intercourse when there is a threat of spontaneous abortion or premature labor

Explain need to avoid routine douching
- *Never* use hand bulb syringe because of danger of air embolism
- If douching is absolutely necessary, bag should not be elevated more than 2 feet above hips, and nozzle should not be inserted more than 3 inches through vulva

Discuss pros and cons of breast-feeding vs. bottle feeding

Discuss special caretaking considerations for working mothers

Evaluation

There are no complications caused by poor compliance

Family is prepared for role transitions and new infant care duties

PREGNANCY-INDUCED HYPERTENSION (PIH; PREECLAMPSIA)

Syndrome of hypertension, edema, and proteinuria occurring during the second half of pregnancy, characteristically in primigravidas; resolves within 10 days postpartum

Assessment

Observations/findings

GENERAL OBSERVATIONS

Elevated BP
Proteinuria
Edema
  Face
  Fingers
  Pretibial pitting type
Irritability, emotional tension
Hyperreflexia
Nervousness
Nausea, vomiting
Visual disturbances
Severe generalized headache
Altered level of consciousness
Epigastric pain
Oliguria
Pulmonary edema
Onset of labor
Magnesium blood level above 7.5 mEq/L

MILD PREECLAMPSIA

BP above 140/90 mm Hg or rise in systolic pressure of 30 mm Hg above normal and in diastolic pressure of 15 mm Hg above normal on two occasions at least 6 hr apart

Proteinuria >0.3 g/L/24 hr or 1 g/L in two random specimens collected at least 6 hr apart

SEVERE PREECLAMPSIA

BP above 160/110 mm Hg or systolic pressure of 50 mm Hg above normal diastolic pressure of 35 mm Hg above normal

Proteinuria: more then 5 g daily
Massive generalized edema
Cerebral or visual disturbances
Oliguria: 500 ml or less in 24 hr
Rising plasma creatinine

Laboratory/diagnostic studies

Hct
Liver enzyme (serum glutamic oxidase transaminase [SGOT], serum glutamic pyruvic transaminase [SGPT], lactate dehydrogenase [LDH], creatine phosphokinase [CPK])
Mg^+, Ca^+ levels
Blood urea nitrogen (BUN), creatinine every 4 weeks
Electrolytes as indicated
Ultrasound profile every 4 weeks
Urine (24 hr) for total protein and creatinine
NST and CST as indicated

Lecithin/sphingomyelin (L/S) ratio as indicated
Fetoscope/Doppler for fetal heart tones by 20 weeks gestation
Ultrasound for size and dates as indicated
Biparietal diameter (BPD) at 16-18 weeks gestation
Amniocentesis (p. 718)

Potential complications

Hypertensive crisis
Vascular overload, congestive heart failure
Uteroplacental insufficiency (UPI)
Intrauterine growth retardation (IUGR)
Central nervous system (CNS) disturbances
Cerebrovascular accident (CVA)
Seizures
Fetal loss
Prematurity
Magnesium sulfate toxicity, respiratory arrest
   Flushing
   Thirst
   Diaphoresis
   Anxiety
   Drowsiness
   Lethargy
   Slight slurring of speech
   Ataxia
   Flaccidity
   Hypotension
   Hyporeflexia; disappearance of patellar reflex
Essential hypertension
Disseminated intravascular coagulation (DIC)
Abruptio placenta

Medical management

Laboratory/diagnostic tests as indicated
Bed rest
Daily weights
Vital signs with blood pressure
Seizure precautions
Magnesium sulfate therapy—IV continuous infusion
Electronic fetal monitoring as indicated
IV fluids as indicated
Antihypertensives as indicated
Anticonvulsives as indicated
Oxytocin infusion for delivery as indicated (p. 733)

Nursing diagnoses/goals/interventions

ndx: Alteration in uteroplacental and renal tissue perfusion related to pregnancy-induced hypertension

GOAL: *Patient will not have seizures or change in level of consciousness; fetus will not show signs of distress; physiologic metabolic needs will be minimized, and tissue perfusion will be maximized; blood pressure readings will be maintained or lowered*

Mild preeclampsia

Place patient in quiet, nonstimulating environment—subdued lighting
Maintain bed rest: lateral position is preferred; bathroom privileges may be ordered
Give complete bed bath unless otherwise ordered
Administer medication as ordered
Check urine for pH, protein, blood, glucose, and acetone q shift and more frequently as condition becomes more acute
Limit visitors as indicated by condition; permit brief but frequent visits by toddlers or other children, since they help to reduce patient's anxiety about their welfare
Maintain seizure precautions
   Padded tongue blade or oral airway at bedside
   Padded side rails; crib bumpers can be used
   Suction equipment readily available
   Oxygen ready to use
   Call light within easy reach
   Magnesium sulfate, calcium antidote, and hydralazine readily available
Collect 24 hr urine specimens as ordered
Auscultate FHR for a full minute q8h and prn or use electronic fetal monitor for 20 to 40 min q8h
Provide diversionary activities
   Watching television
   Painting
   Reading
   Doing needlework

Severe preeclampsia

Continue with ongoing care of mild preeclampsia and *increase* frequency of nursing functions as condition progresses
Place patient in quiet, darkened room
Maintain padded side rails up at all times
Maintain complete bed rest—no visitors
Check BP, and P qh and prn
Auscultate chest for breath sounds prn
Maintain seizure precautions
Connect indwelling catheter to closed gravity drainage system as ordered
Have emergency delivery pack available
Measure intake and output q4h and prn; report output <60 ml/hr
Check urine protein q4h as ordered
Administer parenteral fluids as ordered

Administer magnesium sulfate as ordered
  Observe patient for progressing signs of magnesium sulfate toxicity
  Check deep tendon reflexes q4h to 8h and prior to each dose of magnesium sulfate or qh if patient is receiving continuous magnesium sulfate infusion
  Assess need for respiratory support with vital signs if magnesium sulfate is administered with a respiratory rate below 12/min
  Check respiratory rate q30 min for four times and prn after administration
  Have calcium antidote at bedside
  Check deep tendon reflexes (DTRs) with vital signs; if patellar reflex is absent, withhold next dose of magnesium sulfate until magnesium blood level is drawn, and notify physician
Administer hydralazine 5 mg IV bolus when diastolic blood pressure reaches 110 mm Hg as ordered
  If diastolic pressure is not lowered to 90 to 100 mm Hg in 20 min, administer hydralazine 10 mg IV bolus as ordered
  Take BP q5 min and report to physician
  Do not leave patient unattended at any time
Never leave patient alone when convulsion is pending
Note and report symptoms of
  Extremely high BP
  Severe headache
  Extreme irritability
  Acute anxiety
  Visual disturbances

Delivery care

See Oxytocin Infusion: Augmentation or Induction of Labor (p. 733) if labor is induced
Maintain separate IV lines for concurrent administration of oxytocin and magnesium sulfate
Ensure that cross-matched blood is immediately available from blood bank if cesarean section is performed
Prepare for neonatal stimulation and resuscitation
Notify pediatrician to be present at time of delivery
Notify admitting nursery that mother had magnesium sulfate

Postdelivery care

Continue with ongoing care of severe preeclampsia and decrease frequency of nursing functions as patient's condition improves
NOTE: Delivery is considered the "treatment" for PIH; however, symptoms may not subside for 2 to 7 days, and an eclamptic seizure is possible during that time

ndx: Alteration in fluid volume: excess volume related to pregnancy-induced hypertension

GOAL: *Patient will not have signs and symptoms indicating congestive heart failure; edema is minimal, and circulating fluid volume is adequate*

Weigh patient daily at same time with same clothing and scale
Check BP and P q4h and prn—same arm and in same position
Measure intake and output
Check urine protein as ordered
Maintain diet as ordered
Administer medication as ordered
Maintain availability of blood products for immediate use if necessary
Administer IV fluids as ordered
Maintain separate IV lines for concurrent administration of magnesium sulfate and oxytocin
Document use of pump and infusion rates per hospital policy

ndx: Knowledge deficit regarding care for pregnancy-induced hypertension

GOAL: *Patient will be compliant to plan of care and will assist in interventions as able; patient and fetus will have good delivery outcome*

Undelivered patient

Discuss symptoms of recurrence or progression to report to physician
Discuss procedure for urine collection and appropriate storage based on type of laboratory test, if ordered
Emphasize importance of planned rest periods

Signs of labor

Emphasize importance of keeping physician's appointments
Teach name of medication, dosage, time of administration, purpose, and side effects
Explain need to avoid taking over-the-counter medications without checking with physician
Explain need for bed rest as indicated
Discuss symptoms indicating maternal and fetal distress

Delivered patient

See appropriate standard, depending on method of delivery: Cesarean Delivery (p. 743), or Postpartum Care (p. 739)

Emphasize importance of sixth postnatal week physician's appointment to rule out chronic hypertension
Discuss conception control methods to use until no longer indicated by physician

Evaluation

Complications are avoided
Patient delivers a healthy infant
Fluid overload is avoided
Patient complies with plan of care

ECLAMPSIA

Progression of preeclampsia characterized by tonic and clonic convulsions

Assessment

Observations/findings

Seizure
    Twitching and blinking of eyes
    Crying or screaming
    Loss of consciousness
    Tachypnea
    Description of seizure
      Tonic
        Rigid body
        Jaws fixed
        Hands clenched
        Legs inverted
        Cyanosis
        Breath-holding
      Clonic
        Twitching of facial muscles
        Frothing at mouth; may be blood tinged
        Biting of tongue
        Urinary or fecal incontinence
Postseizure
    Altered level of consciousness
    Headache
    Oliguria
    Amnesia of events preceding seizure
    Nausea and/or vomiting
    Muscle soreness: backache
    Aspiration: choking

Laboratory/diagnostic studies

Magnesium sulfate levels
Blood chemistries as indicated
Ultrasound/x-ray examination as indicated
Electronic fetal monitoring
Cardiac monitoring

Potential complications

Respiratory distress
    Difficulty in breathing
    Diminished breath sounds
    Cyanosis
    Tachycardia, tachypnea
Fetal distress (p. 734)
Signs of onset of labor
See Pregnancy-Induced Hypertension (PIH) (p. 713)

Medical management

Anticonvulsives as indicated
Magnesium sulfate therapy as indicated (for 24 hr after delivery)
Neuro checks with vital signs
Sedatives as indicated
Antihypertensives
IV fluids as indicated
NPO
Delivery of infant when stabilized
Oxygen therapy

Nursing diagnosis/goal/intervention

ndx: Potential for injury related to seizure control

GOAL: *Patient will be protected from injury to self and fetus*

During and after seizure

Prevent injury by
    Removing surrounding furniture if on floor
    Supporting and protecting head; turn head to side if possible
    Gently restraining limbs
    Never leaving patient unattended
Insert oral airway or padded tongue blade when able; *never attempt to force jaws open*
Loosen constrictive clothing
Suction oropharynx and nasopharynx prn
Administer oxygen per nasal cannula or face mask at 10 to 12 L/min for 10 min as ordered when possible
Maintain NPO
Give mouth care when reactive
Auscultate FHR q1h to 2h and prn or monitor FHR with electronic monitor
Connect indwelling urinary catheter to closed gravity drainage system
    Measure urinary output qh
    Report output <30 ml/hr to physician
Maintain parenteral fluids as ordered
Monitor central venous pressure (CVP) or pulmonary artery wedge pressure (PAWP) (p. 141) as ordered

Measure intake and output
Do neuro check immediately after seizure and prn
   Pupillary size and reaction to light
   Level of consciousness
Check BP and P q15 min for six times and prn; leave BP cuff on arm continuously
Do not take temperature unless necessary; take axillary temperature
Do not move patient unnecessarily
Reorient patient to environment when conscious
Provide emotional support
Administer medication as ordered: anticonvulsives, sedatives, hypotensives
Protect from extraneous stimuli
   Keep room darkened; light only enough to make observations and provide care
   Avoid sudden noises
   Avoid jarring bed
   Converse only if absolutely necessary
Observe for onset of labor
Reinforce physician's explanation of what has happened and maternal and fetal prognosis to both patient and spouse or significant other
See interventions for severe preeclampsia (p. 714)
See Pregnancy-Induced Hypertension (PIH) (p. 713)

Evaluation

There are no complications or injuries

HYPEREMESIS GRAVIDARUM

Excessive vomiting during pregnancy, potentially resulting in dehydration and/or starvation

Assessment
Observations/findings

Nausea and vomiting usually in morning and/or after meals
Epigastric pain
Hiccups
Heartburn
Thirst; may be severe
Weight loss
Oliguria
Concentrated urine
Dry skin
Emesis of food, mucus, and/or bile

Laboratory/diagnostic studies

Blood chemistries/electrolytes
Hgb/Hct

CVP monitoring as indicated
Cardiac monitoring

Potential complications

Dehydration
Jaundice
Tachycardia
Elevated temperature
Alkalosis
Starvation
Emotional disturbances regarding pregnancy and family relationships
Withdrawal
Depression

Medical management

IV fluids as indicated
Total parenteral nutrition (TPN)/intralipids as indicated
Central venous catheter as indicated
Frequent small meals
Continuous nasogastric tube feedings as indicated

Nursing diagnoses/goals/interventions

ndx: Fluid volume deficit related to hyperemesis (more acute) and alteration in nutrition related to dehydration and hyperemesis

GOAL: *Patient will not lose weight and will be less than 10% dehydrated*

Acute care

Maintain complete bed rest
Maintain NPO status for 24 to 48 hr
Administer parenteral fluids with B complex vitamins and vitamin C as ordered
Administer eletrolyte replacement or TPN as ordered
Dipstick urine for pH, protein, blood, glucose, acetone, and specific gravity q shift
Maintain feeding/parenteral nutrition as ordered
Maintain patent IV access
Measure intake and output q2h to 4h
Administer medications as ordered; may include antihistiminics, antiemetics, anticholinergics, and sedatives
Administer oral hygiene q2h and prn
Check BP, T, P, and R q4h and prn
Monitor CVP readings as ordered
Provide private room if possible
Allow no visitors for first 24 hr; inform family of patient's progress by phone
Have same person care for patient each shift, if possible

Encourage verbalization
Request psychiatric evaluation if indicated

Convalescent care

Continue with acute care and decrease frequency of nursing functions as patient's condition improves
Encourage activity as tolerated
Serve small, frequent feedings of solid foods high in carbohydrate, such as crackers, dry toast, and cereal 5 to 6 times each day
Serve small amounts of liquids such as hot tea, crushed ice, carbonated beverages, and cold fruit juices an hour after each meal
Increase amounts of solid food and fluids slowly according to tolerance
Serve food attractively and at proper temperature
Provide foods patient craves; avoid foods and fluids high in fat content
Remove meal tray from bedside as soon as patient has finished
Avoid exposing patient to odors that are nauseating
   Certain foods
   Room deodorizers
   Colognes and perfumes
   Mouthwash solutions

ndx: Knowledge deficit regarding care for hyperemesis

GOAL: *Patient will be able to adjust to special needs and will be able to demonstrate self-care*

Explain need for well-balanced diet with adequate fluid intake at scheduled times
Discuss symptoms of recurrence to report to physician
Emphasize importance of planned rest periods
Reinforce physician's explanation of effect of condition on fetus
Explain that symptoms nearly always disappear by fourth month of pregnancy
Teach name of medication, dosage, time of administration, purpose, and side effects
Explain need to avoid taking over-the-counter medications without checking with physician
Emphasize importance of ongoing outpatient care
Relate that referral to Visiting Nurse's Association may be indicated
Relate that termination of pregnancy may be indicated for unwanted pregnancy
Explain that therapeutic abortion may be indicated for deteriorating physical and/or mental condition, such as that caused by persistent elevated temperature despite adequate hydration, tachycardia, jaundice, retinal hemorrhage, profound depression, or delirium

Evaluation

There are no complications
Patient maintains adequate nutrition and hydration
Patient is able to demonstrate self-care

AMNIOCENTESIS

Withdrawal of amniotic fluid through a needle inserted through the maternal abdominal and uterine wall to assess fetal health, genetic karyotype, maturity, and/or sex

Assessment
Potential complications

Fainting
Abdominal pain
Nausea
Premature labor
Fetal hyperactivity or hypoactivity
Fetal tachycardia: above 160 beats/min
Fetal bradycardia: below 120 beats/min
Maternal hemorrhage
Amnionitis
   Tachycardia
   Elevated temperature
   Foul odor of amniotic fluid

Medical management

Obtain consent
Laboratory tests as indicated

Nursing diagnosis/goal/interventions

ndx: Potential for injury related to invasive procedure/amniocentesis

GOAL: *Patient will have no injury (complications) to self or fetus*

Auscultate FHR
Empty bladder prior to procedure
Explain that procedure is usually not harmful to mother or fetus
Explain that procedure is virtually painless

Postprocedure care

Apply adhesive bandage to site of injection
Palpate fundus for fetal activity
Monitor FHR with electronic monitor if possible or auscultate FHR q15 min twice
Check BP, P, and R
Position on left side if patient experiences profuse diaphoresis, fainting, or nausea
Reinforce physician's explanation of reason for procedure

Assessment of fetal maturity and health
Diagnosis of genetic defects
Sex determination
Discuss symptoms to report to physician
  Any vaginal drainage or discharge
  Fetal hyperactivity, diminished activity, or absence of fetal movement
  Any signs of infection
  Elevated temperature
  Chills
  Abdominal pain
  Cramps

Evaluation

There are no complications, and there is no injury to mother or fetus
Diagnostic information is obtained

CARE OF DIABETIC MOTHER DURING LAST TRIMESTER OF PREGNANCY

Diabetic mothers are frequently hospitalized during the last trimester of pregnancy to monitor insulin needs, which are usually higher than during the previous two trimesters, and to monitor fetal well-being because of the increased fetal and neonatal morbidity and mortality associated with maternal diabetes

Assessment

Observations/findings

Large weight gain
Presence of risk factors
  Previously diagnosed glycosuria
  Insulin dependent
  Positive family history
  Obesity > 200 lb
  Previous large-for-gestional-age (LGA) baby
  Previous stillbirth
  Previous congenital anomalies
  Habitual abortion
  Maternal age ≥25 years

Laboratory/diagnostic studies

Blood glucose screening
Urine glucose/acetone
NST/CST
Blood chemistries as ordered

Potential complications

Hypoglycemia (p. 450)
Diabetic ketoacidosis (p. 437)

PIH (p. 713)
  Hypertension
  Edema (especially of face and hands)
  Proteinuria
Anxiety
Spontaneous abortion
Hydramnios
Worsening diabetes: increasing insulin requirements
Pyelonephritis
Increased congenital anomalies in infant
  Cardiac defects
  Neural tube defects
  Caudal regression syndrome
  See Infant of Diabetic Mother (IDM) (p. 759)

Medical management

Glucose screening tests as indicated
Insulin as indicated on sliding scale
IV fluids as indicated
American Dietetic Association (ADA) diet as indicated
Monitored weight gain
Fractional urine testing as indicated

Nursing diagnoses/goals/interventions

ndx: Potential for injury to mother and fetus related to hypoglycemia/hyperglycemia

GOAL: *Patient will achieve and maintain euglycemia; there will be no injuries (complications) to mother or fetus*

Maintain patient on NPH or other long-acting insulin as ordered; as EDC approaches, patient's insulin may be regulated by home monitoring of blood glucose and regular insulin on a sliding scale
Test blood and fractional urine using Testape or Dipstix qid and prn
Replace foods not eaten with appropriate exchange; see Diabetic Food Replacement (p. 880)
Auscultate FHR tid and prn
Check BP and P qid and prn
Weigh patient daily at same time with same clothing and scale
Measure intake and output
Collect 24 hr urine specimens for estriol, protein, etc., testing as ordered
Check blood glucose levels and glucose tolerance levels periodically as ordered
Assist physician with amniocentesis
Maintain bed rest with bathroom privileges or activity as ordered
Encourage diversional activities

Reading
Doing needlework
Painting
Writing
Doing handicrafts

Encourage verbalization about concerns for fetus and self

Reinforce physician's explanation of status of fetus and reasons for laboratory studies

Explain procedure for and implications of nonstress testing or oxytocin challenge test

ndx: Knowledge deficit regarding changes in diabetic regimen during pregnancy

GOAL: *Patient and significant other will verbalize understanding of diabetic regimen during pregnancy*

Discuss need for compliance with diabetic regimen
Discuss maternal perception of fetal movement
Explain need for antepartum surveillance
Explain potential need for planning delivery if cesarean section
Explain procedure for 24 hr urine collection and storage if ordered
Discuss symptoms of hypoglycemia and appropriate treatment
Discuss symptoms of diabetic ketoacidosis and appropriate treatment (p. 437)
Discuss symptoms to report to physician
  Diminished fetal activity
  Signs of PIH
  Signs of labor
  Signs of uncontrolled diabetes
Demonstrate and have patient and/or significant other return-demonstrate
  Home glucose monitoring
  Use of sliding scale insulin injections
  See Insulin Therapy Teaching Guide (p. 444)

Evaluation

Complications are avoided
There is good infant outcome at delivery
Patient remains euglycemic
Patient complies with diabetic regimen

CARE OF DIABETIC MOTHER DURING LABOR AND DELIVERY

Insulin needs vary during labor and delivery, necessitating careful patient observation and monitoring of glucose levels

Assessment

Observations/findings

Hypoglycemia
  Hunger
  Perspiration
  Palpitation
  Tachycardia
  Weakness
  Tremor
  Pallor
See Care of Mother in First Stage of Labor (p. 728)
See Care of Mother during Delivery (p. 732)

Laboratory/diagnostic studies

Blood glucose monitoring
Electrolytes as ordered
Electronic fetal monitoring
Real-time ultrasound

Potential complications

See Care of Diabetic Mother during Last Trimester of Pregnancy (p. 719)
Hypoglycemia of mother and infant following delivery
See Infant of Diabetic Mother (IDM) (p. 759)

Medical management

Decreased insulin
Continuous IV infusion of insulin if blood glucose is >420 mg/dl
Capillary blood glucose monitoring q1h to 2h
IV fluids as indicated
NPO as indicated
For elective cesarean section
  No insulin in morning
  Early morning delivery (8 to 9 AM preferred because of glucose levels)
  Monitoring of glucose following delivery
  Observation for insulin reaction
  Family planning counseling and implications for future pregnancies

Nursing diagnoses/goals/interventions

ndx: Potential for injury to mother and fetus related to hypoglycemia/hyperglycemia and possible uteroplacental insufficiency during labor

GOAL: *Mother will maintain euglycemia, and fetus will not experience distress*

Labor and delivery care

Administer parenteral fluids; electrolyte solutions may be ordered
Monitor fetus internally if possible

Check blood glucose as ordered q1h to 3h
Be aware that regular insulin is preferred to long-lasting insulin
See Care of Mother in First Stage of Labor (p. 728)
See Care of Mother during Delivery (p. 732)
See Fetal Distress (p. 734)
See Care of Mother on Fetal Monitor (p. 735)

Postdelivery care

See Postpartum Care (p. 739)
Observe for symptoms of hypoglycemia
Be aware that insulin dosage will be adjusted to prepregnant state needs
Use regular insulin based on blood glucose tests for first 24 to 48 hr as ordered
Progress to NPH or other long-acting insulin after first 24 to 48 hr as ordered, when patient is maintaining stable diet
Check blood glucose levels periodically if ordered
Administer perineal care with antiseptic solution after each elimination

ndx: Knowledge deficit regarding changes in diabetic regimen during labor

GOAL: *Patient and significant other will demonstrate knowledge of diabetic regimen changes*

Explain need for NPO status during labor
Explain need for changes in insulin requirements
Explain that insulin and dietary needs may vary because of lactation postpartum
Discuss changes in administration of insulin
Explain need for more frequent capillary glucose monitoring
Explain need to avoid persons with infections, especially upper respiratory infections (URIs), during puerperium
See Care of Diabetic Mother during Last Trimester of Pregnancy (p. 719)

Evaluation

Complications are avoided
Patient maintains euglycemia
Injury to mother and fetus is minimal
Patient adapts to changing regimen

PREMATURE RUPTURE OF MEMBRANES (PROM)

Rupture of the bag of waters (RBOW) prior to the onset of labor

Assessment

Observations/findings

Fluid leaking from vagina
Positive nitrazine paper test

Laboratory/diagnostic studies

Nitrazine paper test
"Fern" pattern on dried microscope slide
Fluid cultures as indicated

Potential complications

Bleeding
Amnionitis
   Foul odor of vaginal discharge
   Maternal elevated temperature
   Maternal tachycardia
   Maternal leukocytosis
Meconium-stained amniotic fluid
Umbilical cord protruding from introitus
Fetal tachycardia: above 160 beats/min
Fetal bradycardia: below 120 beats/min
Variable decelerations on electronically monitored patient
See Care of Mother in First Stage of Labor (p. 728)

Medical management

Oxytocin augmentation of labor as indicated
Electronic fetal monitoring
Blood specimens for ruling out infection
Cervical culture
Fetal maturity testing
IUPC (intrauterine pressure catheter) as indicated

Nursing diagnosis/goal/interventions

ndx: Potential for infection related to premature rupture of membranes

GOAL: *Patient will be treated for infection or will not have symptoms of infection*

Maintain complete bed rest
Check T, P, and R q4h
Auscultate FHR or use electronic FHR monitor q1h to 4h and prn
Avoid vaginal examinations
Observe drainage of amniotic fluid for color, amount, and odor q2h to 4h and prn
Administer perineal care with antiseptic solution after each elimination, q2h to 4h, and prn
Keep patient clean and dry
Palpate fundus for uterine activity q1h to 2h and prn
Administer antibiotics if ordered
Prepare for labor and method of delivery

Prepare oxytocin induction as ordered if labor does not begin within 24 hr of PROM *and* if patient is near EDC

Administer clear fluids as ordered until labor ensues

Discuss with patient that because amniotic fluid is continually produced, she will not experience a "dry" labor

Continue with acute care and decrease frequency of nursing functions as patient's condition stabilizes

Carefully clean perineal region; wipe from front to back after elimination

Change pad under buttocks q2h to 4h and prn

Report any signs of onset of labor; labor usually begins within 24 hr after rupture of membranes

Make note of PROM on infant's chart so that nursery will observe infant for possible respiratory distress, meconium aspiration, and pneumonia at delivery and after

Evaluation

There are no complications

Risk of infection is minimized, or infection is treated

PLACENTA PREVIA

Total, partial, or low implantation of the placenta over the internal cervical os (Figure 14-1); occurs most often in multiparas; total and partial placenta previa prohibits vaginal delivery (the fetus is delivered by cesarean section); with low implantation the fetus can sometimes be delivered vaginally with the presenting part acting as a tamponade against the placenta

Assessment

Observations/findings

Painless vaginal bleeding: intermittent to constant flow

Soft, relaxed uterus

Laboratory/diagnostic studies

Ultrasound of placenta placement
Amniography
Speculum vaginal examination
Hgb/Hct; complete blood cell count (CBC)
Amniocentesis for fetal maturity as indicated
Clotting studies
Electronic fetal monitoring: continuous

Potential complications

Fetal bradycardia: below 120 beats/min
Monitored fetus: late decelerations
Absence of fetal heart tones
Maternal shock
Fetal hyperactivity, hypoxia
Neonatal anemia, shock (hypovolemic)
Cesarean section

Medical management

Cesarean section for fetal distress or to control hemorrhage

Tocolytic agents as indicated

IV fluids as indicated

Type and cross match 2 to 4 units of fresh whole blood and/or other blood products as available

Nursing diagnoses/goals/interventions

ndx: Alteration in tissue perfusion related to malaligned placenta and bleeding

GOAL: *Patient will not hemorrhage, and fetus will not show signs of distress*

NOTE: *Amount of bleeding and position of placenta determines care and frequency of vital sign checks*

Maintain complete bed rest

Never do vaginal or rectal examination

Avoid rectal stimulation; no enemas

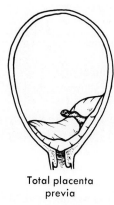
Total placenta previa

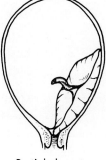
Partial placenta previa

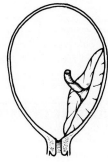
Low implantation

FIGURE 14-1. Placenta previa (abnormal implantation).

Place patient in high Fowler's or lateral position if membranes are ruptured; avoid supine position
Place patient in position of comfort if membranes are not ruptured
Check BP, P, and FHR q¼h to 2h and prn
Observe amount, color, and character of vaginal drainage q15 min to 2h and prn depending on amount of bleeding
Check random pulse oximeter oxygen saturation if respiratory complications are present or impending
Report saturation of more than one perineal pad q30 min
Weigh pads and linen to estimate blood loss as ordered
Administer transfusions as ordered
Report any sign of onset of labor to physician immediately
Monitor FHR electronically as indicated
Administer perineal care with antiseptic solution after every elimination and/or q4h and prn
Prepare for double setup and/or delivery as indicated
Encourage verbalization of fears and how condition affects fetus
Administer oxygen by mask as indicated
Continue with care and decrease frequency of nursing functions as patient's condition stabilizes
Explain and prepare for diagnostic tests if ordered
  Ultrasonography
  Amniography
  Placenta scan
Prepare for delivery as ordered
See Cesarean Delivery (p. 743) or Postpartum Care (p. 739)

ndx: Fluid volume deficit related to blood loss

GOAL: *Patient will maintain adequate BP and/or CVP levels*

Measure intake and output
Administer IV fluids as ordered
Administer transfusions and volume expanders as ordered
Report saturation of more than 1 perineal pad q30 min or less
Monitor IV site with vital signs to ensure patency at all times at least q2h to 4 h and prn

Evaluation

Complications are avoided
Fetal well-being is maintained
Patient has no fluid volume deficit
Viable infant is delivered

ABRUPTIO PLACENTAE

Premature separation of the placenta occurring before the third stage of labor (Figure 14-2)

Assessment
Observations/findings

Uterus
  Extreme tenderness
  General or localized pain
  Pain: may be absent to severe
  Sudden enlargement: symmetric or asymmetric
  Progressive decrease of relaxation between contractions developing into continuous boardlike rigidity
  Uterine tachysystole and hypertonus on monitored patient
  Low back pain
  Hyperactive fetus
Vaginal bleeding may or may not be present
Hemorrhage: usually concealed
Rising uterine fundus
FHR

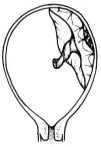
Partial separation (concealed hemorrhage)

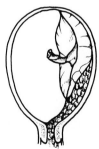
Partial separation (apparent hemorrhage)

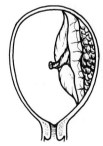
Complete separation (concealed hemorrhage)

FIGURE 14-2. Abruptio placentae (premature separation).

Bradycardia: below 120 beats/min
Heart tones: may be absent
Monitored fetus: may have late decelerations
Absence
Extreme anxiety
Hypovolemia

Laboratory/diagnostic studies

CBC, coagulation profile (platelets, fibrinogen, prothrombin time [PT], partial thromboplastin time [PTT], fibrin split products)
Continuous external fetal monitoring

Potential complications

Fetal distress (p. 734)
DIC (p. 196)
Hypofibrinogenemia
Hypoprothrombinemia
Bleeding from mucous membranes
Bruising; ecchymosis
Oliguria progressing to anuria
Shock (p. 104)
Maternal hemorrhagic shock
Renal failure

Medical management

Cesarean delivery for compromised fetus or hemorrhage
IV fluids as indicated
NPO
Volume expander or blood transfusion as indicated
Oxygen 8 to 10 L/min as indicated

Nursing diagnoses/goals/interventions

ndx: Fluid volume deficit related to bleeding from abrupted placenta before delivery

GOAL: *Patient's Hbg/Hct will be kept at her previous levels*

Initiate and maintain parenteral fluids as ordered
Monitor CVP as ordered
Maintain patent IV line
Measure intake and output q1h (urine flow at least 30 ml/hr)
Administer transfusions and/or volume expanders as ordered
Connect indwelling catheter (Foley) to closed gravity system
Maintain NPO status as ordered

ndx: Alteration in tissue perfusion related to hemorrhage of abrupted placenta

GOAL: *Patient will not develop hemorrhagic shock*

Administer oxygen as ordered
Remain with patient at all times
Maintain complete bed rest in position of comfort
Palpate fundus for presence of uterine contractions and relaxation
Prepare for immediate delivery and neonatal resuscitation
Order type and cross match of 2 to 4 units of packed cells if ordered by physician
Assist with amniotomy if done by physician
Monitor fetus internally with spiral electrode if possible
Check BP, P, and FHR q5 to 10 min
Perform tilt test prn
Administer transfusions or volume expanders as ordered
Administer oxygen as ordered
Control pain carefully as ordered; small doses of analgesics are preferred
Weigh pads and linens to estimate blood loss as ordered
Allay anxiety as much as possible
Explain all actions taken
Ask patient to verbalize any changes in feeling and sensorium
Reinforce physician's explanation for cesarean section if done
Notify postpartum nurses to observe patient for
Incisional hematoma
Disparate intake and output
See Cesarean Delivery (p. 743) or Postpartum Care (p. 739)

Evaluation

Complications are avoided
Fluid levels are adequate for both mother and baby
Maternal and fetal well-being are maintained

PROLAPSED UMBILICAL CORD

Protrusion of the umbilical cord in advance of the presenting part; this should be suspected following amniotomy or spontaneous gross rupture of membranes and should be ruled out by vaginal examination

Assessment

Observations/findings

Umbilical cord: may or may not be visible at introitus
Meconium-stained amniotic fluid
Fetal bradycardia: below 120 beats/min
Slowing pulsations of visible cord
Severe, variable decelerations of FHR

Laboratory/diagnostic studies

Vaginal examination for prolapse verification

Potential complications

Fetal distress (p. 734)
Fetal hypoxia, compromise
Fetal death, stillborn

Medical management

Bed rest (knee-chest position for acute episode)
Cesarean section
Oxygen therapy as indicated
IV therapy as indicated

Nursing diagnosis/goal/interventions

ndx: Potential for injury related to prolapse of umbilical cord

GOAL: *Patient will not be injured, and fetal compromise will not occur*

Maintain absolute bed rest
Never attempt to replace a prolapsed cord into vagina
Avoid cord compression
    Elevate presenting part until delivery
    Pressure of examiner's sterile gloved hand (cord between two spread fingers)
    Knee-chest or exaggerated Trendelenburg's position
    Do not manipulate cord
Prepare for immediate delivery; cesarean section is usually done
Check FHR q2 to 5 min
Administer oxygen (10 to 12 L/min) by face mask as ordered
Gently cover exposed cord with sterile saline compress
Stay with patient at all times
Allay anxiety as much as possible by explanation to patient about importance of maintaining special position and not bearing down or pushing with contractions
Teach patient panting and blowing techniques for use during uterine contractions
Reinforce physician's explanation of need to do immediate delivery
See Postpartum Care (p. 739) or Cesarean Delivery (p. 743)

Evaluation

There are no complications
Danger of injury to fetus is minimized
Fetal compromise does not occur

PRETERM (PREMATURE) LABOR

Physiologic process by which the fetus is expelled from the uterus prior to the end of the thirty-seventh week of gestation

Assessment

Observations/findings

Uterine contractions
    Every 10 min or less
    Lasting 30 sec or more
Progressive cervical dilation: ≥80% effacement or ≥2 cm dilatation
Complaints of back pain or pressure

Laboratory/diagnostic studies

Electronic fetal monitoring (EFM)
Fetoscope/Doppler as indicated
Urinalysis
CBC
Cervical cultures, including group B streptococcus
Amniocentesis to assess fetal lung maturity and presence of infection
Maternal and fetal baseline ECG
Hemogram as ordered
Electrolytes
Blood glucose

Potential complications

Compromised infant at birth
    Prematurity
    Small-for-gestational-age infant
    Respiratory distress syndrome
Tocolysis (magnesium sulfate or ritodrine)
Magnesium sulfate therapy
    Maternal effects
        Flushing, sense of warmth
        Headache
        Dizziness
        Respiratory depression
        Hypotension
        Hyporeflexia
        Nystagmus
        Nausea, vomiting
        Lethargy
        Pulmonary edema
    Fetal/neonatal effects
        Decreased muscle tone
        Respiratory depression
        Lethargy, drowsiness
        Lower apgar scores with prolonged maternal treatment

Ritodrine therapy
    Maternal effects
        Tachycardia
        Palpitations
        Hypotension
        Arrhythmias
        Hypokalemia
        Chest pain
        Pulmonary edema
        Tremors
        Agitation
        Headache
        Elevated blood glucose
        Hyperlipidemia
    Fetal/neonatal effects
        Fetal distress
        Tachycardia
        Bradycardia if severe maternal hypotension
        Neonatal hypotension
        Neonatal hypoglycemia
        Neonatal hypocalcemia
        Neonatal irritability

Medical management

Bed rest in lateral position
Continuous EFM and uterine contraction monitoring for a minimum of 1 hr
Laboratory tests as indicated
IV fluids as indicated
Intake and output
Ultrasound for evaluation of placenta, fetal/uterine anomalies, and gestational age confirmation
Glucocorticoids as indicated
Tocolysis as indicated (magnesium sulfate or ritodrine hydrochloride)

Nursing diagnoses/goals/interventions

ndx: Potential for injury to fetus and mother related to preterm labor and tocolysis therapy

GOAL: *Mother and fetus will be uninjured, and infant will not be compromised at birth*

Maintain complete bed rest in side-lying position
Administer IV fluids as ordered
Note frequency, duration, and strength of contractions q15 min and prn; monitor uterine activity with tocotransducer (tocodynamometer) if available
Auscultate FHR q15 to 30 min or electronically monitor with ultrasound
Measure intake and output as ordered
Assist with amniocentesis and/or ultrasound if ordered
Administer any other medications, including corticosteroids, in exact dose, time, and route as ordered
Decrease frequency of nursing functions as patient's preterm labor is arrested

Continuous labor

See Care of Mother in First Stage of Labor (p. 728)
In addition
    Prepare for high-risk infant
        Notify neonatologist or pediatrician
        Have resuscitative equipment ready for use
        Plan to have infant's blood cross matched if less than 32 weeks' gestation
    Monitor FHR electronically if possible
    Assist physician with fetal blood sampling as indicated
    Consider plotting labor dilation and descent on square-ruled graph paper (labor is usually rapid, but a high frequency of abnormal labors occur as well—Friedman curve)
    Provide comfort measures prior to administering minimal doses of analgesics as ordered
    Retain placenta for pathology as ordered
    See Care of Premature Infant (p. 755)

Tocolytic therapy

Magnesium sulfate
    Maintain patent IV access
    Administer 2 to 4 g IV in a 10% solution over 15 to 30 min for initial dose as ordered
    Continue and monitor IV infusion titrated according to uterine response and side effects (i.e., 2 g/hr)
    Watch for symptoms of toxicity, discontinue, administer oxygen therapy, and notify physician if toxicity occurs
        Respiratory depression
        Hypotension
        Absence of deep tendon reflexes
    Monitor and decrease dosage after 24 hr or when uterine contractions subside as ordered
    Check vital signs and DTRs q30 min to 1 hr
    Continue to monitor uterine activity
    Monitor intake and output q1h; should be at least 30 ml urine per hour
    Auscultate lungs q4h to 8 h for presence of fluid
    Monitor fetus with EFM as ordered
    Check fetal heart tones (FHTs) with vital signs if no EFM is done
    Monitor magnesium sulfate levels
    Obtain baseline electrolytes and calcium levels by venipuncture

Ritodrine hydrochloride
  Obtain laboratory data as ordered (may include CBC, electrolytes, and glucose)
  Administer ritodrine (usually 50 µg/min) via infusion pump or controller with drug piggybacked into main IV line, being careful not to exceed maximum dosage of 350 µg/min
  Monitor rate and dosage and increase by 50 µg/min q10 min based on maternal and fetal responses as ordered
  Do not increase dose and/or discontinue ritodrine
    If patient demonstrates unacceptable side effects
    If maternal heart rate exceeds 140 beats/min
    If fetal tachycardia of 180 beats/min or greater persists
    If systolic blood pressure is <90 mm Hg or more than a 20% decrease, or diastolic BP is <40 mm Hg
  Check BP, P, and FHR q10 min while increasing dosage, then q30 min while patient is receiving IV ritodrine maintenance dose
  Monitor FHR and uterine contractions continuously if possible
Measure intake and output
Place in left lateral position during infusion
Monitor maternal electrocardiogram (ECG) as ordered
Report undesirable side effects, including headache and palpitations, to physician
Continue to maintain IV infusion for 12 hr after arrest of labor, using smallest dose possible to maintain tocolysis
Auscultate lungs q8h to check for fluid overload
Monitor intake and output q1h
Initiate oral therapy 30 min prior to discontinuing IV therapy as ordered
Decrease frequency of nursing functions as preterm labor is arrested

ndx: Alteration in self-concept, role performance, and identity related to perceptions and expectations of pregnancy and delivery

GOAL: *Patient will verbalize positive expressions of self-worth*

Encourage patient to verbalize fears and concerns
Note and document
  Minimal eye contact
  Self-defeating statements and/or behaviors
  Overt expressions of guilt or blame
  Negativity or inadequacy in actions or verbal communications
  Demonstrations of anger

Include significant other in discussions
Provide factual information about placement of blame for initiation and continuation of uterine contractions
Provide positive feedback and encouragement to patient for seeking early interventions

ndx: Alteration in comfort: pain related to uterine contractions

GOAL: *Patient will verbalize decreasing or more tolerable discomfort*

Use nonpharmacologic measures when appropriate
  Positioning
  Muscular relaxation techniques
  Breathing techniques
  Distraction techniques
Eliminate or minimize other factors that could contribute to pain
  Encourage frequent voiding
  Explain all procedures before executing them
  Answer all questions if possible
  Offer choices to allow for control as patient is able
  Keep patient and significant other informed of changes in labor and fetal status
Explain reasons why analgesic agents may not be appropriate
  Effect on fetal heart rate
  Possible masking of contractions
  Combined side effects of tocolytic agents and analgesia
Provide positive reinforcement and touch as appropriate
Plan nursing care to provide rest periods to promote comfort, sleep, and relaxation
Assess and document stress-contributing factors to perception of pain
Assess and document q30 min
  Frequency and length of contractions
  Location of pain
  Intensity and duration of pain

ndx: Knowledge deficit regarding potential premature labor and delivery

GOAL: *Patient will demonstrate self-care, and patient and significant other will verbalize understanding of premature labor and purpose of treatment*

Explain arrested labor
Emphasize importance of maintaining bed rest in side-lying position with bathroom privileges as ordered
Explain need to avoid kneeling or sitting in bed

Emphasize importance of avoiding intercourse or douching
Teach name of medication, dosage, frequency of administration, purpose, and toxic side effects
Emphasize importance of having supportive person to perform housekeeping, cooking, and child care tasks
Discuss signs of labor to report to physician
Provide patient and significant other opportunities to verbalize concerns
Explain rationale behind procedures
Discuss manner in which procedures are to be done
Explain reasons for close observation by staff
Emphasize importance of follow-up medical care
Discuss development and gestational stage of fetus
Discuss possible needs for hospitalization

Evaluation

Complications are avoided
Preterm labor is arrested or infant is born with good outcome
Maternal/fetal injury is avoided
Patient complies with care plan
Patient is comfortable
Patient's self-worth is reestablished or maintained

CARE OF MOTHER IN FIRST STAGE OF LABOR

Physiologic process by which the fetus is expelled from the uterus
early labor *Dilation of 0 to 4 cm with mild to moderate irregular contractions*
active labor *Dilation of 4 cm with moderate to strong regular contractions q2 to 5 min*
transitional labor *Dilation of 8 cm to complete dilation with strong contractions*

Assessment
Observations/findings

Behavior
   Surge of energy and activity
   Talking frequently
   Anxious
   Fear of isolation
Rupture of membranes
Uterine contractions: regular with increasing intensity and frequency
Transitional labor
   Nausea, vomiting
   Irritability
   Loss of coping mechanisms
   Hiccups and/or belching
   Trembling and/or shaking of legs
   Chilling
   Perspiration
   Rectal pressure
   Urge to push
   Hypersensitive abdomen

Laboratory/diagnostic studies

Baseline laboratory tests
   CBC with differential
   Hgb/Hct
   VDRL serology
   Chemistries
Urinalysis
Cultures as indicated by history of signs and symptoms
Ultrasound/x-ray examination as indicated
Electronic fetal monitoring
Fetal scalp pH testing

Potential complications

Fetal distress (p. 734)
   Fetal tachycardia: above 160 beats/min
   Fetal bradycardia: below 120 beats/min
   Meconium-stained amniotic fluid
   Foul-smelling amniotic fluid
Fetal hyperactivity
Monitored labor (p. 735)
   Severe variable decelerations: <70 beats/min for more than 30 sec
   Late decelerations of any magnitude
   Absence of variability
   Prolonged deceleration
   Unstable FHR; sinusoidal pattern
Supine hypotension: BP above 140/90 mm Hg
Inadequate uterine relaxation
   Contractions lasting longer than 90 sec
   Relaxation between contractions less than 30 sec
Arrest of labor
Amnionitis
Elevated temperature
Distended bladder
Dehydration
Hemorrhage

Medical management

Laboratory tests as indicated
IV fluids as indicated
Prenatal chart and previous medical chart ordered to labor and delivery unit
Vital signs q1h and prn as condition changes
Initiation of labor record documentation
Vaginal examination
Analgesia as indicated

Preparation for selected/indicated anesthesia by anesthesiologist/nurse anesthetist

Continuous fetal heart rate–uterine contraction (FHR-UC) monitoring or intermittent FHR-UC monitoring if low-risk criteria is met

Nursing diagnoses/goals/interventions

ndx: Potential for injury to mother related to complications of labor

GOAL: *Patient will have minimal or no complications and will meet criteria for early discharge/low-risk delivery*

Check temperature q2h after rupture of membranes
Consider plotting cervical dilation and fetal descent over time on square-ruled graph paper (Friedman curve)
Have patient shower if indicated and ordered
Administer perineal shave and preparation if ordered
Give enema if ordered
Administer clear liquids as ordered
Measure intake and output
Have patient void q2h and prn
Check urine for glucose and protein
Maintain complete bed rest in position of comfort if membranes are ruptured, especially if presenting part is not yet engaged; otherwise, patient may ambulate as tolerated
Maintain bed rest with side rails up
Allow patient up to bathroom if presenting part is well applied to cervix as ordered
Avoid intake of solid foods
Administer parenteral fluids as ordered
Check BP and P qh and prn
Check T and R q2h to 4h and prn
Auscultate FHR immediately after uterine contractions, q15 to 30 min, if not electronically monitored
Note frequency, duration, and strength of contractions q15 to 30 min and prn
Have patient void q1h to 2h and prn
Initiate lactated Ringer's solution or other IV solution as ordered
Maintain dosing of prelabor medications or drugs as ordered (i.e., anticonvulsants, antihypertensives, or methadone)
Turn to left lateral position, administer 100% oxygen by face mask, and notify physician immediately if mother is in distress
See ASPO (Lamaze) review sheet (Figure 14-3)

ndx: Potential for fetal compromise related to uterine contractions of labor and/or uteroplacental insufficiency*

GOAL: *Patient will deliver an infant in good condition at birth with Apgar score ≥ 8 at 5 min of age*

Note frequency, duration, and strength of contractions q30 to 60 min and prn
Auscultate FHR immediately after uterine contractions, if not electronically monitored
Check BP and P qh and prn
Check T, P, and R q2h to 4h and prn
Auscultate FHR immediately after membranes rupture or amniotomy is done
Turn mother to left-lateral position, administer 100% oxygen by face mask, and notify physician immediately if fetal distress is evident by auscultation or electronic fetal monitoring
See Care of Mother on Fetal Monitor (p. 735)

ndx: Knowledge deficit regarding process of labor

GOAL: *Patient will demonstrate self-care and cooperation in management of labor*

Teach breathing techniques to be used in active labor to patient and spouse or significant other (Figure 14-3)
Allay anxiety as much as possible by doing the following
  Explain reason for performing all procedures
  Encourage spouse or significant other to remain with patient to provide support during labor
  Let spouse or significant other listen to fetal heart tones with stethoscope, fetoscope, or ultrasound stethoscope
  Provide supportive care based on patient's knowledge of labor process
  Inform waiting family members and friends of patient's progress and let patient know that they are interested in her
  Reduce environmental stimuli that may contribute to anxiety and tension; provide relaxed, restful atmosphere
  At appropriate intervals reassure patient that labor is progressing and that both patient and infant are doing fine
  Instruct spouse or significant other when and where to change into scrub suit, cap, and mask to be ready to go into delivery room

---

*Not a NANDA-approved nursing diagnosis.

THE PROCESS	WOMAN	BREATHING	LABOR COACH

Beginning
  Loss of mucus plug
  Rupture of membranes
  Contractions
    Regular or irregular
    Closer together
    More intense
	Rest
	Relax
	Sugar foods
			Time contractions
			Inform doctor
			Rest
			Eat

Progress
  Effacement
  Dilatation
  Contractions
    Closer together
    Stronger
	Relax and focus
	Slow chest breathing as needed
		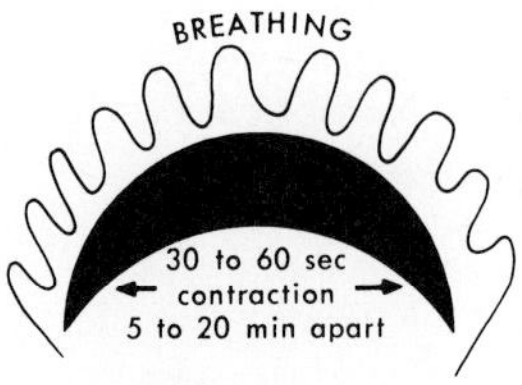 BREATHING
		30 to 60 sec contraction
		5 to 20 min apart
		Cleansing breath
		6-9 breaths per min, in through nose, out through mouth
		Effleurage
		Cleansing breath
			Prep room time
			  45 min to 1 hr
			Check for comfort
			  Positioning
			    Side position—top leg bent, supported with pillow—either side
			    Tailor sit—head supported
			    Reclining chair—head of bed up, knees bent—pillow under each arm
			    Head up 90 degrees—lean on overbed table with pillow
			    All fours—on hands and knees during contractions—relax to side between
			  Effleurage
			  Counter pressure in back or groin
			Release tension

Labor more active—increasing dilatation	Accelerated, decelerated breathing as needed	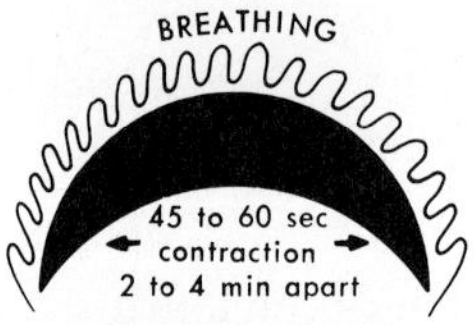 BREATHING
		45 to 60 sec contraction
		2 to 4 min apart
		Cleansing breath
		Accelerating short, shallow pants through nose or mouth, decelerating as contraction fades
		Effleurage
		Cleansing breath
			Time contractions
			  Begins
			  Half over
			  Ends
			Breathe with her if needed
			Give verbal support
			Between contractions
			  Ice chips
			  Water
			  Lollipops
			  Washcloth

Transition
  Dilatation going to completion
  Possible signs
    Irritability
    Hiccups
    Belching
    Trembling
    Nausea
    Perspiration or chills
  Contractions
    Longest
    Strongest
    2-3 peaks
  Rectal pressure
  Urge to push
	Transition breathing as needed
	Blow with urge to push
		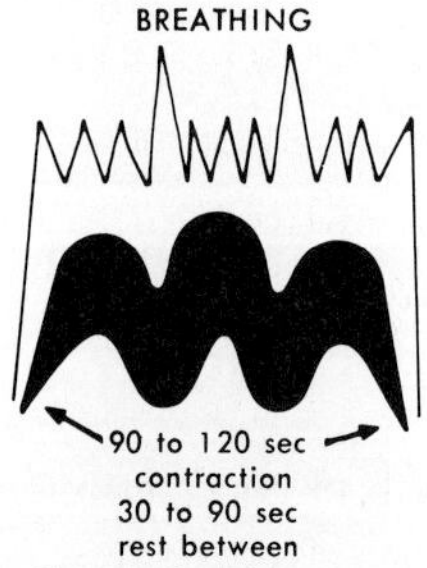 BREATHING
		90 to 120 sec contraction
		30 to 90 sec rest between
		Cleansing breath
		8 or 6 or 4 or 2 fast, shallow pants, blow. Repeat. Blow if urge to push occurs
		Cleansing breath
			Back labor 25% to 30%
			Off back use position numbers 1,2,4, and 5
			Counter measure
			  Fists, tennis balls, rolling pin, massage, pelvis rock
			Great need for firmness, direction, and support
			Take one contraction at a time
			Keep blowing in control
			Call nurse when first feels like pushing
			Check for hyperventilation

FIGURE 14-3. ASPO (Lamaze) review sheet. (Prepared by the teachers of the American Society for Psychoprophylaxis in Obstetrics of Los Angeles, Inc., with permission of the Board of Directors of ASPO of Los Angeles, Inc.)

THE PROCESS	WOMAN	BREATHING	LABOR COACH

Birth
  Good pushing routine may take several contractions
  Pushing may not feel good for 3 or 4 contractions
 	
First baby—push in labor room until baby's head shows
Second baby—to delivery room as soon as completely dilated
 	
As head comes to outlet may experience burning or stinging sensation on perineum, extreme pressure on anus—may feel as if it's "turning inside out"
	Push with contractions
	Stop pushing as directed by doctor or nurse
	
	2 cleansing breaths
	Perform gentle pushing
	2 cleansing breaths
	Stop pushing
	Be sure to follow doctor's directions, stop pushing when directed—blow, then pant, pant blow.
		BREATHING / CONTRACTION (diagram)	Labor room
			  Elevate bed as desired
			  Remind her of technique
			  Pushing position after 2 cleansing breaths, elbows into bed, push gently during contraction, think vagina, forceful pushing will alleviate discomfort, 2 cleansing breaths after contraction
			Coach dress for delivery now
			
			Delivery room
			  Take 2 pillows
			  Encourage
			  Push as before, support her head and shoulders as she pulls herself up
			
			Push as before, support her head and shoulders as she pulls herself up
			Be sure she follows doctor's directions
			Listen for doctor's command —stop pushing, etc., and repeat to her

Expulsion of the placenta—placenta, membranes, umbilical cord are delivered	Enjoy baby with your husband!	Push as directed.	Enjoy baby with your wife!

CONGRATULATIONS

FIGURE 14-3, cont'd. For legend see opposite page.

ndx: Alteration in comfort related to labor contractions

GOAL: *Patient will have maximum comfort; discomfort will be minimized after interventions*

Prehydrate with 500 to 1000 ml of fluid prior to anesthetic procedure as ordered

Measure intake and output q2h; report signs of dehydration to physician

Administer perineal care after vaginal examinations, after use of bedpan, and prn

Administer oral hygiene qh and prn between contractions

  Suck on ice chips, wet washcloth, or sour lollipops unless contraindicated

  Rinse mouth with water and/or mouthwash

Apply petroleum jelly or antichapping lipsticks to dry lips prn

Give back rub qh and prn between contractions

Apply pressure to sacrum as needed prn during contractions

Apply cool compress to forehead prn

Change pad under buttocks when moist q30 to 60 min and prn

Assist with breathing techniques (Figure 14-3)

Change gown and linen as necessary

Turn off bright overhead lights when not needed

Clip call bell to bottom sheet within easy reach

Relieve discomfort with medication as ordered; never leave sedated patient alone

Assist physician with local or regional anesthetic; take BP and P q10 min for three times after anesthetic and until stabilized

Avoid talking to patient during contractions

Reposition patient q30 min and prn; lateral position is preferred

Place pillow or folded blanket under right hip to displace the uterus to the left
Continue with active labor care
Encourage deep ventilation prior to and after each contraction
Avoid urge to push by panting and/or blowing in rapid sequence with contractions until completely dilated
Have emesis basin readily available
Have patient void to ensure empty bladder
Cover feet with blanket or have patient wear socks if chilling occurs
Tell patient that the transition stage usually lasts no more than 1 to 2 hr and then she will be allowed to push and deliver infant
Palpate abdomen very lightly and only as often as necessary if abdomen is hypersensitive
Avoid having persons in labor room who are not directly caring for patient
Accept aggression or other coping behaviors; avoid negative comments
Avoid unnecessary talking or expression of feelings to meet own needs
Focus on patient and support her
  Calm voice
  Touch
  Positive reinforcement after contractions

Evaluation

Complications are avoided
Mother and fetus avoid injury and/or compromise
Infant is delivered in good condition
Discomfort during labor is minimized

CARE OF MOTHER DURING DELIVERY: SECOND STAGE OF LABOR

Expulsion of the fetus, placenta, and membranes from the mother at birth

Assessment
Observations/findings

Involuntary bearing down
Pushing
Grunting sounds
Extreme anxiety
Increase in bloody show
Patient stating, "Baby is coming"
Desire to defecate; fear of "making a mess"
Prolonged second stage
  More than 1 hr for multigravidas
  More than 2 hr for primigravidas

Laboratory/diagnostic studies

Electronic fetal monitoring
Cord blood: gases, pH, and other tests as ordered

Potential complications

High-risk delivery
Birth asphyxia
Difficult delivery
  Shoulder dystocia
  Breech presentation
  Cephalopelvic disproportion
Forceps delivery
Vacuum extraction
Cesarean section
Infant bruising, fractures
See Care of Newborn (p. 751)

Nursing diagnosis/goal/interventions

ndx: Potential alteration in health maintenance related to delivery process

GOAL: *Health of fetus and patient will be maintained throughout delivery*

Delivery care

Auscultate FHR q5 min and/or after each push if electronic monitor is not used
Check BP and P q5 to 10 min
Pad stirrups
Administer oxygen mask at 10 to 12 L/min as ordered
Understand that low- to semi-Fowler's position with lateral tilt is preferred while pushing
Assist with breathing techniques
  Deep ventilation prior to and after each contraction
  Breathing technique and pushing with contractions
Observe perineum while pushing
Notify physician if second stage is prolonged
Prepare perineum according to hospital procedure
Request patient not to touch sterile drapes if used
Place nurse, spouse, and/or labor coach at head of delivery table to encourage patient during delivery process
Encourage long, sustained pushing rather than frequent short pushes
Encourage complete relaxation between contractions
Reassure patient that she is doing well and is advancing infant with each push
Apply cool moist cloth to forehead as needed
Have DeLee suction catheter available and ready to use if meconium-stained amniotic fluid is present
Plan for suctioning of naso-oropharynx following de-

livery of fetal head and prior to delivery of thorax to prevent meconium aspiration

Assist physician or nurse-midwife as needed

Immediate postdelivery care

Permit mother to inspect infant as soon as possible

Place infant on maternal abdomen to provide skin-to-skin contact if delivery room is warm

See Care of Newborn (p. 751)

Defer neonatal eye therapy for 1 to 2 hr after birth to promote eye contact with mother

Check BP and P q5 to 10 min for four times and prn

Add oxytocic drug as ordered to parenteral fluids

Administer injection of antilactation drug as ordered if mother is not breast-feeding

Palpate fundus, noting location and tonus q5 min for four times

Administer perineal care prior to removing legs from stirrups

Place sterile perineal pad and/or pad under buttocks prior to transporting patient to recovery area

Place ice pack on epistiotomy unless otherwise ordered

Assist with infant's warm water bath if infant's temperature is stable as indicated (Leboyer deliveries)

Maintain mother's warmth with blankets as needed

Place radiant heat warmer over upper part of mother's bed or place dry, warmly blanketed infant next to mother so that she can visually inspect, touch, and/or breast-feed nude infant while preventing neonatal heat loss

Let mother and spouse and/or labor coach be with infant in delivery area, providing them with as much privacy as feasible unless this is contraindicated by maternal or fetal pathologic condition

Encourage mother to freely express her feelings about herself and her infant

Explain that behaviors manifested in labor are normal and there is no reason to apologize if mother is apologetic for behavior while in labor

See Postpartum Care (p. 739)

Evaluation

Health is maintained

Complications are avoided

Infant is delivered in good condition, and mother is in good condition

OXYTOCIN INFUSION: AUGMENTATION OR INDUCTION OF LABOR

Oxytocin infusion may be used to either begin the labor process or to augment a labor that is progressing slowly because of inadequate uterine activity

Assessment

Observations/findings

Dysfunctional labor signs
  Prolonged latent phase
  Protracted active phase
  Secondary arrest
  Prolonged deceleration phase
  Protracted descent
  Arrest of descent
Absence of cephalopelvic disproportion

Laboratory/diagnostic studies

FHR-UC monitoring
Cephalopelvic disproportion (CPD) measurements
Ultrasound as ordered

Potential complications

Fetal distress
  Hyperactive fetus
  Fetal tachycardia: above 160 beats/min
  Fetal bradycardia: below 120 beats/min
  Late decelerations
    Prolonged deceleration
    Severe
Uterine hyperstimulation
  Contractions longer than 90 sec
  Contractions occurring more frequently than q2 min
  Peak pressure of contraction above 90 mm Hg pressure
  Inadequate uterine relaxation: less than 30 sec between contractions
  Intrauterine resting tone above 15 mm Hg pressure between contractions
  Sustained tetanic uterine contraction
Meconium-stained amniotic fluid
Maternal hypertension
Water intoxication
  Rising BP
  Edema of face, fingers, and around eyes
  Shortness of breath
  Difficulty in breathing
  Urinary output <30 to 50 ml/hr
Abruptio placentae: sudden, severe uterine pain (p. 723)
Precipitate delivery
Hemorrhage
Shock
Uterine rupture

Medical management

Baseline FHR-UC recording

Oxytocin infusion at a rate of 0.5 mU/min and increasing for desired results at 15 to 20 min intervals in increments of 1 to 2 mU/min not to exceed 20 mU/min

Continuous FHR-UC monitoring

Nursing diagnoses/goals/interventions

ndx Potential for injury related to augmentation of labor

GOAL: *Mother and fetus will not be injured as a result of complications of oxytocin infusion*

See Care of Mother in First Stage of Labor (p. 728)
Maintain complete bed rest
Ensure that physician is immediately available
Apply fetal monitoring; obtain baseline strip prior to start of IV oxytocin
Place patient in position of comfort; lateral position is preferred
Always piggyback oxytocin solution into main IV line (10 U oxytocin in 1000 ml IV fluid = 10 mU/ml)
Administer oxytocin via infusion pump as ordered
Monitor dose in mU/min q15 min and prior to each increase
Increase rate of oxytocic solution as ordered to produce contractions q2 to 3 min of 30 to 60 sec duration
Check BP, P, and FHR q15 to 30 min or as ordered
Observe contractions for frequency, duration, strength, and relaxation q5 min for five times, then q15 to 30 min and prn
Control pain as ordered
Assist in breathing and relaxation techniques (p. 730)
Measure intake and output q2h
Prepare for delivery as indicated
Reinforce physician's explanation of reason for augmentation or induction of labor

ndx Knowledge deficit regarding unfamiliarity with oxytocin infusion procedure

GOAL: *Patient and significant other will verbalize understanding of procedure, indications for it, and expected effects*

Reinforce physician's explanations
Discuss indications for procedure
Explain methodology of administration
Discuss expected effects of oxytocin induction/augmentation of labor
Explain differences between induction/augmentation and normal, spontaneous contractions

ndx Alteration in comfort: pain related to uterine contractions

See Care of Mother in First Stage of Labor (p. 728)

Evaluation

Complications are avoided
Mother and fetus sustain no injuries
Fetus is not compromised
Patient and significant other understand oxytocin infusion procedure, indications for it, and expected effects
Patient is comfortable during infusion procedure

FETAL DISTRESS

Compromise in fetal well-being

Assessment

Observations/findings

Fetal tachycardia: above 160 beats/min
Fetal bradycardia: below 120 beats/min
Meconium-stained amniotic fluid
Fetal hyperactivity or hypoactivity
Monitored fetus
  Nonreassuring FHR patterns
    Progressive increase or decrease in baseline FHR
    Tachycardia: 160 beats/min or greater; progressive decrease in baseline variability
  Ominous FHR patterns
    Severe variable deceleration; FHR below 70 beats/min for longer than 30 sec with
      Rising baseline FHR
      Decreasing variability
      Slow return to baseline (may be with overshoot)
    Late decelerations of any magnitude
    Absence of variability
    Prolonged deceleration
    Severe bradycardia
    Unstable FHR; sinusoidal pattern

Laboratory/diagnostic studies

Electronic fetal monitoring
Amniocentesis
Cord blood studies
Fetal scalp sampling: pH < 7.2

Potential complications

Fetal death
Neonatal death

CNS disorders
Meconium aspiration syndrome (p. 774)
Intracranial hemorrhage
Hypoxia
Hypoglycemia

Medical management

Discontinue tocolytic therapy as applicable
Administer oxygen to patient
Deliver infant as indicated
Fetal blood sampling as indicated
IV fluids as indicated
Laboratory tests as indicated
Neonatal resuscitation required at delivery

Nursing diagnoses/goals/interventions

ndx: Potential fetal compromise related to episode(s) of fetal distress*

GOAL: *Fetus will have minimal compromise, and fetus/infant will be delivered in good condition*

Intervene methodically; it is not necessary to proceed with subsequent steps if intervention corrects FHR pattern
Change maternal position
Correct maternal hypotension: elevate legs; increase rate of maintenance IV infusion
Discontinue oxytocin if infusing
Administer oxygen at rate of 10 to 12 L/min or as ordered
Perform vaginal and/or speculum examination
Assist physician with fetal blood sampling as indicated
Prepare for termination of labor as indicated
Explain briefly to patient the reasons for actions taken

ndx: Anxiety/fear related to uncertain infant outcome and unfamiliarity with fetal distress

GOAL: *Patient and significant other will verbalize understanding of fetal distress and will be able to verbalize fears and concerns regarding infant*

Explain all interventions to mother and significant other, such as
  Reasons for procedure
  How procedures are to be done
  Available choices and options
  Expected results from procedure
Simplify explanations and repeat as necessary
Provide realistic, factual information regarding infant status

Provide information regarding availability of neonatal intensive care unit
Reassure patient that emergency equipment and experienced personnel are available for delivery
Encourage patient to express concerns
Offer choices where feasible
Provide information regarding
  Known possible causes of fetal distress
  Misconceptions
Postdelivery
  Allow parents to see infant before transport to nursery
  Allow mother to stroke infant if possible
  Give realistic information on possible expectations for infant condition

Evaluation

There are no complications
There is no injury to fetus or mother
Anxiety/fears are minimized

CARE OF MOTHER ON FETAL MONITOR

Use of electronic fetal monitoring device to observe fetal heart rate and uterine activity and evaluate fetal distress

Assessment

Observations/findings

Decelerations: early, variable, late
Fetal tachycardia
Fetal bradycardia
Variability
  Long term, short term
  Absent, minimal, average, increased
Periodic changes affected by
  Dilation and station
  Vaginal examinations
  Status of membranes
  Medication and anesthetics
  Vital signs
  Monitoring mode and changes
  Equipment adjustments
  Patient position and repositioning
  Interventions for fetal distress

Potential complications

See Fetal Distress (p. 734)
Uterine hyperstimulation
  Contractions longer than 90 sec
  Contractions occurring more frequently than q2 min

---

*Not a NANDA-approved nursing diagnosis.

Peak pressure of contraction above 90 mm Hg pressure
Inadequate uterine relaxation
  Less than 30 sec between contractions
  Intrauterine resting tone >15 mm Hg pressure between contractions
Positional discomfort
Loss of signal source
Fear of fetal jeopardy

Medical management

Continuous or intermittent monitoring
External or internal monitoring

Nursing diagnoses/goals/interventions

ndx: Potential for fetal compromise related to labor and delivery experience*

GOAL: *Fetus will not be compromised*

Maintain complete bed rest
Position patient comfortably
  Encourage lateral position if bed is flat or modify this if patient is in semi-Fowler's position to prevent supine hypotension syndrome
Test FHR q4h and prn
Chart all nursing and patient care activities on strip chart
  Dilation and station
  Vaginal examinations
  Status of membranes
  Medication and anesthetics
  BP, T, P, and R
  Mode of monitoring and changes
  Adjustments of equipment
  Patient's position and repositioning
  Intervention for fetal distress

ndx: Knowledge deficit regarding electronic fetal monitoring procedure

GOAL: *Patient and significant other will adjust appropriately to use of fetal monitor during labor and delivery*

Explain that fetal status via FHR can be continuously assessed even during contractions
Explain that lower activity on strip chart shows uterine activity; upper panel shows FHR
Reassure patient and significant other that prepared childbirth techniques can be implemented without difficulty

---

*Not a NANDA-approved nursing diagnosis.

Explain that effleurage performed during external monitoring can be done on sides of abdomen or upper thighs
Relate that breathing patterns based on timing and intensity of contractions can be enhanced by observation of uterine activity panel of strip chart for onset of contractions
  Note peak of contraction; knowing that contraction will not get stronger and is half over is usually helpful
  Note diminishing intensity
  Coordinate with appropriate breathing and relaxation techniques
Reassure patient and significant other that use of internal mode of monitoring does not restrict patient movement
Explain that use of external mode of monitoring usually requires patient cooperation in positioning and movement
Reassure patient and significant other that use of monitor does not imply fetal jeopardy

Evaluation

Complications are avoided
Early detection and intervention of fetal distress are achieved
Infant is born in good condition

External Monitoring
ULTRASOUND TRANSDUCER

Monitors FHR with high-frequency sound waves

Tap transducer prior to use to ensure sound transmission
Apply ultrasound transmission gel to maternal abdomen; clean abdomen and transducer and reapply gel q2h and prn
Massage reddened skin areas and reposition belt q2h and prn
Auscultate FHR with stethoscope or fetoscope if in doubt as to validity of strip chart
Position and reposition transducer prn to ensure clear, interpretable FHR data

PHONOTRANSDUCER

Monitors FHR with a microphone technique

Clean and dry maternal abdomen prior to application and prn
Tape transducer in place to avoid unwanted sounds
Adjust sensitivity to ensure clarity of signal source as needed

Avoid use if there is frequent maternal movement or environmental noises

ABDOMINAL ECG TRANSDUCER

Monitors fetal ECG via maternal abdomen and converts it to FHR

Prepare skin sites with alcohol swabs prior to each application of pregelled disposable electrodes
Avoid use if signal source is inadequate because of maternal obesity, less than 34 weeks gestational age, or maternal muscular activity and tension

TOCOTRANSDUCER

Monitors uterine activity via a pressure-sensing device placed on the maternal abdomen

Position and reposition qh and prn on the fundus where least maternal tissue is in evidence
Maintain abdominal strap snugly
Adjust penset *between* contractions to print between 20 and 25 mm Hg on strip chart
Palpate fundus q30 to 60 min to gauge strength of contraction; only frequency and duration of contractions can be assessed with tocotransducer
Do not assess patient's need for analgesic based on uterine activity displayed on strip chart
Massage reddened areas under transducer and belt qh and prn

Internal Monitoring
SPIRAL ELECTRODE

Obtains fetal ECG from presenting part and converts it into FHR

Ensure that color-coded wires are appropriately attached to push post on leg plate
Apply electrode paste to leg plate q2h and prn
Observe FHR panel of strip chart for long- and short-term variability
Turn electrode counterclockwise to remove; never pull straight out from presenting part
Administer perineal care after voiding and q2h prn

INTRAUTERINE CATHETER

Fluid-filled catheter internally monitors intrauterine pressure

Flush catheter with sterile water prior to insertion and prn
Ensure that black mark on catheter is visible at introitus
Maintain height of strain gauge at miduterine level
Turn stopcock off to patient, then with pressure valve of strain gauge released, flush strain gauge, remove syringe, and set stylus to 0 line on chart paper; test further according to manufacturer's instructions q3h to 4h and prn
Check proper functioning by tapping catheter, asking patient to cough, or applying fundal pressure; observe appropriate inflection on strip chart
Maintain catheter taped to patient's leg to prevent dislodgment

NONSTRESS TEST (NST)

Basis for NST is that the healthy fetus will exhibit acceleration of FHR with movement

Assessment
Observations/findings

Accelerations of FHR
Other periodic changes in FHR
Baseline changes in FHR
Evidence of fetal movement on strip chart
    Blips
    Spikes
    Momentary increases in uterine pressure

Laboratory/diagnostic studies
INTERPRETATION OF RESULTS

Reactive: two or more accelerations of FHR with an amplitude of 15 beats/min lasting 15 sec or more associated with fetal movement in a *10 min period or* five or more FHR accelerations in a 20 min period
Nonreactive: either less than two accelerations of FHR with an amplitude below 15 beats/min or lasting less than 15 sec, *or* absence of accelerations associated with fetal movement in a 10 min period, *or* less than five FHR accelerations in a 20 min period
Suspicious: definite accelerations of FHR associated with fetal movement; however, number of accelerations or amplitude and duration do not meet criteria of reactive or nonreactive test
Unsatisfactory: quality of FHR recording is not adequate for interpretation

Potential complications

Identification of fetal compromise
Detection of uteroplacental insufficiency

Medical management

Begun at 32 to 34 weeks in high-risk patients
If nonreactive, CST (p. 738)

If reactive, repeat 1 to 2 times per week until delivery or until nonreactive

Nursing diagnosis/goal/interventions

ndx: Potential identification of fetal compromise related to uteroplacental insufficiency*

GOAL: *Patient will be prepared for procedure*

Explain general use of equipment and procedure to patient and significant other

Give full liquid meal (if not taken prior to test) to reduce bowel sounds if ordered

Request patient to void

Assist patient with assuming semi-Fowler's position with lateral uterine tilt

Monitor FHR and uterine activity externally until test can be interpreted

Confirm fetal movement by palpation or patient confirmation

Reinforce implications of reactive and nonreactive tests

Evaluation

Patient cooperates with procedure
Complications are avoided

CONTRACTION STRESS TEST (CST)

Assessment of uteroplacental reserve by means of "stressing" the fetus with contractions and observing the resultant FHR pattern

Assessment

Observations/findings

Periodic changes in FHR
  Accelerations
  Decelerations: early, late, variable
Baseline changes in FHR
  Tachycardia
  Bradycardia
  Absent or minimal variability
  Sinusoidal pattern

Laboratory/diagnostic studies

INTERPRETATION OF RESULTS

Negative: three contractions > 40 sec duration in a 10 min period without late decelerations; there is usually a good baseline variability and acceleration of FHR with fetal movement

Positive: persistent and consistent late decelerations occurring with more than half the contractions
Hyperstimulation: contractions occurring more often than q2 min and/or lasting longer than 90 sec
  Uterine hypertonus; rise of baseline uterine tone
  Late decelerations occurring during or after excessive uterine activity
Suspicious: late decelerations occurring with less than half the uterine contractions once an adequate contraction pattern has been established
Unsatisfactory: inadequate contraction pattern or tracing too poor to interpret; test is not interpretable and cannot be used for clinical management

Potential complications

Uterine hyperstimulation
Elevated BP
Onset of labor
Supine hypotension syndrome
Clarity of strip chart tracing
Fetal compromise
Emergency delivery

Medical management

Following nonreactive NST

If positive CST, imminent delivery
If negative CST, repeated per hospital protocol until delivery or until CST becomes positive

Nursing diagnosis/goal/intervention

ndx: Potential for fetal compromise related to uteroplacental insufficiency*

GOAL: *Patient will be prepared for procedure and potential outcomes, and fetus will not be compromised*

Explain general use of equipment and procedure to patient and significant other

Give full liquid meal (if not taken prior to test) to reduce bowel sounds if ordered

Request patient to void

Assist patient with assuming semi-Fowler's or lateral tilt position

Understand that contractions can be stimulated by dilute IV oxytocin or by nipple stimulation

Nipple-stimulated contractions

Monitor FHR and uterine activity externally to determine baseline until at least 10 min of interpretable data are obtained

---

*Not a NANDA-approved nursing diagnosis.

*Not a NANDA-approved nursing diagnosis.

Check BP and P q15 min

Defer nipple stimulation if three unstimulated contractions of greater than 40 sec duration occur within a 10 min period

Apply warm, moist washcloth to both breasts for several minutes

Instruct patient to massage and/or roll nipple of one breast for 10 min; if uterine contractions do not occur, stimulate both breasts for 10 min

Restimulate breasts intermittently as needed to maintain uterine contractions

If nipple stimulation does not produce desired uterine activity, proceed to oxytocin-stimulated contraction stress test

Oxytocin-stimulated contractions (oxytocin challenge test; OCT)

Administer parenteral fluids with oxytocin piggybacked into main IV line; deliver with infusion pump in mU/min

Check BP and P q15 min

Monitor FHR and uterine contractions externally to determine baseline uterine activity until 10 min of interpretable data are obtained prior to administration of oxytocin

Defer oxytocin infusion if three unstimulated contractions of greater than 40 sec duration occur within a 10 min period; interpret the results

Increase dosage of oxytocin q15 to 20 min as ordered

Discontinue oxytocin when three uterine contractions of greater than 40 sec duration have occurred within a 10 min period

Postprocedure care

Continue to monitor FHR and uterine contractions until uterine activity is diminished to pretest baseline

Interpret results of test

Teach patient signs of onset of labor; labor almost never begins within 48 hr if fetus is less than 38 weeks gestational age

Evaluation

Complications are absent or minimized
Patient complies with procedure instructions

POSTPARTUM CARE

Care after delivery of a fetus through the vaginal canal throughout the maternal recovery period to 6 weeks after birth

Assessment

Observations/findings

Skin
  Mask of pregnancy
  Striae
Breasts
  Colostrum
  Breast milk
Abdomen
  Uterine involution
    Firm
    Midline
    1 to 2 finger breadths below umbilicus and decreasing
  Relaxed abdominal muscles
Lochia
  Color: rubra, serosa, or alba
  Flow: heavy, moderate, light, or scant
Perineum: episiotomy
Transition to parenthood; "postpartum depression"

Laboratory/diagnostic studies

Hgb/Hct
Medication blood levels as ordered
CBC with differential if indicated
Electrolytes if indicated

Potential complications

Hemorrhage; soft, relaxed fundus
Postanesthesia headache
Infection
  Elevated temperature
  Diaphoresis
  Chilling
  Nausea, vomiting
  Tachycardia
  Foul odor of lochia
  After pains
  Drainage from episiotomy
  Edema, redness, or discoloration at incisions or lacerations
  Gaping sutures at incisions or lacerations
Bladder distention
Painful hemorrhoids
Constipation
Thrombophlebitis
Pulmonary embolus
Engorged breasts; sore nipples
Behavioral changes
  Depression
  Withdrawal
  Lack of contact with, or care of, newborn

Child abuse
Child neglect

Medical management

Postpartum assessment with vital signs
Vital signs q15 min for 1 to 2 hr, then q30 min twice, then q4h for 24 hr, then q8h and prn; neuro checks with vital signs if regional anesthesia is received
IV fluids
Oxytocics as indicated
Pain medications, stool softeners, antiflatulents as indicated
Breast binder if indicated
Lactation suppression drugs
Ice bag to perineum as indicated
Topical anesthetic to episiotomy prn
Foley catheter if indicatd
Progressive ambulation as tolerated
Laboratory tests as indicated
Regular diet as tolerated, encourage po fluid and snacks
Intake and output
Anti-Rh globulin as indicated

Nursing diagnoses/goals/interventions

***ndx**:* Potential alteration in health maintenance related to postpartum transition

GOAL: *Patient will avoid complications; vital signs and postpartum progress will remain within normal parameters*

Check the following q15 min for 1 to 2 hr, then q30 min for four times, then q4h for 24 hr
   Fundus location and tone
   Episiotomy condition
   Lochia amount, color, and consistency
   BP, P, and R
   Level of consciousness
   Spinal dermatomes if regional anesthesia was given
Maintain bed rest in quiet environment; keep side rails up
Recover mother and infant in same bed under radiant heat warmer, if possible, to promote visual inspection, skin contact, and bonding
Encourage spouse or significant other to remain at bedside
Place patient in position of comfort
Maintain parenteral fluids with oxytocics as ordered
Initiate diet as ordered
Encourage fluids po unless contraindicated
Measure intake and output for 24 hr or as ordered
Avoid distended bladder; encourage voiding within 6 to 8 hr after delivery or catheterize as ordered
Administer perineal care after elimination and prn
Change perineal pads q30 to 60 min and/or as needed; report excessive bleeding to physician
Avoid unnecessary massage of fundus, which can cause uterine relaxation and hemorrhage
Note time when sensation has returned to lower extremities after spinal anesthetic
Administer oral hygiene, sponge bath, back rub, and linen change prior to transfer to room
Manage pain; administer medication as ordered
Apply ice bag to perineum as ordered
Maintain warmth with blankets; avoid drafts in patient care unit
Allow patient to sleep undisturbed as much as possible
Remain with patient during the first time out of bed
Use voiding measures as needed
Administer perineal care after each elimination
Change perineal pad from front to back after each elimination
Use perineal light tid if ordered
Use sitz bath tid and prn if ordered
Administer anesthetic spray to episiotomy and hemorrhoids prn
Apply anesthetic ointment to hemorrhoids prn
Administer stool softeners, mild laxatives, or suppositories as ordered
Ambulate qid; activity as tolerated
Assist with holding and inspecting infant as soon as possible and before 6 hr after delivery and prn until mother is able to become actively involved in infant care
Permit mother to have infant at bedside as little or as much as she desires
Meet mother's needs during "taking hold" phase (about 10 days)
   Reassure mother that she is performing well in all aspects of self-care and infant care
   Avoid intervening between mother and infant regardless of how awkward her skills seem
   Positively reinforce all tasks done well
   Avoid negative criticism at all times, unless solicited by parent
Administer rubella vaccine just prior to patient's discharge if ordered
Assist and teach mother to perform all infant care tasks: bathing, feeding, diapering, cord care, cuddling, etc.
Teach mother and visitors proper handwashing technique
Involve spouse or significant other in infant care and teaching

ndx: Alteration in comfort related to episiotomy, afterbirth pains, and/or breast discomfort

GOAL: *Patient's pain will be relieved or minimized, patient's uterine fundus will be firm and pain-free, and patient will demonstrate proper breast care*

Maintain planned rest periods once or twice daily and prn
  No phone calls or visitors
  Care for infant out of mother's hearing
Care for infant at night to assure mother adequate rest as requested
Meet mother's dependency needs during "taking in" phase (first 2 to 3 days)
  Encourage verbalization; mothers are usually extremely talkative, repeatedly relating experience of labor and delivery
  Understand that enthusiastic listening by nurse helps experience become more meaningful to parents
Shower or bathe daily; avoid washing nipples of breast-feeding mothers at any other time
Have mother wear supportive bra at all times
Check breasts q4h to 8h and prn
If breast-feeding
  Manually express breasts q4h and after nursing
  Place warm moist towel packs on engorged breasts for 15 to 30 min q1h to 3h, then massage and manually express breasts or have infant nurse
  See Breast-Feeding (p. 747)
If bottle-feeding
  Never massage or manually express engorged breasts
  Have mother wear snug-fitting breast binder over bra and use ice bags q1h to 3h for 15 min on each side if breasts are engorged
Anticipate need for pain relief
Massage fundus if boggy; teach mother self-massage
Administer pain medication as ordered and document effectiveness
If bladder is distended, encourage patient to void
Instruct mother to squeeze buttocks together when sitting down if episiotomy is painful with ambulation
Encourage mother to use relaxation techniques learned in labor for afterbirth pains during breast-feeding

ndx: Potential for infection related to incision and/or lacerations

GOAL: *Episiotomy and/or lacerations will heal without evidence of infection*

Instruct patient on perineal care per hospital policy
Instruct patient on use of sitz bath
Watch for elevated temperature or other changes in vital sign parameters
Note and report any abnormal, foul-smelling drainage or discharge
Administer antibiotics as ordered

ndx: Potential alteration in elimination (bowel or urinary) patterns related to childbirth experience

GOAL: *Patient will demonstrate measures that prevent constipation and will void spontaneously without any discomfort*

Give stool softeners or laxative as ordered
Encourage patient to ambulate as tolerated, increasing progressively
Maintain regular diet with between-meal snacks; increase amount of fruit and roughage
Encourage daily fluids to 3000 ml daily unless contraindicated
Encourage patient to void q4 to 6h as able
Employ techniques to assist voiding as needed

ndx: Potential fluid volume deficit related to postpartum bleeding

GOAL: *Patient will not have symptoms of hypovolemic or hemorrhagic shock and will not hemorrhage*

Note any changes in quality and quantity of lochia
Check postdelivery Hgb and Hct for abnormal values and report to physician
Watch for symptoms of DIC (p. 196)
Check for uterine tone with vital signs
If soft and/or relaxed, massage until firm
Teach mother self-massage of uterine fundus
Teach mother normal parameters of lochia and instruct her to call physician if there is abnormally heavy flow
Encourage increased fluid intake (2000 to 3000 ml) daily unless contraindicated
Maintain IV fluids if ordered
Monitor oxytocics as ordered

ndx: Potential alteration in parenting related to transition to parenthood

GOAL: *Mother will demonstrate adequate infant caretaking skills*

Assist with newborn care and feeding q3h to 4h and prn

Observe mother-infant interaction; report to physician
  Mother not holding infant while feeding
  Lack of eye contact between mother and infant
  Absence of verbalization of mother to infant
  Lack of physical contact with infant
Encourage verbalization about role of mothering, impact of new family member, and sibling rivalry, if applicable
Encourage visits by healthy siblings unless contraindicated
See Care of Newborn (p. 751)

ndx: Alteration in self-concept: disturbance in body image related to birth experience

GOAL: *Mother will demonstrate effective emotional adjustment and healthy self-esteem*

Encourage discussion of real and perceived problems
Help mother validate the reality of her labor and delivery experience
Give reassurance concerning her ability as a mother
Help patient accept emotional ups and downs of postpartum period and explain that these feelings and changes are common during this time
Encourage rest periods throughout the day
Provide opportunity for parent/infant interactions and involve father or significant other as possible
Support and encourage parents and/or significant other in interactions and caring for infant

ndx: Knowledge deficit regarding postpartum care

GOAL: *Patient will demonstrate postpartum self-care and will demonstrate care of infant*

Caution patient to avoid coitus or douching for 4 to 6 weeks or as indicated by physician
Demonstrate breast care and manual expression if mother is breast-feeding
Emphasize importance of nutritious diet
Caution patient to avoid lifting anything heavier than the infant for 2 to 3 weeks
Explain need for planned rest periods
Explain need to carefully clean perineal region
  Wipe from front to back after urinating
  Administer perineal self-care
  Apply perineal pad from front to back
  Wash vulva and perineum, including sutures, before washing anal area when showering
Relate that absorbable sutures do not need to be removed
Relate that sitz bath and perineal light may be used at home prn
Instruct patient to use anesthetic spray and/or ointment to perineal area and/or hemorrhoids
Caution patient to avoid constipation; stool softeners or mild laxatives may be necessary
Discuss symptoms to report to physician
  Temperature above 100° F (37.8° C)
  Foul odor of lochia
Relate that shower or tub bath may be taken
Explain that lochia may continue for 3 to 4 weeks, changing from red to brown to white
Relate that menses will return 6 to 8 weeks after delivery, often despite breast-feeding
  Explain that some nursing mothers do not menstruate until they wean infant from breast, whereas others resume menstruation at various times while nursing
  Emphasize that pregnancy is possible 4 to 6 weeks after delivery, whether mother is breast-feeding or not; discuss availability of nonprescription methods of contraception
Explain need for mild exercise initially
  Do not start vigorous exercise until approved by physician
  Explain that Kegel exercises can be begun during early puerperium
Discuss normalcy of postpartum "blues"
Discuss need to plan for needs of other children at home and discuss possible behavioral changes as a result of new family member
Teach name of medication, dosage, time of administration, purpose, and side effects
Emphasize importance of ongoing outpatient care, including postpartum checkup
Emphasize the normalcy of feelings that may be disturbing
  Initial lack of feeling of love for infant
  Variations from prenatal expectations of what infant would look like; disappointment in sex, weight, or appearance
  Frustration caused by increased demands on time
  Feelings of being trapped
  Unsettled feelings about being a mother and parent
  Feelings of tension, nervousness, and fatigue
Discuss how to contact available community resources
  Housekeeping agencies
  Nursing care agencies
  Diaper services
  Family planning organizations
  Breast-feeding organizations: La Leche League*

---

*La Leche League International, 9616 Minneapolis Ave., Franklin Park, Ill.

Parenting groups
Publications on infant care
   Growth and development
   Parenting
   Health care
Discuss proper principles and practice of infant care
See Care of Newborn (p. 751)

Evaluation

Complications are avoided
Health will be maintained
Patient will demonstrate self-care and infant care appropriately
Infection does not occur
Pain is relieved or minimized
Proper postpartum self-care is demonstrated
Postpartum hemorrhage is avoided

CESAREAN DELIVERY

Delivery of a fetus through a uterine incision; most common is the transverse lower segment incision, with the classic vertical cesarean incision done less frequently

Assessment

Observations/findings
INDICATIONS

CPD in previous or current pregnancy
Fetal distress
Failure to progress in labor
Malposition of fetus
   Breech presentation
   Transverse lie
   Abnormal vertex presentation
Umbilical cord prolapse
Abruptio placentae
Placenta previa
High-risk pregnancy due to maternal conditions such as cardiac defects and diabetes

Preoperative laboratory/diagnostic studies

Electronic fetal monitoring for fetal well-being
ECG monitoring
CBC with differential
Electrolytes
Hgb/Hct
Type and cross match for blood
Urinalysis
Amniocentesis for fetal lung maturity as indicated
X-ray examination as indicated
Ultrasound as ordered

Potential complications

Hemorrhage; soft, relaxed uterine fundus
Shock
Anemia
DIC
Infection
   Elevated temperature
   Tachycardia
   Foul odor of lochia
Site of incision
   Redness
   Pain
   Swelling
   Drainage
Cystitis
Engorged breasts
Pneumonia
Paralytic ileus
Thrombophlebitis
Pulmonary embolus
Behavioral changes
   Guilt
   Depression
   Withdrawal
   Lack of contact with or care of newborn
Anesthesia reaction: malignant hyperthermia
Fetal injury during surgery
Fetal blood loss during surgery
Neonatal depression/resuscitation at birth
Infant respiratory distress syndrome (p. 773)

Medical management

IV fluids as indicated
Anesthesia: regional or general
Permission for attendance at cesarean section of significant other
Laboratory/diagnostic tests as indicated
Oxytocic administration as indicated
Vital signs per recovery room protocol
Abdominal surgery skin preparation
Consent form signed
Foley catheter insertion

Nursing diagnoses/goals/interventions

***ndx*:** Potential alteration in health maintenance related to cesarean section delivery

GOAL: *Patient will have optimal health maintenance during postoperative period*

Provide surgical patient–teaching information as appropriate prior to procedure

Immediate postoperative care

See Care of Patient in Recovery Room (p. 30)
Check following q15 min for 2 to 3 hr, then q30 min for four times, then q4h for 24 hr
  Site of incision
  Fundus location and tone
  Lochia amount, color, and consistency
  BP, P, and R
Change and/or reinforce abdominal dressing as necessary
Change perineal pad q1h to 2h and prn
Administer perineal care q2h to 4h and prn
Manage pain; administer medication as ordered
Maintain NPO; administer mouth care q2h and prn
Maintain parenteral fluids with oxytocics as ordered
Connect indwelling catheter to closed gravity drainage system
See Postpartum Care (p. 739) and Care of Newborn (p. 751)

ndx: Knowledge deficit regarding procedure and post-cesarean delivery care

GOAL: *Patient will verbalize rationale for cesarean delivery and perform self-care activities during postpartum period*

Discuss with mother and significant other the reason for cesarean section
Explain "normal" preoperative procedures and potential variations for current situation
Witness consent form and obtain baseline vital signs
Draw blood for CBC, electrolytes, type, and screen
Obtain urine for urinalysis
Insert Foley catheter
Choose type of anesthesia (general or epidural) if options are appropriate
Maintain NPO status
Perform abdominal preparation per hospital policy and aseptic technique principles
Administer IV fluids as ordered
Remove contact lenses and jewelry
Discuss presence of husband/significant other in operating room as appropriate
Encourage parents to attend preparatory classes specifically for cesarean delivery if cesarean is elective
Inform father that immediately postdelivery, he may hold infant close to mother's face and arms unless contraindicated
Discuss the following with mother and significant other during the postpartum period
  Need to avoid coitus or douching for 4 to 6 weeks or as indicated by physician
  Breast care and manual expression if breast-feeding (p. 747)
  Need to avoid sitting for long periods of time with knees bent
  Care of incision
  Symptoms of wound infection to report to physician
  Importance of nutritious diet
  To avoid lifting anything heavier than infant for 4 to 6 weeks
  Importance of planned rest periods
  Need to avoid constipation; stool softeners or mild laxatives may be necessary
  That showers may be taken
  That lochia may continue for 3 to 4 weeks, changing from red to brown to white
  That menses will return 6 to 8 weeks after delivery unless breast-feeding
    Explain that some nursing mothers do not menstruate until weaning infant from breast
    Explain that others resume menstruation at various times while nursing
    Explain that pregnancy is possible whether mother is breast-feeding or not, 4 to 6 weeks after delivery; discuss availability of nonprescription methods of contraception
  Importance of exercise; do not start vigorous exercise until approved by physician
  Name of medication, dosage, time of administration, purpose, and side effects
  Importance of follow-up outpatient care, including postpartum checkup
  Normalcy of postpartum "blues"
  Need to plan for needs of other children at home and discuss possible behavioral changes as a result of new family member
  Normalcy of feelings that may be disturbing to mother
    Initial lack of feeling of love for infant
    Variations from prenatal expectations of what infant would look like: disappointment in sex, weight, or appearance
    Frustration resulting from increased demands on time
    Feelings of being trapped
    Unsettled feelings about being a mother and parent
    Feelings of tension, nervousness, and fatigue
  How to contact available community resources
    Housekeeping agencies
    Nursing care agencies
    Diaper services
    Family planning organizations

Breast-feeding organizations: La Leche League,
   Lactation Institutes
Cesarean birth groups (such as C/Sec. Inc.)
Parenting groups
Publications on infant care
   Growth and development
   Parenting
   Health care
   Infant stimulation
See Care of Newborn (p. 751)

Breast-feeding

Discuss, demonstrate, and return-demonstrate breast-feeding principles related to cesarean delivery as follows
   If desired, breast-feeding is possible
   Feed only breast milk to baby
   Do not supplement with formula or water routinely (see Breast-feeding, p. 747)
   Take pain medication 20 to 30 min prior to nursing
   Proper positioning prevents and relieves discomfort
Instruct mother
   When lying on either side
      Put baby on his side facing you
      Pull baby's buttocks toward abdomen
      Use pillows to support your back and protect abdomen
   When sitting up in bed
      Use pillows under both knees to support them
      Place a pillow under each arm and another over abdomen
      Put baby on his side toward you in "crook" of your arm, with his face and belly facing toward you
      Pull baby in close
   If your abdomen is very sore after delivery, or your baby is under 6 lb, you can feed sitting up, using "football hold" (Figure 14-4); place baby facing up on pillow at your side and supported under your arm, his head toward foot of bed, feet toward head of bed

ndx: Anxiety/fear related to potential or actual fetal distress

GOAL: *Mother will verbalize concerns regarding infant*

Note any display of
   Ambivalence
   Inability to communicate
   Resentment
   Disappointment
   Expressed fear
   Restlessness

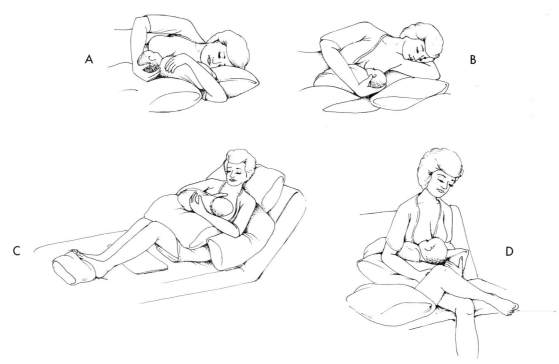

FIGURE 14-4. Comfortable breast-feeding positions following cesarean delivery. **A** and **B**, Side-lying position. **C**, Sitting in bed. **D**, "Football" hold.

Tearfulness
Trembling
Anger
Encourage parents to verbalize their concerns
Provide parents with realistic information regarding infant condition
Inform parents that pediatrician/neonatal resuscitation team will be present during cesarean section and that emergency equipment will be available
Encourage husband/significant other to be present for delivery as indicated

ndx: Alteration in self-concept: disturbance in body image related to interruption of anticipated childbirth experience

GOAL: *Mother will verbalize expressions of continued self-worth*

Encourage mother to verbalize fears and feelings of guilt and/or blame
   Sense of failure at not delivering "normally"
   Feelings of being cheated or disappointed
   Feelings of intrusion from surgical procedure
Provide support through reassurance and open communication
Include husband/significant other in discussions
Provide positive feedback to mother and significant other

ndx: Potential for injury or infection and postoperative complications related to surgical procedure

GOAL: *Incision will be clean and dry, without any signs or symptoms of infection; uterine involution will progress normally*

Monitor for elevated temperature or tachycardia as signs of infection
Observe incision for signs of infection with vital signs
   Redness
   Tenderness
   Swelling at incision site
   Reports of pain
   Unusual discharge
   Elevated temperature
Change dressing prn or as ordered
Assess fundus, lochia, and bladder with vital signs as ordered
Evaluate vital signs for symptoms of infection or hemorrhage q4h and prn
Massage fundus if boggy or does not remain firm
Notify physician of deviations from normal parameters
   Boggy, displaced uterus
   Uterine tenderness on palpation
   Persistent discharge of lochia rubra or return of lochia rubra
   Hemorrhage symptoms
   Foul-smelling lochia

ndx: Alteration in comfort related to postoperative condition

GOAL: *Patient will verbalize decrease or absence of pain following relief measures*

Anticipate need for pain medications and/or additional methods of pain relief
Note, document, and identify
   Reports of pain at incisional site: abdomen
   Facial grimace of pain
   Decreasing mobility
   Relief/distraction behavior
Administer pain medication as ordered and evaluate its effectiveness
Provide other comfort measures that may be helpful, such as repositioning or supporting with pillows

ndx: Impaired tissue perfusion related to postoperative immobility

GOAL: *Patient will not have respiratory congestion and will have no signs or symptoms of pulmonary embolism or deep vein thrombosis during hospitalization*

Assess respiratory status with vital signs
Document and report increased respiratory rate, nonproductive cough, audible rhonchi, rales, or upper airway congestion
Encourage patient to cough, turn, and deep breathe q2h during first postoperative day, then prn
Demonstrate splinting to support incision
Encourage use of incentive spirometer
Encourage early ambulation
Discuss elevating feet prn and not crossing legs
Check Homan's sign with vital signs
Note symptoms of
   Deep vein thrombosis formation
   Localized tenderness
   Calf pain
   Redness
   Swelling
   Elevated temperature
   Positive Homan's sign
   Pulmonary embolus
   Restlessness
   Chest pain
   Diaphoresis
   Dyspnea

Tachycardia
Change in BP
Auscultation abnormalities

ndx: Potential alteration in urinary and bowel elimination patterns related to postoperative cesarean section

GOAL: *Patient will void spontaneously without discomfort and will have a bowel movement within 3 to 5 days after surgery*

Encourage voiding q4h to 6h if possible
Employ techniques to encourage voiding as needed
Explain perineal care procedures per hospital policy
Note reports of bladder distention and inability to void
Encourage mother to
   Ambulate as tolerated
   Increase intake of fluids (2000 to 3000 ml daily)
   Increase fruit and roughage in diet
Give stool softener/laxative as ordered
Administer antiflatulents as ordered
Monitor intake and output until eliminating adequately
See Postpartum Care (p. 739)

Evaluation

There are no complications
Health is maintained throughout surgical course
Patient demonstrates self-care postoperatively
Breast-feeding is successful as desired by mother
Fears and anxieties are verbalized
Self-concept and self-esteem remain intact
There are no postoperative infections
Pain is minimized by relief measures

BREAST-FEEDING

Assessment

Observations/findings

Breasts
   Hardness
   Tenderness
   Pain
   Redness
Dehydration
Infant
   Nursing more frequently than q2h
   Voiding less than six times daily

Potential complications

Engorgement
Nipple problems
   Cracked nipples
   Inverted nipples
   Sore nipples
Mastitis
Nipple confusion of infant
Another pregnancy

Medical management

Antibiotics for mastitis as indicated
Referral to lactation specialist/consultant
Increase of caloric intake by 500 calories/day
Increase of fluid intake by 3000 ml daily unless contraindicated
Contraception counseling
Family planning counseling referrals as indicated

Nursing diagnoses/goals/interventions

ndx: Potential fluid volume deficit in infant related to inadequate breast-feeding

GOAL: *Infant will receive adequate intake for weight gain*

Instruct mother to
   Feed baby when hungry
   Begin feeding infant on one side for 10 to 30 min or until he begins to slow down
   Break suction of baby's mouth on nipple by placing finger inside mouth between gums
   Avoid pulling infant off breast without releasing suction
   Burp baby in a sitting position after nursing at each breast
   Place infant on opposite breast for 10 to 30 min or until he begins to slow down
   Change back to other breast again until infant seems satisfied and falls asleep
   Replace nursing bra after nursing is completed
Remind mother that during newborn period total feeding time can range from 20 min to 1 hr each
Remind mother that best way to tell if baby is getting enough milk is to listen for swallowing while sucking
Explain that adequate intake and nutrition is judged by six to eight wet diapers per day, baby sleeps 1 to 2 hr between feedings, and is gaining weight by time of newborn examination with first visit to health care provider

ndx: Potential alteration in comfort related to improper positioning and/or complications of breast-feeding

GOAL: *Patient will have minimal or no discomfort with breast-feeding*

See Figure 14-5 on hand expression of breast milk
See Figures 14-6 and 14-7 on proper body and nipple positioning
Encourage daily fluid intake to 3000 ml daily unless contraindicated
Initiate breast-feeding as soon as mother and infant are in good condition (this may be on delivery table); manually express both breasts q4h until infant can be nursed
Remain with mother for at least her first two breast-feeding experiences
Have mother assume most comfortable position for her; may be sitting or lying on side
Alternate breast that is used first at each feeding; place safety pin on bra as reminder

Apply small amount of hydrous lanolin to nipples to prevent dryness and cracking if necessary as ordered; it does not need to be washed off before next feeding
Have mother shower daily for breast and general cleanliness
Do not remove protective oils from breasts before each feeding by washing with any solution except water
Avoid using nipple shield; if necessary, use only long enough to draw nipple out so that infant may grasp and suckle
Encourage correct positioning
Discuss symptoms of complications and how to report them to health care provider
Request support or help from community resources for special problems

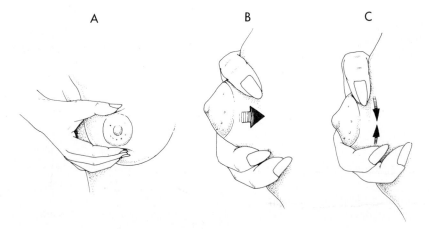

FIGURE 14-5. Hand expression of breast milk. **A,** Place thumb and fingers about 1 to 1½ inches behind nipple, forming C shape. **B,** Press in toward body. **C,** Firmly press fingers together on lacteal sinuses to express milk.

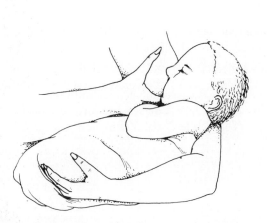

FIGURE 14-6. Correct body position for breast-feeding. Head of infant is in crook of mother's arm with front of infant facing front of mother.

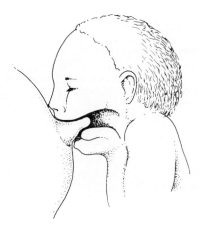

FIGURE 14-7. Correct latch-on position. Infant's mouth compresses milk-collecting sinuses in areola.

ndx: Knowledge deficit regarding principles of breast-feeding

GOAL: *Patient will demonstrate successful breast-feeding techniques*

Discuss and assist mother with the following
   Breast-feeding reflex: "let-down" reflex
   Handwashing before breast-feeding
   Body position (Figure 14-6)
   Nipple position (Figure 14-7)
   Inversion of nipples as indicated
Explain that supply of milk is related to demand
   Giving formula only decreases milk supply
   No need to supplement
   Need for feeding often on demand (often up to every 1½ to 2 hr; later about every 3 hr—breast-fed babies usually eat every 3 hr)
Emphasize importance of drinking at least six to eight glasses of liquid each day (water, juice, and milk) and eating a balanced diet, including meat, milk, vegetables and fruits, grains and cereals
Advise patient to limit visitors and household duties for the first month postpartum
Suggest that patient have relatives or friends assist with household chores, shopping, and meals prn
Explain need for planned rest periods and napping when able
Demonstrate hand expression of milk (Figure 14-5)
   Wash hands well before starting
   Cup breast with either hand (left hand for left breast, right hand for right breast)
   Place thumb above and fingers below nipple, 1 to 1½ inches behind nipple on areola (forming the letter "C")
   Press in toward back, then roll fingers down toward nipple, while gently pressing thumb and finger together
   Do not let fingers slide on skin
   Move fingers completely around areola to reach all milk sinuses
   Alternate between breasts every few minutes
Relate that milk can be expressed into clean glass containers or into plastic disposable bottle liners
Explain that mother's daily fluid intake should be a minimum of 3000 ml unless contraindicated; a full 8 oz glass of fluid prior to each nursing session will help ensure adequate maternal hydration
Discuss adjustment of dietary intake to meet infant's needs
   Eat well-balanced, high-protein diet
   Avoid foods that cause infant distress (colicky, crying, wakeful); do not arbitrarily omit foods usually eaten
Explain that breast milk normally has a thin, watery appearance
Explain that milk supply will be adequate if infant nurses regularly; the more infant nurses the more milk is produced
Explain that six wet diapers daily of pale-colored urine is indicative that infant is properly hydrated
Explain that four to six bowel movements daily is normal in breast-fed infant
Explain that it may be necessary to keep infant awake during feedings by unwrapping blanket and gently rubbing back or feet
Tell patient not to routinely give prepared formula
Explain that for several days after delivery it is normal to experience uterine cramping while nursing
Explain that milk flowing from opposite breast while nursing is normal
Caution patient to avoid plastic-coated breast shields in bra between feedings; a clean ironed handkerchief or Woolwich shield from La Leche League is preferred
Discuss treatment for engorged breasts
   Place very warm towel packs on breasts for 15 min
   Massage from outer breast to areola
   Manually express milk or nurse infant
Caution patient that a breast-feeding woman can become pregnant and should be aware of contraceptive methods other than oral contraceptives, which are usually contraindicated for at least the first 3 months
Relate that breast milk normally leaks during coitus
Discuss how to contact local breast-feeding organizations for further information while at home
   La Leche League
   Lactation Institute
   Lactation Specialists/Consultants in private practice
   Breast-feeding clinics

Evaluation

Complications are avoided
Mother is comfortably able to breast-feed her infant
Infant has adequate and progressive weight gain

POSTPARTUM HEMORRHAGE

Maternal blood loss postdelivery due to uterine atony, lacerations, and retained products of conception

Assessment
Observations/findings

Uterine atony
   Relaxed fundus
   Dark bleeding

Boggy, distended uterus
Expulsion of clots
Genital lacerations
    Constant trickle of bright red blood
    Firm fundus
Retained placental tissue
    Dark bleeding
    Boggy, distended uterus
    Abdominal pain

Laboratory/diagnostic studies

Vaginal examination
Clotting studies
Hgb and Hct
CVP monitoring

Potential complications

Shock
    Pallor
    Restlessness
    Weak, rapid pulse
    Decreased BP
    Chills
    Difficulty in breathing
    Air hunger
See Hypovolemic Shock (p. 104)
DIC
Postpartum infection
Anemia
Transfusion hepatitis
Hysterectomy

Medical management

Dilatation and curettage (D & C)
Insertion of uterine packing as indicated
IV fluids as indicated, including volume expanders, blood products, and oxytocin
NPO
Strict intake and output
Vital signs as indicated
Antiembolic stockings as indicated
Oxygen therapy as indicated
Medications as indicated
Oxytocin infusion as indicated
Vaginal packing as indicated

Nursing diagnoses/goals/interventions

ndx: Actual fluid volume deficit related to postpartum hemorrhage

GOAL: *Patient will receive adequate fluid replacement with no untoward effects and will not have symptoms of hemorrhagic/hypovolemic shock*

Never leave patient unattended during active bleeding
Massage relaxed, boggy fundus until firm; *do not overmassage or push hard on a relaxed fundus*
Administer oxygen at 10 to 12 L/min if ordered
Administer parenteral fluids with oxytocics as ordered
Administer volume expanders or blood as ordered
Check BP, P, and R q15 min until stable, then as ordered
Palpate fundus and observe amount of vaginal bleeding q15 min until stable, then qh for four times, then q8h or according to hospital policy
Maintain NPO status
Measure intake and output
Weigh pads and linens to estimate blood loss
Apply antiembolic stockings to legs to enhance venous return
Maintain warmth with blankets
Allay anxiety as much as possible by remaining with patient and offering simple, brief explanations of care
Be aware that physician may order prostaglandin IM to control atony
Continue with acute care and decrease frequency of nursing functions as patient's condition improves
Observe for side effects of iron therapy if ordered
Reinforce physician's explanation of the following, if done
    Vaginal examination
    Insertion of uterine packing
    D & C

ndx: Alteration in comfort: pain related to uterine massage and uterine contraction

GOAL: *Patient will verbalize decreasing or more tolerable discomfort*

Encourage frequent voiding
Apply ice pack to perineum prn
Promote comfort by frequent position changes
Encourage rest periods between examinations
Provide emotional support, especially if pain medication is contraindicated
Administer medications as ordered by physician and check for any reactions
Explain purpose of frequent postpartum assessments
    Palpation of fundus for height, position, and tone
    Uterine massage if necessary
    Lochia flow
Encourage patient to palpate fundus and learn what good uterine tone feels like
Encourage patient to check fundus periodically and to massage as needed

Minimize other factors that could be contributing to discomfort, such as distended bladder, episiotomy pain, or "afterbirth" pain

ndx: Knowledge deficit regarding postpartum blood loss prevention/precautions

GOAL: *Patient will verbalize symptoms to report and will demonstrate self-care as taught*

Discuss symptoms to report to physician or nurse practitioner
    Passage of large or several clots
    Large amount of bleeding: more than a menstrual period
    Pain
    Foul odor of vaginal drainage
See Postpartum Care (p. 739)
Teach name of medication, dosage, time of administration, purpose, and side effects

Evaluation

Patient demonstrates self-care
Hypovolemic/hemorrhagic shock is avoided
Fluid deficit is replaced
Pain perception is minimized
There are no complications

Newborn

CARE OF NEWBORN

Assessment
Observations/findings
GENERAL

Apgar scores
Quality of cry and respirations
Skin color
Apical pulse and heart rate
Respiratory rate
Muscle tone
Reflexes
Thermal control
Cord condition
Feeding and sucking pattern
Stool pattern
Voiding pattern
Congenital defects

SPECIFIC

Apgar scores
Heart rate; presence of murmur
Respiratory effort
Muscle tone
Reflex irritability
Color
Abnormalities or malformations
Head circumference: normal, 33 to 35 cm
Chest circumference: normal, 30 to 33 cm
Birth-related trauma: presence of caput, cephalohematoma, and forceps marks
Amount of subcutaneous fat
Cry
    Lusty
    Feeble
    High-pitched
    Absent
    Asymmetric facies
Umbilical cord
    Drainage
    Bleeding
    Number and type of vessels
    Presence or absence of Wharton's jelly
Unusually high or low temperature: normal, 97.7° F (36.5° C) axillary
Edema (except for presenting part)
Color
    Jaundice
    Pallor
    Gray, dusky
    Cyanosis
    Plethora
GI system
    Hard and soft palate intact
    Refusal to feed
    Excessive mucus
    Regurgitation; vomiting
    Abdominal distention
    Imperforate anus
    Stools
        Meconium
        Bloody
        Diarrhea
        Absent
Neurologic system
    Moro's reflex: absent or asymmetric
    Sucking reflex: strong or weak
    Rooting reflex: good or poor
    Tremors
    Twitching
    Seizure activity
    Loss of motion of an extremity
State of consciousness
    Sleep states (deep, light)
    Awake (drowsy, quiet alert, active alert, crying)

Respiratory rate: normal, 40 to 60/min
  Tachypnea
  Shallow or periodic breathing
  Nasal flaring
  Retractions
  Expiratory grunt
Cardiovascular rate: normal, 120 to 160 beats/min
  Tachycardia
  Bradycardia
  Blood pressure: normal, 60/30 to 90/50 mm Hg
Musculoskeletal system
  Muscle tone
  Muscle strength
  Limpness
  Weakness
  Rigidity
  Asymmetry
  Swelling of skull or spine
  Abnormal position or posture of extremity
Skin
  Pustules
  Abrasions
  Rash
  Petechiae
  Ecchymosis
  Condition of circumcision
Genitourinary system
  Hypospadias
  Epispadias
  Undescended testicles
  Indeterminate sex
  Failure to void

Laboratory/diagnostic studies

Cord blood samples
Phenylketonuria (PKU; newborn screening examination)
Hct

Potential complications

Altered thermoregulation
Birth injuries
Congenital defects
Need for resuscitation at delivery

Medical management

Vitamin K IM injection
Newborn screening examination (PKU)
Eye prophylaxis
Feeding schedule
Cord care protocol
Chemstrip

Hct
Daily weights
Rectal temperature once, then axillary temperature per protocol

Nursing diagnoses/goals/interventions

ndx: Potential alteration in health maintenance related to normal newborn care

GOAL: *Infant will maintain normal parameters of vital signs and body functions and will be discharged with mother in good condition*

See Figure 14-8
Take apgar scores at 1, 5, and 10 min after delivery
Apply clamp to umbilical cord
Identify infant according to facility policy: bracelet, necklace, and/or footprints
Perform congenital defects screening examination
Assist with infant's warm water bath as indicated (Le-Boyer deliveries)
Show warmed infant to parents; identify sex and check identification bracelets initially and at each visit to mother and at discharge
Allow parents to hold infant as condition of infant and parents permit to promote bonding and family-centered care
Perform the following according to facility policy
  Weigh infant
  Measure length and head circumference
  Administer medication as ordered
    Eye prophylaxis
    Vitamin K therapy
  Do resuscitation documentation
  Do newborn admitting assessment
  Perform cord care
Perform neurologic assessment as indicated
Give sponge bath daily until umbilical cord falls off, then bathe daily, washing hair two to three times per week
Perform neonatal behavioral assessment and share infant responses with parents
Administer circumcision care; apply petrolatum gauze to penis
Perform newborn assessments as required by policy and/or infant condition; particularly note the following
  Note time of first voiding and meconium stool
  Auscultate heart rate qh twice and prn
    Report rate above 180 or below 100 beats/min to physician
    Report heart sounds heard on right side of chest
    Report murmur

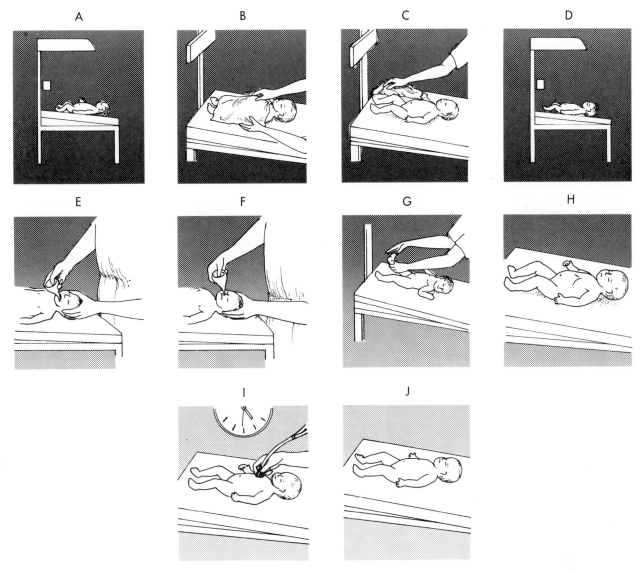

FIGURE 14-8. Immediate stabilization of newborn at delivery—sequence of interventions for assessment at delivery. **A,** Place infant under radiant heat warmer in slight Trendelenburg position. **B,** Dry immediately. **C,** Remove wet linens. **D,** Position infant with head and neck in "sniffing" position. **E and F,** Suction oropharynx, then nasopharynx with bulb syringe as needed. *Not shown:* Suction oropharynx, trachea, and stomach as necessary with 10-French catheter connected to wall suction of 80 to 100 mm Hg per gauge. **G,** Tactile stimulate by slapping twice on sole of foot. **H,** Assess respirations. **I,** Assess heart rate by apical pulse. **J,** Assess color. Resuscitate as indicated by assessment.

Check respiratory rate q30 min for four times and prn

Assess quality of respirations and report if abnormal

Perform heel puncture for blood glucose testing if infant is at risk for hypoglycemia or hypothermia

Provide for sucking needs with pacifier as indicated (be aware that homemade pacifiers are unsafe)

Check rectal temperature one time to determine patency of anus

Administer eye prophylaxis and vitamin K therapy as ordered

Administer sterile water at 4 to 6 hours of age, followed a few minutes later by 5% glucose water, breast-feeding, or formula per facility policy or as ordered

Administer feedings as ordered

Apply alcohol or triple dye to cord according to facility policy; remove cord clamp when cord is dry (usually about 48 hr after birth)

ndx: Potential alteration in body temperature related to immature thermoregulation in newborn

GOAL: *Infant will maintain normal axillary temperature of 97.7° to 98.6°F (36.5° to 37°C)*

Recover mother-baby couple together under radiant heat warmer if possible; otherwise provide neutral thermal environment for infant with warmed blankets, etc.

Observe infant nude, if possible, for 1 to 2 hr postdelivery while maintaining neutral thermal environment

Maintain axillary temperature at 97.7°F (36.5°C); check every 30 min for 2 hr and until stable

Avoid bathing for first hour and until axillary temperature is stable at 97.7°F (36.5°C) and other vital signs are stable

Return to radiant warmer after bath until axillary temperature restabilizes to 97.7°F (36.5°C)

Check axillary temperature daily and as per facility policy

ndx: Potential for ineffective airway clearance related to coordination of suck-swallow-gag reflexes

GOAL: *Infant will maintain patent airway*

Keep bulb syringe in crib at all times; suction prn

Hold infant for feedings: *never prop bottles* (be aware that although demand feedings are preferred, infant may need to be awakened if longer than 4 to 5 hr intervals occur between feedings)

Reposition infant q2h and prn; place on right side or abdomen after feedings for at least 30 min

Perform "football hold" and use obstructed airway maneuvers recommended by American Heart Association as needed for choking

ndx: Potential alteration in parenting related to transition to parenthood

GOAL: *Parents and/or significant other will be able to adjust to new parenting roles*

Avoid separation of mother and infant

Promote acquaintance process between parent and infant

Encourage opportunities for mother to perform infant care as her condition and desires permit

Assist mother in performing all infant care tasks: bathing, feeding, diapering, cord care, cuddling, suctioning, temperature taking, circumcision care

Give positive reinforcement to parents when handling infant

Demonstrate gentle handling of infant, avoiding abrupt or jerking movements

Discuss eye contact at 8 to 10 inches from infant's face for optimal infant vision when performing caretaking tasks and interactions

Identify physical characteristics and behaviors that reflect infant's uniqueness

ndx: Knowledge deficit regarding infant care and role transition to parenthood

GOAL: *Parents and/or significant other will demonstrate adequate caretaking of infant and will demonstrate adjustment to parenting roles*

Teach principles of, demonstrate and have parents return-demonstrate, and document in patient teaching plan
  Infant care: bathing, feeding and burping, diaper change, cord care, circumcision care, temperature taking (rectal and axillary)
  Instructions for formula preparation, pumping and storage of breast milk (p. 747)
Breast/formula feeding
Review
  Importance of dressing according to temperature of day; avoid overheating
  Importance of natural home environment; avoid unnatural quietness and overheating of home
  How to seek assistance for infant problems and concerns of parenthood (e.g., pediatrician's phone number, support groups, etc.)
Discuss conflicts of parental roles
  Idealized versus realistic role of parenting
  Love, resentment, or indifference toward infant
  Personal needs and demands of parenting
Describe how to obtain emergency care if required
Identify abnormal signs and symptoms to report to physician
Jaundice
Fever lasting longer than 24 hr
Infant pulling on ears
Productive cough
Vomiting
Refusal to feed
Diarrhea
Lethargy
See appropriate standard if indicated: Postpartum Care (p. 739); Cesarean Delivery (p. 743); Breast-feeding (p. 747)

Evaluation

Infant achieves and continues health maintenance through discharge

Infant maintains normal axillary temperature in open crib

Infant maintains patent airway

Parents successfully perform infant caretaking skills in transition to parenting roles and have successful transition to parenthood

Parents can demonstrate adequate ability to perform infant caretaking duties

CARE OF PREMATURE INFANT

premature infant *Infant who is born before the end of the thirty-seventh week of gestation*

Observations/findings

Respiratory distress syndrome (p. 773)
    Nasal flaring
    Tachypnea
    Retractions
    Expiratory grunt
Aspiration
Recurrent apnea
Irregular respiratory and cardiac rates
Decreased neonatal heart rate (NHR) variability
Hypoglycemia
    Twitching
    Diaphoresis
    Jitteriness
    Tremors
    Cyanosis
    Lethargy; limpness
    Irregular respiratory rate
    Apnea
    Weak, high-pitched crying
    Convulsions
Difficulty in feeding
Hypocalcemia
Hypothermia
Decreased muscle tone
Weak or absent sucking, swallowing, and gag reflexes
Easily fatigued
Edema

Laboratory/diagnostic studies

Blood glucose monitoring for hypoglycemia
Blood gas monitoring as needed
Blood chemistries as needed
X-ray examinations as needed
Cord blood and placenta saved at delivery for diagnostic tests

Potential complications

Skin breakdown
Jaundice
Neonatal sepsis (p. 765)
Physiologic anemia (third to seventh week)
Iatrogenic anemia
Necrotizing enterocolitis (p. 769)
Congenital defects
Respiratory distress syndrome
Transient tachypnea of newborn (TTN)
Hypovolemic shock
Patent ductus arteriosus (PDA) resulting in congestive heart failure
Poor thermoregulation
Retrolental fibroplasia with oxygen therapy
Meconium aspiration syndrome
Hypoglycemia

Medical management

Gestational age assessment
See Family-Centered Care of High-Risk Infant (p. 779)

Nursing diagnoses/goals/interventions

ndx: Alteration in health maintenance related to delivery of premature infant

GOAL: *Infant will achieve normal parameters of vital signs, weight gain, and body functions, and will be discharged in good condition*

See Care of Newborn (p. 751)

Administer eye prophylaxis and vitamin K therapy as ordered

Conserve infant's energy with planned rest periods and resting after each feeding and procedure

Give sponge bath daily

Clean skin and reapply conductive gels to skin as necessary for electrodes

Use flotation pad or sheepskin

Use pressure diapers to prevent externally rotated and hyperextended hips

Perform gestational age assessment

Administer IM injections with tuberculin syringe and 25-gauge needle into mid-anterior thigh; *do not give injections into buttocks*

Perform heel puncture for Dextrostix or Chemstrip testing q30 to 60 min for 3 hr and prn; if any results are below 45 mg/100 ml, perform immediate blood glucose as ordered

Measure head circumference and length of body weekly

Weigh infant at same time and on same scale daily before feeding

ndx: Alteration in fluids and electrolytes related to water loss and inadequate nutritional replacement

GOAL: *Infant will maintain adequate fluids and electrolytes for growth and weight gain*

Administer parenteral fluids as ordered via peripheral line or umbilical catheterization

Monitor blood gases, electrolytes, and Hct as ordered; monitor amount of blood withdrawn

Initiate oral feedings as ordered (general guidelines follow)
- Encourage mother to provide breast milk for all feedings
- Feed infants under 3 lb q2h to 3h and prn
- Feed infants over 3 lb q3h to 4h and prn
- Do not nipple feed if respiratory rate is above 60 breaths/min
- Use soft preemie nipple
- Provide oral gavage feedings or gavage feedings as ordered, alternating with nipple feedings to prevent tiring; try nipple feeding when infant sucks on gavage tube

Measure intake and output, including passage of stool

Check specific gravity of urine as ordered

Weigh daily

For alterations in parenting, see Family-Centered Care of High-Risk Infant (p. 779)

ndx: Potential ineffective breathing pattern related to prematurity

GOAL: *Infant will not have respiratory distress and will maintain optimal respiratory functioning*

Maintain respiratory and cardiac monitors until infant is stable
- Take apical pulse, counting for a full minute q2h to 4h and prn
- Check respiratory rate q2h and prn

Administer warmed and humidified oxygen by route and percentage as ordered

Chart oxygen concentration q2h and prn

Calibrate oxygen analyzer to room air q8h

Monitor arterial blood gases as ordered

Gently stimulate when apneic by rubbing chest or wiggling leg (connect loose ankle restraint to long piece of gauze and tie to tongue blade outside top hole of incubator)

Reposition q2h; avoid positioning very small infants or those with respiratory distress on abdomen

Maintain head position of incubator or radiant warmer slightly elevated

Diaper or clothe infant as indicated by condition

Provide neutral thermal environment

Maintain axillary temperature at 97.7° F (36.5° C)
- Regulate temperature by skin sensor
- Avoid taking rectal temperatures

Organize nursing functions so that portholes do not have to be opened frequently, causing temperature fluctuations and increasing metabolic rate

ndx: Knowledge deficit regarding role of caring for premature infant

GOAL: *Parents and/or significant other will verbalize understanding through interactive discussion and will successfully demonstrate adequate special infant caretaking skills*

Discuss and identify
- Need to verbalize feelings of emotional unpreparedness for the parenting role
- Need to plan for infant's physical needs, such as crib, clothes, etc., since they may be unprepared because of premature delivery
- Symptoms to report to pediatrician
  - Elevated temperature
  - Yellow skin
  - Poor feeding
  - Vomiting
  - Loose stools
  - Lethargy
  - Productive cough
- Need to dress infant according to temperature of the day
- Need to maintain constant room temperature
- Need to wake infant for every feeding and feed amount of formula ordered
- Need to avoid crowds and persons with infections, especially URIs
- Need to count from due date as birth date in anticipating growth and development patterns
- Need to keep follow-up outpatient care appointments

Teach parents how to take infant's temperature

Explain the following to parents
- Infant receives care in incubator, which simulates uterine environment in providing warmth
- Temperature, oxygen, and humidity are regulated to meet infant's needs
- Infant is not cold, even though unclothed or only diapered; this permits closer observation

Gavage feedings are done until infant is able to suck from a nipple

Disproportionately large head is normal for infant's stage of development

Lanugo will disappear as infant matures

Breast-feeding mothers can manually express breasts to maintain a supply of breast milk; see Breast-feeding (p. 747)

See Care of Newborn (p. 751) and Family-Centered Care of High-Risk Infant (p. 779)

Evaluation

Infant is discharged in good condition as evidenced by appropriate weight gain and stable vital signs

Infant maintains euglycemia, eucalcemia, and normothermia

Infant has an effective and adequate breathing pattern and recovers well from any apneic episodes

Parents can verbalize new knowledge and demonstrate adequate parenting skills

SMALL FOR GESTATIONAL AGE (SMALL FOR DATE, LOW BIRTH WEIGHT, INTRAUTERINE GROWTH RETARDATION, DYSMATURITY)

Infant whose weight and size at birth falls below the tenth percentile of appropriate for gestational age of infant whether delivered at term or earlier than or later than term

Assessment
Observations/findings

Physical characteristics
  Alert; appearance normal
  Cries for and has large capacity for feedings
  Reduced subcutaneous fat
  Loose and dry skin
  Diminished muscular mass, especially over buttocks and cheeks
  Sunken (scaphoid) abdomen
  Thin, yellow, and dry umbilical cord
  Irregular respiratory rate
  Apnea
  Weak, high-pitched cry
  Difficulty in feeding
  Eye rolling
  Tachypnea
  Intercostal retractions
  Expiratory grunt
  Nasal flaring
  Tachycardia
  Twitching
  Jitteriness
  Tremors
  Cyanosis
  Lethargy, limpness
  Convulsions

Laboratory/diagnostic studies

Glucose monitoring
TORCH titers as indicated
Chromosomal studies as indicated
Hct
Electrolyte monitoring
See Care of Premature Infant (p. 755)

Potential complications

Temperature instability
Hypothermia
Meconium aspiration
Respiratory distress
  High oxygen consumption
  Polycythemia
  Plethora
Hyperbilirubinemia
Hypoglycemia
Congenital infections
Chromosomal anomaly
Congenital defects

Medical management

Feeding frequency increased as indicated

Nursing diagnosis/goal/interventions

ndx: Alteration in health maintenance related to small-for-gestational-age infant needs

GOAL: *Optimal health of infant will be promoted, and infant will be discharged in good condition*

See Care of Newborn (p. 751), Care of Premature Infant (p. 755), Family-Centered Care of High-Risk Infant (p. 779), and Large for Gestational Age (p. 758)

Monitor for hypoglycemia and report ≤45 mg% to physician

Monitor electrolytes as ordered

Provide neutral thermal environment; maintain axillary temperatures at 97.7°F (36.5°C)
  Check temperature q15 min until stabilized, then q2h to 4h and prn
  Regulate temperature by skin sensor
  Change sensor site daily and prn

Check apical pulse and respiratory rate q30 to 60 min and prn

Monitor Hgb and Hct as ordered

Initiate feedings with sterile water at 2 to 3 hr of age and follow a few minutes later with formula or glucose water as ordered; feed q3h or as ordered

Do not give formula or glucose water just prior to blood being drawn for testing of blood sugar level

Weigh infant daily unclothed, at same time with same scale

Measure intake and output

Continue with immediate care and decrease frequency of nursing functions as patient's condition improves

Evaluation

Infant is discharged to home in good and stable condition

LARGE FOR GESTATIONAL AGE (DYSMATURITY, HIGH BIRTH WEIGHT)

Neonate whose size and weight at birth fall above the ninetieth percentile of appropriate for gestational age of infant; often born to diabetic mother, multipara, or mother with a genetic predisposition for excessive birth weight

Assessment

Observations/findings

Greater than 9 lb at birth
Birth injuries

Laboratory/diagnostic studies

Blood glucose monitoring
Hgb, Hct
Blood chemistries if indicated
CBC if indicated

Potential complications

Hypoglycemia
  Twitching
  Jitteriness
  Tremors
  Cyanosis
  Lethargy, limpness
  Convulsions
  Irregular respiratory rate
  Apnea
  Weak, high-pitched cry
  Difficulty in feeding
  Eye rolling
  Hyperthermia
Cephalhematoma
Respiratory distress
Polycythemia
Aspiration pneumonia
Erythroblastosis fetalis
Transposition of the great vessels
Brachial paralysis
  Arm abducted
  Internally rotated arm
  Wrist flexed
  Palm limp
  Absence of Moro's reflex on affected side
Fractured clavicle
  Decreased or absent movement of arm
  Overt deformity
  Passive movement of arm produces cries of pain
Phrenic nerve paralysis
  Cyanosis
  Diminished breath sounds
  Labored respirations
  Absence of abdominal bulging on inspiration
  Tachypnea
  Weak cry
Facial paralysis—on affected side
  Asymmetric contour and movement
  Flattened cheek
  Eye open
  Poor suck with drooling on affected side
Neurologic deficit
  Convulsions
  Bulging fontaneles
  Hypotonia or hypertonia
  Hyperreflexia; absence or asymmetry of reflexes
See Postterm Infant (p. 759)

Medical management

Blood glucose monitoring protocol
Gestational age assessment
Feeding schedule

Nursing diagnosis/goal/interventions

ndx: Potential for injury related to birth trauma

GOAL: *Patient will not have unidentified/untreated birth-related injury*

Report symptoms of birth injuries to pediatrician
Document assessment findings on nursing notes and update with changes each shift
Change position side to side q2h and prn
Implement and maintain splints, special diapering, etc., as ordered
See Care of Newborn (p. 751) and Infant of Diabetic Mother (p. 759)

Evaluation

There are no complications

Patient has no unidentified/untreated injuries, no neurologic sequelae, and maintains normal levels of fluids and electrolytes

POSTTERM INFANT (POSTMATURITY)

Infant born after the end of the forty-second week of gestation who has been subjected to placental insufficiency regardless of birth weight

Assessment
Observations/findings

Malnourished appearance
Reduced subcutaneous tissue
Loose, dry skin
Peeling skin, particularly creases and folds
Disproportionate head and chest circumference
Meconium-stained skin
Open-eyed and alert appearance
Absence of vernix caseosa
Deep sole creases over entire foot
Long fingernails
Thick pale skin
Absence of lanugo
Descended testes
Inability to displace cranial bones
Marked flexion of limbs
Neuro check after 24 hr reveals
   Elbow does not reach midline (scarf sign)
   Holds head when pulled up to sit
   May turn head from side to side
   Raises head above back when prone
Intrauterine history of
   Oligohydramnios
   Meconium-stained amniotic fluid, membranes, and umbilical cord

Laboratory/diagnostic studies

Blood glucose monitoring
Blood chemistries as indicated
Blood gases as indicated
Hct, Hgb
Placental/genetic studies

Potential complications

Hypoglycemia
   Twitching
   Jitteriness
   Tremors
   Cyanosis
   Lethargy, limpness
   Irregular respiratory rate; apnea
   Weak, high-pitched cry
   Difficulty in feeding
   Eye rolling
   Hyperthermia
Respiratory distress
Aspiration pneumonia
Meconium aspiration
Hypocalcemia: serum calcium <7 mg/100 ml
   Irritability
   Tachypnea
   Vomiting
Congenital anomalies
   Anencephaly
   Trisomy 16-18
   Seckel's dwarfism
See Large for Gestational Age (p. 758), Small for Gestational Age (p. 757), Meconium Aspiration Syndrome (p. 774), and Respiratory Distress Syndrome (p. 773)

Nursing diagnosis/goal/interventions

ndx: Knowledge deficit regarding mismatched parental expectations of infant

GOAL: *Parents and/or significant other will be able to care for infant's needs*

Share information with parents and/or significant other about
   Peeling skin not harmful to infant
   Importance of keeping fingernails trimmed
   Appetite and nutritional needs despite size or appearance
   Appropriate weight gain, growth, and development
   Importance of regular feedings
See Care of Newborn (p. 751)

Evaluation

There are no complications
Parents demonstrate ability to care for infant

INFANT OF DIABETIC MOTHER (IDM)

Infant has increased risk of illness and death due to uteroplacental insufficiency, respiratory distress syndrome, hypoglycemia, hypocalcemia, hyperbilirubinemia, birth trauma, and congenital anomalies; generally large for gestational age if mother is class A, B, or C diabetic, although infant born to mother with cardiovascular complications and class D, E, F, or R diabetes is usually average or small for gestational age

Assessment

Observations/findings

Macrosomia
Puffy, plethoric facies (tomato face)
Large for gestational age (p. 758)
Intrauterine history of maternal diabetes and polyhydramnios
Murmur related to cardiac defect
Cyanosis related to cardiac defect

Laboratory/diagnostic studies

Blood glucose monitoring
Blood chemistries as indicated
Blood gases as indicated
Hgb, Hct
Blood typing/Coombs' tests

Potential complications

Hypoglycemia
   Twitching
   Jitteriness
   Tremors
   Cyanosis
   Lethargy, limpness
   Seizure activity
   Irregular respiratory rate
   Apnea
   Weak, high-pitched cry
   Difficulty in feeding
   Eye rolling
Hypocalcemia: serum calcium <7 mg/100 ml
   Irritability
   Apnea; tachypnea
   Cyanosis
   Vomiting
Hyperbilirubinemia: jaundice
Hypermagnesemia
Hyperkalemia
Polycythemia
Respiratory distress syndrome (p. 773)
Cephalhematoma
Brachial palsy
Fractured clavicle
Phrenic nerve paralysis
Facial palsy
Prematurity (p. 755)
Congenital anomalies
   Cardiac defects
   Renal anomalies
   Neural tube defects

Medical management

Blood glucose monitoring protocol
Electrolyte monitoring
Total/direct/indirect bilirubin tests as indicated
Blood gases as indicated for respiratory distress
Transcutaneous oxygen or pulse oximeter monitoring as indicated
Parenteral glucose administration through IV, umbilical venous catheter (UVC), or umbilical arterial catheter (UAC) as ordered
Parenteral glucose boluses as indicated by Chemstrip protocol
ECG
Chest x-ray examination as indicated
Gastric aspirate as indicated
Hydrocortizone 5 mg/kg/day IM in two doses if parenteral glucose administration is not effective

Nursing diagnoses/goals/interventions*

ndx: Potential for neurologic sequelae related to altered blood glucose and fluid and electrolytes†

GOAL: *Patient will maintain fluids and electrolytes in normal range and will achieve and maintain euglycemia*

Perform heelstick blood glucose monitoring per facility protocol no less than q30 min twice, then q1h three times; report values below 45 mg/100 ml and do immediate serum glucose test as ordered
Perform blood glucose monitoring prior to administering feedings
Observe for signs and symptoms of respiratory distress
Monitor electrolyte and Hct levels as ordered
Initiate feedings with sterile water at 2 to 3 hr of age, followed a few minutes later by formula or 5% to 10% dextrose water as ordered; follow feeding schedule as ordered
Assess changes in level of consciousness with vital signs q4h and prn
Observe for symptoms of intracranial hemorrhage and seizures
Maintain parenteral glucose administration as ordered; hydrocortizone administration may be ordered if glucose is not effective
Provide neutral thermal environment as indicated
Maintain axillary temperature at 97.7° F (36.5° C)
Administer electrolyte supplements as ordered

---

*See Care of Newborn (p. 751), Large for Gestational Age (p. 758), and Care of Premature Infant (p. 755).
†Not a NANDA-approved nursing diagnosis.

ndx: Knowledge deficit regarding care of infant of diabetic mother

GOAL: *Parents and/or significant other will be able to verbalize symptoms of hypoglycemia in an infant and will be able to meet infant's special needs*

Discuss symptoms of hypoglycemia to report to physician
Teach heelstick glucose monitoring if indicated
Emphasize importance of regular feedings
Emphasize importance of early and good prenatal care for future pregnancies
Teach administration of medications if indicated (include name, dosage, time of administration, purpose, and side effects)
Discuss risk of congenital defects

Evaluation

There are no complications
Patient has no neurologic sequelae
Patient achieves and maintains euglycemia
Parents adequately care for infant and can verbalize an understanding of symptoms of hypoglycemia and implications for future pregnancies

HYPERBILIRUBINEMIA

Elevation of unconjugated serum bilirubin concentration demonstrated by jaundice; due to hemolytic disorders (Rh-ABO incompatibility), infection, enzymatic deficiencies, maternal ingestion of sulfonamides or salicylates, or polycythemia

Assessment
Observations/findings

Jaundice
  Head
  Trunk
  Extremities
  Palms and soles
  Sclera
  Roof of mouth
Pallor
Lethargy
Poor feeding
Dark, concentrated urine
Light stools
Thermal instability
Polycythemia
ABO incompatibility
Rh incompatibility

Laboratory/diagnostic studies

Serum bilirubin, direct and indirect: rising bilirubin levels—above 12 mg/100 ml
Blood typing—mother and infant—cord blood serology
Smear morphology
Direct Coombs' test on infant
Hct
CBC with differential
Reticulocyte count
Serum albumin
Liver function and thyroid tests as indicated
TORCH titers as indicated

Potential complications

Nonphysiologic vs. physiologic jaundice
Breast milk jaundice
Kernicterus
  Depression
    Coma
    Lethargy
    Diminished or absent Moro's reflex
    Hypotonia
    Absent sucking and rooting reflexes
  Excitation (follows depression)
    Twitching
    Generalized seizure activity
    Downward rolling of eyes
    Opisthotonos
    Hypertonia
    High-pitched cry
    Apnea
Hypoglycemia
Sepsis
Respiratory distress

Medical management

Phototherapy
Partial exchange transfusions as indicated
Parenteral and po supplemental fluids

Nursing diagnoses/goals/interventions

ndx: Potential for neurologic sequelae related to toxic bilirubin blood levels*

GOAL: *Patient's bilirubin levels will return to normal*

Administer phototherapy as ordered (see Phototherapy, p. 762)
Measure intake and output; observe urine and stool characteristics

*Not a NANDA-approved nursing diagnosis.

Note and document skin color from head, sclera, and trunk progressively for jaundice at least every shift
Provide neutral thermal environment as needed during phototherapy
Maintain axillary temperature of 97.7° F (36.5° C); avoid cold stress
Monitor vital signs q4h and more often prn for temperature instability
Reposition frequently, at least q2h
Administer feedings as ordered, being conscious of time away from phototherapy
Maintain parenteral fluid therapy as ordered
Observe for abnormal neurologic findings and report to physician
Observe skin color in daylight or under white fluorescent lights
Monitor direct and indirect bilirubin blood levels as ordered
Obtain blood samples with phototherapy lights off for accurate levels
See Exchange Transfusion (p. 763)
See Care of Newborn (p. 751)

ndx: Knowledge deficit regarding altered infant needs

GOAL: *Parents and/or significant other will be able to identify and meet infant's needs*

Emphasize importance of phototherapy regimen and monitoring of bilirubin levels
Emphasize importance of adequate fluid intake and hydration
Explain relationship between breast-feeding and jaundice if infant has physiologic jaundice
Explain need to report diarrhea stools to physician
Emphasize importance of periodic blood chemistries and Hct as ordered
Stress need for follow-up care following hospitalization or home phototherapy
Discuss limit of time out from phototherapy for optimal removal of bilirubin

Evaluation

There are no complications
Parents can verbalize important points of infant care

PHOTOTHERAPY

Blue light therapy decomposes bilirubin by photooxidation

Assessment

Observations/findings

Loose, watery green stools (characteristic)
Lethargy
Skin rash
Priapism
Jaundice
Green urine

Laboratory/diagnostic studies

Bilirubin levels

Potential complications

Dehydration
Hyperthermia
Hypothermia
Apnea
Conjunctivitis

Medical management

Single- or double-light phototherapy with cool white fluorescent lamps
Bilirubin tests repeated as indicated and 4 hr after phototherapy is discontinued

Nursing diagnoses/goals/interventions

ndx: Potential fluid volume deficit related to insensible water loss and dehydration from phototherapy

GOAL: *Patient will maintain adequate hydration and normothermia*

Do not clothe or diaper infant; disposable face mask may be used as "bikini" to prevent excessive skin breakdown potential and soiling, and to minimize unexposed surface area
Maintain neutral thermal environment and axillary temperature at 97.7° F (36.5° C)
Check axillary temperature at least q2h and prn
Avoid exposure of skin temperature probe to phototherapy lights
Weigh infant daily unclothed at same time on same scale before feeding
Offer pacifier prn
Measure accurate intake and output
Check urine specific gravity every shift
Cover *closed* eyelids with eye shields; avoid pressure on nose, allowing maximal light exposure
Maintain parenteral fluid therapy for hydration as ordered
Hold infant during feedings, turn off phototherapy lights, and remove eye shields, keeping track of time not under lights

If holding infant is contraindicated, elevate head, talk to, and stroke infant during and after feedings

Inspect eyes with lights off at least q8h

Change eye pads at least twice a day

Measure distance of lights from infant every shift and maintain at prescribed levels

Use bilimeter to measure footcandles at head, trunk, and foot levels, average together, and document level on nursing shift assessment; if not within prescribed limits, adjust until appropriate

Check lamp use hours and have them changed if greater than 2000 hours for maximum effectiveness

See Hyperbilirubinemia (p. 761) and Care of Newborn (p. 751)

ndx: Alteration in parenting related to disruption of parent-infant interaction for phototherapy

GOAL: *Parent will perform infant care activities as able*

Explain need to provide adequate fluid intake; to offer water between feedings

Discuss signs and symptoms to report to physician
- Recurrence of jaundice
- Persistence of diarrhea
- Emphasize importance of having laboratory tests done as ordered
- Emphasize importance of follow-up outpatient care

Encourage parent participation in infant care activities (feeding, changing soiled linens, etc.)

Review care of infant with hyperbilirubinemia (p. 761) as needed with parents

Permit siblings to visit according to hospital policy

Turn off lights and remove eye shields when parents visit according to time period ordered by physician

Reinforce explanations of phototherapy, reasons for particular interventions, and plan of care

Reinforce limited planned times out from under phototherapy

Designate duties parents can do or assist with

See Care of Newborn (p. 751)

Evaluation

There are no complications
Patient is not dehydrated
Patient's bilirubin levels are returning to normal
Parents are adapting to infant's special needs

EXCHANGE TRANSFUSION

Replacement of 75% to 85% of circulating blood by alternating repeated withdrawal of small amounts of infant's blood and replacing it with equal amounts of donor blood to remove accumulated bilirubin, replace coagulation factors in DIC, and remove antibodies (Rh, ABO) and sensitized red blood cells (RBCs), producing hemolysis of RBCs

Assessment

Observations/findings

Progressively increasing jaundice

Laboratory/diagnostic studies
PRIOR TO PROCEDURE

Bilirubin level
Hgb level and Hct
Blood culture
Calcium level
Random blood glucose test
Donor blood culture
Serum albumin level

AT END OF PROCEDURE (LABORATORY TESTS WITH LAST AMOUNT OF BLOOD REMOVED FROM INFANT AS ORDERED)

Bilirubin level
Calcium level
Random blood sugar test
Hgb level and Hct
Type and hold or type and cross match

Potential complications
DURING PROCEDURE

Bradycardia below 100 beats/min or sudden tachycardia
Cyanosis
Hypothermia
Vomiting
Aspiration
Apnea
Pallor of a limb
Air embolus
Abdominal distention
Sudden hypotension
Cardiac arrest

FOLLOWING PROCEDURE

Tachycardia or bradycardia
Cardiac arrhythmias
Cardiac arrest
Tachypnea or bradypnea
Hypothermia
Lethargy or jitteriness
Increasing jaundice
Dark color of urine

Cyanosis
Edema
Convulsions
Bleeding from cord
Long-term complications
    Hemorrhage
    Heart failure
    Hypocalcemia
    Hypoglycemia
    Sepsis
    Acidosis
    Shock
    Hyperkalemia
    Hypernatremia
    Thrombus formation
    Thrombocytopenia
    Serum hepatitis
    Necrotizing enterocolitis

Medical management

Blood amount (160 ml/kg for two-volume exchange; 25 to 80 ml/kg packed RBCs for partial exchange)
Albumin as indicated
Umbilical catheterization (p. 765)
Permission for parents to attend (unless contraindicated)
Blood warmer (80.6° to 98.6° F [27° to 37° C])

Nursing diagnosis/goal/interventions

ndx: Potential for injury related to exchange transfusion

  GOAL: *Patient will not sustain injury (complications) during or as a result of procedure, and bilirubin levels will return to normal range*

Prior to procedure

Prepare radiant heat warmer, cardiac and respiratory monitors, and pacifier
Maintain NPO status 3 to 4 hr prior to exchange transfusion or aspirate stomach contents prior to procedure
Have resuscitative equipment readily available: oxygen, mask, bag, suction apparatus, and drugs such as sodium bicarbonate, glucose, calcium, and epinephrine
Recheck date of blood, since it should not be more than 48 hr old
Warm blood as ordered
Restrain all four extremities; keep extremities visible to detect any color changes
Assist physician with insertion of umbilical venous line if not already in place
See Umbilical Catheterization (p. 765)
Check laboratory work as ordered
Administer albumin as ordered
Mix blood in amounts as ordered with fresh frozen plasma or plasmanate when fresh whole blood is not used
Place infant under phototherapy lights as ordered
Reinforce parents and/or significant other's understanding of care to be given with primary disease process that necessitates exchange transfusion

During procedure

Note respiratory and cardiac rate q5 min
Check auxillary temperature q15 to 30 min
Suction when necessary
Observe for abnormal behavior or symptoms
Observe all blood tubing connections for integrity periodically
Record amount of blood withdrawn and infused, noting the color
Notify physician when each 100 ml of blood is exchanged

After procedure

Handle infant gently and minimally for 2 to 4 hr
Maintain neutral thermal environment
Monitor respiratory and cardiac rates q15 min for eight times, then q30 to 60 min for 24 to 48 hr or as ordered
Check axillary temperature q1h to 3h for 48 hr
Measure intake and output
Observe cord for bleeding q5 to 15 min for 1 to 2 hr
Perform heel puncture for Dextrostix or Chemstrip testing as ordered until infant feeds or IV therapy is established
Order laboratory tests including blood gases and electrolytes as ordered
Resume feedings 4 to 6 hr after transfusion as ordered
    Ensure adequate intake by using soft nipple with large hole
    Feed slowly or gavage as ordered
Turn and reposition after each feeding
Reinforce physician's explanation of reason for doing exchange transfusion
Encourage parents to see infant after procedure and involve them in as much of infant's care as possible
See Family-Centered Care of High-Risk Infant (p. 779)

Evaluation

There are no complications
Bilirubin levels return to normal range

UMBILICAL CATHETERIZATION

Passage of a radiopaque catheter through one of the umbilical arteries or vein to provide parenteral fluid therapy and/or obtain blood samples or through the umbilical vein for exchange transfusion or emergency administration of drugs, fluids, or volume expanders

Assessment

Observations/findings

Arterial or venous site
IV pump for continuous infusion

Laboratory/diagnostic studies

Chest/abdominal x-ray examination to confirm low or high placement
Hct as indicated
Blood sampling as indicated

Potential complications

Vasospasm
  Blanching or mottling of leg
  Absence of peripheral pulses
  Darkening of legs or toes
Infection at insertion site
  Redness
  Edema
  Drainage
Sepsis
Hemorrhage via connections or oozing from site of insertion
Thromboembolism: progressive cyanosis and blackness of toes; oliguria or anuria
Necrotizing enterocolitis (p. 769)
  Abdominal distention
  Vomiting
Dislodgment of catheter
  Ventricular fibrillation (from electrocution)

Medical management

IV solutions and infusion rate as indicated
Flush solutions as indicated

Nursing diagnosis/goal/interventions

ndx: Potential for injury related to umbilical catheterization

GOAL: *Patient will not experience any injury (complications) related to umbilical catheter*

Validate position of catheter tip by x-ray examination within 1 hr of insertion
Provide neutral thermal environment
Monitor cardiac and respiratory rates qh
Check axillary temperature q2h to 3h
Deliver parenteral fluids by infusion pump
  Note rate of flow qh
  Never permit IV bottle to empty
  Flush solutions as per facility protocol
Check all connections to umbilical line q30 to 60 min
Use only grounded electrical equipment on or near infant
Observe condition of cord q2h to 3h and prn
Retape IV tubing at cord prn per facility policy
If umbilical line is displaced, apply pressure with sterile 4 × 4 inch gauze, and have another person notify physician immediately
Administer cord care as ordered
  Change dressing as ordered
    Apply antibiotic or antiseptic ointment to cord if ordered
Check pedal pulses q2h to 4h and prn
Reposition infant q2h and prn
Reinforce physician's explanation as to reason for umbilical line
Encourage parents to visit nursery and involve them in infant's care as much as possible
Keep running totals of blood losses until replaced by transfusion
Monitor Hct periodically with blood withdrawn qd
Measure intake and output on flow sheet
See Care of Newborn (p. 751) and Family-Centered Care of High-Risk Infant (p. 779)

Evaluation

There are no complications
Solutions are administered as ordered
Blood samples are obtained as ordered
There is no catheter-related infection

NEONATAL SEPSIS

Generalized infection in the newborn, often caused by antepartal or intrapartal asymptomatic maternal infection; acquired postnatal infection is usually due to contact with personnel or contaminated equipment

Assessment

Observations/findings
EARLY SIGNS

Lethargy, especially after first 24 hr
Poor sucking
Anorexia

Regurgitation of feedings
Irritability
Pallor
Hypotonia
Hyporeflexia
Weight loss
Jaundice
Hypothermia
Jitteriness

OTHER SIGNS

Hyperthermia
Grunting
Bradypnea
Apneic spells
Tremors
Seizure activity
Vomiting
Abdominal distention
Dehydration (p. 46)
Cool, clammy skin
Pallor
Cyanosis
Diarrhea
Hypoglycemia
Rashes
Omphalitis
Immediate maternal history: maternal amnionitis and/ or prolonged premature rupture of membranes
Low birth weight
Meconium-stained skin
Birth out of asepsis (BOA)

Laboratory/diagnostic studies

Lumbar puncture
   No. 1 tube: sugar protein
   No. 2 tube: culture and Gram stain
   No. 3 tube: cells and differential
CBC with differential
   Decreased WBC
   Decreased neutrophils
   Platelet count: decreased
Cultures
   Urine by suprapubic tap
   Blood
   Nasopharynx
   Skin lesions
   Gastric aspirate
Maternal blood/amniotic fluid cultures as ordered
Sedimentation rate: increased
Chest x-ray examination

Potential complications

Meconium aspiration syndrome (p. 774)
Pneumonia
Respiratory distress syndrome (p. 773)
Osteomyelitis
Septic arthritis
Overwhelming sepsis
Death

Medical management

Septic workup (obtaining all specimens for diagnosis confirmation)
Antibiotics
Feeding schedule/IV fluids as indicated
Antipyretics as indicated

Nursing diagnoses/goals/interventions

ndx Potential for complications related to neonatal sepsis*

GOAL: *Patient will receive therapy as ordered; repeat cultures after medical treatment will show "no growth" or other complications*

Maintain isolation: isolette care
Turn and position q2h and prn
Observe vital signs q2h, noting changes and reporting to physician as needed
Monitor vital signs with decreasing frequency as condition stabilizes and infant improves
Maintain neutral thermal environment in order to monitor febrile periods
Check axillary temperatures q2h with vital signs
Maintain strict handwashing procedure
Teach handwashing and gowning technique to parents prior to handling infant
Administer oxygen as ordered
Use apnea monitor if indicated
Perform periodic ABGs as ordered
Plan rest periods; avoid unnecessary handling
Give cool sponge baths as indicated
Gently stimulate when apneic by rubbing chest, tapping incubator, or wiggling leg (connect loose ankle restraint to long piece of gauze and tie to tongue blade outside top hole of incubator)
Maintain resuscitation equipment nearby
Observe for focal signs of convulsions
   Suction nose and mouth as necessary
   Turn head to side

---

*Not a NANDA-approved nursing diagnosis.

Protect from banging head against side of incubator or falling from radiant warmer
Give oxygen as necessary
Assist physician with septic workup as indicated
Administer antibiotics as ordered
Reinforce parents and/or significant other's understanding of
    Name of medication, dosage, time of administration, purpose, and side effects
    Importance of ongoing outpatient care
    Symptoms of recurrence to report to physician
See Family-Centered Care of High-Risk Infant (p. 779) and Care of Newborn (p. 751)

ndx: Alteration in nutrition: less than body requirements related to neonatal sepsis

GOAL: *Patient will not lose weight, but will demonstrate a progressive weight gain*

Administer parenteral fluids as ordered
Keep bulb syringe at bedside for emesis/obstructed airway management
Measure intake and output
Urine specific gravity twice per shift
Weigh infant daily
Administer gavage feedings as ordered
Accurately chart infant's activity and feeding behavior
Insert nasogastric tube periodically as necessary to relieve abdominal distention if infant is unable to burp and is nipple feeding
Observe coordination of suck/swallow reflexes with feedings
Provide for sucking needs with pacifier as indicated

Evaluation

There are no complications
Patient's laboratory test values return to normal levels
Patient becomes afebrile
Patient gains weight

INFANTS OF ADDICTED MOTHERS

Withdrawal symptoms usually occur within the first 24 hr of life and are most commonly due to maternal antepartal dependence on heroin, methadone, diazepam (Valium), PCP, cocaine, and alcohol

Assessment
Observations/findings

Muscle tremors
Irritability
Hyperactive reflexes
High-pitched, shrill cry
Increased muscle tone; twitching
Sneezing, nasal stuffiness
Frantic sucking of fists
Regurgitation, vomiting
Frequent yawning
Increased mucus production
Respiratory distress
Restlessness
Inability to sleep
Poor feeding
Uncoordinated sucking and swallowing
Excessive sweating
Increased lacrimation
Elevated temperature
Abrasions of nose and knees
Diarrhea; dehydration
Cyanosis and/or apnea
Pallor
Convulsions
Maternal history of drug/substance abuse
Previous sibling with symptoms of neonatal withdrawal syndrome

Laboratory/diagnostic studies

Positive maternal/neonatal urine toxicology screens
Abnormal BNBAS (Brazelton examination)
Auditory screening examination as ordered

Potential complications

Child abuse
Child neglect
Failure-to-thrive syndrome
Delayed growth and development
Seizures
CNS damage
Respiratory distress: meconium aspiration syndrome (p. 774)
Long-term consequences
    Mental retardation
    Loss of fine motor control
    Poor social/interaction skills
    Abnormal sleep-wake cycles
Difficult foster care requirements

Medical management

Paragoric/phenobarbital therapy as needed
Neonatal Abstinence Scales for assessment of symptoms and drug dosing
Special discharge planning as indicated

Feeding routine
Parent-infant interaction documentation
Police hold as indicated
Social services referral as indicated

Nursing diagnoses/goals/interventions

ndx: Alteration in nutrition: less than body requirements related to neonatal withdrawal symptoms

GOAL: *Patient will have normal weight gain pattern on growth curve chart*

Give small, frequent feedings as ordered
Swaddle in soft warm clothes and blanket for comfort
Suction infant as needed
Monitor vital signs q2h and decrease frequency as patient's condition improves
Weigh infant q12h unclothed, at same time with same scale or as ordered
Administer parenteral fluids as ordered; see Umbilical Catheterization if applicable (p. 765)
Administer medications as ordered: phenobarbitol or paragoric
Offer pacifier prn
Position infant on side or abdomen
Monitor intake and output
Note episodes of diarrhea/loose stools
Note bowel sound hyperactivity with vital signs
Take axillary temperature with vital signs at least q4h and prn

ndx: Potential alteration in level of consciousness related to CNS effects of drugs on infants*

GOAL: *Patient will not have seizures*

Maintain regular assessments on neonatal abstinence scale as available in facility
Maintain administration of anticonvulsive medications as ordered
Allow for routine rest periods as permitted; do not disturb for routine nursing care during sleep
Maintain quiet environment with minimal visual, auditory, and tactile stimulation during peak withdrawal time
Hold infant securely and close to one's own body when handling
Perform BNBAS as offered by facility

ndx: Potential impairment of skin integrity related to frantic muscular activity and diarrhea during withdrawal

---
*Not a NANDA-approved nursing diagnosis.

GOAL: *Patient will have no skin breakdown or will have minimal skin breakdown*

Cover hands with mitts of infant shirt
Administer judicious skin care
  Clean neck folds, ears, etc., after each regurgitation or vomiting, q4h, and prn
  Clean buttocks and perineum after each diarrheal stool and prn
Reapply paste of zinc oxide ointment q2h to 4h and prn to excoriated buttocks with diaper changes
Expose excoriated skin areas to air and/or heat lamp prn
Protect against abrasions of face and bony prominences, such as heels, head, sacrum, knees, and ankles; if flailing, swaddle infant and pad sides of crib
Observe for developing skin lesions due to high incidence of gonococcal and herpes type 2 infection in gravid drug-addicted women

ndx: Potential alteration in parenting related to altered parent-infant interaction secondary to withdrawal syndrome and life-style of parents

GOAL: *Ability of mother to perform infant care duties will be demonstrated; mother and significant other will be able to adequately care for infant*

See Care of Newborn (p. 751)
Encourage mother to become involved in infant's care as soon and as much as possible
Keep mother informed of infant's condition and progress
Be honest and straightforward in answering mother's questions
Avoid getting into arguments with mother should she try to manipulate, accuse, and challenge nursing care
Do everything possible to promote maternal-infant attachment
Assist mother in exploring her own feelings about her relationship with her mother
Avoid situations that promote separation and isolation of mother and infant
Encourage visits and communication with infant's father and/or significant others
Do not force unwanted infant on a mother who cannot cope with her addiction and the responsibilities of motherhood
Involve social service worker and/or visiting nurse in predischarge planning for home care
Ensure that parents and/or significant other demonstrates positive parenting behaviors as related to

bonding and the "taking hold" phase
Holds infant while feeding
Manages routine infant care
Has eye-to-eye contact with infant
Ensure that parents and/or significant other knows and understands
That infant restlessness and irritability may be present during the first few months of life
That narcotics will pass through breast milk and promote infant drug addiction but may also relieve some signs and symptoms of withdrawal
Availability of community resources to assist with parenting, foster care, and drug rehabilitation
Resource phone numbers and name of contact individual if possible
Importance of ongoing treatment
Postpartum care (p. 739)

Evaluation

There are no complications
There is a normal weight gain pattern
There are no uncontrollable seizures
Skin integrity is maintained
Parenting skills are demonstrated by parents and/or significant other

NECROTIZING ENTEROCOLITIS (NEC)

Ischemia of the intestinal tract and invasion of the mucosa with enteric pathogens; occurs most frequently in small and asphyxiated preterm infants, in those with Hirschsprung's disease, after exchange transfusion, or with an aggressive feeding schedule

Assessment

Observations/findings

Onset or increase in amount of feeding residuals
Abdomen
    Distention; increasing circumference
    Increasing bowel sounds
    Skin: shiny, dry, and tender
    Increase in visible vascularity
    Dependent edema
Lethargy
Apnea, bradycardia, or other respiratory distress
Decrease in bowel sounds after prolonged apnea and bradycardia
Pallor
Temperature instability
Vomiting
Increased number of stools: may progress to diarrhea
Blood in stools (hematochezia)

Laboratory/diagnostic studies

Hematest of stools and emesis: occult blood—positive stools and/or gastric contents
Hct: decreased
Platelet count: decreased
Coagulation studies: increased bleeding time
CBC with differential
Radiographic findings
    Dilation of the intestine, progressing to free air in the abdomen following perforation
Blood, stool, and urine cultures as ordered

Potential complications

Sepsis
Hyperbilirubinemia
Shock
DIC
Abscess
Metabolic acidosis
Paralytic ileus
Recurrent bowel obstruction
Hyponatremia
Hyperkalemia

Medical management

Parenteral fluids: hyperalimentation and intralipid therapy
Hematest of stools
Antibiotics
Volume expanders as indicated
NPO initially for 7 to 10 days then slowly progressive feeding schedule
Nasogastric tube to gravity drainage or intermittent low suction as indicated
Oxygen administration as indicated
No rectal temperatures or rectal probes
Abdominal girth measurements q8h and prn
Intake and output
Bowel resection if more conservative measures are unsuccessful

Nursing diagnoses/goals/interventions

ndx: Alteration in nutrition: less than body requirements related to ischemia and malabsorption of intestinal tract

GOAL: *Patient will not lose weight but will resume normal oral feeding schedule after treatment*

Auscultate bowel sounds with vital signs q2h to 3h and prn

Measure accurate intake and output
Measure and record abdominal girth q4h and prn
Take vital signs as indicated by patient condition at least q2h during acute phase and then with decreasing frequency as condition improves
Continue with acute care and decrease frequency of nursing functions as patient's condition improves
Administer parenteral fluids, total parenteral nutrition (TPN), and/or fat emulsion as ordered
Maintain NPO for 7 to 14 days after absence of Hematest-positive stools and abdominal distention
Progress with oral intake as ordered: give one or two feedings of plain water followed by dilute mother's or donor breast milk
Encourage mother to continue to lactate (although infant is NPO during acute phase) and explain importance of breast milk
  Avoid abdominal trauma by application of skin probes and monitor electrodes

ndx: Alteration in bowel elimination related to bowel resection*

GOAL: *Patient will follow normal feeding and weight gain pattern postoperatively*

Perform care as described in Medical Management and as above
Maintain respiratory assistance as needed
Auscultate chest for breath sounds q2h and prn
Observe site of incision for redness, swelling, and drainage
Administer ostomy care (p. 391)
Take axillary temperatures
Avoid any rectal stimulation
Manage pain as ordered
Turn q2h and prn
Change dressings as needed
Administer formula based on infant's intolerance as ordered if breast milk is unavailable
Look for symptoms of protein intolerance—give predigested protein formula as ordered
Look for symptoms of fat and/or sugar intolerance—give monosaccharide, triglyceride formula as ordered

ndx: Knowledge deficit regarding special infant care procedures

GOAL: *Parents and/or significant other will perform infant care duties; patient will be discharged in good condition*

See Care of Newborn (p. 751)
Parent will discuss, verbalize, demonstrate, and return-demonstrate ostomy and incisional care (p. 391)
Discuss symptoms of wound infection to report to physician
Discuss other symptoms to report to physician
  Diarrhea
  Suspected weight loss
  Diet: type, frequency, and amount
  Importance of follow-up outpatient care

Evaluation

There are no complications
There is no significant weight loss
Patient resumes a normal feeding pattern and growth/development
Parents perform all infant care duties

CONGENITAL SYPHILIS

Fetal infection with Treponema pallidum after sixteenth week of gestation, often resulting in a deformed, congenitally afflicted, and premature infant

Assessment
Observations/findings

Edema
  Generalized
  Joints
Severe anemia
Elevated temperature
Poor feeding
Irritability
Copper-colored rash on face, palms, and soles
Red rash
  Perioral area
  Perineal area
Serous nasal discharge
  Snuffles
  Excoriated lips
  Oral fissures
  Hoarseness
Jaundice
Birth history of large, boggy placenta
Positive serology
Spirochetes in drainage
Lymphadenopathy
Hepatosplenomegaly

Laboratory/diagnostic studies

Cultures of any lesions
Cord blood studies as ordered

---

*Resection of necrotic bowel is indicated following bowel perforation and in the infant whose condition rapidly deteriorates.

Rapid plasma reagin (RPR) with titer
FTA-ABS with titer
IgM-FTA-ABS
Elevated cord serum IgM
X-ray examination of long bones for evidence of metaphysical demineralization or periosteal new bone formation
Darkfield examination of any nasal discharge
Lumbar puncture
Maternal
  RPR
  FTA-ABS
  Pathology examination of placenta

Potential complications

Stillbirth
Intrauterine growth retardation
Prematurity
Failure-to-thrive syndrome
Ascites
Unexplained hydrops fetalis
Intractible rash
Hyperbilirubinemia
Anemia
Nephrosis
Meningitis
Delayed effects on nervous system, joints, teeth, and eyes

Medical management

Laboratory tests as indicated
Septic workup as indicated
Lumbar puncture if treatment is indicated by laboratory findings
Antibiotics (penicillin) as indicated

Nursing diagnoses/goals/interventions

ndx: Potential or actual infection related to maternal history of syphilis

GOAL: *Patient will receive adequate treatment for infection*

Maintain isolation of infant in isolette
Maintain isolation technique including rubber gloves
Maintain careful handwashing
Maintain careful disposal of items in contact with cutaneous and mucosal lesions for period of time indicated by infection control guidelines
Check axillary temperature q3h to 4h and prn
Assist physician with obtaining samples from lesions
Administer antibiotics as ordered
Administer eye prophylaxis medication as ordered
Measure intake and output

Keep bulb syringe and suction catheter with mucous trap in crib or readily available at all times
Suction nasopharynx prior to feedings and prn
Use soft nipple with large hole for feedings
Administer gavage feedings as indicated if infant is lethargic; intermittent gavage and nipple feedings may be alternated if ordered
Offer pacifier prn
Change position q1h to 2h and prn
Observe for pressure points; provide skin care prn
See Care of Newborn (p. 751)

ndx: Knowledge deficit regarding isolation due to infection

GOAL: *Family will care for infant's needs*

See Care of Newborn (p. 751)
Explain that specific tests for treponemal antibody may remain positive for years despite adequate therapy
Explain that infant will not be contagious to anyone after adequate therapy
Emphasize importance of follow-up outpatient care, which may include periodic laboratory tests

Evaluation

There are no complications
Patient receives full course of therapeutics as ordered
Parents demonstrate adequate infant care skills

TORCH INFECTIONS

Refers to several infectious agents that can infect fetuses and cause similar congenital malformations or developmental abnormalities: T, toxoplasmosis; O, other; R, rubella; C, cytomegalovirus; H, herpesvirus

Assessment
Observations/findings

Maternal: history of consistent contact with cat feces, poorly cooked infected meats, exposure to rubella or other infectious agents during pregnancy; rashes, oral/genital lesions; multiple blood transfusions during pregnancy; renal transplant patient
Infant
  See Genital Herpes (p. 598)
  Lethargy
  Febrile episodes
  Mottled skin
  Poor feeding
  Seizures
  Vesicular lesions on skin and scalp
  Neurologic involvement

Temperature instability
Hepatosplenomegaly
Diarrhea
Jaundice
Cataracts

Laboratory/diagnostic studies

Serologic tests
  IgM titers: elevated
  Fluorescent antibody testing
Fluid cultures as ordered: abnormal cerebrospinal fluid (CSF) values
Urine screens/cytology as ordered
TORCH antibody screening
Viral cultures for cytomegalovirus (CMV) and herpes
Cultures of lesions as indicated
Abnormal liver function studies
Abnormal coagulation studies

Potential complications

Microcephaly
Hydrocephaly
Cerebral calcifications
Chorioretinitis
Encephalitis
Seizures
Sepsis
Respiratory distress/pneumonia
Prematurity
Hepatitis
DIC
Skin lesions
Congenital blindness
Glaucoma
Cardiac defects
Deafness
Retinopathy

Medical management

Drug therapy as indicated by findings
Isolation as indicated
Other therapy as indicated by infant condition
See Care of Newborn (p. 751) and Care of Premature Infant (p. 755)

Nursing diagnoses/goals/interventions

ndx: Actual infection related to antenatal TORCH exposure

GOAL: *Patient will not develop complications and will be discharged in good condition*

Congenital syphilis
See p. 770

Herpesvirus
PREDELIVERY CARE

Avoid internal fetal monitoring
Avoid frequent vaginal examinations
Prepare for cesarean delivery prior to rupture of membranes or within 4 to 6 hr if membranes have spontaneously ruptured prior to patient's hospital admission—no need to isolate infant if cesarean delivery is done prior to rupture of membranes

POSTDELIVERY CARE

Perform active genital herpes or positive culture cytology for herpes
Place patient in private room per facility policy
Maintain strict handwashing routine
Wear gown and gloves prior to having contact with contaminated area or articles
Double-bag perineal pads and other contaminated waste
Infant can be brought to mother if strict technique is followed
  Supervise mother in handwashing procedure
  Place clean gown on mother
  Assist mother with sitting in chair
  Bring infant to mother
  Do not lay infant on mother's bed
See Neonatal Sepsis (p. 765)

SUSPECTED/AFFECTED INFANT

Isolate infant in nursery per hospital policy
Maintain strict handwashing
Wear gown and gloves prior to contacting contaminated area or articles
Take infant to mother under supervised conditions
Double-bag contaminated articles
Be aware that incubation period for neonatal herpes is 2 to 12 days
Observe infant for symptoms of sepsis, convulsions, and other signs of neurologic involvement

Inactive herpes

Provide routine maternal and neonatal care if mother has no active lesions but a known history of genital herpes
Do not isolate mother or infant

Nongenital herpes present

Isolate mother postdelivery per hospital policy
Isolate newborn *only* after newborn has left nursery to go out to mother

Expedite drying or crusting to reduce virus titer by topical application of ethyl ether, povidone-iodine, or tincture of benzoin as ordered
Follow sequence for infant visitation as described in Active Genital Herpes section
Instruct mother to wear a mask or dressing to cover lesions when performing infant caretaking activities

Nongenital herpes absent

Provide routine maternal and neonatal care
See Care of Newborn (p. 751) and Postpartum Care (p. 739)

ndx: Knowledge deficit regarding infant care and isolation techniques to prevent spread of infection

GOAL: *Parents and/or significant other will verbalize understanding of infant care and isolation techniques through interactive discussion and actual return demonstration*

See Congenital Syphilis (p. 770)
Reinforce physician's teaching and discuss with parents and/or significant other
   Implications for infant's future growth and development
   Incidence of complications
   Maintenance of therapy
   Importance of regular follow-up
   Isolation practices
   Infant care duties
See Care of Newborn (p. 751) and Care of Premature Infant (p. 739)

Evaluation

There are no complications
Infant is discharged in good condition
There is no spread of infection
Parents and/or significant other can perform infant care duties

RESPIRATORY DISTRESS SYNDROME (HYALINE MEMBRANE DISEASE)

Condition of decreased pulmonary gas exchange producing retention of carbon dioxide usually due to deficiency of surfactant in immature lungs

Assessment

Observations/findings

Tachypnea >60 respirations/min
Nasal flaring
Expiratory grunt
Cyanosis
Pallor
Absence of and/or abnormal breath sounds
Retractions: intercostal, suprasternal, substernal
Seesaw breathing
Hypothermia
Skin pale or ashen
Pitting edema of hands or feet
Hypoactive, flaccid, or motionless
White, frothy mucus in respiratory tract
Fatigue
Bradycardia or tachycardia
Jaundice
Hypotension: mean BP, 35 to 40 mm Hg

Laboratory/diagnostic studies

Chest x-ray examination
Blood gas sampling
Oxygen saturation values by pulse oximeter
Transcutaneous oxygen/CO_2 monitor readings
CBC with differential
Coagulation studies
Hgb/Hct
Blood chemistries as ordered

Potential complications

Mechanical ventilation
Respiratory infection/pneumonia
Hyperbilirubinemia (p. 761)
Shock
Alveolar rupture
Intracranial hemorrhage
Patent ductus arteriosus
Long term
   Bronchopulmonary dysplasia (p. 777)
   Retrolental fibroplasia
   Neurologic impairment
   Altered parent-infant relationship (bonding and attachment)

Medical management

Supplemental oxygen therapy as indicated
Mechanical ventilation as necessary
Ventilator support: q2h with ventilator setting changes and prn
Hood oxygen 40% to 50% q4h and prn with changes
Incubator oxygen: q8h and prn
Continuous positive airway pressure (CPAP) as required
Neutral thermal environment
IV fluids as indicated
Antibiotics as indicated

Sodium bicarbonate for documented metabolic acidosis
Strict intake and output

Nursing diagnosis/goal/interventions

ndx Ineffective breathing pattern related to respiratory distress syndrome

GOAL: *Patient will not have metabolic acidosis but will have adequate ventilation to keep blood gas values within normal limits*

Provide neutral thermal environment
Maintain axillary temperature of 97.7° F (36.5° C); regulate temperature by skin sensor
Position with head slightly hyperextended
Reposition q2h
Administer warmed and humidified oxygen as ordered
Have resuscitative equipment available at all times: oxygen, suction, bagging apparatus, drugs
Maintain on respiratory and cardiac monitors; note rates and variability 60 min and prn
Maintain ventilatory support as ordered
Auscultate chest for breath sounds q1h to 2h and prn
Suction q2h and prn
Perform postural drainage and percussion as ordered
Maintain umbilical arterial and/or venous line; see Umbilical Catheterization (p. 765)
Administer parenteral fluids as ordered
Administer sodium bicarbonate as ordered; never give undiluted
Monitor electrolytes, Hct, and glucose as ordered
Perform blood gas determinations as ordered
Administer antibiotics as ordered
Analyze oxygen q2h and before drawing blood gases, correlate with O_2 saturation and/or transcutaneous O_2/CO_2 monitors
Check blender setting for oxygen concentration q2h and prn
Calibrate oxygen analyzer q8h
Measure intake and assess output as indicated
Omit normal hygiene at times
  Plan care to allow for rest periods
  Avoid exhausting infant
Discuss with parents and/or significant others and document
  General use of monitoring and life-support equipment and any postdischarge sequelae
  Parenting skills
  Infant caretaking skills
See Care of Newborn (p. 751), Care of Premature Infant (p. 755), and Care of Newborn on a Ventilator (p. 776)

Evaluation

There are no complications
Blood gas values are corrected and maintained within normal range
Respiratory distress is resolved

MECONIUM ASPIRATION SYNDROME

Fetal hypoxia frequently causes relaxation of the anal sphincter, passage of meconium, and gasping respiratory efforts, resulting in meconium aspiration; suspected in a meconium-stained neonate, postmature infant, or an infant large or small for gestational age

Assessment

Observations/findings

Respiratory distress
  Tachypnea
  Tachycardia
  Nasal flaring
  Pallor
  Dusky
  Cyanosis
  Expiratory grunt
  Retractions
Meconium-stained gastric aspirate; fingernails and/or skin; umbilical cord
Rotund appearance of chest and/or abdomen
Palpable liver
Meconium in amniotic fluid
Meconium visualized below vocal cords

Laboratory/diagnostic studies

Chest x-ray examination shows hyperinflation (within hours of delivery)
Serum glucose levels
Hct
Blood gas analysis
Cultures as indicated

Potential complications

See Respiratory Distress Syndrome (p. 773)

Medical management

See Respiratory Distress Syndrome (p. 773)

Nursing diagnosis/goal/interventions

ndx Ineffective airway clearance related to meconium aspiration

GOAL: *Patient will have all meconium removed from airway, and respiratory distress/infection will not develop*

At delivery, suction meconium-colored fluid from oral and nasopharynx with DeLee mucous trap or wall suction after head is delivered, prior to delivery of shoulders

After delivery of infant and cord is clamped, take infant to radiant warmer and assist with intubation to visualize vocal cords for suction of meconium *before* initial stimulation and breaths are taken

Follow immediate stabilization of newborn at delivery procedure (Figure 14-8)

Resuscitate as indicated by assessment

Empty stomach of meconium and mucus by suctioning with DeLee mucous trap or wall suction to 80 mm Hg and 10 French catheter

Provide ventilatory support as ordered (can range from supplemental oxygen to full mechanical respirator support)

Perform postural drainage and percussion q2h to 6h as ordered; position to promote maximum drainage from affected area

Change position at least q2h and prn

Administer antibiotics as ordered

Assist with x-ray examination as ordered

See Respiratory Distress Syndrome (p. 773) for other routine care, Care of Newborn on a Ventilator (p. 776), and Care of Newborn with Endotracheal Tube (p. 775)

Evaluation

There are no complications

Patient does not develop respiratory infection and does not have respiratory distress

CARE OF NEWBORN WITH ENDOTRACHEAL TUBE

Assessment

Observations/findings

Entire or partial expulsion of tube
Loose tape securing tube
Disconnected or loose adapter on endotracheal tube
Obstruction of tube
  Kink in tube or in adapter on tube
  Increased retractions
  Uneven chest excursion
  Sucking of tube
  Coughing
  Restlessness
  Cyanosis
  Mucous plug
Pressure areas on nares or side of mouth near endotracheal tube

Laboratory/diagnostic studies

Abnormal arterial or capillary blood gas values

Potential complications

Respiratory infections
Unintended extubation
Airway obstruction
Skin breakdown
Long term complications
  Tracheal stenosis
  Abnormal oral-motor development
  Inhibition of normal reflexes of sucking/feeding

Medical management

See Respiratory Distress Syndrome (p. 773), Care of Newborn on a Ventilator (p. 776), and Meconium Aspiration Syndrome (p. 774)

Nursing diagnosis/goal/interventions

ndx Potential for ineffective airway clearance related to endotracheal intubation

GOAL: *Patient will maintain a patent, functioning airway*

Observe position of tube q30 min and prn
Maintain patency
  Check for kinks in tube or adapter prn
  Suction q2h and prn—¼ cm beyond end of endotracheal tube
  Check connections qh and prn
Resecure tube with tape prn
Measure length of exposed tube q2h and prn
Measure suction catheter to extend just beyond end of endotracheal tube
Provide oral care of shift and prn
When suctioning
  Hyperoxygenate with 15% more oxygen than infant is receiving for 1 min before (2 min for dusky infant) and during suctioning
  Instill 0.2 to 0.5 ml normal saline solution into endotracheal tube before suctioning
  Allow two to three mechanical or manual breaths to distribute solution down tube
  Insert suction catheter to carina (meets resistance), re-

move 0.5 cm, note demarcation line on suction catheter for future suctioning, and suction no longer than 5 sec; twirl catheter as removing if holes on catheter are not alternated
Auscultate breath sounds after suctioning for effect and potential extubation
Take extreme care not to dislodge tube when repositioning
Maintain tube in anatomically correct alignment with trachea
Maintain nasogastric tube as ordered

Evaluation

There are no complications
Patent airway is maintained

CARE OF NEWBORN ON A VENTILATOR

Assessment
Observations/findings

Newborn
 Restlessness
 Audible cry
 Rapid onset of cyanosis
 Excessive sucking
 Excessive mucus from mouth or nose
 Gasping respirations
 Absent or abnormal breath sounds
 Tachycardia or bradycardia
 Tachypnea or bradypnea
 Apnea
 Gastric distention
Ventilator
 Rise or fall in peak pressure on pressure gauge
 Fall in positive end expiratory pressure (PEEP)
 Low fluid level in nebulizer or humidifier
 Condensation in tubing

Laboratory/diagnostic studies

Periodic blood gas analysis to monitor adequate ventilation
Transillumination of chest wall for pneumothorax
See Respiratory Distress Syndrome (p. 773)

Potential complications

Pneumothorax
 Rapid general deterioration
 Cyanosis
 Shift of apical impulse
 Unequal percussion sounds
 Asymmetric thorax
Bronchiopulmonary dysplasia
See Respiratory Distress Syndrome (p. 773)

Medical management
Ventilator settings: FIO_2, PIP/PEEP, IMV, or CPAP
See Respiratory Distress Syndrome (p. 773)

Nursing diagnosis/goal/interventions

ndx: Potential for ineffective breathing pattern related to mechanical ventilation therapy

GOAL: *Patient will maintain a patent airway and will be weaned from ventilator support*

Maintain care of nasal prongs (CPAP)
 Change nasal prongs/sponge q24h
 Clean internal and external nares with applicator prn
 Clean nasal prongs prn
 Check nasal prongs q2h and prn for patency
 Suction nose gently when prongs are removed for checking
 Maintain orogastric tube at all times
 Lubricate prongs prior to insertion with antibiotic or steroid ointment as ordered
Maintain care of mask assembly (CPAP)
 Alternate mask sizes q2h; massage reddened skin areas q30 min if unable to alternate mask size
 Apply gentle massage to reddened skin areas q2h and prn
 Keep nasogastric tube inserted at all times
Maintain care of endotracheal tube (p. 775)
Maintain patient on cardiac monitor at all times
Auscultate chest for breath sounds q1h to 2h, before and after suctioning, and prn
Record respiratory and cardiac rates qh during acute phase, decreasing frequency as patient's condition improves
Observe pressure reading q30 min
Record responses to changes in oxygen concentration and ventilator settings
Check all connections for security qh
Drain condensation in tubing prn
Maintain excess ventilator tubing within warmed environment
Administer oxygen as ordered; analyze oxygen q2h
Monitor blood gases as ordered
Calibrate oxygen analyzer q8h
Refill nebulizer or humidifier prn
Reposition infant q2h and prn
 Take extreme care not to dislodge endotracheal tube

Maintain endotracheal tube in anatomically correct position with trachea
Protect infant's skin from contact with ventilator tubing frame
Maintain nasogastric or orogastric tube as ordered for gastric distention
Change oxygen tubing and equipment q24h to 48h to prevent gram-negative rods ("waterbugs")
Have syringe and butterfly needle with three-way stopcock in-between readily available for physician to use in event pneumothorax occurs (emergency aspiration of pneumothorax)
Have bag and mask immediately available at all times
Suction q2h and prn; see Care of Newborn with Endotracheal Tube (p. 775)
Perform postural drainage and percussion as ordered; avoid for at least 1 hr after feedings
Place infant with head raised 15 to 30 degrees during and after feedings
Restrain arms; pin soft arm restraints to diaper if necessary
Administer parenteral fluids and medications as ordered
Share information with family as appropriate

Evaluation

There are no complications
Patent airway is maintained
Ventilator support is discontinued

BRONCHOPULMONARY DYSPLASIA

Chronic lung condition with obstructive bronchiolitis, hyperinfiltration, and pulmonary fibrosis secondary to treatment for respiratory distress syndrome, including high oxygen concentrations delivered by positive pressure ventilation

Assessment

Observations/findings

Tachycardia
Respiratory distress
Cyanosis
Difficult weaning from oxygen and/or ventilator
Tachypnea
Retractions
Grunting, nasal flaring increasing with activity
Diminished breath sounds
Crepitant rales
Difficult maintenance of oxygenation during and after suctioning procedures
Repeated episodes of respiratory infections
Poor weight gain per growth chart

Laboratory/diagnostic studies

Confirmation by chest x-ray findings of hyperaeration, enlarged heart, and chronic lung disease changes
Blood chemistries for fluid/electrolyte imbalances
Urine specific gravities every shift
Arterial/capillary blood gases
Routine Hgb, Hct

Potential complications

Frequent upper and lower respiratory infections
Developmental lags
Failure to thrive syndrome
Congestive heart failure
Cor pulmonale
Chronic hypertension
Hypercapnea
Retrolental fibroplasia

Medical management

Antibiotics for respiratory infections
Diuretics for fluid balance as indicated
Nasogastric or gastrostomy feedings for nutrition
Antihypertensives as indicated
Bronchodilators as indicated
Vitamins as indicated
Electrolyte supplements as indicated
Oxygen as indicated
Mechanical ventilation as indicated (early weaning from an endotracheal tube and low peak inspiratory pressures for ventilation can be expected to decrease complications and improve outcome)
Sedatives as indicated
Anticonvulsants as indicated

Nursing diagnoses/goals/interventions

ndx Ineffective breathing pattern related to chronic lung disease

GOAL: *Patient's blood gas values will remain within specific limits (specify), and respiratory assessment findings will remain within specific limits (specify)*

Monitor vital signs as ordered
Space interventions to promote maximum respiratory efficiency
Plan daily routine to promote rest periods
Avoid sensory stimuli during planned rest periods
Elevate head of bed 20 to 30 degrees
Use infant seat at 30 to 45 degrees intermittently with bed rest

Maintain oxygen therapy as ordered
Perform oral/nasal/endotracheal tube suctioning prn for secretions
Perform chest percussion prior to suctioning prn
Administer brochodilators as ordered
Monitor theophylline levels and bring nontherapeutic levels to physician's attention

ndx: Alteration in nutrition: potential for more or less than body requirements related to poor intake or fluid retention

GOAL: *Patient will maintain weight gain of 15 to 30 g/day; weight loss will be avoided, and fluid retention or overload will not occur*

Provide orogastric, nasogastric, or gastrostomy feedings as ordered; progress from continuous to bolus feedings is desirable
Provide caloric supplements as ordered
Weigh daily or q12h as ordered
Maintain po intake to specified calories/kg/day and document on flow sheet as indicated
Auscultate lungs for "wet" rales with vital signs at least q4h and with decreasing frequency as condition stabilizes
Observe parent-infant interactions for feeding assessment and document in nursing notes
Monitor intake and output
Observe and document emesis, stool descriptions, and other output
Measure urine specific gravity every shift—done before diuretics are given

ndx: Potential impairment of skin integrity related to diarrhea and pharmacotherapeutics

GOAL: *Patient will not have perineal area skin breakdown*

Monitor amount of stool and note amount and description of stool on flow sheet
Monitor perineal skin condition with initial assessment at least every shift and prn with diaper changes
Give good skin cleansing with diaper changes
Apply topical ointments as ordered
Use heat lamp at 18 inches and with area open to air for 30 min q4h or more as time allows; 30 min qh is maximum for heat lamp
Report multiple episodes of diarrhea to physician
Test stool pH and blood once each shift
Monitor administration of bronchodilators and antibiotics

ndx: Knowledge deficit regarding prolonged hospitalization and respiratory support required for infant

GOAL: *Parents and/or significant other will understand about infant needs and will become progressively involved in caretaking activities*

Discuss long-term follow-up needs of infant
Emphasize importance of maintaining oxygen therapy if ordered by physician
Explain that infant is more susceptible to URIs and discuss when to report to physician
Teach administration of oxygen and medications
Teach suctioning of infant
Discuss special feeding needs
Teach infant stimulation
Provide infant cardiopulmonary resuscitation training
See Care of Newborn (p. 751), Care of Premature Infant (p. 755), and Care of Newborn on a Ventilator (p. 776)

Evaluation

Patient has achieved and maintains adequate oxygenation
Patient maintains an acceptable weight gain without compromising respiratory status
Patient does not have perineal skin breakdown
Parents feel comfortable in giving care for infant

INTERMITTENT GAVAGE FEEDING

Feeding via a tube passed into the stomach through the nose or mouth; for infant with weak sucking, uncoordinated suck and swallow, respiratory distress and/or respiratory rate above 60/min, repeated apneic spells, or fatigue in sucking on "preemie" nipple (inadequate oral intake)

Assessment

Observations/findings

Cyanosis
Choking
Gagging
Spitting
Regurgitation
Vomiting
Rate of flow: excessively slow or fast
Large amount of residual for size of neonate

Potential complications

Aspiration of formula
Insertion of gavage tube into trachea
Tissue trauma with poor ingestion technique

Nursing diagnosis/goal/interventions

ndx: Alteration in nutrition: less than body requirements related to inadequate nipple-feeding intake

GOAL: *Infant will gain weight and will receive adequate Kcal/kg/day*

Use 8 French feeding tube (5 to 6 French if infant is very small)
Place infant with head raised 15 to 30 degrees during feeding and on right side or abdomen after feeding
Hold infant during feeding by mother (or nurse) if possible
Restrain only if necessary
Measure tube length before insertion from tip of nose to earlobe to xiphoid process; mark with a small piece of tape before insertion
Check placement of tube
  Place end of tube in water; will bubble with expiration if misplaced in respiratory tract
  Aspirate; evaluate contents, return to stomach or discard, and record gastric residual as ordered
  Subtract residual amount from feeding as ordered; feeding may be skipped if residual is over amount specified by physician
  If no residual, instill air into stomach and auscultate stomach for air sounds
Hold syringe 6 to 8 inches above infant's head
Initiate flow with slight pressure on plunger; gravity flow is preferred (remove plunger)
Feed infant slowly; stroke skin during feeding
Offer pacifier during feeding to promote gravity flow, calm infant, and reinforce relationship of sucking and full stomach
Do not allow air to enter stomach when feeding is complete; immediately pinch off and withdraw tubing when feeding is complete
Burp gently by rubbing or patting back
Turn head to right side after feeding or position infant on right side
Avoid postural drainage and percussion for at least 1 hr after feeding
Indicate the following on nursing care plan
  Amount and type of feeding
  Size of catheter
  Time of feeding
See Family-Centered Care of High-Risk Infant (p. 779)
Discuss the following with parents and/or significant other
  Explanation of need for gavage feedings
  That nipple feedings may be resumed when infant shows signs of the following
    Sucking on gavage tube and/or pacifier
    Rooting actively
    Good suck and swallow coordination
    Effort does not outweigh caloric intake in nipple feeding
    Not tiring when nipple feeding
    Gaining weight in excess of 3 lb
    Respiratory rate below 60/min
See appropriate standard of care, depending on infant's condition: Care of Premature Infant (p. 755), Respiratory Distress Syndrome (p. 773), or Care of High-Risk Infant (p. 779)

Evaluation

Infant receives adequate nutrition for weight gain, growth, and development
Complications are avoided

FAMILY-CENTERED CARE OF HIGH-RISK INFANT

Philosophy and interventions promoting bonding and attachment, and a method of assessing parent-infant interaction in helping to provide individualized, need-specific parent teaching and continuity of care

Assessment
Observations/findings

Sensory deprivation of newborn and parents
Anticipatory grief and emotional separation

Laboratory/diagnostic studies

Parent-infant interaction scales
Nursing Child Assessment Satellite Training (NCAST) assessment tools*
BNBAS (Brazelton) assessment scale

Potential complications

Poor parenting/infant care skills of caretakers
Lack of bonding and noninitiation of attachment process
Long-term complications
  Child abuse and/or neglect
  Poor growth and development

Medical management

Interdisciplinary team conferences
Patient care rounds
Parent-infant interaction documentation
Social services consult
Specific discharge planning needs

---

*NCAST Program, University of Washington, CDMRC RES-110-WJ10, Seattle, Washington 91895.

Nursing diagnosis/goal/interventions

ndx: Potential alteration in parenting related to birth of high-risk neonate

GOAL: *Parents will participate as able in infant care and will demonstrate appropriate interactions and parenting skills*

Explain to parents what infant looks like and what equipment they will see prior to visiting nursery
Have mother visit nursery and visually examine and touch infant before 12 hr of age
Encourage parents' questions and explain equipment usage
Involve parents in infant's care as much as possible
At mother's or parent's visit to nursery, do the following
    Welcome parent by name
    Personalize comments about infant's status
    Tell mother that she is mothering better than the nurses, since she is able to become involved in infant's care
    Leave a note in infant's incubator or crib, such as "Hi Mom, I've been waiting to see you" at least daily as appropriate
    Encourage mother to come back to nursery soon, that it is important for her infant to get to know her
Play radio with soft music in nursery prn
Place decals outside incubator on adjacent walls
Hang mobiles within viewing distance of infant
Encourage parents to bring in brightly colored toys or music box for their infant
Assign same nurse each shift if possible
Provide infant with experiences similar to those of normal infants, including sound, touch, and smell of primary caretaker
Talk to infant during nursing care procedures
Offer pacifier prn when infant does not tire from sucking
Respond to infant's crying
Stroke infant's head and chest; hold arm or leg during nursing procedures
Hold and cuddle infant close to body as soon as able
Promote eye contact between mother and infant by repositioning infant to face mother; for infants receiving phototherapy, turn lights off and remove eye patches when mother visits
Allow siblings to view infant through nursery window if feasible
Ascertain what parents think is going to happen to infant and reinforce physician's explanation of care plan and prognosis at parents' pace and level of understanding
Maintain records of parents' visits and phone calls
    Report to physician fewer than two phone calls or visits weekly
    Call parents when appropriate
For parents who have been physically and/or emotionally separated from their infant
    Provide private room close to nursery nursing staff for mother to spend 1 to 2 hr daily for 2 or 3 days with infant prior to discharge
    Provide mother with supplies to feed and bathe infant and assure her that she will not be disturbed unless she calls for assistance
Help parents anticipate equipment and time required and caretaker's physical ability to cope with infant's needs well in advance of discharge
Refer to Visiting Nurse's Association as indicated for predischarge and/or postdischarge home visit
See Care of Newborn (p. 751) and Care of Premature Infant (p. 755)

Evaluation

There are no complications
Parents demonstrate appropriate infant interaction and caretaking skills

15 Chapter

Pediatrics

Basic Standards of Care

INFANT AGE-GROUP CARE

Usual age: 1 month to 1 year
Placement: with infants or toddlers according to diagnosis

Hygiene

Give complete bed bath daily
Change diaper prn with diaper area care: soap and water wash, careful drying
Use Desitin or A & D ointment prn
Administer hair care
Give shampoo q3 days and prn
Trim nails prn
Clean outer ear gently qod

Sleep

Sleep 16 to 18 hr daily
Take morning and afternoon nap

Diet and fluids

Institute intake and output sheet
Know fluid requirement: 120 to 150 ml/kg daily
Know calorie requirement: 115 kcal/kg daily
Give appropriate diet for age
  1 to 3 months
    20 kcal/oz formula or breast-feeding
  3 to 6 months
    20 kcal/oz formula or breast-feeding
    Diluted juices ad lib
    Introduce foods in following order
      Cereal and fruit
      Yellow vegetables
      Green vegetables
      Meat
      Mixed puree dinners
  6 to 9 months
    Formula: 20 kcal/oz three times daily and at bedtime or breast-feeding
    Juices ad lib
    Solids: all purees by spoon three times daily
    Begin adding junior foods and cup training
  9 to 12 months
    20 kcal/oz formula three times daily and at bedtime or breast-feeding
    Solids: all chopped table foods by spoon three times daily
    Begin adding table foods; increase cup training

Elimination

Record and describe all stools on intake and output sheet
  1 week to 3 months: approximately q3h to 8h
  3 months to 1 year: approximately one to three times daily
Record urinary output on intake and output sheet
  Record amount if measured
  Record "wet" if not measured
  Average urinary output
    10 to 20 ml/hr
    240 to 500 ml daily

Activity

Hold for bottle and solid feeding; many leave bottle with infant when able to hold
Provide high chair for meals when able to sit
Provide toys for visual, auditory, and developmental stimulation
Encourage activity appropriate for age

Emotional development

Respond to infant's expressed needs for warmth, physical contact, comfort, and social playtime
Bundle for sleep and nap time
Involve parents in infant's care as much as possible
Comfort infant when mother leaves, if distressed

Environmental safety

Keep side rails up at all times
Keep bed free of loose linen and absorbent pads
Allow no toys with sharp edges and points
Allow no pillows

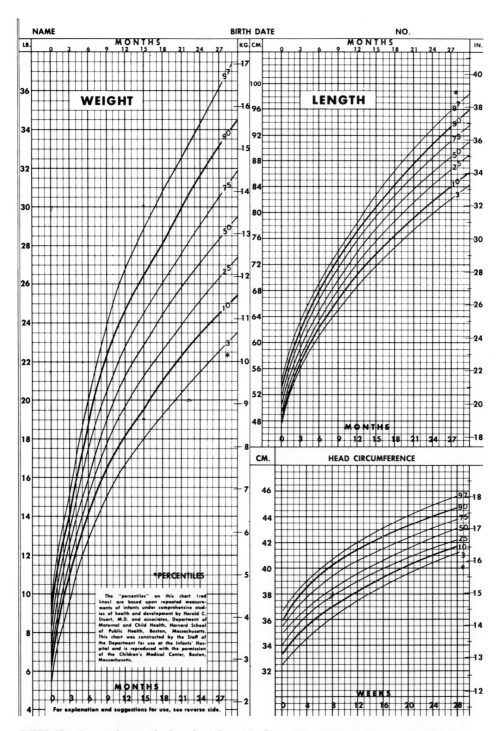

FIGURE 15-1. Percentile growth chart for infant girls. (From The Children's Hospital Medical Center, Boston, Mass. Reprinted by permission.)

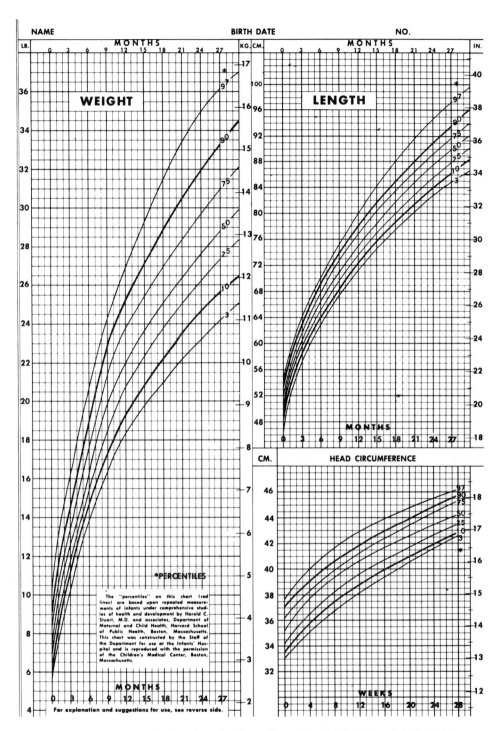

FIGURE 15-2. Percentile growth chart for infant boys. (From The Children's Hospital Medical Center, Boston, Mass. Reprinted by permission.)

TODDLER AGE-GROUP CARE

Usual age: 1 to 3 years
Placement: with infants and toddlers according to diagnosis

Hygiene

Give complete bed or tub bath daily
Initiate dental care in older toddlers
Not toilet trained
  Change diaper prn with diaper area care: soap and water wash, careful drying
  Use Desitin or A & D ointment prn
Toilet trained
  Do not use diapers
  Follow toilet training schedule as done at home
Administer hair care prn
Clean outer ears gently qod
Use pillow if desired
No top covers on bed during day; cover with blanket at nap and bedtime

Sleep

Sleep 13 hr daily
Take morning and afternoon nap (1 hr each or 2 hr afternoon nap)

Diet and fluids

Know fluid requirement: 90 to 120 ml/kg daily
Know calorie requirement: approximately 1300 kcal
Give appropriate diet for age
  1 year to 18 months
    Junior foods to finger foods, gradual introduction to regular diet
    Avoid carrot sticks, nuts, etc.
    Milk and juices by cup
  18 months to 3 years
    Regular table food, all fluids by cup
    Avoid carrot sticks, nuts, etc.

Elimination

Record and describe all stools: usual frequency, one to two times daily
Record urinary output if on intake and output
  Average urinary output
    20 to 25 ml/hr
    500 to 600 ml daily

Activity

Allow free movement in crib when possible
Understand that toddler overestimates ability to perform safely
Do not leave younger toddlers unsupervised in chairs, etc.
Apply restraints as necessary

Emotional development

Be aware of dual stage of development: feelings of autonomy vs. dependence
Encourage child to do those things he can do safely for himself; be prepared to do for him or comfort him when he needs to be dependent
Do not reinforce normal negativism
Involve parents in care as much as possible
Comfort child when mother leaves
Protect favorite toy or blanket

Environmental safety

Keep side rails up at all times
Prevent climbing over side rails with canopy-type crib or overbed net
Allow no toys with sharp edges and points

PRESCHOOL-AGE CHILD CARE

Usual age: 3 to 6 years
Placement: with preschool age or older children, according to diagnosis

Hygiene

AM care
  Give complete bed or tub bath daily
  Administer hair care
  Shampoo weekly and prn
  Administer nail care
  Administer mouth care: including teeth brushing
HS care
  Wash face and hands
  Brush teeth
  Wash hands after using bathroom
  Place top covers on bed; pillow may be used

Sleep

Sleep 11 to 13 hr nightly
Take 2 hr afternoon nap

Diet and fluids

Know fluid requirement: 90 to 120 ml/kg daily
Know calorie requirement: approximately 1000 kcal daily
Understand that need for calorie intake decreases as growth rate increases—may have periods of disinterest in food
Maintain regular diet

Cut up and prepare food; allow child to feed himself
Understand that child will eat better if portions are smaller and meal is presented one item at a time
Measure intake and output when indicated by diagnosis

Elimination

Record and describe all stools: usual frequency, once daily
Record urinary output if on intake and output
    Average urinary output
        20 to 40 ml/hr
        600 to 1000 ml daily
    May still be bed-wetting; *do not chastise*

Activity

Understand that this is a period of great need for physical activity
Allow child to sit up and ambulate as much as condition allows
Involve child in care and planning as much as possible
Provide diversionary activities

Emotional development

Understand that child likes playing with other children
Understand that child needs to feel in some control of environment
Understand that child likes music and familiar stories
Understand that child needs repetitive, simple explanation for reassurance
Explain procedures honestly just prior to performance
Involve parents in care as much as possible

Environmental safety

Be aware that child is more coordinated, but over-estimates abilities
Keep side rails up
Be aware that child is capable of putting away toys—takes pride in straightening up
Sit only in low chairs

SCHOOL-AGE CHILD CARE

Usual age: 6 to 12 years
Placement: with other school-age children according to diagnosis

Hygiene

AM care
    Give complete bed bath daily (tub or shower when feasible)—self-care advisable
    Administer hair care
    Shampoo weekly and prn
    Administer mouth care, including teeth brushing
    Administer back care, if on bed rest
HS care
    Wash face and hands
    Brush teeth
    Administer back care, if on bed rest
    Wash hands after using bathroom
    Place top covers on bed; pillow(s) may be used

Sleep

Sleep 8 to 10 hr at night
Maintain quiet rest period in afternoon—need not sleep

Diet and fluids

Know fluid requirement: 60 to 90 ml/kg daily
Know calorie requirement: 2100 to 2500 kcal daily
Maintain regular diet
Understand that food likes and dislikes are highly developed
Discourage between-meal snacks if not eating meals well
Understand that child is self-sufficient in preparing own food
Offer food choices whenever possible

Elimination

Record and describe all stools: usual frequency, once daily
Record urinary output if on intake and output
    Average urinary output
        30 to 50 ml/hr
        900 to 1200 ml daily

Activity

Encourage intellectual pursuits, schoolwork
Understand that child is well-coordinated and more safety conscious
May ambulate freely, bed in low position, and side rails down during the day

Emotional development

Involve child in planning care
Give child careful explanation of events with adequate time to prepare himself emotionally
Accept occasional lapses into dependence; encourage gradual return to independence
Be aware that time awareness is good
Understand that child enjoys group and competitive play

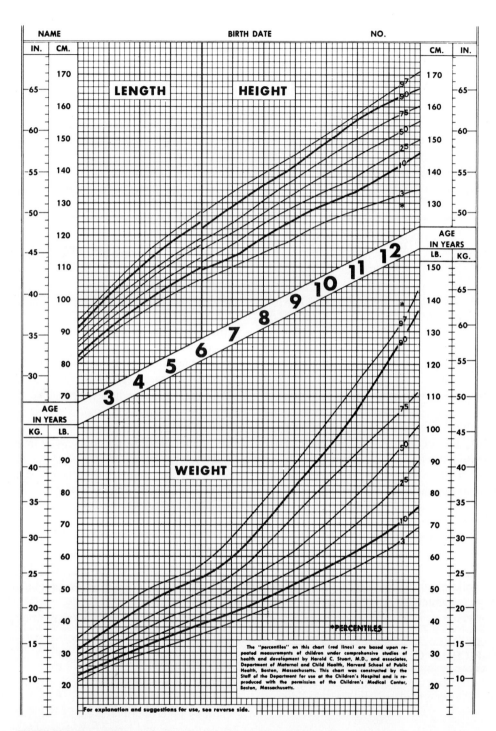

FIGURE 15-3. Percentile growth chart for girls. (From The Children's Hospital Medical Center, Boston, Mass. Reprinted by permission.)

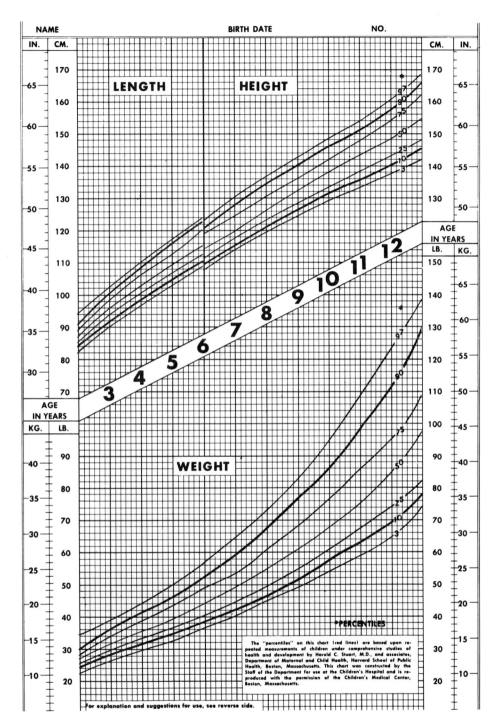

FIGURE 15-4. Percentile growth chart for boys. (From The Children's Hospital Medical Center, Boston, Mass. Reprinted by permission.)

Be aware that child is modest and proud
　Do not cause embarrassment or feeling of inferiority
　Respect modesty
　Keep covered and screened when necessary
Understand that child's concept of himself is important
　Do not tease, belittle, or compare him unfavorably with other children
　Be aware that he may engage in belittling other children to build his own ego
Understand child's need to control environment
Give responsibility for child's own immediate environment and belongings

Environment

Be aware that child is more conscious of environment outside room; allow child to explore and become oriented to remainder of unit when possible

ADOLESCENT AGE-GROUP CARE

Usual age: 12 to 18 years
Placement: with other adolescents, according to diagnosis

Hygiene

AM care
　Give complete bath: bed, self-care, tub, or shower
　Administer hair care
　Shampoo as desired
　Administer mouth care, including teeth brushing
　Administer back care
　Administer perineal care
HS care
　Wash face and hands
　Brush teeth
　Offer back rub
　Place top covers on bed; pillow(s) may be used

Sleep

Sleep 8 hr at night
Maintain quiet rest period in afternoon if desired

Diet and fluids

Know fluid requirement: 60 to 90 ml/kg daily
Know calorie requirement: 2500 to 3000 kcal daily
Maintain regular diet
Understand that increased need for calories is related to increasing growth rate
May need double portions
Serve frequent between-meal and bedtime snacks
Offer food choices whenever possible

Elimination

Record and describe all stools; usual frequency, daily or qod
Record urinary output if on intake and output
　Average urinary output
　　50 to 70 ml/hr
　　1200 to 1680 ml daily

Activity

Encourage intellectual pursuits, schoolwork
Ambulate freely with bed in low position and side rail down during day

Emotional development

Understand that adolescent considers himself adult
Understand that adolescent must have adequate explanation and involvement in planning care
Be aware that involvement with peers is of utmost importance
Understand that adolescent needs accepting attitude concerning appearance and teenage behavior
Understand that adolescent wants nurse to be an understanding adult who sets good example
Accept labile mood swings; adolescent may swing between being communicative and noncommunicative, cheerful and depressed, sensitive and cruel, etc.

Environment

Be aware of need for control of environment
Give responsibility for adolescent's own immediate environment and belongings
Do not be compulsive

Respiratory System

CROUP: LARYNGOTRACHEOBRONCHITIS

An acute viral (predominantly parainfluenza virus) infection of the larynx, trachea, and bronchi, which results in varying degrees of respiratory tract obstruction

Usual age: infant or toddler; most common in males
Seasonal occurrence: fall/winter

Assessment
Observations/findings
See Respiratory Assessment (p. 219)
Restlessness
Apprehension
Cyanosis
Nasal flaring

Retractions (suprasternal, substernal, intercostal)
Audible inspiratory stridor
Cough (brassy or barking character) with history of worsening at night
Hoarse voice
Tachypnea
Ausculated stridor, bilateral decreased breath sounds
Rhonchi, rales
Increasing tachycardia
Low-grade fever
History of cold for 1 to 2 days

Laboratory/diagnostic studies

X-ray examination (lateral neck) to rule out foreign body
White blood cell count (WBC): usually normal
Blood cultures: negative

Potential complications

Complete laryngeal obstruction
Secondary bacterial infection causing pneumonia, bronchiolitis, otitis media, or epiglottitis

Medical management

Cool, highly humidified environment with oxygen via mist tent
Racemic epinephrine via nebulizer for severe respiratory distress
Cardiac monitor
Vital signs qh with acute symptoms to include pulse rate and respiratory assessment; temperature q4h and prn
NPO if in acute distress
Parenteral fluids
Corticosteroids IV (use is controversial)
Antipyretics prn for fever
Endotracheal intubation (or tracheostomy) with laryngeal obstruction

Nursing diagnoses/goals/interventions

ndx: Ineffective breathing pattern related to inflammation and swelling of the trachea, larynx, and bronchi

GOAL: *Patient will have clear breath sounds and age-appropriate respiratory rate prior to discharge*

Monitor vital signs with respiratory assessment as ordered and prn
Maintain cool, moist, oxygenated environment via mist tent
Initiate oxygen as ordered or prn for respiratory distress
Allow patient to assume position of comfort when possible
Elevate head of bed
Use nebulized mist inhaler with racemic epinephrine as ordered
Administer antiinflammatory drugs if ordered
Keep endotracheal intubation (ET) or tracheostomy equipment at bedside and assist with intubation procedure if necessary (ET size approximately that of patient's pinky finger)

ndx: Anxiety related to air hunger, hospitalization, and separation from parents

GOAL: *Child will experience a nonstressful environment that promotes normal respiratory patterns and normal child-parent relationships*

Provide nonstressful environment
  Postpone routine care while respiratory distress is severe
  Bed rest
  Allow parents to participate in child's care and encourage rooming-in
  Alleviate parental anxiety by explaining
    Need for cool, moist environment
    Need for undisturbed rest
    Precautionary reasons for emergency intubation equipment at the bedside
    That their anxiety is transmitted to their child; therefore it is imperative that they remain calm
  Allow parents to play with child in mist tent when necessary
  Provide age-appropriate play activities as child's condition improves

ndx: Potential fluid volume deficit related to insensible loss in the presence of fever, hyperventilation, and inability to tolerate fluids po

GOAL: *Patient will remain hydrated and will be able to tolerate age-appropriate fluid volume po*

Maintain NPO status in the presence of respiratory distress and administer maintenance fluids parenterally as ordered
Record intake and output and monitor specific gravity
As respiratory status improves, urge fluids as tolerated (assess child's likes and dislikes and use of bottle vs. cup)
Give lukewarm clear liquids because they are tolerated best
Provide cooling measures prn and administer antipyretics as ordered

TABLE 15-1. Childhood Diseases

Disease	Causative agents	Transmission	Incubation	Communicability	Observations
Rubella (German measles)	Rubella virus	Droplet or direct contact with infected persons or articles freshly contaminated with nasopharyngeal secretions, feces, or urine	14-21 days after exposure	7 days before to 5 days after rash appears	Low-grade fever, headache, lymphadenopathy (postauricular and cervical), malaise, conjunctivitis, anorexia, sore throat, rash (maculopapular exanthema, generalized) Duration 3-5 days
Congenital rubella	Rubella virus	Transplacental during first trimester of pregnancy	Virus only dangerous to fetus	Infants may be infectious for months	Any combination possible—growth retardation, mental retardation, microcephaly, deafness, cataracts, strabismus, retinopathy, congenital heart disease, thrombocytopenic purpura, behavioral abnormalities
Rubeola (measles)	Measles virus	Direct contact with droplets	10-20 days	4 days before to 5 days after rash appears	Fear, malaise, coryza, cough, conjunctivitis, Koplik's spots (small red spots with bluish white center seen on buccal mucosa opposite molars), lymphadenopathy, rash (maculopapular, erythema followed by desquamation)
Roseola infantum (exanthema subitum)	Presumably virus	Unknown; occurs between 6 mo and 2 yr	Unknown	Unknown	Fever of 104°-105° F (40°-40.5° C) for up to 3-4 days, anorexia, irritability, rash (maculopapular appearing when fever suddenly drops)
Chickenpox (varicella)	Varicella-zoster	Highly communicable via direct contact, indirect contact, droplet spread, airborne	14-21 days after exposure	Onset of fever until last vesicle is dried (5-7 days)	Malaise, fever, rash (macule to papule to vesicle)—appears first on head and mucous membranes, then concentrates on body, sparse on extremities, severe itching
Whooping cough (pertussis)	*Bordetella pertussis*	Direct contact, droplet spread, indirect contact with contaminated articles	5-21 days	7 days after exposure to 3 weeks after onset of paroxysms	See Pertussis: Whooping Cough (p. 795)

Complications	Treatment	Ongoing care	Prevention
In adolescent and adults: arthritis, encephalitis, purpura	Symptomatic: antipyretics, analgesics	Prevent exposure of nonimmune pregnant women in first trimester; provide comfort measures as necessary	12 mo or older: rubella vaccine or in combination with measles and mumps
As pertains to defect present	As pertains to defect present	Strict isolation of neonates with rubella until throat culture is free of virus; select nursing personnel who are not at risk for rubella infection; provide care as pertains to defect present	Determination of rubella titer and administration of rubella vaccine to women before pregnancy occurs
Otitis media, pneumonia, laryngitis, mastoiditis, encephalitis	Bed rest, antipyretics, vaporizer, antibiotics may be necessary	Isolate from onset of inflammation of mucous membranes through fifth day of rash; provide cooling measures for fever, especially if prone to seizures; dim lights if photophobia is present; cleanse eyelids with warm saline solution, prevent rubbing of eyes; maintain skin cleanliness with tepid baths; encourage fluids and soft, bland foods	15 mo: measles vaccine; may be in combination with mumps and rubella vaccine
Convulsions due to high fever	Symptomatic: antipyretics	Control high fever with cooling measures—tepid baths, antipyretics	None
Rare in normal children; encephalitis, pneumonia, bacterial skin infection possible; Reye's syndrome; severe when contracted by immunosuppressed individuals; scarring from scratching	Symptomatic: antipyretics, antihistamines for itch	Isolate until all lesions have crusted (5-7 days); prevent scratching—apply mitts, pat lesions with mixture of baking soda and warm water, keep fingernails short and clean; skin care—daily bath, change clothes and linens daily	No active immunization available; for high-risk susceptible children VZIG should be given within 72 hr of exposure; may modify varicella
Pneumonia, atelectasis, emphysema	See Pertussis: Whooping Cough (p. 795)	See Pertussis: Whooping Cough (p. 795)	DTP (diphtheria-tetanus-pertussis) at 2 mo, 4 mo, 6 mo, 18 mo, 4-6 yr

Continued.

TABLE 15-1. Childhood Diseases—cont'd

Disease	Causative agents	Transmission	Incubation	Communicability	Observations
Diphtheria	*Corynebacterium diphtheriae*	Direct contact with infected person, carrier, or contaminated articles	2-5 days	Variable: until bacilli are no longer present (three negative cultures)—usually 2 wk, may be up to 4 wk	Mucopurulent nasal discharge, malaise, anorexia, sore throat, tachycardia, low-grade fever, white or gray membrane in pharynx, hoarseness, apprehension, cyanosis
Mumps	Mumps virus	Direct contact with droplet or droplet spread	14-21 days	7 days before to 9 days after swelling appears	Headache, anorexia, malaise, fever, parotid gland swelling
Scarlet fever (scarlatina)	Group A β-hemolytic streptococci	Direct contact or droplet, indirect contact with contaminated articles, or ingestion of contaminated food	2-4 days	Approximately 10 days; may persist for months	High fever, tachycardia, vomiting, headache, chills, malaise, abdominal pain, enlarged tonsils, red strawberry tongue, red pinhead-sized lesions becoming generalized with flushed face followed by desquamation
Tetanus	*Clostridium tetani*	Direct or indirect contact with wound	3 days to 3 weeks	None	Stiffening of striated muscles; usually jaw, spastic rigidity
Poliomyelitis	Enterovirus	Direct contact via fecal-oral and pharyngeal routes	7-14 days	In throat—1 week after onset; in stool—4-6 weeks after onset	Headache, lethargy, anorexia, vomiting, fever, muscle pain and stiffness; CNS—loss of deep tendon reflexes, positive Kernig's and Brudzinki's signs, weakening of muscles and paralysis

ndx: Knowledge deficit regarding home care needs

GOAL: *Parents and/or significant other will demonstrate understanding of home care and follow-up instructions through interactive discussion*

Discuss diet
Explain need to encourage fluids
Discuss symptoms of recurrence to report to physician
   Increasingly labored respirations
   Poor appetite
   Restlessness
   Increasing, persistent stridor
   Fever
Explain that normal course of disease is worse at night, with improvement during waking hours
Discuss use of cool vaporizer at nap and bedtime
Teach cooling measures

Complications	Treatment	Ongoing care	Prevention
Toxemia, septic shock, airway obstruction, myocarditis, neuritis	Antitoxin, antibiotics, complete bed rest, respiratory support, tracheostomy as necessary	Strict isolation until two to three cultures are negative; maintain bed rest; observe for signs of respiratory obstruction; suction prn; provide humidified air	DTP (diphtheria-tetanus-pertussis) at 2 mo, 4 mo, 6 mo, 18 mo, 4-6 yr
Meningoencephalitis, deafness, orchitis (after puberty)	Symptomatic: analgesics, antipyretics, parenteral fluids if refuses to drink	Isolation; encourage fluids and soft, bland foods; apply warm compresses to neck; maintain bed rest; observe for neurologic symptoms	15 mo: mumps vaccine, usually with measles and rubella
Glomerulonephritis, rheumatic fever	Antibiotics: usually penicillin, analgesics, bed rest	Isolate until 24 hr after initiating therapy; maintain bed rest; relieve sore throat; encourage fluids and soft diet	None available
Laryngospasms, asphyxia	Antibiotics, debridement of wound, tetanus antitoxin	Suction; minimize spasticity with medication and quiet, dark room; administer adequate fluid and nutrition—parenteral fluids, tube feeding; supply respiratory support as necessary	Tetanus vaccine (usually with diptheria and pertussis) at 2 mo, 4 mo, 6 mo, 18 mo, 4-6 yr
Respiratory paralysis, hypertension	Supportive: analgesics, bed rest, respiratory support as necessary	Enteric isolation; maintain bed rest; administer physical therapy; administer sedation as necessary; maintain body alignment; observe for respiratory paralysis	TOPV (trivalent oral-polio vaccine) at 2 mo, 4 mo, 18 mo, 4-6 yr

Teach name of medication, dosage, time of administration, purpose, and side effects

Evaluation

Breath sounds are clear at rest
Respiratory rate is age appropriate
Parent-child relationship is promoted
Prehospitalization diet is tolerated
Parents state understanding of disease, treatment, and home care needs

EPIGLOTTITIS

A severe, rapidly progressing infection of the epiglottis and surrounding areas; most commonly associated with Haemophilus influenzae but may result from other bacteria or virus

Usual age: 2 to 7 years; most common in males
Seasonal occurrence: none

Assessment

Observations/findings

Rapid onset and progression of respiratory difficulty within several hours
Sore throat; dysphagia
Drooling
Hoarseness or aphonia
Inspiratory stridor
Tachypnea
Retractions (suprasternal, substernal, intercostal)
Bilateral, decreased breath sounds
Rhonchi
Pallor or cyanosis
Increasing tachycardia
Restlessness
Disorientation
Lethargy
Fever greater than 101.3° F (38.5° C)

Laboratory/diagnostic studies

WBC: usually elevated
Chest x-ray examination for differential diagnosis
Throat culture to isolate organism (only done *after* intubation)

Potential complications

Respiratory arrest
Septicemia

Medical management

Laryngoscopy to visualize the epiglottis (characteristically edematous and cherry red)
Endotracheal intubation or tracheostomy
Throat culture obtained after an airway has been established
Cool, highly humidified environment with oxygen
Postural drainage to mobilize copious secretions
Cardiac monitor
Vital signs qh with acute symptoms to include pulse rate and respiratory assessment; temperature q4h and prn
NPO
Maintenance parenteral fluids
Antibiotic therapy
Corticosteroid therapy
Antipyretics prn for fever

Nursing diagnoses/goals/interventions

ndx: Ineffective airway clearance related to edema, copious secretions, and altered anatomic structure of airway (endotracheal tube)

GOAL: *Patient will have a patent airway and clear breath sounds with an age-appropriate respiratory rate prior to discharge; color will be pink*

Recognize signs and symptoms of epiglottitis (see observations above) and assist with establishing an artificial airway immediately (have three endotracheal tubes ready: size that approximates size of patient's pinky finger, one larger, and one smaller)
Maintain intubation (p. 272)
Maintain a patent airway with postural drainage and tracheal suctioning as ordered
Maintain cool, moist, oxygenated environment
Initiate oxygen as ordered or prn for respiratory distress
Monitor vital signs with respiratory assessment qh and prn for signs of respiratory difficulty (tachycardia, tachypnea, retractions, restlessness, cyanosis)
Postpone routine care while respiratory distress is severe
Allow child to assume position of comfort: usually high-Fowler's position
Administer antiinflammatory drugs if ordered
Administer antibiotic therapy as ordered
Implement measures to reduce anxiety
  Have parents participate in the care of their child
  Keep child and parents informed and explain all procedures

ndx: Potential fluid volume deficit related to insensible loss in the presence of fever, hyperventilation, inability to tolerate fluids po and/or NPO status

GOAL: *Patient will remain hydrated and will be able to tolerate age-appropriate fluid volume po prior to discharge*

Maintain NPO while intubated
Administer maintenance parenteral fluids as ordered
Record intake and output and specific gravity
Administer antipyretic therapy as ordered
Anticipate beginning oral fluids after extubation
Resume age-appropriate diet as tolerated

ndx: Knowledge deficit regarding home care needs

GOAL: *Parents and/or significant other will demonstrate understanding of follow-up instructions through interactive discussion*

Discuss diet
Explain need to encourage fluids
Teach fever management

Explain that epiglottitis rarely recurs
Teach name of medication, dosage, purpose, time of administration, and side effects

Evaluation

Extubation occurs after 36 hr
Patient's airway is patent with clear breath sounds and age-appropriate respiratory rate
Prehospitalization diet is resumed
Parents understand home care needs

PERTUSSIS: WHOOPING COUGH

An acute infection of the respiratory tract caused by Bordetella pertussis and characterized by a series of repeated spasmodic coughs ending in forced, prolonged inspiration (the "whoop") and vomiting

Usual age: nonimmunized children under 4 years
Seasonal occurrence: spring and summer
Strict isolation: highly contagious and transmitted by direct contact, droplet spread, or indirectly from freshly contaminated articles

Assessment

Observations/findings

See Respiratory Assessment (p. 219)
1- to 2-week history of upper respiratory infection (URI) symptoms (catarrhal stage)
Worsening of cough to spasmodic episodes followed by vomiting (paroxysmal stage)
    Paroxysms of coughing
    Frequency usually increasing to several times an hour
    Coughing followed by vomiting of thick mucus
    Degree of respiratory distress during a spasm, particularly color change during spasm (bright red face or cyanotic)
Nutritional assessment
    Calorie intake
    Nutritional state
    Weight loss
    Dehydration (p. 866)

Laboratory/diagnostic studies

WBC: elevated
Nasopharyngeal swab or sputum sample to isolate *Bordetella*

Potential complications

Pneumonia, atelectasis, emphysema, otitis media
Respiratory arrest
Neurologic complications: seizures from anoxia; intracranial hemorrhages
Nutritional deficit: weight loss, dehydration from excessive vomiting
Hernia
Prolapsed rectum

Medical management

Oxygen for dyspnea and cyanosis following paroxysms
Cool, humidified environment via mist tent
Gentle suctioning prn to clear airway of thick mucus
Parenteral fluids when vomiting is severe enough to cause nutritional deficit
Antibiotics
Pertussis immune globulin (sometimes recommended in children less than 2 years of age)
Emergency intubation in the event of severely decreased oxygenation

Nursing diagnoses/goals/interventions

ndx: Ineffective airway clearance related to thick pulmonary secretions

GOAL: *Child's airway will remain patent and clear of mucus, and child will be supported during paroxysms to prevent complications related to anoxia*

Place child in a room amenable to close observation
Be in attendance during all paroxysms to provide a calm, reassuring environment
Monitor vital signs q2h and prn
Assess respiratory status during and immediately following a coughing episode: color, respiratory rate, nasal flaring, retractions, breath sounds
Assess child's ability to clear secretions on own
Use gentle suction prn to keep airway clear (bulb suctioning is preferred, since deep nasopharyngeal suctioning can aggravate spasms)
Administer humidified oxygen prn for cyanosis
Maintain cool, humidified environment via mist tent
Elevate head of bed
Reduce child's exposure to smoke, dust, temperature changes, and excessive excitement, since they may precipitate a coughing episode
Keep child occupied with age-appropriate, quiet activities (preoccupation is associated with fewer paroxysms)

ndx: Potential fluid volume deficit related to excessive vomiting

GOAL: *Patient will be able to tolerate age-appropriate fluid volume (p. 866) and will maintain weight*

Offer small, frequent volumes of clear liquids after a coughing/vomiting episode
Offer fluids child likes via appropriate method (cup vs. bottle)
Weigh child daily
Administer parenteral fluids if ordered

ndx: Potential alteration in nutrition: less than body requirements related to excessive vomiting

GOAL: *Patient will tolerate an age-appropriate diet reflecting appropriate caloric requirements and will maintain weight*

Calculate caloric requirements for age and weight (p. 866)
Ensure feedings of 20 kcal/oz formula or milk, despite episodes of vomiting
  Offer small, frequent feedings after a coughing/vomiting episode
  Offer items high in calories (items child likes)
  If feeding is vomited, prevent aspiration by suctioning prn
  Allow child to rest briefly, then refeed

ndx: Knowledge deficit regarding home care needs and disease process

GOAL: *Parents and/or significant other will be able to state and demonstrate how to support their child during paroxysms and will state that they feel comfortable caring for their child at home*

Teach parents about stages of disease process (catarrhal stage, paroxysms stage, convalescent stage)
Explain that coughing paroxysms will continue in less severe form for several weeks after discharge
Teach parents and have them demonstrate techniques to support infant during paroxysms
Have parents demonstrate use of bulb syringe in clearing nasal and oral passages of secretions
Explain importance of refeeding if vomiting occurs
Explain need to maintain good nutritional diet
Explain need to weigh child frequently to ensure adequate hydration and nutrition
Teach name of medication, dosage, time of administration, purpose, and side effects
Emphasize need for follow-up care
Emphasize that child should avoid contact with other susceptible children
Explain to parents that the most effective treatment is prevention with the pertussis vaccine (ensure that other children are immunized)
Reassure parents that disease will not recur, because a single attack gives lifetime immunity

Evaluation

Paroxysms have decreased in severity and frequency
No complications related to anoxia have occurred
Weight is maintained
Child remains hydrated and well nourished
Parents demonstrate care of child during paroxysms
Parents state they feel comfortable caring for their child at home

PNEUMONIA

An inflammatory process of the lungs classified by the area involved or causative agent

Types or areas involved	Causative agents
Lobar	Bacterial
Bronchopneumonia	Viral
Interstitial	Mycoplasma
Bronchiolitis	Aspiration
Bilateral	Chemical
Right upper lobe (RUL)	Hypostatic
Right middle lobe (RML)	
Right lower lobe (RLL)	
Left upper lobe (LUL)	
Left lower lobe (LLL)	

NOTE: Nursing care is based on degree of respiratory distress and age of patient rather than on type of pneumonia

Usual age: any
Placement: respiratory isolation with staphylococcal pneumonia until treated for 48 hr with antibiotics

Assessment
Observations/findings

See Respiratory Assessment (p. 219)
Signs and symptoms of respiratory distress
  Cyanosis
  Nasal flaring
  Retractions
  Tachypnea
  Tachycardia
  Restlessness
  Malaise

Quality and frequency of cough
Sputum production
Color and character of sputum
Chest pain in older children
Auscultated rales, rhonchi, decreased breath sounds
Fever
Anorexia
Vomiting
Abdominal pain
Abdominal distention
Nutritional assessment

Laboratory/diagnostic studies

WBC: very elevated with bacterial pneumonia; slightly elevated with viral pneumonia
Nasopharynx, throat, and blood culture to isolate organism
Blood gases
Sputum culture when possible
Chest x-ray examination to localize area of infiltration, rule out pleural effusion and empyema, and locate pneumatoceles if staphylococcal pneumonia
Blood and urine for countercurrent immunoelectrophoresis (CIE) to detect specific bacterial antigens

Potential complications

Pleural effusion (with pneumococcus or group A streptococcus)
Empyema (with *Hemophilus influenzae* or staphylococcus)
Otitis media
Meningitis
Pericarditis
Septicemia
Respiratory arrest

Medical management

Vital signs q2h and prn with respiratory assessment
Oxygenated, cool, humidified environment
Chest physiotherapy and suctioning q2h to 4h
Parenteral fluids
Antipyretic therapy prn for fever control
Antibiotic therapy for bacterial pneumonia: penicillin G (pneumococcal and streptococcal pneumonia); methicillin (staphylococcal pneumonia)

Nursing diagnoses/goals/interventions

ndx Ineffective airway clearance related to thick mucous production in lungs and ineffective cough

GOAL: *Patient will have a patent airway, clear breath sounds, and age-appropriate respiratory rate prior to discharge*

Vital signs q2h to 4h
Initiate humidified oxygen as ordered or prn for respiratory distress via age-appropriate method (mist tent, nasal prongs, mask, or hood)
Encourage effective, sputum-raising cough
Perform postural drainage as indicated
Perform chest percussion as ordered
Auscultate lungs q2h to determine need for suctioning and/or positioning
Allow patient to assume posture of most comfort: 30-degree elevation of head or placement in infant seat is most comfortable
Change infant's position frequently, at least q2h
Administer antibiotic therapy as ordered

ndx Activity intolerance related to fatigue from increased respiratory effort

GOAL: *Patient will experience a nonstressful environment and will be able to engage in age-appropriate activities*

Plan frequent rest periods for conservation of energy
Promote a nonstressful environment by
  Minimizing nursing care activities during severe respiratory distress
  Placing child in environment with minimal stimulation (quiet, dim lights)
  Encouraging parents to participate in care of their child
  Gradually increasing activity as tolerated, encouraging quiet bedside activities

ndx Potential fluid volume deficit related to fever, insensible water loss from tachypnea, and poor fluid intake from dyspnea

GOAL: *Patient will be afebrile, have age-appropriate respiratory rate, and will tolerate age-appropriate fluid volume intake and diet (see standard for age under Basic Standards of Care, pp. 781-788)*

Record intake and output and specific gravity
Assess hydration status
Encourage fluids as tolerated; give at room temperature; give cautiously to avoid aspiration
Administer parenteral fluids as ordered
Conduct cooling measures prn
Maintain cool environment
Administer antipyretic therapy as ordered
As condition improves, gradually advance to appropriate diet for age

ndx: Knowledge deficit regarding disease process and home care interventions

GOAL: *Patient and/or parents will demonstrate understanding of follow-up instructions through interactive discussion and actual return demonstration*

Explain need for rest
Explain need for nourishing diet for age and extra fluids
Discuss signs and symptoms of respiratory distress
Emphasize need to avoid exposure to other persons with URIs
Demonstrate and have parents demonstrate procedure for postural drainage and percussion
Teach name of antibiotic and antipyretic, dosage, time of administration, purpose, and side effects

Evaluation

Patient is afebrile
Respiratory rate is age appropriate, airway is patent, and breath sounds are clear
Child's prehospital activity tolerance has resumed
Child has resumed previous diet and fluid intake
Parents understand child's need for rest, fluids, diet, and follow-up care

ASTHMA

An acute spasm of smooth muscle in the bronchi and bronchioles; most frequent cause is allergic hypersensitivity to foreign substances, but it may be triggered by infection, or physical or psychologic stress; characterized by bilateral wheezing and trapped secretions

Usual age: any

Assessment

Observations/findings

See Respiratory Assessment (p. 219)
Family history of asthma
Known allergies of child
Compliance to management regimen
Posture is upright with shoulders hunched over
Nasal flaring
Cyanosis
Air hunger
Retractions
Prolonged expiratory phase with pursed lips
"Tight" cough
Dyspnea
Orthopnea
Audible expiratory wheeze
Auscultated inspiratory/expiratory wheeze; note pitch (higher pitch indicates progressive obstruction)
Rales
Rhonchi
Decreased breath sounds with increased airway resistance to airflow ("tight" chest)
Diaphoresis
Fatigue
Increasing tachycardia
Restlessness
Apprehension
Disorientation
Abdominal pain
Vomiting
Anorexia
Psychobehavioral assessment
Determination of child's asthma allergens

Laboratory/diagnostic studies

Sputum examination: eosinophilia with allergic reactivity
Complete blood cell count (CBC) with differential: leukocytosis, eosinophilia, above-average hemoglobin (Hgb) and hematocrit (Hct) with chronic hypoxemia
Blood gas evaluation
   Rising PCO_2: if 50 to 60, may need ventilatory assistance
   Rapidly falling pH and respiratory acidosis
Chest x-ray examination
   Overexpansion of lungs
   Rule out pneumothorax, atelectasis, pneumonia, pneumomediastinum
Pulmonary function tests

Potential complications

Atelectasis
Emphysema with chronic hyperinflation
Pneumothorax
Cor-pulmonale with right-sided failure
Cardiac arrythmias
Emotional/behavioral problems
Respiratory failure requiring mechanical assistance
Associated URI
Side effects from corticosteroid use

Medical management

Cool, humidified, oxygenated environment
Bronchodilators (sympathomimetics and methylxanthines) via IV line and nebulization
Monitoring for therapeutic levels of theophylline

Postural drainage, percussion, and suctioning as tolerated to clear airway (Begin *only after* airway opens and secretions become mobile)
Corticosteroids IV
IV hydration
Clear liquids or NPO depending on severity of respiratory distress
Treatment of coexisting bacterial infection with antibiotics

Nursing/diagnoses/goals/interventions

ndx: Ineffective airway clearance, ineffective breathing pattern, and impaired gas exchange related to bronchospasm and increased pulmonary secretions

GOAL: *Child will have an age-appropriate respiratory rate, will state that he can breathe better, will be able to mobilize secretions, and will maintain a patent airway*

Monitor vitals signs, including respiratory assessment q2h and prn
Initiate oxygen as ordered and prn for respiratory distress and/or cyanosis
NOTE: Avoid use of high levels of oxygen, since it may significantly *depress* respirations
Administer bronchodilators via nebulizer as ordered and assess respiratory status before and after administration
Administer constant infusion of bronchodilators intravenously as ordered
Administer corticosteroids as ordered
Ensure that patient receives maximum fluids for age and weight via parenteral and/or oral route
Allow patient to assume position of most comfort
Initiate postural drainage, percussion, and suctioning prn as tolerated *only after* patient's condition has improved and he is able to tolerate it; if initiated too soon, it can aggravate symptoms
Check theophylline levels and administer bolus dosages of bronchodilators intravenously as ordered to maintain therapeutic drug levels
Monitor blood gases
Monitor for signs and symptoms of respiratory failure and prepare for emergency intubation if any of the following occur: rapid, shallow respirations; decreased breath sounds; severe retractions; cyanosis; poor capillary refill; tachycardia; decreased level of consciousness

ndx: Anxiety related to breathlessness, air hunger, and fear

GOAL: *Child's anxiety will be minimized*

Minimize nursing routines until child's respiratory status improves
Allow child to assume position of greatest comfort
Encourage use of relaxation techniques (e.g., abdominal breathing exercises, guided imagery)
Provide emotional support to child and parents by explaining all procedures to them
Allow parents to participate in care of their child *if* they can remain calm and supportive
Recognize that disorientation and panic intensify as patient becomes hypoxemic

ndx: Potential fluid deficit related to side effects of medications and respiratory distress

GOAL: *Child will remain well hydrated*

Assess for anorexia, nausea, vomiting, and abdominal pain
Monitor blood levels of theophylline to determine toxicity
Keep NPO and administer maximum fluid requirements parenterally during severe respiratory distress
Administer small, frequent feedings of lukewarm clear fluids when tolerated
Advance to regular diet for age as tolerated
Monitor intake and output

ndx: Potential alteration in activity tolerance related to precipitation of or worsening of respiratory symptoms with increased activity

GOAL: *Child will be able to tolerate progressive increases in activities*

Encourage bed rest with severe respiratory symptoms
Gradually increase activity while encouraging quiet bedside activities: books, games, play dough, etc.
Teach diaphragmatic breathing exercises to increase strength of respiratory muscles
Refer child to physical therapy or asthma camp (through local American Lung Association) for physical training
Encourage moderate exercise with at least a 15 min "warm-up" session (swimming is excellent exercise and readily tolerated)
Teach proper use of physical and mental relaxation techniques to ward off an impending attack
For child with exercise-induced asthma, instruct child in proper use of inhalers prior to exercise

ndx: Potential anxiety related to ineffective parent-child relationship

GOAL: *Harmful parent-child conflict will be identified and appropriate referral made*

Assess whether child's symptoms improve when separated from parents
Assess parent-child interactions; if relationship has adverse effect on child, recommend counseling or psychiatric assistance
Consider involving parents in an ongoing parent group

ndx: Knowledge deficit regarding disease process and treatment

GOAL: *Patient and/or parents will demonstrate understanding of disease and treatment through interactive discussion and actual return demonstration*

Teach child and/or parents to avoid known allergens
Teach parents and child early warning signs of an impending attack and encourage intervention with rest, increased fluids, and medication
Teach diaphragmatic breathing exercises
Teach parents and child how to control symptoms by proper administration of medications
Caution against overuse of bronchodilators via inhalers
Discuss possible triggers with child and/or parents and encourage them to keep records of child's activity prior to, during, and after attacks
Warn against exposure to known environmental irritants: smoking, URIs, cold weather, and excessive humidity
Allow parents and/or child to administer inhalation therapy at least once during hospitalization
Give parents verbal and written instructions about medications including name, action, dosage, time of administration, and side effects
Schedule medication administration just before bedtime with sufficient fluid intake; this may decrease severity of nighttime symptoms and promote needed rest
Provide guidance for parents in promoting normal growth and development; allergens should be avoided but not to the extent that child's development is inhibited or excessive family conflict is created
Tell parents that even with careful management occasional attacks may occur
Discuss desensitization when appropriate

Evaluation

Respiratory rate is age appropriate
Airway is patent
Child feels and appears relaxed
Parents are supportive and interact appropriately to promote relaxation in their child
Child's preadmission activity level is resumed
Age-appropriate diet is resumed
Growth and development are promoted
Parents and/or child shows understanding of disease and management through discussion and demonstration
Appropriate ongoing referrals are made

BRONCHIOLITIS

A lower respiratory tract infection with obstruction at the bronchiolar level; usually of viral origin; consists of hypersecretion, edema, and inflammatory reaction of small bronchioles

Usual age: infant
Seasonal occurrence: winter and early spring

Assessment
Observations/findings

Spasmodic hacking cough
Nasal flaring
Cyanosis
Tachypnea
Prolonged expiratory phase
Retractions
Expiratory wheeze
Rales
Rhonchi
Decreased breath sounds
Increasing tachycardia
Low-grade fever
Fatigue
Irritability
Poor feeding related to increased respiratory distress with sucking

Laboratory/diagnostic studies

Chest x-ray examination: may show segmental collapse or hyperinflation
Blood gas evaluation to monitor for respiratory acidosis
Viral studies of nasal aspirates

Potential complications

Respiratory acidosis
Respiratory arrest

Congestive heart failure (p. 857)
Atelectasis
Prolonged illness with persistent abnormal respiratory function
Asthma in childhood

Medical management

Humidified, oxygenated environment via mist tent or oxygen hood
Monitoring of blood gases
Postural drainage, percussion, and suctioning prn as tolerated to clear airway when respiratory status improves
Ribovarin via oxygen hood if RSV (respiratory syncytial virus) is suspected or isolated
Antipyretics prn
Antibiotic therapy if bacterial infection is suspected
With severe respiratory distress
  NPO
  Maintenance parenteral fluids or small, frequent nasogastric feedings
  Intubation with assisted ventilation if necessary

Nursing diagnoses/goals/interventions

ndx: Impaired gas exchange related to increased pulmonary secretions and inadequate ventilation

GOAL: *Infant will have a patent airway, age-appropriate respiratory rate, normal blood gases, and pink color*

Monitor pulse, respiratory rate, and breath sounds q1h to 2h and prn
Maintain a humidified, oxygenated environment
Have oxygen via mask available at bedside for cyanosis
Minimize nursing care activities to conserve infant's energy
Elevate head of bed
Administer postural drainage, percussion, and suctioning prn as tolerated
Bulb suction nares prn to clear airway (infants are nose breathers)
Administer antibiotic therapy if ordered
Administer ribovarin as ordered via oxygen hood for RSV
Monitor for signs and symptoms of cardiac failure (p. 857)

ndx: Potential fluid volume deficit related to decreased oral intake increased insensible loss, and fever

GOAL: *Infant will remain well hydrated and will maintain weight*

Maintain NPO during severe distress
Provide maintenance fluids parenterally as ordered
NOTE: Intravenous fluids are administered cautiously; unresolved bronchiolitis can lead to cardiac failure
Monitor intake and output
Weigh infant daily
Monitor electrolytes and replace as ordered intravenously
Administer antipyretic therapy prn as ordered
Conduct cooling measures prn

ndx: Potential alteration in nutrition: less than body requirements related to fatigue and increased respiratory distress with sucking

GOAL: *Infant will tolerate age/weight–appropriate caloric intake by mouth prior to discharge*

Begin small, frequent nasogastric feedings as soon as tolerated
Introduce pacifier during nasogastric feedings to assess sucking strength and degree of respiratory distress with sucking, and to promote sucking reflex
Begin small, frequent oral feedings of clear liquids, then dilute formula as tolerated when infant is able to suck without severe respiratory distress
Gradually increase concentration and volume of feedings to age-appropriate amount as tolerated
Clear nasal passage prior to feedings

ndx: Potential for parental anxiety related to decreased parent-infant contact with mist tent therapy, bed rest, and prolonged hospitalization

GOAL: *Infant will be cared for by parents as much as possible*

Provide emotional support and reassurance to parents
Encourage touching, holding, and cuddling by parents as tolerated by infant
Help parents feel calm so they can provide needed comfort to their child
Involve parents actively in care of their infant as soon as feasible

ndx: Knowledge deficit regarding disease process and home care management

GOAL: *Parents and/or significant other will demonstrate understanding of home care instructions through interactive discussion and actual return demonstration*

Teach parents to use a vaporizer at night and during daytime naps

Tell parents to avoid exposure to URIs
Explain action of medication, dosage, time of administration, and side effects
Teach parents how to manage feedings during respiratory distress
Have parents demonstrate use of nasal bulb suction

Evaluation

Infant has age-appropriate respiratory rate with patent airway
Color is indicative of adequate perfusion
Infant is well hydrated
Infant is gaining weight
Age-appropriate diet is tolerated
Parent-child contact is promoted
Parents understand home care needs

CYSTIC FIBROSIS

An autosomal recessive disease involving a generalized dysfunction of exocrine glands and characterized by an increased production of thick mucus that causes a varying degree of obstruction in several organs; most commonly affected are the lungs, sweat glands, tear glands, paranasal sinuses, salivary glands, pancreas, liver, intestines, and reproductive tract

Usual age: any; onset most common in infants and toddlers

Assessment
Observations/findings
NEWBORN PERIOD

Meconium ileus: vomiting, absence of stools, abdominal distention, dehydration
"Salty" taste to skin
Poor weight gain
Failure to thrive
Listless

EXPECTED FINDINGS

Gastrointestinal (GI) system
   Poor weight gain with voracious appetite
   Thin extremities with abdominal distention
   Stool
     Increased frequency
     Loose consistency (diarrhea)
     Bulky
     Greasy; float in toilet
     Foul smelling
   Anorexia with infections and respiratory distress
Pulmonary system
   See Respiratory Assessment (p. 219); expect increase in respiratory distress symptoms with pulmonary infections and advanced lung damage
   History of chronic pulmonary disease
   Chronic sinusitis
   Nasal polyps
   Initially dry, nonproductive chronic cough; loose productive cough with infection and advancing lung damage
   Thick, tenacious mucus
   Nasal flaring
   Tachypnea
   Prolonged expiratory phase through pursed lips
   Shortness of breath with increased activity
   Barrel chest
   Clubbing of fingers and toes
   Cyanosis
   Rales
   Wheeze
   Decreased breath sounds
Biliary or hepatic duct obstruction
   Jaundice
   Splenomegaly
   Hepatomegaly
   Ascites
   Portal hypertension (p. 399)
   Esophageal varices with GI bleeding
Additional observations
   See Cardiovascular Assessment (p. 67): at risk for CHF (p. 857)
   Dehydration (p. 866)
   Hyponatremia (p. 46)

Laboratory/diagnostic studies

Increased sweat chloride test by pilocarpine iontophoresis (greater than 60 mEq/L is abnormal)
Decreased or absence of trypsin, lipase, and amylase from duodenal contents
Fresh stool samples studied for trypsin and fat (trypsin is minimal or absent: fat is elevated—steatorrhea)
Increased albumin content in stools: azotorrhea (greater than 20 mg%
Chest x-ray examination
   Confirms chronic lung disease with emphysema
   Assists in identifying pulmonary complications
Pulmonary function tests
   Decreased vital capacity and tidal volume
   Increased airway resistance
   Decreased forced expiratory volume
Blood gases: reveal varying degree of respiratory acidosis

Potential complications

Lobar atelectasis
Lung abscesses
Spontaneous pneumothorax
Chronic cor pulmonale
Hemoptysis
Intestinal obstruction
Prolapsed rectum
Anemia
Diabetes mellitus

Medical management

Inhalation therapy to liquefy mucus and prevent and treat infections
Postural drainage, percussion, and vibration two to four times a day; increased frequency with infections
Suctioning may be ordered in infants and toddlers who cannot expectorate mucus on their own
Oxygen therapy
Bronchodilators, mucolytics, and/or expectorants via ultrasonic nebulization
IV antibiotics to treat pulmonary infections
Antibiotics via nebulization are sometimes ordered to treat microorganism directly
Pancreatic enzyme replacement
Twice recommended daily allowance of water-miscible vitamins
Daily iron supplement
Salt tablet supplements during hot weather
Diagnosis and treatment of complications

Nursing diagnoses/goals/interventions

ndx: Ineffective airway clearance related to mucopurulent secretions

GOAL: *Patient will have a patent airway; secretions will be mobilized and removed*

Administer inhalation therapy via ultrasonic nebulization as ordered prior to postural drainage
Perform postural drainage, percussion, and vibration q2h to 4h as ordered
Schedule respiratory treatments before meals and at bedtime
Have patient cough up and spit out mucus if able
Suction prn
Note color, amount, and consistency of sputum
Administer oxygen as ordered and prn
CAUTION: High levels of oxygen should be avoided, since they may depress respirations!
Assess vital signs with respiratory assessment q2h and prn

Encourage oral fluids or increase intravenous flow rate to ensure adequate hydration for liquifecation of secretions
Administer intravenous antibiotics as ordered
Administer antibiotics via nebulization if ordered *after* postural drainage routine
Protect child from contact with others who may transmit additional respiratory infections

ndx: Potential alteration in nutrition: less than body requirements related to increased caloric and protein needs secondary to impaired intestinal absorption, and loss of fat and fat-soluble vitamins in stool

GOAL: *Patient will remain hydrated, will gain weight, and will take a well-balanced diet*

Administer pancreatic enzymes with each meal and with snacks
A low-fat, high-protein, high-calorie diet may be encouraged; however, do not enforce severe restrictions, since this may impede psychologic adjustment
Monitor food intake and stool frequency, character, and consistency
Alter pancreatic enzyme therapy as needed to promote normal bowel movements
Allow older child to regulate his own diet and determine need for enzyme adjustment or dietary restrictions
Record intake and output
Weigh patient daily
Administer lipid-soluble vitamins in water-miscible liquid as ordered
Encourage generous use of added salt in diet
Administer salt tablet supplements as necessary during hot weather

ndx: Alteration in bowel elimination: diarrhea or constipation related to insufficient or excessive replacement of pancreatic enzymes

GOAL: *Patient will have normal bowel elimination patterns*

Keep accurate stool record, noting color, consistency, amount, and frequency of stools
Keep accurate record of dietary intake to identify certain foods that may contribute to altered stool patterns
Avoid known dietary irritants
Adjust pancreatic enzyme replacement as necessary in accordance with food intake and stool pattern
Encourage parents and/or child to alter diet and enzyme therapy as needed to promote growth and normal bowel movements

ndx: Activity intolerance related to dyspnea

GOAL: *Patient will be able to tolerate physical activity and participate in age-appropriate play*

Teach patient breathing exercises to help aerate lungs to maximum capacity

In young child encourage bubble blowing or blowing out candles

In older child teach abdominal breathing exercises

Encourage daily exercises to promote and maintain posture

Encourage participation in swimming or hydrotherapy, since this helps strengthen muscles of respiration and promotes good breathing habits

Avoid environmental irritants such as smoke and pollutants

Perform respiratory treatments prior to participation in physical activity

ndx: Potential for ineffective individual and/or family coping related to chronicity of illness, financial burden, and/or disruption of family functioning

GOAL: *Individual and family will adjust to ramifications of the disease; their need for additional support will be identified, and appropriate referrals will be made*

Encourage parents and child to communicate their feelings and concerns to you and each other

Have parents and child talk with another family who has a child with cystic fibrosis

Assess family's coping abilities and problem-solving abilities

Discuss with family the need for everyone to participate in the care of the child with cystic fibrosis

Encourage parents to foster family life by spending time with each individual member and carrying on "normal" activities

Encourage parents to promote normal growth and development in their child with cystic fibrosis

Discuss financial burden with parents

Make appropriate referral for counseling and financial assistance if necessary

ndx: Knowledge deficit regarding chronic nature of disease and home care needs

GOAL: *Patient and/or parents will demonstrate understanding of home care and follow-up instructions through interactive discussion and actual return demonstration*

Teach child and/or parents use of nebulizer and other respiratory equipment that will be used at home: oxygen, suction, humidifier

Teach child and/or parents postural drainage, percussion, and vibration

Have child and/or parents demonstrate postural drainage routine prior to discharge

Set up home schedule to meet life-style of individual family

Teach breathing exercises and have child demonstrate them before discharge

Involve child in ongoing exercise program, because activity increases respiratory effort and movement of mucus in airways

Tell child and/or parents to avoid persons with URIs and known respiratory irritants such as smoke, air pollutants, and humidity

Teach need to monitor weight and stools

Encourage a high-calorie, moderate fat diet

Teach parents to mix supplemental pancreatic enzymes with carbohydrate foods such as applesauce; protein foods will cause enzymes to break down immediately

Teach name of medications, dosage, time of administration, purpose, and side effects

If child has received repeated therapy with drugs known to be ototoxic, discuss need for hearing test evaluation

Yearly influenza immunizations are strongly recommended

Discuss need for salt replacement requirements during hot weather

Alert parents to symptoms of deterioration to report to physician
  Fever
  Weight loss
  Poor appetite
  Respiratory distress
  Fatigue
  Failure to raise sputum following respiratory therapy techniques
  Excessive number of large, bulky, foul-smelling stools

Make appropriate referrals to community resources (Cystic Fibrosis Foundation)

Make appropriate referral for genetic counseling

Evaluation

Child has patent airway
Cough is productive, and mucus is cleared from airway
Child eats well-balanced diet
Child gains weight

Stools are formed, and normal pattern is established
Child participates in ongoing exercise program
Child and/or parents demonstrate and state their ability to accept and adjust to life with cystic fibrosis
Parents, child, and family have ongoing community support
Parents and child understand disease and its ramifications, and parents are able to care for child at home

Gastrointestinal System

CLEFT LIP REPAIR

Surgical repair of congenital interruption in the development of the upper lip; may be unilateral or bilateral

Usual age: infant

Assessment
Observations/findings
AT BIRTH

Separation of lip may range from notch in vermilion border of lip to complete extension to floor of nose
May or may not be associated with cleft palate
May or may not be associated with other congenital anomalies

PREOPERATIVE

Infant's ability to take fluids using modified feeding techniques as preferred by surgeon (Lamb's nipple, flanged nipple, Breck feeder)
Infant's tolerance of side-lying and supine position
Parents' perception of their infant

POSTOPERATIVE

Excessive bleeding, signs of infection, or separation at incision site
Security of Logan bow
Respiratory stridor, distress, or obstruction
Skin irritation under elbow restraints
Tolerance of modified feeding techniques
Fluid and caloric intake
Degree of discomfort
Parents' response to surgical repair

Laboratory/diagnostic studies
Ongoing evaluation includes
    Hearing tests
    Speech evaluation
    Orthodontal and prosthodontal evaluation of teeth malposition and structural changes of maxillary arches

Potential complications
Respiratory distress postoperatively
Infection of incision
Repeated otitis media with hearing loss
Malocclusion of teeth
Speech impairment

Medical management
Surgical correction of defect
Modified feeding technique
Type of feeding preferred (generally no milk products)
Elbow restraints
Cleaning and care of suture line
Antibiotic therapy is preferred by some surgeons
Mild sedation is preferred by some surgeons

Nursing diagnoses/goals/interventions

ndx Potential for infection of suture line related to undue stress on incision, direct trauma to site, or interference with scar formation

GOAL: *Patient's suture line will remain intact and free of infection*

Prevent crying by anticipating needs of infant; hold, cuddle, and use tactile, visual, and auditory stimulation to comfort infant
Use elbow restraints at all times to prevent direct trauma to area from infant's hands
Keep Logan bow in place
Position infant supine or in modified side-lying position so infant will not cause trauma to site if he turns his head
Cleanse suture line after every meal and prn
Keep suture line moist with prescribed ointment
Offer small amount of water after feedings to cleanse lip and mouth
Administer antibiotics if ordered
Administer sedative if ordered

ndx Potential alteration in nutrition: less than body requirements related to altered feeding techniques and inability to suck effectively

GOAL: *Infant will receive age-appropriate caloric intake (p. 866), will gain weight, and will remain hydrated*

Administer parenteral fluids until oral intake is adequate

Introduce altered feeding technique preoperatively so infant can adjust to it

Do not allow nipple or pacifiers in mouth

Administer clear liquids and advance diet as tolerated and ordered

Avoid use of milk products

Feed in upright position

Burp infant after each ounce

Position in infant seat or side-lying position after feedings

Measure intake and output

Weigh infant daily

ndx: Alteration in physical mobility related to use of elbow restraints

GOAL: *Infant's elbow range of motion (ROM) will be maintained, and normal growth and development will be promoted*

Remove elbow restraints, one at a time, at least q8h

Check skin under restraints for signs of irritation

Perform ROM exercises to arms

Promote age-appropriate development through auditory, visual, and tactile stimulation

ndx: Potential alteration in parenting related to infant's physical disfigurement

GOAL: *Parent-infant relationship will be promoted, and bonding will occur*

Repair of lip should be performed as soon after birth as possible

Discuss with parents their perception of their infant, feelings around the time of birth, and feelings about feeding modifications

Point out positive things about their infant

Involve parents in care and feeding of their infant immediately

Have parents meet with other family whose child had cleft lip, if necessary

ndx: Knowledge deficit regarding home care needs and follow-up care

GOAL: *Parent and/or significant other will demonstrate understanding of home care and follow-up instructions through interactive discussion and actual return demonstration*

Teach parents how to use alternative feeding technique

Have parents feed child several times prior to discharge

Teach lip care

Teach application of elbow restraints and need for ROM exercises

Tell parents dietary restrictions if any (usually milk products)

Discuss symptoms of incision infection to report to physician
  Redness
  Swelling
  Drainage
  Bleeding
  Separation of incision

Teach name of medication, purpose, dosage, time of administration, and side effects

Ensure that parents understand need for ongoing evaluation of child's hearing, speech, and dental development

Evaluation

Suture line is clean and intact

Infant has sufficient caloric intake for growth

Infant is gaining weight

Infant is hydrated

ROM of elbows is maintained

Parents have positive feelings about infant

Parents are able to care for child at home

Parents state need for ongoing evaluation of speech, hearing, and teeth formation

CLEFT PALATE REPAIR

Surgical repair of congenital interruption of development of the oral palate; may involve the hard or soft palate, or both

Usual age: toddler

Assessment

Observations/findings

AT BIRTH

Separation of hard or soft palate, or both

Regurgitation of oral feedings through nose

Associated cleft lip, if present

Associated congenital anomalies, if present

PREOPERATIVE

Toddler's experience with Breck feeder and/or ability to drink from cup

Toddler's tolerance of prone position

Toddler's developmental status

POSTOPERATIVE

Degree of respiratory distress as a result of increased mucous secretions and swelling of incision site

Excessive bleeding
Intact sutures
Degree of discomfort
Tolerance of feeding techniques
Fluid and caloric intake

Laboratory/diagnostic studies

See Cleft Lip Repair (p. 805)

Potential complications

Airway obstruction
See Cleft Lip Repair (p. 805)

Medical management

Surgical correction of defect
Mist tent
Diet and restrictions if any (usually milk products are avoided)
Elbow restraints
Parenteral fluids immediately postoperatively until oral intake is adequate
Antibiotics are preferred by some surgeons
Mild sedation is preferred by some surgeons
Analgesic (usually acetaminophen) for discomfort

Nursing diagnoses/goals/interventions*

ndx Potential for ineffective airway clearance related to increased oral secretions and swelling of incisional area

GOAL: *Patient's airway will remain patent*

Administer mist tent therapy as ordered
Position child in prone, head-down position to promote drainage of oral secretions
Do not suction
Monitor respiratory status qh for first 24 to 48 hr postoperatively

ndx Potential alteration in nutrition: less than body requirements related to discomfort and altered feeding techniques

GOAL: *Patient will tolerate age-appropriate caloric intake (p. 866)*

Introduce modified feeding technique prior to surgery to familiarize child and parent
Administer parenteral fluids as ordered until child is able to tolerate adequate oral intake
Administer liquids and purees via Breck feeder or cup
Feed in high chair
Allow parent to feed child as soon as possible

---

*See Cleft Lip Repair (p. 805).

Monitor intake and output
Weigh child daily
Administer analgesics prior to feeding

ndx Potential for infection of suture site related to trauma to area and interference with healing process

GOAL: *Suture line will remain clean and intact, and patient will be afebrile*

Monitor temperature q4h and prn
Use elbow restraints at all times
Avoid use of straws or feeding utensils; use cup or Breck feeder *only*
Give child small amount of water after each feeding to cleanse suture line and prevent accumulation of food on incisional area
Assess child for excessive bleeding, drainage, and foul mouth odor
Administer antibiotics if ordered
Administer sedative if ordered

ndx Knowledge deficit regarding home care needs and follow-up care

GOAL: *Parents and/or significant other will demonstrate understanding of home care and follow-up instructions through interactive discussion and actual return demonstration*

Teach feeding techniques
Tell parents dietary restrictions if any (usually milk products are avoided)
Demonstrate use of elbow restraints and ROM exercises
Discuss signs of infection
  Elevated temperature
  Drainage
  Excessive bleeding
  Foul mouth odor
Teach name of medication, purpose, dosage, time of administration, and side effects
Have parents demonstrate
  Modified feeding techniques
  Application of elbow restraints
  ROM exercises
  Administration of medications
Ensure that parents understand need for ongoing evaluation of hearing, speech, and teeth formation

Evaluation

Airway is clear
Age-appropriate caloric intake is tolerated
Suture site is clean and intact
Patient is afebrile

Parents demonstrate ability to care for child at home
Parents state need for follow-up care

TRACHEOESOPHAGEAL FISTULA

A congenital anomaly usually consisting of esophageal atresia combined with a connection of the esophagus with the trachea by way of a fistula (Figure 15-5)

Usual age: newborn; high incidence of prematurity and low birth weight

Assessment
Observations/findings

History of maternal polyhydramnios
Low weight for gestational age
Excessive salivation
Persistent drooling of salivary mucus
Bubbling from nostrils
Normal swallow with feedings followed by sudden cough and regurgitation of feeding through nose and mouth
Cyanosis, coughing, and choking with feedings
Inability to pass nasogastric tube into stomach
Abdominal distention

May have history of repeated pneumonia during first few months of life (**H** type)

Laboratory/diagnostic studies

X-ray studies: radiopaque catheter is inserted into esophagus and followed by chest films; diagnosis is confirmed by failure of catheter to reach stomach or passage of catheter through abnormal channels; GI gas is also observed on x-ray examination

Potential complications

Aspiration pneumonia
Apnea/respiratory arrest
Dehydration
Inanition
Pathologic food aversion if surgery is delayed until toddlerhood
Esophageal strictures (postsurgical complication)
Additional congenital anomalies (cardiac, renal, and/or gastrointestinal)

Medical management
Postdiagnosis

NPO
Maintenance parenteral fluids and electrolyte replacement

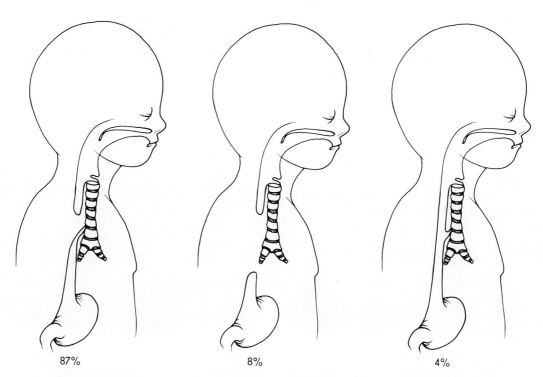

FIGURE 15-5. Three most commonly encountered forms of esophageal atresia and tracheoesophageal fistula, in order of frequency.

Suctioning of nose and pharynx prn
Humidified oxygen therapy
Drainage of pouch via catheter
External warming device
Endotracheal intubation and assisted ventilation with severe respiratory distress
Antibiotic therapy
Insertion of gastrostomy tube (usually done with patient under local anesthesia preoperatively to allow escape of air from stomach, thus decreasing possibility of gastric reflux into fistula)

Surgery

Palliative surgery with ligation of fistula and insertion of gastrostomy tube *or*
Corrective surgery with ligation of fistula, anastomosis of esophagus, and gastrostomy placement; type of surgery done is determined by type of tracheoesophageal fistula and length of esophagus available for anastomosis

Postgastrostomy

Evaluation of respiratory status
Gastrostomy tube connected to gravity drainage or to low, intermittent suction
Continuation of pouch drainage
Continuation of maintenance parenteral fluids; hyperalimentation may be ordered
Replacement of gastrostomy drainage with parenteral fluids
Monitoring and replacement of fluids and electrolytes
Continuation of warm, humidified, oxygenated environment

Nursing diagnoses/goals/interventions (preoperative)

ndx: Ineffective airway clearance related to secretions of esophageal pouch, regurgitation of all feedings, and risk of aspiration

GOAL: *Patient's airway will remain patent, and respiratory distress will be recognized and treated promptly*

Maintain NPO status
Keep infant in warm, humidified, oxygenated environment
Suction frequently to clear nares and mouth of mucus
Keep pouch catheter (usually sump tube) connected to low, continuous suction as ordered
Monitor respiratory status qh and prn
Place infant in head-elevated position of at least 30 degrees
Keep infant calm and quiet by stroking, handling gently, and using pacifier; crying causes gastric regurgitation
Turn q2h
Administer antibiotics if ordered
Prepare for insertion of gastrostomy tube for gastric decompression
Postgastrostomy: maintain gastrostomy tube connected to gravity drainage or to low, intermittent suction as ordered

ndx: Potential fluid volume deficit related to inability to tolerate oral feedings

GOAL: *Patient will remain hydrated*

Monitor for signs of dehydration (p. 866)
Maintain NPO status
Administer parenteral fluids and electrolytes as ordered
Replace gastrostomy drainage with parenteral fluids as ordered
Measure intake and output and specific gravity
Weigh infant daily

ndx: Potential alteration in body temperature related to age, an inability to raise body temperature through shivering and/or use of external warming devices

GOAL: *Infant's body temperature will remain between 98.6° and 100.4° F (37° and 38° C)*

Place infant under or in an external warming device
Keep infant partially dressed; especially use cap to prevent loss of warmth through head
Keep snuggly wrapped in blankets if feasible
Keep infant in *warm*, humidified environment
Monitor temperature q4h and prn and regulate temperature of environment accordingly

ndx: Knowledge deficit regarding condition and treatment

GOAL: *Parents and/or significant other will state accurate understanding of the condition and its treatment*

Prepare parents for necessary preoperative procedures
Explain surgical procedure to parents
Carefully explain existing problem and reason for NPO status
Provide parents with visual explanation of defect
Allow parents to continue to parent their child
Assess parents' coping ability and provide resources as necessary

Evaluation

Infant's airway is patent and free of secretions

Infant remains hydrated

Infant's vital signs remain within age-appropriate norms

Parents have clear understanding of defect and required surgical correction

TRACHEOESOPHAGEAL FISTULA REPAIR

Usual age: newborn

Preoperative Care

See Tracheoesophageal Fistula (p. 808)

Postoperative Care

(After surgical anastomosis of esophagus/gastrostomy placement)

Assessment

Observations/findings

Respiratory status (see Respiratory Assessment, p. 219)

Type and amount of chest tube drainage (saliva in chest tube indicates anastomotic leak)

Signs and symptoms of anastomotic leak or perforation
  Severe respiratory distress
  Asymmetric movement of chest
  Respiratory failure (p. 261)
  Fever
  Shock (p. 104)

Tolerance to gastrostomy and oral feedings when started

Laboratory/diagnostic studies

Barium swallow under fluoroscopy may be done prior to oral feedings

Esophagoscopy may be performed for direct observation of anastomosis

Potential complications

Respiratory failure (p. 261)
Perforation of anastomosis
Shock (p. 104)
Hyponatremia (p. 46)
Dehydration (p. 866)
Hypothermia (p. 329)

Medical management

Insertion of chest tube and connection to underwater seal

Determination of distance a catheter can be inserted for safe suctioning to ensure patent airway and prevent trauma to anastomosis

Warm, humidified environment

Oxygen therapy prn

NPO

Parenteral fluids: hyperalimentation may be ordered until sufficient oral and/or gastrostomy feedings are tolerated

Gastrostomy tube connected to gravity drainage or to low, intermittent suction

Gastrostomy replacement fluids

Small, frequent feedings via gastrostomy tube begun 7 to 10 days after insertion, *without* clamping of tube following feedings; diet advanced via gastrostomy tube as tolerated

Oral feedings begun 1 to 2 weeks after anastomosis

Removal of gastrostomy tube

Prophylactic antibiotics may be ordered

Analgesics to control pain

Nursing diagnoses/goals/interventions

ndx: Potential for ineffective airway clearance related to anesthesia, gastric regurgitation through fistula, and/or anastomotic leak or perforation

GOAL: *Patient will have age-appropriate respiratory rate (p. 866); color will be pink, airway patent, and breath sounds clear; early signs of possible anastomotic leak will be recognized and treated promptly*

Maintain NPO

Maintain gastrostomy tube connected to gravity drainage or to low, intermittent suction

Maintain chest tube connected to underwater seal; note amount and type of drainage qh

Monitor vital signs with respiratory assessment q1h and prn

Maintain warm, humidified environment

Administer oxygen prn as ordered

Keep infant in head-up position

Avoid hyperextension of neck to prevent pull on sutured esophagus

A suction catheter should be marked by surgeon indicating maximum length that it can be inserted when performing nasopharyngeal suctioning; prior to suctioning, measure suction catheter to be used against premeasured catheter

Suction *gently* and frequently to maintain airway, vigorous suctioning will traumatize tissue and increase edema already present from operation

Turn q2h
Perform postural drainage and percussion prn
Administer antibiotics if ordered

ndx: Potential fluid volume deficit related to NPO status, inability to tolerate oral feedings, and gastric suctioning

GOAL: *Infant will remain hydrated*

Maintain NPO status
Administer parenteral fluids as ordered
Administer gastric replacement solution parenterally as ordered
Monitor intake and output and specific gravity
Weigh daily
Begin gastrostomy feedings as ordered

ndx: Alteration in nutritional status: less than body requirements related to inability to tolerate age-appropriate caloric intake orally

GOAL: *Infant will tolerate diet reflecting age-appropriate caloric requirements (p. 866) via gastrostomy tube and/or orally prior to discharge*

Begin small, frequent clear liquid feedings via gastrostomy tube and advance amount and strength as ordered and tolerated
Check gastric residual prior to each feeding
Refeed gastric residual; amount of feeding to be given is determined by taking amount of formula ordered and subtracting amount of residual
Give feeding by gravity drip
Keep gastrostomy tube open to air (*do not clamp after feedings*); a 10 ml syringe barrel suspended no more than 6 inches above infant's abdomen may be used (Figure 15-6)
Give pacifier until oral feeding is begun
Begin oral feedings as ordered
Observe infant's ability to swallow without choking
Supplement oral feedings with gastrostomy feedings if necessary until infant is able to tolerate full feedings orally

ndx: Alteration in comfort related to surgical incision

GOAL: *Infant will be calm and easily consolable, without evidence of discomfort (irritability, excessive crying, disturbed sleep pattern)*

Assess infant for signs of pain
Provide comforting measures; allow parents to hold and cuddle infant; use quiet voices, soft music, and dim lights

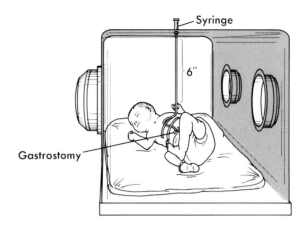

FIGURE 15-6. Feeding by gastrostomy tube.

Keep infant warm and dry
Administer analgesics as ordered

ndx: Knowledge deficit regarding home care needs and follow-up care

GOAL: *Parents and/or significant other will demonstrate understanding of home care and follow-up instructions through interactive discussion and actual return demonstration*

Teach feeding techniques: if surgery was palliative, infant will go home receiving gastrostomy feedings; with corrective surgery, gastrostomy tube will be discontinued prior to discharge, and infant will go home receiving oral feedings
Discuss signs of respiratory difficulty
    Tachypnea
    Retractions
    Nasal flaring
Discuss signs of esophageal stricture
    Difficulty in feeding
    Vomiting
    Coughing
    Gagging
    Dysphagia
Discuss symptoms of wound infection
    Fever
    Redness
    Drainage
    Swelling
    Tenderness
Have parents demonstrate
    Feeding techniques
    Care of gastrostomy tube (if infant will be discharged with one)

Evaluation

Infant's airway is patent, color is pink, and respiratory rate is normal for age
Breath sounds are clear
Patient is well hydrated
Patient is able to tolerate diet reflecting caloric requirements
Patient has no sign of incisional discomfort
Parents demonstrate understanding of home care and follow-up instructions

PYLORIC STENOSIS

A congenital obstruction of the gastric pylorus caused by hypertrophy of the circular pyloric musculature; it is most frequent in males, and symptoms usually occur in the second or third week of life

Assessment
Observations/findings

History of formula changes without resolution of symptoms
Expected findings
  Nonbilious vomiting following soon after feeding, becoming progressively more severe and projectile
  Vomitus may be blood tinged
  Eager acceptance of second feeding soon after vomiting episode
  Presence of abdominal peristaltic waves from left to right
  Palpable olive-shaped pyloric mass
  Weight loss or no weight gain since birth
  Decreased stool frequency
  Hunger
  Irritability
  Dehydration (p. 866)

Laboratory/diagnostic studies

Hypochloremic alkalosis
  Low serum chloride
  Increased pH
  Increased bicarbonate
Elevated Hct and Hgb with hemoconcentration
NOTE: Because of hemoconcentration from extracellular fluid depletion, decreased serum levels of sodium and potassium may be masked
Upper GI series
  Delayed gastric emptying
  Elongated, threadlike pyloric channel
Palpation of "tumor" immediately after vomiting

Potential complications

Dehydration
Aspiration of vomitus

Medical management
Preoperative

NPO
Rehydration with parenteral fluids
Replenishment of potassium stores and correction of alkalosis with parenteral electrolyte administration
NOTE: Replacement therapy may delay surgery 24 to 48 hr
Nasogastric tube connected to gravity drainage may be preferred by some surgeons for gastric decompression and lavage

Surgery

Surgical correction of pyloric obstruction by pyloromyotomy

Postoperative

Nasogastric tube may or may not be ordered postoperatively
Maintenance parenteral fluids until infant is able to retain age-appropriate feedings
Feedings may begin as soon as 4 to 6 hr postoperatively
Small, frequent clear liquid feedings, advancing volume and strength as tolerated

Nursing diagnoses/goals/interventions

ndx: Fluid volume deficit preoperatively related to severe vomiting

GOAL: *Infant will be well hydrated with normal electrolyte values prior to surgery*

Monitor improvement of symptoms of dehydration (p. 866)
Maintain NPO if ordered
Provide maintenance fluids parenterally as ordered
Maintain nasogastric tube if ordered; check drainage q2h to 4h and replace with parenteral fluids as ordered
Monitor serum electrolyte values and replace parenterally as ordered
Monitor intake and output

ndx: Potential fluid volume deficit postoperatively related to inability to tolerate age-appropriate volume of feedings

GOAL: *Infant will tolerate fluid requirements orally without vomiting*

Maintain NPO status as ordered

Maintain nasogastric tube connected to low, intermittent suction if ordered; empty and measure drainage q2h to 4h and replace as ordered

Administer parenteral fluids; decrease as oral intake increases

Assess infant's readiness for oral feedings: alert, bowel sounds present, flatus and/or stool, eager sucking of pacifier without being content

Monitor intake and output

Begin small, clear liquid feedings (usually electrolyte solution) q3h as ordered; increase volume as ordered and tolerated

Monitor for vomiting

NOTE: Some vomiting is expected for 24 to 48 hr postoperatively

ndx: Alteration in nutrition: less than body requirements related to preoperative vomiting and inability to tolerate age-appropriate diet

GOAL: *Infant will tolerate feedings sufficient to meet caloric requirements (115 calories/kg) prior to discharge and will gain weight*

Weigh infant daily

Gradually and progressively increase volume and strength of feedings as ordered and tolerated

Advance to previous formula or breast milk as soon as feasible

Keep infant prone or propped on right side after feedings

Burp infant frequently during feedings

Involve parents in care and feeding as soon as possible

Observe infant's response to feedings and feeding techniques

ndx: Potential for infection related to surgical incision

GOAL: *Infant will remain afebrile, and incision will remain clean and intact*

Observe incision for signs of infection: redness, pain, swelling, drainage

Keep incision clean and dry

Monitor temperature with vital signs q4h

ndx: Knowledge deficit regarding home care and follow-up needs

GOAL: *Parents and/or significant other will demonstrate understanding of home care and follow-up instructions through interactive discussion and actual return demonstration*

Teach feeding schedule and techniques

Have parents feed infant prior to discharge

If infant vomits during postoperative feedings
  Discuss with parents their feelings and fears about vomiting/feeding
  Inform parents that some vomiting is expected 24 to 48 hr after surgery

Discuss symptoms of wound infection

Ensure that parents understand need for follow-up care

Evaluation

Infant is well hydrated

Infant tolerates age-appropriate diet reflecting fluid and caloric requirements

Infant begins to gain weight

Infant's surgical incision remains clean and intact

Parents are able to feed and care for child and understand home care instructions

RUPTURED (PERFORATED) APPENDIX

An obstruction of the appendiceal lumen progressively causes inflammation, distention, decreased blood supply, necrosis, and perforation of the appendix; perforation causes generalized peritonitis or a localized abscess

Usual age: any

Assessment

Observations/findings

Abdominal pain: sudden relief from pain with perforation, followed by increased diffuse pain

Rigidity

Guarding

Side-lying position with knees flexed for maximum comfort

Progressive abdominal distention

Vomiting

Diarrhea or constipation

Decreased or absent bowel sounds

Fever

Tachypnea

Shallow respirations

Tachycardia

Chills

Pallor or flushing

Irritability
Restlessness
Dehydration (p. 866)

Laboratory/diagnostic studies
WBC count elevated
Urinalysis to rule out urinary tract infection (UTI)
Abdominal x-ray examination to rule out other causes for pain (e.g., fecal impaction)
Chest x-ray examination to rule out pneumonia

Potential complications
Dehydration (p. 866)
Sepsis
Electrolyte imbalance
Pelvic abscess
Pneumonia (p. 243)

Medical management
Preoperative
NPO
Parenteral fluids to stabilize hydration and electrolyte status
Nasogastric tube connected to low, intermittent suction
Antibiotic therapy

Surgery
Surgical removal of appendix (appendectomy)

Postoperative
NPO
Parenteral fluids
Nasogastric tube drainage replacement with parenteral fluids
Nasogastric tube connected to low, intermittent suction or sump tube to low, continuous suction
Determination of volume of nasogastric tube irrigation solution
Discontinuation of nasogastric tube
Initiation of oral feedings and advancement from clear liquids to regular diet for age
Incentive spirometer
Determination of type of incisional care
Advancement and discontinuation of Penrose drain
Antibiotics
Analgesics
Antipyretics

Nursing diagnoses/goals/interventions

ndx Potential fluid volume deficit related to fever, nasogastric suctioning, and/or inability to take oral fluids

GOAL: *Patient will remain hydrated and afebrile, and will tolerate sufficient amount of oral fluids to maintain hydration prior to discharge*

Maintain NPO status
Administer parenteral fluids as ordered
Maintain nasogastric suction as ordered
Empty and measure nasogastric tube drainage q4h and prn
Administer gastric replacement fluids parenterally as ordered
Irrigate nasogastric tube as ordered; when measuring nasogastric tube drainage, adjust volume to reflect results of irrigation
Measure intake and output, and specific gravity
Begin clear liquid diet as ordered
Conduct cooling measures prn

ndx Alteration in nutrition: less than body requirements related to increased nutritional requirements for wound healing, dietary restrictions, pain

GOAL: *Patient will tolerate regular diet for age prior to discharge*

Assess for return of peristalsis
  Flatus
  Stooling
  Decrease in quantity of gastric drainage
  Bowel sounds
  Hunger
Begin clear liquid diet and assess patient's tolerance
Advance diet gradually to regular diet for age
Encourage ambulation to promote return of peristalsis
Gradually reduce pain medication as tolerated so it will not contribute to constipation
Monitor weight
Observe for return of prehospitalization bowel pattern

ndx Potential for ineffective breathing pattern related to anesthesia, postoperative immobility, pain

GOAL: *Patient's breath sounds will remain clear, and respiratory rate will be age appropriate (p. 866)*

Monitor vital signs q4h and prn
Monitor respiratory status q2h and prn
Assist and teach patient to turn, cough, and deep breathe, and to use incentive spirometer q2h
Position patient in 45-degree head-up position
Ambulate at least q3h to 4h as tolerated
Administer pain medication if necessary prior to ambulation and vigorous respiratory treatments

ndx: Alteration in comfort: pain related to surgical intervention

GOAL: *Patient will be pain-free prior to discharge*

Assess for symptoms of pain (children may not verbalize pain because they fear the injection)
- Facial grimacing
- Crying
- Poor appetite
- Guarding
- Refusal to increase physical activity

Administer analgesics as ordered
Change to oral preparation of analgesics as soon as patient is tolerating oral fluids
Institute other comfort and pain control measures
- Relaxation
- Breathing exercises
- Splinting of incision with rolled blanket
- Position for comfort; avoid extension of abdominal musculature

ndx: Alteration in skin integrity related to surgical intervention

GOAL: *Patient's surgical incision will heal without signs of infection*

Monitor wound for signs of infection
- Fever
- Redness
- Swelling
- Copious or foul drainage

Administer incisional care as ordered
Observe color, amount, and characteristics of drainage from Penrose drain
Administer antibiotic therapy as ordered
Encourage proper nutrition

ndx: Knowledge deficit regarding home care and follow-up needs

GOAL: *Patient and/or parents will demonstrate understanding of home care and follow-up instructions through interactive discussion and actual return demonstration*

Teach wound care if any
Discuss symptoms of wound infection to report to physician
- Redness
- Pain
- Edema
- Drainage

Discuss diet
Explain need for exercise to tolerance with planned rest periods
Caution patient to avoid strenuous exercise for several weeks
Teach name of medication, purpose, dosage, time of administration, and side effects

Evaluation

Patient is hydrated
Prehospitalization diet and bowel patterns have returned
Breath sounds are clear
Wound is clean and healing
Comfort is achieved
Patient is afebrile
Patient and/or parents understand home care and follow-up instructions

HIRSCHSPRUNG'S DISEASE: AGANGLIONIC MEGACOLON

A congenital condition characterized by greatly dilated colon proximal to an area of narrowing, usually in the rectum or rectosigmoid, resulting from absence of parasympathetic ganglion cells and peristalsis

Usual age: under 1 year; predominantly males

Assessment

Observations/findings

EARLY INFANCY

Failure to pass meconium within 24 to 48 hr of life
Partial or complete intestinal obstruction
- Vomiting of bilious or fecal matter
- Abdominal distention
- Constipation
- Diarrhea: most ominous sign

Poor feeding
Weight loss

LATER INFANCY: LESS SEVERE TYPE

Gradually increasing constipation
Small pellet or ribbonlike stool
Abdominal distention
Fecal mass palpable: left lower quadrant
Disturbed nutrition
- Failure to grow
- Loss of subcutaneous tissue

Anemia
Nutritional assessment

Laboratory/diagnostic studies

Rectal examination: tight internal sphincter with explosive, foul-smelling watery stool

Barium enema: retention of barium and visualization of dilated proximal colon and narrowed distal segment

Rectal biopsy: confirms lack of ganglion cells

Anorectal manometry: normal contraction of external sphincter with failure of internal sphincter to relax or contract

Potential complications

Enterocolitis (p. 819)
Septic shock (p. 104)
Dehydration (p. 866)
Hypokalemia (p. 46)
Hyponatremia (p. 46)
Hypoproteinemia (p. 46)
Metabolic acidosis (p. 46)

Medical management

Surgical creation of a loop or double-barrel colostomy just above determined level of ganglionic bowel

Corrective surgery via abdominoperineal pull-through procedure (p. 817)

Parenteral fluids for hydration

NPO initially; po begun after defecation through colostomy

Nasogastric tube connected to low, intermittent suction (discontinued after defecation through colostomy)

Antibiotics

Nursing diagnoses/goals/interventions

ndx: Alteration in nutrition: less than body requirements related to imposed dietary restriction secondary to surgery for creation of colostomy

GOAL: *Patient will tolerate age-appropriate diet (see requirements for age, p. 866) prior to discharge*

Maintain NPO status as ordered
Maintain nasogastric tube connected to **gravity** drainage or to low, intermittent suction as ordered
Irrigate nasogastric tube q2h and prn to ensure patency
Note color, amount, and characteristic of nasogastric drainage
Administer parenteral fluids as ordered
Administer nasogastric replacement fluids as ordered
Monitor intake and output and specific gravity
Weigh patient daily
Assess abdomen for
 Distention (measure girth with vital signs)
 Return of bowel sounds
 Passage of flatus and stool through colostomy

ndx: Alteration in bowel elimination: constipation or diarrhea related to altered bowel evacuation via colostomy

GOAL: *Patient will develop normal bowel pattern and will remain hydrated*

Observe color and consistency of colostomy drainage
Measure amount of colostomy drainage; if volume is large and watery, consider increasing fluid replacement to compensate for fluid loss via colostomy
Observe rectal discharge; mucus and stool may be present, especially if loop colostomy was performed
Follow special diet if ordered (usually low-residue diet)
Observe dietary intake influence on stool pattern and avoid items that cause increase in loose stools or increased gas

ndx: Knowledge deficit regarding colostomy care at home and need for follow-up care

GOAL: *Parents and/or significant other will demonstrate understanding of colostomy care and home care needs through interactive discussion and actual return demonstration*

Teach and have parents demonstrate colostomy care (p. 393)
Reassure parents that they will not hurt child by touching stoma
Explain special diet as ordered
Emphasize importance of adequate fluid intake
Teach observation of colostomy drainage
Discuss need for corrective surgery
Discuss financial burden
NOTE: If conservative dietary management is employed, patient will not have a colostomy and will be treated at home until corrective surgery is scheduled
Teach parents how to give normal saline enemas
Teach name of laxative medication, purpose, dosage, time of administration, and side effects
Discuss low-residue diet
Discuss signs and symptoms to report to physician
 Abdominal distention
 Fever
 Vomiting
 Abdominal pain
 Irritability
 Dyspnea

Evaluation

Patient tolerates age-appropriate diet
Patient is hydrated
Patient has developed normal bowel elimination pattern

Parents demonstrate their ability to care for colostomy
Parents understand home care and follow-up instructions

ABDOMINOPERINEAL PULL-THROUGH PROCEDURE

A corrective procedure for Hirschsprung's disease: Swenson, Duhamel, or Soave

Usual age: any, usually by 1 year of age or 20 lb

Postoperative assessment for potential complications

Enterocolitis
   Frequent green, liquid stools
   Dehydration (p. 866)
   Hyponatremia (p. 46)
   Hypokalemia (p. 46)
   Magnesium deficiency
      Disorientation
      Hyperreactivity to stimuli
      Muscular twitching
      Convulsions
      Bulging anterior fontanel (if still open)
Prolonged paralytic ileus
   Abdominal distention
   Increased amount of gastric drainage
   Bilious gastric drainage
Ventilatory problems
   Tachypnea
   Tachycardia
   Decreased breath sounds
   Rales
Pelvic abscess
   Fever
   Palpable pelvic mass
   Anal discharge, purulent or bloody
   Septic shock (p. 104)

Medical management

Preoperative

Clear liquid diet orally for 48 to 72 hr
Colonic irrigations with normal saline
If colostomy is present, irrigation of distal loop and rectum with normal saline
Night before operation
   Antibiotic irrigation of colostomy to cleanse bowel of bacteria; oral antibiotics may be ordered 1 day before surgery
   Parenteral fluids
   NPO

Postoperative

NPO
Parenteral fluids
Nasogastric tube connected to low, intermittent suction
Irrigation of nasogastric tube q2h to 4h
Nasogastric replacement fluids
Foley catheter may be present for 1 to 2 days postoperatively
May have Penrose drain for rectal drainage
Abdominal dressing
Respiratory care: postural drainage and percussion prn
Vital signs q2h; *no rectal temperatures*
Antibiotics
Analgesics
Oral feedings begun with return of peristalsis; advancement from clear liquid diet to age-appropriate diet as tolerated

Nursing diagnoses/goals/interventions

ndx: Alteration in nutrition: less than body requirements related to imposed dietary restrictions and/or chronic poor feeding

GOAL: *Patient will tolerate age-appropriate diet prior to discharge*

Maintain NPO status immediately postoperatively
Administer parenteral fluids as ordered
Administer hyperalimentation solution as ordered if prolonged ileus occurs
Assess abdomen for return of peristalsis
   Presence of bowel sounds
   Nondistended abdomen (measure girth)
   Passing of flatus and/or stool
   Decrease in amount of nasogastric drainage
Discontinue nasogastric tube as ordered
Begin clear liquid diet, advancing to diet for age as ordered and tolerated (may be low-residue diet)
Observe child/parent behavior around feeding time
Do not force child to eat or make an issue out of eating
Make referral for nutritional/feeding strategy counseling as necessary

ndx: Potential fluid volume deficit related to gastric drainage, NPO status, and/or frequent loose stools

GOAL: *Patient will remain hydrated*

Maintain NPO immediately postoperatively
Maintain nasogastric tube to low, intermittent suction
Ensure patency of nasogastric tube by irrigating q2h as ordered

Measure nasogastric drainage q4h and prn, and replace with parenteral fluids as ordered
Measure intake and output
Monitor specific gravity

***ndx*:** Alteration in bowel elimination: diarrhea related to poor sphincter control and/or as expected sequela of surgery

GOAL: *Patient will eventually develop normal bowel pattern and will eventually be toilet trained*

Observe frequency, consistency, color, and volume of stools
Anticipate that child may have as many as 5 to 15 loose stools per day
Assist in identifying possible dietary irritants
Ensure dietary restrictions if ordered
Anticipate and teach parents that child will be slow to toilet train

***ndx*:** Potential for ineffective breathing pattern related to anesthesia, postoperative immobility and/or pain

GOAL: *Patient's breath sounds will remain clear, and respiratory rate will be age appropriate*

Monitor vital signs q4h and prn
Monitor respiratory status q2h and prn
Assist patient with turning and coughing q2h
Administer postural drainage and percussion if necessary
Elevate head of bed; encourage parents to hold child; sit child in padded high chair; ambulate if developmentally able
Administer pain medication if necessary prior to vigorous respiratory treatments or ambulation

***ndx*:** Alteration in comfort: pain related to surgical intervention

GOAL: *Patient will be pain-free prior to discharge*

Assess for symptoms of pain
    Facial grimacing
    Crying
    Poor appetite
    Withdrawn behavior
    Refusal to increase physical activity
Administer analgesics as ordered
Institute other comfort measures
    Cuddling, sucking of pacifier, minimal auditory and visual stimulation
    Position for comfort; avoid extension of abdominal musculature

Gently cleanse anal area with soap and water; warm water squirted on area with syringe or perineal bottle is soothing

***ndx*:** Alteration in skin integrity related to surgical intervention and expected frequent loose stools postoperatively

GOAL: *Patient's surgical incision will heal without signs of infection, and skin of anal/perineal area will remain intact*

Monitor wound for signs of infection
    Fever
    Redness
    Swelling
    Copious or foul drainage
Administer incisional care as ordered
Prevent contamination of abdominal wound with urine by pinning diaper below dressing; a Foley catheter may be used immediately postoperatively for urinary diversion
Observe color, amount, and characteristic of drainage from rectal Penrose drain if present
Cleanse anal area gently with soap and water after each bowel movement
Apply protective ointments to anal and perineal area q2h and prn
Encourage proper nutrition

***ndx*:** Knowledge deficit regarding home care and follow-up needs

GOAL: *Parents and/or significant other will demonstrate understanding of home care and follow-up instructions through interactive discussion and actual return demonstration*

Explain appropriate diet with restrictions if any
Teach care of anal/perineal area
Discuss symptoms of wound infection to report to physician: redness, pain, swelling, drainage
Teach name of medications, purpose, dosage, time of administration, and side effects
Have parents demonstrate
    Anal/perineal care
    Feeding strategies
Discuss toilet training expectations
Discuss availability of community health services for support and follow-up

Evaluation

Patient tolerates age-appropriate diet
Patient is hydrated

Patient is beginning to establish normal stool pattern via rectum
Patient's breath sounds are clear
Patient is pain-free
Patient's anal/perineal area is clean and irritation is controlled
Parents demonstrate ability to care for child at home

GASTROENTERITIS

A condition characterized by vomiting and diarrhea resulting from infection, allergy, intolerance for specific food substances, or ingestion of toxins

Usual age: any
Complications are most severe in infants
Child should be placed on enteric isolation precautions

Assessment
Observations/findings

Frequent loose stools
   Yellow-green, green
   May be mucoid
   May be bloody
Weight loss or failure to gain weight
Decreased appetite
Abdominal pain and/or cramping
Abdominal distention
Hyperactive bowel sounds
Vomiting
Fever
Irritability
Increasing lethargy
Excoriated buttocks
Dehydration (p. 866)
   Depressed anterior fontanel
   Sunken eyes
   Loss of skin turgor
   Dry mucous membranes
   No tears with crying
   High urine specific gravity
   Oliguria
Some degree of electrolyte imbalance:
   Hyponatremia or hypernatremia (p. 47)
   Hypokalemia or hyperkalemia (p. 47)
   Metabolic acidosis (p. 47)
See Gastrointestinal Assessment (p. 339)
Nutritional assessment

Laboratory/diagnostic studies

WBC differential: increased bands with shigellosis
Stool specimens
   May have increased leukocytes or clumps of pus with enteroinvasive organisms
   May be positive for occult blood
   May be positive for reducing substance (sugar in stool) with disaccharide intolerance
Serum electrolytes
CBC: elevated Hct

Potential complications

Hypovolemic shock (p. 104)

Medical management

NPO until rehydrated
Parenteral fluids and electrolyes (potassium is added to parenteral solution only after renal function is ensured by passage of urine)
With chronic diarrhea, hyperalimentation may be necessary
Replacement of stool output with parenteral fluids as necessary to maintain adequate hydration
Use of oral rehydration therapy (p. 821) may be considered if child is less than 10% dehydrated, vomiting is minimal, and stool losses are less than 10 ml/kg/hr
Intake and output; specific gravity
Antibiotic therapy
Tests of stools for occult blood, pH, and reducing substance
Vital signs q1h to 2h
Small, frequent feedings of clear liquids begun, with gradual advancement of diet as tolerated

Nursing diagnoses/goals/interventions

ndx: Fluid volume deficit related to inability to tolerate oral fluids without vomiting and diarrhea

GOAL: *Patient will have tears, moist mucous membranes, normal skin turgor, and adequate urinary output for age (see standard for age under Basic Standards of Care, pp. 781-788), and will gain weight*

Monitor vital signs q1h to 2h as ordered and prn
Monitor cardiac activity until fluid and electrolyte imbalances are corrected
Maintain NPO status as ordered
Administer parenteral fluids with added electrolytes as ordered
Weigh patient daily
Monitor intake and output
Determine specific gravity on each voided specimen
Describe frequency and character of stools
Describe frequency and character of vomitus (if present)

Monitor for resolving or persistent signs of dehydration

Administer stool replacement fluids if ordered

Monitor serum electrolytes

Begin small, frequent feedings of electrolyte solution as ordered and monitor patient's tolerance to it; advance diet gradually as tolerated

ndx: Alteration in bowel elimination: diarrhea related to ingestion of an irritant, infectious process, or intestinal malabsorption

GOAL: *Patient will resume prehospitalized bowel pattern*

Maintain NPO status until stools decrease in number and volume to prevent further gastric irritation

Describe frequency, character, and color of stools

Collect stool specimens as ordered

Test each stool for occult blood, pH, and reducing substance

Begin small, frequent feedings of electrolyte solution as ordered

Give liquids at room temperature; cold liquids increase bowel motility

Advance to breast milk feedings or gradually advance formula from quarter strength, half strength, and full strength as tolerated and ordered (infants)

Assess patient's tolerance to each dietary change and reduce strength of formula if stool volume increases significantly

In an older child, diet may be advanced from clear liquids to BRAT (bananas, rice, applesauce, toast) diet with elimination of all milk products (see Diet for Control of Diarrhea, below)

ndx: Alteration in skin integrity related to frequent loose stools with irritation of anal area and buttocks

GOAL: *Patient's skin will heal, no further excoriation will occur, and no secondary infection will be introduced*

Keep diaper area clean and dry

Check and change diaper q1h and prn

Wash skin with mild soap and water after each stool; rinse well with water only (soap can be an irritant) and dry thoroughly

Leave diaper area exposed to air as much as possible

Use cloth diapers against skin

Avoid use of heat lamp, since it can cause thermal burns and further skin irritation

Apply protective ointments after each diaper change

Ensure proper nutrition as soon as feasible to promote tissue healing

Wear gloves and wash hands before and after changing diapers

ndx: Knowledge deficit regarding home care needs and procedure to follow should diarrhea recur

GOAL: *Patient and/or parents will demonstrate understanding of home care and follow-up instructions through interactive discussion and actual return demonstration*

Explain reasons for NPO order and slow, gradual advancement of diet with restrictions

Explain need for isolation to prevent transmission of illness

Teach good handwashing techniques before and after diaper changes

Teach care of diaper area

Explain need to report recurrence of symptoms to physician

If symptoms recur, instruct parents to prevent dehydration by

Giving ad lib breast milk feedings (if breast feeding)

Avoiding lactose-containing formulas or cow's milk for 1-2 days

Giving child oral electrolyte solution (Infalyte-Mix as directed on package), not to exceed 150 ml/kg/day

Giving breast milk, clear liquids, or free water if child is still thirsty

Instruct patient or parents to begin BRAT diet as tolerated; as stools continue to firm, more foods should be gradually added from regular diet

Teach name of medication, purpose, dosage time of administration, and side effects

Evaluation

Patient is hydrated

Patient is gaining weight

Urinary output is at least 1 ml/kg/hr in child or 2 ml/kg/hr in infant

Stools have decreased in frequency and are firm

Patient is tolerating advances in diet

Skin of buttocks is healed or healing

Patient and/or parents understand dietary management, and parents are able to care for child at home

DIET FOR CONTROL OF DIARRHEA

Clear liquids
 Water
 Tea
 Carbonated beverages (served flat)

Gelatin
Flavored ice pops
Bouillon broth
Electrolyte solution (only if recommended by physician)
Apple juice (diluted to half strength—some children may not tolerate half strength; therefore, this may be eliminated from diet until stool pattern has returned)
BRAT diet
　Breast milk
　Bananas
　Rice
　Applesauce
　Toast
　Soup (not creamed)
　Soda crackers
　Pretzels
　Dry sweetened cereals (no milk)
After stools begin to firm, add the following
　Formula as ordered
　Boiled or broiled chicken
　Apples
　Cottage cheese
　Tapioca
　Mashed potatoes
As stools continue to firm, gradually add more foods from regular diet

ORAL REHYDRATION THERAPY

The intestinal tract is used to provide adequate fluid intake for rehydration and to avoid the use of intravenous therapy; this therapy is also useful for preventing dehydration and hospitalization if initiated in the early stages of gastroenteritis

Criteria for use

Vomiting is absent or minimal
Child is less than 10% dehydrated
Stool losses are less than 10 ml/kg/hr

Oral electrolyte solution contents*

Glucose 2%: 111 mmol/L
Sodium: 50 to 60 mmol/L
Potassium: 20 to 30 mmol/L
Chloride: 30 to 50 mmol/L
Bicarbonate: 30 mmol/L

Rehydration therapy

If patient is 10% dehydrated or more, intravenous fluids must be used

If patient is vomiting, give 10 to 15 ml of electrolyte solution q15 min for four times, then increase to 30 ml q30 min twice, then
　Give 15 to 20 ml/kg/hr until rehydrated *or*
　Give entire deficit plus one third of maintenance requirements for 24 hr period plus ongoing losses over the next 8 hr (e.g., for a 10 kg child with 5% dehydration, you would give 500 ml deficit plus 333 ml maintenance plus ongoing stool losses, *all* over the next 8 hr)

Maintenance therapy

Use same oral electrolyte solution as above and give at rate of 150 ml/kg/day; give any additional fluids ad lib as breast milk or free water; lactose-free solids can be started after child is rehydrated and is not vomiting (see BRAT diet at left)
NOTE: Criterion for continuing oral feeding is based on how well child is doing, not necessarily how stools are; it is not recommended that child be made NPO in presence of ongoing or increasing diarrhea

INCARCERATED INGUINAL HERNIA

An obstruction of an intestinal loop, which has passed through the inguinal ring into the inguinal canal

Usual age: under 1 year

Assessment

Observations/findings

Red, firm, tender, globular, irreducible swelling in groin
Fretfulness resulting from pain
Anorexia
Nausea, vomiting
Abdominal distention
Absence of bowel movements
Dehydration (p. 866)
If bowel loop is ischemic or gangrenous
　Shock (p. 104)
　Fever
　Absence of bowel sounds
　Metabolic acidosis (p. 47)

Laboratory/diagnostic studies

WBC: elevated if loop is gangrenous
Serum electrolytes

Potential complications

Shock (p. 104)
Gangrenous bowel loop

---

*Infalyte-Mix with 1 L of water added

Medical management

Manual reduction of hernia if possible
Surgical reduction of hernia (see Abdominal Herniorrhaphy, p. 390)
Correction of hydration and electrolyte imbalances
Analgesics

Nursing diagnosis/goal/interventions (preoperative)*

ndx: Alteration in comfort: pain related to intestinal obstruction

GOAL: *Patient will show signs of comfort: decreased crying and increased ability to sleep without disturbance*

Prevent crying and straining, since this increases intestinal protrusion
Apply ice to affected side
Administer sedation as ordered
Position for comfort

INTUSSUSCEPTION

An intestinal obstruction resulting from one section of intestine invaginating (telescoping) into an adjacent section

Usual age: 3 to 24 months

Assessment
Observations/findings

FIRST 12 HR

Intermittent abdominal pain
Vomiting
Passage of one normal stool

AFTER FIRST 12 HR

Increasing vomiting
Severe pain with screaming and drawing up of knees to chest
Passage of red, jellylike stool (blood and mucus)
Abdominal tenderness
Abdominal distention
Sausage-shaped "tumor" may be visible in right or left upper quadrant

Laboratory/diagnostic studies

Barium enema: demonstrates obstruction to flow of barium and is used as a nonsurgical technique to reduce telescoping of intestine

---

*See Abdominal Herniorrhaphy (p. 390) and Ruptured (Perforated) Appendix (p. 813) for postoperative nursing diagnoses, goals, and interventions; alter interventions appropriately for age (see standard for age under Basic Standards of Care, pp. 781-788).

Potential complications

Shock (p. 104)
Perforation of bowel

Medical management

Nonsurgical hydrostatic reduction by barium enema
See Ruptured (Perforated) Appendix (p. 813) for general abdominal surgery management

Nursing diagnoses/goals/interventions

See Ruptured (Perforated) Appendix (p. 813) for nursing concerns after abdominal surgery

Central Nervous System

HYDROCEPHALUS

Excessive cerebrospinal fluid (CSF) within the ventricular and subarachnoid spaces
noncommunicating hydrocephalus *CSF flow is blocked somewhere within the ventricular system*
communicating hydrocephalus *CSF is not absorbed from the subarachnoid space, but there is no interference within the ventricular system*

Usual age: first year of life but can be diagnosed at any age

Assessment
Observations/findings

See Neurologic Assessment (p. 283)
History of meningitis, intracranial infections or hemorrhage, perinatal anoxia, and/or intrauterine infection
Gradual increase in head size
Widening suture lines
Widening, bulging, nonpulsating anterior fontanel
"Bossing" of brow
Shiny scalp
Dilated scalp veins
Macewen's sign (cracked-pot sound with percussion of skull)
Visible sclera above iris: "sun setting"
Strabismus
Irritability
Lethargy
Poor suck or feeding difficulty
High-pitched cry
Opisthotonos
Persistant primitive reflexes
Delayed development
Ataxia
Increased intracranial pressure (ICP)
  Alterations in consciousness and responsiveness

Vomiting, especially associated with position change
Headache on awakening
Seizures
Bradycardia
Bradypnea
Hypothermia
Associated neurologic defects (myelomeningocele)

Laboratory/diagnostic studies

Diagnosis made on basis of abnormal head circumference and neurologic signs
Computed tomography (CT) scan: confirms presence of dilated ventricles and assists in identifying possible cause (neoplasms, cysts, congenital malformation such as Arnold-Chiari malformation or intracranial hemorrhages)
Ventricular puncture (taps) are sometimes used to measure ICP, remove CSF to reduce pressure, and obtain CSF for culture

Potential complications

Associated anomalies
Mental retardation
Neurologic disabilities

Medical management

Determination of type of hydrocephalus
Insertion of shunt to carry excess CSF away from lateral ventricle to an extracranial site (usually peritoneum in infants and young children, or atrium in adolescent) where it can then be reabsorbed
Small frequent feedings to ensure adequate nutrition

Nursing diagnoses/goals/interventions

ndx: Potential sensory/perceptual alterations related to increased ICP secondary to CSF accumulation in ventricles

GOAL: *Patient will be assessed for increased neurologic deterioration*

Monitor level of consciousness and responsiveness q1h to 2h
Assess vital signs q1h to 2h
Monitor blood pressure q2h to 4h
Measure head circumference q shift
Weigh patient daily

ndx: Potential alteration in skin integrity of scalp related to inability of infant to turn head secondary to increased head size and weight

GOAL: *Infant's skin will remain intact*

Change position q2h; may consider changing position of head q1h
Avoid loose linen in bed
Lay head on foam rubber pad or use water bed if available
Assess head for pressure points at least q2h
Stimulate circulation to area with each position change
Maintain nutrition as ordered

ndx: Knowledge deficit regarding disorder and treatment

GOAL: *Parents and/or significant other demonstrate understanding of treatment of hydrocephalus through interactive discussion and will make informed decisions about treatment*

Explain disorder to parents
Prepare parents for surgery
Teach parents how to handle child and support child's head

Evaluation

Skin of scalp remains intact
Neurologic status is evaluated
Parents are prepared for surgical intervention

VENTRICULAR SHUNT INSERTION

Treatment for noncommunicating hydrocephalus involving surgical placement of device that bypasses cranial obstruction and carries CSF to an extracranial site where it is then reabsorbed

Usual age: infant; reinsertion or revisions can occur at any age

Assessment

Observations/findings
PREOPERATIVE

See Hydrocephalus (p. 822)
Assessment of neurologic status, especially behavior, developmental ability, and presence or absence of developmental reflexes, for postoperative comparison
Pupillary reaction
Response to auditory and visual stimulation
Head circumference
Fontanel size, protrusion, and pulsability (usually nonpulsating)
Level of consciousness
Respiratory and cardiac rate and quality
Motion present in extremities
Degree of irritability
Cry and sucking quality

POSTOPERATIVE

Reassess neurologic status for improvement or deterioration
Assess for signs and symptoms of increased ICP (p. 331)
Fever
Sites of incision
 Leakage of CSF
 Swelling
 Redness
 Drainage
 "Tracking" along shunt

Potential complications

Shunt malfunction
Shunt infection
With ventriculoperitoneal shunt
 Peritonitis (p. 372)
 Abdominal distention
 Paralytic ileus (p. 377)
 Abdominal pain
With ventriculoatrial shunt
 Shunt block by blood clot
 Pulmonary embolus (p. 247)

Medical management

Insertion of mechanical shunt
Monitoring of neurologic status q1h to 2h following shunt insertion
Antibiotics prophylactically or for treatment of shunt infection
Gradual increase in elevation of head ordered after close assessment of neurologic improvement and signs and symptoms of increased ICP
Change of surgical incision dressings and order for dressing changes
Parenteral fluids with gradual advance in diet as tolerated

Nursing diagnoses/goals/interventions

ndx Potential sensory/perceptual alterations related to possible shunt malfunction or shunt infection

GOAL: *Patient will be assessed for neurologic baseline; shunt disorders will be assessed and treated promptly*

Measure head circumference q4h
Assess fontanel for size and bulging; level of consciousness; pupil size, position, and reaction; extraocular movements and ability to fix and follow; muscle tone; and quality of cry qh
Assess vital signs qh and prn
Assess temperature q4h and prn
Monitor blood pressure q1h to 2h

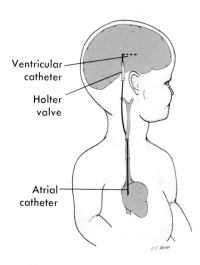

FIGURE 15-7. Ventriculoatrial shunt.

Maintain position on nonoperative side of head; *do not position on shunt* (Figure 15-7)
Keep child flat as ordered; only advance elevation of head as ordered to prevent rapid decrease in ICP

ndx Potential for infection related to surgical intervention

GOAL: *Child will remain afebrile with no signs of skin infection*

Prevent contamination of surgical sites by keeping them covered with sterile dressing and by washing hands thoroughly before touching area
Monitor temperature q4h and prn
Assess surgical incisions q2h for redness, swelling, drainage, intactness of sutures, and "tracking" along shunt
Administer antibiotics as ordered

ndx Potential alteration in skin integrity related to decreased mobility, increased head size, and weight

See goal and interventions under Hydrocephalus (p. 823)

ndx Knowledge deficit regarding home care and follow-up needs

GOAL: *Parents and/or significant other will demonstrate understanding of home care and follow-up instructions through interactive discussion and actual return demonstration*

Explain purpose of shunt insertion
Discuss symptoms of shunt failure or infection and increasing ICP to report to physician

Poor feeding
Vomiting
Change in behavior
Increased lethargy
Irritability
"Sun setting" eyes
Fever
Signs of skin infection around incision
   Redness
   Swelling
   Drainage
Emphasize need for ongoing assessment and care on outpatient basis
Have parents demonstrate how to pump shunt, if ordered

Evaluation

Patient is alert and interactive, and behaves in age-appropriate manner
Skin remains intact
No signs of incisional infection are present
Parents can state symptoms of shunt infection or malfunction

MYELOMENINGOCELE

A congenital defect in the spinal vertebrae resulting in motor and sensory dysfunction of the trunk and lower extremities below the level of deformity and accompanied by nonfunctional bowel and bladder sphincters; malformed cord and roots are contained in a sac and covered by a thin vascular membrane

Usual age: diagnosed in newborn period

Assessment

Observations/findings
NEWBORN PERIOD

Meningeal sac
   Location
   Increasing tension
   Leakage of CSF
   Malodorous drainage
   Rupture
Presence or absence of associated hydrocephalus (p. 822)
Parents' reaction to diagnosis

ANY AGE

Level of spinal defect
Degree of neurologic impairment
Spastic or flaccid lower extremities
Bilateral clubfoot
Bilateral or unilateral hip dislocation
Constant dribbling of urine
Distended or flaccid bladder
Frequent small, loose stools or constipation
Progress in bowel and bladder training
Method of mobility (braces, wheelchair)
Integrity of skin
Patient and family's adjustment to diagnosis

Laboratory/diagnostic studies

Culture of CSF in presence of fever and signs of central nervous system (CNS) infection
Urinalysis and cultures in presence of urinary tract infection (UTI)
Blood urea nitrogen (BUN) and creatinine to assess renal function

Potential complications

Hydrocephalus (p. 822)
Meningitis (p. 828)
Seizure disorder (p. 291)
UTI (p. 291)
Renal failure (p. 557)
Decubitus ulcers (p. 619)
Progressive kyphoscoliosis
Death

Medical management
Newborn period

Assessment of degree of neurologic involvement
Moist, sterile normal saline dressings to sac (may also use antibacterial solution)
Dislocated hips in position of abduction
Parenteral fluids as necessary to ensure hydration and electrolyte balance
Honest information to parents about anomalies to assist them in making appropriate decisions about treatment in newborn period
Surgical closure of protruding sac
Insertion of mechanical shunt if hydrocephalus is present (see Ventricular Shunt Insertion, p. 823)

Ongoing management

Correction of orthopedic deformities; casting/bracing as necessary
Ongoing exercise regimen (physical therapy referral)
Shunt revisions as necessary
Anticonvulsants if seizure disorder is present
Assessment of renal function
Antibiotics for UTIs
Laxatives, stool softeners, and/or suppositories as necessary for bowel training

Minimal restrictions on child's activities to promote growth and development
Assessment of child and/or family's adjustment

Nursing diagnoses/goals/interventions: newborn period

ndx: Potential for infection related to open sac with draining, protruding spinal contents

GOAL: *Patient will remain free of CNS infection related to contamination of sac*

Prevent contamination of sac from stool or urine by placing infant prone and undiapered, and securing a pad below sac
Change diapers promptly as necessary
Use aseptic technique in caring for sac
Change sterile dressing with sterile solutions as ordered
Avoid exposure to persons with known infections
Preserve intact skin around sac; avoid use of tape
Avoid pressure on sac; use protective donut as necessary
Use sterile towel while holding infant
Check temperature q4h and prn
Measure head circumference daily

ndx: Impaired physical mobility related to lack of nerve innervation to lower extremities (degree dependent on level of involvement)

GOAL: *Infant will maintain present level of physical ability*

Position infant
　Keep infant prone with entire body in slightly head-up position, head turned to either side
　Place linen roll under ankles to keep foot in neutral position
　Keep legs positioned in moderate abduction
Perform passive ROM exercises as recommended by physical therapy
Turn q2h

ndx: Potential alteration in skin integrity related to decreased mobility and decreased sensation to lower extremities

GOAL: *Infant's skin will remain intact and clean*

Assess skin q2h and prn for pressure areas, redness, and blanching
Use water bed if available
Turn q2h and prn

Keep skin clean and dry
Ensure adequate fluid intake for hydration
Ensure adequate dietary intake of protein and carbohydrate

ndx: Potential alteration in bowel and bladder control related to lack of nerve innervation for appropriate defecation and urination

GOAL: *Patient will establish bowel and bladder regimen to prevent constipation and urinary retention*

Assess voiding and stooling pattern
Voiding
　Note color, volume, presence of constant dribbling, and presence of distended bladder after spontaneous void
　Perform Crede's maneuver on bladder q2h to 4h as necessary to promote bladder emptying (p. 537)
Stools
　Note frequency and consistency of stool
　Note constant dribbling of loose stool; may indicate stooling around an area of constipation
　Assess abdomen for distention or palpable stool in left lower quadrant
　Administer suppositories as ordered prn

ndx: Knowledge deficit regarding condition and treatment

GOAL: *Parents and/or significant other will make an informed decision about treatment*

Ensure that parents are given *all* the facts about myelomeningocele; *do not* allow them to receive one-sided information
Organize an ethical committee of physicians, social workers, nurses, and other parents of children with myelomeningocele; have the committee meet with the parents of the newborn to present factual information to them
If necessary, have parents who have a child with myelomeningocele meet with parents of infant
Also consider having parents of infant meet with family who chose other alternatives
Allow parents sufficient time to make an informed decision
Realize that parents are grieving and decision making is difficult for them at this time

Nursing diagnoses/goals/interventions: ongoing concerns

ndx: Potential for injury related to decreased perception of pain, touch, and temperature in lower extremities

GOAL: *Patient and/or parents will be aware of how to protect patient from injury; no preventable injury will occur*

Teach patient or parents how to assess for skin irritations
Explain need to alter position of child (shift weight) as often as q30 min
Caution patient or parents to avoid use of hot baths; to check water temperature with inner aspect of forearm or with thermometer
Explain need to keep skin of feet warm, dry, and soft
Discuss age-appropriate safety precautions

ndx: Impaired physical mobility related to neurologic dysfunction of lower extremities (also loss of abdominal musculature control with thoracic defects)

GOAL: *Patient will obtain optimal mobility through use of his physical abilities and use of assistive devices*

Perform ROM exercises; as child gets older teach him how to do this
Position patient in alignment
    Support calf with pillows
    Avoid prolonged periods in one position; change q2h
If braces are used
    Assess correct positioning of braces
    Assess for skin irritation under braces
    Have patient demonstrate application of braces
If wheelchair is used
    Use soft cushion in chair
    Support legs on pillows
    Remember to change patient's position q2h and prn
Encourage progressive mobilization
    Exercise upper extremities: push-ups, pull-ups, throwing balls, weight lifting
    Encourage self-care activities: combing hair, bathing self, dressing self
    Guide patient's legs as patient transfers self from bed to wheelchair
    Encourage independence

ndx: Altered bowel elimination: constipation related to decreased nerve innervation, decreased abdominal muscle innervation, decreased sense of need to defecate, and decreased mobility

GOAL: *Patient will learn dietary habits and use of medications to promote regular bowel function*

Meet age-appropriate fluid requirements (p. 866)
Administer well-balanced high-bulk diet: fruit, fruit juices, vegetables, bran, whole-grain breads and cereals, nuts
Involve patient in daily exercise regimen
Encourage mobilization
For individuals eligible for bowel training
    Observe stool pattern and identify normal defecation pattern
    Establish time for defecation after a meal
    Ensure privacy
    Sit patient on commode or toilet (if feasible)
    Administer suppositories or laxatives as ordered

ndx: Alteration in urinary elimination: incontinence/retention related to decreased nerve innervation

GOAL: *Patient will establish a pattern of micturition*

Assess present voiding pattern
    Any sensation
    Timing in relation to fluid intake
    Constant dribbling or large volume at one time
    Amount voided
    Bladder distention after voiding
    Amount of residual urine after voiding
Maintain hydration by meeting age-appropriate fluid
Teach intermittent catheterization to patient and family
    Explain reasons for catheterization
    Demonstrate clean technique
    Explain need to empty bladder at set times because of danger of overdistention of bladder and its contribution to bladder infections
    Explain relationship between fluid intake and frequency of catheterization
Keep skin clean and dry
Administer antibiotics as ordered for UTI

ndx: Potential alteration in skin integrity related to immobility, decreased sensation, and/or urinary/bowel incontinence

GOAL: *Patient's skin will be intact, clean, and dry*

Turn patient at least q2h and prn
Assess skin frequently for redness or blanching
Use water beds if available
Position patient for comfort; eliminate wrinkles in sheets
Keep patient clean and dry
When using soap, be sure to rinse it off thoroughly
Apply lotions to keep skin soft
Also refer to nursing diagnosis of *potential for injury*, above

ndx: Potential alteration in nutrition: more than body requirements related to imbalance between intake and energy expenditure

GOAL: *Patient will eat a diet sufficient to promote growth and development but will not become obese*

Calculate caloric requirements (p. 866); keep in mind that actual caloric requirements for someone immobile will be less than recommended
Discuss balance between intake and energy expenditure with parents early in care of child
Assess family's eating habits
Assist family with identifying well-balanced diet
Assist family with identifying high-calorie foods and encourage them to eliminate them from family's diet
Have patient drink glass of water prior to meals
Increase amount of socialization and diversionary activity to distract patient from thoughts of food
Encourage patient to be involved in routine physical activity
Promote physical exercise as recommended by physical therapist
Allow patient to do as much for self as possible
Monitor weight

ndx: Altered self-concept related to prolonged debilitation, inability to complete developmental tasks, and/or social isolation

GOAL: *Patient will identify things patient likes about self*

Provide child with opportunity to discuss fears, concerns, grief, and anger
Ask patient to identify things patient likes about self
If patient is unable to do so, tell patient things you like about him
Encourage patient to look at self in mirror
Encourage grooming, including alternating hair styles, wearing makeup, and experimenting with different clothes, hats, jewelry, etc.
Encourage independence and reward patient for efforts to become independent
Allow patient sufficient time to accomplish a task; it may take a little longer
Encourage interaction with other children; take patient to playroom, have patient play a quiet game with roommate, etc.
Set aside time for school friends to visit child in hospital
Continue contact with school and schedule time for schoolwork so child does not fall behind
Involve child in ongoing community support group consisting of children with similar limitations

ndx: Altered family process related to chronic nature of disease and adjustment requirements for all family members

GOAL: *Family will verbalize feelings, will care for ill family member, will support each other, and will use resources appropriately*

Discuss financial stress with parents
Discuss social stigma associated with disability
Discuss unresolved anger, guilt, jealousy, or grief
Assess how each family member is coping with disease
Assess ways in which child's disease has altered family functioning
Identify ways that each family member can participate in care of ill family member
Give family members insight into feelings of disabled child
Involve family in ongoing counseling
Increase community resources as necessary to assist family with stress
Have family meet regularly with other families with a child with myelomeningocele

Evaluation

Patient functions at highest level of physical ability
Skin remains intact and clean
Bowel and bladder regimen is established and maintained
Diet-exercise relationship is sufficient to prevent obesity
Child has positive self-image
Family and/or child understand complexities of ongoing care
Family members have adjusted to life with a child requiring extensive care

MENINGITIS

Inflammation of the meninges, usually due to an infectious agent: bacterial, viral, tubercular, or mycotic

Usual age: any; most common in infants and toddlers
Placement: patients with all types of bacterial meningitis are placed on respiratory isolation until treated for 48 hr with antibiotics
Meningococcal meningitis warrants strict isolation until treated for at least 48 hr
Viral (aseptic) meningitis warrants respiratory isolation for duration of hospitalization

Assessment

Observations/findings

History of preexisting infection
Irritability
Headache
Bulging anterior fontanel
Photophobia
High-pitched cry
Nuchal rigidity
Opisthotonos
Hyperactive deep tendon reflexes
Brudzinski's sign: flexing neck causes knees and hips to bend upward
Kernig's sign: leg flexed at hip cannot be straightened at knee
Disturbances in sensorium
    Delirium
    Stupor
Poor feeding
Vomiting
Tachypnea
Tachycardia
Petechiae, purpuric spots with meningococcal meningitis

Laboratory/diagnostic studies

Lumbar puncture
    Bacterial
        May or may not be cloudy
        Low glucose, high protein
        High WBC: predominantly polymorphonuclear leukocytes
        Culture and sensitivities: identify specific organism and appropriate antibiotics
    Viral
        Normal glucose, normal or slightly elevated protein level
        Slightly elevated WBC: predominantly mononuclear leukocytes
Blood culture: may indicate septicemia
CBC: elevated WBC
Serum electrolytes: may be altered; serum sodium is monitored to assess for syndrome of inappropriate antidiuretic hormones (SIADH)
Urine electrolytes: to monitor for SIADH
CT scan: may be indicated to evaluate for complications

Potential complications

Cerebral edema
Hydrocephalus
Brain abscess formation
Seizure disorder
Coma
Neurologic loss: changes in behavior and motor development
Hearing loss, visual loss
SIADH
Shock (p. 104)
Disseminated Intravascular Coagulation (DIC) (p. 196)
Respiratory arrest (p. 261)
Death

Medical management

Determination of causative organism
Respiratory or strict isolation depending on organism
Parenteral fluids given below maintenance requirements until resolution of SIADH
NPO initially, advancing diet from clear liquids to age-appropriate diet as tolerated; fluid restrictions may still prevail when diet is started; parenteral fluids are decreased as oral fluids increase
Intake and output with specific gravity
High doses of intravenous antibiotics specific to isolated organism
Antipyretics
Anticonvulsants if necessary
Repeat lumbar puncture to assess effectiveness of therapy

Nursing diagnoses/goals/interventions

ndx Sensory-perceptual alterations related to increased sensitivity to visual, auditory, and tactile stimulation

GOAL: *Patient will experience reduced environmental stimulation until neurologic sensitivity is decreased, age-appropriate stimulation will be tolerated prior to discharge and permanent alterations in vision or hearing, if any, will be identified*

Assess child's level of consciousness, behavior, and level of irritability q1h to 2h
Check pupil response, ability to fix and follow, extraocular movements, response to sound, muscle tone, and reflexes q2h
Assess vital signs q2h and prn
Keep child isolated in quiet room with door closed to reduce environmental noise
Keep lights dimmed to prevent aggravation of photophobia
Talk to child in quiet, soothing tone
Allow patient to assume position of comfort with minimal handling

Encourage parents to provide comforting measures
Postpone nursing routines to decrease stimulation and allow for undisturbed sleep
Administer anticonvulsants if ordered and monitor serum levels
Gradually resume normal handling as status improves
Encourage preillness activity as muscular rigidity decreases
Assess patient's preillness development
Assess improvements in neurologic status and compare with preillness abilities
Assess return of vision and hearing; identify sensory losses, if any, and make appropriate referrals for follow-up care
Have oxygen and suction available in the event that seizures occur

ndx: Hyperthermia related to inflammatory response to CNS infection

GOAL: *Patient's temperature will maintain age-appropriate temperature range*

Assess temperature q2h and prn
Provide cooling measures prn; avoid cooling to point of shivering
Administer antibiotics as ordered
Administer parenteral fluids as ordered
Administer antipyretics as ordered
Control exposure to extremes in temperature
Keep room temperature moderately warm
Dress child in minimal clothing

ndx: Potential fluid volume excess related to inappropriate release of antidiuretic hormone by pituitary (SIADH) unrelated to plasma osmolality

GOAL: *Patient's neurologic status will not be complicated by cerebral edema related to fluid retention*

Monitor for signs and symptoms of SIADH
　Serum sodium below 130 mEq/L
　Decreased serum osmolality
　Decreased urinary output with rising specific gravities
　Elevated urine electrolytes and osmolality as compared with serum levels
　Weight gain
　Weakness and lethargy
Maintain strict measure of intake and output
Administer fluid-restrictive parenteral fluids as ordered
Gradually decrease parenteral fluid rate as oral intake increases to maintain fluid restrictions

Measure head circumference and assess fontanels for bulging q2h to 4h and prn

ndx: Knowledge deficit regarding nature of illness, home care, and follow-up needs

GOAL: *Patient and/or parents will demonstrate understanding of treatment, and home care and follow-up instructions through interactive discussion and actual return demonstration*

Explain reasons for restrictive activity, environmental stimulation, and fluids
Instruct parents to allow child to resume activity as tolerated with scheduled periods for rest
Discuss recurrence of symptoms to report to physician
　Poor feeding
　Vomiting
　Lethargy
　Irritability
　Fever
Explain need for follow-up assessment of child's visual and hearing development
Teach name of medication, purpose, dosage, time of administration, and side effects

Evaluation

Patient is alert and has resumed preillness developmental ability
Fever is controlled
Resolution of fluid retention with liberalization of administered fluids
Parents understand possible neurologic sequelae and need for follow-up assessment

Genitourinary System

ACUTE GLOMERULONEPHRITIS

An inflammatory process of the kidneys involving an antigen-antibody reaction secondary to an infection elsewhere in the body; most common precipitating factor is group A beta-hemolytic streptococcus

Usual age: any; peak age is 5 years

Assessment
Observations/findings

Evidence of antecedent streptococcal infection
Hematuria: grossly bloody to smoky, brownish hue
Oliguria
Edema: facial, periorbital, slightly generalized
Weight gain
Headache

Anorexia
Vomiting
Fever
Diarrhea
Flank pain
Hypertension
Anemia
Lethargy

Laboratory/diagnostic studies

Urinalysis: proteinuria, elevated specific gravity, red blood cell casts, white blood cells
Blood studies
    Elevated BUN and creatinine
    Decreased serum complement activity
    Increased antistreptolysin titer
    Mild leukocytosis
    Increased erythrocytic sedimentation rate
    Mild anemia
Chest x-ray examination: pulmonary edema, pleural fluid, cardiac enlargement (seen with cardiac decompensation)
Electrocardiogram (ECG) if hyperkalemic

Potential complications

Hypertensive encephalopathy: headaches, drowsiness, restlessness, diplopia, dizziness, seizures, coma
Acute cardiac decompensation caused by hypervolemia: tachycardia, tachypnea, systolic murmur, pulmonary edema, orthopnea, abdominal distention
Acute renal failure (p. 557)
Chronic glomerulonephritis

Medical management

Antihypertensives
Diuretics
Antibiotics with persistent streptococcal infection
Prophylactic antibiotics during convalescent period
Intake and output
Daily weight
Blood pressure q2h
Sodium-restricted diet
Potassium restriction until urine output is greater than 200 to 300 ml/day
Determination of fluid administration; may need to restrict if urine output is significantly scant; with restrictions, fluids are determined by urine output plus estimated insensible losses

Nursing diagnoses/goals/interventions

ndx Fluid volume excess related to sodium and water retention secondary to decreased glomerular filtration rate

GOAL: *Patient will maintain normal fluid balance, urine output will return to normal, and edema will disappear*

Assess vital signs with BP q2h and prn
Assess edema: color and texture of skin, areas of edema, degree of pitting
Weigh patient daily at same time with same clothing and scale
Measure intake and output
Determine specific gravity on all voided specimens
Check character and quantity of urinary output; initiate daily specimen for visual comparison
Administer fluids based on urinary output plus estimated insensible loss if ordered
Administer diuretics if ordered
Anticipate diuresis in 3 to 4 days with increased urinary output and clearing of urine color

ndx Alteration in nutrition: less than body requirements related to anorexia, fatigue, and dietary restrictions

GOAL: *Patient will have an adequate nutritional intake to meet metabolic requirements*

Monitor electrolyte values to determine discontinuation of dietary restrictions
Maintain diet as ordered
    Low-protein diet with severe azotemia
    Low-potassium diet if documented hyperkalemic and during oliguric stage
    Regular diet with *no added salt*
Offer foods child likes
Have parents bring in favorite food from home if possible
Promote socialization during mealtime; have child eat with other children or with family when possible

ndx Activity intolerance related to lethargy, anemia, and/or fatigue

GOAL: *Patient will resume preillness activity level prior to discharge*

Maintain bed rest as ordered
Encourage quiet diversional play activities
Encourage educational activity appropriate for age
Encourage ambulation after diuresis occurs and blood pressure and weight have stabilized
Let child determine appropriate level of activity with guidance (usually children restrict their own activity voluntarily)
Schedule rest periods throughout the day

ndx: Potential alteration in sensory/perceptual ability related to altered level of consciousness secondary to hypertensive encephalopathy

GOAL: *Patient's blood pressure will be age appropriate, and patient will be alert and oriented*

Assess sensorium, mental responsiveness, and vision prn
Be prepared to intervene if seizure activity occurs
Administer antihypertensive medication as ordered
Evaluate blood pressure q2h and prior to administering antihypertensives
Regulate fluids as ordered
Administer diuretics if ordered
Keep patient on bed rest with quiet activities as ordered

ndx: Knowledge deficit regarding home care and follow-up needs

GOAL: *Patient and/or parents will demonstrate understanding of home care and follow-up instructions through interactive discussion and actual return demonstration*

Explain need for planned rest periods and avoidance of fatigue
Caution patient and/or parents that outdoor games and sports and strenuous activity are to be avoided until there is no microscopic evidence of disease
Explain that clinical symptoms resolve in 7 to 10 days; however, laboratory findings persist for several weeks to months
Reassure patient and/or parents that recurrence is uncommon
Discuss diet: usually regular with no restrictions
Explain need to avoid individuals with known infections
Emphasize need for continued schooling
Emphasize need for continued peer contact
Teach name of medication, purpose, dosage, time of administration, and side effects
Emphasize need for ongoing outpatient care

Evaluation

Urinary output is good, and urine is clear
Blood pressure is normal for age
Edema has resolved
Weight has decreased, reflecting correction of fluid retention
Appetite has improved
Preillness activity tolerance has resumed (with restrictions)
Patient is alert and oriented
Patient and/or parents demonstrate ability to care for child at home

NEPHROSIS (NEPHROTIC SYNDROME)

A syndrome resulting from degenerative changes in the kidneys without inflammation

Usual age: any; most commonly 2 to 4 years

Assessment

Observations/findings

Edema: severe, generalized, dependent
Oliguria
Dark, frothy urine
Weight gain: weight may double
Normal blood pressure
Anorexia
Lassitude
Irritability
Malnutrition
Ascites
Diarrhea
Vomiting
Pallor, with or without anemia
Decreased activity tolerance

Laboratory/diagnostic studies

Urine
    Proteinuria, mainly albumin
    Increased specific gravity
Creatinine clearance test: normal
Serum
    Hypoalbuminemia
    Hyperlipidemia

Potential complications

Umbilical and inguinal hernias
Rectal prolapse
Respiratory distress
Sepsis
Peritonitis
Malnutrition
Relapse
Renal failure

Medical management

Corticosteroid therapy
For patient who is steroid resistant, cyclophosphamide in combination with steroid therapy is used
Diuretics may be used in some cases, even though the edema does not usually respond to diuretic therapy
Salt-poor albumin may be used

High-protein diet; avoidance of highly salted foods
Prophylactic broad-spectrum antibiotics to decrease risk of infection until child is on tapering dose of steroids
Eye irrigations/ophthalmic creams for eye irritation from severe edema

Nursing diagnoses/goals/interventions

ndx: Alteration in fluid volume: excess volume in interstitial spaces related to shifting of fluid from plasma to interstitial spaces, glomerular permeability to protein, and sodium and water retention; potential for fluid deficit—hypovolemia related to shifting of fluid from vascular space to interstitial spaces

GOAL: *Patient will have decreased edema and increased urinary output with decreasing specific gravities, and will show no signs of dehydration*

Weigh patient daily
Measure intake and output
Determine specific gravity on all voided specimens
Assess degree of edema
Measure abdominal girth to monitor degree of ascites
Administer corticosteroids as ordered (p. 467)
Administer diuretics if ordered
Administer salt-poor albumin if ordered
Administer fluids orally as desired; *do not restrict*
Anticipate diuresis in 3 to 4 days with weight loss, increased urinary output, and decreased specific gravities
Be aware that dehydration from hypovolemia can occur in spite of excess fluid retention
Monitor for signs of hypovolemia, especially pulse quality and rate, and blood pressure

ndx: Alteration in nutrition: less than body requirements related to anorexia, fatigue, and/or dietary restrictions

GOAL: *Patient will consume adequate caloric intake to meet metabolic requirements*

Plan meals and dietary approach with team consisting of nurse, dietitian, parents, and child
Anticipate that high-protein diet may not be desirable to child
Make meals attractive
Give small portions more frequently
Honor food likes and dislikes
Use creative play techniques to encourage eating (games, rewards, and special treats)
Have parents feed child
Make mealtime a social time; have child eat with other children or with parents
Record food intake for calorie count evaluation
Administer diet as ordered: *no added salt*

ndx: Alteration in skin integrity related to generalized edema

GOAL: *Patient's skin will remain intact*

Assess color and texture of skin and degree of pitting (especially around eyes and dependent areas)
Elevate head on pillows to decrease periorbital edema
Keep skin warm and dry; pay particular attention to creases, fingers, and toes; use dry cloth or cotton to keep fingers and toes separated; *do not* use powders
Turn patient q2h and prn while on bed rest
Administer skin care to pressure areas q1h to 2h
Place pillows under and between legs to avoid pressure
Provide scrotal support, especially when ambulatory
Administer warm saline eye irrigations q2h to 4h
Use ophthalmic ointments as ordered

ndx: Potential for infection related to increased susceptibility secondary to edema and corticosteroid therapy

GOAL: *Patient will remain free of infection*

Assess temperature, pulse, and respirations q4h and prn
Assess for signs of pulmonary and skin infections
Avoid persons with infections, especially URIs
Administer prophylactic antibiotics as ordered
Tell parents that child should not receive immunizations until he is no longer receiving steroids and is free of proteinuria

ndx: Activity intolerance related to fatigue

GOAL: *Patient will resume preillness activity level prior to discharge*

Maintain bed rest as ordered
Encourage quiet diversional play activities
Encourage educational activity appropriate for age
Encourage ambulation after diuresis occurs and blood pressure and weight have stabilized
Let child determine appropriate level of activity with guidance (usually children restrict their own activity voluntarily)
Schedule rest periods throughout the day

ndx: Potential disturbance in body image related to rapid changes in body size and side effects of steroid therapy

GOAL: *Patient will have a positive, realistic self-image*

Encourage patient to express feelings about self
Encourage patient to ask questions about diagnosis and treatment
Give patient encouraging information: altered body changes are temporary and reversible
Avoid reference to patient's weight or size
Promote social interaction
Promote physical activity within tolerance
Allow child access to mirror to provide visualization of self
Point out improvements in degree of edema as they occur

ndx: Knowledge deficit regarding home care and follow-up needs

GOAL: *Patient and/or parents will demonstrate understanding of home care and follow-up instructions through interactive discussion and actual return demonstration*

Explain nature of disease
Explain need for normal activity with planned rest periods
Discuss diet: well-balanced, adequate protein; fluids as desired, no restrictions
Explain need to avoid persons with URIs
Emphasize importance of encouraging social interaction
Discuss symptoms of recurrence to report to physician
  Weight gain
  Increasing edema
  Decreasing or absent urine output
Teach name of medications, purpose, dosage, time of administration, and side effects
  Side effects of corticosteroids to anticipate: round face, increased appetite, increased hair, abdominal distention, mood swings
Have parents and/or patient demonstrate urine testing for albumin if ordered

Evaluation
Patient is hydrated
Weight has decreased, urinary output has increased, and edema has resolved
Patient is able to tolerate moderate activity
Patient is consuming well-balanced diet
Skin remains clean and intact
Patient is free of infection
Patient has a realistic perception of self
Patient and/or parents understand home care instructions

Hematology

ACUTE LEUKEMIA

A disease characterized by uncontrolled proliferation of leukocyte precursors in blood, bone marrow, and reticuloendothelial tissues

Usual age: any; best prognosis is in child between 2 and 9 years of age

Assessment
Observations/findings
INSIDIOUS ONSET

Moderate pallor
Anorexia
Weight loss
Irritability
Abdominal pain
Malaise
Joint pains
Persistent low-grade fever
Bleeding from gums
Epistaxis
Tendency to bruise
Fatique
Shortness of breath with exertion

ABRUPT ONSET

Fever
Tachypnea
Tachycardia
Abdominal pain
Drop in Hgb
Marked pallor
Purpura
Bone pain
Lymphadenopathy
Hemorrhagic episodes from any orifice
Buccal mucosa ulcerations
Hemorrhagic skin eruptions
Hepatomegaly
Splenomegaly
CNS leukemic infiltration
  Nausea
  Vomiting
  Headache
  Lethargy
  Irritability
  Dizziness
  Ataxia
  Convulsions
  Nuchal rigidity
Infection

Laboratory/diagnostic studies

Bone marrow aspiration/biopsy: to identify presence of blasts in marrow, to identify specific cell type involved, and to isolate null cell, T cell, and B cell markers

Lumbar puncture: to confirm presence or absence of CNS leukemic infiltrates

Chest x-ray examination: to identify mediastinal masses

CBC with differential
  WBC: normal, depressed, or elevated
  Presence of blasts in peripheral circulation
  Thrombocytopenia
  Platelet count <40,000/mm^3

Identification of prognostic factors: *best* prognosis
  Age: between 2 and 9 years
  WBC <10,000/mm^3
  Leukemia type: acute lymphoid leukemia (ALL)

Potential complications

Severe systemic infection
Hemorrhage
Relapse
Permanent side effects from chemotherapy/radiation: cardiomyopathy, learning disabilities
Death

Medical management

Identification of specific type of leukemia
Determination of combination of chemotherapeutic agents to use based on type, prognostic factors, and stage of treatment (induction, consolidation, maintenance, reinduction)
Xanthine-oxidase inhibitor (allopurinol)
Corticosteroids
Determination of CNS prevention or treatment approach: cranial irradiation, intrathecal chemotherapeutic agents, or both
Testicular biopsies in males
Bone marrow transplantation may be considered
Treatment of complications of myelosuppression
  Protective isolation during neutropenia
  Blood products as necessary: packed red blood cells (PRBCs), platelets, granulocytes
  Antibiotics for ongoing infection
  Antiemetics
  Nystatin for oral *Candida albicans*
  Parenteral fluids to ensure adequate hydration when patient is receiving chemotherapeutic agents that may cause hemorrhagic cystitis
  Hyperalimentation for nutritional deficit
Childhood immunizations are withheld with bone marrow depression

Nursing diagnoses/goals/interventions

ndx: Potential for infection related to neutropenia

GOAL: *Patient will be protected from infectious organism*

Monitor temperature closely (*no rectal temperatures*)
Be aware that common signs of infection (redness, swelling, pus) may be missing because WBCs necessary for such responses are lacking
Administer antibiotics as ordered
Administer granulocyte transfusions as ordered
Avoid unnecessary exposure to potential sources of infection
  Scrupulous handwashing by all individuals prior to contact with patient
  Place in private room when patient is neutropenic
  Avoid exposure to individuals with known infections
  Use aseptic technique in caring for puncture sites
  Change intravenous tubing every day
Ensure adequate nutritional intake
Do *not* administer immunizations during neutropenia
If child is exposed to communicable diseases, gamma globulin may be ordered

ndx: Activity intolerance related to anemia

GOAL: *Patient will participate in age-appropriate activity*

Observe for signs of anemia: pallor, irritability and intolerance of normal activity, low Hgb levels
Determine patient's tolerance for activity
  Allow independence as tolerated and desired by patient
  Accept need for dependence when demonstrated
Encourage quiet bedside activities
Have planned rest periods throughout the day
Change position and provide back and pressure point care prn
Consider use of water bed or air mattress
Transfuse with PRBCs as ordered

ndx: Potential for injury: bleeding related to decreased platelet counts

GOAL: *Patient will not suffer from preventable injury*

Postpone use of intramuscular injections and suppositories
Avoid play activity that may result in physical injury
Do not allow toys with sharp edges or points
Apply pressure for 5 to 10 min after venipuncture sticks

If nosebleed occurs, pinch nostrils against nasal septum, applying constant pressure for at least 10 min

Do not use aspirin or aspirin-containing products

Administer platelet transfusion as ordered

Administer maximum intravenous fluids prior to, during, and after cyclophosphamide administration and have patient void frequently to prevent hemorrhagic cystitis

ndx: Alteration in oral mucous membrane: stomatitis/thrush related to side effects of chemotherapeutic agents

GOAL: *Patient's mucous membranes will be pink, intact, and free of lesions*

Administer oral hygiene using half-normal saline and half-hydrogen peroxide solution q2h and prn, especially after meals

Use soft toothbrush or sponge toothettes

Administer systemic or topical anesthetics as ordered for severe pain

Allow patient to suck on ice cubes to lessen pain from sores

Administer nystatin mouth rinse as ordered

Avoid use of lemon glycerin swabs since they are drying to mucous membranes

ndx: Alteration in nutrition: less than body requirements related to anorexia, malaise, nausea and vomiting side effects of chemotherapy, and/or stomatitis

GOAL: *Patient will tolerate adequate nutrition to meet metabolic demands*

In the presence of stomatitis offer nonirritating, bland foods at moderate temperature

Monitor intake and output and dietary intake; if insufficient amounts are consumed, administer parenteral fluids or hyperalimentation as ordered

Administer antiemetics prior to giving chemotherapy and during administration of chemotherapy as ordered

Anticipate that child will have alternating periods of hunger and anorexia

Encourage intake of high-quality, high-calorie foods during periods of hunger

Do not force or make an issue out of eating during times of anorexia; liquids may be the only thing tolerated

    Allow child to participate in preparation of food if possible

    Serve creative, appealing food items in small, frequent servings

    Allow child choices in choosing what and when he wants to eat

    Allow parents to bring favorite foods from home if feasible

    Consult dietitian for assistance in obtaining appealing foods and nutritional supplementation

Monitor weight daily

ndx: Alteration in comfort related to bone pain

GOAL: *Patient will be as comfortable as possible*

Postpone routine nursing activities to minimize handling of patient

Maintain proper body alignment

Consider use of water bed or air mattress

Use methods of distraction such as relaxation, breathing techniques, soft music, and guided imagery

Administer analgesics as ordered

Analgesics should be given on a round-the-clock schedule to *prevent* pain

When intravenous infusions of analgesics are used, the dose should be slowly titrated until maximum pain control is achieved

Alleviate any parenteral fears about addiction

ndx: Disturbance in body image related to alopecia and/or rapid changes in body appearance ranging from weight loss to weight gain secondary to treatment

GOAL: *Patient will maintain a positive self-image*

Encourage patient to express feelings about self

Encourage patient to ask questions about diagnosis and treatment

Give patient encouraging information: hair will grow back, weight loss and weight gain fluctuations are a result of treatment and will resolve once therapy is discontinued

Promote social interaction, especially peer contact, on a regular basis

Explore possibility of wearing wigs, caps, scarves, or no head covering at all to enhance self-image

ndx: Potential for ineffective coping: individual and family related to diagnosis and uncertain outcome

GOAL: *Patient and family will have adequate internal and external resources to cope effectively with diagnosis*

Provide consistency in care by limiting number of people caring for patient

Develop a trusting relationship with patient and family

Give them honest, accurate information

Clarify any misconceptions

Have a positive approach when possible

Determine patient and/or family's knowledge of condition and prognosis; be sensitive to their need to verbalize feelings

Recognize that parents may need to verbalize feelings of guilt, hostility, grief, or fear

Assess coping mechanisms, problem-solving abilities, and use of religious or counseling assistance

Involve parents in care of their child to the extent that *they wish* to be involved

Encourage parents to continue normal interactions with their child

Make appropriate referrals to support groups and community services

Assist patient and/or parents in explaining the disease to other family members, friends, teachers, etc.

ndx: Knowledge deficit regarding disease process, home care, and follow-up needs

GOAL: *Patient and/or parents will demonstrate understanding of disease process, and home care and follow-up instructions through interactive discussion*

Explain nature of disease and treatment

Explain that patient and parents can anticipate at least 2 to 3 years of treatment

Explain need for planned rest periods

Explain need to return to normal activities as tolerated

Explain need to avoid individuals with known infections

Explain need for high-quality dietary intake

Explain need for continued social contact and home teaching if activity is restricted to home environment

Explain need for good oral hygiene

Explain need for ongoing follow-up care

Discuss symptoms to report to physician
  Fever
  Increased fatigue
  Bleeding or bruising
  Pain

Teach name of medication, purpose, dosage, time of administration, and side effects

Evaluation

Patient is protected from infectious organisms

Progressive physical activity is tolerated

Bleeding is controlled

Mucous membranes are clear and intact

Patient is able to tolerate regular diet

Patient is comfortable

Patient can state positive things about self

Patient and/or parents feel capable of coping with diagnosis and treatment implications and are knowledgeable about home care needs

SICKLE CELL CRISIS

Episodes in patients with sickle cell disease involving acute sickling of erythrocytes, which causes occlusion of small blood vessels with distal ischemia and infarction

Usual age: any

Assessment

Observations/findings

Swelling of hands and feet

Joint, back pain

Fever

Fatigability

Ventilation-oxygenation
  Tachypnea
  Nasal flaring
  Tachycardia
  Anemia
  Epistaxis

GI system
  Vomiting
  Anorexia
  Abdominal pain

Urinary system
  Hematuria
  Polyuria
  Enuresis

Neurologic system
  Irritability
  Headache
  Meningism

Heart murmurs

Laboratory/diagnostic studies

CBC with differential
  Sickled cells in peripheral blood smear
  Hbg: may be decreased
  WBC: may be elevated

With hemolytic crisis
  Hyperbilirubinemia
  Hyperplastic bone marrow with pancytopenia

With aplastic crisis
  Decreased reticulocyte count

Hemoglobin electrophoresis: specific for detecting sickle cell disease or sickle cell trait

Potential complications

Cerebral vascular accidents
Subarachnoid hemorrhage
Cranial nerve palsies
Massive liver necrosis
Renal failure
Myocardial infarctions
Osteomyelitis
Visual changes

Medical management

Rigorous hydration using parenteral fluids
Oxygenation
Bed rest
Analgesics
Antipyretics
Antibiotics to treat existing infections if any
Transfusion of PRBCs with aplastic crisis
Exchange tranfusions for aplastic, hyperhemolytic, and sequestration crises
Folic acid

Nursing diagnoses/goals/interventions

ndx: Alteration in peripheral tissue perfusion related to viscous blood and thrombus formation secondary to sickling

GOAL: *Patient will have improved peripheral circulation*

Keep metabolic demands minimal and reduce sickling by
  Maintaining bed rest
  Avoiding strenuous physical activity
  Postponing routine nursing activities
  Allowing frequent rest periods
  Decreasing emotional stress (do not make unnecessary demands)
  Monitoring temperature and administering antipyretics prn as ordered to keep patient afebrile
  Monitoring vital signs q2h
  Keeping skin dry and warm
  Promoting adequate ventilation and oxygenation
    Administer oxygen via mist tent or nasal prongs as ordered
    Assist patient with turning, coughing, and deep breathing q2h
Administer maximum amount of fluids for age parenterally as ordered
Encourage oral fluids if desired and tolerated
Measure intake and output
Avoid persons with known infections
Treat existing infections with antibiotics as ordered

ndx: Alteration in comfort: pain related to tissue hypoxia and swelling of joints

GOAL: *Patient will show evidence that pain is alleviated or controlled*

Protect painful joints with pillows
Maintain anatomic alignment
Administer back care and pressure point care q2h
Apply warm soaks to joints prn for comfort
Move patient using slow, gentle movements
Administer analgesics orally or by constant intravenous infusion as ordered
Analgesics should be given to *prevent* pain
When intravenous infusions of analgesics are used, the dose should be slowly titrated until maximum pain control is achieved

ndx: Activity intolerance related to pain, anemia, and decreased tissue oxygenation

GOAL: *Patient will tolerate precrisis activity level prior to discharge*

Maintain bed rest during severe pain
Turn patient q2h
Initiate active ROM exercises as joint pain decreases
Encourage ambulation to level of tolerance
Allow child to determine own tolerance level

ndx: Knowledge deficit regarding home care, follow-up, and preventive care needs

GOAL: *Patient and/or parents will demonstrate understanding of home care, follow-up, and preventive care instructions through interactive discussion and actual return demonstration*

Discuss conditions that precipitate a crisis
  Infection
  Dehydration
  Decreased oxygenation
Teach preventive measures, including the following
  Maintain child's general health
  Avoid strenuous exercise
  Eat well-balanced, high-calorie, high-protein diet
  Drink maximum amount of fluids for age (p. 866)
  Avoid persons with known infections, especially URIs
Discuss symptoms of recurrence to report to physician
  Joint pain
  Abdominal pain
  Fever
  Hematuria
Teach name of medication, purpose, dosage, time of administration, and side effects

Emphasize need for ongoing medical care
Have parents demonstrate active ROM to involved joints

Evaluation

Patient is hydrated, and vital signs are stable
Patient is afebrile
Patient is comfortable and tolerating increased physical activity and movement of joints without pain
Patient and/or parents understand preventive measures and need for follow-up care

Endocrine System

DIABETES MELLITUS (INSULIN DEPENDENT/TYPE 1)

A complex disorder of energy metabolism resulting from deficient insulin secretion by the pancreas

Usual age: any

Assessment
Observations/findings

Glycosuria
Polyuria
Polydipsia
Polyphagia
Weight loss
Ketoacidosis
    Lethargy
    Obtunded
    Coma
    Nausea, vomiting
    Abdominal pain
    Ketonuria
    Sweet, fruity odor to breath
    Hyperpnea
    Hypokalemia
Hypoglycemia, hyperinsulinism
    Personality change
    Irritability
    Dizziness
    Hunger
    Cold, clammy skin
    Fast, thready pulse
    Convulsions

Laboratory/diagnostic studies

Blood glucose: elevated
Urinalysis: glycosuria, ketonuria
Electrolytes: may have hypokalemia, decreased serum carbon dioxide (bicarbonate), and decreased pH with ketoacidosis
Glucose tolerance test: confirms diagnosis
Hemoglobin A_1 levels: elevated in poorly controlled diabetes

Potential complications

Hypoglycemia or hyperglycemia
Cardiac arrest with hypokalemia
Cardiovascular disease
Retinopathy
Nephropathy
Urinary tract infection
Neuropathy

Medical management
During ketoacidosis

NPO
Parenteral fluids to correct dehydration; glucose and electrolytes (fluids are administered with caution to prevent cerebral edema)
Insulin by continuous infusion given 0.1U/kg/hr until blood sugar falls to 200 mg/dl (blood sugar should not be dropped any faster than 100 mg/dl/hr because of danger of cerebral edema)
Fingerstick glucose monitoring q1h
Administration of bicarbonate if pH is significantly low
Administration of regular insulin begun, using a sliding scale based on blood glucose results
Indwelling catheter
Intake and output
Urine testing for sugar and acetone
Clear liquid diet begun and advanced to food exchange diet as tolerated
Determination of daily dose of insulin (usually combination of short-acting regular and long-acting NPH insulins)

Ongoing management

Adjustment of insulin as necessary
Evaluation of patient's and/or parents' understanding about disease and treatment
Evaluation and treatment of any complications

Nursing diagnoses/goals/interventions: ketoacidosis

ndx: Fluid volume deficit related to polyuria secondary to elevated serum glucose levels

GOAL: *Patient will be hydrated with balanced intake and output*

Maintain NPO status if patient is obtunded, lethargic, or comatose

Rehydrate slowly by administering accurate parenteral fluids as ordered using volume controller device

Administer continuous insulin infusion as ordered; begin q4h administration of regular insulin using sliding scale as ordered; begin daily dose of regular and long-acting insulin as ordered

Monitor blood glucose levels q1h using bedside glucose monitoring strips (Dextrostix, Chemstrip)

Test urine for acetone as ordered (some physicians may still order urine glucose testing, but insulin adjustments are usually based on serum glucose results)

Begin clear liquids when patient is alert as ordered

Record intake and output

Weigh patient daily

ndx: Electrolyte imbalance related to increased renal excretion of potassium and sodium, and metabolic acidosis

GOAL: *Patient will have normal serum electrolyte values*

Monitor vital signs q1h and prn

Place patient on cardiac monitor (a depressed ST segment, a flattened T wave, and a prominent U wave are present)

Monitor serum electrolyte values

Administer sodium and potassium replacements as ordered with careful monitoring of cardiac rhythm patterns and blood levels to avoid rebound hyperkalemia

Administer bicarbonate if ordered

ndx: Knowledge deficit regarding management of the disease at home

GOAL: *Patient and/or parents will demonstrate understanding of home management through interactive discussion and actual return demonstration*

Begin teaching during acute stage; explain test results, treatment, and signs and symptoms as they relate to the disease

Teach nature of disease and treatment

Teach names and types of insulins to be used, purpose, dosage, time of administration, and side effects

Teach home glucose monitoring (p. 443)

Teach urine testing for sugar and acetone (p. 443)

Teach insulin injection (p. 444)

Teach use of portable insulin infusion pump if ordered

Explain site rotation

Explain food exchange diet (p. 880) and need to give three meals and three snacks a day

Explain glucagon usage and teach technique for administration

Explain record keeping

Explain need to anticipate hyperglycemia and increased insulin requirements during an illness

Discuss symptoms of diabetic ketoacidosis to report to physician
- Continual elevated blood sugar (not isolated case)
- Presence of acetone in urine
- Polyuria
- Polydipsia
- Weight loss
- Drowsiness

Discuss symptoms of hypoglycemia to report to physician
- Decreased blood sugar
- Excessive hunger
- Jitteriness
- Cold, clammy perspiration
- Labile emotional reactions

Explain relationship between diet, exercise, insulin, and blood glucose levels

Explain need to avoid giving injection in limb used for exercise (legs if running, arms if swimming) to prevent rapid absorption of insulin and subsequent hypoglycemia

Emphasize need to encourage and allow pursuit of normal activities for age

Emphasize need for ongoing communication and outpatient follow-up with physician

Explore need for public health nurse visitations to provide support and reinforce teaching during first few weeks at home

Obtain necessary prescriptions for home equipment
- Insulin
- Syringes
- Needles
- Automatic fingerstick device and reagent kit
- Urine testing kit including Clinitest and acetone tablets
- Glucagon kit
- Insulin pump if ordered

Have patient and/or parents demonstrate prior to discharge
- How to draw up insulin correctly in syringe
- How to draw up two insulins in same syringe
- Injection into an orange for practice (may consider having parents inject nurse with saline prior to injecting their child)

Actual administration of insulin to child
Site rotation
Understanding of food exchange diet
Urine testing
Blood testing
Record keeping
How to intervene if a hypoglycemic or hyperglycemic reaction occurs

Evaluation

Patient's blood sugar and electrolyte values are stable at normal levels
Urine is negative for sugar and acetone
Patient is eating a regular diet
Patient and parents understand home care management, use of equipment, and need for ongoing outpatient care

FAILURE TO THRIVE (FTT)

A general term indicating a child who fails to grow (falls more than two standard deviations below the mean height and weight for age and sex or a child who fails to maintain a previously established growth pattern) and is developmentally delayed as part of a disease process; in its simplest sense it is a presenting symptom of an organic problem; in its most complex form it is a syndrome involving psychosocial disruption

Usual age: infant or toddler

Assessment

Observations/findings

Child admitted with this symptom is granted a thorough assessment of all body systems; a possible organic cause for failure to thrive is thoroughly investigated, and nurse assists with various specimen collections and testings that are done; in addition, varying degrees of psychosocial disruption occur, even with an organic cause; therefore, nurse will assess for nonorganic indices as follows
Weight, height, head circumference below fifth percentile
Delayed physical and social development
Dull affect; apathy
Poor hygiene
Withdrawal behavior
No fear of strangers
Avoidance of eye contact: "radar gaze"
Minimal smiling or babbling
Stiffening on being held close or flaccidity and unresponsiveness
Eating disorders: self-induced vomiting, anorexia, pica, voracious appetite

Observations during mealtime

Child's reaction to food: resists and becomes irritable; spits food out; is easily distracted; is passive during meals
Mother's behavior during mealtime: tries to keep child too clean; offers too much or too little; is easily frustrated; forces child to eat

Assessment of mother-child interaction

Does child recognize mother as different from others?
Does child seek out mother?
Does mother respond? How?
Is mother sensitive to needs of her child?
Child's temperament: passive, active, fussy
Self-stimulating behaviors: head banging, thumb sucking, rocking, biting of lower lip
Is child held close, at arm's distance, turned out, or toward mother?
Does mother have realistic expectations for child?
Does mother play and talk with child?
Mother's perception of child: what does she say?

Additional assessment

Is mother-father relationship intact? Good or stressed?
Was pregnancy planned or unplanned?
How is the development of the other children?
What are their financial resources?
Who feeds child at home—consistent person or many different people?
Care giver's eating habits and knowledge of infant/toddler nutrition
Prenatal history, including reaction to pregnancy, stressors during pregnancy, and feelings toward baby
Mother's feelings about herself; be *alert* to the following
  Maternal deprivation as child
  Low self-concept
  Stressful life with limited support system
  Negative verbalizations about infant: ugly, smells, spits up, is irritable
  Unrealistic expectations of infant
  Poor interaction with infant: poor eye contact, little verbalization, no enthusiasm
  Not responsive to needs of child: does not recognize when infant is tired, hungry, or soiled
  Insists that something physical is wrong with child
  Negative statements about role as mother
After admission, mother visits infrequently, misses meetings, etc.

Laboratory/diagnostic studies

CBC: often anemic

X-ray examination of long bones: determines skeletal age of bone (often delayed)

Development screening tests: identify delays in motor and social development

Several diagnostic studies are performed to identify organic cause for failure to thrive (see Failure to Thrive: Organic Workup, p. 843)

Potential complications

Child abuse
Metabolic dysfunction
Temporary placement in foster care

Medical management

Organic cause for growth delay ruled out
Treatment of organic cause if identified
Close community follow-up
Monitoring and evaluation of growth and development

Nursing diagnoses/goals/interventions

ndx: Alteration in nutrition: less than body requirements related to maternal deprivation

GOAL: *Child will maintain age-appropriate diet reflecting adequate caloric intake and will show progressive weight gain*

Weigh child daily: before meals, same time, same scale, naked

Keep calorie count

Keep stool record

Assign consistent care givers

Consult dietitian: meet with family for nutritional teaching

Calculate caloric and fluid requirements (p. 866)

Consider the following feeding interventions
- Promote a positive, nurturing environment, especially during mealtime
  - Keep stimulation to a minimum to avoid distraction; feed in private room if available
  - Always hold infant for bottle feeding
  - Talk softly to child and encourage eye contact
  - Avoid conversation with others while feeding; this is *child's* time
- Set 30 min time limit for meal
- Give bottle at end of meal; take bottle away after 20 min or if child is playing with it but not drinking it
- If child is hungry between meals, give water only
- Avoid excessive stimulation for 1 hr after meals; use soft music, vocalizations, and holding
- Some children may benefit from small, frequent meals and frequent burping until able to tolerate volume of food required to meet daily metabolic requirements

ndx: Altered growth and development related to insufficient stimulation at home from primary care giver

GOAL: *Child will show signs of increased physical and emotional development as recorded on standardized developmental screening tests (Denver Developmental Screening Test [DDST] is frequently used)*

Assist child in responding meaningfully to environment
- Respond to child's cues: pick him up when he cries; verbalize to child when he babbles, etc.
- Respond to child with vigor and enthusiasm

Coordinate child's daily schedule to include four to five stimulation sessions per day; each session should last only 10 to 15 min and should not be scheduled immediately before or after meals

Identify very specific developmental goals; each stimulation session should focus on one specific goal; for example
- At 10 AM child is scheduled for gross motor stimulation
- A specific goal might be: child will sit without support
- For the next 15 min, stimulation is geared toward improving back and stomach muscles and balance

Consult physical therapists and/or occupational therapists as needed

Teach parents age-appropriate growth and development

Teach parents appropriate stimulation to promote growth and development

ndx: Alteration in parenting related to inadequate support system, difficulty in coping with stress, and/or lack of parenting skills

GOAL: *Parents will improve their coping abilities, will be able to identify and respond appropriately to their child's needs, and will verbalize positive feelings regarding infant*

Assess parent-child interactions, reinforcing any improvements in the parents' ability to identify their child's needs

Keep record of parental visiting and calling patterns

Realize that parents are under a great deal of stress at home and that this is complicated by their child's hospitalization

Establish rapport with parents; encourage sharing of feelings toward parenthood and child

Have parents discuss stressors in their life right now: financial, relationships, housing, difficulty in adjusting to new baby, recent losses, etc.

Be aware that mother, in particular, may have poor self-concept; give her positive feedback in her attempts to mother her child

Contract with parents; set up times for them to come in or call hospital (if they are unable to find transportation to hospital) to discuss care

   Discuss child's progress with them

   Encourage them to be involved in their child's care

   Allow parents to participate in planning of child's schedule

   Explain reasons for such routines

Assess parents' understanding of infant care; do not assume that they are just neglectful—they may not have learned skills

Give parents verbal and written information about infant's diet, growth and development, and age-appropriate stimulation

If parents are unable to cope with care of their child because of stressors in their home environment and no improvement is seen in their ability to relate to their child, then temporary placement in a foster home may be necessary; reinforce to parents that this is *temporary* and done as a means to assist them with their crisis; make certain that parents are referred appropriately in order to receive the assistance they need; make appropriate referrals to improve the support system

   Visiting Nurse's Association

   Early intervention/developmental programs

   Social service agencies

   Psychiatric services

Make certain a primary physician is identified to follow child's progress on an outpatient basis

Evaluation

Child is gaining weight

Dietary intake has improved

Child shows improvement in growth and development and is more interactive with environment

Parental stressors and coping abilities are identified

Parents show improvement in care of their child, or appropriate placement in foster care occurs

Plans for follow-up care and assessment are made

Failure to Thrive: Organic Workup

General diseases states
- Infection
  - CBC
  - Red blood cell indices
  - Erythrocyte sedimentation rate
  - Purified protein derivative or tuberculin test
  - Serology
  - Nose, throat, stool, and urine cultures
  - Chest x-ray examination
  - Coccidioidomycosis and histoplasmosis skin tests
- Infestation
  - Scabies
  - Pediculosis
  - Stool ovum slides
  - Parasite and ameba
  - Pinworm slides
- Nutrition: diet testing
- Metabolism
  - Random blood sugar
  - BUN
  - Amino acid assays
  - Carbon dioxide level
  - Sodium level
  - Potassium level
  - Chloride level
  - Calcium level
  - Phosphorus level

Chronic intoxication: lead level

Malfunction of organ system
- Central nervous system
  - Skull x-ray examination
  - Electroencephalogram (EEG)
  - CT scan
- GI system
  - Stool fat and trypsin
  - Stool pH and reducing substances
  - Occult blood
  - D-Xylose tolerance tests
  - GI series
  - Barium enema
  - Liver function tests
- Genitourinary system
  - Urinalysis
  - Urine concentration tests
  - Intravenous pyelogram
- Cardiovascular system: ECG
- Endocrine system
  - Protein-bound iodine level
  - Triiodothyronine level (T_3)
  - Thyroxine level (T_4)

17-Ketosteroid level
Glucose tolerance test
Growth hormone
Hematopoietic system
Sickle cell prep
Serum iron level
Bilirubin level
Respiratory system
Sweat test
Pulmonary function tests
Chromosomal or genetic disorder
Buccal smear
Karyotyping
Urine for amino acids
Prenatal infection
Rubella titer
Cytomegalovirus culture
Toxoplasmosis test
Herpes

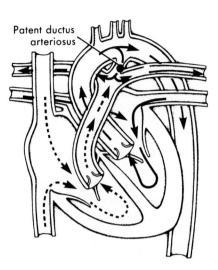

FIGURE 15-8. Patent ductus arteriosus (PDA). (From Whaley, L.F., and Wong, D.L.: Essentials of pediatric nursing, ed. 2, St. Louis, 1985, The C.V. Mosby Co.)

Cardiovascular System

CONGENITAL HEART DEFECTS

Noncyanotic (Acyanotic)
PATENT DUCTUS ARTERIOSUS (PDA) (Figure 15-8)

Persistence of blood flow through the fetal ductus arteriosus, between the aorta and the main pulmonary artery

Assessment
Observations/findings
INFANT

Prematurity
Respiratory distress syndrome
Congestive heart failure (CHF) (p. 857)
Tachycardia
Bounding pedal pulses
Hepatomegaly
Splenomegaly

OLDER CHILD

Exertional dyspnea
Physical underdevelopment
Widened pulse pressure

ANY AGE

Loud, continuous "machinery" heart murmur heard throughout systole and diastole: mid to upper left sternal border

Laboratory/diagnostic studies

ECG: normal or left ventricular hypertrophy
X-ray examination: prominent pulmonary arteries, enlarged left ventricle
Echocardiogram: detects presence of PDA
Cardiac catheterization: confirms presence of defect: provides visualization of size; demonstrates increased pressures in pulmonary artery and right ventricle and presence of oxygenated blood in pulmonary artery

Potential complications

Pulmonary hypertension
After corrective surgery
Phrenic nerve injury
Subacute bacterial endocarditis (p. 93)

Medical management

Treatment of CHF (p. 857) with fluid restriction, diuretics, and digitalization
In premature infant indomethacin is used to enhance PDA closure (this pharmacologic approach does not work in older children)
Closed heart surgical intervention: ligation of PDA
PDA "plug" during cardiac catheterization may be used; this technique remains experimental
Antibiotic prophylaxis with dental work or other surgical procedures

ATRIAL SEPTAL DEFECT (ASD) (Figure 15-9)

An abnormal opening between two atria; may result from persistence of blood flow through the fetal foramen ovale (ostium secundum) or a defect in the intraatrial septum (a low-septum is called ostium primum ASD and is often associated with a cleft mitral valve); results in some degree of left-to-right blood shunting

Assessment
Observations/findings

Symptoms vary according to size of defect
Most children are asymptomatic
   Normal growth and development
   Normal exercise tolerance
   Soft systolic ejection murmur over second to third interspace along left sternal border is heard on examination
Ostium primum ASDs with associated valve abnormalities: CHF (p. 857)

Laboratory/diagnostic studies

ECG: right ventricular hypertrophy (RVH); prolonged PR interval possible; varying degrees of heart block possible
Radiology: enlarged right atrium, right ventricle, and pulmonary artery
Echocardiogram: location of defect, size of shunt, right ventricular enlargement

Cardiac catheterization: confirms diagnosis and location of defect; oxygen content of right atrium is higher than that of superior vena cava

Potential complications

If ASD remains undetected until adulthood
   CHF (p. 101)
   Pulmonary vascular disease
After corrective cardiac surgery
   Transient pulmonary edema
   Heart block
   Hemorrhage
   Subacute bacterial endocarditis (p. 93)

Medical management

CHF management (p. 857) for children with ostium primum ASD with associated valve abnormalities
Open-heart surgical intervention: closure of ASD with suture of small defect or Dacron patch on large defect
Nonoperative closure may be attempted using an ASD "umbrella," which is inserted during cardiac catheterization; this technique is presently experimental
Antibiotic prophylaxis with dental work or other surgical procedures

VENTRICULAR SEPTAL DEFECT (VSD) (Figure 15-10)

An abnormal opening between ventricles; results in left-to-right shunting of blood; often associated with

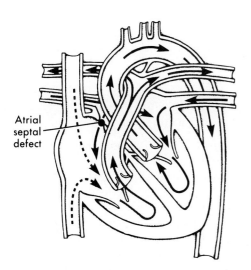

FIGURE 15-9. Atrial septal defect (ASD). (From Whaley, L.F., and Wong, D.L.: Essentials of pediatric nursing, ed. 2, St. Louis, 1985, The C.V. Mosby Co.)

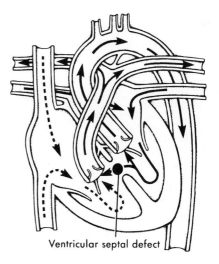

FIGURE 15-10. Ventricular septal defect (VSD). (From Whaley, L.F., and Wong., D.L.: Essentials of pediatric nursing, ed. 2, St. Louis, 1985, The C.V. Mosby Co.)

other defects; can occur in either the membranous (usually moderate to large defects) or the muscular portion (usually small) of the ventricular septum

Assessment
Observations/findings

Dependent on amount of blood flow through defect
Minimal blood flow: asymptomatic
With large VSDs seen in infants
    Dyspnea
    Tachypnea
    Tachycardia
    Recurrent pulmonary infection
    Feeding difficulties
    Poor growth
    Profuse diaphoresis
    CHF (p. 857)
Rumbling or harsh pansystolic murmur is heard best at left lower sternal border and may radiate throughout precordium (not necessarily indicative of severity of defect)

Laboratory/diagnostic studies

ECG: left ventricular hypertrophy or bilateral ventricular hypertrophy
Radiology: cardiomegaly
Echocardiogram: presence of defect and quantity of shunting
Cardiac catheterization: exact size and location of defect and quantity of shunting

Potential complications

Pulmonary artery hypertension: if it progresses to degree that right ventricular pressure is greater than left ventricular pressure, blood will flow right-to-left (Eisenmenger's complex)
Pneumonia
After corrective surgery
    Heart block
    Residual shunt
    Subacute bacterial endocarditis (p. 93)

Medical management

CHF management (p. 857)
Palliative closed-heart surgery done with severe VSDs or those with associated complex lesions: pulmonary artery banding (PAB)—reduces diameter of pulmonary artery to decrease blood flow through pulmonary artery to lungs
Corrective open-heart surgery: closure of ventricular septal defect either with suture of small defect or Dacron patching of large defect
Antibiotic prophylaxis with dental work or other surgical procedures

COARCTATION OF AORTA (Figure 15-11)

Narrowing of the aorta, usually occurring beyond the left subclavian artery at the area of the ductus insertion; often associated with patent ductus arteriosus and aortic valve defects

Assessment
Observations/findings

NEONATE

Decreased or absent femoral pulses
Poor perfusion
Elevated blood pressure in upper extremities
Decreased blood pressure in lower extremities
Bounding pulses in upper extremities
CHF (p. 857)

OLDER CHILD (MOST COMMON PRESENTATION)

Decreased femoral pulses
Cold feet
Increased BP in upper extremities
Decreased BP in lower extremities
Epistaxis
Headache

ANY AGE

Systolic murmur possible and variable

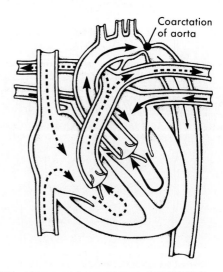

FIGURE 15-11. Coarctation of aorta. (From Whaley, L.F., and Wong, D.L.: Essentials of pediatric nursing, ed. 2, St. Louis, 1985, The C.V. Mosby Co.)

Laboratory/diagnostic studies

ECG: usually normal
Radiology: dilated ascending aorta, cardiomegaly or normal heart size
Echocardiogram: may visualize segment of coarctation
Cardiac catheterization: confirms diagnosis, visualization of defect, and degree of narrowing

Potential complications

Damage to aorta: becomes thin and calcified as a result of persistently high pressures
Aneurysms in intercostal arteries
Cerebral hemorrhage
CHF (p. 857)
Subacute bacterial endocarditis (p. 93)
After corrective surgery
  Hypertension
  Restenosis
  Phrenic nerve injury

Medical management

With significant hypertension in older child
  Antihypertensives
  Exercise restriction
CHF management (p. 857)
In infants who depend on patency of ductus arteriosus to provide adequate systemic blood flow, prostaglandins are used to keep ductus open until surgical correction is possible
Closed-heart surgery
  End-to-end anastomosis *or*
  Insertion of graft replacement *or*
  Subclavian arterioplasty (infants): take down subclavian artery and use as live tissue patch for aorta
  Gore-Tex patch: patch is placed over top of aorta, allowing growth of live aortic tissue as child grows
In some children who have spontaneous recurrence of coarctation, nonoperative dilation may be done by angioplasty (balloon is inflated in narrowed area during cardiac catheterization); this procedure is still experimental
Antibiotic prophylaxis with dental work or other surgical procedures

AORTIC STENOSIS (Figure 15-12)

Narrowing or stricture of the aortic valve; stricture may be valvar, supravalvar, or subvalvar

Assessment
Observations/findings

Dependent on degree of outflow obstruction
Severe obstruction

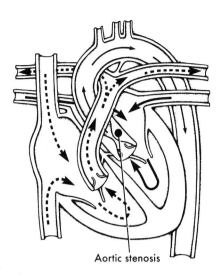

FIGURE 15-12. Aortic stenosis. (From Whaley, L.F., and Wong, D.L.: Essentials of pediatric nursing, ed. 2, St. Louis, 1985, The C.V. Mosby Co.)

  Symptoms occur in infancy
  Poor growth
  Poor perfusion
  Faint peripheral pulses
  Narrow pulse pressures
  CHF (p. 857)
Minimal obstruction in older child
  May be asymptomatic
  Chest pain
  Syncope
  Exercise intolerance
  Dyspnea
  Fatigue
  Narrow pulse pressures
Harsh systolic ejection murmur: best heard in aortic area

Laboratory/diagnostic studies

ECG: left ventricular hypertrophy (LVH); can be normal
Radiology: LVH and enlargement of ascending aorta
Echocardiogram: thickening of aortic valve visualized; level of lesion is identified; quantitative analysis of left ventricular pressure
Cardiac catheterization: confirms diagnosis; demonstrates magnitude and site of pressure gradient from left ventricle to aorta

Potential complications

Sudden death with idiopathic hypertrophic subaortic stenosis (IHSS)

After corrective surgery
　Persistent stenosis
　Restenosis
　Aortic valve insufficiency
　Subacute bacterial endocarditis (p. 93)

Medical management

Open-heart surgical intervention: aortic commissurotomy; valve is dilated, and commissures of valve are incised

Valve replacement may be necessary in older child in whom commissurotomy would create significant aortic insufficiency

Coumadin therapy postoperatively with valve replacement

Antibiotic prophylaxis with dental work or other surgical procedures

PULMONIC STENOSIS (Figure 15-13)

An obstructive lesion that interferes with the blood flow from the right ventricle; stricture may be valvar, supravalvar, or subvalvar

Assessment

Observations/findings

Dependent on degree of outflow obstruction
Minimal obstruction: mild exercise intolerance
Severe obstruction in older children
　Chest pain
　Dizziness
　Dyspnea on exertion
　Fatigue

Ejection or crescendo-decrescendo systolic murmur: soft in mild obstruction; loud in severe obstruction; best heard in upper left sternal border and may be transmitted to back and across left chest

Laboratory/diagnostic findings

ECG: RVH
Radiology: right ventricular and main pulmonary artery enlargement
Echocardiogram: detects thickness and decreased motion of pulmonic valve
Cardiac catheterization: confirms diagnosis; identifies nature of stenotic valve and severity of stenosis; gradient measured—repair of pulmonic stenosis is recommended if pressure gradient is 60 mm Hg or more across pulmonic valve

Potential complications

Sudden death (rare)
Cyanosis and CHF (rare)
After corrective surgery
　Pulmonary regurgitation
　Transient arrythmias
　Subacute bacterial endocarditis (p. 93)

Medical management

Monitoring of progression of stenosis as child grows
Nonoperative intervention: pulmonic valvotomy involving dilation of stenotic area during cardiac catheterization
Open-heart surgical intervention: pulmonic valvotomy—stenosis relieved by incising fused commissures as widely as possible
Antibiotic prophylaxis with dental work or other surgical procedures

Cyanotic

TETRALOGY OF FALLOT (Figure 15-14)

Includes four defects: (1) VSD, (2) right ventricular outflow obstruction (valvar and subvalvar pulmonic stenosis most common), (3) overriding aorta, and (4) RVH; results in dominant right-to-left blood flow

Assessment

Observations/findings

Cyanosis: occurs at 3 to 6 months of age (may occur only with crying/feeding in neonate because of patent ductus arteriosus)
Dyspnea
Tachypnea
Tachycardia
Delayed physical growth

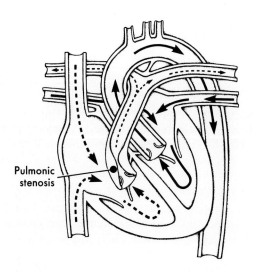

FIGURE 15-13. Pulmonic stenosis. (From Whaley, L.F., and Wong, D.L.: Nursing care of infants and children, ed. 3, St. Louis, 1987, The C.V. Mosby Co.)

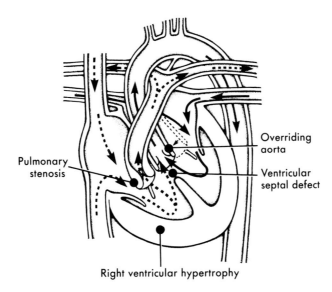

FIGURE 15-14. Tetralogy of Fallot. (From Whaley, L.F., and Wong, D.L.: Essentials of pediatric nursing, ed. 2, St. Louis, 1985, The C.V. Mosby Co.)

Clubbing of fingers and toes
Paroxymal dyspneic attacks, "blue" spells
   Severe dyspnea
   Severe cyanosis
   Hyperpnea
   Gasping
In an older child (though rare today because of early recognition and surgical intervention)
   Squatting
   Fainting
Pansystolic murmur: most intense at left sternal border

Laboratory/diagnostic studies

ECG: right axis deviation and RVH
Radiology: "boot-shaped" cardiac silhouette
Echocardiogram: demonstrates aortic override, large aorta, VSD, and thick right ventricular wall
Cardiac catheterization: actual visualization of all defects; systolic hypertension in right ventricle with sudden fall in pulmonary artery pressure
CBC: polycythemia
Blood gases: decreased PaO_2 and oxygen saturation

Potential complications

Thrombus formation
Cerebral emboli
Seizures
Brain abscess
After surgical correction
   Persistent right ventricular failure
   Heart block
   Ventricular arrhythmias
   Subacute bacterial endocarditis (p. 93)

Medical management

Adequate fluid administration to prevent dehydration
Treatment of "tet" spells
Oxygen prn
Propranolol
Knee-chest position
Morphine sulfate: relaxes right ventricular infundibulum, increases pulmonary blood flow, and decreases right-to-left shunt
Prostaglandins are used in neonates to keep ductus arteriosus patent until surgery is possible
Palliative closed-heart surgical interventions
   Blalock-Taussig shunt: end-to-side anastomosis of right subclavian artery to right pulmonary artery or left subclavian artery to left pulmonary artery
   Modified Blalock-Taussig: Gore-Tex graft is used instead of end-to-side anastomosis
Corrective open-heart surgical intervention: complete repair of defects—closure of ventricular septal defect and correction of overriding aorta and pulmonic valvotomy
Antibiotic prophylaxis with dental work or other surgical procedures

TRANSPOSITION OF GREAT VESSELS (TGV)
(Figure 15-15)

Pulmonary artery leaves left ventricle, and aorta leaves right ventricle, resulting in complete separation of pulmonary and systemic circulation; life beyond birth is possible only if mixing of pulmonary and systemic circulations occurs through patent ductus arteriosus, atrial septal defect, and/or ventricular septal defect

Assessment
Observations/findings

With minimal mixing of circulations
   Severe cyanosis
   Tachypnea
   Severe hypoxia
   Rapid onset of CHF (p. 857)
   Rapid deterioration if PDA closes
With significant mixing of circulations
   Less severe cyanosis
   Increased cyanosis with feeding/crying
   Progressive hyperpnea
   CHF
Heart murmur dependent on associated defects

Laboratory/diagnostic studies

ECG: right axis deviation, RVH
Radiology: progressive cardiomegaly
Echocardiogram: identification of aorta anterior to pulmonary artery and to the right of it

Cardiac catheterization: visualization of all defects; right ventricular hypertension; higher oxygen concentration in pulmonary artery than in aorta

Potential complications

Metabolic acidosis
After corrective surgery
   Baffle obstruction
   Baffle leaks
   Atrial dysrhythmias
   Tricuspid regurgitation
   Subacute bacterial endocarditis (p. 93)

Medical management

In neonate
   CHF management (p. 857) with digoxin and diuretics
   Correction of metabolic acidosis: may give sodium bicarbonate
   Arterial oxygenation using palliative nonoperative interventions
   Balloon atrial septostomy during cardiac catheterization to allow mixing
   Administration of prostaglandins to maintain patency of ductus arteriosus
Corrective open-heart surgery
   Mustard procedure: atrial septum is taken down and baffle placed to redirect pulmonary and systemic circulations
   Senning procedure: similar to Mustard procedure except right atrial wall and interatrial septum are used as baffle
Antibiotic prophylaxis with dental work or other surgical procedures

CONGENITAL HEART SURGERY

Preoperative Preparation
Assessment

Obtain baseline vital signs
Ensure that child does not have infection
Ensure that laboratory studies are complete
   Chest x-ray examination
   ECG
   CBC
   Urinalysis
   Type and cross match for blood
   Electrolytes
   Coagulation studies
   Renal function tests

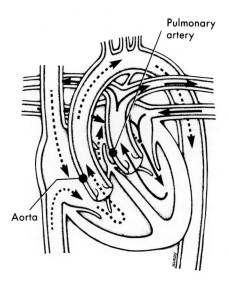

FIGURE 15-15. Transposition of great vessels (TGV). (From Whaley, L.F., and Wong, D.L.: Essentials of pediatric nursing, ed. 2, St. Louis, 1985, The C.V. Mosby Co.)

Nursing diagnosis/goal/interventions

ndx: Knowledge deficit regarding preparation for surgery

GOAL: *Patient and/or parents will demonstrate understanding of surgical procedure and postoperative care through interactive discussion*

Reinforce physician's explanation of procedure
Encourage questions that will establish true understanding of surgery and alleviate fears
Gear teaching to parents and to child, depending on child's age and ability to understand
Provide diagram of heart and explain procedure
Obtain history of child's developmental status, usual daily routine, likes and dislikes, favorite toy, position in family, dietary habits, and sleep pattern in order to meet child's needs postoperatively
Explain preoperative procedures
   NPO
   Laboratory tests
   Transport to operating room by way of crib or stretcher
   Room where parents can wait during surgery
Reassure parents that surgeon will contact them after surgery
Describe operating room environment
   Physicians and nurses wear gowns, hats, and masks
   Allow child to try on operating room attire
Discuss anesthesia: "special sleep during which child will feel no pain"; reassure child that he will not wake up during surgery
Answer questions about operating room
   Physicians and nurses are present all the time
   Child will be helped to breathe by respirator and tube in throat
   Child will wake up soon after surgery
Describe postoperative environment
   Child will be in recovery room or intensive care unit (ICU)
   Provide visit to care unit prior to surgery
   Equipment
      Respiratory assistance to continue until respiration is stabilized
      Child will be unable to talk with tube in throat
      Nasogastric tube
      Monitor to chest
      Beep noises of monitor
      Chest tube(s)
      Presence of several monitoring lines
         Arterial line
         Central venous pressure (CVP) line
         Right atrial (RA) line (open heart)
         Left atrial (LA) line (open heart)
         Pacemaker wires present (open heart)
      Chest dressing or sutures
      Intravenous lines for fluid administration
      Urinary catheter
   Physicians and nurses will be present at all times
Explain that postoperative nursing care will include
   Frequent vital signs
   Coughing and deep breathing
   Pain management: explain availability of pain medication
Allow child to express self through play
   Mask, gown, cap
   Oxygen mask
   Syringe
   Doll
   Practice coughing and deep breathing
Do not overload young child with too much factual information that may be frightening; focus teaching on what child will see, hear, smell, and feel, rather than on details of surgery
Reassure child and parents concerning visitation
Allow ample time for questions and encourage feedback to ensure understanding

Evaluation

Patient and/or parents have expressed their concerns, fears, and anxieties about surgery and demonstrate understanding appropriate to their developmental ability

Palliative Procedures

Procedures done to either increase or decrease pulmonary blood flow as the defect demands

BALLOON SEPTOSTOMY (NONOPERATIVE)

Enlargement of foramen ovale to increase pulmonary blood flow; performed during cardiac catheterization

Assessment

Postprocedure observations

Assess for adequate mixing of blood by monitoring arterial blood gases (ABGs) and oxygen saturation
Decreased cyanosis
Increased activity tolerance
Improved feeding
Decreased oxygen requirement
Decreased respiratory effort

Potential complications (rare)

Cardiac perforation
Conduction abnormalities

BLALOCK-TAUSSIG SHUNT

Anastomosis of subclavian artery to pulmonary artery to increase pulmonary blood flow

Assessment
Postoperative observations

See Closed-Heart Surgery (below)
Decreased cyanosis
Decreased oxygen requirement
Decreased respiratory effort
Machinery-like murmur
Weak or absent BP in arm on operative side; do not draw blood or start IV in arm on operative side
Increased activity tolerance
Improved feeding

Potential complications

Thrombus formation in shunt
    Return to preoperative state of cyanosis
    Disappearance of shunt murmur

PULMONARY ARTERY BANDING (PAB)

Application of constrictive band to main pulmonary artery in order to decrease pulmonary blood flow

Assessment
Postoperative observations

See Closed-Heart Surgery (below)
With adequate restriction of blood flow
    Decreasing evidence of CHF
        Improved urinary output
        Relief of edema
        Stabilization of weight
        Improved respiratory function
        Decreased need for digoxin and diuretics
        Improved feeding
With inadequate restriction of blood flow: little or no relief from CHF

Potential complications

Insufficient blood flow restriction

Corrective Surgery
CLOSED-HEART SURGERY
Assessment
Observations/findings

Respiratory status
    Patent airway
    Equality of chest movements and breath sounds
    Signs of respiratory distress: tachypnea, dyspnea, nasal flaring, cyanosis, retractions
    Presence of adventitious sounds: stridor, rales, rhonchi
    Subcutaneous emphysema (crepitus)
    Chest tube function (p. 271)
Cardiovascular status
    Peripheral perfusion: warmth, color, capillary refill, pulses in extremities
    Heart rate and rhythm
    Murmur status
    BP
        Coarctation repair: continued hypertension
        Patent ductus ligation: mild hypertension
        Blalock-Taussig operation: absent or faint in arm on operative side
Renal status
    Urinary output (minimum 1 ml/kg/hr)
    Specific gravity
Neurologic status
    Level of consciousness
    Age-appropriate developmental ability
GI status: return of bowel sounds

Laboratory/diagnostic studies

ABGs
Hgb
Hct
Creatinine
Electrolytes
Chest x-ray examination: to evaluate presence of postoperative complications

Potential complications

See specific defect under Congenital Heart Defects
Atelectasis (p. 257)
Pneumothorax (p. 252)
Tension pneumothorax (p. 254)
CHF (p. 857)

Medical management

Ventilatory assistance: wean from ventilatory support
Oxygen
Postural drainage, percussion, and suctioning
Order dressing changes if any
Maintenance parenteral fluids
Digitalis
Diuretics
Antibiotics
Analgesics
Antipyretics
Removal of chest tube
Removal of sutures

Nursing diagnoses/goals/interventions

ndx: Potential alteration in cardiac output: decreased output related to inadequate myocardial contractility

GOAL: *Patient will have adequate cardiac output as evidenced by improved peripheral perfusion, increased urinary output, alertness, and clear breath sounds*

Assess extremities for perfusion: warm, pink color, rapid capillary refill, good pulses
Maintain continuous ECG monitoring
Assess apical rate and rhythm qh
Assess level of consciousness qh
Assess breath sounds qh
Assess adequacy of urinary output (minimal 1ml/kg/hr)
Administer digoxin if ordered
Administer diuretics if ordered

ndx: Potential for ineffective breathing pattern related to anesthesia, incisional pain, and/or increased pulmonary secretions

GOAL: *Patient will have age-appropriate respiratory rate and clear breath sounds*

Assess respiratory status qh
Initiate care of endotracheal tube if in place (p. 272)
Maintain ventilatory settings as ordered
Maintain airway patency
Administer humidified oxygen as ordered
Perform postural drainage, percussion, and suctioning q2h to 4h
Teach and/or assist patient to turn, cough, and deep breathe q2h
Use incentive spirometer in children who are old enough to use it
Administer analgesics prior to pulmonary treatments
Initiate care of chest tube (p. 271)
Monitor blood gases

ndx: Potential fluid volume excess related to decreased cardiac output and compensatory kidney mechanisms

GOAL: *Patient will have minimum urinary output of 1 ml/kg/hr*

Maintain parenteral fluids as ordered
Measure urinary output qh
Record accurate intake and output
Observe for signs of volume excess: decreased urinary output, loose cough, pulmonary congestion, periorbital edema

ndx: Potential for infection related to surgical incision and/or invasive lines

GOAL: *Child will be afebrile with clean, intact surgical incision and puncture sites*

Monitor temperature q2h and prn
Use good handwashing technique
Use strict asepsis for all dressing changes
Perform aseptic dressing change as ordered
Check incision site and puncture sites for redness, swelling, and drainage
Perform Foley catheter care as per hospital policy
Administer antibiotics as ordered
Assist in collecting specimens to determine site of infection with temperature elevation

ndx: Potential alteration in sensory-perceptual ability related to anesthesia and/or cerebral hypoxia

GOAL: *Patient will return to preoperative development ability*

Assess level of consciousness and motor, sensory, and developmental ability qh
Review preoperative baseline assessment
Encourage parental participation in care and stimulation

ndx: Alteration in nutrition: less than body requirements related to imposed NPO status postoperatively

GOAL: *Patient will tolerate age-appropriate diet reflecting adequate caloric intake to meet metabolic requirements*

Maintain NPO status immediately postoperatively
Assess return of bowel function
Begin clear liquid feedings and advance gradually as ordered
Monitor child's ability to consume increasing amounts of oral feedings

ndx: Potential for ineffective coping related to stress of child with chronic illness, stress of frequent hospitalizations, and separation from child

GOAL: *Parents will demonstrate increased coping ability as evidenced by increased verbalization that they feel confident in their ability to care for their child*

Discuss parents' feelings of fear, guilt, grief, anger, etc.
Have parents participate in care of their child as soon as possible
Encourage them to continue to do activities they normally would do with child at home: bathe, feed, dress, change diaper, hold, cuddle, play
Have parents meet with other parents with children with congenital heart disease
Involve parents in ongoing support group

Explore parents' feelings regarding overprotecting child and restricting activity of child—the "vulnerable child" feelings

Discuss ways in which parents can gradually increase child's independence

Refer to community agencies as necessary for ongoing support and follow-up

ndx: Knowledge deficit regarding home care and follow-up needs

GOAL: *Parents and/or significant other will demonstrate understanding of home care and follow-up instructions through interactive discussion and actual return demonstration*

Explain congenital heart defect and surgical intervention

Explain that if surgery was palliative, they can expect corrective surgery in the future

Explain need for nutritious diet
  Age-appropriate type and amount
  May be salt and/or fluid restricted

Explain need for exercise to tolerance; some children will continue to be exercise restricted

Discuss symptoms to report to physician
  Fever
  Fatigue
  Increased respiratory rate
  Incisional redness, swelling, or drainage

Teach name of medication, purpose, dosage, time of administration, and side effects

Emphasize importance of follow-up care with surgeon, cardiologist, and pediatrician

Have parents demonstrate measuring and administration of medication

Evaluation

Patient has clear breath sounds and age-appropriate heart and respiratory rates

Patient is afebrile

Nutritional intake is age appropriate

Urinary output exceeds 1 ml/kg/hr

Parents understand home care needs and feel confident in their ability to care for their child at home

OPEN-HEART SURGERY
Assessment
Observations/findings

Assessments are guided by an understanding of potential complications specifically associated with corrective surgery for specific defects (see Congenital Heart Defects, p. 844)

Review preoperative status, intraoperative course, duration of cardiopulmonary bypass, and normal growth and physiologic parameters of pediatric patient

Cardiovascular status
  Peripheral perfusion
    Warmth and color of extremities
    Capillary refill
    Peripheral pulses
  Heart rate and rhythm
    Dysrhythmias are common
    Cause of rhythm disturbance must be identified: check acid-base balance, presence of hypoxia, electrolyte imbalance, and digoxin level
  Murmur status
  Presence of pacer wires
  Blood pressure
  Central venous pressure (CVP)
  Right atrial pressure (RAP)
  Left atrial pressure (LAP)
  Arterial pressure (A line)

Respiratory status
  Presence or absence of spontaneous respirations
  Equality of chest movements
  Equality of breath sounds (note any areas of decreased breath sounds)
  Presence of adventitious sounds
  Signs of respiratory distress: nasal flaring, cyanosis, retractions, restlessness, bradycardia
  Endotracheal intubation (p. 272)
  Ventilatory assistance (p. 277)
  Chest tube function and drainage (p. 271)

Renal status
  Hourly urinary output (minimum in infants is 1 ml/kg/hr)
  Specific gravity
  Presence of hemoglobinuria, pH

Neurologic status
  Level of consciousness
  Neuromuscular/developmental ability
  Presence of localized or generalized neurologic abnormalities
  Presence of "postoperative psychosis": disorientation, inappropriate behavior for age, restlessness, agitation

GI status
  Nasogastric drainage: monitor amount, type, pH, and for presence of blood
  Return of bowel sounds
  Abdominal girths

Temperature
  Hyperthermia
  Hypothermia: may result from surgical hypothermia

Fluid status
  Dehydration (p. 866)
  Overhydration

Laboratory/diagnostic studies

Electrolytes: monitor sodium, potassium, and calcium levels
Base deficit or excess: serum pH
ABGs: PaO_2, $PaCO_2$, pH
CBC: hematocrit, hemoglobin
Coagulation studies
BUN: elevated with renal failure
Creatinine: elevated with renal failure
Urine osmolality: elevated with renal failure
Chest x-ray examination: evaluation of lung complications
12-lead ECG: evaluation of dysrhythmia

Potential complications

Cardiac
  Dysrhythmias
  Decreased cardiac output (cardiogenic shock) (p. 104)
  Cardiac tamponade (p. 100)
Pulmonary
  Atelectasis (p. 257)
  Pulmonary edema (CHF) (p. 245)
  Pneumothorax (p. 252)
  Tension pneumothorax (p. 254)
Renal
  Acute renal failure (p. 557)
  Hemoglobinuria
Metabolic
  Acidosis (p. 46)
  Electrolyte disturbances
  Hypovolemia/hypervolemia
Hematologic
  Coagulation abnormalities
  Hypotension
  Surgical bleeding
Neurologic
  Cerebral bleeding from embolization
  Focal or diffuse CNS dysfunction
  "Postoperative psychosis"
Gastrointestinal
  Paralytic ileus
  GI bleeding

Medical management

Validation of dysrhythmia and determination of pharmacologic treatment
Cardiovascular medications
Diuretics
Initiate temporary pacing if necessary
Treatment of hypovolemia with volume expanders (PRBCs, whole blood, colloid, fresh frozen plasma [FFP], etc.)
Fluid restriction imposed until risk of hypervolemia is passed, then advancement to maintenance
Accurate intake and output
Low-dose dopamine for increased renal perfusion
Monitoring of electrolytes and replacement as necessary
Monitoring of ABGs
Order for ventilatory settings and weaning of child off ventilatory support
Postural drainage, percussion, and suctioning
Provision of caloric requirements via parenteral fluids, then orally as tolerated
Hyperalimentation with prolonged complicated postoperative course
Analgesics
Antibiotics
Antacids
Antipyretics

Nursing diagnoses/goals/interventions

ndx: Potential alteration in cardiac output: decreased output related to inadequate contractility of heart, decreased preload, inadequate heart rate, and/or increased vascular resistance

GOAL: *Patient will have adequate cardiac output as evidenced by age-appropriate heart rate and blood pressure, with warm, pink extremities and strong peripheral pulses*

Assess peripheral perfusion qh
Determine oxygen saturation using oximeter qh
Monitor heart rate and rhythm continuously with ECG monitor
Assess apical rate and rhythm qh
Look for underlying cause of rhythm disturbances if present: hypoxia, acid-base imbalance, electrolyte imbalance, digoxin toxicity
Monitor blood pressure qh: note decreased pulse pressure, pulsus paradoxus, or pulsus alternans
Monitor RAP, LAP, CVP, and arterial pressure qh
Assess for signs and symptoms of hypovolemia
Measure urinary output hourly; be alert for decreased urinary output
Assess for postoperative bleeding
Be alert to excessive bloody chest tube drainage
Monitor coagulation studies
Assess respiratory status qh; be alert for increased pulmonary secretions and increased respiratory distress

Be alert to changes in behavior or level of consciousness
Administer volume expanders as ordered (colloid, plasma, PRBCs)
Administer cardiovascular medications as ordered
Administer electrolytes as ordered
Administer diuretics as ordered
Maintain temporary pacing as ordered

ndx: Potential for impaired gas exchange: ineffective breathing pattern related to increased pulmonary secretions, hypoventilation, and/or pain

GOAL: *Patient will have clear breath sounds, normal ABGs, and spontaneous effective respirations*

Perform respiratory assessment (p. 219) qh
Perform postural drainage, percussion, and suctioning q2h and prn with manual administration of 100% oxygen before and after suctioning
Change position q2h
Maintain endotracheal tube if present (p. 272)
Monitor ventilatory settings as ordered (p. 277); assist in making necessary changes as ordered
Monitor ABGs and respiratory status frequently to determine effectiveness of ventilatory changes
Monitor chest tube drainage qh (p. 271)
Administer analgesics as ordered prior to vigorous pulmonary treatments to promote cooperation in deep breathing and coughing routines
In child who is not intubated, use incentive spirometers, and coughing and deep-breathing exercises to promote lung expansion

ndx: Potential alteration in renal tissue perfusion secondary to decreased cardiac output

GOAL: *Patient will show evidence of adequate renal perfusion by maintaining urinary output of at least 1 ml/kg/hr*

Record accurate hourly intake (includes parenteral fluids, fluids used to flush lines, and oral intake) and output (urinary output, nasogastric drainage, chest tube drainage, bloods drawn for studies) measurements
Monitor urinary output; should be at least 1 ml/kg/hr
Measure specific gravity qh
Assess for presence of hemoglobinuria
Be alert to early signs of acute renal failure
 Monitor serum BUN and creatinine: increased
 Monitor electrolytes: hyperkalemia
 Monitor urine osmolality: increased

Ensure normovolemia by administering parenteral fluids as ordered
Administer electrolytes as ordered
Administer diuretics as ordered
Administer low-dose dopamine if ordered to improve renal perfusion

ndx: Potential sensory-perceptual alterations related to intraoperative hypoxia, embolus, or decreased cardiac output

GOAL: *Patient will exhibit age-appropriate developmental behavior*

Assess level of consciousness, pupil response, motor and sensory function, and return of developmental abilities qh
Assess for focal (localized weakness, poor motor function, partial seizures) or diffuse neurologic dysfunction (changes in behavior or level of consciousness)
Assess for presence of "postoperative psychosis": agitation, restlessness, combativeness, disorientation
Reassure child, orient to surroundings, and decrease stimulation as much as possible
Control pain
Provide frequent uninterrupted opportunities for sleep
Encourage parents to stay with child as much as possible
Have parents bring in familiar objects from home: favorite toy, tape player, books, etc.

ndx: Potential alteration in nutrition: less than body requirements related to dietary restriction following surgery

GOAL: *Patient will tolerate age-appropriate diet*

Maintain gastric decompression postoperatively with nasogastric tube
Irrigate nasogastric tube q2h to 4h to ensure patency
Evaluate nasogastric drainage for volume, pH, and presence of blood
Initiate antacid therapy as ordered if drainage is positive for blood
Measure abdominal girth q2h
Assess abdomen for return of peristalsis
 Decreased nasogastric drainage
 Presence of bowel sounds
 Decreased gastric distention
 Passing of flatus or stool
Administer parenteral fluids or hyperalimentation as ordered
Begin clear oral feedings with return of bowel function
Advance diet gradually as ordered

ndx: Potential for hypothermia related to cooling measures used during cardiopulmonary bypass procedure

GOAL: *Patient will maintain his body temperature at 99.5° F (37.5° C)*

Assess temperature qh
Use external warming devices to elevate child's temperature slowly
Continue use of warming devices as necessary to maintain temperature
Keep environmental temperature warm
Keep child partially dressed: hat, socks, blanket draped over extremities, etc.

ndx: Potential for infection related to surgical incision, use of cardiopulmonary bypass, and/or multiple invasive lines

GOAL: *Child will be afebrile with clean, intact surgical incision and puncture sites*

Monitor temperature q2h and prn
Be aware that good handwashing is crucial
Maintain strict asepsis for all dressing changes
Perform aseptic dressing change as ordered
Check incision site and puncture sites for redness, swelling, and drainage
Perform Foley catheter care as per hospital policy
Administer antibiotics as ordered
Assist in collecting specimens to determine site of infection with temperature elevation
Monitor CBC for increased WBC count

ndx: Knowledge deficit regarding home care and follow-up needs

GOAL: *Patient and/or parents will demonstrate understanding of home care and follow-up instructions through interactive discussion and actual return demonstration*

Explain congenital heart defect and surgical repair performed
Explain dietary needs: specific amount (minimal), type of formula, how often
Explain need for exercise to tolerance
Review restriction in exercise if any
Explain that child should gradually resume normal activity level and be treated as a normal child
Emphasize importance of good incisional care and hygiene if ordered
Discuss symptoms to report to physician
　Fever
　Incisional redness, swelling, drainage
Teach name of medication, purpose, dosage, time of administration, and side effects
Emphasize importance of follow-up care with cardiac surgeon, cardiologist, and pediatrician
Have patient and/or parents demonstrate
　Care of child
　Administration of medications

Evaluation

Patient is alert
Heart rate and rhythm are normal with improved peripheral perfusion
Respiratory rate is normal, and breath sounds are clear
Urinary output is adequate
Infant or child is able to maintain body temperature
Infant or child is tolerating age-appropriate diet
Child and/or parents understand home-care and follow-up instructions

CONGESTIVE HEART FAILURE (CHF)

A state in which the cardiac output is inadequate to meet the body's metabolic needs; in infants and young children it occurs bilaterally

Assessment

Observations/findings

Signs and symptoms of decreased cardiac output
　Restlessness, fussiness
　Mottled, pale skin
　Cool extremities
　Decreased urinary output
　Diaphoresis
　Exercise intolerance
　Poor feeding or inability to take po feedings
Increasing respiratory distress
　Nasal flaring
　Cyanosis
　Tachypnea
　Retractions
　Grunting
　Rales
　Tachycardia
Systemic venous congestion
　Rapid weight gain
　Edema: periorbital
　Abdominal distention
　Hepatosplenomegaly

Laboratory/diagnostic studies

Chest x-ray examination: cardiac enlargement and pulmonary congestion

Arterial blood gases: acidosis

Serum glucose: hypoglycemia often occurs in infants with CHF

Serum electrolytes
  Sodium: hyponatremia may occur with water retention
  Potassium: hypokalemia or hyperkalemia

Serum calcium: normal levels essential for myocardial contractility

CBC
  Anemia
  WBC elevation may occur

Medical management

Improvement of cardiac contractility and reduction of volume overload through use of
  Digitalization (see Pediatric Digitalis Therapy p. 859)
  Diuretics
  Fluid restriction
  Postural drainage, percussion, and suctioning in infants

Nursing diagnoses/goals/interventions

ndx: Alteration in cardiac output: decreased output related to ineffective contractility of the heart—excessive preload or afterload

GOAL: *Patient will experience improved cardiac output as evidenced by increased urinary output, decreased heart rate, decreased respiratory rate, and clear breath sounds*

Assess resting apical and respiratory rates q1h to 2h and prn

Administer digoxin accurately as ordered; do not give if heart rate is less than 100 beats/min or if rhythm is irregular

Administer diuretics as ordered

Monitor serum electrolyte levels

Restrict fluids as ordered

Monitor accurate intake and output

Weigh daily or bid at same times, unclothed, before feedings

Observe for resolution of CHF: decreased heart and respiratory rates, increased urinary output, decreased periorbital edema, decrease in and stabilization of weight, increased activity tolerance, improved feeding activity

ndx: Activity intolerance related to dyspnea and fatigue

GOAL: *Patient will experience minimal dyspnea and fatigue and will tolerate gradual increases in activity*

Reduce cardiac demands
  Plan frequent rest periods
  Avoid unneccessary handling of infant to prevent fatigue
  Anticipate needs to prevent crying
  Keep infant warm and comfortable; avoid overdressing or cold stress
Avoid overfatigue during feedings
  Feed in oxygen-enriched environment
  Give small, frequent feedings
  Gavage feedings in infants if sucking causes increased respiratory distress
Avoid exposure to individuals with known infections

ndx: Impaired gas exchange related to increased pulmonary secretions

GOAL: *Patient will have improved gas exchange as evidenced by clear breath sounds, decreased respiratory rate, and normal blood gases*

Maintain warm, humidified, oxygenated environment via mist tent or oxygen hood

Monitor respiratory status q1h to 2h; especially note changes in color, respiratory rate, use of accessory muscles, and presence of rales

Monitor arterial blood gases

Monitor oxygen saturation with oximeter

Elevate head of bed: use infant seat for infants; elevate older child on pillows

Perform postural drainage and percussion prn as ordered

Remove increased mucus via suctioning prn; suction *only* if infant needs it; avoid excessive suctioning, since it increases cardiac demands

ndx: Alteration in nutrition: less than body requirements related to dyspnea and fatigue

GOAL: *Patient will tolerate diet reflecting adequate caloric intake to meet metabolic needs*

Determine caloric requirements (p. 866)

Increase calories in formula to meet requirements yet remain within fluid restriction and patient's tolerance

Avoid overfatigue during feedings

Feed patient in oxygenated environment

Limit handling prior to feeding to prevent overexhaustion
Feed smaller amounts more frequently
Use gavage feeding in infants who cannot take adequate po feedings
Burp frequently during feedings to decrease gastric distention

ndx: Knowledge deficit regarding home care and follow-up needs

GOAL: *Parents and/or significant other will demonstrate understanding of home care and follow-up instructions through interactive discussion and actual return demonstration*

Explain need for planned rest periods
Discuss type of formula, amount, and how often
Teach name of medications (digoxin and diuretics), purpose, dosage, time of administration, and side effects (see Pediatric Digitalis Therapy, below)
Discuss symptoms of recurrence to report to physician
  Poor feeding
  Fatigue
  Increased respiratory rate
  Loose cough
  Cyanosis
  Puffiness around eyes
  Decreased urinary output
Confirm dates and times of follow-up appointments with surgeon, cardiologist, and pediatrician
Have parents demonstrate
  Proper measuring and administration of medications
  Ability to feed desired volume of formula

Evaluation

Patient shows evidence of resolving CHF: decreased respiratory and heart rates, decreased oxygen requirements, clear breath sounds, stabilized weight, increased urinary output, increased activity tolerance, increased ability to take oral feedings
Parents understand home care and follow-up instruction

PEDIATRIC DIGITALIS THERAPY

Assessment
Observations/findings
DIGITALIS EFFECT: DESIRED RESULT

Slower heart rate
Improved myocardial contractility: increased cardiac output
Slowed impulses through conduction system

DIGITALIS TOXICITY: UNDESIRABLE RESULT
Cardiac dysrhythmias: most common sign
Nausea, vomiting
Anorexia
Diarrhea
NOTE: There is an increased risk of digoxin toxicity associated with renal failure, hypoxia, acidosis, hypokalemia, and hypercalcemia

Laboratory/diagnostic studies
Serum digoxin level
Potassium and calcium levels

Nursing responsibility

To promote safe, accurate administration of digoxin
  Ensure completeness of physician's order
    Name of preparation
    Dosage written in micrograms and milliliter equivalents
    Route of administration
    Intervals of administration
    Pulse rate under which drug is to be withheld
  Administration
    Have two people licensed to administer medications calculate dosage and volume, and double-check amount after measured
    Check resting apical pulse for rate and rhythm prior to each administration (count for full minute or according to hospital policy)
    If toxic symptoms are present, withhold dose, place child on cardiac monitor, and notify physician
    Monitor for dysrhythmias; check serum electrolytes if toxicity is suspected
    If child vomits and you are unsure if child received dose, *do not repeat dose*
    Determine best method of ensuring complete administration of oral dose: spoon, syringe, nipple, or dropper
    Never dilute with anything

Nursing diagnosis/goal/interventions

ndx: Knowledge deficit regarding proper administration of medication

GOAL: *Patient and/or parents will demonstrate proper measuring and administration of digoxin and will verbally explain its purpose and side effects*

Teach name of medication, purpose, dosage, and time of administration
Discuss signs and symptoms of toxicity

Explain need to withhold dose and notify physician if toxic symptoms occur
Explain need to give complete dose; caution parents not to mix with formula or food
Teach method of administration: before meals
Caution parents not to repeat dose if unsure if child vomited it
Explain need to keep medication out of reach of children
Explain need for ongoing evaluation by cardiologist
Have patient and/or parents demonstrate
  Measurement of dosage
  Proper administration of medication

Evaluation

Patient does not exhibit signs of digitalis toxicity
Patient and/or parents understand digitalis therapy

TEMPORARY ARTIFICIAL PACEMAKER

Assessment
Observations/findings
PACEMAKER FAILURE

Bradycardia (asystole)
Possible ECG pattern changes
  Absence of pacemaker artifact
  No ventricular response: absence of QRS complex after pacemaker artifact
  Competition: presence of pacer response complex *and* patient's own complex
  Runaway pacer: pacer artifact appears at several hundred per minute
Hypotension: Stokes-Adams syndrome
  Faintness
  Convulsions
  Coma
Pallor or cyanosis
Decreased urinary output
Fatigability
Signs of decreased cardiac output

INFECTION

Site of insertion
  Redness
  Pain
  Swelling
  Drainage
Fever

Laboratory/diagnostic studies
Continuous ECG monitoring

Potential complications
Pacemaker failure

Medical management

Determination of pacemaker settings
Treatment of pacemaker malfunctions
Discontinuation of temporary pacemaker when feasible

Nursing diagnoses/goals/interventions

ndx: Potential alteration in cardiac output: decreased output related to pacemaker malfunction

GOAL: *Patient will maintain adequate cardiac output; pacemaker failure will be identified, and prompt treatment will occur*

Place patient on continuous ECG monitoring
Check heart rate qh
Monitor BP q4h and prn
Maintain settings on pacemaker as ordered
Protect pacemaker from falls and moisture
Prevent pull on catheter
Monitor intake and output
Position for most effective cardiac pacing

ndx: Potential for infection related to insertion of pacemaker wires

GOAL: *Patient will have clean, intact skin without evidence of infection*

Observe for signs of infection at insertion site
Change insertion site dressing daily using aseptic technique and ointment if ordered
Keep wires safely taped to chest after temporary pacemaker is discontinued

Evaluation

Pacemaker is functioning properly
Child maintains adequate cardiac output
There are no signs of infection
Pacer wires remain in place after removal of temporary pacemaker

Other aspects of pediatrics

CHILD ABUSE

Physical, sexual, or emotional maltreatment or neglect of children by parents, guardians, or other care givers

Assessment
Observations/findings
PHYSICAL ABUSE

Injuries are unexplained, recurrent, and/or inappropriate to history given

Bruises and welts
  In various stages of resolution
  Clustered
  Outlining shape of article used
  On different surface areas
  Circumferential on extremity
Burns
  Cigarette marks
  Scalded: socklike, glovelike, doughnut shape on buttocks and genitalia
  Having shape of instrument: iron, heater, etc.
  Infected: treatment delayed
Fractures
  Multiple
  Various stages of healing
  Frequently long bones or skull
Lacerations and abrasions
  Multiple
  Neglected
  Bite marks
  Scalp bald spots
Hemorrhage
  Intraabdominal
  Renal
Neurologic injuries
  Coma
  Subdural hematoma
Optic injuries
  Hyphema
  Detached retina
  Black eyes
Genitalia
  Edematous
  Excoriated

PHYSICAL NEGLECT

See Failure to Thrive (p. 841)
Evidence of poor hygiene
No immunizations appropriate for age
Prescribed medications not given
Exposure to unsafe environment
Poor adult supervision
Abandoned
Abdominal distention
Inappropriate clothing for weather
Diaper rash
Irritable

SEXUAL ABUSE

Venereal disease
Pain or itching in genital area
Pain on urination
Poor sphincter tone
Vaginal or penile bleeding or lacerations

EMOTIONAL ABUSE

See Failure to Thrive (p. 841)
Disruptive behavior
Hyperactivity
Speech disorders

BEHAVIOR

Fearful of adults
Depressed
Withdrawn
Accepting of painful procedures
Cries excessively and inconsolably
Seeks constant reassurance
Compulsive
Aggressive or compliant
Frightened of parents
Seeks parents' approval
Exhibits clinging, grabbing, or lap-hungry behavior
Chronically truant
Manipulative (p. 25)
Poor self-concept
Apprehensive when other children cry
Overanxious to please
Evasive when asked about accident
Poor peer relationships
Delinquent or runaway
Attempted suicide (p. 20)
Sleep disorders
Overly adaptive behavior
Developmental lags
Psychoneurotic reactions
Habit disorders (sucking, biting, rocking)
Sophisticated sexual knowledge
Irritable when handled

PARENT OR PRIMARY CARE GIVER

Evidence of dysfunctional attachment process in new mother
Hostile and depressed
Unrealistic expectations for child given developmental age
Overconcerned or underconcerned about child's injury
Asks few or no questions of care givers
Behavior toward crying or injured child is aloof, not comforting or affectionate
Explains need for physical punishment because of "badness" in victim
Seductive toward child of opposite sex
Refuses to allow child to be hospitalized

Laboratory/diagnostic studies

See Failure to Thrive (p. 841)
Appropriate to suspected injury
Long bone survey: to document other skeletal injuries

Potential complications

Fatal traumatic injuries
Behavioral disorders
Malnutrition
Venereal disease
Pregnancy in young adolescent

Medical management

Dependent on type and extent of injury
Thorough documentation of injuries
Report of case to appropriate authorities

Nursing diagnoses/goals/interventions*

ndx: Alteration in parenting related to stressors that contribute to abuse of a child: lack of support system, poor financial resources, abusive relationship with own parents, lack of knowledge about parenting, etc.

GOAL: *Child will no longer experience abuse from parents; parents will obtain adequate resources to prevent further abuse of their child and will seek assistance for abusive behavior*

Do not exhibit judgmental behavior toward parents
Assist parents in identifying their stresses
Explore more effective ways of dealing with stress
Discuss ways to use resources during times of stress to avoid injuring themselves or their child
Notify authorities of suspicion or fact of abuse or neglect as mandated by law
Make referral to social agency for purpose of
    Assessing home environment
    Providing additional support services as necessary
    Having ongoing contact with family once they return to home environment
    Having ongoing advocate for protection of child
Cooperate with authorities in decisions made
    Understand that court order forbidding discharge of child to parents may occur
    Child may be discharged to foster home pending final decisions by legal authorities

ndx: Anxiety in child related to abuse by parents and separation from parents

GOAL: *Child will show evidence of decreased anxiety by increased verbalization, increased interaction with other children, increased interest in play, and decreased crying*

Perform functions slowly with sensitivity, observing child closely for emotional reactions
Have consistent care givers so child learns sense of trust
Encourage parents to visit and participate in care of their child
Observe child's reaction to parents when they visit
If child is old enough, encourage child to talk about what happened
Reinforce that child was not injured because he was "bad"
Have child participate in play activities as soon as feasible
Encourage doll play with discussion of incident so child can express feelings and fears regarding assault
Prevent further injury if possible

Evaluation

All injuries are identified and documented thoroughly
Patient shows improvement specific to type of injury
Authorities are aware of abuse incident
Appropriate referrals are made
Parents show improvement in care of their child, or child is placed in foster home
Child has expressed some of his anxiety and fears verbally or through play

ANOREXIA NERVOSA

A disorder characterized by emaciation occurring as a result of self-inflicted starvation; etiology appears to be primarily psychologic, but it may include underlying organic factors

Usual age: adolescence; predominantly females
Peak ages: 12 to 13 years and 19 to 20 years

Assessment

Observations/findings
USUAL FAMILY PROFILE

Middle- to upper-class socioeconomic level
Conservative philosophy, high personal standards
Often dependent, seductive relationship with a warm, passive father
Often dependent relationship with dominant, solicitous, chronically depressed mother
Family members closely fused
Personal boundaries not respected
Mind reading prevalent
Sense of independence sabotaged

---

*Dependent on type and extent of injury.

Expressions of anger, anxiety, or aggressiveness blocked
Arguments not allowed
Togetherness prized
Loyalty exaggerated
Excellence as the standard
Anorectic seeks love and approval, becomes perfectionist, cannot achieve it, develops physical complaints
Family attention focuses on and reinforces weight loss and poor eating

PRODROMAL PERIOD

Increasing irritability
Eczema may develop
Abdominal discomfort
Headaches
Hyperactivity
Depression
Anxiety
Social withdrawal from friends
High level of investment in schoolwork and high-energy sports
Often was previously overweight

ORGANIC SYMPTOMS

Severe weight loss
Secondary amenorrhea
Bradycardia
Lowered body temperature
Decreased BP
Cold intolerance
Dry skin
Brittle nails
Lanugo hair
Decreased appetite
Feelings of satiety
Breasts atrophied
Axillary and pubic hair reduced
Sleep disturbances
Constipation
Increased susceptibility to infection

AFFECT/BEHAVIOR

Academically high achiever
Conforming behavior
Conscientious
Increased energy levels
Relentless pursuit of thinness and fear of fatness
Anorexia frequently precipitated by adolescent crisis
History of being overweight
Fear of developing feelings of sexuality

Disturbed body image of delusional proportions
　Defends emaciation as normal
　Feels rewarded by achieving and maintaining emaciated state
　Is fearful of weight gain
　Interprets others' concerns as attempts to make her fat
　Admires emaciated self in mirror
Inaccurate and confused perception and interpretation of inner stimuli
　Does not recognize signs of nutritional need
　Is unable to assess amount of food taken
　Derives pleasure from refusal of food
　Hides food; may flush it down toilet secretly
　May induce vomiting after eating
　May use laxatives to speed passage of food
　Is preoccupied with food and related activities; may plan and prepare meals for others, collect recipes, count calories, etc.
　Increases activity to counteract weight gain
　May conceal weights on body before weighing
　May hoard food, especially candy and nonnutritive foods
Paralyzing sense of ineffectiveness
　Behaves with defiance and rebellion but is overwhelmed by sense of ineffectiveness
　Feels she responds only to demands and wishes of others
　Doubts ability of, or right to, self-assertion

Laboratory/diagnostic studies

CBC with differential: leukopenia, lymphocytosis, anemia
Blood serum studies
　Hypoglycemia, hypocholesteremia, hypoproteinemia
　Decreased estrogen levels
Urine studies: decreased urinary 17-ketosteroids

Potential complications

Cardiac arrhythmias

Medical management

Determination of extent of nutritional deprivation
If severe, nasogastric feedings are ordered if food is refused by patient
Parenteral fluids/hyperalimentation for dehydration or life-threatening malnutrition
Behavior modification therapy
Daily weight
Reference to psychotherapist with family therapy approach to care

Nursing diagnoses/goals/interventions

ndx: Alteration in nutrition: less than body requirements related to anorexia, self-induced vomiting, laxative abuse, and/or distorted perception of body

GOAL: *Patient will tolerate a diet reflecting appropriate caloric requirements (p. 866) to meet metabolic demands*

Allow choice of foods (low-calorie foods not allowed)
Structure mealtimes to a time limit (e.g., 40 min)
Diminish distractions (e.g., conversation, television) during mealtimes
State time to eat, present food, and state time limit; inform patient that if food is not consumed during a set time, a nasogastric tube will be inserted for a tube feeding
If food not taken, insert nasogastric tube and feed as ordered in a matter-of-fact, nonpunitive manner; do not allow bargaining
Reinsert nasogastric tube each time tube feeding is necessary (tube left in place allows child opportunity to drain stomach contents and causes discomfort when encouraged to eat meals)
Withdraw attention during mealtime if patient refuses to eat
Do not allow hoarding of food
Monitor intake and output
   Keep records at nurses' station
   Observations should be done as unobtrusively as possible
Parenteral fluids may be necessary; administer as ordered; accompany patient to bathroom to prevent emptying of intravenous fluids
Minimize attention paid to eating, or behavior will be reinforced

Behavior modification therapy

Patient obtains or loses privileges based on established desired weight gain per day
   Separation from family for a period is helpful
   Deprive patient of pleasurable activities
   Restrict nursing intervention to technical nature
   Isolate socially
   Communication should be utilitarian, not supportive
   Reward patient only for weight gain
      Time with nurse
      Increased visitor time
      Social activities with other children
      Access to TV, radio, stereo, and/or telephone
Maintain consistency of treatment
   One staff member per shift should have final word on decisions
Prevent manipulation of staff
   Set and maintain strict limits
   Communicate limits and consequences of exceeding those limits clearly and in nonpunitive manner
   See Manipulative Behavior (p. 25)
Obtain accurate weights
   Weigh patient daily before morning meal
   Weigh patient in gown only; prevent concealment of weight on body
   Establish allowable privileges if weight is gained
   Encourage feeling of responsibility for weight gain

ndx: Disturbance in body image related to inaccurate perception of self as fat: poor self-esteem

GOAL: *Patient will begin to verbalize positive things about self and will begin to accurately perceive self as thin*

Give positive support and praise for things well done
Foster successful experiences
Begin with tasks easily accomplished
Focus on positive traits
Encourage patient to verbalize thoughts
Have patient draw picture of self and discuss perception of self
Encourage good hygiene and grooming for feeling of well-being
Respond factually and consistently to child's questions concerning diet and nutrition
Encourage and reinforce constructive physical activity: bed making, helping other children

ndx: Ineffective individual coping related to feelings of loss of control, fear of growing up, and/or personalized response to family dysfunction

GOAL: *Patient will exhibit non-food-related coping skills by maintaining weight during stressful times, verbalizing her thoughts; and seeking appropriate resources to assist her in coping*

Encourage ventilation of feelings
Observe and record responses to stress
Encourage coming to staff when stressed
Discourage (withdraw your attention from) rituals or emotional associations with meals, food, etc.
Support patient's attempts at self-determination, especially when with family

ndx: Ineffective family coping related to inability to communicate and inability to meet the needs of all family members

GOAL: *Family will demonstrate effective coping by recognizing the needs of each member, improving their listening skills, working toward meeting the needs of each member, and seeking assistance as necessary*

Encourage child and family to verbalize thoughts, perceptions, and feelings

Point out areas where child and family members disagree

Check out each family member's perception of what another has said to reinforce listening skills

Emphasize with child and family members importance of using "I" and taking responsibility for self

With family members present, be child's advocate and support child's attempts at self-determination

Redirect control conflicts between child and parents away from food and onto developmental issues related to curfews, school activities, etc.

Refer family for ongoing psychiatric care

Evaluation

Child shows progressive weight gain

Child had improved self-concept

Child begins to show evidence of using non-food related coping behaviors

Family has accepted problem and has agreed to participate in ongoing psychiatric care

VITAL SIGNS

Temperature

When

Routinely according to hospital policy
 As ordered by physician
 As indicated by standard of care for disease or operation

How

Rectally: first newborn temperature
Orally: 3 years or over if no contraindication
Axillary: newborns and under 3 years

Normal values

Rectal: approximately 97.5° to 99.5° F or 36.5° to 38° C
Oral: approximately 97° to 99° F or 36° to 37.5° C
Axillary: approximately 96.5° to 98.5° F or 35.5° to 37° C

Blood Pressure

When

Routinely according to hospital policy
As ordered by physician
As indicated by standard of care for disease or operation

How

Cuffs of several sizes should be available; cuff bladder should cover no more or less than two-thirds length of upper arm; essential that size cuff being used on each child be noted in nursing care plan so that there is consistency in all pressures taken

Too large a cuff will result in lower than actual pressure

Too small a cuff will result in higher than actual pressure

Normal values

See Table 15-2

Heart Rate

When

Routinely according to hospital policy
As ordered by physician
As indicated by standard of care for disease or operation

TABLE 15-2. Normal BP Values for Age*

Age	Systolic / Diastolic
Neonate: to 1 mo	80 ± 16 / 46 ± 16
Infant: 1-12 mo	96 ± 30 / 65 ± 25
Preschool: 2-6 yr	60 to 110 / 40 to 75
School age: 8-10 yr	105 ± 15 / 60 ± 10
Adolescent: 11-16 yr	85 to 130 / 45 to 85
Adults	90 to 140 / 60 to 90

*Wide ranges of normal result in questionable value of one BP reading; greatest value of BP readings in children is in serial BP (when indicated by condition) to show upward or downward trend.

How

Apically: under 10 years of age
Radially: over 10 years of age
Apical pulse in young children will usually provide more information about quality and rhythm of heart rate than will radial pulse

Normal values

See Table 15-3

Respirations

When

Routinely according to hospital policy
As ordered by physician
As indicated by standard of care for disease or operation

How

With child quiet, at lowest activity level
Count for a full minute

Normal values

See Table 15-4

NUTRITION

See Tables 15-5 and 15-6 for fluid and caloric requirements

Dehydration checklist

Change in behavior
  Fussy
  Too quiet
  Thirsty
  Nauseated
  Weak cry
Change in appearance
  Pale
  Ashen-gray
  Wrinkled brow
  "Worried" look
  Sunken eyeballs
  Sunken fontanelles
Tissue turgor
  Loose skin
  Skin picks up easily
  Skin does not bounce back
Mucous membranes
  Dry mouth
  Dry tongue
  Absence of salivation
  Mucus thick, tenacious
  No tears

TABLE 15-3. Normal Heart Rate Values for Age*

Age	Approximate beats/min
Neonate: to 1 mo	120-160
Infant	
1-6 mo	130
6-8 mo	120
8-12 mo	115
12 mo	100-140
Preschool	
2 yr	85-125
2-6 yr	90-110
6 yr	65-100
School age: 6-10 yr	85-100
Adolescent	
10-14 yr	80-90
11-16 yr	75-90
18 yr	
Males	70
Females	75
Adults	72

*Most accurate heart rates will always be those taken with child quiet, at lowest activity level, and counted for a full minute.

TABLE 15-4. Normal Respiration Values for Age

	Approximate rate/min
0-12 mo	30-50
1-5 yr	20-30
5-12 yr	15-25
12-18 yr	12-20

TABLE 15-5. Maintenance Fluid Requirement Calculation

Child's weight	ml/kg formula
Up to 10 kg	100 ml/kg/24 hr
11-20 kg	1000 ml + 50 ml/kg over 10 kg/24 hr
21-30 kg	1500 + 25 ml/kg over 20 kg/24 hr

TABLE 15-6. Caloric Requirement Calculation*

Age (yr)	Calories
0-1	115/kg
1-3	1300 daily
3-6	1000 daily
6-9	2100 daily
9-12	2200-2400 daily
12-15	2500-3000 daily
15-18	2300-3400 daily

*These figures are approximate; each child's needs will depend on diagnosis and current nutritional state.

TABLE 15-7. Pediatric Emergency Drugs*

Drug	Indication	Dosage
Albumin	Shock; provide serum protein	0.5-1.0 g/kg IV
Aminophylline	Bronchoconstriction	4-6 mg/kg IV q6h
Atropine	Bradycardia not secondary to hypoxia	0.01 mg/kg subcutaneously
Desferoxamine mesylate (Desferal)	Iron poisoning	15 mg/kg/hr IV *or* 80 mg/kg IM q8h, 3 times
Dexamethasone (Decadron)	Cerebral edema	4 mg IM or IV stat and 0.5-1.5 mg q4h
50% dextrose	Hypoglycemia	5-10 ml IV push
Diazepam (Valium)	Seizures (status epilepticus)	0.1-0.2 mg/kg IV slowly
Diazoxide (Hyperstat)	Hypertensive crisis	2-10 mg/kg rapid IV push
Digoxin (Lanoxin)	Congestive heart failure; paroxysmal atrial tachycardia	Digitalizing dose: divided into three doses; given at q8h intervals Infants: 0.06-0.08 mg/kg Children: 0.04-0.06 mg/kg
Dopamine (Intropin)	Hypotension	2-5 μg/kg/min IV drip to start; may go up to 50 μg/kg/min
Epinephrine (Adrenalin); aqueous 1:10,000	Cardiac arrest; bradycardia and/or hypotension; refractory congestive heart failure	0.01-0.02 ml/kg intracardiac 1 ml/100 5% dextrose in water at 5-10 microdrops/min IV
Ethacrynic acid (Edecrin)	Severe congestive heart failure	1 mg/kg IV push
Furosemide (Lasix)	Pulmonary edema	1 mg/kg IV or IM
Hydralazine (Apresoline)	Hypertensive crisis (with reserpine)	1.7-3.5 mg/kg/day IV or IM divided q4h or q6h
Hydrocortisone sodium succinate (Solu-Cortef)	Asthma	3-5 mg/kg IV q6h
Isoproterenol (Isuprel)	Bradycardia and/or hypotension	0.2 mg (1 ml) in 100 ml at 3-5 microdrops/min (0.05-4.0 μg/min)
Glucagon	Hypoglycemic reactions	0.025-0.1 mg/kg IV or IM
Levarterenol (Levophed)	Hypotension secondary to paroxysmal tachycardia	1 mg/250 ml (4 μg/ml) IV drip with monitoring of BP; start at 0.1 μg/kg/min
Lidocaine (Xylocaine) (2% solution or 20 mg/ml), 1 g vial	Runs of premature ventricular contractions or ventricular tachycardia	Bolus: 1 mg/kg slow IV push, may be repeated one time only; IV drip 20-40 μg/kg/min; 1 g vial/100 ml D5W = 10 μg/ml
Mannitol (25% ampule or 20% in IV bottle)	Acute cerebral edema	1-2 g/kg in 20 min
Metaraminol (Aramine, Metaramine)	Hypotension (with or without paroxymal atrial tachycardia)	0.3-2 mg/kg in 500 ml 5% dextrose in water, IV drip while monitoring BP
Methylprednisolone (Solu-Medrol)	Septic shock	15-30 mg/kg IV
Naloxone (Narcan)	Narcotic toxicity	0.01 mg/kg IV; 0.4 mg/ml, 0.02 mg/ml: neonatal
Paraldehyde	Grand mal seizure	0.15 ml/kg po or IM or 0.3 ml/kg per rectum (mixed with equal volume vegetable oil)
Phenobarbital	Anticonvulsant	5-15 mg/kg IM or slow IV
Procainamide (Pronestyl)	Ventricular tachycardia or runs of premature ventricular contractions	2 mg/kg (maximum 100 mg) IV slowly over 5 min with ECG monitoring

*Prepared by Howard W. Switzky, B.S., R.Ph., Pediatric Clinical Pharmacist Specialist, Kaiser Permanente Medical Center, Los Angeles, Calif., and Clinical Instructor, University of Southern California, School of Pharmacy, Los Angeles, Calif. *Continued.*

TABLE 15-7. Pediatric Emergency Drugs—cont'd

Drug	Indication	Dosage
Propranolol (Inderal)	Cardiac arrhythmias; tetralogy hypercyanotic spells	0.1-0.2 mg/kg slow IV (maximum dose 3 mg)
Pyridoxine	Seizures due to pyridoxine deficiency or dependency	50 mg IM or IV, then 10-25 mg daily po
Reserpine (Serpasil)	Hypertensive crisis	0.07 mg/kg IM
Sodium bicarbonate	Acidosis	2-4 mEq/kg IV; 1-2 mEq/kg intracardiac; repeat q5-10 min
Urea	Promote diuresis	0.5-1.5 g/kg as 30% solution IV slowly over 30 min

Weight change: severe drop from normal weight
Urinary output
  Decreased amount and frequency
  Concentrated
  Increased specific gravity
Respirations
  Rapid
  Shallow
Heart rate: rapid
Body temperature: subnormal *or* fever
Neurologic status
  Weak
  Depressed
  Twitching
  Convulsions

DRUGS

See Table 15-7 on pediatric emergency drugs
Atropine: see Table 15-8
Pentobarbital (Nembutal): 1 mg/lb of body weight
Meperidine: 60% to 75% of body weight (pounds) in milligrams
All drugs given IM (unless otherwise ordered)

TABLE 15-8. Average Dosage of Atropine

Weight (lb)	Atropine
3 to 20	0.1 mg
20 to 30	0.15 to 0.2 mg
30 to 40	0.2 to 0.3 mg
40 to 50	0.3 to 0.4 mg
50 to 100	0.4 mg
Over 100	0.6 mg

BIBLIOGRAPHY

GENERAL CARE

Carpentino, L.J.: Nursing diagnosis, Philadelphia, 1983, J.B. Lippincott Co.

Doenges, M.E., Jeffries, M., and Moorhouse, M.: Nursing care plans: Nursing diagnoses in planning patient care, Philadelphia, 1984, F.A. Davis Co.

Kim, M.J., McFarland, G.K., and McLane, A.M.: Pocket guide to nursing diagnoses, St. Louis, 1987, The C.V. Mosby Co.

North American Nursing Diagnosis Association (NANDA): Classification of nursing diagnoses: proceedings of the sixth conference, edited by M.E. Hurley, St. Louis, 1986, The C.V. Mosby Co.

BEHAVIORAL DYSFUNCTIONS

American Psychiatric Association: Diagnostic and statistical manual of mental disorders, ed. 3, Washington, D.C., 1980, The Association.

Burgess, A.W., and Baldwin, B.A.: Crisis intervention: theory and practice, Englewood Cliffs, N.J., 1981, Prentice-Hall, Inc.

Doenges, M.: Nurse's pocket guide: Nursing diagnoses with interventions, Philadelphia, 1984, F.A. Davis Co.

Engel, G.: Grief and grieving, Am. J. Nurs. 64(9):93, 1964.

Haber, J., et al.: Comprehensive psychiatric nursing, ed. 3, New York, 1987, McGraw-Hill Book Co.

Kolb, L.: Disturbance in body image. In Arieti, S., and Reiser, M., editors: American handbook of psychiatry, ed. 2, New York, 1975, Basic Books, Inc., Publishers.

North American Nursing Diagnosis Association (NANDA): Classification of nursing diagnoses: proceedings of the sixth conference, edited by M.E. Hurley, St. Louis, 1986, The C.V. Mosby Co.

Roy, C.: Introduction to nursing: an adaptation model, ed. 2, Englewood Cliffs, N.J., 1984, Prentice-Hall, Inc.

Sullivan, H.S.: The interpersonal theory of psychiatry, New York, 1953, W.W. Norton & Co., Inc.

Thompson, J.M., et al.: Clinical nursing, St. Louis, 1986, The C.V. Mosby Co.

Wilson, H., and Kneisl, C.: Psychiatric nursing, ed. 2, Menlo Park, Calif., 1983, Addison-Wesley Publishing Co., Inc.

NUTRITION/PARENTERAL THERAPY

Guthrie, P., and Turner, W.: Peripheral and central nutrition, NITA 9:393, Sept./Oct. 1986.

Haynes-Johnson, V.: Tube feeding complications: causes, prevention and therapy, Nutr. Support Serv. 6(3):17, 1986.

Hinson, L.: Nutritional assessment and management of the hospitalized patient, Crit. Care Nurse 5(2):53, 1985.

Jones, D., et al.: Medical surgical nursing: a conceptual approach, New York, 1980, McGraw-Hill Book Co.

Kaminski, M.: Hyperalimentation: a guide for clinicians, New York, 1985, Marcel Dekker, Inc.

Metheny, N.: 20 ways to prevent tube-feeding complications, Nursing '85, p. 47, Jan. 1985.

Moore, C.L., et al.: Nursing care and management of venous access ports, Oncol. Nurs. Forum 13(3):35, 1986.

Nestle, M.: Nutrition in clinical practice, Irvine, Calif., 1985, Jones Medical Publications.

Recker, D., and Metzler, D.: Use of the multi-lumen catheter, Crit. Care Nurse 4(3):92, 1984.

Rutherford, C.: Peripheral parenteral nutrition, NITA 9:232, May/June 1986.

Scholl, D.: Nutrition and diet therapy, Oradell, N.J., 1986, Medical Economics Co., Inc.

Weldy, N.J.: Body fluids and electrolytes, ed. 5, St. Louis, 1988. The C.V. Mosby Co.

CARDIOVASCULAR SYSTEM

Abels, L.F.: Mosby's manual of critical care, St. Louis, 1979, The C.V. Mosby Co.

Allen, J.A., and Throm, L.: Percutaneous transluminal coronary angioplasty: a new alternative for ischemic heart disease, Crit. Care Nurse 2(1):24, 1982.

American Heart Association: Guidelines for cardiac rehabilitation, ed. 2, Los Angeles, 1982, American Heart Association, Greater Los Angeles Affiliation.

American Heart Association: Standards and guidelines for cardiopulmonary resuscitation and emergency cardiac care, JAMA 225:2841, 1986.

American Nurses' Association, Division of Medical-Surgical Nursing Practice, and American Heart Association, Council on Cardiovascular Nursing: Standards of cardiovascular nursing, Kansas City, Mo., 1981, American Nurses' Association.

Andreoli, K., et al.: Comprehensive cardiac care, ed. 6, St. Louis, 1987, The C.V. Mosby Co.

Budassi, S.A., and Barber, J.M.: Emergency nursing: principles and practice, ed. 2, St. Louis, 1985, The C.V. Mosby Co.

Canobbio, M.M.: Cardiovascular system. In Thompson, J.M., et al.: Clinical nursing, St. Louis, 1986, The C.V. Mosby Co.

Cobey, J.C., and Covey, J.H.: Chronic leg ulcers, Am. J. Nurs. 74:258, 1974.

Conover, M.H.: Exercises in diagnosing ECG tracings, ed. 3, St. Louis, 1984, The C.V. Mosby Co.

Conover, M.H.: Pocket nurse guide to electrocardiography, St. Louis, 1986, The C.V. Mosby Co.

Costrini, N.V., and Thomson, W.M.: Manual of medical therapeutics, ed. 22, Boston, 1977, Little, Brown & Co., Inc.

Dasling, M.C., et al.: Surgery of the aorta, CCQ 8:25, 1985.

Dillman, P.A.: The biophysical responses to shock trousers, JEN 3:21, 1977.

Dorr, K.S.: Intra-aortic balloon pump, Crit. Care Update, p. 12, 1978.

Doyle, J.E.: Treatment modalities in peripheral vascular disease, Nurs. Clin. North Am. 21(2):241, 1986.

Fardy, P.A., et al.: Cardiac rehabilitation: implication for the nurse and other health professionals, St. Louis, 1980, The C.V. Mosby Co.

Foreman, M.D.: Arterial prosthetic graft infections: the pathophysiologic basis of nursing care, Focus Crit. Care 12:23, 1985.

Fowkes, W.C., and Hunn, V.K.: Clinical assessment for the nurse practitioner, St. Louis, 1973, The C.V. Mosby Co.

Frazee, S., and Nail, L.: New challenge in cardiac nursing: the intra-aortic balloon, Heart Lung 2:526, 1973.

Gershan, J.A., and Jiricka, M.K.: Percutaneous transluminal coronary angioplasty: implications for nursing, Focus Crit. Care 11:28, 1984.

Giles, I.D.: Principles of vasodilator therapy for left ventricular congestive heart failure, Heart Lung 9(2):271, 1980.

Goldberger, A.L., and Goldberger, E.: Clinical electrocardiography: a simplified approach, ed. 3, St. Louis, 1986, The C.V. Mosby Co.

Goldberger, E.: Textbook of clinical cardiology, St. Louis, 1982, The C.V. Mosby Co.

Guzzetta, E.E., and Dossey, D.M.: Cardiovascular nursing: body-mind tapestry, St. Louis, 1984, The C.V. Mosby Co.

Herman, J.A.: Nursing assessment and nursing diagnosis in patients with peripheral vascular disease, Nurs. Clin. North Am. 21:219, 1986.

Isaacson, J., et al.: Post pump psychosis, Crit. Care Nurse 14:83, 1982.

Johanson, B.C., et al.: Standards for critical care, St. Louis, ed. 2, 1985, The C.V. Mosby Co.

Katsaros, C., and Bobb, J.: Shock—the critical hour, JEN 4:45, 1978.

Khan, M.I.G.: Manual of cardiac drug therapy, London, 1984, Baillière Tindall.

Kim, H.S., and Chung, E.K.: Torsade de pointes: polymorphous ventricular tachycardia, Heart Lung 12(3):296, 1983.

King, O.: Care of the cardiac surgical patient, St. Louis, 1975, The C.V. Mosby Co.

Kossowsky, W.A., Lyon, A.F., and Spain, D.M.: Repraisal of the postmyocardial infarction Dressler's syndrome, Am. Heart J. 102(5):954, 1981.

Kurtz, K., Kempema, J., and Birnbaum, M.R.: Coping with acute abdominal crisis and more: multisystem failure, Nursing '78 8:22, 1978.

Lasater, M.G.: Torsade de pointes: etiology and treatment, Focus Crit. Care 13(5):17, 1986.

Loan, T.: Nursing interaction with patients undergoing coronary angioplasty, Heart Lung 15(4):369, 1986.

Long, G.D.: Managing the patient with abdominal aortic aneurysm, Nursing '78 8:20, 1978.

Lundin, D.V.: You can inject heparin subcutaneously, RN 41:51, 1978.

Massey, J.A.: Diagnostic testing for peripheral vascular disease, Nurs. Clin. North Am. 21:207, 1986.

Massie, B.M., and Chatterjee, K.: Vasodilator therapy of pump failure complicating acute myocardial infarction, Med. Clin. North Am. 63:25, 1979.

McCarthy, J.J., and Williams, L.R.: Femoral artery reconstruction, CCQ 8:39, 1985.

McCauley, K., and Weaver, T.E.: Cardiac and pulmonary disease: nutritional implications, Nurs. Clin. North Am. 18(1):81, 1983.

Michaelson, C.: Bedside assessment and diagnosis of acute left ventricular failure. In Canobbio, M., editor: Issues in cardiology, CCQ 4(3):1, 1981.

Miller, D.C., and Roon, A.J.: Diagnosis and management of peripheral vascular disease, Menlo Park, Calif., 1982, Addison-Wesley Publishing Co., Inc.

Moore, K., and Maschak, B.J.: How patient education can reduce the hazards of anticoagulation, Nursing '77 7:24, 1977.

Moore, S.J.: Pericarditis after acute myocardial infarction: manifestations and nursing implications, Heart Lung 3(3):551, 1979.

Nurse's Reference Library: Drugs, Horsham, Pa., 1982, Intermed Communications, Inc.

Ott, B.B.: Percutaneous transluminal coronary angioplasty and nursing implications, Heart Lung 11(4):294, 1982.

Riedinger, M.S., and Shellock, F.G.: Technical aspects of the thermodilution method for measuring cardiac output, Heart Lung 13(3):215, 1984.

Sadler, D.: Nursing for cardiovascular health, East Norwalk, Conn., 1984, Appleton-Century-Crofts.

Sexton, D.L.: The patient with peripheral arterial occlusive disease, Nurs. Clin. North Am. 12:89, 1977.

Spann, J.F.: Pericarditis: diagnosis and complications. In Chest pain: problems in differential diagnosis, vol. 6, Kansas City, Mo., 1981, Biomedical Marion Laboratories, Inc.

Spillall, J.A.: Office diagnosis of occlusive arterial disease, J. Cardiovasc. Med., p. 107, 1984.

Webb, P.H.: Neurological deficit after carotid endarterectomy, Am. J. Nurs. 79(4):654, 1979.

Weiland, A.P., and Walker, W.E.: Physiologic principles and clinical sequelae of cardiopulmonary bypass, Heart Lung 15(1):34, 1986.

Whitman, G.: Intra-aortic balloon pumping and cardiac mechanics: a programmed lesson, Heart Lung 7:1034, 1978.

Young, J.R.: Thrombophlebitis and chronic venous insufficiency, Geriatrics 28:63, 1973.

HEMATOLOGIC SYSTEM

Benson, M.L., and Benson, D.M.: Autotransfusion is here—are you ready, Nursing '85 3:36, 1985.

Carnevali, D.L.: Nursing care planning: diagnosis and management, ed. 3, Philadelphia, 1983, J.B. Lippincott Co.

Carpenito, L.J.: Handbook of nursing diagnosis, ed. 2, Philadelphia, 1987, J.B. Lippincott Co.

Carpenito, L.J.: Nursing diagnosis: application to clinical practice, ed. 2, Philadelphia, 1987, J.B. Lippincott Co.

Christie, D., et al.: Quinine-induced thrombocytopenia following intravenous use of heroin, Arch. Intern. Med. 143:1174, 1983.

Curtin, L.L.: What we say/what we do, Nurs. Manage. 1:7, 1984.

Daugherty, C.M., editor: Symposium on nursing: diagnosis, Nurs. Clin. North Am., 1985.

Doenges, M.E., Jeffries, M.F., and Moorhouse, M.F.: Nursing care plans: nursing diagnoses in planning patient care, Philadelphia, 1984, F.A. Davis Co.

Eddy, J.L., Selgas-Cordes, R., and Curran, M.: Cutaneous T-cell lymphoma, Am. J. Nurs. 2:202, 1984.

Hamilton, H.K.: Diseases, Nurses Reference Library Series, Springhouse, Pa., 1983, Intermed Communications, Inc.

Hamilton, H.K.: Definitions, Nurses Reference Library, reprint, Springhouse, Pa., 1984, Springhouse Corp.

Hood, G.H., and Dincher, J.R.: Total patient care: foundation and practice, ed. 7, St. Louis, 1980, The C.V. Mosby Co.

Hussar, D.A.: New drugs, Nursing '84 6:65, 1984.

Johanson, B.C., et al.: Standards for critical care, ed. 2, St. Louis, 1985, The C.V. Mosby Co.

Kim, M.J., McFarland, G.K., and McLane, A.M.: Pocket guide to nursing diagnoses, ed. 2, St. Louis, 1987, The C.V. Mosby Co.

Koch, P.M.: Thrombocytopenia: don't let it make a big problem out of nothing, Nursing '84 10:54, 1984.

Martens, K.: Let's diagnose strengths, not just problems, Am. J. Nurs. 2:192, 1986.

McConnell, E.A.: Leukocyte studies: what the counts can tell you, Nursing '86 3:42, 1986.

McKnight, P.: Decision tree for distinguishing nursing diagnosis, clinical nursing problems, clinical medical problems, and relegation to relevent domains of nursing, NANDA 3:5, 1985.

Michael Reese Hospital and Medical Center: Nursing care plans: nursing diagnosis and intervention, edited by M. Gulanick, A. Klopp, and S. Galanes, St. Louis, 1986, The C.V. Mosby Co.

Michaels, R.M., editor: Cardiac damage following radiotherapy for Hodgkin's disease, Am. J. Nurs. **5:**650, 1984.

Millar, S., editor: Taking action against reaction, Nursing '86, **3:**94, 1986; from AACN procedure manual for critical care, Philadelphia, 1985, W.B. Saunders Co.

Montefusco, C.M., Goldsmith, J., and Veith, F.J.: Cyclosporine immunosuppression in organ graft recipients: nursing implications, Crit. Care Nurse 3/4:117, 1984.

North American Nursing Diagnosis Association (NANDA) Classification of Nursing Diagnoses: proceedings of the sixth conference, edited by M.E. Hurley, St. Louis, 1986, The C.V. Mosby Co.

Nuscher, R., et al.: Bone marrow transplantation, Am. J. Nurs. **6:**764, 1984.

Potter, O.D., editor: Emergencies, Nurses Reference Library, Springhouse, Pa., 1985, Springhouse Corp.

Ptachcinski, R.: Sandimmune (cyclosporine) development and trials: symposium, 1983, Sandoz, Inc.

Querin, J.J., and Stable, L.D.: 12 simple sensible steps for successful blood transfusion, Nursing '83 **11:**34, 1983.

Rahr, V.: Giving intrathecal drugs, Am. J. Nurs. **7:**829, 1986.

Rice, H.V.: Acute blood-loss anemia, Nursing '83, **6:**162, 1983.

Roy, Sr.C.: Introduction to nursing: an adaptation model, Englewood Cliffs, N.J., 1984, Prentice-Hall, Inc.

Sauter, G., et al.: Acute myelogenous leukemia: maintenance therapy after early consolidation treatment does not prolong survival, Lancet **1:**379, 1984.

Smith, L.G.: Reactions to blood transfusions, Am. J. Nurs. **9:**1096, 1984.

Swearingen, P.L.: Manual of nursing therapeutics: applying nursing diagnoses to medical disorders, Menlo Park, Calif., 1986, Addison-Wesley Publishing Co., Inc.

Taylor, D.L.: Immune response: physiology, signs and symptoms, Nursing '84, **5:**52, 1984.

Thompson, J.M., et al.: Clinical nursing, St. Louis, 1986, The C.V. Mosby Co.

Ulrich, C., Canale, S., and Wendell, S.: Nursing care planning guides: a nursing diagnosis approach, Philadelphia, 1986, W.B. Saunders Co.

Williams, L.: Hemapheresis procedures: textbook of hematology, ed. 3, New York, 1983, McGraw-Hill Book Co.

Wintrobe, M.M., et al.: Clinical hematology, ed. 8, Philadelphia, 1981, Lea & Febiger.

Young, M.S., and Lucas, C.M.: Nursing diagnosis: common problems in implementation, Top. Clin. Nurs. **1:**68, 1984.

RESPIRATORY SYSTEM

Abels, L.: Critical care nursing: a physiologic approach, St. Louis, 1986, The C.V. Mosby Co.

Berte, J.: Critical care: the lung, ed. 2, East Norwalk, Conn., 1986, Appleton-Century-Crofts.

Brenner, B.: Comprehensive management of respiratory emergencies, Rockville, Md., 1985, Aspen Publishers, Inc.

Clayton, B., Stock, Y., and Squire, V.: Squire's basic pharmacology for nurses, ed. 8, St. Louis, 1985, The C.V. Mosby Co.

Davido, J.: Pulmonary rehabilitation, Nurs. Clin. North Am. **16**(2):275, 1981.

Farzan, S.: A concise handbook of respiratory diseases, Reston, Va., 1985, Reston Publishing Co., Inc.

Halloway, N.M.: Nursing the critically ill adult, Menlo Park, Calif., 1980, Addison-Wesley Publishing Co., Inc.

Hodgkin, J., Zorn, E., and Connors, G.: Pulmonary rehabilitation: guidelines to success, Boston, 1984, Butterworth Publishers.

Kenner, C.V., Guzzetta, C.E., and Dossey, B.M.: Critical care nursing: body-mind-spirit, Boston, 1985, Little, Brown & Co., Inc.

Kim, M.J., McFarland, G.K., and McLane, A.M.: Pocket guide to nursing diagnoses, ed. 2, St. Louis, 1987, The C.V. Mosby Co.

Lehrer, S.: Understanding lung sounds, Philadelphia, 1984, W.B. Saunders Co.

Luckmann, J., and Sorensen, K.: Medical-surgical nursing, ed. 3, Philadelphia, 1987, W.B. Saunders Co.

McDonald, G.: Symposium on respiratory care: a home care program for patients with chronic lung disease, Nurs. Clin. North Am. **16:**259, 1981.

Murray, J.: The normal lung: the basis for diagnosis and treatment of pulmonary diseases, ed. 2, Philadelphia, 1986, W.B. Saunders Co.

Op'T Holt, T.: Assessment-based respiratory care, New York, 1986, John Wiley & Sons, Inc.

Perry, A.G., et al.: Shock: comprehensive nursing management, St. Louis, 1983, The C.V. Mosby Co.

Peterson, G.: Symposium on respiratory care: application and assessment of oxygen therapy, Nurs. Clin. North Am. **16:**241, 1981.

Robinson, S., and Russo, R., editors: Providing respiratory care, Nursing '83, 1983.

Sweetwood, H.: Nursing in the intensive respiratory care unit, New York, 1979, Springer Publishing Co., Inc.

Tisi, G.: Pulmonary physiology in clinical medicine, ed. 2, Baltimore, 1985, Williams & Wilkins.

Ulrich, S., Canale, S., and Wendell, S.: Nursing care planning guides, Philadelphia, 1986, W.B. Saunders Co.

Wade, J.: Comprehensive respiratory care, ed. 3, St. Louis, 1983, The C.V. Mosby Co.

Weinberger, S.: Principles of pulmonary medicine, Philadelphia, 1986, W.B. Saunders Co.

Wilkins, R., Shelden, R., and Krider, S.: Clinical assessment in respiratory care, St. Louis, 1985, The C.V. Mosby Co.

Zschoche, D., editor: Mosby's comprehensive review of critical care, ed. 3, St. Louis, 1986, The C.V. Mosby Co.

NEUROLOGIC SYSTEM

Adams, H.P.: Current status of antifibrinolytic therapy for treatment of patients with aneurysmal subarachnoid hemorrhage, Curr. Concepts Cerebrovasc. Dis. **16**(5):23, 1981.

Aita, J.F.: Why patients with Parkinson's disease fall, JAMA **247**(4):515, 1982.

Alter, M.: Amyotrophic lateral sclerosis, Med. Times **110**(10):42, 1982.

Barry, K., and Texerian, S.: The role of the nurse in the diagnostic classification and management of epileptic seizures, J. Neurosurg. Nurs. **15**(4):243, 1983.

Blount, M., Kinney, A.B., and Stove, M.: Plasma exchange in management of myasthenia gravis, Nurs. Clin. North Am. **14**(1):173, 1979.

Budassi, S., and Barber, J.: Mosby's manual of emergency care: practices and procedures, ed. 2, 1984, The C.V. Mosby Co.

Campbell, V.G.: Neurological system. In Thompson, J.M., et al.: Clinical nursing, St. Louis, 1986, The C.V. Mosby Co.

Campion, H.R., et al.: Trauma scare, Crit. Care Med. **9**(9):672, 1981.

Conway, B.L.: Carini and Owens' neurological and neurosurgical nursing, ed. 8, St. Louis, 1982, The C.V. Mosby Co.

Cuddy, P.G.: Management of acute opioid intoxication, CCQ **4:**65, 1982.

Dau, P.C., et al.: Plasmapheresis and immunosuppressive drug therapy in myasthenia gravis, N. Engl. J. Med. **297**(21):1134, 1977.

Davis, J., and Niason, C.: Neurologic critical care, New York, 1979, Van Nostrand Reinhold Co., Inc.

Department of Health, Education and Welfare: Guidelines for stroke care, Washington, D.C., 1976, U.S. Government Printing Office.

Essentials of the neurological examination, Philadelphia, 1974, Smith Kline & French.

Goodman, G.: The pharmacological basis of therapeutics, ed. 7, 1985, MacMillan Publishing Co.

Hart, R.G., and Sherman, D.G.: The diagnosis of multiple sclerosis, JAMA **247**(4):498, 1982.

Hickey, F.: The clinical practice of neurological and neurosurgical nursing, ed. 2, Philadelphia, 1986, J.B. Lippincott Co.

Johanson, B.C., et al.: Standards for critical care, St. Louis, ed. 2, 1985, The C.V. Mosby Co.

Knoben, J.E., Anderson, P.O., and Watanabe, A.S.: Handbook of clinical drug data, ed. 4, Hamilton, Ill., Drug Intelligence Publication.

Krenzel, J.R., and Rohrer, L.M.: Handbook of care of paraplegic and quadriplegic individuals, Chicago, 1972, National Association of Paraplegia and Quadriplegia.

Krenzelok, E.P.: Phencyclidine—a contemporary drug of abuse, CCQ **4:**55, 1982.

Krupp, M.A.: Current medical diagnosis and treatment, Los Altos, Calif., 1981, Lange Medical Publications.

Lewis, S.M., and Collier, I.C.: Medical surgical nursing: assessment and management of clinical problems, New York, 1983, McGraw-Hill Book Co.

Mauss, N., and Mitchel, P.: Increased intracranial pressure, an update, Heart Lung **5:**919, 1976.

Mosby's medical and nursing dictionary, ed. 2, St. Louis, 1986, The C.V. Mosby Co.

Myasthenia gravis: a manual for physicians, New York, 1971, Myasthenia Gravis Foundation.

Nikas, D., and Konkoly, L.: Nursing responsibilities in arterial and intracranial pressure monitoring, J. Neurosurg. Nurs. **7:**116, 1975.

Nursing the multiple sclerosis patient, Chicago, 1969, National Multiple Sclerosis Society.

Phipps, W.J., Long, B.C., and Woods, N.F.: Medical-surgical nursing: concepts and clinical practice, ed. 3, St. Louis, 1986, The C.V. Mosby Co.

Purchase, G.: Neuromedical, neurosurgical nursing, London, 1977, Baillière Tindall.

Redelman, K., editor: Neurological injuries, CCQ **2**(1), 1979.

Ricci, M.: Educational core curriculum for neuroscience nursing, vol. 2, ed. 2, Park Ridge, Ill., 1984, American Association of Neuroscience Nurses.

Richmond, T.S., editor: Neurotrauma, Nurs. Clin. North Am. **21**(4):549, 1986.

Rimel, R., John, J., and Edlich, R.F.: Assessment of recovery following head trauma. In Redelman, K., editor: Neurological injuries, CCQ **2**(1):97, 1979.

Snyder, M.: A guide to neurological and neurosurgical nursing, New York, 1983, John Wiley & Sons, Inc.

Taylor, J., and Ballenger, S.: Neurological dysfunction and nursing intervention, New York, 1980, McGraw-Hill Book Co.

Teasdale, G., and Jennett, B.: Assessment of coma and impaired consciousness: a practical scale, Lancet **2:**81, 1974.

Thompson, J.M., et al.: Clinical nursing, St. Louis, 1986, The C.V. Mosby Co.

Tongs, T.G.: "The alcohols" in poisonings and overdose, CCQ **1**(4), 1982.

Turner, M.: Intracranial hypertension. In Redelman, K., editor: Neurological injuries, CCQ **2**(1):67, 1979.

Tyson, G.W., et al.: Acute care of the spinal cord injured patient. In Neurological injuries, CCQ **2**(1):45, 1979.

Vogt, G., Miller, M., and Esluer, M.: Mosby's manual of neurological care, St. Louis, 1985, The C.V. Mosby Co.

Walton, Sir J.N.: Brain diseases of the nervous system, ed. 9, New York, 1985, Oxford University Press, Inc.

William, A.: Classification and diagnosis of epilepsy, Nurs. Clin. North Am. **9:**747, 1974.

Wing, S.: Cervical spine injuries: treatment and related nursing care, J. Neurosurg. Nurs. **9:**138, 1977.

DIGESTIVE SYSTEM

Baker, W.L.: Hypophosphatemia, Am. J. Nurs. **85**(9):999, 1985.

Biblehimer, H.L.: Dealing with a wound that drains 1.5 liters a day, RN **49**(8):21, 1986.

Boarini, J.: The ostomy: what can go wrong? Am. J. Nurs. **85**(12):1358, 1985.

Brozenec, S.: Caring for the postoperative patient with an abdominal drain, Nursing '85 **15**(4):55, 1985.

Cargile, N.D.: Buying time when you face a bowel obstruction, RN **48**(8):40, 1985.

Carolan, J.: Clearing up gastric suction setbacks, RN **48**(6):38, 1985.

Carpenito, L.J., et al.: Nursing diagnosis: application to clinical practice, ed. 2, Philadelphia, 1987, J.B. Lippincott Co.

Casedonte, L.B.: The patient with a fistula, a colostomy, and an ileal conduit, RN **47**(9):42, 1984.

Decker, S.I.: The life-threatening consequences of a GI bleed, RN **48**(10):18, 1985.

DiCicco-Bloom, B., et al.: The homebound alcoholic, Am. J. Nurs. **86**(2):167, 1986.

Dodd, R.P.: Ascites: when the liver can't cope, RN **47**(10):26, 1984.

Doenges, M.E., Jeffries, M., and Moorhouse, M.: Nursing care plans: Nursing diagnoses in planning patient care, Philadelphia, 1984, F.A. Davis Co.

Dolinger, R.: How radiation complicates stoma care, RN **49**(9):32, 1986.

Doyle, J.T.: "You swallowed your what!" RN **48**(7):40, 1985.

Given, B.S., and Simmons, S.J.: Gastroenterology in nursing, ed. 4, St. Louis, 1984, The C.V. Mosby Co.

Greifzu, S.: Colorectal cancer: when a polyp is more than a polyp, RN **49**(9):23, 1986.

Jermier, B.J., and Treloar, D.M.: Bringing your patient through gallbladder surgery, RN **49**(11):18, 1986.

Johanson, B.C., et al.: Standards for critical care, ed. 2, St. Louis, 1985, The C.V. Mosby Co.

Jones, S.: Simpler and safer tube-feeding techniques, RN **47**(10):40, 1984.

Kearns, P.C.: Exercises to ease pain after abdominal surgery, RN **49**(7):45, 1986.

Kim, M.J., McFarland, G.K., and McLane, A.M.: Pocket guide to nursing diagnoses, ed. 2, St. Louis, 1987, The C.V. Mosby Co.

King, R.C.: Dealing with poisonings, RN **47**(12):45, 1984.

LaSala, C.: Transhepatic biliary decompression catheter, Nursing '85 **15**(2):53, 1985.

The Merck manual, ed. 14, Rahway, N.J., 1983, Merck, Sharp, & Dohne Research Laboratories.
Michael Reese Hospital and Medical Center: Nursing care plans: nursing diagnosis and intervention, edited by M. Gulanick, A. Klopp, and S. Galanes, St. Louis, 1986, The C.V. Mosby Co.
Montanari, J.: Documenting your postop assessment findings, Nursing '85 **15**(8):31, 1985.
Nemer, F.D., and Rolstad, B.S.: The role of the ileoanal reservoir in patients with ulcerative colitis and familial polyposis, J. Enterostom. Ther. **12**(3):74, 1985.
Neuberger, G.B., and Reckling, J.B.: A new look at wound care, Nursing '85 **15**(2):34, 1985.
Nichols, R.R.: Simple remedies for postop gas pain, RN **49**(2):42, 1986.
Penninger, J.I., et al.: After the ostomy: helping the patient reclaim his sexuality, RN **48**(4):46, 1985.
Peternel, E.: A high-tech approach to a GI problem, RN **48**(6):44, 1985.
Schaefer, K.M.: Easing the torment of an irritable bowel, RN **49**(4):34, 1986.
Thompson, J.M., et al.: Clinical nursing, St. Louis, 1986, The C.V. Mosby Co.
Vargo, J.: Viral hepatitis: how to protect patients—and yourself, RN **47**(7):22, 1984.

ENDOCRINE SYSTEM

American Diabetes Association: Foot care for the diabetic, Southern California Affiliate, Inc., American Diabetes Association, 1982.
Andreoli, J., et al., editors: Cecil essentials of medicine, Philadelphia, 1986, W.B. Saunders Co.
Diabetic teaching manual, Los Angeles, 1981, rev. ed., 1987, Southern California Kaiser Permanente Medical Center.
Gordon, M.: Nursing diagnosis: process and application, New York, 1987, McGraw-Hill Book Co.
Guthrie, D.W., and Guthrie, R.A.: Nursing management of diabetes mellitus, ed. 2, St. Louis, 1982, The C.V. Mosby Co.
Hardy, J.: Hardy's textbook of surgery, Philadelphia, 1983, J.B. Lippincott Co.
Honigman, R.E.: Thyroid function tests, Nursing '82, **12**:68, April 1982.
Jones, D., Dunbar, C., and Jirovec, M.: Medical-surgical nursing, New York, 1982, McGraw-Hill Book Co.
Jones, S.G.: Adrenal patient: proceed with caution, RN **45**(1):67, 1982.
Jones, S.G.: Bilateral adrenalectomy: postop dangers to watch for, RN **45**(3):66, 1982.
Jones, S.G.: Kid-glove care in pheocromocytoma, RN **45**(2):67, 1982.
Martyn, P.A.: If you guessed cardiovascular disease, guess again, Am. J. Nurs. **82**(8):1238, 1982.
Nemchik, R.: A very different diet: a new generation of oral drugs, RN **45**(11):41, 1981.
Potter, D.O., editorial director: The nurses reference library assessment, Springhouse, Pa., 1982, Intermed Communications, Inc.
Thompson, J., et al.: Clinical nursing, St. Louis, 1986, The C.V. Mosby Co.
Ulrich, S., Canale, S., and Wendell, S.: Nursing care planning guides: a nursing diagnosis approach, Philadelphia, 1986, W.B. Saunders Co.
Williams, R.H., editor: Textbook of endocrinology, Philadelphia, 1981, W.B. Saunders Co.

MUSCULOSKELETAL SYSTEM

Beil, A.V.: Osteoporosis: how to avoid its crippling effects, RN **49**(8):14, 1986.
Bourne, B.A., and Kutcher, J.L.: Amputation: helping a patient face the loss of a limb, RN **48**(2):38, 1985.
Campbell, E.B., and others: After the fall—confusion, Am. J. Nurs. **86**(2):151, 1986.
Carpenito, L.J.: Nursing diagnosis, ed. 2, Philadelphia, 1987, J.B. Lippincott Co.
Doenges, M.E., Jeffries, M., and Moorhouse, M.: Nursing care plans: nursing diagnoses in planning patient care, Philadelphia, 1984, F.A. Davis Co.
Evers, J.A., and Werpachowski, D.: Dealing with fractures, RN **47**(11):53, 1984.
Farrell, J.: Illustrated guide to orthopedic nursing, ed. 2, Philadelphia, 1982, J.B. Lippincott Co.
Hennig, L.M., and Burrows, S.K.: Keeping up on arthritis meds, RN **49**(2):32, 1986.
Ingersoll, G., and others: Caring for the quadriplegic patient with ankylosing spondylitis, Nursing '85 **15**(10):45, 1985.
Kim, M.J., McFarland, G.K., and McLane, A.M.: Pocket guide to nursing diagnoses, ed. 2, St. Louis, 1987, The C.V. Mosby Co.
Maier, P.: Take the work out of range-of-motion exercises, RN **49**(9):46, 1986.
The Merck manual, ed. 14, Rahway, N.J., 1983, Merck, Sharp, & Dohne Research Laboratories.
Mims, B.C.: Back surgery: helping your patient get through it, RN **48**(5):27, 1985.
Orthopedic reference manual, Ann Arbor, Mich., 1984, Catherine McAuley Health Center.
Thompson, J.M., et al.: Clinical nursing, St. Louis, 1986, The C.V. Mosby Co.
Tompkins, J.S., and Brown, M.D.: Dissolving a lifetime of lower back pain with chemonucleolysis, Nursing '85 **15**(7):47, 1985.
Watts, V., et al.: When your patient has jaw surgery, RN **48**(10):44, 1985.

GENITOURINARY SYSTEM

Abels, L.: Critical care nursing: a physiologic approach, St. Louis, 1986, The C.V. Mosby Co.
Allen, A., and Gorman, S., editors: The post anesthesia review for certification, Richmond, Va., 1985, American Society of Post Anesthesia Nurses (ASPAN).
Carpenito, L.: Nursing diagnosis: application to clinical practice, ed. 2, Philadelphia, 1987, J.B. Lippincott Co.
Gerber, A.: The Kock continent ileal reservoir: an alternative to the conventional urostomy, J. Enterostom. Ther. **12**(1):15, 1985.
Gruendemann, B., and Huth-Meeker, M.: Alexander's care of the patient in surgery, ed. 8, St. Louis, 1987, The C.V. Mosby Co.
Lerner, J., and Khan, A.: Mosby's manual of urologic nursing, St. Louis, 1982, The C.V. Mosby Co.
Lippincott manual of nursing practice, ed. 4, Philadelphia, 1986, J.B. Lippincott Co.
Luckmann, J., and Sorensen, K.: Medical-surgical nursing, ed. 7, Philadelphia, 1984, J.B. Lippincott Co.
Nursing '81 books: Nursing photobook implementing urologic procedures, Springhouse, Pa., 1981, Intermed Communications, Inc.
Nursing '84 books: Nurses' clinical library: renal and urologic disorders, Springhouse, Pa., 1984, Springhouse Corp.
Pawlowski, J.: Percutaneous nephrolithotripsy—a nursing care plan, AORN J. **39**(5):779, 1984.

Puderbaugh-Ulrich, S., Weyland-Canale, S., and Wendell, S.: Nursing care planning guides: a nursing diagnosis approach, Philadelphia, 1986, W.B. Saunders Co.

Richard, C.: Comprehensive nephrology nursing, Boston, 1986, Little, Brown & Co., Inc.

Rogers-Kinney, M., et al.: AACN's clinical reference for critical-care nursing, New York, 1981, McGraw-Hill Book Co.

Short-Googe, M., and Mook, T.: The inflatable penile prosthesis: new developments, Am. J. Nurs., p. 1044, July 1983.

Swearingen, P., editor: Manual of nursing therapeutics applying nursing diagnoses to medical disorders, Reading, Mass., 1986, Addison-Wesley Publishing Co., Inc.

Thomas-Harwood, C.: Pulverizing kidney stones: what you should know about lithotripsy, RN, p. 32, July 1985.

Wyngaarden, J., and Smith, L., editors: Cecil textbook of medicine, ed. 17, Philadelphia, 1985, W.B. Saunders Co.

Young, M.: Lithotripsy: a revolutionary technique with implications for nursing care, J. Nephrol. Nurs. 3(1):34, 1986.

FEMALE REPRODUCTIVE SYSTEM

Carpenito, L.J., et al.: Nursing diagnosis: application to clinical practice, ed. 2, Philadelphia, 1987, J.B. Lippincott Co.

Coyne, C.M., Woods, N.F., and Mitchell, E.S.: Premenstrual tension syndrome, JOGNN 14(6):446, 1985.

Fogel, C.I., and Woods, N.F.: Health care of women: a nursing perspective, St. Louis, 1981, The C.V. Mosby Co.

Frank, E.P.: What are nurses doing to help PMS patients? Am. J. Nurs. 86(2):136, 1986.

Johanson, B.C., et al.: Standards for critical care, ed. 2, St. Louis, 1985, The C.V. Mosby Co.

Kim, M.J., McFarland, G.K., and McLane, A.M.: Pocket guide to nursing diagnoses, ed. 2, St. Louis, 1987, The C.V. Mosby Co.

Michael Reese Hospital and Medical Center: Nursing care plans: nursing diagnosis and intervention, edited by M. Gulanick, A. Klopp, and S. Galanes, St. Louis, 1986, The C.V. Mosby Co.

O'Laughlin, K.M.: Changes in bladder function in the woman undergoing radical hysterectomy for cervical cancer, JOGNN 15(5):380, 1986.

Thompson, J.M., et al.: Clinical nursing, St. Louis, 1986, The C.V. Mosby Co.

Ulrich, S., Canale, S., and Wendell, S.: Nursing care planning guides: a nursing diagnosis approach, Philadelphia, 1986, W.B. Saunders Co.

INTEGUMENTARY SYSTEM

Doenges, M.E., Jeffries, M., and Moorhouse, M.: Nursing care plans: nursing diagnoses in planning patient care, Philadelphia, 1984, F.A. Davis Co.

Carpentino, L.J.: Nursing diagnosis, ed. 2, Philadelphia, 1987, J.B. Lippincott Co.

Kim, M.J., McFarland, G.K., and McLane, A.M.: Pocket guide to nursing diagnoses, ed. 2, St. Louis, 1987, The C.V. Mosby Co.

Thompson, J.M., et al.: Clinical nursing, St. Louis, 1986, The C.V. Mosby Co.

OPTIC AND AUDITORY SYSTEMS

Campbell, S.L.: Some sound advice for managing a hearing-impaired patient, Nursing '84 14(12):46, 1984.

Carden, R.G.: The ins and outs of contact lenses, RN 48(2):48, 1985.

Carpenito, L.J., et al.: Nursing diagnosis: application to clinical practice, ed. 2, Philadelphia, 1987, J.B. Lippincott Co.

Doenges, M.E., Jeffries, M., and Moorhouse, M.: Nursing care plans: nursing diagnoses in planning patient care, Philadelphia, 1984, F.A. Davis Co.

Kim, M.J., McFarland, G.K., and McLane, A.M.: Pocket guide to nursing diagnoses, ed. 2, St. Louis, 1987, The C.V. Mosby Co.

Lent-Wunderlich, E., and Ott, M.J.: Helping your patient through eye surgery, RN 49(6):43, 1986.

The Merck mannual, ed. 14, Rahway, N.J., 1983, Merck, Sharp, & Dohne Laboratories.

Michael Reese Hospital and Medical Center: Nursing care plans: nursing diagnosis and intervention, edited by M. Gulanick, A. Klopp, and S. Galanes, St. Louis, 1986, The C.V. Mosby Co.

Radocy, L.: What lasers can do for your glaucoma patient, RN 48(10):28, 1985.

Thompson, J.M., et al.: Clinical nursing, St. Louis, 1986, The C.V. Mosby Co.

Tooke, M.C., et al.: Corneal transplantation, Am. J. Nurs. 86(6):685, 1986.

ONCOLOGY

Aveilanet, C.: Cancer prevention: cancer risk factors, Cancer Nurs. 5:295, 1982.

Beck, S.: Impact of a systematic oral care protocol on stomatitis after chemotherapy, Cancer Nurs. 2:185, 1979.

Becker, T.M.: Cancer chemotherapy: a manual for nurses, Boston, 1981, Little, Brown & Co., Inc.

Bouchard-Kurtz, R., and Speese-Owens, N.: Nursing care of the cancer patient, ed. 4, St. Louis, 1981, The C.V. Mosby Co.

Cancer chemotherapy guidelines and recommendations for nursing education and practice, Pittsburgh, 1984, Oncology Nursing Society.

A cancer source for nurses, New York, 1981, American Cancer Society.

Carter, S., Gladstein, E., and Livingson, R.B., editors: Principles of cancer treatment, New York, 1982, McGraw Hill Book Co.

Chemotherapy and you: a guide to self-help during treatment, Bethesda, Md., 1981, U.S. Department of Health and Human Services, Public Health Service.

Cornelius, J.: Screening for head and neck cancers, Nurs. Pract. 4:14, 1979.

DeVita, V.T., Hellman, S., and Rosenberg, S.A.: Cancer principles and practice of oncology, Philadelphia, 1982, J.B. Lippincott Co.

Dodd, M.J.: Cancer patients' knowledge of chemotherapy: assessment and informational intervention, Oncol. Nurs. Forum 9:39, 1982.

Dodd, M.J.: Suggestions for managing the side effects of chemotherapy, East Norwalk, Conn., Appleton & Lange. (In press.)

Donovan, M.I., and Pierce, S.: Cancer care: A guide for patient education, New York, 1981, Appleton-Century-Crofts.

Dorr, R.T., and Fritz, W.L.: Cancer chemotherapy handbook, New York, 1980, Elsevier Science Publishing Co., Inc.

Eating hints: recipes and tips for better nutrition during cancer treatment, Bethesda, Md., 1982, U.S. Department of Health and Human Services, National Institutes of Health.

Eddy, D.M.: Appropriateness of cervical cancer screening, Gynecol. Oncol. 12:188, 1981.

For men only: testicular self-exam, New York, 1984, American Cancer Society.

Frank-Stromborg, M.: Nursing's contribution to case finding and the early detection of cancer. In Marino, L.B., editor: Cancer nursing, St. Louis, 1981, The C.V. Mosby Co.

A guide to proper nutrition for the patient undergoing cancer therapy, Evansville, Ind., 1979, Mead Johnson & Co.

Guidelines for the cancer related check-up: recommendation and rationale, New York, 1980, American Cancer Society.

Leahy, I.M., St. German, J.M., and Varricehio, C.G.: The nurse and radiotherapy: a manual for daily use, St. Louis, 1979, The C.V. Mosby Co.

Leffall, L.D., and Stearns, M.W.: Early diagnosis of colorectal cancer, pamphlet 3311, New York, 1974, American Cancer Society.

Manual for staging of cancer, Philadelphia, 1983, J.B. Lippincott Co.

Marino, L.B., Cancer nursing, St. Louis, 1981, The C.V. Mosby Co.

Nunnally, C.: Taste alteration. In Yasko, J., editor: Guidelines for cancer care: symptom management, Reston, Va., 1983, Reston Publishing Co.

Outcome standards for cancer nursing education, fundamental level, New York, 1982, Oncology Nursing Society (ONS) Education Committee.

Outcome standards for cancer nursing practice, New York, 1979, ONS and ANA Division of Medical Surgical Nursing Practice.

Outcome standards for cancer patient education, New York, 1982, ONS Education Committee.

Outcome standards for public cancer education, New York, 1983, ONS Education Committee.

Pilapil, F., and Studva, K.V., editors: Programmed instruction: understanding cancer and chemotherapy, New York, 1979, Masson Publishing USA, Inc.

Pizzo, P., and Young, R.: Management of the infections of the cancer patient. In DeVita, V.T., editor: Cancer principles and practices of oncology, Philadelphia, 1982, J.B. Lippincott Co.

Research report: cancer of the lung, Bethesda, Md., Aug. 1980, National Cancer Institute.

The University of Rochester School of Medicine and Dentistry: Clinical oncology for medical students and physicians: a multidisciplinary approach, Rochester, N.Y., 1978, American Cancer Society.

Vredevoe, D.L., et al.: Concepts of oncology nursing, Englewood Cliffs, N.J., 1981, Prentice-Hall, Inc.

Yasko, J.M., editor: Bone marrow depression related to treatment with chemotherapy, 1983, Adria Laboratories, Inc.

Yasko, J.M., editor: Cutaneous manifestations related to treatment with chemotherapy, 1983, Adria Laboratories, Inc.

Yasko, J.M., editor: Gastrointestinal manifestations related to treatment with chemotherapy, 1983, Adria Laboratories, Inc.

Yasko, J., and Nunnally, C.: Infection. In Yasko, J., editor: Guidelines for cancer care: symptom management, Reston, Va., 1983, Reston Publishing Co.

PERINATAL/NEONATAL

American Academy of Pediatrics/American College of Obstetricians and Gynecologists (AAP/ACOG): Guidelines for perinatal care, Washington, D.C., 1983.

Cloherty, J., and Stark, A.: Manual of neonatal care, Boston, 1983, Little, Brown & Co., Inc.

Cole, C.: The Harriet Lane handbook, ed. 10, Chicago, 1984, Year Book Medical Publishers, Inc.

Cropley, C., and Bloom, R.: Neonatal resuscitation, Los Angeles, 1986, Charles R. Drew Postgraduate Medical School.

Doenges, M., Jeffries, M., and Moorhouse, M.: Nursing care plans: nursing diagnoses in planning patient care, Philadelphia, 1984, F.A. Davis Co.

Fletcher, M., MacDonald, M., and Avery, G.: Atlas of procedures in neonatology, Philadelphia, 1983, J.B. Lippincott Co.

Frantz, K.: Managing nipple problems, reprint No. 11, Oak Park, Ill., 1982, La Leche League International.

Freeman, R., and Garite, T.: Fetal heart rate monitoring, Baltimore, 1981, Williams & Wilkins.

Friedman, M.: Family nursing, New York, 1986, Appleton-Century-Crofts.

Gordon, M.: Manual of nursing diagnosis, New York, 1987, McGraw-Hill Book Co.

A guide to successful breastfeeding, Los Angeles, 1986, Southern California Kaiser Permanente Medical Centers.

Jensen, M.D., and Bobak, I.M.: Maternity and gynecologic care, ed. 3, St. Louis, 1985, The C.V. Mosby Co.

Klaus, M., and Fanaroff, A.: Care of the high-risk neonate, ed. 2, Philadelphia, 1979, W.B. Saunders Co.

Oxorn, H.: Human labor and birth, ed. 5, East Norwalk, Conn., 1986, Appleton-Century-Crofts.

Perinatal Advisory Council of Los Angeles Communities: Neonatal protocols, Los Angeles, 1986, The Council.

Perinatal Advisory Council of Los Angeles Communities: Prenatal and intrapartum protocols, Los Angeles, 1986, The Council.

Queenan, J., and Hobbins, J.: Protocols for high-risk pregnancies, Oradell, N.J., 1983, Medical Economics Books.

Rivlin, M., Morrison, J., and Bates, G.: Manual of clinical problems in obstetrics and gynecology, Boston, 1984, Little, Brown & Co., Inc.

PEDIATRICS

Carpenito, L.J.: Handbook of nursing diagnosis, ed. 2, Philadelphia, 1987, J.B. Lippincott Co.

Curley, M.A.Q.: Pediatric cardiac dysrhythmias, Bowie, Md., 1985, Brady Communications Co., Inc.

Finberg, L., et al.: Oral rehydration for diarrhea, J. Pediatr. 101(4):497, 1982.

Fried, E.: Acute epiglottitis, Issues Compr. Pediatr. Nurs. 4:29, 1980.

Larter, N.: Cystic fibrosis, Am. J. Nurs., p. 527, March 1981.

Rifas, E.: Teaching patients to manage acute asthma, Nursing '83, p. 77, April 1983.

Simkins, R.: Croup and epiglottitis, Am. J. Nurs., p. 527, March 1981.

Smith, J.B.: Pediatric critical care, New York, 1983, John Wiley & Sons, Inc.

Waskerwitz, M.: Special nursing care for children receiving chemotherapy, J. Assoc. Pediatr. Oncol. Nurses 1(1):16, 1984.

Waskerwitz, M., and Ruccione, K.: An overview of cancer in children in the 1980's, Nurs. Clin. North Am. 20(1), 1985.

Whaley, L.F., and Wong, D.L.: Essentials of pediatric nursing, St. Louis, 1985, The C.V. Mosby Co.

Appendix A

Medical-Surgical Care

Mass Equivalents for Medications (Metric and Apothecary System)

Apothecary (grains)	Metric (mg)	Metric (g)
1/200	0.3	0.0003
1/150	0.4	0.0004
1/100	0.6	0.0006
1/60	1	0.001
1/30	2	0.002
1/20	3	0.003
1/15	4	0.004
1/10	6	0.006
1/8	8	0.008
1/6	10	0.010
1/4	15	0.015
1/3	20	0.020
1/2*	30	0.030
3/4	50	0.050
1	60	0.060
1½	100	0.100
2	120	0.12
2½	150	0.15
3	200	0.2
4	250	0.25
5	300	0.3
7½	500	0.5
10	600	0.6
15	1000	1.0
30	2000	2.0

*From ½ to 5 grains the following more accurate "approximate equivalents" are also acceptable.

¼ grain = 16 mg	2½ grains = 160 mg
½ grain = 32 mg	3 grains = 200 mg
1 grain = 65 mg	4 grains = 260 mg
1½ grains = 100 mg	5 grains = 325 mg
2 grains = 130 mg	

Liquid Equivalent for Medication

Apothecary and customary*	Metric (ml)
1 minim	0.06
5 minims	0.3
10 minims	0.6
15 minims	1
60 minims (1 fluid dram or 1/8 fl oz)	4
75 minims (1¼ fluid drams)	5.0
240 minims (4 fluid drams or ½ fl oz)	15
1 fl oz	30
2 fl oz	60
3 fl oz	90
4 fl oz	120
6 fl oz	180
8 fl oz	240
12 fl oz	360
16 fl oz (1 pt)	480
32 fl oz (1 qt)	960
35 fl oz	1000 (1 L)
64 fl oz	1825
128 fl oz (1 gal)	3650

*Minims, fluid drams, or fl oz.

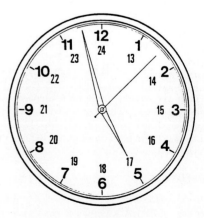

24 hr clock.

METRIC CONVERSIONS*

LENGTH

1 inch (in)	= 2.5 centimeters (cm)
1 foot (ft)	= 30 cm
1 yard (yd)	= 0.9 meters (m)
1 mile	= 1.6 kilometers (km)

MASS (WEIGHT)

1 ounze (oz)	= 28 grams (g)
1 pound (lb)	= 0.45 kilogram (kg)
1 short ton (2000 lb)	= 0.9 tonne

VOLUME

1 teaspoon (tsp)	= 5 milliliters (ml)
1 tablespoon (tbsp)	= 15 ml
1 fluid ounce (fl oz)	= 30 ml
1 cup	= 0.24 liters (L)
1 pint (pt)	= 0.47 L
1 quart (qt)	= 0.95 L
1 gallon (gal)	= 3.8 L

*Appropriate conversions to metric measures.

24 Hr Clock System

Conventional 12 hr time	24 hr clock time
12 midnight	0000
12:01 AM	0001
1:00 AM	0100
1:30 AM	0130
2:00 AM	0200
3:00 AM	0300
4:00 AM	0400
5:00 AM	0500
6:00 AM	0600
7:00 AM	0700
8:00 AM	0800
9:00 AM	0900
10:00 AM	1000
11:00 AM	1100
12 noon	1200
1:00 PM	1300
2:00 PM	1400
3:00 PM	1500
4:00 PM	1600
5:00 PM	1700
6:00 PM	1800
7:00 PM	1900
8:00 PM	2000
9:00 PM	2100
10:00 PM	2200
11:00 PM	2300
	2400

Linear Equivalents

Inches	Centimeters (cm)	Meters (m)
0.5	1.25	0.0125
1	2.5	0.025
2	5.1	0.051
3	7.6	0.076
4	10.2	0.10
5	12.7	0.13
6	15.2	0.15
7	17.8	0.18
8	20.8	0.20
9	23.0	0.23
10	25.4	0.25
12	30.5	0.30
18	45.7	0.46
24	61.0	0.61
30	76.2	0.76
36	91.4	0.91
42	106.7	1.07
48	121.9	1.22
54	137.2	1.37
60	152.4	1.52
66	167.6	1.63
72	182.9	1.83

Centigrade-Fahrenheit Equivalents*

Centigrade (C)	Fahrenheit (F)
36.0	96.8
36.5	97.7
37.0	98.6
37.5	99.5
38.0	100.4
38.5	101.3
39.0	102.2
39.5	103.2
40.0	104.0
40.5	104.9
41.0	105.8
41.5	106.7
42.0	107.6

*CONVERSION
F to C: subtract 32, then multiply by 5/9.
C to F: multiply by 9/5, then add 32.

Kidney Function Test

Laboratory test	Normal value
Acetone	Negative
Albumin (random)	Negative
Amylase	35-260 Somogyi U/hr
Bilirubin (random)	Negative
Blood (occult)	Negative
Creatinine	0.8-2.0 g/24 hr
Glucose (random)	Negative
pH	4.6-8.0
Sodium	80-180 mEq/24 hr
Specific gravity	1.010-1.025
Urea nitrogen	6-17 g/24 hr

Normal Hematology Laboratory Values

Laboratory test	Normal value
Coagulation studies	
Bleeding time (Duke)	1-3 min
Clotting time	3-9 min
Factor V	75%-125%
Factor VIII	50%-200%
Fibrinogen	200-400 mg/100 ml
Partial thromboplastin time (PTT)	20-45 sec
Prothrombin time (PT)	12-15 sec (>25%)
Erythrocyte sedimentation rate	0-20 mm/hr
Complete blood count (CBC)	
Hematocrit (Hct)	
Males	40%-54%
Females	38%-47%
Hemoglobin (Hgb)	
Males	13.5-18.0 g/100 ml
Females	12.0-16.0 g/100 ml
Red blood cells	
Males	4.8-5.5 mil/mm^3
Females	4.4-5.0 mil/mm^3
White blood cells	5000-10,000/mm^3
Erythrocyte indices	
Mean corpuscular Hgb (MCH)	29-32 pg
Mean corpuscular Hgb concentration (MCHC)	30-36 g/100 ml packed cells
Mean corpuscular volume (MCV)	82-96 μ^3
Platelet count	150,000-300,000/mm^3

Normal Chemistry Laboratory Values (Serum, Plasma, Whole Blood)

Laboratory test	Normal value
Amylase	60-160 Somogyi U/100 ml
Bicarbonate	21-28 mmol/L
Bilirubin	
Total	0.2-0.8 mg/100 ml
Direct	0-0.3 mg/100 ml
Blood gases	
pH	7.38-7.44 mm Hg
PCO_2 (arterial)	35-45 mm Hg
PO_2 (arterial)	95-100 mm Hg
Blood urea nitrogen (BUN)	7-15 mg/100 ml
Calcium	5-6 mEq/L
Chloride	98-106 mEq/L
Creatinine phosphokinase (CPK)	
Males	55-170 U/L
Females	30-135 U/L
Creatinine	0.4-1.2 mg/100 ml
C-reactive protein (CRP)	<1+
Glucose (fasting)	60-90 mg/100 ml
Iron	65-150 μg/100 ml
Iron-binding capacity	250-450 μg/100 ml
Lactic acid (whole blood)	5-20 mg/100 ml
LE (lupus erythematosus) preparation	No cells present
Lactic dehydrogenase (LDH)	71-207 IU/L
Lipids	
Total	400-800 mg/100 ml
Cholesterol	150-250 mg/100 ml
Triglycerides	10-190 mg/100 ml
Phospholipids	150-380 mg/100 ml
Fatty acids	9.0-15.0 mmol/L
Magnesium	1.65-2.5 mEq/L
Parathyroid	163-347 pg/ml
pH	7.35-7.45
Phosphorus	2.5-4.8 mg/100 ml
Potassium	4.1-5.6 mEq/L
Protein	
Total	6.0-7.8 g/100 ml
Albumin	3.2-4.5 g/100 ml
Globulin	2.3-3.5 g/100 ml
Serum glutamic oxaloacetic transaminase (SGOT)	4-40 U/ml
Serum glutamic pyruvic transaminase (SGPT)	1-36 U/ml
Sodium	136-143 mEq/L
T_3 (resin uptake)	25%-38% relative uptake
Urea nitrogen (BUN)	8-18 mg/100 ml
Uric acid	2.1-7.8 mg/100 ml

Diabetic Food Replacement

Food	Amount	Total available glucose (g)	Amount orange juice or lemon-lime soft drink (oz)	Amount milk (oz)	Food	Amount	Total available glucose (g)	Amount orange juice or lemon-lime soft drink (oz)	Amount milk (oz)
Apple	1 whole	10	4	4½	Milk (regular)	1 cup	18	7	8
Apple juice	½ cup	10	4	4½	Milk (skim)	1 cup	17	7	8
Apricot	1 whole	10	4	4½	Mixed vegetables	120 g	8	3	3½
Beets	120 g	8	3	3½					
Bread	1 slice	16	6	7	Pea soup	1 bowl	25	10	11
Broth		0			Peach	½	10	4	4½
Butter	1 pat	4	1½	1½	Pears	1 small dish	10	4	4½
Carrots	120 g	8	3	3½					
Cereal (cold)	1 box	16	6	7	Peas	120 g	8	3	3½
Cereal (cooked)	½ cup	16	6	7	Peas and carrots	120 g	8	3	3½
Cheese	1 slice	4.5	2	2	Pineapple juice	½ cup	10	4	4½
Cherries	1 serving	10	4	4½	Plums	3	15	6	7
Corn	120 g	16	6	7	Flavored ice pop	1 whole	16	6	7
Cottage cheese	½ cup	9	3½	4	Potatoes	120 g	16	6	7
Egg	1	4.5	2	2	Prune juice	¼ cup	10	4	4½
Gelatin	65 g	16	6	7	Prunes	1 small dish	10	4	4½
Grape juice	¼ cup	10	4	4½					
Grapefruit juice	½ cup	10	4	4½	Rice	120 g	16	6	7
					Squash	120 g	8	3	3½
Macaroni	120 g	16	6	7	Sugar	1 pkg	4.2	1½	1½
Meat	60 g	9	3½	4	Sugar	1 tsp	4.2	1½	1½

Conversion Factors to SI Units for Some Biochemical Components of Blood*

Component	Normal range in units as customarily reported	Conversion factor	Normal range in SI units, molecular units, international units, or decimal fractions
Acetoacetic acid (S)	0.2-1.0 mg/dL	98	19.6-98.0 μmol/L
Acetone (S)	0.3-2.0 mg/dL	172	51.6-344.0 μmol/L
Albumin (S)	3.2-4.5 g/dL	10	32-45 g/L
Ammonia (P)	20-120 μg/dL	0.588	11.7-70.5 μmol/L
Amylase (S)	60-160 Somogyi units/dL	1.85	111-296 U/L
Base, total (S)	145-160 mEq/L	1	145-160 mmol/L
Bicarbonate (P)	21-28 mEq/L	1	21-28 mmol/L
Bile acids (S)	0.3-3.0 mg/dL	10	3-30 mg/L
		2.547	0.8-7.6 μmol/L
Bilirubin, direct (S)	Up to 0.3 mg/dL	17.1	Up to 5.1 μmol/L
Bilirubin, indirect (S)	0.1-1.0 mg/dL	17.1	1.7-17.1 μmol/L

*This is a selected (not a complete) list of biochemical components. The ranges listed may differ from those accepted in some laboratories and are shown to illustrate the conversion factor and the method of expression in SI molecular units.

Conversion Factors to SI Units for Some Biochemical Components of Blood*—cont'd

Component	Normal range in units as customarily reported	Conversion factor	Normal range in SI units, molecular units, international units, or decimal fractions
Blood gases (B)			
PCO_2 arterial	35-40 mm Hg	0.133	4.66-5.32 kPa
PO_2 arterial	95-100 mm Hg	0.133	12.64-13.30 kPa
Calcium (S)	8.5-10.5 mg/dL	0.25	2.1-2.6 mmol/L
Chloride (S)	95-103 mEq/L	1	95-103 mmol/L
Creatine (S)	0.1-0.4 mg/dL	76.3	7.6-30.5 µmol/L
Creatinine (S)	0.6-1.2 mg/dL	88.4	53-106 µmol/L
Creatinine clearance (P)	107-139 mL/min	0.0167	1.78-2.32 mL/s
Fatty acids (total) (S)	8-20 mg/dL	0.01	0.08-2.00 mg/L
Fibrinogen (P)	200-400 mg/dL	0.01	2.00-4.00 g/L
Gamma globulin (S)	0.5-1.6 g/dL	10	5-16 g/L
Globulins (total) (S)	2.3-3.5 g/dL	10	23-35 g/L
Glucose (fasting) (S)	70-110 mg/dL	0.055	3.85-6.05 mmol/L
Insulin (radioimmunoassay) (P)	4-24 µIU/mL	0.0417	0.17-1.00 µg/L
	0.20-0.84 µg/L	172.2	35-145 pmol/L
Iodine, BEI (S)	3.5-6.5 µg/dL	0.079	0.28-0.51 µmol/L
Iodine, PBI (S)	4.0-8.0 µg/dL	0.079	0.32-0.63 µmol/L
Iron, total (S)	60-150 µg/dL	0.179	11-27 µmol/L
Iron-binding capacity (S)	300-360 µg/dL	0.179	54-64 µmol/L
17-Ketosteroids (P)	25-125 µg/dL	0.01	0.25-1.25 mg/L
Lactic dehydrogenase (S)	80-120 units at 30° C	0.48	38-62 U/L at 30° C
	Lactate → pyruvate		
	100-190 U/L at 37° C	1	100-190 U/L at 37° C
Lipase (S)	0-1.5 U/mL (Cherry-Crandall)	278	0-417 U/L
Lipids (total) (S)	400-800 mg/dL	0.01	4.00-8.00 g/L
Cholesterol	150-250 mg/dL	0.026	3.9-6.5 mmol/L
Triglycerides	75-165 mg/dL	0.0114	0.85-1.89 mmol/L
Phospholipids	150-380 mg/dL	0.01	1.50-3.80 g/L
Free fatty acids	9.0-15.0 mM/L	1	9.0-15.0 mmol/L
Nonprotein nitrogen (S)	20-35 mg/dL	0.714	14.3-25.0 mmol/L
Phosphatase (P)			
Acid (units/dL)	Cherry-Crandall	2.77	0-5.5 U/L
	King-Armstrong	1.77	0-5.5 U/L
	Bodansky	5.37	0-5.5 U/L
Alkaline (units/dL)	King-Armstrong	1.77	30-120 U/L
	Bodansky	5.37	30-120 U/L
	Bessey-Lowry-Brock	16.67	30-120 U/L
Phosphorus, inorganic (S)	3.0-4.5 mg/dL	0.323	0.97-1.45 mmol/L
Potassium (P)	3.8-5.0 mEq/L	1	3.8-5.0 mmol/L
Proteins, total (S)	6.0-7.8 g/dL	10	60-78 g/L
Albumin	3.2-4.5 g/dL	10	32-45 g/L
Globulin	2.3-3.5 g/dL	10	23-35 g/L
Sodium (P)	136-142 mEq/L	1	136-142 mmol/L
Testosterone			
Males (S)	300-1,200 ng/dL	0.035	10.5-42.0 nmol/L
Females	39-95 ng/dL	0.035	1.0-3.3 nmol/L
Thyroid tests (S)			
Thyroxine (T_4)	4-11 µg/dL	12.87	51-142 nmol/L
T_4 expressed as iodine	3.2-7.2 µg/dL	79.0	253-569 nmol/L
T_3 resin uptake	25%-38% relative uptake	0.01	0.25%-0.38% relative uptake
TSH (S)	10 µU/mL	1	$<10^{-3}$ IU/L
Urea nitrogen (S)	8-23 mg/dL	0.357	2.9-8.2 mmol/L
Uric acid (S)	2-6 mg/dL	59.5	0.120-0.360 mmol/L
Vitamin B_{12} (S)	160-950 pg/mL	0.74	118-703 pmol/L

Some Hematology Values*

Component	Normal range in units as customarily reported	Conversion factor	Normal range in SI units, molecular units, international units, or decimal fractions
Red cell volume (male)	25-35 mL/kg body weight	0.001	0.025-0.035 L/kg body weight
Hematocrit	40%-50%	0.01	0.40-0.50
Hemoglobin	13.5-18.0 g/dL	10	135-180 g/L
Hemoglobin	13.5-18.0 g/dL	0.155	2.09-2.79 mmol/L
RBC count	$4.5\text{-}6 \times 10^6/\mu L$	1	$4.6\text{-}6 \times 10^{12}/L$
WBC count	$4.5\text{-}10 \times 10^3/\mu L$	1	$4.5\text{-}10 \times 10^9/L$
Mean corpuscular volume	80-96 μm^3	1	80-96 fL

*The International Committee for Standardization in Hematology recommends that the numbers remain the same but that the units change, so that hemoglobin is expressed as grams per deciliter (g/dL) even though other measurements are expressed as units per liter (U/L).

Equivalent Values of kPa and mm Hg Units

kPa	0.1	0.2	0.3	0.4	0.5	0.6	0.7	0.8	0.9
mm Hg	0.750	1.50	2.25	3.00	3.75	4.50	5.25	6.00	6.75

kPa	mm Hg	kPa	mm Hg
1	7.50	21	158
2	15.0	22	165
3	22.5	23	172
4	30.0	24	180
5	37.5	25	188
6	45.0	26	195
7	52.5	27	202
8	60.0	28	210
9	67.5	29	218
10	75.0	30	225
11	82.5	31	232
12	90.0	32	240
13	97.5	33	248
14	105	34	255
15	112	35	262
16	120	36	270
17	128	37	278
18	135	38	285
19	142	39	292
20	150	40	300

From World Health Organization: The SI for the health professions, Geneva, 1977, The Organization, p. 40.

APPENDIX B

Guidelines for Patient Care Planning

Patient Care Standards can be used to plan individualized, goal-directed nursing care through the use of the nursing process. In planning the patient's care, the nurse should mutually set goals with the patient and/or family. The goals should be realistic, measurable, and based on the nursing assessment. The plan of care should be made in conjunction with the prescribed medical care in order to restore, promote, or maintain the patient's well-being.

In order to ensure quality and appropriateness of care, it is imperative that any standard care plan be individualized to meet the patient's unique needs. Although the standards contained in this book include the nursing diagnoses, goals, and interventions one would most likely encounter in a given situation, it is expected that the nurse would individualize the plan by any number of methods, including but not limited to the following:

1. Noting the patient's name, other identification data, the date and time of initiation of the care plan, and adding the nurse's signature.
2. Crossing through or deleting those nursing diagnoses, goals, and interventions that are not appropriate and initialing same.
3. Adding nursing diagnoses, goals, and interventions that are appropriate, as well as the date initiated and the nurse's initials.
4. Evaluating the plan on a daily basis, penciling in the current date and the nurse's initials if the interventions are still applicable. This can be done in a "review" or "evaluation" column adjacent to the nursing interventions. This provides an accountability mechanism to ensure currency of the plan on a daily basis.
5. Discontinuing the part of the plan that is no longer appropriate because of achievement of patient-centered goals. This can be done in a "discontinued/resolved" column.

It is possible that a preprinted, standard care plan will meet the needs of some individuals without any changes. Therefore to demonstrate that the nurse has used the nursing process, it is important that the care plan be initiated, evaluated, and eventually discontinued by the nurse, who demonstrates accountability by dating and signing (or initialing) these items.

Documentation in the patient's record should reflect the plan of care by including nursing interventions and the patient's response to them. In addition, instructions given to the patient and/or family regarding postdischarge self-care should be documented, as well as their understanding of these instructions. A predischarge summary statement should include information about the patient's outcome, a guide for which can be found in the Evaluation sections included with most of the standards in this text.

In summary, the nurse should use the nursing process to assess, plan, intervene, and evaluate nursing care for the patient from admission through discharge from the hospital. The plan of care should be individualized to meet each patient's needs, and documentation of care should reflect the patient's status.

A sample patient case study, accompanied by an individualized patient care plan, is provided here for your review.

CASE STUDY

Mr. Allen is a 60-year-old man admitted to the hospital with complaints of weakness, confusion, and diminishing urine output over the past week. Mr. Allen shows a history of hypertension and glomerulonephritis. On admission his vital signs are BP, 180/90; heart rate, 80 and irregular; respirations, 20; and temperature, 99.5° F (37.5° C). He is also nauseated and vomiting. Mr. Allen reports that his shoes are tight. His ankles show 2+ edema bilaterally. Mr. Allen's lungs have bilateral basal crackles. Mr. Allen's daughter states that Mr. Allen has not been taking his medications regularly and that he has not been complying with his prescribed diet. Mr. Allen has not been able to work for 2 years. He reports feeling depressed at times and has an outburst of anger in the emergency room because his toothbrush was left at home.

Laboratory findings are potassium, 5.7; blood urea nitrogen (BUN), 100; creatinine, 5.

Mr. Allen is placed on bed rest and NPO status. A Foley catheter is inserted and drains 10 ml of dark yellow, concentrated urine. An IV infusion of D5W is started at keep-open rate. Fluids are restricted to 1200 ml/24 hr. A polystyrene sulfonate (Kayexalate) enema is ordered. Furosemide (Lasix) is administered for diuresis and prazosin (Minipress) for hypertension. Blood samples for electrolyte, BUN, and creatinine studies are to be redrawn in 4 hr.

He is diagnosed as having renal failure.

Care Plan Format

Initiation date	Nursing diagnosis/problem	Goal(s)	Review/ evaluation date	Interventions	Resolution/ discontinue date
10/1	Alteration in urinary elimination (oliguria) related to decreased renal function	Patient will maintain present level of urinary elimination or better (as near normal as possible) as evidenced by balanced intake and output, and normal laboratory values for BUN and creatinine within 2 weeks	10/1	Catheter care q8h: 0600, 1400, 2200 Measure urine output qh Monitor urine specific gravity q8h: 0600, 1400, 2200 Note character of urine and report abnormalities Measure intake and output accurately Administer IV D5W as ordered (keep-open rate) Restrict fluids as ordered to 1200 ml/24 hr; 500 ml, days; 400 ml, evenings; 300 ml, nights) Monitor serum BUN, creatinine, and electrolytes as ordered and report abnormalities	10/3
10/1	Fluid volume excess related to decreased ability of kidneys to extract water	Patient will show no signs of fluid volume excess within 1 week as evidenced by balanced intake and output, weight loss of 5 kg, usual mental status, clear breath sounds, and absence of pitting peripheral edema		Maintain NPO status Monitor for and report elevated BP Weigh patient on bed scale at 0600 with same scale and clothing Assess level of consciousness q4h; note and report changes in mental status at 0600, 1000, 1400, 1800, 2200, and 0200	

Care Plan Format—cont'd

Initiation date	Nursing diagnosis/problem	Goal(s)	Review/ evaluation date	Interventions	Resolution/ discontinue date
				Assess heart sounds for presence of S_3 and/or S_4	
				Assess breath sounds for rales q4h	
				Assess for peripheral edema	
				Assess for distended neck veins	
				Administer diuretic as ordered (Lasix 80 mg IV bid)	
				Provide ice chips to control thirst	
	Electrolyte imbalance (hyperkalemia) related to decreasing renal ability to regulate and excrete electrolytes	Patient will maintain safe serum potassium level as evidenced by serum potassium ≤ 4.5 and absence of signs and symptoms of hyperkalemia within 2 days		Monitor serum electrolytes q4h as ordered and report abnormalities	
				Monitor and report symptoms of potassium imbalance (irritability, nausea, diarrhea, intestinal colic, arrythmias, and peaked T-wave on ECG)	
				Restrict potassium as ordered	
				Administer Kayexalate enema as ordered	
	Grieving related to loss of function of major organ system, changes in life-style, and life-threatening prognosis	Patient will progress through grieving process as evidenced by expression of feelings to care giver or significant other, utilization of support systems, and effective coping mechanisms, and by compliance with treatment plan and participation in self-care activities		Be sensitive to changes and restrictions in patient's life-style	
				Encourage patient to express feelings of frustration, anger, fear, and uncertainty	
				Actively listen	
				Observe for behavioral and emotional signs of grieving (denial, anger, crying, withdrawal, noncompliance, dependency, etc.)	
				Be patient and empathetic as patient experiences emotional changes and develops coping mechanisms	
				Set limits on maladaptive coping mechanisms if they interfere with patient's well-being	

Continued.

Care Plan Format—cont'd

Initiation date	Nursing diagnosis/problem	Goal(s)	Review/ evaluation date	Interventions	Resolution/ discontinue date
				Support adaptive behaviors that suggest progression and resolution of grieving process Support realistic hope; answer questions honestly, providing requested information Arrange for visitation by clergy Teach and reteach about disease process and management Involve family and significant others in teaching program	

DOCUMENTATION

10/1

- **S:** "I have been urinating less and less every day"; "I've been drinking large amounts of water at home"; patient admitted to 7W from ER
- **O:** Patient has history of diminishing urine output over past 1 week and history of glomerulonephritis; Foley catheter inserted on admission and drained 10 ml of dark yellow, concentrated urine; IV D5W started in left arm—infusing well at keep-open rate; Lasix 80 mg given IV stat with no further urine output noted; BUN, 100; creatinine 5; admission weight, 90 kg
- **A:** Alteration in urinary elimination (oliguria) related to decreased renal function
- **P:** Measure urine output qh
  Monitor urine specific gravity q8h
  Note character of urine and report abnormalities
  Measure intake and output accurately
  Continue IV D5W at keep-open rate
  Restrict fluids to 1200 ml/24 hr
  Monitor serum BUN, creatinine, and electrolytes and report abnormalities

- **S:** "I'm so thirsty—I've been drinking large amounts of water"; "I haven't urinated at all today"; "My shoes are really tight"; "I think I've gained some weight"; "I'm not sure what it is—I keep forgetting things"; "I'm very tired"
- **O:** Patient awake, lethargic, oriented to person and place but requires frequent reorientation to time; elevated BP of 180/90; bilateral neck vein distention noted; lungs show bilateral basal crackles—do not clear with cough; patient shows 2+ pitting edema in ankles bilaterally; heart tones S_3 noted; IV D5W started at keep-open rate in left arm—infusing well; patient is on NPO status; placed on 1200 ml/day fluid restriction; Lasix 80 mg given IV stat; no urine output noted; patient's weight is 90 kg on admission; potassium, 5; patient complaining of thirst
- **A:** Fluid volume excess related to decreased ability of kidneys to extract water
- **P:** Weigh patient daily at same time with same clothing and scale
  Monitor for elevated BP
  Assess level of consciousness; note changes in mental status
  Assess heart sounds for presence of S_3 and/or S_4
  Assess breath sounds for rales
  Obtain chest x-ray film as ordered

S, Subjective assessment; O, objective assessment; A, assessment (nursing diagnosis); P, plan.

Assess for peripheral edema
Assess for distended neck veins
Restrict fluids as ordered
Administer diuretics as ordered
Maintain NPO status except for ice chips to control thirst

S: "I'm feeling nauseated"; "Sometimes I feel my heart skip a beat"; "I don't know why I can't get comfortable and rest"

O: Patient awake and restless; nauseated—vomited scant amount of green secretion; NPO at present; cardiac monitor shows frequent premature ventricular beats; apical heart rate, 80 and irregular; Kayexalate enema given—large amount of liquid brown return noted; serum potassium on admission, 5; serum potassium redrawn in 4 hr, 4.7

A: Electrolyte imbalance (hyperkalemia) related to decreasing renal ability to regulate and excrete electrolytes

P: Monitor serum electrolytes q4h as ordered
Report abnormal serum electrolyte values to physician
Dialyze as ordered
Monitor for signs and symptoms of irritability, nausea, diarrhea, intestinal colic, arrythmias, and peaked T wave on ECG
Restrict dietary potassium as ordered
Administer Kayexalate as ordered

S: "I haven't worked in 2 years because of my kidney problems"; "I can't even go to church on Sundays anymore"; "I can't stand this much longer"; "The doctor better get me well this time"; "I can't believe my daughter left my toothbrush at home—she can't do anything right"; "So, I don't take my pills all of the time—what's the difference? No one cares"

O: Patient exhibiting anger at staff and family; daughter reports patient has been depressed at home and noncompliant with medications and treatment regimen; patient is Catholic—verbalizes desire to attend church

A: Grieving related to loss of function of major organ system, changes in life-style, and life-threatening prognosis

P: Be sensitive to changes and restrictions in patient's life-style
Encourage patient to express feelings of frustration, anger, fear, and uncertainty
Actively listen
Observe for behavioral and emotional signs of grieving (denial, anger, crying, withdrawal, noncompliance, dependency, etc.)
Be patient and empathetic as patient experiences emotional changes and develops coping mechanisms
Set limits on maladaptive coping mechanisms if they interfere with patient's well-being
Support adaptive behaviors that suggest a progression and resolution of grieving process
Support realistic hope; answer questions honestly, providing requested information
Arrange for visitation with clergy
Teach and reteach about disease process and management
Involve family and significant others in teaching process

INDEX

A

Abdominal ECG transducer, 737
Abdominal herniorrhaphy, 390-391
Abdominal hysterectomy, total, and bilateral salpingo-oophorectomy, 606-608
Abdominal tubal ligation, 604-605
Abdominoperineal pull-through procedure, 817-819
Abortion, 603-604
Abruptio placentae, 723-724
Abscess, brain, 323
Abuse
  chemical substance, 326-329
  child, 860-862
  drug, 325-329
  substance, 325-329
Acceptance by dying patient, 34
Acetabulum, diseased, surgical repair of, 493
Acetazolamide for seizure disorders, 292
Acetest, 443, 444
Acetohexamide for diabetes, 446
Acetone tests, 444
Achalasia, 343-344
Acid-base imbalances, 44-46
Acidosis
  metabolic, 46-47
  respiratory, 44-45
Acoustic neuromas, 301
ACTH; see Adrenocorticotropic hormone
Actinomycin D; see Dactinomycin
Active labor, 728
Activity, reduction or limitation in, 2-3
Activity intolerance, actual or potential, 2
Activity progression program in cardiac rehabilitation, 116-119
Adaptive behaviors, 19
Addicted mothers, infants of, 767-769
Addisonian crisis, 457
Adenomas, pituitary, 301
ADH; see Antidiuretic hormone
Adolescent age-group care, 788
Adrenal cortex, 420, 421
Adrenal crisis, 457
Adrenal gland(s), surgical removal of, 465-467
Adrenalectomy, 465-467

Adrenalin; see Epinephrine
Adrenocortical insufficiency, 457-460
Adrenocorticotropic hormone, 421
  excessive secretion of, 460
Adria flaré, 703
Adriamycin; see Doxorubicin
Adrucil; see 5-Fluorouracil
Adult respiratory distress syndrome, 263-266
Adult-onset glaucoma, 632-633
Adventitious breath sounds, 222-223
Aerolone; see Isoproterenol
Aerosol therapy, humidity and, 229-230
Afterloader, radium therapy sealed in, care of patient receiving, 614-616
Aganglionic megacolon, 815-817
Aggressive behavior, 21
Aging, 31
Aging patient, assessment of, 31-32
Aging process, normal variations during, 31-32
Air in pleural space, 252
Airway(s)
  artificial, 272-275
  nasopharyngeal, 272-273
  oropharyngeal, 272
Albumin
  for child, 867
  serum, normal, 214
    reactions to transfusion of, 217
Albuterol for asthma, 235
Alcohol
  intoxication with, 325-326
  serum levels of, and effects of, 327
Aldosterone, 421
Aldosteronism, primary, 462-464
Alignment, body positions to maintain, 297
Alkaloids, vinca, 676-679
  hazards associated with, 671
Alkalosis
  metabolic, 46-47
  respiratory, 44-45
Alkeran; see Melphalan
Alkylating agents, 672-675
  hazards associated with, 670
ALL; see Lymphoblastic leukemia, acute

Alopecia from chemotherapy, 702-703
ALS; *see* Amyotrophic lateral sclerosis
Altered consciousness, 288
    care of patient with, 288-291
Alupent; *see* Metaproterenol
Alveolar spaces, inflammation of, 243
Alveoli
    abnormal accumulation of fluid in, 245
    collapse of, 257
Alzheimer's disease, 309-310
Ambulatory peritoneal dialysis, continuous, 562-563
American Parkinson Disease Foundation, 312
American Psychiatric Association Diagnostic and Statistical Manual, Third Edition (DSM III), 10
Amethopterin; *see* Methotrexate
Aminophylline, 4
    for asthma, 235
    for child, 867
AML; *see* Myelogenous leukemia, acute
Amniocentesis, 718-719
Amphetamines, abuse of, 325
Amphotericin B for meningitis, 323
Ampicillin
    plus gentamicin for endocarditis prophylaxis, 95
    for meningitis, 323
Amputation of leg, 499-501
AMSA; *see* Amsacrine
Amsacrine, 684-685
Amyotrophic lateral sclerosis, 319-321
Anal reservoir, anastomosis of ileum to, 387-388
Anaphylactic shock, 104; *see also* Vasogenic shock
Anastomosis of ileum to anal reservoir, 387-388
Androgens, 421
Anemia
    aplastic, 168-173
    with chemotherapy, 689-690
    hemolytic, 165-167
    hypochromic, 163-165
    hypoplastic, 168
    iron deficiency, 163-165
    macrocytic, hyperchromic, 161-163
    microcytic, 163-165
    pernicious, 161-163
Anesthesia
    general, care of patient in recovery room following, 30
    spinal, care of patient in recovery room following, 30-31
Anger
    in dying patient, 34
    vs. hostility, 21
Angina, Prinzmetal's variant, drug for, 92-93

Angina pectoris, 85-87
    drugs for, 91-93
Angioplasty, transluminal, percutaneous, 138-140
Ankle
    arthroplasty of, 495, 497
    and foot, burns of, positioning with, 629
Ankylosing spondylitis, 491-492
Anorexia nervosa in child, 862-865
Antepartum assessment, 711-713
Anterior pelvic exenteration, 612
Antibiotic coverage for endocarditis prophylaxis, 95
Antibiotic therapy in meningitis, 323
Antibiotics for chemotherapy, 678-683
    hazards associated with, 671
Anticipatory grief, 18
Anticoagulant, 151
Anticoagulant therapy, 151-154
Antidiuretic hormone, 421
    insufficient secretion of, 456
Antimetabolites, 674-677
    hazards associated with, 670-671
Antineoplastic chemotherapy, 666-684
Antithyroid medications, 429
Anus, ileal reservoir at, construction of, 386-387
Anxiety, 14
    mild, 14
    moderate, 14-15
    severe, 15-16
Aorta, coarctation of, 846-847
Aortic stenosis, 847-848
Aortic valve replacement, 111
Aortofemoral bypass graft, 81-83
Aplastic anemia, 168-173
Apnea, posthyperventilation, in neurologic dysfunction, 284
Apneustic respirations in neurologic dysfunction, 284
Appendix, ruptured (perforated), 813-815
Applicator, Ernst, radium therapy sealed in, care of patient receiving, 614-616
Apresoline; *see* Hydralazine
Ara-C; *see* Cytarabine
Aramine; *see* Metaraminol
ARDS; *see* Adult respiratory distress syndrome
Arrest, sinus, 121-122
Arrhythmia, sinus, 121, 122
Arterial insufficiency, chronic, 77-80
Arterial system, 68
Artery
    coronary
        bypass graft of, 111
        graft of, 110

INDEX

Artery—cont'd
  coronary—cont'd
    spasm of, drug for, 92-93
  pulmonary, banding of, 852
Arthritis
  gouty, 480-481
  pyogenic, acute, 474-475
  rheumatoid, 472-474
Arthroplasty
  cup, 493
  joint, total, 495-499
  Keller, 510
  Mayo, 510
Arthroscopic surgery of knee, 501-502
Artificial airways, 272-275
Artificial pacemaker, temporary, in child, 860
Artificial urinary sphincter, 531-534
Ascites
  continuous peritoneal-jugular shunt for, 403-405
  paracentesis for, care of patient undergoing, 405-406
ASD; see Atrial septal defect
Asparaginase, 682-683, 703
  hazards associated with, 671
L-Asparaginase; see Asparaginase
Aspiration of secretions, 226-227
Aspirin and nutrition, 4
ASPO review sheet, 730-731
Assaultive behavior, 21-22
Asthma, 233-236
  pediatric, 798-800
Astrocytomas, 300
Ataxic breathing in neurologic dysfunction, 284
Ataxic respiration, 220
Atelectasis, 257-258
Atonic bladder, 537
Atresia, esophageal, 808
Atrial beats, premature, 122
Atrial catheter, Silastic, 57-58
Atrial contractions, premature, 122-123
Atrial fibrillation, 124, 125
Atrial flutter, 123, 124
Atrial origin, ECG rhythms of, 122-125
Atrial septal defect, 845
Atrial tachycardia, paroxysmal, 124-125
Atrioventricular block
  first-degree, 129
  Mobitz type I, 129-130
  Mobitz type II, 130
  second-degree, 129, 130

Atrioventricular block—cont'd
  third-degree, 130-131
Atrioventricular junctional rhythms, 132
Atropine
  abuse of, 325
  for child, 867, 868
Auditory system, 638-645
  and optic system, 631-645
Auditory-impaired patient, 643-645
Augmentation of labor with oxytocin infusion, 733-734
Automatic bladder, 537
Autonomous bladder, 537
Axilla, chest, and arm burns, positioning with, 629
Azacytidine, 676-677
t-Azacytidine; see Azacytidine
Azathioprine, hazards associated with, 671

B

Back pain, low, 482-483
Balanced suspension with Thomas' splint and Pearson's attachment, 511, 512
Balloon pump, 145-148
Balloon septostomy, 851
Banding, pulmonary artery, 852
Barbiturates
  abuse of, 325
  and nutrition, 4
Bargaining by dying patient, 34
Base bicarbonate
  deficit of, 46-47
  excess of, 46-47
Basophil, 159
BBB; see Bundle-branch block
BCNU; see Carmustine
Beats, atrial, premature, 122
Bed, circle, care of patient on, 333-334
Behavior(s)
  adaptive, 19
  aggressive, 21
  assaultive, 21-22
  demanding, 26-27
  dependent, 28
  manipulative, 25-26
  suicidal, 20
  withdrawn, 27-28
Behavioral dysfunctions, standards of care and nursing diagnoses related to, 10-28
Bennett MA-1 ventilator, 277
Bennett PR2 ventilator, 277
Benzyl penicillin for meningitis, 323

Beta-2; see Isoetharine
Bicarbonate
  base
    deficit of, 46-47
    excess of, 46-47
  deficit of, 44-45
  excess of, 44-45
Bilateral salpingo-oophorectomy, total abdominal hysterectomy and, 606-608
Biliary cirrhosis, 399-401
Biliary decompression catheter, transhepatic, 398-399
Biliary obstruction, 394-396
Biliary surgery, 396-397
Biopsy, liver, 412
Biot's respiration, 220
  in neurologic dysfunction, 284
Bird Mark 7 ventilator, 277
Birth weight
  high, 758-759
  low, 757-758
Bladder
  atonic, 537
  automatic, 537
  autonomous, 537
  cancer of, detection and prevention of, 656-657
  cord, 537
  damage to, from chemotherapy, 698-699
  flaccid, 537
  hyperreflexive, 537
  hypertonic, 537
  hypotonic, 537
  infection of, 522
  lower motor neuron, 537
  neurogenic, 537-540
  reflex, 537
  tabetic, 537
  upper motor neuron, 537
Blalock-Taussig shunt, 852
Bleeding, gastric, 355-357
Bleeding esophageal varices, 344-346
Blenoxane; see Bleomycin sulfate
"Bleo"; see Bleomycin sulfate
Bleomycin sulfate, 678-679, 703
  hazards associated with, 671
Block
  atrioventricular
    first-degree, 129
    Mobitz type I, 129-130
    Mobitz type II, 130
    second-degree, 129, 130

Block—cont'd
  atrioventricular—cont'd
    third-degree, 130-131
  bundle-branch, 131-132
Blood
  or blood components, 212-214
    removal of, 209
    transfusion of, reaction to, 215-217
  loss of, signs and symptoms of, 161
  in pleural space, 255
  whole, 212-213
    reactions to transfusions of, 215-216, 217
Blood cells
  human, 159
  red, 159, 212
    defective production of, 161-165
    increased numbers of, 173-175
    rapid destruction of, 165-167
    reactions to transfusions of, 215, 216
  white, 159
    pheresis of, 211
Blood chemistry laboratory values, normal, 879
Blood components
  blood or, 212-214
    removal of, 209
    transfusion of, reaction to, 215-219
  SI units for, conversion factors for, 880-881
Blood pressure of child, 865
Blood transfusions, 218
  reactions to, 214-217
Body cast, care of patient in, 515
Body image, 10-11
  altered, 10-11
Body positions to maintain correct alignment, 297
Body temperature, potential alteration in, 7-8
Bone marrow study, 209
Bone marrow transplantation, 181-196
  schedule for, 182
Bourns Bear 1 ventilator, 277
Bowel
  irritable, 370-372
  short, syndrome of, 373-374
Bowel elimination, alteration in, 5-6
Bowel training, 332-333
Boys
  infant, percentile growth chart for, 783
  percentile growth chart for, 787
Bradycardia, sinus, 119, 120, 121
Brain abscess, 323

INDEX

Brain implants for cancer, 708
Brain tumors, 300-302
Breast cancer, detection and prevention of, 658-660
Breast implants for cancer, 708
Breast milk, hand expression of, 748
Breast self-examination, 659
Breast-feeding, 747-749
    following cesarean delivery, 745
    correct body position for, 748
Breath and voice sounds, 222-223
Breathing
    ataxic, in neurologic dysfunction, 284
    cluster, in neurologic dysfunction, 284
    intermittent positive pressure, 280-281
Brethine; *see* Terbutaline
Bricanyl; *see* Terbutaline
Bricker procedure for urinary diversion, 542
Bronchial mucous membrane, inflammation of, 236
Bronchial sounds, 222
Bronchiectasis, 238-239
Bronchiolitis, 800-802
Bronchitis, 236-238
Bronchodilators, 235
Bronchophony, 223
Bronchopulmonary dysplasia, 777-778
Bronchoscope, 224
Bronchoscopy, therapeutic, 224-225
Bronchovesicular sounds, 222
Bronchus, chronic dilation of, 238
Bronkaid Mist; *see* Epinephrine
Bronkephrine; *see* Ethylnorepinephrine
Bronkodyl; *see* Theophylline
Bronkometer; *see* Isoetharine
Bronkosol; *see* Isoetharine
Brooke formula for fluid replacement for burns, 630
Bryant's traction, 511, 512, 513
Buckling, scleral, 633
Bundle-branch block, 131-132
Bunionectomy, 510-511
Burns
    ankle and foot, positioning with, 629
    care of patient with, 625-630
    chemical, of esophagus, 342
    chest, axilla, and arm, positioning with, 629
    classification of, 625
    fluid replacement for, calculation of, 630
    hand, positioning with, 629
    head and neck, positioning with, 628
    surface of, calculation of percentage of, 626
Busulfan, 672-673

Butazolidin; *see* Phenylbutazone
Bypass
    gastric, 359, 360
    jejunoileal, 359, 360, 361
Bypass graft
    aortofemoral, 81-83
    coronary artery, 111
    femoropopliteal, 78

C

Calcitonin, 422
Calcium
    deficit of, 38-39
    excess of, 38-41
Calculi, renal, 553-557
Caloric requirement calculation for child, 866
Cancer; *see also* Carcinoma; Oncology
    bladder, 656-657
    breast, 658-660
    cervical, 661-662
    colorectal, 655-656
    detection and prevention of, 651-665
    of esophagus and stomach, 654-655
    head and neck, 652-653
    of kidney, 656-657
    lung, 653-654
    ovarian, 660-661
    of pelvis, 656-657
    prostate, 658
    radiotherapy for, 705-708
    skin, 652
    staging of, utilizing TNM classification, 665
    testicular, 657-658
    of ureter, 656-657
    of urethra, 656-657
    uterine, 662
    vaginal, 660
Cannabis, abuse of, 325
Cantor tube, 388, 389
    care of patient with, 388-390
CAPD; *see* Continuous ambulatory peritoneal dialysis
Capillary wedge pressure, pulmonary, 141, 144, 145
Captopril, 93
    potential complications of, 90
Carbamazepine for seizure disorders, 292
Carbon dioxide tension
    decreased, 44-45
    elevated, 44-45
Carcinoma; *see also* Cancer; Oncology
    esophageal, 347-349

Carcinoma—cont'd
  gastric, 364-365
  hepatic, 410-412
  intestinal, 376-377
  of large intestine, 376
  pancreatic, 417-418
  of small intestine, 376
Cardiac catheterization, 138
Cardiac cycle, 120
Cardiac injury, syndrome following, 114-115
Cardiac output, thermodilution method of measuring, 145
Cardiac rehabilitation, 115-119
Cardiac surgery, 108-114
  classification of, 108
Cardiac tamponade, 100-101
Cardiogenic shock, 104, 105-106
  drugs for, 90
Cardiotoxicity from chemotherapy, 696-697
Cardiovascular assessment, 67-73
Cardiovascular reconditioning
  initial postdischarge activities for, 118-119
  program of, 119
Cardiovascular risk factor profile, 87
Cardiovascular system, 67-156
  of child, 844-860
  hematologic assessment of, 159
Cardioversion, 150
Carmustine, 674-675
Carotid endarterectomy, 80-81
Cast, care of patient in, 514-516
Cataract removal with or without intraocular lens transplant, 633
Catheter(s)
  atrial, Silastic, 57-58
  central venous, 55
    care of patient with, 55-59
  intrauterine, 737
  nasal, for oxygen therapy, 229
  pulmonary, triple-lumen balloon-tipped, 144
  subclavian, multilumen, 56-57
  Swan-Ganz, 141, 143, 144, 145
  transhepatic biliary decompression, 398-399
  urethral, indwelling, 541
    care of patient with, 540-542
Catheterization
  cardiac, 138
  umbilical, of newborn, 765
Cavity
  oral, disruption of, 1-2
  peritoneal, inflammation of, 372

Cavity—cont'd
  pleural, pus in, 256
CCNU; see Lomustine
CCPD; see Continuous cycling peritoneal dialysis
Celestin tube, 350
  care of patient with, 350-352
Cells
  blood; see Blood cells
  Reed-Sternberg, 202
Cellulitis, 621-622
Celontin; see Methsuximide
Centigrade-Fahrenheit equivalents, 877
Central diabetes insipidus, 456-457
Central line, total parenteral nutrition administered through, 52
Central nervous system
  of child, 822-830
  surgical intervention of, 307-309
Central neurogenic hyperventilation in neurologic dysfunction, 284
Central venous catheter, 55
  care of patient with, 55-59
Central venous nutrition, 53
Cerebellum, tumors of, 300
Cerebrovascular accident, 294, 296-300
Cerebrovascular circulation, alterations in, 293
Cerebrovascular disruptions, 293-296
Cerubidin; see Daunomycin
Cervical cast, care of patient in, 515
Cervical cord injuries, 304
Cervical spine, fracture or dislocation of, 489-491
Cervical traction, 511, 512
Cervix
  cancer of, detection and prevention of, 661-662
  cold-knife conization of, 602
  surgical removal of, 606, 608
Cesarean delivery, 743-747
Cesium implants, gynecologic, 708
Cesium therapy; see Radium therapy
Chemical substance abuse, 326-329
Chemonucleolysis, 492-493
Chemotherapeutic drugs, 672-685
  administration of, 669-670
  extravasation of, 704-705
  handling of, safety in, 670, 684
  hazards associated with, 670-671
Chemotherapy, 666
  antineoplastic, 666-684
  complications in, 684-705
  radioactive, unsealed, 709-710

INDEX

Chest
　axilla, and arm, burns of, positioning with, 629
　flail, 260-261
Chest tubes, 271-272
　removal of, 272
Chest wall
　landmarks of, 70
　surgical excision of, 269
Cheyne-Stokes respirations, 220
　in neurologic dysfunction, 284
CHF; see Congestive heart failure
Chickenpox, 790-791
Child(ren)
　abuse of, 860-862
　cardiovascular system of, 844-860
　central nervous system of, 822-830
　diabetes mellitus in, 839-841
　emergency drugs for, 867-868
　endocrine system of, 839-844
　gastrointestinal system of, 805-822
　genitourinary system of, 830-834
　hematology of, 834-839
　nutrition and, 866
　preschool-age, 784-785
　respiratory system of, 788-805
　school-age, 785, 788
　vital signs of, 865-866
Childhood diseases, 790-793
Chloral hydrate, abuse of, 325
Chlorambucil, 672-673
Chloramphenicol for meningitis, 323
Chlorothiazide, 4
Chlorpropamide for diabetes, 446
Cholecystectomy, 396
Choledochojejunostomy, 396
Choledocholithotomy, 396
Choledyl; see Oxtriphylline
Cholinergic crisis, 317-318
Choriocarcinoma, 601
Chymodiactin; see Chymopapain injection
Chymopapain injection, 492
Circle bed, care of patient on, 333-334
Circulation, cerebrovascular, alterations in, 293
Circulatory system of heart, 69
Cirrhosis, 399-401
Cisplatin, 682-683, 703
　hazards associated with, 671
Cleaning fluid, abuse of, 325
Cleft lip repair, 805-806
Cleft palate repair, 806-808
Climacteric, 599-600

Clinitest, 443, 444
Clonazepam for seizure disorders, 292
Clonopin; see Clonazepam
Closed menisectomy, 509
Closed-heart surgery, 108
　in child, 852-854
Closure, ileostomy, 387-388
Closure sounds from heart valves, transmission of, 71
Cluster breathing in neurologic dysfunction, 284
Coagulation, intravascular, disseminated, 196-198
Coarctation of aorta, 846-847
Coarse crackles, 222
Cocaine, abuse of, 325
Coccidioides immitis meningitis, antibiotic therapy for, 323
Codeine, abuse of, 325
Cognition, disruptions in, 23-24
COLD; see Obstructive lung disease, chronic
Cold-knife conization of cervix, 602
Colectomy, 386-387
Colitis, ulcerative, 370-372
Colon, diverticular disease of, 378-380
Colorectal cancer, detection and prevention of, 655-656
Colostomy, 368
　irrigation of, 393
Colpostat, radium therapy sealed in, care of patient receiving, 614-616
Coma, hyperosmolar hyperglycemic nonketotic, 440-442
Coma Scale, Glasgow, 288
Comfort, alteration in (pain, chronic or acute), 8-9
Comminuted fracture of head, 302
Communicating hydrocephalus, 822
Communication, 25
　dysfunctional, 25
Compartmental syndrome, 506-507
　diagnosis of, 507-509
Complete fracture, 484
Complete heart block, 130-131
Compound fracture, 483
　of head, 302
Concussion, 302
Conditioning phase of bone marrow transplantation, 184-187
Conduit, ileal, 542
Congenital heart defects, 844-850
Congenital heart disease, repair for, 110, 111
Congenital heart surgery, 850-857
Congenital rubella, 790-791
Congenital syphilis, 770-771
Congestive heart failure
　in child, 857-859

Congestive heart failure—cont'd
  drugs for, 90-93
Conization of cervix, cold-knife, 602
Consciousness, altered, 288
  care of patient with, 288-291
Constipation from chemotherapy, 695
Contact lens removal, 637
Continent ileal reservoir, 542, 543
Continent ileostomy, 382-386
Continuous ambulatory peritoneal dialysis, 562-563
Continuous cycling peritoneal dialysis, 563
Continuous drip narcotics, intravenous, 64-65
Continuous mechanical ventilation, 277-280
  care of patient on, 277-279
Continuous passive motion device, 517
Continuous peritoneal-jugular shunt for ascites, 403-405
Contraceptives, oral, and nutrition, 4
Contraction stress test, 738-739
Contractions
  atrial, premature, 122-123
  ventricular, premature, 125-126
    multifocal, 126
Contusion, 302
COPD; see Obstructive pulmonary disease, chronic
Coping, individual, ineffective, 19-20
Cord
  spermatic, torsion of, 588-589
  spinal, injuries to, 304-307
    paralysis from, 335-338
  umbilical, prolapsed, 724-725
Cord bladder, 537
Cord injuries, 304
Corneal transplant, 633
Coronary artery bypass graft, 111
Coronary artery graft, 110
Coronary artery spasm, drug for, 92-93
Cortex, adrenal, 420, 421
Corticosteroid therapy, 467-469
Corticosteroids and nutrition, 4
Cortisol, 421
Cosmegen; see Dactinomycin
Cough, whooping, 790-791, 795-796
Counterpulsation, intraaortic balloon, 145-148
Countershock, direct current, 150-151
Coup-contracoup phenomenon, 302
Crackles, 222
Cranial nerves, functions of, 286
Craniectomy, 307
Craniocerebral trauma, 302-304
Craniotomy, 307

Crises, 19
Crohn's disease, 370-372
Croup, 788-789, 792-793
Crutch-walking gaits, 516
Crutch-walking procedure, 516-517
Cryopexy, retinal, 633
Cryoprecipitate, 213
Cryptococcal meningitis, antibiotic therapy for, 323
CST; see Contraction stress test
CTX; see Cyclophosphamide
Cup arthroplasty, 493
Curettage, dilation and, 601-602
Cushing's disease, 460
Cushing's syndrome, 460-462
Cutaneous ureterostomy, 542, 543
CVA; see Cerebrovascular accident
Cyanotic heart defects, 848-850
Cycling peritoneal dialysis, continuous, 563
Cyclophosphamide, 672-673
  before bone marrow transplantation, 184
  hazards with, 670
Cystic fibrosis, 802-805
Cystitis, 522
  hemorrhagic, from chemotherapy, 698-699
Cystolithotomy, 554
Cytarabine, 674-675
  before bone marrow transplantation, 184
  hazards associated with, 670
Cytomegalovirus in neonate, 771
Cytosar; see Cytarabine
Cytoxan; see Cyclophosphamide

D

D & C; see Dilation and curettage
Dacarbazine, 682-683, 704
  hazards associated with, 671
Dactinomycin, 680-681, 704
  hazards associated with, 671
Daunomycin, 680-681
  hazards associated with, 671
Daunorubicin, 680-681, 704
  hazards associated with, 671
Decadron; see Dexamethasone
Decision making, compromised, 24
Decompression, global, 634
Decompression catheter, transhepatic biliary, 398-399
Decubitus ulcer, 619-621
Defibrillation, 150-151
Deficiency
  iron, anemia of, 163-165

Deficiency—cont'd
  vitamin B$_{12}$, 161
Degrees of patient position, 74
Dehydration; see Hypovolemia
Delivery
  care of mother during, 732-733
  cesarean, 743-747
  immediate stabilization of newborn at, 753
  labor and, care of diabetic mother during, 720-721
Demanding behavior, 26-27
Demerol; see Meperidine
Denial and shock by dying patient, 33-34
Depakene; see Valproic acid
Dependent behavior, 28
Depressants
  abuse of, 326-327
  commonly abused, 325
Depressed fracture of head, 302
Depression in dying patient, 34
Dermatologic toxicity from chemotherapy, 703-704
Desferal; see Desferioxamine mesylate
Desferioxamine mesylate for child, 867
Dexamethasone for child, 867
Dextrose 50% for child, 867
Diabetes insipidus, 440
  central, 456-457
Diabetes mellitus, 437, 440
  in child, 839-841
  insulin-dependent, 839-841
  mother with
    care of
      during labor and delivery, 720-721
      during last trimester of pregnancy, 719-720
    infant of, 759-761
  patient with
    personal care and, 449-450
    sick day rules for, 446-448
    skin, foot, and leg care of, 448-449
    teaching of, 442-450
    travel tips for, 450
    urine testing with, teaching guide for, 443-444
Diabetic flow sheet, 446
Diabetic food replacements, 880
Diabetic ketoacidosis, 437-440
Diabinese; see Dymelor
Diagnoses, nursing; see Nursing diagnoses
Diagnostic procedures, neurologic, 288
Dialysis, peritoneal, 562-567
  continuous ambulatory, 562-563
  continuous cycling, 563

Dialysis, peritoneal—cont'd
  intermittent, 562
Diamox; see Acetazolamide
Diarrhea
  from chemotherapy, 694-695
  diet for control of, 820-821
Diastix, 444
Diazepam
  for child, 867
  for seizure disorders, 292
Diazoxide for child, 867
DIC; see Disseminated intravascular coagulation
Diet
  for control of diarrhea, 820-821
  low-bacterial, 195
Digestive system, 339-418
  diagram of, 340
Digital replantation, 504-506
Digitalis, 154
Digitalis therapy, 154-156
  pediatric, 859-860
Digoxin for child, 867
Dilantin; see Phenytoin
Dilation and curettage, 601-602
Dilaudid; see Hydromorphone
Dilor; see Dyphylline
Diphenylhydantoin; see Phenytoin
Diphtheria, 792-793
Direct current countershock, 150-151
Disc
  herniated, 482
  surgical removal of, 487
Discase; see Chymopapain injection
Discectomy, 487
Disease
  Alzheimer's, 309-310
  childhood, 790-793
  concurrent
    in cardiovascular assessment, 69
    in peripheral vascular assessment, 73
  Crohn's, 370-372
  Cushing's, 460
  diverticular, of colon, 378-380
  graft vs. host, 189
    clinical grading of severity of, 189
    proposed clinical stage of, 188
  Graves', 427
  heart
    congenital, repair of, 110, 111
    valvular, 94-98

Disease—cont'd
  Hirschsprung's, 815-817
  Hodgkin's, 202-205, 663-664
    staging of, 202
  hyaline membrane, 773-774
  inflammatory, pelvic, 596-597
  kidney, polycystic, 548-551
  "Lou Gehrig's," 319
  lung, chronic obstructive, 230-233
  Parkinson's, 310-313
  peptic ulcer, 354-355
  pulmonary, chronic obstructive, 230-233
    disability scale for, 242
  sickle cell, 837
Dislocation of cervical spine, 489-491
Disorientation, 23-24
Dissection, neck, radical, 266-269
Disseminated intravascular coagulation, 196-198
Disseminated sclerosis, 313-315
Dissolution, kidney stone, percutaneous, 554
Distress
  fetal, 734-735
  spiritual, potential for, 6-7
Diuril; see Chlorothiazide
Diversion, urinary, 542-548
Diverticular disease of colon, 378-380
Diverticulitis, 378-380
Diverticulosis, 343-344, 378
DMT, abuse of, 325
DNR; see Daunomycin
Dopamine for child, 867
Doriden; see Glutethimide
Dorsal root rhizotomy, microsurgical, 487
Doxorubicin, 680-681, 703, 704
  hazards associated with, 671
Dressler's syndrome, 114
Drip rates, IV, regulation of, 55
Drop rate–calibrated infusion controllers, 60
Drop rate–calibrated infusion pumps, 60
Drops, eye, instillation of, 637-638
Drug(s)
  abuse of, 325-329
  antithyroid, 429
  chemotherapeutic; see Chemotherapeutic drugs
  effect of, on nutritional status, 4
  emergency, pediatric, 867-868
  liquid equivalents for, 876
  mass equivalents for, 876
  to be taken with food, 4
  used in seizure disorders, 292

Drug(s)—cont'd
  vasodilator, 89-93
    potential complications of, 90
Drug delivery system, Port-A-Cath implantable, 58
DSM III, 10
DTIC; see Dacarbazine
Ductus arteriosus, patent, 844
Duhamel procedure, 817
Dumping syndrome, 358-359
Duodenostomy; see Enteral nutrition
Duodenostomy-jejunostomy, 367, 368
Duodenum
  endoscopy of, 352
  ulcers of, 354
Dyflex; see Dyphylline
Dying, stages of care during, 33-34
Dying patient, emotional care of, 32-34
Dymelor; see Acetohexamide
Dyphylline for asthma, 235
Dyrenium; see Triamterene
Dysfunctional grieving, 18-19
Dysmaturity, 757-759
Dysplasia, bronchopulmonary, 777-778

E

Ear
  assessment of, 638-639
  diagram of, 638
Early labor, 728
ECG changes, miscellaneous, 133
ECG complex, normal, 119
ECG intervals, meaning and significance of, 119
ECG rhythms, 119-134
  of atrial origin, 122-125
  nursing diagnoses/goals/interventions for, 134
  of sinus origin, 119-122
  of ventricular origin, 125-129
ECG transducer, abdominal, 737
Eclampsia, 716-717
Edecrin; see Ethacrynic acid
Edema, pulmonary, 245-246
Effusion, pleural, 258-259
Egophony, 223
Elbow
  arthroplasty of, 495, 496
  and shoulder, range-of-motion exercises for, 299
Eldesine; see Vindesine
Electrical nerve stimulation, transcutaneous, 65-66
Electrocardiogram in cardiovascular assessment, 72
Electrode, spiral, for fetal monitoring, 737

Electrolyte imbalances, 36-44
    and fluid imbalance, observation of, 36-48
Electronic infusion devices, 60
Elimination
    bowel, alteration in, 5-6
    urinary, alteration in, 5-6
Elixophyllin; *see* Theophylline
Elspar; *see* Asparaginase
Embolism, pulmonary, 247-248
Emergency drugs, pediatric, 867-868
Emerson ventilator, 277
Emotional abuse of child, 861
Emotional care of dying patient, 32-34
Emphysema, 239-242
Empyema, thoracic, 256-257
Encephalitis, 323
Endarterectomy, carotid, 80-81
Endocarditis
    antibiotic coverage for prophylaxis with, 95
    infective, 93-94
Endocrine glands, 420, 421-422
Endocrine system, 419-469
    assessment of, 419-424
    of child, 839-844
    diagram of, 420
Endolymphatic hydrops, 639-640
Endoscopic removal of kidney stone, 554
Endoscopy, esophageal, gastric, duodenal, 352
Endotracheal tube, 273-275
    newborn with, care of, 775-776
    removal of, care during/after, 274-275
Endoxana; *see* Cyclophosphamide
End-to-end jejunoileal bypass, 359, 360, 361
Engstrom ventilator, 277
Enteral nutrition, 34-51
Enteritis, regional, 370-372
Enterocolitis, necrotizing, 769-770
Enucleation, 633
Eosinophil, 159
Ephedrine for asthma, 235
Epidural hematoma, 303
Epidural method of ICP monitoring, 330
Epiglottitis, 793-795
Epilepsy Foundation of America, 293
Epinephrine, 421
    for asthma, 235
    for child, 867
Ernst applicator, radium therapy sealed in, care in patient
        receiving, 614-616
Erythema from chemotherapy, 703
Erythrocytes; *see* Red blood cells

Erythromycin for endocarditis prophylaxis, 95
    vancomycin plus, 95
Escherichia coli meningitis, antibiotic therapy for, 323
Esophageal atresia, 808
Esophageal reflux, hiatal hernia with, 346-347
Esophagitis, 343-344
Esophagogastrectomy, 349
Esophagostomy, 367, 368; *see also* Enteral nutrition
Esophagus, 342-354
    cancer of, detection and prevention of, 654-655
    carcinoma of, 347-349
    endoscopy of, 352
    inflammation of, 343-344
    stricture of, 343-344
    surgery on, 349-350
    trauma to, 342-343
    varices of, bleeding of, 344-346
Estrogen, 422
ESWL; *see* Extracorporeal shock wave lithotripsy
Ethacrynic acid for child, 867
Ethosuximide for seizure disorders, 292
Ethylnorepinephrine for asthma, 235
Etoposide, 678-679
    hazards associated with, 671
Exanthema subitum; *see* Roseola infantum
Exchange transfusion of newborn, 763-764
Exenteration, pelvic, 612-614
Exercise program, prescribed, for cardiac rehabilitation,
        118-119
Exercises
    isometric, 517
    range-of-motion (ROM), 517
        of shoulder and elbow, 299
        of wrist and hand, 299
    terminology for, 517
Expression of breast milk, hand, 748
External fetal monitoring, 736-737
External fixation for complicated fractures, 502-504
Extracellular fluid volume
    deficit, 46-49
    excess of, 46-47
Extracorporeal shock wave lithotripsy, 554-555
Extraction, surgical kidney stone, 554
Extravasation of chemotherapeutic drugs, 704-705
Eye
    assessment of, 631-632
    diagram of, 631
    surgery on, 633-635
Eye drops or ointment, instillation of, 637-638
Eye globe, surgical removal of, 633

F

Facet joint rhizotomy, 487
Fahrenheit-centigrade equivalents, 877
Failure to thrive, 841-844
Fallopian tubes, surgical removal of, 606, 608
Fallot, tetralogy of, 848-850
Family-centered care of high-risk infant, 779-780
Feeding
  by gastrostomy tube, 811
  of newborn, gavage, intermittent, 778-779
  tube, teaching about, 50-51
Female reproductive system, 594-617
  assessment of, 594-596
  diagram of, 595
Femoropopliteal bypass graft, 78
Ferrous sulfate, 4
Fetal distress, 734-735
Fetal monitor, care of mother on, 735-737
Fetal monitoring
  external, 736-737
  internal, 737
Fever, scarlet, 792-793
Fibrillation
  atrial, 124, 125
  ventricular, 127-128
Fibrosis, cystic, 802-805
Fine crackles, 222
Finger
  arthroplasty of, 495, 497
  replantation of, 504
Finger puncture sites, 443
First-degree AV block, 129
Fistula, tracheoesophageal, 808-810
  repair of, 810-812
Fixation
  external, for complicated fractures, 502-504
  of hip, internal, 493
  maxillomandibular, 485-486
Flaccid bladder, 537
Flagyl; *see* Metronidazole
Flail chest, 260-261
Flaré, Adria, 703
Fluid(s)
  in alveoli, abnormal accumulation of, 245
  maintenance, calculation of, for child, 866
  in pleural space, 258
  replacement of, for burns, calculation of, 630

Fluid imbalances, 46-49
  and electrolyte imbalances, observation of, 36-48
Fluorouracil; *see* 5-Fluorouracil
5-Fluorouracil, 676-677
  hazards associated with, 670
Flutter, atrial, 123, 124
Follicle-stimulating hormone, 421
Food, drugs to be taken with, 4
Food safeness, temperature for, 196
Foot and ankle burns, positioning with, 629
Foot, leg, and skin care teaching guide for diabetic patient, 448-449
"Football" hold for breast-feeding, 745
Foreign bodies, esophageal, 342
Fracture(s), 483-485
  of cervical spine, 489-491
  complete, 484
  compound, 483
  external fixation for, 502-504
  of head, 302
  hip, surgical repair of, 493
  incomplete, 484
  jaw, repair of, 485-486
  simple, 483
Frame, Stryker, 334
Frontal lobe brain tumors, 300
5-FU; *see* 5-Fluorouracil
Full-thickness burns, 625
Furosemide for child, 867
Fusion, spinal, 487

G

Gaits, crutch-walking, 516
Gallbladder, 394-399
  infection of, 394-396
  stones in, 394-396
  surgery on, 396-397
Gas in pleural space, 252
Gastrectomy, dumping syndrome following, 358
Gastric bypass, 359, 360; *see also* Stomach
Gastroenteritis, 819-820
Gastrointestinal ostomy, tube, or prosthetic valve, care of patient with, 367-370
Gastrointestinal system
  assessment of, 339-342
  of child, 805-822
  hematologic assessment of, 157, 159
Gastroplasty/partitioning, 359, 360
Gastrostomy 367, 368; *see also* Enteral nutrition
Gastrostomy tube, feeding by, 811

Gavage feeding of newborn, intermittent, 778-779
General anesthesia, care of patient in recovery room following, 30
General care and nursing diagnoses, 1-66
General preoperative care/teaching, 29-30
Genital herpes, 598-599
Genitourinary system, 518-593
   assessment of, 518-522
   of child, 830-834
   diagram of, 519-520
   hematologic assessment of, 160
Gentamicin
   ampicillin plus, for endocarditis prophylaxis, 95
   for meningitis, 323
German measles; see Rubella
Gestational age
   large for, 758-759
   small for, 757-758
Girl
   infant, percentile growth chart for, 782
   percentile growth chart for, 786
Gland(s), 420, 421-422; see also specific gland
Glasgow Coma Scale, 288
Glaucoma
   acute (narrow-angle), 632
   adult onset, 632-633
   chronic (wide-angle), 632
Gliomas, 300
Global decompression, 634
Glomerulonephritis, 551-553
   acute, 830-832
Glucagon, 421
   for child, 867
Glucocorticoids, 421
   deficiency of, 457
   excess of, 460
Glucose monitoring, home, teaching guide for, 443
Glucose tests, 444
Glue, abuse of, 325
Glutethimide, abuse of, 325
Gonadal dysfunction from chemotherapy, 696
Gonorrhea, 524-526
Gouty arthritis, 480-481
Graft
   aortofemoral bypass, 81-83
   bypass, coronary artery, 111
   coronary artery, 110
   femoropopliteal bypass, 78
   skin, skinning vulvectomy with, 609, 610

Graft vs. host disease, 189
   clinical grading of severity of, 189
   proposed clinical stage of, 188
Graves' disease, 427
Great vessels, transposition of, 850
Grief, 18
   anticipatory, 18
   dysfunctional, 18-19
   normal stages of, 18
Grieving, dysfunctional, 18-19
Growth chart, percentile
   for boys, 787
   for girls, 786
   for infant boys, 783
   for infant girls, 782
Growth hormone, 421
Growth retardation, intrauterine, 757-758
Guillain-Barré syndrome, 321-323
Gynecologic cesium implants, 708

H

Haemophilus influenzae meningitis, antibiotic therapy for, 323
Hallucinogens
   abuse of, 327
   commonly abused, 325
Hallux valgus, correction of, 510
Halo traction, 333, 511, 512-513
Hand
   burns of, positioning with, 629
   and wrist, range-of-motion exercises of, 299
Hand expression of breast milk, 748
Harrington rod instrumentation for scoliosis, 487
Hashish, abuse of, 325
Head
   fractures of, 302
   and neck
      burns of, positioning with, 628
      cancer of, detection and prevention of, 652-653
Head and neck implants for cancer, 708
Heart
   circulatory system of, 69
   damage to, from chemotherapy, 696-697
   injury to, syndrome following, 114-115
   oxygen saturation in, normal values for, 142
   surgery on, 108-114
      classification of, 108
Heart defects
   congenital, 844-850
   cyanotic, 848-850
   noncyanotic, 844-848

Heart disease
    congenital, repair of, 110, 111
    valvular, 94-98
Heart failure, 101-104
    congestive
        in child, 857-859
        drugs for, 90-93
    vasodilator drugs commonly used for, potential complications of, 90
Heart rate of children, 865-866
Heart surgery, congenital, 850-857
Heart valve, 71
    closure sounds from, transmission of, 71
    replacement of, 110, 111
Height and weight, desirable, 4
Hematologic system, 157-218
    assessment of, 157-161
    disorders of, approach to, clues that might be found for, 161
Hematology
    of child, 834-839
    laboratory values for, normal, 878, 882
Hematoma
    epidural, 303
    subdural, 302
Hemodialysis, 567-571
Hemodynamic monitoring, 141-145
Hemolytic anemia, 165-167
Hemorrhage, postpartum, 749-751
Hemorrhagic cystitis from chemotherapy, 698-699
Hemothorax, 255-256
Heparin
    home record for, 154
    subcutaneous injection of, 152-154
Hepatic; see Liver
Hepatitis
    infectious, 401
    non-A, non-B, 401
    serum, 401
    viral, 401-403
Hepatotoxicity from chemotherapy, 701-702
Hernia
    hiatal, with esophageal reflux, 346-347
    inguinal, incarcerated, 821-822
Herniated disc, 482
Herniorrhaphy, abdominal, 390-391
Heroin, abuse of, 325
Herpes, genital, 598-599
Herpes type 1 viral infection, 622-623
Herpes zoster, 623-625

Herpesvirus in neonate, 771, 772-773
Hespan, 214
Hetastarch, 214
Hiatal hernia with esophageal reflux, 346-347
High birth weight, 758-759
High-risk infant, family-centered care of, 779-780
Hip
    arthroplasty of, 495, 496
    fracture of, surgical repair of, 493
    surgery on, 493-495
Hip spica cast, care of patient in, 515
Hirschsprung's disease, 815-817
HN_2; see Mechlorethamine
Hodgkin's disease, 202-205, 663-664
    staging of, 202
Home glucose monitoring teaching guide, 443
Hopelessness, 16-18
Hormone
    adrenocorticotropic, 421
        excessive secretion of, 460
    antidiuretic, 421
        insufficient secretion of, 456
    follicle-stimulating, 421
    growth, 421
    interstitial cell-stimulating, 421
    luteinizing, 421
    luteotrophic, 421
    parathyroid, 422
        deficiency of, 432-434
        excess of, 434-436
    thyroid
        excess of, 427-430
        lack of, 424-427
    thyroid-stimulating, 421
Hostility
    vs. anger, 21
    excessive, 21-22
Human blood cells, 159
Humerus, traction on, 511, 512
Humidifiers, 230
Humidity and aerosol therapy, 229-230
Hyaline membrane disease, 773-774
Hydatidiform mole, 600-601
Hydralazine, 92
    for child, 867
    and nutrition, 4
    potential complications of, 90
Hydrocephalus, 822-830
    communicating, 822
    noncommunicating, 822

Hydrocortisone sodium succinate for child, 867
Hydromorphone, abuse of, 325
Hydrops, endolymphatic, 639-640
Hyperbilirubinemia in newborn, 761-762
Hypercalcemia, 38-41
Hyperchromic macrocytic anemia, 161-163
Hyperemesis gravidarum, 717-718
Hyperglycemia, 437-440
Hyperglycemic nonketotic coma, hyperosmolar, 440-442
Hyperkalemia, 36-37
Hypermagnesemia, 42-43
Hypernatremia, 40-41
Hyperosmolar hyperglycemic nonketotic coma, 440-442
Hyperparathyroidism, 434-436
Hyperpyrexia from chemotherapy, 703
Hyperreflexive bladder, 537
Hypersensitivity reactions to chemotherapy, 703
Hyperstat; see Diazoxide
Hypertension
 drugs for, 92-93
 portal, portacaval-splenorenal shunts for, 407-410
 pregnancy-induced, 713-716
Hypertensive crisis, 83-85
 drug for, 90
Hyperthyroidism, 427-430
Hypertonic bladder, 537
Hypertrophy, prostatic, 579-580
Hyperuricemia from chemotherapy, 699-700
Hyperventilation, neurologic, central, in neurologic dysfunction, 284
Hypervolemia, 46-47
Hypocalcemia, 38-39
Hypochromic anemia, 163-165
Hypoglycemia, 450-453
Hypoglycemic therapy, oral, teaching guide for, 446
Hypokalemia, 36-39
Hypomagnesemia, 42-45
Hyponatremia, 40-43
Hypoparathyroidism, 432-434
Hypoperfusion, prerenal, 557
Hypophysectomy, 454-456
Hypopituitarism, 453-454
Hypoplastic anemia, 168
Hypothermia, 329-330
Hypothyroidism, 424-427
Hypotonic bladder, 537
Hypoventilatory respiratory failure, 261
Hypovolemia, 46-49
Hypovolemic shock, 104-105, 106
Hypoxemia, oxygen for, 227

Hypoxic respiratory failure, 261
Hysterectomy
 abdominal, total, and bilateral salpingo-oophorectomy, 606-608
 radical, 608-609
 modified, 616-617

I

^{131}I; see Radioactive iodine
ICP; see Intracranial pressure
Identity, personal, 13
 disturbance in, 13-14
IDM; see Infant of diabetic mother
Ileal conduit, 542
Ileal reservoir
 at anus, construction of, 386-387
 capacity of, methods for increasing, 385
 continent, 542, 543
Ileoanal reservoir, 386-388
Ileostomy, 368
 closure of, 387-388
 continent, 382-386
 temporary, 386-387
Ileum, anastomosis of, to anal reservoir, 387-388
Ileus, paralytic, 377-378
Image, body, 10-11
 altered, 11
Imbalance(s)
 acid-base, 44-46
 electrolyte, 36-44
 fluid, 46-49
Implant
 penile, 584-588
 radioactive, for cancer, 708
Implantable drug delivery system, Port-A-Cath, 58
Implanted port, 58-59
Imuran; see Azathioprine
Incarcerated inguinal hernia, 821-822
Incentive spirometer, 281
Incomplete fracture, 484
Incontinence, urinary, 526-528
 female, surgery for, 528-531
Increased intracranial pressure, 331-332
Inderal; see Propranolol
Individual coping, ineffective, 19-20
Indocin; see Indomethacin
Indomethacin, 4
Induction of labor with oxytocin infusion, 733-734
Indwelling urethral catheter, 541
 care of patient with, 540-542

Ineffective individual coping, 19-20
Infant; *see also* Newborn
   of addicted mothers, 767-769
   of diabetic mother, 759-761
   high-risk, family-centered care of, 779-780
   large for gestational age, 758-759
   postterm, 759
   premature, 755
     care of, 755-757
   small for gestational age, 757-758
Infant age-group care, 781
Infant boys, percentile growth chart for, 783
Infant girls, percentile growth chart for, 782
Infarction, myocardial, 87-89
Infection(s)
   of gallbladder, 394-396
   neurologic, 323-325
   TORCH, 771-773
   urinary tract, 522-524
   viral, herpes type 1, 622-623
Infectious hepatitis, 401
Infectious polyneuritis, acute, 321
Infective endocarditis, 93-94
Inflammation
   of alveolar spaces, 243
   of bronchial mucous membrane, 236
   of peritoneal cavity, 372
Inflammatory disease, pelvic, 596-597
Inflatable penile prosthesis, 585
Infusion
   oxytocin, 733-734
   saline or prostaglandin, for abortion, 603-604
Infusion controllers
   drop rate–calibrated, 60
   volumetric, 60
Infusion devices, electronic, 60
Infusion pumps, 60
Inguinal hernia, incarcerated, 821-822
Injection
   chymopapain, 492
   heparin, subcutaneous, 152-154
   insulin, sites for, 444-445
     rotation of, 445
Injury
   cardiac, syndrome following, 114-115
   cervical cord, 304
   cord, 304
   esophageal, 342
   lumbar cord, 305
   potential for, 3

Injury—cont'd
   spinal cord, 304-307
     paralysis from, 335-338
   thoracic cord, 305
Inpatient program for cardiac rehabilitation, 115-118
Insertion
   pacemaker, 134-138
   ventricular shunt, 823-825
Insufficiency
   adrenocortical, 457-460
   arterial, chronic, 77-80
Insulin, 421
   action of, 447
   conventional, 447
   human, 447
   purified, 447
   types of, 445-446
Insulin injection sites, 444-445
   rotation of, 445
Insulin therapy teaching guide, 444-446
Insulin-dependent diabetes mellitus, 839-841
Integumentary system, 618-630
   assessment of, 618-619
   hematologic assessment of, 157
Interaction, social, impaired, 24-28
Interferon, 684-685
Intermittent gavage feeding of newborn, 778-779
Intermittent peritoneal dialysis, 562
Intermittent positive pressure breathing, 280-281
   ventilators for, 279, 280
Intermittent positive pressure ventilator, 280
Internal fetal monitoring, 737
Internal fixation of hip, 493
Interstitial cell-stimulating hormone, 421
Intestinal tube, naso-oral, care of patient with, 388-390
Intestine(s), 370-394
   carcinoma of, 376-377
   obstruction of, 374-376
   surgery on, 380-382
Intolerance, activity, actual or potential, 2
Intoxication, alcohol, 325-326
Intraaortic balloon counterpulsation, 145-148
Intracranial pressure
   increased, 331-332
   monitoring of, 290, 330-331
Intraocular lens transplant, cataract removal with or without, 633
Intrarenal syndrome, 557
Intrauterine catheter, 737
Intrauterine growth retardation, 757-758

Intravascular coagulation, disseminated, 196-198
Intravenous continuous drip narcotics, 64-65
Intravenous drip rates, regulation of, 55
Intraventricular ICP monitoring, 330
Intron A; see Interferon
Intropin; see Dopamine
Intussusception, 822
Iodine, radioactive, 709-710
IPPB; see Intermittent positive pressure breathing
Iridectomy, 633
Iridencleisis, 633
Iron deficiency anemia, 163-165
Irrigation, colostomy, 393
Irritable bowel syndrome, 370-372
Islets of Langerhans, 420, 421
Isoetharine for asthma, 235
Isometric exercises, 517
Isoniazid for meningitis, 323
Isoproterenol
  for asthma, 235
  for child, 867
Isosorbide dinitrate, 91
Isuprel; see Isoproterenol

J

Jaw fracture, repair of, 485-486
Jejunoileal bypass, 359, 360, 361
Jejunostomy; see Enteral nutrition
Jejunostomy-duodenostomy, 367, 368
Jet nebulizers, 229
Joint, facet, rhizotomy of, 487
Joint arthroplasty, total, 495-499
Junctional escape rhythms, 132

K

Keller arthroplasty, 510
Keratophakia, 633
Keratotomy, radial, 633
Ketoacidosis
  in child, 839
  diabetic, 437-440
Keto-Diastic, 444
Ketostix, 444
Kidney
  cancer of, detection and prevention of, 656-657
  damage to, from chemotherapy, 698
  disease of, polycystic, 548-551
  stones in, 553-557
  surgical removal of, 571
  transplant of, 575-579

Kidney failure, 557-562
Kidney function test, normal values for, 877
Knee
  arthroplasty of, 495, 496
  arthroscopic surgery of, 501-502
  meniscus of, surgical removal of, 509
Knowledge deficit, 9-10
Kock's pouch, 382-386, 542, 543
kPa and mm Hg units, equivalent values of, 882
Kwashiorkor, 60

L

La Leche League International, 742
Labor
  active, 728
  augmentation or induction of, with oxytocin infusion, 733-734
  and delivery, care of diabetic mother during, 720-721
  early, 728
  first stage of, care of mother in, 728-732
  preterm (premature), 725-728
  second stage of, care of mother in, 732-733
  transitional, 728
Laboratory studies in cardiovascular assessment, 72
Lamaze review sheet, 730-731
Laminectomy, 487
Langerhans, islets of, 420, 421
Lanoxin; see Digoxin
Large for gestational age infant, 758-759
Large intestine, carcinoma of, 376
Laryngectomy, 266-269
Laryngotracheobronchitis, 788-789, 792-793
Larynx, removal of, 266
Lasix; see Furosemide
Latch-on position for breast-feeding, 748
Lateral sclerosis, amyotrophic, 319-321
Lead, V_1 monitoring, modified, 134
Left ventricular failure, 101, 102
Leg
  amputation of, 499-501
  foot, and skin, teaching guide for care of, by diabetic patient, 448-449
Lens
  contact, removal of, 637
  intraocular, transplant of, cataract removal with or without, 633
  surgical removal of, 633
Lesions, motor neuron, 305
Leukapheresis, 211

Leukemia, 662-663
    acute, 177-181
        in child, 834-837
    lymphoblastic, acute, 177-178
    lymphocytic, acute (ALL), 177-178
    myelogenous, acute, 178
Leukeran; see Chlorambucil
Leukocyte concentrate, 213
    reactions to transfusion of, 217
Leukocytes
    in acute leukemia, 177
    pheresis of, 211
Leukopenia with chemotherapy, 684-687
Levarterenol for child, 867
LeVeen shunt, 403-405
Levine tube, 365, 366
Levophed; see Levarterenol
LH; see Luteinizing hormone
Lidocaine for child, 867
Ligation
    and stripping, vein, 76-77
    tubal, 604-605
Linear equivalents, 877
Linear fracture of head, 302
Linton tube, 352, 353
    care of patient with, 352-354
Lip, cleft, repair of, 805-806
Liquid equivalents for medications, 876
Lithotripsy
    extracorporeal shock wave, 554-555
    percutaneous ultrasonic, 555
Liver, 399-412
    biopsy of, 412
    carcinoma of, 410-412
    damage to, from chemotherapy, 701-702
    surgery on, 406-407
Lobe(s) of lung, removal of, 269
Lobectomy, 269-271
Lomustine, 674-675
Long-term venous access devices, 57-59
Lou Gehrig's disease, 319
Low birth weight, 757-758
Low-bacterial diet, 195
Lower motor neuron bladder, 537
Lower motor neuron lesions, 305
LSD, abuse of, 325, 327
Lufyllin; see Dyphylline
Lumbar cord injuries, 305
Lumbar puncture, 329
Luminal; see Phenobarbital

Lung
    cancer of, detection and prevention of, 653-654
    disease of, chronic obstructive, 230-233
    lobe(s) of, removal of, 269
    removal of, 269
Lupus erythematosus, systemic, 476-479
Lupus Foundation of America, Inc., 479
Luteinizing hormone, 421
Luteotrophic hormone, 421
Lymphadenectomy, vulvectomy with, 609, 610-611
Lymphangiography, 208
Lymphatic system
    diagram of, 158
    x-ray visualization of, 208
Lymphoblastic leukemia, acute, 177-178
Lymphoblasts, proliferative, 177-178
Lymphocyte, 159
Lymphocytic leukemia, acute (ALL), 177-178
Lymphoma
    malignant, 205-206
    non-Hodgkin's, 205
Lymphosarcoma, 205

M

Macrocytic anemia, hyperchromic, 161-163
Macrodantin; see Nitrofurantoin
Magnesium
    deficit of, 42-45
    excess of, 42-43
Maintenance fluid requirement calculation, pediatric, 866
Malignant lymphoma, 205-206
Malnutrition, 59-60
Manipulative behavior, 25-26
Mannitol for child, 867
Marasmic kwashiorkor, 60
Marasmus, 60
Marijuana, abuse of, 325
Marrow, bone
    study of, 209
    transplantation of, 181-196
        schedule for, 182
Marshall-Marchetti-Kranz procedure for urinary incontinence, 528
Mask, oxygen, for oxygen therapy, 229
Mass equivalents for medications, 876
MAST; see Military antishock trousers
Matulane; see Procarbazine
Maturational crises, 19
Maxillomandibular fixation, 485-486
Mayo arthroplasty, 510

Measles; *see* Rubella; Rubeola
Mechanical ventilation, continuous, 277-280
    care of patient on, 277-279
Mechlorethamine, 672-673, 704
    hazards with, 670
Meconium aspiration syndrome, 774-775
Medical-surgical care, 876-882
Medications; *see* Drug(s)
Medium crackles, 222
Megacolon, aganglionic, 815-817
Melphalan, 674-675
Membrane
    mucous; *see* Mucous membrane
    premature rupture of, 721-722
Menière's syndrome, 639-640
Meningiomas, 301
Meningitis, 323, 828-830
    antibiotic therapy in, 323
Meningiococcal meningitis, antibiotics for, 323
Menisectomy
    closed, 509
    open, 509-510
Menopause, 599-600
Meperidine
    abuse of, 325
    for child, 868
Mephenytoin for seizure disorders, 292
Meprobamate, abuse of, 325
Mercaptopurine, 676-677
6-Mercaptopurine, 676-677
Mesantoin; *see* Mephenytoin
Mescaline, abuse of, 325, 327
Metabolic acidosis, 46-47
Metabolic alkalosis, 46-47
Metaprel; *see* Metaproterenol
Metaproterenol for asthma, 235
Metaramine; *see* Metaraminol
Metaraminol for child, 867
Methadone, abuse of, 325
Methicillin for meningitis, 323
Methimazole, 429
Methotrexate, 676-677
    hazards associated with, 671
    and nutrition, 4
Methsuximide for seizure disorders, 292
Methyl CCNU; *see* Semustin
Methylphenidate, abuse of, 325
Methylprednisolone for child, 867
Metric conversions, 877
Metronidazole, 4

Mexate; *see* Methotrexate
MI; *see* Myocardial infarction
Microcytic anemia, 163-165
Microsurgical dorsal root rhizotomy, 487
Mild anxiety, 14
Military antishock trousers, 148-150
Milk, breast, hand expression of, 748
Miller-Abbott tube, 388, 389
    care of patient with, 388-390
Mineral oil and nutrition, 4
Mineralocorticoids, 421
    deficiency of, 457
    overproduction of, 462
Minocycline for meningitis, 323
Mithracin; *see* Mithramycin
Mithramycin, 680-681, 704
    hazards associated with, 671
Mitomycin, 680-681, 704
    hazards associated with, 671
Mitomycin C; *see* Mitomycin
Mitral regurgitation, 95, 96
Mitral stenosis, 95, 96
Mitral valve replacement, 111
mm Hg and kPa units, equivalent values for, 882
Mobility, physical, impaired, 2-3
Mobitz type I block, 129-130
Mobitz type II block, 130
Moderate anxiety, 14-15
Modified radical mastectomy, 616-617
Modified V_1 monitoring lead, 134
Mole, hydatidiform, 600-601
Monitor, fetal, care of mother on, 735-737
Monitoring
    fetal
        external, 736-737
        internal, 737
    glucose, home, teaching guide for, 443
    hemodynamic, 141-145
    intracranial pressure, 290, 330-331
    tissue pressure, 507-509
Monitoring lead, V_1, modified, 134
Monocyte, 159
Mothers
    addicted, infants of, 767-769
    care of, 711-751
    diabetic
        care of
            during labor and delivery, 720-721
            during last trimester of pregnancy, 719-720
        infant of, 759-761

Mothers—cont'd
    on fetal monitor, care of, 735-737
    in first stage of labor, care of, 728-732
    in second stage of labor, care of, 732-733
Motor neuron lesions, 305
Mould, radium therapy sealed in, care of patient receiving, 614-616
Moxalactam for meningitis, 323
MTX; see Methotrexate
Mucositis, 692
    from chemotherapy, 692-693
Mucous membrane
    bronchial, inflammation of, 236
    oral, alteration in, actual or potential, 1-2
Multifocal premature ventricular contractions, 126
Multilumen subclavian catheters, 56-57
Multiple myeloma, 198-202
Multiple sclerosis, 313-315
Mumps, 792-793
Murmurs, valvular heart disease, 95
Musculoskeletal system, 470-517
    assessment of, 470-472
    hematologic assessment of, 160
Mustargen; see Mechlorethamine
Mutamycin; see Mitomycin
Myasthenia gravis, 315-317
Myasthenia gravis crisis, 317-318
Myasthenia Gravis Foundation, Inc., 317
Mycobacterium tuberculosis, 248
Myelitis, 323
Myeloblasts, proliferation of, 178
Myelogenous leukemia, acute, 178
Myeloma, multiple, 198-202
Myelomeningocele, 825-828
Myelosuppression from chemotherapy, 684-690
Myleran; see Busulfan
Myocardial infarction, 87-89
Myringotomy with tube insertion, 641-642
Mysoline; see Primidone
Myxedema, 424-427

N

Nafcillin for meningitis, 323
Naloxone for child, 867
Narcan; see Naloxone
Narcotics
    abuse of, 326-327
    commonly abused, 325
    continuous drip, intravenous, 64-65
Narrow-angle glaucoma, 632

Nasal catheter for oxygen therapy, 229
Nasogastric tube, 365, 366
    care of patient with, 365-367
Nasogastric tube feeding; see Enteral nutrition
Naso-oral intestinal tube, care of patient with, 388-390
Nasopharyngeal airway, 272-273
Nasotracheal tube, 273-275
National Parkinson's Foundation hotline, 312
Nausea and vomiting from chemotherapy, 690-692
NCAST Program, 779
Nebulizers
    jet, 229
    ultrasonic, 229-230
NEC; see Necrotizing enterocolitis
Neck
    dissection of, radical, 266-269
    and head
        burns of, 628
        cancer of, detection and prevention of, 652-653
        implants of, for cancer, 708
Necrotizing enterocolitis, 769-770
Neglect, child, 861
Nembutal; see Pentobarbital
Neomycin and nutrition, 4
Neonatal/perinatal standards, 711-781
Neonate; see Newborn
Nephrectomy, 554, 571-575
Nephrolithotomy, 554
Nephrolithotripsy, 554
Nephrosis, 832-834
Nephrostomy, percutaneous, 554
Nephrotic syndrome, 832-834
Nephrotoxicity from chemotherapy, 698
Nerve(s)
    cranial, functions of, 286
    damage to, from chemotherapy, 700-701
Nerve stimulation, transcutaneous electrical, 65-66
Nervous system, diagram of, 284
Neurogenic bladder, 537-540
Neurogenic hyperventilation, central, in neurologic dysfunction, 284
Neurologic diagnostic procedures, 288
Neurologic dysfunction, patterns of respiration in, 284
Neurologic infections, 323-325
Neurologic patient, general rehabilitative care of, 334-335
Neurologic system, 283-338
    assessment of, 283-287
    hematologic assessment of, 160
Neuromas, acoustic, 301
Neurotoxicity from chemotherapy, 700-701

Neutrophil, 159
Newborn, 751-780; *see also* Infant
   care of, 751-755
   with endotracheal tube, care of, 775-776
   exchange transfusion of, 763-764
   hyperbilirubinemia in, 761-762
   immediate stabilization of, at delivery, 753
   intermittent gavage feeding of, 778-779
   phototherapy for, 762-763
   respiratory distress syndrome (hyaline membrane disease) in, 773-774
   sepsis in, 765-767
   TORCH infection in, 771-773
   umbilical catheterization of, 765
   on ventilator, care of, 776-777
Nifedipine, 92-93
   potential complications of, 90
Nitrates, 91-92
   potential complications of, 90
Nitrofurantoin, 4
Nitrogen mustard; *see* Mechlorethamine
Nitroglycerin, 91
   potential complications of, 90
Nitrosoureas, 674-675
Non-A, non-B hepatitis, 401
Noncommunicating hydrocephalus, 822
Noncyanotic heart defects, 844-848
Non-Hodgkin's lymphoma, 205
Nonrebreathing mask for oxygen therapy, 229
Nonstress test, 737-738
Nonvolumetric devices, 60
Norepinephrine, 421
Norisodrine; *see* Isoproterenol
North American Nursing Diagnosis Association, 1
NST; *see* Nonstress test
Nursing care
   general, and nursing diagnoses, 1-66
   of patient
      with central venous catheter, 55-59
      in recovery room, 30-31
   during stages of labor, 33-34
   standards of
      related to behavioral dysfunction/nursing diagnoses, 10-28
      related to nursing diagnoses, 1-10
Nursing Child Assessment Satellite Training Program, 779
Nursing diagnoses
   general care and, 1-66
   NANDA-approved, 1-28
   related to behavioral dysfunctions, 10-28

Nursing diagnoses—cont'd
   standards of care related to, 1-10
Nutrition
   alterations in, 3-5
   for child, 866
   enteral, 34-51
   knowledge deficit related to, 64
   parenteral, total, 51-55
   venous
      central, 53
      peripheral, 51, 53
Nutritional status, drug effects on, 4

O

Obesity, surgical intervention for, 359-364
Obstruction
   biliary, 394-396
   intestinal, 374-376
Obstructive lung disease, chronic, 230-233
Obstructive pulmonary disease, chronic, 230-233
   disability scale for, 242
Occipital lobe brain tumors, 300
Ohio 560 ventilator, 277
Ointments, eye, instillation of, 637-638
Oncology, 646-710
   assessment in, 646-651
Oncovin; *see* Vincristine sulfate
Open menisectomy, 509-510
Open-heart surgery, 108-114
   in child, 854-857
Opiates, abuse of, 326-327
Opium, abuse of, 325
Optic system, 631-638
   and auditory system, 631-645
Oral cavity, disruption of, 1-2
Oral contraceptives and nutrition, 4
Oral hypoglycemic therapy teaching guide, 446
Oral mucous membrane, alteration in, actual or potential, 1-2
Oral rehydration therapy, 821
Orchiectomy for testicular tumor, 591-593
Orchiopexy, 589-591
Organic solvents, commonly abused, 325
Orinase; *see* Tolbutamide
Orogastric tube feeding; *see* Enteral nutrition
Oropharyngeal airway, 272
Orthopedic sepsis, 474-475
Osteomyelitis, acute, 474-475
Osteoporosis, 481-482
Osteosarcoma, 475-476

Ostomy, 391
    management and care of, 391-393
    upper GI, care of patient with, 367-370
Ovary(ies)
    cancer of, detection and prevention of, 660-661
    dysfunction of, from chemotherapy, 696
    as endocrine organ, 420
    surgical removal of, 606, 608
Overflow incontinence, 526
Oxtriphylline for asthma, 235
Oxycodone, abuse of, 325
Oxygen mask for oxygen therapy, 229
Oxygen saturation in heart, normal values for, 142
Oxygen therapy, 227-229
Oxytocin, 421
    infusion of, 733-734

P

^{32}P; see Phosphorus, radioactive
PAB; see Pulmonary artery banding
PAC; see Premature atrial contractions
Pacemaker, 134
    artificial, temporary, in child, 860
    insertion of, 134-138
    permanent, 136, 137
    temporary, 134, 135, 136, 137
    ventricular, 135
Pain
    back, low, 482-483
    chronic or acute, 8-9
Painful respiration, 220
Palate, cleft, repair of, 806-808
Pancreas, 413-418
    carcinoma of, 417-418
    inflammation of, 413-414
    surgery on, 414-416
Pancreatectomy, 414
Pancreatitis, acute or chronic, 413-414
Pancreatoduodenectomy, 414
Pancytopenia from aplastic anemia, 168
Panic, 16
PAP; see Pulmonary artery pressure
Paracentesis, 405
    for ascites, care of patient undergoing, 405-406
Paradione; see Paramethadione
Paragangliomas, 464
Paraldehyde for child, 867
Paralysis from spinal cord injury, 335-338
Paralytic ileus, 377-378
Paramethadione for seizure disorders, 292

Paraplegia, 335-336
Parathyroid glands, 420, 422
    surgical removal of, 436-437
Parathyroid hormone, 422
    deficiency of, 432
    excess of, 434-436
Parathyroidectomy, 436-437
Parenteral nutrition, total, 51-55
Parietal lobe brain tumors, 300
Parkinson's disease, 310-313
Paroxysmal atrial tachycardia, 124-125
Partial placenta previa, 722
Partial rebreathing mask for oxygen therapy, 229
Partial-thickness burns, 625
Passive motion device, continuous, 517
PAT; see Paroxysmal atrial tachycardia
Patent ductus arteriosus, 844
Patient care planning, guidelines for, 883-887
Patient position, degrees of, 74
PCWP; see Pulmonary capillary wedge pressure
PDA: see Patent ductus arteriosus
Pearson's attachment, Thomas' splint and, balanced suspension with, 511, 512
Pectoriloquy, whispered, 223
Pediatrics, 781-868
Pelvic exenteration, 612-614
Pelvic inflammatory disease, 596-597
Pelvic traction, 511, 512
Pelvis, cancer of, detection and prevention of, 656-657
Penicillin
    for endocarditis prophylaxis, 95
    and nutrition, 4
Penicillin G for meningitis, 323
Penile implant, 584-588
Pentobarbital for child, 868
Peptic ulcer disease, 354-355
Percentile growth chart
    for boys, 787
    for girls, 786
    for infant boys, 783
    for infant girls, 782
Percutaneous kidney stone dissolution, 554
Percutaneous nephrostomy, 554
Percutaneous transluminal angioplasty, 138-140
Percutaneous ultrasonic lithotripsy, 555
Pereya procedure for urinary incontinence, 528
Perforated appendix, 813-815
Pericardiocentesis, 99-100
Pericarditis, 98-99
Perinatal/neonatal standards, 711-781

INDEX

Peripheral vascular assessment, 73-74
Peripheral venous nutrition, 51, 53
Peritoneal cavity, inflammation of, 372
Peritoneal dialysis, 562-567
    continuous ambulatory, 562-563
    continuous cycling, 563
    intermittent, 562
Peritoneal-jugular shunt for ascites, continuous, 403-405
Peritonitis, 372-373
Permanent pacemaker, 136, 137
Pernicious anemia, 161-163
Personal identity, 13
    disturbances in, 13-14
Pertussis, 790-791, 795-796
Phencyclidine, abuse of, 325, 327
Phenobarbital
    for child, 867
    for seizure disorders, 292
Phenomenon
    coup-contracoup, 302
    Wenckebach's, 129-130
Phenylbutazone, 4
Phenytoin, 4
    for seizure disorders, 292
Pheochromocytoma, 464-465
Pheresis, 209-218
    red cell, 214
Phlebitis, 74
Phlebothrombosis, 74
Phonotransducer, 736-373
Phosphorus, radioactive, 709
Photocoagulation, retinal, 633
Phototherapy of newborn, 762-763
Physical abuse of child, 860-861
Physical mobility, impaired, 2-3
Physical neglect of child, 861
PID; *see* Pelvic inflammatory disease
PIH; *see* Pregnancy-induced hypertension
Pituitary gland, 420, 421
    adenomas of, 301
    anterior, hormones of, decrease in, 453
    surgical removal of, 454-456
Placenta, premature separation of, 723
Placenta previa, 722-723
Plasma, 213
    pheresis of, 209-211
    reaction to transfusion of, 217
Plasmapheresis, 209-211
Platelet concentrate, 214
Plateletpheresis, 211

Platelets, 159
    pheresis of, 211
    problems with, causing thrombocytopenia, 175
    reactions to transfusions of, 217
Platinol; *see* Cisplatin
Pleura, opening in, 254
Pleural cavity, pus in, 256
Pleural effusion, 258-259
Pleural friction rub, 222
Pleural space
    air or gas in, 252
    blood in, 255
    fluid in, 258
    removal of air or fluid from, 225
Pneumatic trousers, 148-150
Pneumococcal meningitis, antibiotic therapy for, 323
Pneumonectomy, 269-271
Pneumonia, 243-245
    pediatric, 796-798
Pneumothorax, 252-254
    tension, 254-255
Podophyllotoxins, 678-679
    hazards associated with, 671
Poliomyelitis, 792-793
Polycystic kidney disease, 548-551
Polycythemia, 173-175
    relative, 173
    secondary, 173
Polycythemia vera, 173
Polymorphous ventricular tachycardia, 128-129
Polyneuritis, infectious, acute, 321
Polyradiculitis, 321
Port, implanted, 58-59
Port-A-Cath implantable drug delivery system, 58
Portacaval shunts, 407-410
Portal cirrhosis, 399-401
Portal hypertension, portacaval-splenorenal shunts for, 407-410
Position, patient, degrees of, 74
Positive pressure breathing, intermittent, 280-281
Positive pressure ventilator
    intermittent, 280
    pressure-limited, 277, 279
    volume-cycled, 277, 279-280
Post–cardiac injury syndrome, 114-115
Postcardiotomy, 114
Posterior pelvic exenteration, 612
Postgastrectomy syndrome, 358
Posthyperventilation apnea in neurologic dysfunction, 284
Postmaturity, 759

Postmyocardial infarction syndrome, 114
Postnecrotic cirrhosis, 399-401
Postpartum care, 739-743
Postpartum hemorrhage, 749-751
Postrenal syndrome, 557
Postterm infant, 759
Potassium
  deficit of, 36-39
  excess of, 36-37
Pouch, Kock's, 382-386, 542, 543
PR interval, 119
Prazosin, 92
  potential complications of, 90
Prednisolone, 4
Preeclampsia; see Pregnancy-induced hypertension
Preexcitation, ventricular, 132-133
Pregnancy
  last trimester of, care of diabetic mother during, 719-720
  tubal, and salpingectomy, 605-606
Pregnancy-induced hypertension, 713-716
Premature atrial beats, 122
Premature atrial contractions, 122-123
Premature infant, 755
  care of, 755-757
Premature labor, 725-728
Premature rupture of membranes, 721-722
Premature separation of placenta, 723
Premature ventricular contractions, 125-126
  multifocal, 126
Premenstrual syndrome, 599
Preoperative care/teaching, general, 29-30
Preparation phase before bone marrow transplantation, 182-184
Prerenal hypoperfusion, 557
Preschool-age child care, 784-785
Prescribed exercise program for cardiac rehabilitation, 118-119
Pressure
  intracranial
    increased, 331-332
    monitoring of, 290, 330-331
  pulmonary artery, 141, 144, 145
  pulmonary capillary wedge, 141, 144, 145
  tissue, monitoring of, 507-509
Pressure ulcer, 619-621
Pressure wave forms, 144
  problems associated with, 141
Pressure-limited positive pressure ventilator, 277, 279
Preterm labor, 725-728

Primary aldosteronism, 462-464
Primatene; see Epinephrine
Primidone for seizure disorders, 292
Prinzmetal's variant angina, drug for, 92-93
Procainamide for child, 867
Procarbazine, 682-683
Proctocolectomy, 382
Progesterone, 422
Progressive systemic sclerosis, 479-480
Prolactin, 421
Prolapsed umbilical cord, 724-725
PROM; see Premature rupture of membranes
Prone position, 297
Pronestyl; see Procainamide
Propranolol for child, 868
Propylthiouracil, 429
Prostaglandin infusion for abortion, 603-604
Prostate gland
  cancer of, detection and prevention of, 658
  hypertrophy of, 579-580
  infection of, 522
  surgical removal of, 580-584
  transurethral resection of, 580
Prostatectomy, 580-584
  retropubic, 580, 581
    radical, 581
  suprapubic, 580, 581
Prostatitis, 522
Prosthetic valve, upper GI, care of patient with, 367-370
Proventil; see Albuterol
Pseudomonas meningitis, antibiotic therapy for, 323
Psilocybin, abuse of, 325
Psychologic responses in cardiovascular assessment, 69
PTCA; see Percutaneous transluminal angioplasty
PTH; see Parathyroid hormone
PUL; see Percutaneous ultrasonic lithotripsy
Pulmonary artery banding, 852
Pulmonary artery pressure, 141, 144, 145
Pulmonary capillary wedge pressure, 141, 144, 145
Pulmonary catheter, triple-lumen balloon-tipped, 144
Pulmonary disease, chronic obstructive, 230-233
  disability scale for, 242
Pulmonary edema, 245-246
Pulmonary embolism, 247-248
Pulmonary rehabilitation, 242-248
Pulmonary toxicity from chemotherapy, 697
Pulmonary tuberculosis, 248-250
Pulmonic stenosis, 848
Pump
  balloon, 145-148

Pump—cont'd
 infusion, 60
Puncture
 finger, sites for, 443
 lumbar, 329
Pupil response, variations in, 287
Purinethol; see Mercaptopurine
Pus in pleural cavity, 256
PVC; see Premature ventricular contractions
Pyelolithotomy, 554
Pyelonephritis, 522
Pyloric stenosis, 812-813
Pyogenic arthritis, acute, 474-475
Pyridoxine for child, 868

Q

Quadriplegia, 336-338
QRS interval, 119
QT interval, 119

R

Radial keratotomy, 633
Radical hysterectomy, modified, 608-609, 616-617
Radical neck dissection, 266-269
Radical retropubic prostatectomy, 581
Radioactive chemotherapy, unsealed, 709-710
Radioactive iodine, 709-710
Radioactive phosphorus, 709
Radiotherapy for cancer, 705-708
Radium therapy sealed in mould, afterloader, colpostat, or Ernst applicator, care of patient receiving, 614-616
Rales, 222
Range-of-motion exercises, 517
 of shoulder and elbow, 299
 of wrist and hand, 299
Reconditioning, cardiovascular
 initial postdischarge activities for, 118-119
 program of, 119
Recovery room, patient in, care of, 30-31
Rectal surgery, 393-394
Red blood cells, 159, 212
 defective, production of, 161-165
 increased numbers of, 173-175
 pheresis of, 214, 218
 rapid destruction of, 165-167
 reactions to transfusion of, 215, 216
Reed-Sternberg cells, 202
Reflex bladder, 537
Reflex incontinence, 526
Reflex responses, classification of, 285
Reflux, esophageal, hiatal hernia with, 346-347
Regional enteritis, 370-372
Regurgitation
 aortic, 95, 96
 mitral, 95, 96
Rehabilitation
 cardiac, 115-119
 pulmonary, 242-243
Rehabilitative care of neurologic patient, general, 334-335
Rehydration therapy, oral, 821
Rejection, classification of, 575
Relative polycythemia, 173
Renal calculi, 553-557
Renal failure, 557-562
Replantation, digital, 504-506
Reproductive system, female, 594-617
 assessment of, 594-596
 diagram of, 595
Resection of prostate, transurethral, 580
Reserpine, 4
 for child, 868
Resistance, vascular, systemic, calculation of, 107
Respiration
 apneustic, in neurologic dysfunction, 284
 ataxic, 220
 Biot's, 220
  in neurologic dysfunction, 284
 Cheyne-Stokes, 220
  in neurologic dysfunction, 284
 of child, 866
 normal, 220
 painful, 220
 patterns of, 220
  in neurologic dysfunction, 284
 sighing, 220
Respiratory acidosis, 44-45
Respiratory alkalosis, 44-45
Respiratory distress syndrome, 773-774
 adult, 263-266
Respiratory failure, 261-263
Respiratory findings, normal, 221
Respiratory system, 219-281
 assessment of, 219-224
 of child, 788-805
 diagram of, 220
 hematologic assessment of, 160
Response
 pupil, variation in, 287
 reflex, classification of, 285
Retardation, growth, intrauterine, 757-758

Retention, urinary, acute, 534-536
Retinal cryopexy, 633
Retropubic prostatectomy, 580, 581
   radical, 581
Rheumatoid arthritis, 472-474
Rhizotomy
   dorsal root, microsurgical, 487
   facet joint, 487
Rhonchi, 222
Rhythms
   atrioventricular junctional escape, 132
   ECG, 119-134
      of atrial origin, 122-125
      nursing diagnosis/goals/interventions for, 134
      of sinus origin, 119-122
      of ventricular origin, 125-129
   sinus, normal, 119, 120
Rifampin for meningitis, 323
Right ventricular failure, 101, 102
Ritalin; *see* Methylphenidate
Rod, Harrington, for scoliosis, 487
Roferon; *see* Interferon
Role performance, 12-13
   disturbance in, 13
Roles, 12-13
ROM exercises; *see* Range-of-motion exercises
Roseola infantum, 790-791
Rub, pleural friction, 222
Rubella, 790-791
   congenital, 790-791
   in neonate, 771
Rubeola, 790-791
Rubidomycin; *see* Daunorubicin
Rupture of membranes, premature, 721-722
Ruptured appendix, 813-815

S

Safeness, food, temperature for, 196
Salem sump tube, 365, 366
Saline infusion for abortion, 603-604
Salpingectomy, tubal pregnancy and, 605-606
Salpingo-oophorectomy, bilateral, total abdominal hysterectomy and, 606-608
Saphenous vein, ligation and stripping of, 76-77
Sarcoidosis, 250-252
Saturation, oxygen, in heart, normal values for, 142
Scarlatina; *see* Scarlet fever
Scarlet fever, 792-793
School-age child care, 785, 788
Scleral buckling, 633

Scleroderma, 479-480
Sclerosis
   lateral, amyotrophic, 319-321
   multiple (disseminated), 313-315
   systemic, progressive, 479-480
Sclerotomy, 633
Scoliosis, Harrington rod instrumentation for, 487
Scopolamine, abuse of, 325
Secondary polycythemia, 173
Second-degree AV block, 129, 130
Secretions, aspiration of, 226-227
Seizures, 291-293
   classification of, 291
   drugs used for, 292
Self-catheterization procedure, 535-536
Self-concept, 10
   disturbance in, 10-14
Self-directed violence, potential for, 20-21
Self-esteem, 12
Semustin, 674-675
Sengstaken-Blakemore tube, 352, 353
   care of patient with, 352-354
Separation of placenta, premature, 723
Sepsis
   neonatal, 765-767
   orthopedic, 474-475
Septal defect
   atrial, 845
   ventricular, 845-846
Septic shock, 104; *see also* Vasogenic shock
Septostomy, balloon, 851
Serpasil; *see* Reserpine
Serum albumin, normal, 214
   reactions to transfusions of, 217
Serum hepatitis, 401
Severe anxiety, 15-16
Sexual abuse of child, 861
Shingles, 623-625
Shock
   anaphylactic, 104; *see also* Shock, vasogenic
   cardiogenic, 104, 105-106
   denial and, by dying patient, 33-34
   hypovolemic, 104-105, 106
   septic, 104; *see also* Shock, vasogenic
   synchronized, 150
   vasogenic, 104, 105, 106
   warm, 104; *see also* Shock, vasogenic
Shock syndrome, 104-108
   signs of, 104
Shock trousers, 148-150

Shock wave lithotripsy, extracorporeal, 554-555
Short bowel syndrome, 373-374
Shoulder
  arthroplasty of, 495, 496
  and elbow, range-of-motion exercises of, 299
Shunt
  Blalock-Taussig, 852
  continuous peritoneal-jugular, for ascites, 403-405
  LeVeen, 403-405
  portacaval-splenorenal, for portal hypertension, 407-410
  ventricular, insertion of, 823-825
  ventriculoatrial, 824
SI units for blood components, conversion factor for, 880-881
Sibilant wheezes, 222
Sick day rules for diabetic patient, 446-448
Sickle cell crises, 837-839
Sickle cell disease, 837
Side arm traction, 511, 512
Side-lying position, 297
  for breast-feeding, 745
Sighing respiration, 220
Silastic atrial catheter, 57-58
Simple fracture, 483
Simple oxygen mask for oxygen therapy, 229
Sinus arrest, 121-122
Sinus arrhythmia, 121, 122
Sinus bradycardia, 119, 120, 121
Sinus origin, ECG rhythms of, 119-122
Sinus rhythm, normal, 119, 120
Sinus tachycardia, 121
Situational crises, 19
Skeletal traction, 511, 512
Skin
  alteration in, 1
  cancer of, detection and prevention of, 652
  integrity of, impairment of, actual or potential, 1
  reactions of, to chemotherapy, 703-704
  traction on, 511-512
Skin, foot, and leg care teaching guide for diabetic patient, 448-449
Skin graft, skinning vulvectomy with, 609, 610
Skinning vulvectomy with skin graft, 609, 610
Skull tongs, 333
SLE; see Systemic lupus erythematosus
Sleep pattern disturbances, 5
Small for date infant, 757-758
Small for gestational age infant, 757-758
Small intestine, carcinoma of, 376
Soave procedure, 817

Social crises, 19
Social interaction, impaired, 24-28
Sodium
  deficit of, 40-43
  excess of, 40-41
Sodium bicarbonate for child, 868
Sodium diphenylhydantoin; see Phenytoin
Sodium iodide, 429
Sodium nitroprusside, 90
Solu-Cortef; see Hydrocortisone sodium succinate
Solu-Medrol; see Methylprednisolone
Solvents, organic, commonly abused, 325
Somatotropin, 421
Sonorous wheeze, 222
Sounds
  breath and voice, 222-223
  closure, from heart valves, transmission of, 71
Spasm, coronary artery, drug for, 92-93
Spermatic cord, torsion of, 588-589
Sphincter, urinary, artificial, 531-534
Spinal anesthesia, care of patient in recovery room following, 30-31
Spinal cord injuries, 304-307
  paralysis from, 335-338
Spinal column, diagram of, 285
Spinal fusion, 487
Spinal surgery, 487-489
Spinal tap, 329
Spiral electrode for fetal monitoring, 737
Spiritual distress, potential for, 6-7
Spirometer, incentive, 281
Spleen, removal of, 206
Splenectomy, 206-208
Splenorenal shunts, 407-410
Splint, Thomas', and Pearson's attachment, balanced suspension with, 511, 512
Spondylitis, ankylosing, 491-492
Standards of care
  related to behavioral dysfunctions/nursing diagnoses, 10-28
  related to nursing diagnoses, 1-10
Stapedectomy, 640-641
Staphylococcal meningitis, antibiotic therapy for, 323
Stapling of stomach for obesity, 359
Stenosis
  aortic, 95, 96, 847-848
  mitral, 95, 96
  pulmonic, 848
  pyloric, 812-813

Stimulants
    abuse of, 327
    commonly abused, 325
Stimulation, nerve, transcutaneous electrical, 65-66
Stomach, 354-370
    bleeding of, 355-357
    cancer of, detection and prevention of, 654-655
    carcinoma of, 364-365
    endoscopy of, 352
    stapling of, for obesity, 359
    surgery on, 357-358
    ulcers of, 354
Stomatitis, 692
    from chemotherapy, 692-693
Stones
    in gallbladder, 394-396
    kidney, 553-557
Streptococcal meningitis, antibiotic therapy for, 323
Streptomycin for meningitis, 323
Streptozocin, 682-683, 704
Stress incontinence, 526
Stress test, contraction, 738-739
Stricture, esophageal, 343-344
Stripping, vein ligation and, 76-77
Stroke, 294
Stryker frame, 334
ST-T segment changes, 86
Subarachnoid method of ICP monitoring, 330
Subclavian catheters, multilumen, 56-57
Subcutaneous heparin injection, 152-154
Subdural hematoma, 302
Substance abuse, 325-329
    chemical, 326-329
Subtotal thyroidectomy, 430
Suicidal behavior, 20
Suicide, potential for, 20-21
Sulfonylureas for diabetes, 446
Supine position, 297
Suprapubic prostatectomy, 580, 581
Surgery
    biliary, 396-397
    cardiac, 108-114
        congenital, 850-857
    closed-heart, 108
        in child, 852-854
    esophageal, 349-350
    eye, 633-635
    for female urinary incontinence, 528-531
    gastric, 357-358
    hepatic, 406-407

Surgery—cont'd
    hip, 493-495
    intestinal, 380-382
    of knee, arthroscopic, 501-502
    open-heart, 108-114
        in child, 854-857
    pancreatic, 414-416
    rectal, 393-394
Surgical excision of chest wall, 269
Surgical intervention
    of central nervous system, 307-309
    for obesity, 359-364
Surgical removal
    of adrenal glands, 465-467
    of disc, 487
    of disc lamina, 487
    of eye globe, 633
    of kidney, 571
    of larynx, 266
    of lens, 633
    of lobe of lung, 269
    of lung, 269
    of meniscus of knee joint, 509-510
    of parathyroid glands, 436-437
    of part of leg, 499
    of pituitary gland, 454-456
    of prostate gland, 580-584
    of spleen, 206
    of thyroid, 430
    of uterus, cervix, fallopian tubes, and ovaries, 606, 608
    of vulva, 609
Suspension, balanced, with Thomas' splint and Pearson's attachment, 511, 512
Swan-Ganz catheter, 141, 143, 144, 145
Swenson procedure, 817
Sympathomimetics for asthma, 235
Synchronized shock, 150
Syndrome
    compartmental, 506-507
        diagnoses of, 507-509
    Cushing's, 460-462
    Dressler's, 114
    dumping, 358-359
    Guillain-Barré, 321-323
    intrarenal, 557
    irritable bowel, 370-372
    meconium aspiration, 774-775
    Menière's, 639-640
    nephrotic, 832-834
    post–cardiac injury, 114-115

Syndrome—cont'd
  postmyocardial infarction, 114
  postrenal, 557
  premenstrual, 599
  respiratory distress, 773-774
    adult, 263-266
  shock, 104-108
    signs of, 104
  short bowel, 373-374
  toxic shock, 597-598
  Wolff-Parkinson-White, 132-133
Syphilis, congenital, 770-771
Systemic lupus erythematosus, 476-479
Systemic sclerosis, progressive, 479-480
Systemic vascular resistance, calculation of, 107

T

T tube, 397
  care of patient with, 397-398
Tabetic bladder, 537
Tachycardia
  atrial, paroxysmal, 124-125
  sinus, 121
  ventricular, 126-127
    polymorphous, 128-129
Tamponade, cardiac, 100-101
Tap, spinal, 329
Teaching
  of diabetic patient, 442-450
  preoperative, general, 29-30
Tegretol; see Carbamazepine
Temperature
  body, potential alteration in, 7-8
  of child, 865
  for food safeness, 196
Temporal lobe brain tumors, 300
Temporary artificial pacemaker in child, 860
Temporary ileostomy, 386-387
Temporary pacemaker, 134, 135, 136, 137
Teniposide; see VM-26
TENS; see Transcutaneous electrical nerve stimulation
Tension pneumothorax, 254-255
Terbutaline for asthma, 235
Test(s)
  acetone, 444
  glucose, 444
  kidney function, normal values for, 877
  nonstress, 737-378
  stress, contraction, 738-739
Tes-Tape, 444

Testis
  as endocrine organ, 420
  surgical removal of, 591-593
Testicular cancer, detection and prevention of, 657-658
Testicular dysfunction from chemotherapy, 696
Testicular self-examination, 657
Testicular tumor, orchiectomy for, 591-593
Testing, urine, diabetic, teaching guide for, 443-444
Testosterone, 422
Tetanus, 792-793
Tetracycline and nutrition, 4
Tetralogy of Fallot, 848-850
TGV; see Transposition of great vessels
Theolair; see Theophylline
Theophylline for asthma, 235
Therapeutic bronchoscopy, 224-225
Thermodilution method of measuring cardiac output, 145
Thiazides and nutrition, 4
Thioguanine, 676-677
6-Thioguanine, 676-677
Thio-tepa, 674-675
Third-degree heart block, 130-131
Thomas' splint and Pearson's attachment, balanced suspension with, 511, 512
Thoracentesis, 225-227
Thoracic cord injuries, 305
Thoracic empyema, 256-257
Thoracotomy, 269-271
Thought processes, alteration in, 23-24
Thrive, failure to, 841-844
Thrombocytopenia, 175-177
  with chemotherapy, 688-689
Thromboembolism, 74
Thrombophlebitis, 74
Thrombosis, venous, 74-76
Thumb, replacement of, 504
Thymus, 420
Thyroid crisis (storm), 427-430
Thyroid gland, 420, 422
  surgical removal of, 430
Thyroid hormone
  excess of, 427-430
  lack of, 424-427
Thyroidectomy, 430-431
Thyroid-stimulating hormone, 421
Thyrotoxic crisis, 427-430
Thyroxine, 422
Tissue pressure monitoring, 507-509
TMN classifications, 664
  cancer staging utilizing, 665

Tocotransducer, 737
Toddler age-group care, 784
Tolazamide for diabetes, 446
Tolbutamide for diabetes, 446
Tolinase; see Tolazamide
Tongs, skull, 333
TORCH infections, 771-773
Torsade de pointes, 128-129
Torsion of spermatic cord, 588-589
Total abdominal hysterectomy and bilateral salpingo-oophorectomy, 606-608
Total joint arthroplasty, 495-499
Total parenteral nutrition, 51-55
Total pelvic exenteration, 612
Total placenta previa, 722
Total-body irradiation before bone marrow transplantation, 184
Toxic shock syndrome, 597-598
Toxoplasmosis in neonate, 771
TPN; see Total parenteral nutrition
Trabeculectomy, 633
Tracheoesophageal fistula, 808-810
Tracheostomy, 275-277
Tracheostomy tube, 275
Traction, 511-513
　Bryant's, 511, 512, 513
　care of patient in, 513-514
　cervical, 511, 512
　halo, 333, 511, 512-513
　on humerus, 511, 512
　pelvic, 511, 512
　side arm, 511, 512
　skeletal, 511, 512
　skin, 511-512
Transcutaneous electrical nerve stimulation, 65-66
Transducer
　abdominal, ECG, 737
　ultrasound, 736
Transfusion(s)
　blood, 218
　　reactions to, 214-217
　of newborn, exchange, 763-764
Transhepatic biliary decompression catheter, 398-399
Transitional labor, 728
Transluminal angioplasty, percutaneous, 138-140
Transplant
　corneal, 633
　intraocular lens, cataract removal with or without, 633
　renal, 575-579
Transplant phase of bone marrow transplantation, 187-196

Transplantation, bone marrow, 181-196
　schedule for, 182
Transposition of great vessels, 850
Transurethral resection of prostate, 580
Transvenous approach of temporary pacemaker, 135
Trauma
　craniocerebral, 302-304
　esophageal, 342-343
Travel tips for diabetic patient, 450
Triamterene, 4
Tricuspid valve replacement, 111
Tridione; see Trimethadione
Triethylene-thiophosphoramide; see Thio-tepa
Triiodothyronine, 422
Trimethadione for seizure disorders, 292
Triple-lumen balloon-tipped pulmonary catheter, 144
Trousers, shock, 148-150
TSH; see Thyroid-stimulating hormone
TSS; see Toxic shock syndrome
Tubal ligation, 604-605
Tubal pregnancy and salpingectomy, 605-606
Tube
　Cantor, 388, 389
　　care of patient with, 388-390
　Celestin, 350
　　care of patient with, 350-352
　chest, 271-272
　　removal of, 272
　endotracheal, 273-275
　　newborn with, care of, 775-776
　　removal of, care during/after, 274-275
　gastrostomy, feeding by, 811
　intestinal, naso-oral, care of patient with, 388-390
　Levine, 365, 366
　Linton, 352, 353
　　care of patient with, 352-354
　Miller-Abbott, 388, 389
　　care of patient with, 388-390
　nasogastric, 365, 366
　　care of patient with, 365-367
　nasotracheal, 273-275
　Salem sump, 365, 366
　Sengstaken-Blakemore, 352, 353
　　care of patient with, 352-354
　T, 397
　　care of patient with, 397-398
　tracheostomy, 275
　upper GI, care of patient with, 367-370
Tube feedings, teaching about, 50-51
Tube insertion, myringotomy with, 641-642

Tuberculosis, pulmonary, 248-250
Tuberculous meningitis, antibiotic therapy for, 323
Tumor(s)
   brain, 300-302
   classification of, 665
   testicular, orchiectomy for, 591-593
TURP; see Transurethral resection of prostate
Twenty-four hour clock system, 876, 877
Tympanoplasty, 642-643

U

Ulcer(s)
   decubitus, 619-621
   duodenal, 354
   gastric, 354
   peptic, 354-355
   pressure, 619-621
Ulcerative colitis, 370-372
Ultrasonic lithotripsy, percutaneous, 555
Ultrasonic nebulizers, 229-230
Ultrasound transducer, 736
Umbilical catheterization of newborn, 765
Umbilical cord, prolapsed, 724-725
Uninhibited neurogenic bladder, 537
Unsealed radioactive chemotherapy, 709-710
Upper gastrointestinal ostomy, tube, or prosthetic valve, care of patient with, 367-370
Upper motor neuron bladder, 537
Upper motor neuron lesions, 305
Urea for child, 868
Ureter, cancer of, detection and prevention of, 656-657
Ureterolithotomy, 554
Ureterosigmoidostomy, 542, 544
Ureterostomy, cutaneous, 542, 543
Urethra
   cancer of, detection and prevention of, 656-657
   infection of, 522
Urethral catheter, indwelling, 541
   care of patient with, 540-542
Urethritis, 522
Urgency incontinence, 526
Urinary diversion, 542-548
Urinary elimination, alteration in, 5-6
Urinary incontinence, 526-528
   female, surgery for, 528-531
Urinary retention, acute, 534-536
Urinary sphincter, artificial, 531-534
Urinary tract infection, 522-524
Urine testing, diabetic, teaching guide for, 443-444
Urolithiasis, 553-557

Urologic toxicity from chemotherapy, 698-700
Uterus
   cancer of, detection and prevention of, 662
   surgical removal of, 606, 608
UTI; see Urinary tract infection

V

V_1 monitoring lead, modified, 134
Vaginal cancer, detection and prevention of, 660
Valium; see Diazepam
Valproic acid for seizure disorders, 292
Valve
   aortic, replacement of, 111
   heart, 71
   mitral, replacement of, 111
   prosthetic, upper GI, care of patient with, 367-370
   replacement of, 110, 111
   tricuspid, replacement of, 111
Valvular heart disease, 94-98
Valvular heart disease murmurs, 95
Vancomycin plus erythromycin for endocarditis prophylaxis, 95
Vaponefrin; see Epinephrine
Variable pressure limit volumetric infusion pumps, 60
Varicella; see Chickenpox
Varices, esophageal, bleeding, 344-346
Vascular assessment, peripheral, 73-74
Vascular resistance, systemic, calculation of, 107
Vasodilator drugs, 89-93
   potential complications of, 90
Vasogenic shock, 104, 105, 106
Vein ligation and stripping, 76-77
Velban; see Vinblastine sulfate
Venous access devices, long-term, 57-59
Venous catheter, central, 55
   care of patient with, 55-59
Venous nutrition
   central, 53
   peripheral, 51, 53
Venous system, 68
Venous thrombosis, 74-76
Ventilation, mechanical, continuous, 277-280
   care of patient on, 277-279
Ventilator
   newborn on, care of, 776-777
   positive pressure
      intermittent, 280
      pressure-limited, 277, 279
      volume-cycled, 277, 279-280
Ventolin; see Albuterol

INDEX

Ventricular contractions, premature, 125-126
    multifocal, 126
Ventricular failure, 101, 102
Ventricular fibrillation, 127-128
Ventricular origin, ECG rhythms of, 125-129
Ventricular pacemaker, 135
Ventricular preexcitation, 132-133
Ventricular septal defect, 845-846
Ventricular shunt insertion, 823-825
Ventricular tachycardia, 126-127
    polymorphous, 128-129
Ventriculoatrial shunt, 824
Ventriculostomy, 330
Venturi mask for oxygen therapy, 229
Vesicular sound, 222
Vessels, great, transposition of, 850
Vinblastine sulfate, 676-679, 704
    hazards associated with, 671
Vinca alkaloids, 676-679
    hazards associated with, 671
Vincristine sulfate, 678-679, 704
    hazards associated with, 671
Vindesine, 678-679
    hazards associated with, 671
Violence
    directed at others, potential for, 21-22
    potential for, 20-22
    self-directed, potential for, 20-21
Viral hepatitis, 401-403
Viral infection, herpes type 1, 622-623
Visually impaired patient, 635-637
Vital signs, pediatric, 865-866
Vitamin B_{12} deficiency, 161
VM-26, 678-679
    hazards associated with, 671
Voice and breath sounds, 222-223
Voiding measures to facilitate bladder emptying, 535
Volume-cycled positive pressure ventilator, 277, 279-280
Volumetric devices, 60
Volumetric infusion controllers, 60
Volumetric infusion pumps, 60
Vomiting
    excessive, during pregnancy, 717

Vomiting—cont'd
    nausea and, from chemotherapy, 690-692
VP-16; *see* Etoposide
VSD; *see* Ventricular septal defect
Vulva, surgical removal of, 609
Vulvectomy, 609-612
    with lymphadenectomy, 609, 610-611
    skinning, with skin graft, 609, 610

W

Warfarin, 152
Warm shock, 104; *see also* Vasogenic shock
Wave forms, pressure, 144
    problems associated with, 141
Weight
    birth
        high, 758-759
        low, 757-758
    and height, desirable, 4
Wenckebach's phenomenon, 129-130
Wheezes, 222
Whipple procedure, 414
Whispered pectoriloquy, 223
White blood cells, 159
    pheresis of, 211
Whole blood, 212-213
    reaction to transfusion of, 215-216, 217
Whooping cough, 790-791, 795, 796
Wide-angle glaucoma, 632
Withdrawn behavior, 27-28
Wolff-Parkinson-White syndrome, 132-133
Wrist
    arthroplasty of, 495, 497
    and hand, range-of-motion exercises of, 299

X

Xanthine derivatives for asthma, 235
Xylocaine; *see* Lidocaine

Z

Zanosar; *see* Streptozocin
Zarontin; *see* Ethosuximide